Imaging in Trauma
and Critical Care

Imaging in Trauma and Critical Care

STUART E. MIRVIS, MD, FACR
Professor of Radiology
Division Head, Trauma and Emergency Radiology
University of Maryland School of Medicine
Baltimore, Maryland

K. SHANMUGANATHAN, MD
Associate Professor of Radiology
Division of Trauma and Emergency Radiology
University of Maryland School of Medicine
Baltimore, Maryland

SECOND EDITION

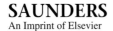

SAUNDERS
An Imprint of Elsevier

SAUNDERS
An Imprint of Elsevier

The Curtis Center
Independence Square West
Philadelphia, Pennsylvania 19106

IMAGING IN TRAUMA AND CRITICAL CARE, SECOND EDITION   ISBN 0-7216-9340-7
Copyright © 2003, Elsevier Science (USA). All rights reserved.

NOTICE

Medicine is an ever-changing field. Standard safety precautions must be followed, but as new research and clinical experience broaden our knowledge, changes in treatment and drug therapy may become necessary or appropriate. Readers are advised to check the most current product information provided by the manufacturer of each drug to be administered to verify the recommended dose, the method and duration of administration, and contraindications. It is the responsibility of the licensed prescriber, relying on experience and knowledge of the patient, to determine dosages and the best treatment for each individual patient. Neither the publisher nor the author assumes any liability for any injury and/or damage to persons or property arising from this publication.

Previous edition copyrighted 1992

International Standard Book Number 0-7216-9340-7

Acquisitions Editor: Allan Ross
Publishing Services Manager: Patricia Tannian
Project Manager: John Casey
Book Design Manager: Gail Morey Hudson
Cover Design : Jack Hannus

Printed in United States of America

Last digit is the print number: 9   8   7   6   5   4   3   2   1

Contributors

JAY CINNAMON, MD
Professor of Radiology
Vice-Chairman and Chief, Division of Neuroradiology
Department of Radiology
Emory University School of Medicine
Atlanta, Georgia

BARRY DALY MD, FRCR
Professor of Radiology
Chief, Section of Abdominal Imaging
Department of Diagnostic Radiology
University of Maryland School of Medicine
Baltimore, Maryland

DAVID R. GENS, MD
Associate Professor of Surgery
Program in Trauma
University of Maryland School of Medicine
Baltimore, Maryland

GEOFFREY S. HASTINGS, MD
Associate Clinical Professor of Radiology
Department of Radiology
San Francisco General Hospital
San Francisco, California

LAWRENCE E. HOLDER, MD
Clinical Professor of Radiology
University of Florida
Shands Jacksonville
Jacksonville, Florida

KAREN L. KILLEEN, MD
Clinical Assistant Professor of Radiology
University of Maryland School of Medicine
Baltimore, Maryland

DAVID M. LEFKOWITZ, MD
Associate Professor of Radiology
Medical Director, MRI
Division of Neuroradiology
University of Maryland School of Medicine
Baltimore, Maryland

STUART E. MIRVIS, MD, FACR
Professor of Radiology
Division Head, Trauma and Emergency Radiology
University of Maryland School of Medicine
Baltimore, Maryland

MICHAEL MULLIGAN, MD
Associate Professor Radiology
Assistant Chief of Musculoskeletal Radiology
Department of Radiology
University of Maryland School of Medicine
Baltimore, Maryland

ROBERT D. PUGATCH, MD
Professor of Radiology
Division of Thoracic Radiology
University of Maryland School of Medicine
Baltimore, Maryland

CHARLES S. RESNIK, MD
Professor of Radiology
Director of Musculoskeletal Imaging
University of Maryland School of Medicine
Baltimore, Maryland

BRADLEY C. ROBERTSON, MD, DDS, FACS
Director, Plastic Surgery
R. Adams Cowley Shock Trauma Center;
Associate Professor
University of Maryland School of Medicine
Baltimore, Maryland

ISMET SARIKAYA, MD
Fellow in Nuclear Medicine
Memorial Sloan-Kettering Cancer Center
New York, New York

THOMAS M. SCALEA, MD
Physician in Chief
R Adams Cowley Shock Trauma Center;
Francis X. Kelly/MBNA Professor of Trauma Surgery
Director, Program in Trauma
University of Maryland School of Medicine
Baltimore, Maryland

K. SHANMUGANATHAN, MD
Associate Professor of Radiology
Division of Trauma and Emergency Radiology
University of Maryland School of Medicine
Baltimore, Maryland

ERIN M. SIMON, MD, OTR
Assistant Professor of Radiology
University of Pennsylvania School of Medicine;
Neuroradiologist, Department of Radiology
The Children's Hospital of Philadelphia
Philadelphia, Pennsylvania

CARLOS J. SIVIT, MD
Professor of Radiology and Pediatrics
Case Western Reserve School of Medicine;
Director of Pediatric Radiology
Rainbow Babies and Children's Hospital
Cleveland, Ohio

JAMES G. SMIRNIOTOPOULOS, MD
Professor of Radiology, Neurology, and Biomedical
  Informatics
Chair, Department of Radiology and Radiological Sciences
Uniformed Services University of the Health Sciences
Bethesda, Maryland

STACY E. SMITH
Assistant Professor of Radiology
Division of Musculoskeletal Radiology
University of Maryland School of Medicine
Baltimore, Maryland

M. J. B. STALLMEYER, MD
Assistant Professor of Radiology
Interventional and Diagnostic Neuroradiology
University of Maryland School of Medicine
Baltimore, Maryland

CHARLES S. WHITE, MD
Professor of Radiology
Director, Thoracic Imaging
University of Maryland School of Medicine
Baltimore, Maryland

JADE J. WONG-YOU-CHEONG, MD
Associate Professor of Radiology
Director of Ultrasound
Department of Diagnostic Radiology
University of Maryland School of Medicine
Baltimore, Maryland

ROBERT A. ZIMMERMAN, MD
Professor of Radiology
University of Pennsylvania School of Medicine;
Vice-Chairman and Neuroradiology
Division Chief, Department of Radiology
The Children's Hospital of Philadelphia
Philadelphia, Pennsylvania

This work is dedicated with
love and deep gratitude to my parents
Erma and Marvin Mirvis
for their continuous guidance and support
and to my loving wife
Linda
and stellar children
Julie and Adam
for their patience and understanding
in sharing me for so long with this textbook

SEM

I would like to dedicate this book to
My parents
for their patience, unconditional love, and guidance.
I am greatly indebted to my mentor
Stu Mirvis
for his tremendous influence on my professional life.
Without his guidance it would not have been possible to complete this book.
I would like to thank
my past teachers in radiology including
Judy Webb, Rodney Reznek, and Audry Tucker
from whom I had the privilege of learning.
I am particularly grateful to
Ruth and John Warren
for inspiring me to pursue a career in radiology

KS

Foreword

Enormous changes in the assessment of trauma patients have occurred since the first edition of *Imaging in Trauma and Critical Care* was published in 1992. I was extremely happy to learn that Stuart Mirvis had decided to embark on the second edition of this remarkable contribution, and it is a great honor to be invited to write the foreword for this new edition. Despite the increasing interest in emergency and trauma medicine and the need for comprehensive information on current imaging of traumatic diseases, it is not surprising that a comparable book in trauma radiology was not published during the past 10 years. The experience that Stu Mirvis has accumulated over many years of tireless work at the University of Maryland Shock Trauma Center is simply unique, and his commitment and devotion to the imaging of the traumatized and acutely ill patient are unmatched.

Keeping the same easily readable and instructive style as the first edition, Stu has done a marvelous job in expanding and reorganizing the text. Each chapter has been revised and updated to include the latest developments and imaging trends in the management of trauma patients. It is noteworthy that helical and multidetector CT were not in clinical use by the time of publication of the first edition, but are now integrally included in this excellent revision. This edition provides a comprehensive review of trauma imaging based on an organ system approach but also keeps in perspective the multisystem nature of the disease. Dr. Mirvis has invited the collaboration of other experts in the field who have brought additional expertise and updates in different subspecialties. Dedicated new chapters in pediatric imaging, penetrating trauma, nuclear medicine applications, angiography and interventional radiology add to the comprehensiveness of this edition. In addition, the chapter on craniocerebral injury incorporates dedicated sections on pediatric brain injury and on the assessment of vascular injuries of the head and neck, where imaging has evolved to play a primary role in management decisions. The chapters on cervical spine and abdominal trauma were considerably revised to adapt to the growing application of various imaging modalities. The first and last chapters, written as clinical perspectives, are excellent and emphasize the need for continued cooperation among the specialists caring for the acutely injured patient.

As I have known Stu for many years I can attest to the fact that this book reflects his passion for the growing field of emergency imaging and his commitment to education and academic radiology. *Imaging in Trauma and Critical Care* is all encompassing. It is an up-to-date, comprehensive, multisystem, multimodality text that will have a prime place as a reference in trauma medicine. It provides an invaluable resource to all of us involved in the care of trauma victims and will unquestionably become "the textbook" in trauma imaging. Allowing for the rapid changes occurring in imaging technology and in trauma care, this book should remain a classic for years to come.

Diego B. Nunez, Jr., MD, MPH
Clinical Professor of Radiology
Yale University School of Medicine;
Chairman, Department of Radiology
Hospital of Saint Raphael
New Haven, Connecticut

Preface

In 1992, the first edition of *Imaging in Trauma and Critical Care* was published. My desire to write this first book with my colleague, Dr. Jeremy Young, was inspired by the wealth of material I saw in my practice at the Shock Trauma Center at the University of Maryland, part of the long- established and highly successful Maryland Institute for Emergency Medical Services system. Medical imaging was playing a more important role in management decisions and in acute trauma and postacute trauma intensive care. I believed a textbook focused on this subject would be a useful tool not only for radiologists, but also for emergency physicians, trauma surgeons, and anesthesiologists, among others, working in the acute care setting.

After publication of the first edition, several events occurred within my practice that led to consideration of a major revision of the original textbook. First, I established an association with a full-time partner, Dr. Kathirkamanthan Shanmuganathan (known to all, thankfully, as simply Dr. Shan). Dr. Shan almost instantly became as fascinated by trauma imaging as I was, establishing himself rapidly as a major contributor to academic radiology. We have enjoyed a successful collaboration based on mutual respect and deep friendship. So for this second edition, and fortunately for me, a lot of preparation fell on Dr. Shan's shoulders.

Second, the trauma center had acquired a new physician-in-chief, Dr. Thomas Scalea, who came to the Shock Trauma Center as a senior trauma surgeon from Brooklyn, New York, at the King's County Hospital. Dr. Scalea brought along a well-developed interest in the use of imaging technology and intervention in the trauma patient based on his previous collaboration with well-known interventionalist Dr. Salvatore Sclafani. Thus we did not need to "teach" Tom the benefits of diagnostic imaging and interventional techniques, since he understood these from the start of our association. Over the course of time, imaging protocols, reflected in this current text, were developed and have evolved to optimize the strengths of imaging in appropriately selected patients. Dr. Scalea's leadership fostered expanded use of imaging services, which in turn provided more experience and teaching material that could be used to prepare the current edition of this textbook. His knowledge of trauma surgery and imaging has assisted us in establishing new opportunities to apply our technology and expe-

rience, such as the use of multidetector row CT for penetrating torso trauma.

Third, advances in computer technology in the 1990s, such as PACS (picture archiving, communication, and storage), much faster and more robust personal computers, and digital image storage and manipulation, have permitted us a far greater ability to identify, organize, and maintain pertinent images for use in this text. Finally, the trauma center has been fortunate enough to be able to provide state-of-the-art imaging equipment such as helical and multidetector row CT with stand-alone workstations, computed radiography, and high-resolution angiography immediately adjacent to the trauma resuscitation unit.

These have provided far better image quality than was routinely available in the early to mid-1990s. High-field magnetic resonance imaging has also been substantially upgraded since the first edition of this book and can be used without major limitations for most clinically stable trauma patients.

The past decade has seen a major influence of diagnostic imaging on the treatment of trauma patients. Since CT has become so much faster and can quickly reconstruct images, it has been more widely used for virtually all body regions. A total picture of body injury can be gleaned relatively quickly and can provide a great deal of information, considering the transport time and scan cost. The value of screening CT for spinal injury, chest trauma, and blunt abdominal trauma is well established. This development has called into question the need for, and role of, traditional radiography in the initial assessment of clinically stable blunt trauma patients. When CT is planned for one body system, it seems expedient to "clear" any other regions that are in question based either on mechanism of injury or physical findings. The interplay between radiography, traditional surgical diagnostic techniques, and CT scanning will continue to evolve for years to come. The greater use of abdominopelvic CT and interventional radiology in blunt trauma care has particularly brought about the decline of nontherapeutic surgical exploration of the abdomen that has occurred over the past decade.

This second edition of *Imaging in Trauma and Critical Care* has been expanded from the previous 11 chapters to 17 chapters. The current edition devotes an entire chapter to the topic of abdominal intensive care imaging. New chapters are now devoted to trauma of the renal system and retroperitoneum and to the CT diagnosis of penetrating torso trauma. Another new chapter describes applications of nuclear medicine for acute and subacute trauma. This edition also introduces a chapter focused on pediatric trauma imaging. The final chapter of this new textbook offers some predictions concerning the future of trauma imaging and intervention. Finally, a revised chapter on craniocerebral trauma is now divided into separate sections discussing adult head trauma, pediatric head trauma, and cervicocranial vascular injury.

The vast majority of images in this new edition are replacements of the previous material. Certain images from the last edition of this book were retained for this edition because they still best reflected the pertinent pathology. Many line drawings from the previous edition were also retained, since these were usually the best available to illustrate the anatomy being described. Multiplanar reformations and more readily available surface contour and volumetric three-dimensional images were added to enhance presentation of pathology in selected cases. The image quality of magnetic resonance studies has improved considerably since the last edition, with the addition of faster sequences, fluid-attenuation inversion recovery, and diffusion-weighted sequences, to cite a few new methodologies.

It is important for the reader to note at the outset that the imaging approaches and algorithms suggested in this textbook represent the current practice at the institutions of the various chapter authors. No attempt was made to offer a uniform diagnostic approach to trauma imaging that will suffice for all centers. The use and order of imaging procedures in trauma patients are site-dependent considerations that vary with equipment, physical layout, and clinical and support personnel, as well as diagnostic expertise and availability. The opening chapter of the text, Clinical Perspective on Trauma Imaging, highlights this important consideration.

I have attempted to keep the material and references as up-to-date as possible given the long production schedule involved in textbook preparation. Although primarily intended for an audience of imaging specialists, I hope that the strong contribution to the text from our surgical and trauma–critical care colleagues will help to better blend the imaging information into a lucid clinical context for the benefit of a less image-oriented audience. I hope that you enjoy reading and learning from this second edition of *Imaging in Trauma and Critical Care* and find it a useful and practical addition to your medical library.

Stuart E. Mirvis, MD, FACR

Contents

1 Clinical Perspective on Trauma Imaging

David R. Gens

OVERVIEW: AN INTEGRATED TEAM APPROACH

Trauma care has been a neglected segment of health care delivery in the United States. The National Academy of Sciences referred to this problem in its "white paper" in 1966, "Accidental Death and Disability: The Neglected Disease of Modern Society."[1] The cover story of the March 1990 issue of the *Bulletin of the American College of Surgeons*, "What's Wrong with Trauma Care?," addressed the same problem, but 34 years later.[2] The essential element necessary to correct the problem is a systematic approach to trauma care, involving not only a well-coordinated emergency medical system, but also a well-coordinated receiving facility. The trauma system delivering health care, whether it is a local emergency department or a tertiary care center, must ensure an integrated approach to the provision of this specialized care. This integrated, coordinated approach is essential to the success of a trauma center.

R Adams Cowley, MD,[3] founder of the Maryland Institute for Emergency Medical Services Systems, was the first to recognize trauma as a disease and the first to recognize the need for a systematic approach to its treatment. Cowley had the insight to recognize that without proper organization (starting from field triage and treatment protocols), precious time may be lost, time that may cost a trauma victim's life. To describe this time, he coined the phrase "the Golden Hour," not necessarily to mean 60 minutes of time, but to imply a certain period within which a trauma victim must receive both diagnosis and appropriate treatment. As the time from injury to diagnosis and treatment shortens, mortality decreases (Fig. 1-1). The ability to decrease this interval involves many factors and includes efficient communications systems, rapid transportation (helicopters), efficient field triage, and an efficient receiving facility. With an "economy of time" from start to finish, from the "first responder" to the definitive treatment and diagnosis, the chance of a successful outcome is improved in terms of both survival and morbidity. Advances in computer technology have resulted in faster CT capabilities with better definition, as well as digital archiving systems (PACS), that enable a clinician to retrieve images remotely without wasting precious time searching for "lost films."

The team approach to the trauma victim is the single most important factor in achieving a successful outcome once the trauma victim reaches the treating facility. Inherent in this approach is the concept of a single "captain of the ship," the traumatologist. This person must understand and integrate multiple services. He or she must work closely with many specialists, especially radiologists and radiology technicians. For a patient with multiple injuries, the traumatologist must conceive a well-organized, integrated approach with the radiology team to provide the best economy of time. Treatment priorities must be established and fully understood not only by the emergency department staff (nurses, physicians, lab technicians), but also by the radiology team (radiologist and technologists). With a complete understanding of the treatment protocols, technologists may make better use of equipment, not only for patients with multiple injuries,

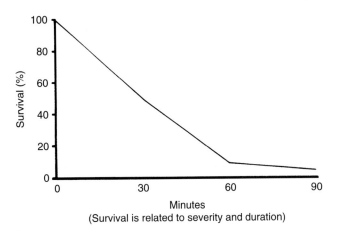

Fig. 1-1
Percentage of patients surviving as a function of time from initial trauma to arrival at medical facility.

but also for multiple trauma admissions. It is frequently necessary to image (using either plain radiography or CT) patients "out of order." Based on experience with trauma patients, the traumatologist must make that decision according to the apparent severity of the injuries of each patient rather than the patients' order of arrival (e.g., a head-injured patient with a dilated pupil, which carries a high probability of a life-threatening brain injury). If the radiology service understands this triage priority and can adapt to the priorities, then the entire trauma team functions in a more coordinated fashion, saving valuable time where it is most appropriate. The traumatologist should speak with the radiology technologist about each patient admitted to establish the priorities of films to be performed, as well as the order in which the patients are to be studied. The performance of "special" radiographic views, which might be desired by consulting subspecialty services, should await the performance of "protocol" radiographs or other required imaging studies that can detect possible life-threatening injury. Direct dialogue between the traumatologist team leader and the radiology team can promote efficient time economy and improve outcome.

PRIORITIES IN TRAUMA PATIENT MANAGEMENT
Field and Receiving Facility

The key to a successful trauma system starts in the field. Once an accident occurs, a cascade of events follows. An observer reports the accident (911 system), and a central alarm system then alerts a paramedic team, which is dispatched to the scene of the accident. This first responder must quickly and correctly assess the trauma victim(s) and make triage decisions. Two types of errors can be committed at this point. First, an incorrect decision may be made regarding the patient: the patient is incorrectly assessed and is more severely injured than thought to be (under-

triage, a serious error), or the patient's injuries are not as severe as first thought (overtriage). The second type of triage error is to incorrectly assess the receiving facility. The patient is correctly assessed, but the receiving hospital is not adequately equipped to handle the patient because the medical staff (physicians, nurses, radiologists, or technicians) is not familiar with trauma patients or the facility is inadequately equipped (CT or technicians not readily available, unstaffed operating rooms). If the field care provider makes the error of underestimating the patient's injuries and then sends that patient to an inadequate facility, the patient may receive inadequate care.

Studies performed in California documented that mortality of those patients reaching a hospitals with an effective trauma care system is lower than in hospitals with no organized trauma system in place. Approximately one third of all deaths related to injuries (exclusive of the central nervous system) within hospitals lacking an organized trauma system are preventable.[4,5] These deaths may be prevented by the establishment of a trauma care system. For this reason, it is imperative that paramedics have well-defined priorities in trauma patient triage and treatment. By adhering to a strict field protocol, fewer mistakes will be made and a better economy of time achieved. Table 1-1 lists some examples of Maryland's emergency medical services system trauma protocols. An effective communication system also must be available to ensure the ability of the paramedic to easily and rapidly communicate with the central alarm system and the receiving facility. A protocol exists also for paramedic communication[6] (Table 1-2).

Besides well-organized field and communication systems, the development of a trauma system must include strict criteria regarding the capabilities of the receiving facility. The paramedic equipped with a set of treatment and triage protocols needs an appropriate emergency department capable of administering trauma care. For this reason, the American College of Surgeons Committee on Trauma established guidelines for the resources necessary to build an efficient trauma system.[7] Preventable trauma deaths can be reduced by dedicating staff and resources to the care of trauma victims. This is attained by avoiding delays in achieving appropriate resuscitation, diagnosis, and definitive therapy. Organizing a trauma center's interventional radiology service has become increasingly important within the last several years as a result of the increased use of angiography for diagnosis and treatment of solid visceral injuries that were formerly handled surgically.

With all three elements (field, communication, and receiving facility) in place and working in synchrony, few if any delays in triage, diagnosis, or treatment occur. Any weak link can break the chain. In trauma care, dedicated personnel, from paramedic to radiographer to attending surgeon, all understanding the concept of economy of time and the importance of following a protocol system, can improve the patient's ultimate outcome.

Table 1-1
General Patient Triage for Trauma

I. Critically ill or injured person who requires immediate attention; delay potentially threatens life or function.
  A. Burns
    1. Age <10 or >50, with second- or third-degree burns potentially over >10% BSA
    2. Other ages, second- and third-degree burns over >20% BSA
    3. Second- or third-degree burns of face, hands, feet, or perineum
    4. Electrical, chemical, or respiratory burns
  B. Multiple trauma patient
  C. Trauma patient with multiple system involvement and any of the following:
    1. Systolic BP <80 mm Hg
    2. MAST applied and inflated
    3. Respiratory distress
    4. Unconsciousness
    5. Uncontrollable bleeding
    6. Penetrating wounds to head
  D. Severe single-system trauma

II. Less serious, requires emergency medical attention, but does not immediately endanger patient's life
  A. Burns
    1. Age <10 or >50, third-degree burns <10% BSA
    2. Other ages, second- or third-degree burns <20% BSA
  B. Trauma patient with moderate blood loss with stable vital signs, bleeding controlled, and no signs or symptoms compatible with shock
  C. Concussions with awakening or agitation
  D. Fractures with neurovascular compromise

III. Nonemergency condition, requires medical attention but not "emergency"
  A. Burns: minor
  B. Trauma
    1. Uncomplicated fractures
    2. Lacerations requiring suturing, with bleeding controlled

IV. Does not require medical attention and may not require transport (e.g., obviously dead)

Table 1-2
Protocol for Paramedic Communication

1. All priority 1 patients require online medical consultation.*

2. All priority 2 patients who have persistent symptoms or need further therapeutic intervention(s) require online consultation.*

3. Notification should be made to the receiving hospital for priority 2 or priority 3 patients, whose symptoms have resolved and whose vital signs are within normal limits.*

4. If medical consultation is genuinely unavailable, or if the time necessary to initiate consultation significantly compromises patient care, the provider shall proceed with additional protocol-directed care as long as transport will not be significantly delayed. "Exceptional Call" must be indicated on the patient care report (PCR).

5. Trauma Communications
   The following information must be communicated to the appropriate trauma center or local hospital:
   a. Patient's age(s), injuries, ETA
   b. Number of victims
   c. Detailed description of the incident

6. Mass Casualty Incident (MCI) Communications
   a. When a local jurisdiction declares an MCI, it is extremely important to maximize patient care resources and reserve EMS communications for emergency situations. Except for extraordinary care intervention, EMS providers may perform all skills and administer medication within protocol during a declared MCI. When the MCI condition is instituted, the "Exceptional Call" box must be checked on the PCR.
   b. During an MCI, the EMS officer-in-charge (OIC) will designate an EMS communicator who will establish appropriate communications.

*See Table 1-1.

Resuscitation Phase

Shock is defined as inadequate delivery of oxygen to the cells. In trauma, this usually is caused by hemorrhage (commonly) or hypoventilation (less commonly). Increasing oxygen delivery immediately, which is of the utmost importance, is achieved by increasing the oxygen-carrying capacity through blood transfusions and increasing oxygen delivery by adding supplemental oxygen (nasal cannula, face mask, or endotracheal intubation). The traumatologist's responsibility is to recognize and treat shock immediately by using a well-defined system in the approach to each patient. Once a patient reaches the admitting area or emergency department, an organized system of initial assessment should proceed. This initial assessment should consist of a primary survey with concomitant resuscitation. A more detailed secondary survey would then follow, depending on the discovery of any life-threatening injuries during the primary survey. It is usually during the secondary survey that the need for an appropriate order of radiographs is determined.[8]

The primary survey is intended to disclose any life-threatening injury requiring immediate treatment. To avoid errors of commission, the "ABCs"—airway, breathing, and circulation—must be adhered to strictly (Table 1-3).

The airway is assessed for patency. Stridorous sounds may indicate foreign material in the hypopharynx (blood or vomitus) or even at the base of the tongue, which has fallen posteriorly. More rarely, stridor or more subtle changes in voice may indicate a fractured larynx or trachea. Before any diagnostic imaging studies are initiated, the treating team must make certain that an adequate airway has been established. Control of the cervical spine must be ensured at all times either by leaving a cervical collar in place until appropriate imaging studies have been performed or by using in-line cervical traction during intubation. After intubation, the cervical collar is reapplied to maintain stability.

Breathing is assessed by observing chest expansion and by auscultation and percussion. Detecting subtle changes in breath sounds or, for that matter, a minimal to moderate pneumothorax, can be extremely difficult in a noisy emergency department; for that reason, most pneumothoraces are diagnosed by chest radiographs. Absent breath sounds in the presence of hemodynamic instability warrant a tube thoracostomy before any radiographs.

Hypoventilation is an emergency and should be addressed immediately, first with a bag-valve device (Ambu bag) and then with orotracheal intubation, which is preferred by the author over nasotracheal intubation.

Adequate circulation can be ascertained simply by checking skin color and texture (sweaty or dry), capillary refill time, or pulse. These measures take seconds to carry out and can be obtained even before blood pressure is known (a palpable radial pulse indicates a systolic blood pressure of at least 80 mm Hg).

Active bleeding must be arrested immediately by direct pressure or by placement of sutures. These relatively non-cosmetic sutures are placed hurriedly and can be replaced later by finer and more cosmetic ones. During the primary survey, stopping exsanguinating hemorrhage, not cosmesis, is the goal.

The neurologic disability assessment is quickly obtained using the AVPU system to ascertain the level of consciousness (Table 1-4). Pupil size and response to light are checked at the same time. A more detailed examination using the Glasgow Coma Scale (GCS) is part of the secondary survey.

The patient should be completely exposed so that any obvious injury is not overlooked. Life-threatening injuries discovered during the primary survey should be addressed as soon as they are found.

The secondary survey, which takes place after the primary survey and once life-threatening injuries have been addressed, includes a more detailed examination of the head, face, neck, thorax, abdomen, and extremities. The need for most plain radiographs is determined at this stage. Following a set protocol of standard radiographs for all trauma patients is extremely important (see below).

The neurologic evaluation of a trauma patient usually determines the sequence of diagnostic and therapeutic

---

Table 1-3
ABCs of Trauma Care

I. Primary survey
   A. Airway
   B. Breathing
   C. Circulation
   D. Disability: neurologic status
   E. Exposed: completely undress patient

II. Secondary survey
   A. Head to toe: complete physical examination
   B. Protocol radiographs: cervical spine, chest, pelvis
   C. Special procedures: DPL, CT, emergency surgery

III. Definitive care phase
   A. Fracture stabilization
   B. Suturing of lacerations
   C. Semiurgent surgical procedures

Table 1-4
Brief Neurologic Evaluation

A—Alert
V—Responds to vocal stimuli
P—Responds to painful stimuli
U— Unresponsive

intervention. The GCS (Table 1-5) is designed to quickly identify patients with brain injuries and to assign patients on a scale from 3 (the worst) to 15 (the best).[9] This number may be computed very quickly during the primary survey or later during the secondary survey. Most patients with GCS scores lower than 9 require endotracheal intubation and hyperventilation (used in moderation and for a limited period) followed immediately by a CT scan of the brain, which supersedes all other radiologic studies. Some patients with GCS scores from 10 to 14 need intubation and require cranial CT (due to agitation or uncooperativeness). At the University of Maryland Shock Trauma Center (UMSTC), most patients with GCS scores of 15 undergo cranial CT if they experience loss of consciousness (LOC). Because brain tissue is extremely fragile and is easily irreversibly damaged by pressure (edema, subdural, epidural, or intracerebral hematomas), a brain-injured patient takes priority over other patients. The lower the GCS score, usually the more severe the brain injury; therefore the GCS score can be used grossly to help prioritize cranial CT scans in brain-injured patients. A patient with a GCS score of 10 certainly would take priority over a patient with a GCS score of 15 with LOC. The traumatologist must communicate with the CT technologist regarding these prioritizations. The traumatologist should delay cranial CT scans for a patient with a GCS score of 14 or 15 if he or she knows that a patient is en route from the field with a probable GCS score of 10 or less (as assessed by a well-trained paramedic and easily communicated to the traumatologist in the trauma resuscitation unit).

Table 1-5
Glasgow Coma Scale

Response	Value
Best Motor Response	
Obeys commands	6
Localizes to pain	5
Withdrawals to pain	4
Flexion to pain	3
Extension to pain	2
None	1
Best Verbal Response	
Oriented	5
Confused	4
Inappropriate words	3
Incomprehensible words	2
None	1
Best Eye Opening	
Spontaneously	4
To speech	3
To pain	2
None	1

PROTOCOLS IN ASSESSING THE TRAUMA VICTIM
Clinical Protocols

Every patient who arrives in the trauma resuscitation unit must be considered acutely ill with potentially life-threatening injuries until proved otherwise. The traumatologist must approach each patient in this fashion and must avoid making any errors. Most serious errors are those of omission. To avoid such mistakes, the trauma resuscitation unit team (nurses, physicians, and other staff) should adhere to a strict set of protocols. Most of these are guidelines established by the American College of Surgeons Committee on Trauma in their Advanced Trauma Life Support course.[8] However, unless the admitting team is constantly reminded of these guidelines, serious errors of omission may occur. The traumatologist must be present for every admission to ensure that these protocols are followed. Most of these protocols have been mentioned earlier in the original ABCs; however, some merit special emphasis.

Brain. All patients with an admitting GCS lower than 9 require intubation to protect the airway and avoid hypoxia. During intubation manual in-line immobilization of the cervical spine is maintained at all times. Alcohol is never assumed to be the cause of neurologic depression: rather, cerebral injury is considered causal until proved otherwise.

Hypotension is to be avoided at all costs. The mortality from head trauma doubles with every incidence of hypotension. For this reason a brain-injured patient should not be transported to diagnostic imaging until aggressive monitoring and resuscitation have been ensured.

Spine. All trauma patients, especially those who have blunt trauma, are assumed to have a spine injury until proved otherwise. Corticosteroids are given to all spine-injured patients with a neurologic deficit[10] if less than 8 hours have elapsed from injury. Steroids may be given for 24 to 48 hours depending on the time of diagnosis from injury.[11] In a trauma patient who is free of alcohol or other drugs, has no distracting injury, and has a normal neurologic examination (spinal cord and brain), no radiographs are necessary and the cervical collar can be removed. Otherwise, a hard cervical collar must be worn at all times until the spine has been evaluated radiographically and interpreted by a radiologist or a competent physician. Only the traumatologist can order the cervical collar to be removed. All obtunded patients must have thoracolumbar spine radiographs taken before being placed erect.

Abdomen. In a neurologically compromised patient, some diagnostic test other than a physical examination must be performed. This also applies to a neurologically normal patient who will be lost to physical examination while under general anesthesia (prolonged orthopedic or neurosurgical procedures). The choice of type of diagnostic examination is discussed later.

Stomach. Orogastric tubes are inserted in all critically injured patients. Nasogastric tubes are avoided in patients with brain injuries and those with severe facial fractures to decrease the likelihood of a subsequent paranasal sinusitis or the possibility of transcranial intubation through a disrupted cribriform plate.

Bladder. Transurethral urinary bladder catheters are placed in all critically injured patients and in patients who are unable to void after approximately 30 minutes. However, if blood is present at the urethral meatus, catheterization is not attempted, and a retrograde urethrogram is obtained along with urologic service consultation.

Laboratory and Pulse Oximetry. Standard blood chemistries and urine analyses are obtained in all trauma patients who have suffered major trauma. (Table 1-6). Serum lactate is a good measure of the level of resuscitation. Pulse oximetry should be measured to ensure adequate oxygen levels especially during transport and while in the radiology suites.

Radiologic Protocols

With the development of a system of clinical protocols comes the necessary development of a radiologic survey by protocol. By adhering to such a protocol, errors of omission tend to decrease.

Cervical Spine. Three cervical spine radiographs (lateral, anteroposterior [AP], and odontoid) are obtained for any patient who is awake and alert and has a normal mental status but has significant distracting pain, neuro-

---

Table 1-6
Minimum Laboratory Analyses

Blood Chemistries
Arterial blood gases
Electrolytes
BUN/creatinine
Amylase
Toxicology
Type and cross-match for blood
PT and PTT
Serum lactate

Urinary
Dipstick for blood, sugar, protein
Toxicology

---

logic deficit, or neck pain or tenderness. In a patient who is unreliable to examination (altered level of consciousness, significant distracting pain, or drugs on board), two radiographs (lateral and AP) are obtained and the cervical collar is left in place until the patient is "reliable." Adequate lateral cervical spine films depict the base of the skull to the upper border of the first thoracic vertebra.

Chest. A supine radiograph is obtained in all patients. Indistinctness of the aortic arch or the aorticopulmonary window warrants an erect chest radiograph when clinically possible (normal cervical or thoracolumbar spine radiographs). Obviously, when the possibility of a thoracic arterial injury is clinically remote, such as a gunshot wound to the head, then an erect radiograph is not necessary.

Pelvis. In a severely injured patient, minimally to moderately severe pelvic fractures may be undetected by physical examination alone, especially posterior fractures that are minimally displaced or are stable to manual manipulation. For this reason, any patient sustaining blunt trauma or penetrating wounds near the pelvis should have an AP pelvic radiograph.

Thoracic and Lumbar Spine. All patients who are neurologically compromised (either because of drugs or as a result of a spinal or head injury) must undergo thoracic and lumbar spine radiographs before being positioned upright or moved from their stretchers. If these studies cannot be obtained for technical or logistic reasons, then injury to the spinal column must be assumed until proved otherwise. In an awake (nonintoxicated) patient, physical examination for pain in the thoracic and lumbar areas will suffice: however, the patient must be completely intact neurologically for this approach to be acceptable.

Injury Pattern. Certain mechanisms of injury warrant special radiographic investigation due to the nature of association of injuries. Axial skeletal surveys are necessary in a trauma victim who has fallen from a height and landed on his or her feet. Injuries to the elbows and wrists should be sought if a patient has fallen on outstretched hands. All extremities that exhibit swelling, lacerations, or ecchymosis should be studied.

Deviations from Radiologic Protocol

To deviate from the radiologic protocol (omission of films), the traumatologist must have a well thought-out justification. For example, a patient who has been transferred from another facility and arrives with adequate radiographs does not need these radiographs repeated. An erect chest radiograph is not necessary if the mechanism of injury, such as a fall from a height of less than 10 feet or nonthoracic penetrating trauma, is not associated with major thoracic vascular injury. If the supine chest radiograph demonstrates normal mediastinal contours in a blunt trauma victim, no erect chest radiograph is obtained.

The traumatologist should question any reason to break the radiologic protocol rather than question which radiographs to obtain. Although this method might appear overly "routinized," it permits the narrowest margin of error and offers the greatest economy of time in recognizing and treating injuries.

TRIAGE IN PERFORMING DIAGNOSTIC IMAGING

The order in which radiographic examinations are performed is based mainly on the number of patients who need studies and the clinical presentation of each patient. As mentioned earlier, the order in which patients arrive is not necessarily the order in which they should receive their imaging studies. Rarely will "first come, first served" be applied or be appropriate. The trauma team (especially the technologist) has to adapt to the potential of sudden alteration in the clinical status of each patient; therefore the order of imaging preference may change constantly. If more than one patient arrives concurrently, the traumatologist must expeditiously determine the order in which patients should undergo radiographic studies. The traumatologist, in consultation with the radiologist when desired, must develop a strategy of imaging priorities for a given patient and the sequence in which patients will be studied. This information must be clearly communicated to the radiology staff.

Infrequently, while several newly arrived patients may be awaiting imaging studies the traumatologist may receive information from the central communication system about additional pending arrivals and their injuries. If any of these new patients have evidence of cerebral injury as determined by field physical examination, then the traumatologist should attempt to maintain or plan for CT availability upon that patient's arrival. In the difficult decisions of imaging prioritization, the traumatologist must be flexible and able to adapt according to the clinical presentations of on-site and pending patients. The traumatologist should consider the most appropriate and expedient use of available diagnostic imaging capability. For instance, a patient originally scheduled for abdominal CT may undergo diagnostic peritoneal lavage (DPL) or abdominal sonography instead of CT to make the CT machine available for a patient with a high likelihood of cerebral injury. Appropriate prioritization of diagnostic imaging studies requires ongoing communication among the field paramedics, traumatologist, and radiology staff. The clinical parameters that best determine patient order are vital signs (blood pressure, heart rate, respirations) and gross neurologic examination.

Vital Signs

Vital signs, both from the field and immediately upon arrival, indicate the "potential" a patient has for life-threatening injuries and therefore the necessity of an emergency workup. The ABCs come first, and a patient must be resuscitated before receiving nonvital radiographs (extremity radiographs). In trauma, hypotension is almost always hemorrhagic, rarely neurogenic, and even more rarely cardiogenic or septic. Therapy (in the form of volume resuscitation) always precedes diagnostic radiography. Few radiographs should be considered critical, and some, such as the chest radiograph, may be obtained while resuscitation efforts are in progress. If the presence of a tension pneumothorax is in question, a chest radiograph may be obtained immediately; however, in the presence of hemodynamic instability and decreased breath sounds, immediate chest decompression should precede the chest radiograph. In the presence of a clinically unstable pelvic fracture, an AP pelvic radiograph may disclose the type of pelvic fracture, which in turn will indicate the possibility of abdominal injuries. The pelvic radiograph indicates whether the pelvic fracture is likely to be amenable to external fixation for the treatment of pelvic hemorrhage or if angiographic evaluation and embolization may be required.

When the patient has been resuscitated and vital signs have become stable, then the trauma team may proceed with the protocol set of radiographs. Vital signs should be considered grossly stable when the pulse remains below 100 beats per minute for at least 15 minutes and systolic blood pressure remains above 120 to 140 mm Hg. However, patients receiving ß-receptor antagonists might not be able to exhibit a tachycardia, and a systolic blood pressure of 120 to 140 mm Hg might represent relative "hypotension" in a patient who is normally hypertensive.

Physical Examination—Neurologic Assessment

A patient who has an apparent life-threatening acute cerebral injury (admission GCS lower than 9, dilated pupil, or decorticate or decerebrate posturing) should undergo cranial CT immediately after acquisition of the protocol radiographs, as described earlier. However, if CT is immediately available, vital signs are stable, and physical examination indicates no evidence of injury to the chest, abdomen, or pelvis, the patient may be sent immediately for cranial CT before obtaining the standard radiographs. Images of the cervical spine, chest, and pelvis may be obtained either by CT after the cranial CT or by plain radiographs in the admitting area. When several patients have an apparent cerebral injury, a triage protocol may be followed based on the admission GCS score. While the patient with the lowest GCS score is undergoing cranial CT, the standard admission protocol radiographs can be obtained in the other patients. These "rules" are broad guidelines, and particular clinical situations may alter this triage scheme.

IMAGING PRIORITIES FOR MAJOR INJURIES IN SPECIFIC BODY REGIONS

Trauma patients who have complex, multiple injuries can have an almost infinite variety of clinical scenarios. Although a patient may have injuries in several body regions, a predominant or primary "focus" of injury usually can be determined in each patient. To guide the reader through the complex decision tree of clinical management and its integration with diagnostic imaging priorities, specific body regions serve as the primary foci of interest. Both clinical and imaging priorities are considered in the context of this focus, as well as the interplay of simultaneous injury to other body systems and varying patient hemodynamic status.

Focus: Cerebral Injury

Choice of Diagnostic Methodology. Controversy persists regarding the best technique for diagnosing cerebral injury. First and foremost was the physical examination. Skull radiographs were able to identify the calcified pineal gland in the AP plane and document a shift away from the midline to indicate a mass lesion. Cerebral angiography could better localize and depict the type of mass effect but was invasive, time consuming, expensive, and required specialized radiologic expertise. CT scan, which is noninvasive, rapid to perform, and readily available in level I trauma centers, is currently the mainstay of diagnosis of acute cerebral injury. It is practically no longer necessary (although preferable) to await the arrival of a neurosurgeon in the resuscitation area before ordering diagnostic CT. In most cases now, CT is completed before the neurosurgeon's arrival. Currently, magnetic resonance imaging (MRI) has no apparent advantage over CT for acute brain trauma. The traumatologist and neurosurgeon need to know grossly what is producing the neurologic change in the patient and if neurosurgical treatment (evacuation of subdural, epidural, and intracerebral hematomas) or nonsurgical therapy (hyperventilation for edema or contusion) is indicated. A study by Snow[12] showed that MRI was of no advantage for acute or subacute brain injury, but it was somewhat useful for evaluation of chronic brain injury.

Priorities in Association with Unstable Vital Signs. As emphasized earlier, diagnostic imaging of brain injuries almost always takes precedence over imaging assessment of other injuries. However, if vital signs are unstable, resuscitation and correction of hemorrhagic shock must precede diagnostic cranial CT. If a patient remains unstable and a source of hemorrhage that requires operation is identified, the patient is taken immediately to the operating suite. During surgery (abdominal, thoracic, or perhaps vascular), an intracranial pressure monitor is placed. After surgery, the patient is transported immediately for a brain CT; this requires timely coordination between the operation room staff and the CT staff.

If both cranial and abdominal CT scans are to be obtained, the cerebral scan takes precedence. If the cranial CT scan reveals a mass lesion (subdural, epidural, or intracerebral hematoma) that requires surgical evacuation, then the abdominal CT scan should be postponed (assuming an operating room is immediately available for emergency craniotomy), and the patient should be transported immediately to the operating suite. Diagnostic peritoneal lavage (DPL) or abdominal sonography (focused assessment with sonography for trauma [FAST]) could be performed at the same time the patient is being prepared for a craniotomy. If either is positive for hemorrhage, then abdominal exploration and craniotomy could be performed at the same time. Rapid availability, interpretation, and communication of diagnostic information to the traumatology team are crucial. If an operating room is not immediately available, then thoracic or abdominal CT may proceed until the operating room becomes available.

Focus: Spinal Trauma

In trauma patients, the traumatologist must assume the presence of a spinal injury (column or cord) until proved otherwise. This is true of all blunt trauma patients, who have an incidence of spinal injury of 4.2%,[13] as well as of some patients with noncervical penetrating injuries who may have fallen after the initial injury. Neck pain appears to be a valuable indicator of spinal injury[14,15]; however, 18% to 33% of all patients will have "unreliable" examination due to intoxication or cerebral injury.[13,14] Each institute needs to develop a policy that addresses the clearing of the cervical spine; general traumatologists, trauma radiologists, orthopedists, and neurosurgeons should all be involved in the development of the cervical spine policy. The following policy has been developed by and is currently used at the UMSTC. It should be noted that this policy differs slightly from the policy adopted by the Eastern Association for the Surgery of Trauma,[16] specifically in the absence of the use of MRI for identifying ligament injury in a comatose patient.

Cervical Spine Evaluation Policy

Reliable Patient Without Neurologic Deficit. Radiographic evaluation of the cervical spine is not necessary in all trauma patients. Patients who are deemed "reliable" (awake, alert, normal mental status, and no significant distracting pain) may be evaluated clinically. In the strict absence of neck pain or tenderness, the cervical spine may be "cleared," and no radiographs of the cervical spine are necessary. Strict adherence to this protocol mandates that there is no distracting injury; if a distracting injury is present, then the patient is deemed "unreliable."

If neck pain or tenderness is present, then three radiographs are obtained: lateral, AP, and odontoid views ("three views"). If these views are normal and the patient is able to flex and extend the neck adequately, then flexion and extension radiographs are obtained; the patient flexes and extends without assistance. With adequate normal flexion and extension films, the patient may wear a soft collar for comfort. If the flexion and extension radiographs are "inadequate," the patient may have an undisclosed ligament injury and should continue to wear the rigid collar and then return for a reevaluation 1 to 2 weeks later. If either the three views or flexion and extension are abnormal, then a spine consultation is warranted.

Reliable Patient with Neurologic Deficit. A reliable patient who has a neurologic deficit (motor or sensory) attributable to the cervical spine will have the three-view radiographs as well as a helical CT scan of the entire spine performed. Spine consultation is obtained in all cases.

Unreliable Patient Without Neurologic Deficit. The approach to an unreliable patient is substantially different from a reliable patient. The protocol addresses the possibility of a significant ligament injury in the absence of a bony injury. In a recent study, 18% of all blunt trauma patients were deemed "unreliable," and 5.5% of these had cervical spine injury.[13] Any alteration of mental status from injury, alcohol, or drugs renders the patient unreliable. If a patient is expected to return to a "normal" mental state within 24 hours, then lateral and AP cervical spine films are obtained; adequate films must depict the base of the occipital bone to the upper border of the first thoracic vertebra. If these films are normal and if the patient's mental status is normal after 24 hours, the "reliable patient" protocol described earlier is resumed. On the other hand, if either of the two radiographs is abnormal, a helical CT of the entire cervical spine is obtained, and spine consultation is requested.

If the treating physicians think that the patient's mental status will not normalize in 24 hours (severe brain injury, multiple severe injuries, and the like), then lateral and AP cervical spine radiographs, as well as helical CT of the entire cervical spine, are obtained. If these images are normal and the patient is still "unreliable," then MRI of the cervical spine is performed on hospital day five. Obtaining an MRI in these critically ill patients (especially in a severely brain-injured patient with elevated intracranial pressure and monitoring devices) can be extremely difficult and time consuming. MRI often is deferred, and the cervical spine collar remains in place for an extended period, causing alopecia over the occiput and skin breakdown over the chin. Although it is rare for an unreliable patient to have a ligamentous injury without radiologic or CT evidence of fracture or malalignment (0.5%),[13] unfortunately, no imaging method other than MRI can disclose this type of injury with the patient maintained in neutral position and with a hard cervical collar in place. If the MRI is normal, the collar can be removed.

When a lateral cervical spine film is obtained, all seven cervical vertebrae and the C7-T1 junction must be viewed. To displace the shoulders, the patient's wrists are pulled caudally while relaxed. If this initial attempt fails, a repeat radiograph centered over the lower cervical spine is obtained with increased exposure. If this radiograph does not demonstrate the lower cervical spine adequately, then several options exist. First, any patient who needs emergency surgery is assumed to have a cervical spine injury, and further workup is deferred until after surgery. Second, if the patient requires CT for another reason, it can be used to evaluate the lower cervicothoracic junction. Third, in an alert, cooperative patient (which excludes most brain-injured or intoxicated patients), the swimmer's view may be of help if performed with fixed three-phase x-ray generators.

In a patient with a neurologic deficit consistent with a cervical cord injury and a normal cervical spine series, the traumatologist must consider other possible injuries not necessarily detected by plain radiographs (e.g., an acutely herniated intervertebral disc, an epidural hematoma, or a focal spinal stenosis and degenerative spondylitis leading to a central cord contusion). This information is needed to select patients who would benefit from surgical intervention. Epidural defects can be appreciated by myelography, but CT with intrathecal contrast (M-CT) offers greater sensitivity and specificity.[17] MRI is now the imaging method of choice for acute spinal cord injury when looking for ligament injury, epidural hematoma, herniated disc, or cord contusion. MRI requires no ionizing radiation or invasive lumbar or transcervical puncture for contrast instillation. However, MRI is somewhat limited in acutely injured trauma patients because of the need for advanced life support and monitoring equipment in close proximity to the strong magnetic field around the magnet.

Focus: Soft Tissue of the Neck

Controversy exists in the surgical literature regarding whether the diagnostic workup of wounds that penetrate the cervical platysma muscle requires surgical exploration or whether it can be carried out through a selective, non-operative approach.

The mandatory exploration approach dictates that any patient with wounds that penetrate the platysma muscle must undergo surgical exploration for diagnosis and possible therapeutic intervention. There are absolute indications for exploration (Table 1-7) to which the traumatologist must strictly adhere. Patients with unstable vital signs should go immediately to the operating room. Depending on the zone of injury in the neck (Fig. 1-2),[18] those with stable vital signs should be transferred either to the operating room for diagnosis of vascular, airway, or digestive system injuries or to the radiology suite for workup of a potential vascular injury. This can be achieved by one of several methods, including conventional angiography, MRA, or contrast-enhanced helical CT.[19] Helical CT has been gaining popularity with good results.[20] Rogers reported a decrease in mean time to diagnosis and less neurologic sequelae when compared with angiography.[21] Those patients with middle-zone (also referred to as zone II) injuries proceed to the operating room for emergency neck exploration, whereas those with high (zone III) or low (zone I) injuries require a diagnostic workup to detail the exact level of possible vascular injury. With this protocol, the surgical approach (thoracotomy or median sternotomy) changes in 29% of those with a positive preoperative angiogram.[18] If angiography is performed, all four principal cerebral vessels should be studied. Fry[22]

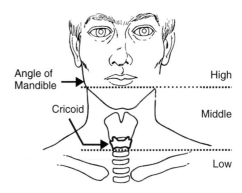

Fig. 1-2
Zones of penetrating cervical trauma, which influence patient management.

found that four-vessel angiography disclosed several unsuspected vertebral artery injuries. The nontherapeutic exploration rate for mandatory exploration is 33% to 63%.[18,23-27]

The selective, nonoperative approach is based on the presence or absence of signs and symptoms of injury to the different structures of the neck (airway, esophagus, arteries, and veins) (Table 1-8). In the absence of clinical signs, most patients may be safely observed; however, most traumatologists believe it is necessary to rule out the presence of asymptomatic vascular, esophageal, and tracheobronchial injuries. An elective radiographic four-vessel study (angiogram, MRA, or spiral CT) is performed to disclose

---

Table 1-7
Absolute Indications for Neck Exploration in Penetrating Trauma

General
All gunshot wounds
Shock

Vascular
Acute hemorrhage
Absent pulse
Expanding hematoma

Airway
Difficult breathing
Stridor
Voice change
Cervical subcutaneous emphysema

Visceral
Dysphagia
Cervical subcutaneous emphysema
Hemoptysis
Hematemesis

Neurologic
Progressive deficit

Table 1-8
Manifestations of Cervical Injuries

Injury	Clinical Presentation
Carotid artery	Decreased level of consciousness Cerebral vascular accident Hematoma, hemorrhage Hypotension Absent pulse
Jugular vein	Hematoma, hemorrhage Hypotension
Larynx or trachea	Stridor, hoarseness Cervical subcutaneous emphysema Dysphonia Hemoptysis
Esophagus or pharynx	Cervical subcutaneous emphysema Hematemesis Dysphagia
Cervical nerves	Recurrent laryngeal: hoarseness Hypoglossal: deviation of tongue Glossopharyngeal: dysphagia Stellate ganglion: Horner's syndrome Spinal accessory: loss of shoulder shrug Phrenic: diaphragmatic paralysis

any carotid or vertebral artery injuries. Esophagography with water-soluble contrast may follow angiography with a false-negative rate of 25% to 50%.[28,29] Others prefer esophagoscopy.[28,29] Neither method is extremely accurate, and if a false-negative examination is suspected, then both should be performed to improve accuracy. Panendoscopy should also be performed for possible hypopharyngeal, tracheal, or major bronchial injuries. Patients at risk of aspiration (e.g., brain injured, uncooperative, intubated) should undergo esophagoscopy under anesthesia. Comparison of these two management protocols reveals that the length of hospital stay and hospital costs for the observed, nonoperated groups are less than or equal to those for the mandatory exploration group. The mortality and morbidity are approximately equal.[23]

Focus: The Mediastinum and Pleural Space

The chest radiograph is one of the baseline studies that should be obtained in all trauma patients. The supine chest radiograph may disclose an unsuspected pneumothorax, hemothorax, lung contusion, or evidence of mediastinal hemorrhage (see below). A "rib series" consisting of oblique chest radiographs is never obtained, since pulmonary complications of thoracic trauma, not the presence or absence of rib fractures, are of greatest importance in directing management. However, demonstration of numerous or displaced ribs on the AP radiograph may have implications regarding pain management.

Of major concern in a patient who has been involved in deceleration trauma is the appearance of the mediastinum. Any patient who has been involved in a decelerating vehicular accident or has fallen from a height greater than 10 feet is at risk. The supine radiograph is evaluated initially. If the contours of the mediastinum are well delineated, then this view will suffice, and no further imaging evaluation of the mediastinum is required. For a patient whose AP supine view is equivocal or inadequate to "clear" the mediastinum, then, if possible, a "true erect" view of the thorax is obtained with the patient leaning slightly forward of the 90-degree vertical position (Fig. 1-3) (to mimic the position used for a PA chest radiograph). Radiographic exposure may be increased to better delineate the mediastinal structures (assuming the lungs were properly exposed on the AP supine view). If the mediastinal contours are normal on this true erect view, then the evaluation of the mediastinum is concluded. However, if the erect view indicates the presence of mediastinal hemorrhage by obscuration or distortion of the mediastinal contour, then a chest CT is obtained.

For selected patients in whom the erect chest radiograph cannot be obtained or for whom radiographic evidence reveals mediastinal hemorrhage, contrast-enhanced helical thoracic CT should be performed to assess the mediastinum, especially if clinical suspicion

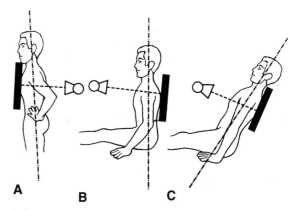

Fig. 1-3
The "true erect" anteroposterior (AP) chest radiograph **(B)** more closely reproduces the appearance of the mediastinum obtained on the standard posteroanterior (PA) view **(A)**. The semi-recumbent **(C)** view distorts and magnifies the mediastinal configuration.

for great vessel injury is low or moderate and if other CT studies are planned. Although some earlier reports suggested that CT scanning may produce false-negative results for detection of great vessel injury,[30,31] more recent reports found helical CT scanning for thoracic injuries to be safe and reliable.[32-34]

If the helical CT demonstrates either a pseudoaneurysm or an intimal flap, the patient is considered for operative repair of the aorta without the need of preoperative aortography. Aortography is reserved for patients with an equivocal CT or for those who have a possible aortic arch injury. These patients require cardiac bypass capabilities and median sternotomy rather than thoracotomy. Patients with a traumatic aortic rupture should be given antihypertensive therapy to decrease the rupture rate.[34] Because of the improved quality of the contrast-enhanced helical CT and therefore better diagnostic capabilities, aortography is obviated in most cases, allowing for rapid diagnosis and treatment.

Endovascular Aortic Stent Grafts. The use of endovascular stent grafts for the treatment of traumatic aortic rupture has been reported in several case reports[35,36] and in one protocol study from Japan.[37] The advantages of this technique are many and compelling: less blood loss, avoidance of a lengthy thoracotomy with the patient in a left thoracotomy position, and less anesthesia time. The patient with multiple injuries (especially brain injury) would most likely benefit the most. More protocol studies need to be done to answer safety issues. As of today, the U.S. Food and Drug Administration has not approved the use of endovascular stent grafts for the treatment of acute traumatic rupture.

Priorities in Association with Craniocerebral Injury. Patients with multiple injuries and stable vital signs in whom the mediastinum is definitely abnormal should proceed to contrast-enhanced helical CT of the chest. Other clinical situations may coexist that also require diagnostic studies. Patients with evidence of cerebral injury should have cranial CT performed before chest or abdominal CT. If a life-threatening intracranial injury is demonstrated, then the chest and abdominal CT may be completed expediently while the operating room is being readied. The images can be reconstructed and read while the patient is being prepared in the operating room. The cranial surgery should precede the thoracic surgery, since the cerebral injury is more likely to be fatal in a shorter period than is a rupture of the thoracic aorta. Abdominal surgery may be performed concomitant with the craniotomy. Hypertension should be avoided at all times.

Priorities in Association with Abdominal Injury. If FAST or DPL is positive and the vital signs remain stable in a patient whose mediastinum is abnormal on the admitting chest radiograph, it is safe to proceed to CT of the chest and abdomen. With continued stable vital signs and demonstration of both aortic and major abdominal injuries, the abdomen should be addressed first followed by repair of the thoracic aorta. If the abdominal injuries appear to be minimal, the thoracotomy should precede an abdominal exploration.

If the vital signs remain unstable despite adequate fluid resuscitation and the supine chest radiograph demonstrates an indistinct mediastinal contour, FAST or DPL should be performed. If FAST or DPL is positive (RBCs >100,000 or gross blood), the patient should be taken directly to the operating room for exploratory celiotomy because of the chance of an abdominal injury causing blood loss. Table 1-9 lists the percentage of therapeutic celiotomies performed relative to DPL cell count. Chest CT should follow immediately postoperatively to determine the presence or absence of aortic injury.

An AP pelvic radiograph should also be obtained (by protocol) to determine if a severe pelvic fracture is the cause of hemorrhagic shock. If pelvic fractures are present and are amenable to orthopedic stabilization, then the orthopedic surgeon should be consulted for possible expedient external fixation before thoracic aortic repair. If there is evidence of continued bleeding, then a pelvic angiogram may be performed in conjunction with con-

firmatory thoracic angiography. An endovascular stent graft of the aorta should be considered in a critical, unstable patient.

Priorities in Association with Delayed Deterioration of Vital Signs. If DPL or FAST is positive and the mediastinum is indistinct on either a supine or erect chest radiograph, then the patient should proceed immediately to the operating room because of unstable vital signs and hemoperitoneum. However, since the need for chest CT is known before surgery, the traumatologist should arrange for the chest CT to be performed immediately at the conclusion of the abdominal surgery.

Hemorrhagic shock caused by abdominal trauma (most likely splenic or hepatic) is usually treatable; however, hemorrhagic shock caused by a ruptured aorta is unlikely to be treatable because total exsanguination occurs rapidly. Therefore a patient who arrives in shock yet is able to be resuscitated is most likely freely bleeding from a source other than the thoracic aorta, especially if the left hemithorax is not opacified with blood on the admitting protocol chest radiograph.

CT Diagnosis of Occult Pneumothoraces and Treatment. With the increased use of both abdominal and chest CT, pneumothoraces not seen on chest radiographs are being diagnosed with increasing frequency. The incidence among patients receiving an abdominal CT for trauma is about 8%.[38] Most traumatologists do not treat these occult pneumothoraces with tube thoracostomy if a patient is stable and is not going to receive positive pressure ventilation. However, if a patient is going to the operating room for a lengthy procedure, a chest tube is placed as a precaution against the development of a tension pneumothorax during surgery.

Focus: The Diaphragm

Diagnosis. The diagnosis of traumatic rupture of the diaphragm is difficult to confidently establish preoperatively. With penetrating trauma, the diagnosis usually is assumed because of the location of the wound. Diaphragmatic injury must be considered with any injury of the thorax below the fourth intercostal space. In most cases of penetrating injury due to gunshot wounds, the diagnosis is established surgically. Stab wounds that potentially penetrate the diaphragm (if they occur on the left side) are usually repaired to prevent possible herniation of abdominal contents later. However, most surgeons do not explore stab wounds on a patient's right side if they occur high on the posterior thorax. The liver is considered protective against herniation, and the wounds are usually more than 2 cm[39] long.

The diagnosis of traumatic diaphragmatic rupture from blunt trauma is often difficult because of associated

Table 1-9 Diagnostic Peritoneal Lavage	
RBCs	**Therapeutic Celiotomy (%)**
>100,000	85
50,000 to 100,000	26
<50,000	4

injuries and few physical signs. In any blunt trauma patient with obscuration of either diaphragm on initial chest radiograph, traumatic rupture must be considered. Gelman et al.[40] found that chest radiography may be diagnostic or at least suggestive of injury in about 60% of patients with left-sided hemidiaphragm injury. This entity is found more commonly on the left side (70%) than on the right (30%).[40-42] The diagnosis in not infrequently made because of concurrent associated intraabdominal injuries. In the review by Gelman et al.,[40] DPL (leading to celiotomy) was positive in four (67%) of six patients with right-sided rupture and in 26 (81%) of 32 patients with left-sided rupture. However, DPL may have a false-negative rate as high as 11% for this entity.[43] Table 1-10 reviews the diagnostic accuracy from a large series.[40]

Several other diagnostic methods can be used to confirm suspected diaphragmatic injury, including DPL by observing the fluid draining from a thoracostomy tube. Useful imaging studies include upper GI contrast studies, including fluoroscopy, CT scanning with sagittal reconstruction, and MRI. CT may show direct discontinuity of the hemidiaphragm in blunt trauma but is limited in penetrating injuries, with reported sensitivities of 0% to 80%.[44] With improvements in CT technology and better sagittal reconstruction, the accuracy should improve. MRI also can be used but technically is difficult in an acute trauma patient.[44,45] If the diagnosis remains uncertain despite the use of the above diagnostic tests, thoracoscopy may be useful for both diagnosis and treatment.[46]

Priorities in Association with Vital Signs. A trauma patient with stable vital signs and an admitting chest radiograph suspicious for diaphragm injury should undergo additional studies as described earlier. Generally, a nasogastric tube is placed, followed by instillation of water-soluble GI contrast (barium will preclude performing an abdominal/pelvic CT) for localization of the stomach. The traumatologist must realize that other entities may closely mimic a ruptured diaphragm (e.g.,

severe atelectasis of the entire left lower lobe that elevates the left hemidiaphragm and stomach so that they appear to be in the lower thorax). Once the diagnosis of ruptured hemidiaphragm is established, the patient should proceed to the operating room for repair; however, this is not an emergency if vital signs are stable.

A trauma patient with unstable vital signs requires resuscitation first and a thorough search for the cause of instability. If the admitting chest radiograph suggests diaphragmatic rupture and the instability persists, then DPL or FAST should be performed immediately and, if positive, the patient should go directly to the operating room for celiotomy without further imaging workup of the diaphragm. Inspection at the time of celiotomy likely will reveal the diagnosis. If, however, DPL or FAST results are negative, the cause of the instability still requires investigation. Pelvic radiographs will detect pelvic fracture patterns likely to be associated with significant extraperitoneal blood loss, and abdominal CT may reveal a hidden source of hemorrhage (retroperitoneal, subcapsular hepatic or splenic hematomas, or renal injuries). A ruptured diaphragm per se usually will not cause cardiovascular instability and does not by itself constitute a reason for immediate celiotomy.

Caution must be exercised in patients who require endotracheal intubation. Positive pressure ventilation may delay herniation of abdominal contents through a torn diaphragm into the thorax. The radiographic appearance of a ruptured diaphragm with herniation may be delayed until the patient is extubated at a later date, at which point herniation, leading to respiratory compromise, occurs.

Focus: The Abdomen

The abdomen (from Latin *abdere*, "to hide") is probably the most controversial region of the body for diagnostic workup for both blunt and penetrating trauma. This workup dilemma is further compounded by the recent

Table 1-10
Diagnostic Methods in Blunt Rupture of the Diaphragm

Side	CXR	DPL	FL	UGI	Sono	CT	MRI
			RESULTS OF STUDY*				
Left (20/44,[†] 46%)	8/44	26/32	1/1	2/2	2/1	1/6	2/2
	18%	81%	100%	100%	0%	17%	100%
Right (1/16, 17%)	1/6	4/6	NA	NA	0/1	0/1	NA
	17%	67%	—	—	0%	0%	—
Total (21/50, 42%)	9/50	30/38	1/1	2/2	0/2	1/7	2/2
	18%	79%	100%	100%	0%	14%	100%

*Number of positive/number of patients studied.
†Leading to diagnosis of rupture.
CXR, Chest x-ray; *DPL,* diagnostic peritoneal lavage; *FL,* fluoroscopy; *UGI,* upper gastrointestinal series; *Sono,* sonography.

advent of more rapid CT capabilities ("multislice" CT), as well as the increased use of ultrasound in trauma centers and emergency departments.

Penetrating Abdominal Trauma

Gunshot Wounds

Anterior abdominal wounds. Any gunshot wound with an entrance at or below the fourth intercostal space should be considered intraabdominal. For all transperitoneal anterior abdominal gunshot wounds, most surgeons agree that immediate exploratory laparotomy is indicated after obtaining AP and lateral radiographs of the abdomen for gross localization of the bullet(s). Approximately 80% of abdominal gunshot wounds penetrate the peritoneum, and 95% cause intraabdominal injury. In the presence of unstable vital signs, evisceration, gastrointestinal bleeding, or signs of peritonitis, the patient is transported immediately to an operating room for expeditious control of hemorrhage. A chest radiograph may be performed if a pneumothorax is a consideration. Localizing radiographs and an IVP/cystogram may be performed in the operating room if deemed necessary after control of hemorrhage to locate urinary system injuries; precious time should not be wasted in the emergency department by performing these radiographs. The surgeon will be able to determine the nature of the injuries and the presence of one or two kidneys while in the operating room. If vital signs are stable, AP and lateral radiographs of the abdomen and thorax should be obtained to localize the bullet(s); knowing the trajectory of the missile makes it slightly easier for the surgeon to find injuries.

Tangential, flank, or back. Abdominal gunshot wounds that appear to be tangential (not transperitoneal by AP and lateral radiographs) deserve special consideration. These patients may be observed but should have a physical examination every 4 to 6 hours. They also may undergo a triple-contrast CT (IV, GI, and rectal) to disclose any intraabdominal or extraperitoneal injuries.[47] More recently, some trauma centers conduct a FAST; if the FAST is positive for fluid, the patient should be transported to the operating room. In a recent study the positive predictive value for FAST was 94%.[48] Laparoscopy in the presence of tangential abdominal gunshot wounds has not gained widespread support.

Patients with possible rectal injuries should undergo preoperative sigmoidoscopy for definitive diagnosis if their vital signs are stable because rectal injuries are extraperitoneal and difficult to view at surgery. Practically all transperitoneal gunshot wounds of the abdomen require surgical exploration; therefore there is little indication for GI contrast studies. If vital signs are unstable, the patient should be transported immediately to the operating room, and, if there is any question about a pos-

sible rectal injury, sigmoidoscopy may be performed at the conclusion of the procedure. Alternatively, a transverse loop colostomy may be performed, obviating the need for sigmoidoscopy if the likelihood of a rectal injury is great.

A small percentage of abdominal gunshot wounds do not penetrate the peritoneal cavity but are tangential. The possibility still exists for intraperitoneal injury due to cavitation effect of the missile, especially if it is of high caliber. Laparoscopy has been used to determine intraperitoneal penetration but has not gained widespread acceptance. CT with triple contrast (IV, GI, and rectal) may be diagnostic, especially if the gunshot wound is tangential through the back or flank area. In a recent study, if the triple-contrast study was equivocal for peritoneal penetration, the authors found 100% accuracy of triple contrast when combined with laparoscopy.[47]

Anterior Stab Wounds. If vital signs are unstable or if peritonitis is obvious, then patients with abdominal stab wounds should be taken to the operating room for control of possible intraabdominal hemorrhage or hollow visceral injury.

If vital signs are stable, four methods of workup exist: mandatory laparotomy (with a potentially high negative laparotomy rate), local wound exploration combined with DPL, triple-contrast CT to detect free intraperitoneal air or fluid (presumptive of bowel injury), or a conservative approach involving repeated physical examinations. It is important to remember that approximately one third of anterior abdominal stab wounds do not penetrate the abdominal cavity, one third penetrate but do not cause significant injury, and the last third penetrate and cause significant injury (Fig. 1-4).

Posterior Stab Wounds. Stab wounds of the flank or back are a special problem because of possible injury to

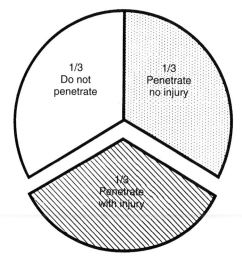

Fig. 1-4
Distribution of injury associated with abdominal stab wounds

retroperitoneal structures, including portions of the ascending or descending colon, kidneys, ureters, pancreas, and portions of the duodenum (all except the first portion). When injuries occur to these organs, they may not originally yield positive peritoneal signs on physical examination.

A patient with unstable vital signs or peritoneal signs is taken to the operation room for exploration. Possible wounds of the retroperitoneal portions of the colon should be sought by proper surgical mobilization. If the urine was positive for blood preoperatively, then the ureters, kidneys, and bladder should be inspected carefully.

In the presence of normal vital signs and normal abdominal physical examination (including a rectal examination negative for blood), a more investigative approach may be taken. Abdominal and pelvic CT with oral, intravenous, and colonic contrast may be performed in a stable patient. Some reports have shown the value of this approach in determining the need for surgical exploration.[49-53] Contrast-enhanced CT (CECT) has been reported to have an accuracy rate of 97% to 100%.[49,52,53] Unfortunately, CECT has not been reliable in diagnosing diaphragmatic injuries. If CECT is "positive" (urine extravasation, pneumoperitoneum or hemoperitoneum, colonic extravasation, or significant retroperitoneal hemorrhage), surgical exploration would be indicated. If CECT reveals no significant injuries, careful clinical observation and frequent physical examination are still needed.

Mandatory Exploratory Celiotomy. Most surgeons do not disagree as to the basic indications for immediate celiotomy (Table 1-11). Shock (which is almost always hemorrhagic), peritonitis (rebound tenderness, guarding, loss of bowel sounds), and gastrointestinal hemorrhage (nasogastric tube drainage positive for blood, or hematochezia) are all absolute indications for surgery after adequate resuscitation. In these clinical circumstances, radiographs are not necessary and should not be performed without good reason. Most surgeons agree that omental evisceration necessitates exploratory celiotomy; however, literature from South Africa advocates that nonexploratory surgery, with amputation of eviscerated

Table 1-11
Indications for Emergency Celiotomy in Abdominal Stab Wound

Shock
Evisceration
Peritonitis
Pneumoperitoneum
Gastrointestinal hemorrhage
Diaphragm laceration

omentum, is safe.[54-56] However, others have found this practice unsafe.[54] Any stab wound to the chest below the fourth intercostal space that penetrates the pleura also lacerates the diaphragm, which requires repair to prevent future herniation of abdominal contents. An exception to this occurs with stab wounds to the right back that injures the portion of the right diaphragm that is covered adequately by the liver. Pneumoperitoneum, a radiologic diagnosis, is also considered an indication for exploratory celiotomy.

Local Wound Exploration and Diagnostic Lavage. With the advent of DPL in 1965 for the diagnosis of blunt abdominal trauma,[57] many surgeons have used this tool for abdominal stab wounds as well. Local exploration of the wound is carried out in the emergency department. If the wound does not penetrate the posterior abdominal fascia, the patient is observed. If the wound does penetrate the posterior abdominal fascia, then DPL is performed. The difficulty with this method lies in determining what lavage RBC is reliable for injury in abdominal stab wounds. Feliciano[58] found DPL to be 95% accurate, with 44% of his patients being observed when an RBC count of <100,000 was deemed negative; however, this figure had a 1.2% false-negative rate. Others, by lowering the acceptable RBC threshold, have decreased the false-negative rate[58-63] (Table 1-12).

Selective Conservatism/Physical Examination. Some surgeons have adopted a policy of mandatory laparotomy for all torso stab wounds. Approximately 15 years ago the therapeutic pendulum in the management of abdominal stab wounds had swung in the direction of selective conservatism, that is, physical examination to identify those patients not requiring immediate exploratory laparotomy and then continued observation to identify those patients who may subsequently require surgery. Shaftan[64] was the first to retrospectively identify the safety of a nonmandatory laparotomy policy. Since then, others have prospectively shown the safety of this policy. Centers that had staunchly maintained a mandatory exploration policy for all abdominal stab wounds reviewed their experiences and had changed to selective conservatism.[65] The incentives to adopt this approach are fewer unnecessary laparotomies, decreased length of stay, less morbidity and mortality and therefore decreased hospital costs.[66] The purist using this management policy would employ physical examination as the sole method to determine the need for exploratory laparotomy.[66] Selective conservatism appears safe, providing careful attention is paid to frequent reexaminations. However, because of the fear of missed injuries, most centers have adopted other methods to raise diagnostic accuracy. DPL is mentioned above, and laparoscopy has never gained widespread

Table 1-12
Diagnostic Peritoneal Lavage in Stab Wounds of the Abdomen

Author	RBC	False Positive(%)	False Negative (%)	Accuracy (%)
Feliciano et al.[58]	100,000	17.1	2.5	91.2
Thal[62]	100,000	9.7	6.5	92.7
Thompson et al.[63]	100,000	9.1	8.6	91.2
Merlotti et al.[60]	10,000	8.3	0.8	98.0
Henneman et al.[61]	5000	24.6	0.0	90.7
Oreskovich and Carrico[59]	1000	32.9	0.0	77.0

acceptance in trauma centers (anesthesia required, difficulty visualizing entire small bowel and retroperitoneal structures, operating room required). Most trauma centers today rely on contrast-enhanced CT.

Focused Assessment with Sonography for Trauma (FAST) after Penetrating Torso Injury. The use of FAST in torso trauma has become increasingly popular since the early 1990s. It was originally used primarily to detect free fluid in patients with blunt abdominal trauma.[67,68] However, recent studies reported the usefulness of FAST in patients with penetrating trauma.[48,69] Patients with a positive FAST would be triaged to the operating room, whereas those with a negative FAST would need either further diagnostic tests, repeat physical examination, or repeat FAST. Also, FAST includes an ultrasonic view of the pericardium and would be beneficial in detecting unsuspected pericardial blood. The drawback of FAST in penetrating trauma is its relatively low sensitivity (Table 1-13), which can be attributed to a relatively smaller quantity of intraperitoneal fluid present in penetrating trauma (especially stab wounds, with a sensitivity reported as low as 18%[48]) than in blunt trauma. A FAST that demonstrates free fluid after either a gunshot wound or stab wound is indicative of abdominal injuries that require surgery, and these patients would be taken to the operating room. FAST may become useful in military trauma or mass casualty situations as a screening tool for surgical triage.

Table 1-13
Accuracy of FAST in Penetrating Abdominal Trauma

Sensitivity (%)	46-67
Specificity (%)	94-98
PPV (%)	90-92
NPV (%)	60-89
Accuracy (%)	68-89

Data from Klein S, Johs S, Fujitani R, et al: *Arch Surg* 123:1173, 1988; and Levitt MA, Criss E, Kobernik M: *Ann Emerg Med* 14:959, 1985.
PPV, Positive predictive value; *NPV*, negative predictive value.

CT for Penetrating Torso Trauma. CT scan for the diagnosis of penetrating intraabdominal injury has gained widespread acceptance since the first reports[50,53,70] in the 1980s. Patients with penetrating wounds to the flank or back may silently harbor injuries to retroperitoneal structures, especially the colon and rectum, without evidence of peritonitis. The cecum and duodenum are partially retroperitoneal, whereas the rectum is totally retroperitoneal. Perforations of these structures may not show clinical signs of injury (peritonitis, fever, elevated WBC) for up to 4 to 8 hours after injury. DPL and FAST are essentially intraperitoneal diagnostic tools and are of little value in this setting. The use of triple-contrast CT may disclose either contrast extravasation (rectum and colon) or peritoneal penetration by the presence of air or fluid. Patients who are hemodynamically stable and without signs of peritonitis can be categorized into three groups depending on the results of the triple-contrast CT study. Group 1 patients have wounds that are obviously subcutaneous and can be discharged. Group 2 patients have wounds that are confined to the retroperitoneum (hematomas) without obvious organ injury. These patients should be observed for up to 72 hours or should undergo a repeat CT. Group 3 patients have obvious peritoneal penetration or retroperitoneal organ injury (pancreas, kidney, ureter). These patients usually require exploratory surgery. The accuracy of triple-contrast CT is reported from 97% to 100%.[47,49,53]

Blunt Abdominal Trauma

Diagnosis. Without doubt, the most difficult patients for a traumatologist to assess are those who have potentially suffered blunt abdominal trauma. Compounding this problem is the fact that a majority of these patients are intoxicated or have a cerebral injury, thus rendering the physical examination less trustworthy and heightening the need for adjunctive tests.[71] Root[57] was the first to describe the use of DPL in evaluation of blunt abdominal trauma patients. The technique has been refined by quantitative analysis.[72,73] Many authors have reported varying degrees of success in evaluating blunt abdominal trauma using DPL[74-77] (Table 1-14).

Table 1-14
Success Rates of DPL in Blunt Abdominal Trauma

Author	Sensitivity (%)	Specificity (%)	Accuracy(%)
Henneman [61]	88	97	95
Parvin et al. [74]	88	88	97
Gill et al. [75]	99	92	95
DuPriest et al. [43]	99	96	98
Engrav et al. [72]	96	99	99
Alyono and Perry [73]	97	100	99
McLellan et al. [77]	76	99	93

In the early 1980s, various articles addressed the use of abdominal CT to diagnose intraabdominal, renal, and other retroperitoneal injuries; other articles merely reported findings,[57] and some compared CT with physical examination.[78]

CT vs. DPL. Much conflict has arisen between the proponents of DPL and those of abdominal CT. To resolve the issue of which test is "best," prospective studies were designed to compare the two methods. The results of these studies are shown in Table 1-15.[79-82] The purpose of these studies was to compare the ability of these two tests to diagnose intraperitoneal injuries, not retroperitoneal injuries (CT versus DPL, not DPL plus IVP for hematuria). Missed injuries (false-negative tests) are of the greatest concern to the trauma surgeon, and each test has a measure of false-negative results. DPL will not assess retroperitoneal structures. Renal injuries may be missed, but IVP should diagnose the majority of renal injuries producing hematuria. Pancreatic injuries (if the retroperitoneum stays intact) also will be missed by DPL, but CT also has limitations in diagnosing pancreatic injuries. CT is excellent in detecting solid visceral injury but has historically had difficulty diagnosing a perforated hollow viscus. CT has become more reliable in this regard since the advent of helical CT. DPL also has limitations in detecting hollow viscus injuries.[82-84]

The conclusions drawn from most of the articles evaluating CT and DPL are that neither should be used exclusively. The methods have practically the same accuracy, and they can be used to complement each other if needed.

FAST for blunt abdominal trauma. The use of FAST to diagnose intraabdominal injury first gained popularity in Europe in the 1980s, and its use eventually spread to the United States in the early 1990s. The first prospective studies were reported by Tso and then by Rozychi.[85,86] Since then its use has gained widespread acceptance in trauma centers as evidenced by the FAST International Consensus Conference in 1997.[87]

FAST has been found to be a reliable test to screen for hemoperitoneum, whether interpreted by a radiologist or nonradiologist[89] (Table 1-16). Shackford recently reviewed the accuracy rates reported from over 20 publications and found that the rate depended on the prevalence of the target disease. If the prevalence was low (fewer patients with intraabdominal injuries), the FAST was more likely to be negative, and the error rate would be low. Conversely, higher prevalence rates yielded higher error rates (Table 1-17).[89]

Recent articles have addressed the accuracy of FAST when performed by the surgeon nonradiologist. "Indeterminate exam" rates (a measure of the sonographist's experience) vary depending on the number of FAST examinations the sonographist has performed. Boulanger[91] reported a 6.7% indeterminate rate when performed by an experienced surgeon sonologist, whereas Tso[85] reported a 12.3% indeterminate rate with the initial experience. The number of FAST examinations

Table 1-15
DPL Versus Abdominal CT in Blunt Trauma

Author	Patients	DPL			CT		
		SE	SP	A	SE	SP	A
Meyer[79]	301	95.9	99.0	98.2	74.3	99.5	92.6
Fabian[80]	91	90.0	100.0	98.0	60.0	100.0	91.0*
Marx[81]	65	100.0	100.0	100.0	40.0	100.0	—

*Initial reading values; values on revised reading were 85 and 97, respectively
SE, Sensitivity; *SP,* specificity; *A,* accuracy.

Table 1-16
Accuracy of FAST in Blunt Abdominal Trauma

	Sensitivity (%)	Specificity (%)	NPV (%)	PPV (%)	Accuracy(%)
Rose[88]	80	98	96	92	96
Shackford[89]	68	98	92	92	92
Rozychi[90]	83.3	99.7	98.9	95.2	—

Data from Rose JS, Levitt MA, Porter J, et al: *J Trauma* 51:545, 2001.

Table 1-17
Error Rate of FAST in Blunt Abdominal Trauma As a Function of Prevalence of Intraabdominal Trauma

Prevalence of Intraabdominal Injury (%)	Error Rate (Avg.) (%)	Sensitivity (Avg.) (%)	Specificity (Avg.) (%)
<10	0.6-3.9 (2.2)	41.7-92.9 (81.1)	97.5-100 (99.0)
10-20	0.3-6.5 (2.6)	81.5-98.1 (88.7)	95.7-100 (99.0)
>20	1.3-14.9 (4.4)	63.2-96.6 (94.4)	93.7-99.0 (96.2)

Data from Shackford SR, Rogers FB, Osler TM, et al: *J Trauma* 46:553, 1999.

required for a nonradiologist to perform to develop competence was originally thought to be 50 to 100. Shackford found this number to be excessive and asserted that nonradiologists required far fewer examinations to achieve competence.[89]

Rose[88] was able to show a decrease in the use of CT when sonography was available; however, he concluded that use of sonography was increased for patients with a low suspicion of injury and that a larger multicenter study was needed. In fact, despite the increased use of FAST by traumatologists, most trauma centers still rely heavily on CT when injury is suspected. The added advantages are imaging of the retroperitoneal structures—kidneys, pancreas, and duodenum.

It has become apparent to this author that the increased use of FAST in fact has accounted for a decreased use of DPL rather than a decrease in the use of CT in blunt abdominal trauma (see below).

Changing Management in Solid Visceral Injury. With the increased availability and use of faster CT scans, nonoperative management of liver and spleen injuries has become the standard of treatment. More recently, angiography with the potential for vessel embolization has become increasingly useful to definitively treat liver and spleen injuries and has improved the ability to successfully manage these injuries nonoperatively.[92] Success rates have been reported from 93% to 97%.[92,93] The success of nonoperative management depends on the grade of injury. Grade I injuries do not require embolization (see Tables 1-18 and 1-19 for grading scale), and grade V injuries should most likely be taken to the operating room. Any injury that demonstrates a contrast blush on CT scan (indicating a pseudoaneurysm or frank extravasation) should be considered for angiography with expectant embolization. Omert et al. concluded that a contrast

Table 1-18
Organ Injury Scales: Spleen

Grade*	Spleen
I	Hematoma, subcapsular, <10% surface area Laceration, capsular tear <1 cm depth

II	Hematoma
	  Subcapsular, 10%-50% surface area
	  Intraparenchymal, <5 cm diameter
	Laceration, 1-3 cm depth, not involving a
	  trabecular vessel

III	Hematoma
	  Subcapsular, >50% surface area or expanding;
	    ruptured subcapsular or parenchymal
	    hematoma
	  Intraparenchymal hematoma >5 cm or
	    expanding
	Laceration >3 cm parenchymal depth or involving
	  trabecular vessels

IV	Laceration, involving segmental or hilar vessels
	  producing major devascularization (>25% of
	  spleen)

V	Laceration, completely shattered spleen Vascular, hilar vascular injury that devascularizes spleen

Data from Bynoe RP, Miles WS, Bell RM: *J Vasc Surg* 14:346, 1991.
*Advance one grade for multiple injuries, up to grade III.

Table 1-19
Organ Injury Scales: Liver

Grade*	Liver
I	Hematoma, subcapsular, <10% surface area Laceration, capsular tear <1 cm depth

II	Hematoma
	  Subcapsular, 10%-50% surface area
	  Intraparenchymal <10 cm diameter
	Laceration, 1-3 cm depth, <10 cm length

III	Hematoma
	  Subcapsular, >50% surface area or expanding;
	    ruptured subcapsular or parenchymal
	    hematoma
	  Intraparenchymal hematoma >10 cm or
	    expanding
	Laceration >3 cm depth

IV	Laceration, parenchymal disruption involving
	  25%-75% of hepatic lobe or 1-3 Couinaud's
	  segments within a single lobe

V	Laceration, parenchymal disruption involving
	  >75% of hepatic lobe or >3 Couinaud's
	  segments within a single lobe
	Vascular, juxtahepatic venous injuries; e.g.,
	  retrohepatic vena cava or central major hepatic
	  veins

VI	Hepatic avulsion

Data from Bynoe RP, Miles WS, Bell RM: *J Vasc Surg* 14:346, 1991.
*Advance one grade for multiple injuries, up to grade III.

blush on CT scan weakly correlated with the need for splenic intervention (surgery or angiographic embolization) but should heighten the traumatologist's awareness for potential intervention.[94]

The potential danger of nonoperative management of solid visceral injuries is a missed hollow viscus injury. The incidence of hollow viscus injury is relatively rare (<1%) in the absence of liver or spleen injury[95]; however, the injury rate increases significantly with the presence of solid visceral injury.[96] Traumatologists must consider the possibility of a hollow viscus injury when managing a patient nonoperatively and need to reexamine the patient continually for signs of increasing abdominal tenderness.

Priorities in Association with Vital Signs. In a blunt trauma victim, the vital signs and physical examination determine the order in which diagnostic tests or therapies are performed. With stable vital signs and abdominal tenderness or evidence of injury (lacerations, contusion, seat belt markings), the traumatologist may use abdominal CT, DPL, or FAST with relatively equal accuracy for intraperitoneal injury. In most instances, CT would be preferable because of added imaging of the retroperitoneal structures and the ability to image other body areas (e.g., brain and spine, which are frequently imaged in blunt trauma patients). Cranial CT, if indicated, should precede the abdominal CT study to detect intracranial injuries requiring surgical treatment. If surgical intracranial lesions are present, the abdominal scan may be aborted and DPL performed in the operating room concomitant with the neurosurgical procedure. CT may be performed immediately postoperatively. In any patient requiring nonabdominal emergency surgery on admission, DPL or FAST should be performed to rapidly assess the peritoneal cavity.

CT and FAST or DPL may be necessary at times in the same patient. If the FAST or DPL is negative yet there is unexplained blood loss (as evidenced by continuing bouts of hypotension), abdominal CT may be performed to look for other "hidden" blood loss, such as a subcapsular liver or spleen hematoma or retroperitoneal hematoma. FAST also may be able to diagnose moderately large liver or spleen subcapsular hematomas. Conversely, CT may be difficult to interpret, or even show equivocal findings suggestive of bowel injury. DPL may provide useful additional information. In a patient with a CT diagnosis of a minor spleen or liver laceration (grade I) and delayed hypotension, DPL or FAST may expediently disclose the presence of a delayed bleed.

Patients with unstable vital signs should be fully resuscitated first. Expedient DPL or FAST will reveal if the abdomen is a likely source of hemorrhage. The protocol chest and pelvis radiographs also will quickly disclose major hemorrhage from either of these two areas. If DPL or FAST is positive, the patient proceeds directly to the operating room for exploratory surgery. Because FAST is easier and quicker to perform, absolutely noninvasive, and complication free, it has practically replaced DPL for diagnosis in blunt abdominal trauma.

The abdominal physical examination also determines which diagnostic study is performed. In the presence of peritonitis (tenderness, guarding, rebound, absent bowel sounds), the patient should be taken to the operating room. Some surgeons may perform confirmation FAST or DPL before surgery. If a patient has orthopedic injuries requiring emergency surgery that will last longer than 1 to 2 hours, then either FST, DPL, or CT should be performed preoperatively because the patient will be "lost" to physical examination during anesthesia and "unexplained" blood loss would not be attributable to the abdomen. FAST may be preferred because it is the most expedient and easiest to perform. In addition, patients with injuries both above and below the abdomen should have some screening diagnostic abdominal test performed.

Traumatologists have to make accurate decisions regarding the appropriate abdominal diagnostic study depending on the spectrum of injuries and vital signs at admission. It is therefore important to know the relative risk of abdominal injury given other injuries. In a review of more that 3200 blunt trauma patients, Roettger and others[97] identified 296 patients with abdominal injuries, 78% of whom underwent therapeutic laparotomies. The authors identified those variables that were risk factors for abdominal injury[97] (Table 1-20). This table provides the traumatologist with some idea of what to anticipate from patients sustaining blunt force injury and therefore should help in the decision-making process regarding use of diagnostic resources.

Focus: Retroperitoneal Injury—Hematuria

Hematuria in a trauma patient is indicative of injury to the kidneys, ureters, bladder, or a combination. Two reasons to investigate hematuria are to verify the presence of two kidneys and to determine the extent of injury to and function of each kidney. Controversy exists as to which patients should undergo urologic radiographic examination and, if so, by which method—IVP or contrast-enhanced CT.

Penetrating Trauma. Of patients with penetrating trauma, approximately 8% of all gunshot wounds and 6% of all stab wounds produce renal injury.[98] The degree of hematuria does not always correlate with the extent of injury.[99] Renal vascular pedicle injuries and ureteral transection produce hematuria in only 23% and 31% of cases.[97] Therefore patients with penetrating wounds whose trajectory indicates likely urologic injury should undergo diagnostic investigation. Neither the amount nor even the presence of hematuria is a reliable predictor of urologic injury in penetrating trauma.[99] All patients with penetrating wounds in locations that increase the risk for urologic injury should undergo a diagnostic study.[100-103] CT scan offers more information regarding other retroperitoneal structures than IVP.

Blunt Trauma. In blunt trauma, there appears to be better correlation between the extent of urologic injury and degree of hematuria. Not all patients with microscopic hematuria need radiographic investigation, because these examinations have been shown to have little effect on ultimate clinical management.[104-108] Klein et al.[104] found that no patient with >10 RBCs per high-power field (HPF) had any renal injuries, and only those with >30 RBCs per HPF had major injury. All patients presenting with >30 RBCs per HPF should undergo diagnostic evaluation. In addition, all patients with microscopic hematuria below this threshold that does not clear within 24 hours should also undergo diagnostic study. Other causes of hematuria unrelated to trauma (e.g., carcinomas of the kidney or bladder) may be disclosed.

The diagnostic study of choice is CT, which has the advantage over IVP of simultaneously imaging other solid viscera, as well as the kidneys, and would be preferred for patients with a greater likelihood of concurrent intraperitoneal injury. CT can provide a better assessment of the extent of renal injury and residual function, the extent of perirenal hematoma, and the presence of urine extravasation than can IVP and can also diagnose renal vascular pedicle injuries with greater specificity than IVP.

A patient who sustains blunt trauma and has hematuria and unstable vital signs requires further investigation by surgical exploration or radiographic study. If the vital signs stabilize with resuscitation, then the patient should go immediately for CT.

If a patient has stable vital signs and gross hematuria or microscopic hematuria of >30 RBCs per HPF, then emergency investigation is warranted. As noted earlier, CT is more sensitive for detection of intraabdominal and retroperitoneal injury and would be the study of choice.

Focus: Pelvic Fractures

The optimal management of patients with pelvic fractures has been evolving over the last three decades, from simple transfusion therapy with expectant tamponade to today's intervention with immediate external bony fixation and arterial embolization under angiographic control. All blunt trauma patients require admitting AP pelvic films by protocol. Once the diagnosis of pelvic fracture is made, the traumatologist must assess the type

---

Table 1-20
Risk Factors for Blunt Abdominal Injuries

Factor	All Patients (%) (N = 5920)	Patients with Abdominal Injury (%)
Blood pressure <90	6	42
Lower rib fracture	7	30
Chest injury	14	27
Pelvic disruption	10	26
Abdominal wall contusion or laceration	17	9
Respiratory insufficiency	27	19
Femoral fracture	12	17

Data from Gill W, Champion H, Long WB, et al: *Br J Surg* 62:121, 1975.

of fracture and determine which therapeutic method may be useful. All patients with pelvic fracture (regardless of fracture type) must have immediate orthopedic consultation. The traumatologist must have a full understanding of pelvic fracture patterns, the relative forces that produce them, and the associated injuries. The pelvic fracture pattern will alert the traumatologist to other potential injuries and guide further diagnostic evaluation.

Young and others[109] described pelvic fractures relative to four principal patterns of force, including AP (anteroposterior, grades I to III), lateral compression (grades I to III), vertical shear, and combined patterns. The diagnosis is based on a combination of radiographic and clinical findings. Radiographs provide the traumatologist with fracture diagnosis, and physical examination provides additional vital information on pelvic stability, which in turn depends on the integrity of the supporting ligaments. Other studies have correlated fracture pattern with specific organ injury pattern, transfusion requirement, and the need for and likelihood of success of therapeutic arterial embolization.[110] With these concepts in mind, the traumatologist, when faced with a patient in shock, will have a better idea of the source of hemorrhage and direct attention toward the correct choice of diagnostic and therapeutic methods. As shown in Table 1-21,[110] a pattern with a lateral compression fracture (type III) is more likely to be bleeding from a pelvic vascular injury than from a ruptured spleen. Therefore angiography (after bony stabilization) would more likely be therapeutic than an exploratory laparotomy.

Although 94% of pelvic fractures may be diagnosed from a high-quality radiograph,[109] in patients with stable vital signs, other views of the pelvis may also be helpful. The inlet view may demonstrate inward compression of the pelvis. The outlet view may demonstrate the degree of vertical displacement seen in a vertical shear fracture.

Pelvic CT is the best method to visualize acetabular, sacral, or sacroiliac fractures-dislocations, especially

when nonemergency internal fixation is contemplated. However, CT is not necessary as an emergency diagnostic study because standard radiographs, as noted above, are both highly accurate and expedient.

In a patient with unstable vital signs and a pelvic fracture, the traumatologist must quickly determine the source of hemorrhage. Physical examination will disclose any gross pelvic ring, bony or ligamentous instability, and obvious, nonspecific abdominal signs of hemorrhage (distention, peritonitis). The protocol AP pelvis radiograph will allow the traumatologist to estimate the severity of pelvic fracture, and FAST or DPL will disclose the presence of hemoperitoneum. If the FAST is negative or the DPL has an RBC count of <100,000, the abdomen probably is not the major source of hemorrhage, and the pelvis, as the most likely source of hemorrhage, is addressed first by immediate external fixation. Orthopedic surgeons, well versed in orthopedic trauma care, can apply external fixation in 30 to 60 minutes. Bony stabilization will decrease bleeding, especially in a patient who needs to be physically moved (stretcher to CT table, stretcher to angiographic table).

After pelvic stabilization and intraabdominal hemorrhage has been excluded, if hypotension continues to be a problem or there is an ongoing need for blood transfusion (more than six units), then pelvic angiography should be performed for possible therapeutic embolization. However, with greater use of external bony fixation, the pelvis will not be able to expand, tamponade will occur at an earlier time, and there will be less need for angiographic embolization.

If FAST is positive or DPL reveals gross blood in the face of unstable vital signs, the patient should go immediately to the operating room for both exploratory laparotomy and pelvic external fixation. In some cases the external fixation may be expediently placed first and "swung down" (caudally) away from the anterior abdomen to allow surgical access for exploratory laparotomy.

In a patient with pelvic fracture and stable vital signs, the abdomen should be assessed by CT. CT can obtain more information about the bony pelvis and intraabdominal and retroperitoneal structures than either FAST or DPL. External fixation, if appropriate, may follow CT.

To adequately manage patients with major pelvic fractures and their associated injuries, the resources of radiology, orthopedic surgery, the operating room staff, and angiography team must be smoothly orchestrated. The order in which these services are needed varies greatly from patient to patient, and the entire team must be able to adapt to a patient's changing needs. The traumatologist should be in charge at all times to determine the order in which diagnoses and therapies proceed.

Table 1-21
Pelvic Fracture Type and Area Injury Pattern

Pelvic Fracture Type	Area Injured and Shock		
	Spleen (%)	Pelvic (%)	Vascular (%)
LC I	13	0	31
LC II	9	9	32
LC III	0	20	40
AP I	9	6	32
AP II	17	10	30
AP III	19	22	67
VS	25	12	63
CMI	13	10	40

Focus: Extremity Injury

The vast majority of orthopedic extremity injuries are not life threatening and should be considered of secondary priority. The initial ABCs of trauma care, as outlined earlier, must always proceed as usual, including the protocol set of admitting radiographs, although there is an obvious orthopedic injury. Priorities of trauma care must be adhered to; if the patient is suffering from a head injury and CT is available, then the orthopedic radiographic survey should wait until the cranial CT is performed. If, however, CT is not available, then the skeletal films should be obtained up to the time that the CT is ready, at which point skeletal radiographs are then discontinued until the patient returns from the CT suite. If the CT discloses a life-threatening neurosurgical lesion, the skeletal films are finished after neurosurgical intervention (perhaps in the operating room, if deemed necessary). A patient with unstable vital signs and hemoperitoneum should go directly to the operating room. In this case, the orthopedic films may be obtained in the operating room after exploratory laparotomy. Patients who have had stable vital signs and whose primary survey is complete may then have extremity radiographs obtained of the areas in question.

Vascular Injury of the Extremity. Controversy still exists regarding the proper workup for penetrating injuries to extremities. Table 1-22 lists the "hard" signs of vascular injury, considered absolute indications for immediate surgical exploration. Most traumatologists agree that angiography is not warranted for patients with hard signs of vascular injury and recommend prompt surgical exploration to obviate any delay. This approach yields positive

---

Table 1-22
Signs of Vascular Injury

Hard Signs
Active hemorrhage
Thrill
Bruit
Expanding hematoma
Pulse deficit
Ischemia

Soft Signs
Peripheral nerve deficit
Small, nonexpanding hematoma
History of hemorrhage (stopped before admission)
Hypotension
Nonpulsatile hematoma

Proximity Alone
Neither hard nor soft signs of injury
Gunshot or stab wound trajectory within 2 cm of major artery

---

exploration in 68% to 91%[111-113] of patients. The management of patients with "soft" signs of vascular injury has become controversial because few will have injury.[114,115] Diagnostic angiography or Doppler duplex scanning has replaced routine exploration, recommended during the Korean War (due to lack of angiography). Some surgeons suggest that if angiography demonstrates an "abnormality" (narrowing, intimal flap), then surgical exploration is mandatory. Since some vascular injuries demonstrated by arteriography may be clinically insignificant, some authors have questioned the necessity of repairing all angiographically demonstrated lesions.[114,116,117] Most surgeons agree that branch arteries do not require repair; however, controversy now surrounds whether it is necessary to repair lesions seen in major vessels angiographically that do not have hemodynamic consequences. More prospective studies like Frykberg's need to be completed to understand the natural history of these injuries.[116]

Another controversy exists concerning the necessity of emergency angiography purely for penetrating injuries in proximity to major vessels without any physical signs of injury. It appears that angiography does not necessarily have to be performed immediately. Frykberg et al.,[114] in a prospective study, found that angiography for proximity wounds may be delayed for up to 24 hours without causing morbidity. The yield of angiography for proximity injuries alone varies from 6% to 20%.[111,112,114,118] Others have studied the association of actual wound location and wounding agent as determinants of the need for angiography in proximity wounds.[117] Some traumatologists use the ankle-to-brachial Doppler pressure index to determine the need for formal study. If the systolic pressure of the injured extremity divided by the systolic pressure of the uninjured extremity is less than 0.9, then either duplex ultrasound or angiography should be performed. The Doppler pressure index has been found to be 72.5% sensitive and 100% specific.[119] Physical examination alone appears accurate for all stab wounds of the extremities and for gunshot wounds to the lateral thigh and lateral arm.[117]

Noninvasive vascular tests are being used as screening tests in an attempt to avoid invasive angiography. Duplex ultrasonography has become increasingly popular and successful.[120] Bynoe[121] found duplex ultrasonography to be 98% accurate when compared with the gold standard of angiography.

Endovascular Grafts. Surgical repair of proximal extremity vascular injuries can be extremely difficult, especially in a patient with multiple injuries. Exposure can be anatomically challenging, which further complicates achieving proximal and distal control of the injured vessel. Dotter[122] first proposed the use of endovascular stent grafts in 1969. Others recently reported on the successful use of endovascular stent grafts in trauma.[123-125] In a patient with stable vital signs, endovascular stent grafts have a distinct advantage over surgical repair. They can be placed in a timely fashion without having to obtain direct access to the injury site, would have less blood loss, and would not require the use of an operating room and general anesthesia. This becomes especially advantageous in a multiply injured blunt trauma patient. However, the operating room and anesthesiology staff should be made aware of the potential need of an operating room if the patient's status changes. Traumatologists, interventional radiologists, and operating room personnel need to work in a coordinated manner to achieve optimal results.

Priorities Associated with Vascular Injury. Patients with hard signs of extremity arterial injury should be surgically explored. Some surgeons would like the luxury of angiography, but this is probably not always necessary (except in very proximal injuries). Certainly the patient with frank ischemia or active uncontrollable hemorrhage needs to be taken immediately to surgery. If angiography is deemed necessary it may be performed in the emergency area by the traumatologist for expediency, realizing that the quality will not be as good as formal angiography performed in the angiography suite. Angiography performed outside of the angiography suite has become rare because of increasing availability and readiness of interventional radiology.

For patients with soft signs of injury, angiography should be performed. Most vascular surgeons repair injuries to major vessels, and some patients may be candidates for endovascular stent graft (see above). Patients with proximity injuries may either be observed or have nonemergency angiography.

CONCLUSION

The success of a trauma system depends on the integrated functioning of the parts that make up the whole. Field activities, from first responder to paramedic to transport and communication teams, have to work in a well-coordinated fashion. The receiving facility must be in a state of preparedness at all times. A designated trauma unit must be 100% dedicated to the care of trauma victims. This requires special allocation of personnel to meet these needs that are so lacking in a major percentage of hospitals in the United States. This dedication cuts across all departments within a hospital. The traumatologist must be well versed in the care of trauma victims and specifically must understand triage priorities regarding use of diagnostic imaging. Likewise, radiologists and technologists must be equally well versed in treatment protocols and priorities. The interventional radiologist takes on an even more important role than in the past

with the advent of life-saving angiographic embolization of liver and spleen injuries, as well as the potential placement of endovascular stent grafts. The advent of more rapid CT imaging with contrast (CT angiography) decreases the time to diagnosis of injuries that previously awaited the angiography team to arrive; in the near future it may significantly decrease the need for diagnostic angiography. MRI has not taken on significant new roles in acute trauma patient management in the past 5 to 10 years.

The traumatology and radiology services form a cohesive team with the common goal of skillful coordination of imaging studies using well thought out strategies based on the clinical status of the patient, the particular imaging capabilities of the center, and the use of quality research results. The ability to adapt to changing clinical circumstances is a key part of this effort. The capacity to apply new technologies to the diagnostic strategy, as they are acquired, is an ongoing process requiring input from many members of the trauma service. Ultimately, the result of this endeavor offers the greatest chance to preserve the lives of acute trauma victims.

REFERENCES

1. National Academy of Sciences and National Research Council: Accidental death and disability: the neglected disease of modern society, Washington, DC, 1966, US Government Printing Office.
2. Trunkey DD: What's wrong with trauma care? *Bull Am Coll Surg* 75:10, 1990.
3. Cowley RA: Trauma center: a new concept for the delivery of critical care, *J Med Soc* 4:979, 1977.
4. West JG, Trunkey DD, Lin RC, Systems of trauma care: a study of two counties, *Arch Surg* 114:455, 1979.
5. Neuman TS, Bockman MA, Moody P, et al: An autopsy study of traumatic deaths, San Diego County, 1979, *Am J Surg* 144:722, 1982.
6. Maryland Institute for Emergency Medical Services Systems: The Maryland medical protocols for cardiac rescue technicians and emergency medical technicians-paramedics. Baltimore, 1990, Maryland Institute for Emergency Medical Services Systems.
7. Committee on Trauma: Hospital resources for optimal care of the injured patient, *Bull Am Coll Surg* 64:43, 1979.
8. Committee on Trauma: *Advanced trauma life for doctors*, ed 6, Chicago, 1997, American College of Surgeons.
9. Teasdale G, Jennett B: Assessment of coma and impaired consciousness: a practical scale, *Lancet* 2:81, 1974.
10. Bracken MB, Shepard MJ, Collins WF: A randomized controlled trial of methylprednisolone or naloxone in the treatment of acute spinal cord injury, *N Engl J Med* 322:1406, 1990.
11. Bracken MB, Shepard MJ, Holford TR: Administration of methylprednisolone for 24 or 48 hours or tirilazad mesylate for 48 hours in the treatment of acute spinal cord injury: results of the Third National Acute Spinal Cord Injury Randomized Controlled Trial, *JAMA* 277:1597, 1997.
12. Snow RB, Zimmerman RD, Gandy Se, Deck MDG: Comparison of magnetic resonance imaging and computed tomography in the evaluation of head injury, *Neurosurgery* 18:45, 1986.
13. Chiu W, Haan J, Cushing BM, et al: Ligamentous injuries of the cervical spine in unreliable blunt trauma patients: incidence, evaluation, and outcome, *J Trauma* 50:457, 2001.

14. Boberge RJ, Wears RC, Kelly M. et al: Selective application of cervical spine radiography in alert victims of blunt trauma: a prospective study, *J Trauma* 28:784, 1988.

15. Bachulis BL, Long WB, Hynes G, Johnson MC: Clinical indications for cervical spine radiographs in the traumatized patient, *Am J Surg* 153:473, 1987.

16. Pasquale M, Fabian TC: Practice management guidelines for trauma from the Eastern Association for the Surgery of Trauma, *J Trauma* 44:941, 1998.

17. Post MJD, Green BA: The use of computed tomography in spinal trauma, *Radiol Clin North Am* 21:327, 1983.

18. Roon AJ, Christensen N: Evaluation and treatment of penetrating cervical injuries, *J Trauma* 19:391, 1979.

19. Mazolewske PJ, Curry JD, Browder T, et al: Computed tomographic scan can be used for surgical decision making in zone II penetrating neck injuries, *J Trauma* 51:315, 2001.

20. Munera F, Soto JA, Velez SM, et al: Diagnosis of arterial injuries caused by penetrating trauma to the neck: comparison of helical CT angiography and conventional angiography, *Radiology* 216:356, 2000.

21. Rogers FB, Baker EF, Osler TM: Computed tomographic angiography as a screening modality for blunt cervical arterial injuries: preliminary results, *J Trauma* 46:380, 1999.

22. Fry WJ: Carotid artery injuries. Paper presented at meeting of the Postgraduate Course in Peripheral Vascular Disease. The American College of Surgeons Seventieth Annual Clinical Congress, San Francisco, 1984.

23. Elerding SC, Manrt FD, Moore EE: A reappraisal of penetrating neck injury management, *J Trauma* 20:695, 1980.

24. Fitchett VH, Pomerantz M, Butsch DW, et al: Penetrating wounds of the neck: a military and civilian experience, *Arch Surg* 99:307, 1969.

25. Flax RL, Fletcher HS, Joseph WL: Management of penetrating injuries of the neck, *Ann Surg* 39:148, 1973.

26. Jones RF, Terrell JC, Salyer KE: Penetrating wounds of the neck: an analysis of 274 cases, *J Trauma* 7:228, 1967.

27. Sandaran S, Walt AJ: Penetrating wounds of the neck: principles and some controversies, *Surg Clin North Am* 57:139, 1977.

28. Sheely CH, Mattox KL, Beall AC, et al: Penetrating wounds of the cervical esophagus, *Am J Surg* 130:707, 1975.

29. Cheadel W, Richardson JD: Options in the management of trauma to the esophagus, *Surg Gynecol Obstet* 155:380, 1982.

30. Miller FB, Richardson JD, Thomas HA, et al: Role of CT in diagnosis of major arterial injury after blunt thoracic trauma, *Surgery* 106:596, 1989.

31. Mirvis SE, Kostrubiak I, Whitley N, et al: Role of CT in excluding major arterial injury after blunt thoracic trauma, *AJR* 149:601, 1987.

32. Richardson P, Mirvis SE, Scorpio R, et al: Value of CT in determining the need for angiography when findings of mediastinal hemorrhage on chest radiographs are equivocal, *AJR* 156:273, 1991.

33. Mirvis SE, Shanmuganathan K: Traumatic aortic injury: diagnosis with contrast-enhanced thoracic CT: five-year experience at a major trauma center, *Radiology* 200:413, 1996.

34. Fabian CC, Davis KA, Gavant ML, et al: Prospective study of blunt aortic injury: helical CT is diagnostic and antihypertensive therapy reduces rupture, *Ann Surg* 227:666, 1998.

35. Singh MJ, Rohrer MJ, Ghaleb M: Endoluminal stent-graft repair of a thoracic aortic transection in a trauma patient with multiple injuries: case report, *J Trauma* 52:376, 2001.

36. Mattisno R, Hamilton IN, Ciraulo CL, et al: Stent-graft repair of acute traumatic thoracic aortic transection with intentional occlusion of the left subclavian artery: case report, *J Trauma* 52:326, 2001.

37. Fujikawa T, Yukioka T, Ishimaru S, et al.: Endovascular stent grafting for the treatment of blunt thoracic aortic injury, *J Trauma* 50:223, 2001.

38. Hill SL, Edmisten T, Holtzman G, et al: The occult pneumothorax: an increasing diagnostic entity in trauma, *Am Surg* 65:254, 1999.

39. Wise L, Conners J, Hwang YA, et al: Traumatic injuries to the diaphragm, *J Trauma* 13:946, 1973.

40. Gelman R, Mirvis SE, Gens DR: Diaphragmatic rupture due to blunt trauma: sensitivity of plain chest radiographs, *AJR* 156:51, 1991.

41. Rodriguez-Morales G, Rodriguez A, Shatney CH: Acute rupture of the diaphragm in blunt trauma patients: analysis of 60 patients, *J Trauma* 26:438, 1986.

42. Morgan AS, Flancbaum L, Esposito T, Cox EF: Blunt injury to the diaphragm: an analysis of 44 patients, *J Trauma* 26:565, 1986.

43. DuPriest RW, Rodriguez A, Khaneja SC, et al: Open diagnostic peritoneal lavage in blunt abdominal trauma, *Surg Gynecol Obstet* 148:890, 1979.

44. Shanmuganathan K, Mirvis S: Advances in emergency radiology. I. Imaging diagnosis of non-aortic thoracic injury, *Radiol Clin North Am* 37:533, 1999.

45. Mirvis SE, Keramati B, Buchman R, Rodriguez A: MR imaging of traumatic diaphragmatic rupture, *J Comput Assist Tomogr* 12:147, 1988.

46. Yamashita J, Iwasaki A, Kawahara K, et al: Thoracoscopic approach to the diagnosis and treatment of diaphragmatic disorders, *Surg Laparosc Endosc* 6:485,1996.

47. Ginzburg E, Carrillo EH, Kopelman T, et al: The role of computed tomography in selective management of gunshot wounds to the abdomen and flank, *J Trauma* 45:1005, 1998.

48. Udobi KF, Rodriguez A, Chiu WC, et al: Role of ultrasonography in penetrating abdominal trauma: a prospective clinical study, *J Trauma* 50:475, 2001.

49. Hauser CJ, Huprich JE, Bosco P, et al: Triple-contrast computed tomography in the evaluation of penetrating abdominal injuries, *Arch Surg* 122:1112, 1987.

50. Phillips T, Sclafani SJA, Goldstein A, et al: Use of the contrast-enhanced CT enema in the management of penetrating trauma to the flank and back, *J Trauma* 26:593, 1986.

51. Fletcher TB, Setiawan H, Harrell RS, et al: Posterior abdominal stab wounds: role of CT evaluation, *Radiology* 173:621, 1989.

52. Kortin OC, Wint D, Thrasher J, et al: Stab sounds to the back and flank in the hemodynamically stable patient: a decision algorithm based on contrast-enhanced computed tomography with colonic opacification, *Am J Surg* 173:189, 1997.

53. Meyer DM, Thal ER, Weigelt JA, Redman HC: The role of CT in the evaluation of stab wounds to the back, *J Trauma* 29:1226, 1989.

54. Burnweit CA, Thal ER: Significance of omental evisceration in abdominal stab wounds, *Am J Surg* 152:670, 1986.

55. Demetriades D, Rabinowitz B: Indications for operation in abdominal stab wounds: a prospective study, *Ann Surg* 205:129, 1987.

56. Hulzinga WKJ, Baker LW, Mitshall ZW: Selective management of abdominal and thoracic stab wounds with established peritoneal penetration: the eviscerated omentum, *Am J Trauma* 153:564, 1987.

57. Root HD, Hauser CW, McKinley CR, et al: Diagnostic peritoneal lavage, *Surgery* 87:533, 1995.

58. Feliciano DV, Bitondo CG, Steed G, et al: Five hundred open taps or lavages in patients with abdominal stab wounds, *Am J Surg* 148:772, 1984.

59. Oreskovich MR, Carrico CT: Stab wounds of the anterior abdomen: analysis of a management plan using local wound exploration and quantitative peritoneal lavage, *Ann Surg* 198:411, 1983.

60. Meriotti GT, Marcet E, Sheaff CM, et al: Use of peritoneal lavage to evaluate abdominal penetration, *J Trauma* 25:22, 1985.

61. Henneman PL, Marx JA, Moore EE, et al: Diagnostic peritoneal lavage: accuracy in predicting necessary laparotomy following blunt and penetrating trauma, *J Trauma* 30:1345, 1990.

62. Thal ER: Evaluation of peritoneal lavage and local exploration in lower chest and abdominal stab wounds, *J Trauma* 17:642, 1977.

63. Thompson JS, Moore EE, Van Duzer-Moore S, et al: The evolution of abdominal stab wound management, *J Trauma* 20:478, 1980.

64. Shaftan GW: Indications for operation in abdominal trauma, *Am J Surg* 99:657, 1960.

65. Sirinek KR, Page CP, Root HD, Levine BA: Is exploratory celiotomy necessary for all patients with truncal stab wounds? *Arch Surg* 125:844, 1990.

66. Nance FC, Cohn I: Surgical judgment in the management of stab wounds of the abdomen: a retrospective and prospective analysis based on a study of 60 stabbed patients, *Ann Surg* 170:569, 1969.

67. Tso P, Rodriguez A, Cooper C, et al: Sonography in blunt abdominal trauma: a preliminary progress report, *J Trauma* 33:39, 1992.

68. Rozychi GS: Abdominal ultrasonography in trauma, *Surg Clin North Am* 75:175, 1995.

69. Boulanger BR, Kearney PA, Tsuei B, et al: The routine use of sonography in penetrating torso injury is beneficial, *J Trauma* 51:320, 2001.

70. Rehm CG, Sherman R, Hinz TW: The role of CT scan in evaluation for laparotomy in patients with stab wounds of the abdomen, *J Trauma* 29:446, 1989.

71. Rodriguez A, DuPriest RW, Shatney CM: Recognition of intraabdominal injury in blunt trauma victims, *Am Surg* 48:456, 1982.

72. Engrav LH, Benjamen CI, Strate RG, et al: Diagnostic peritoneal lavage in blunt abdominal trauma, *J Trauma* 15:845, 1975.

73. Alyono D, Perry JF: Value of quantitative cell count and amylase activity of peritoneal lavage fluid, *J Trauma* 21:345, 1981.

74. Parvin S, Smith DE, Asher WM, Virgillo RW: Effectiveness of peritoneal lavage in blunt abdominal trauma, *Ann Surg* 181:255, 1975.

75. Gill W, Champion H, Long WB, et al: Abdominal lavage in blunt trauma, *Br J Surg* 62:121, 1975.

76. Alyono C, Morrow CE, Perry JF: Reappraisal of diagnostic peritoneal lavage criteria for operation in penetrating and blunt trauma, *Surgery* 92:751, 1982.

77. McLellan BA, Hanna SS, Montoya DR, et al: Analysis of peritoneal lavage parameters in blunt abdominal trauma, *J Trauma* 25:393, 1985.

78. Peitzman AB, Makaroun MS, Slasky BS, et al: Prospective study of computed tomography in initial management of blunt abdominal trauma, *J Trauma* 26:585, 1986.

79. Meyer DM, Thal E, Weigelt JA, et al: Evaluation of computed tomography and diagnostic peritoneal lavage in blunt abdominal trauma, *J Trauma* 29:1168, 1989.

80. Fabian TC, Mangiante EC, White TJ, et al: A prospective study of 91 patients undergoing both computed tomography and peritoneal lavage following blunt abdominal trauma, *J Trauma* 26:602, 1986.

81. Marx JA, Moore EE, Jordan RC, et al: Limitations of computed tomography in the evaluation of acute abdominal trauma: a perspective comparison with diagnostic peritoneal lavage, *J Trauma* 25:933, 1985.

82. Davis JW, Hoyt DB: Complications in evaluating abdominal trauma: diagnostic peritoneal lavage versus computerized axial tomography, *J Trauma* 30:1506, 1990.

83. Sherck JD, Oakes DD: Intestinal injuries missed by computed tomography, *J Trauma* 30:1, 1990.

84. Lilleen KL, Shanmuganathan K, Poletti PA, et al: Helical computed tomography of bowel and mesenteric injuries, *J Trauma* 51:26, 2001.

85. Tso P, Rodriguez A, Copper C, et al: Sonography for blunt abdominal trauma: a preliminary progress report, *J Trauma* 33:39, 1992.

86. Rozychi GS, Ochsner MG, Jaffin JH, et al: Prospective evaluation of surgeon's use of ultrasound in the evaluation of trauma patients, *J Trauma* 34:516, 1993.

87. Scalea TM, Rodriguez A, Chiu WC, et al: Focused assessment with sonography for trauma (FAST): results from an international consensus conference, *J Trauma* 46:466, 1999.

88. Rose JS, Levitt MA, Porter J, et al: Does the presence of ultrasound really affect computed tomographic scan use? A prospective randomized trial of ultrasound in trauma, *J Trauma* 51:545, 2001.

89. Shackford SR, Rogers FB, Osler TM, et al: Focused abdominal sonogram for trauma: the learning curve of nonradiologist clinicians in detecting hemoperitoneum, *J Trauma* 46:553, 1999.

90. Rozychi GS, Ballard RB, Feliciano DV, et al: Surgeon-performed ultrasound for the assessment of truncal injuries: lessons learned from 1540 patients, *Ann Surg* 228:557, 1998.

91. Boulanger BR, Brenneman FD, Kirkpatrick AW, et al: The indeterminate abdominal sonogram in multisystem blunt trauma, *J Trauma* 45:52, 1998.

92. Sclafani SJ, Shaftan GW, Scalea TM: et al: Nonoperative salvage of computed tomography–diagnosed splenic injuries: utilization of angiography for triage and embolization for homeostasis, *J Trauma* 39:818, 1995.

93. Hagiwara A, Yukioka T, Ohta S, et al: Nonsurgical management of patients with blunt splenic injury: efficacy of transcatheter arterial embolization, *AJR* 167:159, 1996.

94. Omert LA, Salyer D, Dunham CM: Implications of the "contrast blush" finding on computed tomographic scan of the spleen in trauma, *J Trauma* 51:272, 2001.

95. Allen GS, Moore FA, Cox CS Jr, et al: Hollow visceral injury and blunt trauma, *J Trauma* 45:69, 1998.

96. Nance ML, Peden GW, Shapiro MB: Solid viscus injury predicts major hollow viscus injury in blunt abdominal trauma, *J Trauma* 43:618, 1997.

97. Roettger RH, Dunham CM, Gens DR: Risk factors associated with abdominal injury in blunt trauma, *Pan Am J Trauma* (in press).

98. Scott R, Carlton CE, Goldman M: Penetrating injuries of the kidney: an analysis of 181 patients, *J Urol* 101:247, 1969.

99. Carroll PR, McAninch JW: Operative indications in penetrating renal trauma, *J Trauma* 25:587, 1985.

100. Prerti JC, Carroll PR, McAninch JW: Ureteral and renal pelvic injuries from external trauma: diagnosis and management, *J Trauma* 29:370, 1989.

101. Liroff SA, Ponter JES, Pierce JM: Gunshot wounds of the ureter: five years of experience, *J Urol* 118:551, 1977.

102. Peterson NE, Pitts JC III: Penetrating injuries of the ureter, *J Urol* 126:587, 1981.

103. Walker JA: Injuries of the ureter due to external violence, *J Urol* 102:410, 1969.

104. Klein S, Johs S, Fujitani R, et al: Hematuria following blunt abdominal trauma: the utility of intravenous pyelography, *Arch Surg* 123:1173, 1988.

105. Fortune JB, Brahme J, Mulligan M, et al: Emergency intravenous pyelography in the trauma patient: a reexamination of the indications, *Arch Surg* 120:1056, 1985.

106. Guice K, Oddhem K, Eida B, et al: Hematuria after blunt trauma: when is pyelography useful? *J Trauma* 23:305, 1983.

107. Levitt MA, Criss E, Kobernik M: Should emergency IVP be used more selectively in blunt trauma? *Ann Emerg Med* 14:959, 1985.

108. Nicolaisen GS, McAninch JW, Marshall GA, et al: Renal trauma: reevaluation of the indications for radiographic assessment, *J Urol* 133:183, 1985.

109. Young JWR, Burgess AR, Brumback RJ, et al: Pelvic fractures: value of plain radiography in early assessment and management, *Radiology* 160:445, 1986.

110. Dalal SA, Burgess AR, Siegel JH, et al: Pelvic fractures in multiple trauma: classification by mechanism is key to pattern of organ injury, resuscitative requirements, and outcome, *J Trauma* 28:981, 1989.

111. Geuder JW, Hobson RW, Padberg FT, et al: The role of contrast angiography in suspected arterial injuries of the extremities, *Am Surg* 51:89, 1985.

112. Sirinek KR, Levine BA, Gaskill HV, et al: Reassessment of the role of routine operative exploration in vascular trauma, *J Trauma* 21:339, 1981.

113. Turcotte JK, Towne JB, Bernhard VM: Is arteriography necessary in the management of vascular trauma of the extremities? *Surgery* 84:557, 1978.

114. Frykberg ER, Crump JM, Vines FS, et al: A reassessment of the role of arteriography in penetrating proximity extremity trauma: a prospective study, *J Trauma* 29:1041, 1989.

115. Feliciano DV, Cruse PA, Burch JM, et al: Delayed diagnosis of arterial injuries, *Am J Surg* 154:579, 1987.

116. Frykberg ER, Vines FS, Alexander RH: The natural history of clinically occult arterial injuries: a prospective evaluation, *J Trauma* 29:577, 1989.

117. Anderson RJ, Hobson RW, Lee BC, et al: Reduced dependency on arteriography for penetrating extremity trauma: influence of wound location and non-invasive vascular studies, *J Trauma* 30:1059, 1990.

118. McCormick TM, Burch BH: Routine angiographic evaluation of neck and extremity injuries, *J Trauma* 19:384, 1979.

119. Massoura ZE, Ivatury RR, Simon RJ, et al: A reassessment of doppler pressure indices in the detection of arterial lesions in proximity penetrating injuries of extremities: a prospective study, *Am J Emerg Med* 14:151, 1996.

120. Coughlin BF, Paushter DM: Peripheral pseudoaneurysms: evaluation with duplex ultrasound, *Radiology* 168:339, 1988.

121. Bynoe RP, Miles WS, Bell RM: Noninvasive diagnosis of vascular trauma by duplex ultrasonography, *J Vasc Surg* 14:346, 1991.

122. Dotter CT: Transluminally placed coil spring endarterial tube grafts: long-term patency in canine popliteal artery, *Invest Radiol* 4:329, 1969.

123. Stecco K, Meir A, Seiver A: Endovascular stent-graft placement for treatment of traumatic penetrating subclavian artery injury, *J Trauma* 48:948, 2000.

124. Marin ML, Veith FJ, Panetta TF, et al: Transluminally placed endovascular stented graft repair for arterial trauma, *J Vasc Surg* 20:466, 1994.

125. Patel AV, Marin ML, Veith FJ, et al: Endovascular graft repair of penetrating subclavian artery injuries, *J Endovasc Surg* 3:382, 1996.

2 | Imaging of Craniocerebral Trauma

Adult Craniocerebral Trauma

James G. Smirniotopoulos,* Stuart E. Mirvis, and
David M. Lefkowitz

Craniocerebral damage is a common accompaniment to both accidental and intentional trauma. Annually in the United States, almost 8 million incidents of head trauma occur, approximately 500,000 of which are considered major.[1] Of this large number of incidents of major head trauma, about 250,000 to 300,000 are severe enough to warrant emergency medical attention and treatment. The overall morbidity rate of craniocerebral injury has been reported from 5% to 60% and, when deaths outside the hospital are included, the overall mortality is 5% to 50%.[2] The overwhelming majority of deaths from motor-vehicle accidents result from head trauma. At the University of Maryland Shock Trauma Center (UMSTC) craniocerebral trauma accounts for 70% of patient deaths. Head trauma occurs twice as frequently among men as among women because, by vocation or avocation, men expose themselves more commonly to violent accidents. For similar reasons, inner-city minorities have twice the incidence (4/1000/year) than nonurban whites (2/1000/year).[1] Almost two thirds of individuals who die from head injury sustain intracranial hemorrhage, either intraaxial (parenchymal or subarachnoid) or extraaxial (subdural,

*The opinions expressed herein are those of the author and are not necessarily representative of the Uniformed Services University of the Health Sciences (USUHS), the Armed Forces Institute of Pathology (AFIP), the Department of the Navy, the Department of Defense (DOD), or the United States government.

epidural).[2] The incidence of types of intracranial lesions varies depending on the selection process used. Autopsy studies show significantly different ratios of lesions, as compared with data from the post-computed tomography (CT) era. Table 2-1 summarizes the incidence of various lesions reported in three large CT series.

GENERAL APPROACH TO CENTRAL NERVOUS SYSTEM TRAUMA

Patients with craniocerebral trauma typically present to the emergency department/trauma center with one of three clinical situations: an acute neurologic deficit (with or without obvious signs or history of trauma), obvious signs of trauma by visual inspection, or a clear history of antecedent trauma. The patient presenting with an acute neurologic deficit deserves special consideration. When a patient experiences a neurologic event, they may lose control of their limbs and/or lose consciousness and then secondarily experience trauma, including craniocerebral trauma. Therefore clinical signs or a documented history of trauma do not prove that trauma is in fact the primary process responsible for the patient's neurologic status, and consideration should be given to other underlying cerebral pathology such as stroke, aneurysm rupture, hypertensive hemorrhage, or seizure disorder, among others (Fig. 2-1).

CHOICE OF NEURORADIOLOGIC EVALUATION

Currently three imaging techniques are applicable to the emergent evaluation of the patient with head trauma or the patient presenting with a sudden neurologic event without clear antecedent trauma: skull radiography, CT, and magnetic resonance imaging (MRI). It has been well demonstrated that MRI is the most sensitive test for documenting the full extent of brain injury in the subacute patient.[3] However, in most circumstances CT is probably the most practical and cost-effective central nervous system (CNS) imaging technique.[4-9] A prospective multi-center study by Masters et al.[5] reviewed the diagnostic imaging findings in more than 7000 patients sustaining head trauma. Their study was intended to evaluate the efficacy and indications for skull radiography, but the conclusions and recommendations included CT scanning. They divided the patient population at risk into three groups (Box 2-1): low (no intracranial injuries), moderate, and high-risk patients. Masters et al.[5] recommended that CT and/or neurosurgical evaluation be performed in the high-risk patients. No significant lesions were noted in the low-risk group, so no imaging was recommended. Those at moderate risk for significant intracranial pathology formed a somewhat more nebulous group. According to the study of Masters et al.,[5] although these patients are at somewhat less risk for intracranial injury, they may still benefit from CT examination. For the moderate-risk group, CT scanning was required, but not necessarily emergently. Although CT is currently the clear choice for initial acute evaluation of the patient with craniocerebral trauma, certain advantages and disadvantages are associated with every imaging modality.[7] A qualified radiologist or radiology trainee should read emergency imaging studies obtained to evaluate traumatic brain injury (TBI).[6]

Radiography

In the past, skull radiographs (a "skull series") have been used as a screening modality for patients with a history of head trauma and/or an acute neurologic deficit. Although certainly less sensitive than CT, radiographs can still demonstrate significant craniocerebral pathology. Skull fractures (excluding those involving the skull base and some fracture in children) are usually quite obvious on routine plain radiographs (Figs. 2-2 and 2-3), and pneumocephalus (secondary to a basilar skull fracture), open fracture, or penetrating trauma can usually be readily detected. Fluid levels in the paranasal sinuses (especially the sphenoid and ethmoids), though nonspecific, suggest basilar skull fractures. Either hemorrhage or cerebrospinal fluid (CSF) can accumulate in the normally air-filled sinuses. The air-fluid level will only be noted when the films are obtained with a "horizontal X-ray beam"—this causes the fluid level to be parallel to the beam. Opacification or fluid levels in the petrous mastoid air cells or in the middle ear may also indicate a basilar fracture with CSF fluid extravasation or hemorrhage. Pneumocephalus can also be found in patients sustaining barotrauma, (i.e., scuba diving).[10] Injuries caused by metallic fragments from missiles (bullets) and other sources of shrapnel are readily visible by radiography and

Table 2-1 Incidence of Intracranial Lesions Observed by CT	
Lesion Observed	Incidence (Mortality)*
EDH	5% to 10%
SDH (acute)	11% to 18%
Contusion (or focal edema)	15% to 25%
Parenchymal hematoma	6% to 11% (58%)
IVH	8%
Diffuse axonal sheer	16% to 68%[†]

Data from references 4, 6, and 62.
*Mortality statistic from Frazee[1] 1986.
[†]High incidence of 68% for DAI based on series of selected patients with a Glasgow Coma Scale score of 8 or less within 24 hours of admission.[6]

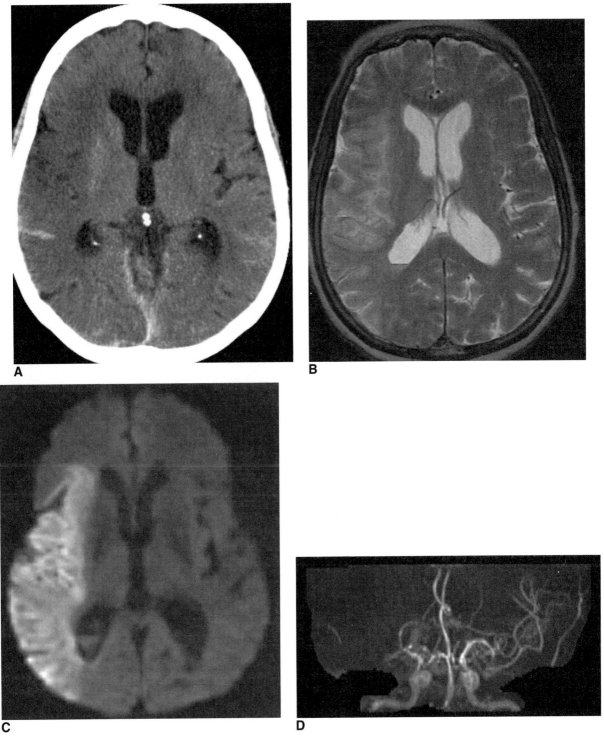

Fig. 2-1
Computed tomography (CT) and magnetic resonance imaging (MRI) of cerebral vascular accident presenting as possible trauma. An 81-year-old woman was found lying down and nonresponsive. **A,** Admission CT shows subarachnoid and peritentorial subdural hematoma (SDH). Decreased density and loss of sulci are appreciated in the right cerebrum, indicating edema. Because of this appearance and lack of history of direct trauma, an MRI was performed. **B,** T2-weighted spin-echo image shows generalized increased signal in the right middle cerebral territory consistent with cerebral edema due to a vascular etiology. **C,** Diffusion-weighted sequence also indicates clear edema pattern in the right middle cerebral artery territory. **D,** Anteroposterior (AP) view of magnetic resonance angiogram confirms proximal right middle cerebral artery occlusion, indicating stroke rather than direct trauma as etiology of depressed mental status.

High Risk
Focal neurologic signs
Penetrating skull injury
Depressed skull fracture (palpable)
Depressed level of consciousness (not clearly related to drugs or metabolic)

Moderate Risk
History of change in level of consciousness at time of injury
 Progressive headache
 Unreliable or poor history
Age less than 2 years old
Possible child abuse
Posttraumatic seizure
Posttraumatic amnesia
Serious facial injury
Physical findings of basilar skull fracture*
Vomiting
Multiple trauma

Low Risk
Asymptomatic
Headache, dizziness
Scalp hematoma, laceration, abrasion, and contusion

Modified from Masters SJ, McClean PM, Arcarese JS, et al: *N Engl J Med* 316:84, 1987.
*Battle's sign, raccoon eyes, hemotympanum, CSF otorrhea/rhinorrhea.

do not produce artifacts, as they commonly do on both CT and MRI studies (Fig. 2-4). Unfortunately, many modern plastics and other synthetic materials, as well as wood and some types of glass, will escape detection on radiographs. Digital and computed radiography may greatly improve the ability to detect these materials. Radiography can (with appropriate true orthogonal [nonrotated] positioning) demonstrate intracerebral mass effects, as evidenced by shift of the calcified pineal from the midline or shift of the calcification in the choroid or glomus of the choroid plexus, but cannot differentiate the etiology of the mass effect.

Most institutions with CT scanning capability no longer use skull radiographs to screen patients with craniocerebral trauma. The presence or absence of a skull fracture may not alter patient management and provides no indication as to whether a lesion requiring surgical treatment is present. But radiographs can be used to demonstrate the intracranial or extracranial location of a radiopaque foreign body or to detect depression of skull fractures, which would then mandate a CT study

(see Figs. 2-3 and 2-4). Skull radiographs obtained immediately after injury or operation may also provide a baseline for the potential early detection of subsequent osteomyelitis.

In our experience, skull radiographs have on many occasions proven more sensitive than CT for the detection of some skull fractures, particularly linear and nondisplaced fractures that are oriented parallel to the axial scan plane. These are "volume averaged" with the normal bone included within the slice thickness. Tsai et al.[11] found skull fractures radiographically in 5 of 12 abused children who had a normal CT of the calvarium. Saulsbury and Alford[12] have noted a major potential for delayed clinical deterioration in children when CT misses skull fractures. Despite these observations, CT remains the examination of choice in suspected or documented child abuse, with MRI suggested for optimal evaluation and prediction of outcome.[13] To optimize CT detection of skull fractures, we routinely perform and recommend review of all CT images in extended windows for bone detail as well as review of a lateral "scout" localizing digital radiograph (see below).

Computed Tomography

CT is the ideal method for the initial examination of patients sustaining head trauma or presenting with acute neurologic deficit. CT is fast, thorough, and sensitive.

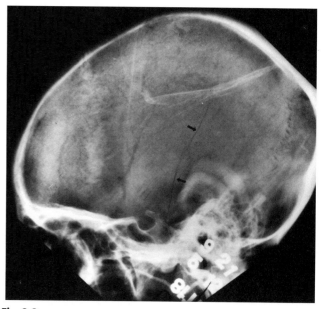

Fig. 2-2
Linear skull fracture on radiography. This lateral radiograph demonstrates a typical linear skull fracture (*arrows*) crossing the temporal-parietal region. The fracture line is relatively radiolucent. The location of the fracture would suggest a possible epidural hematoma from laceration of the proximate middle meningeal artery (MMA).

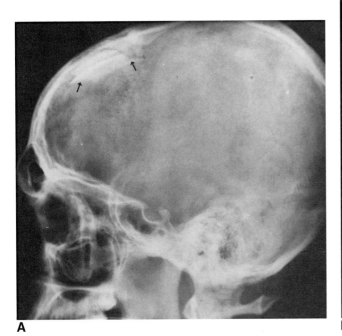

A

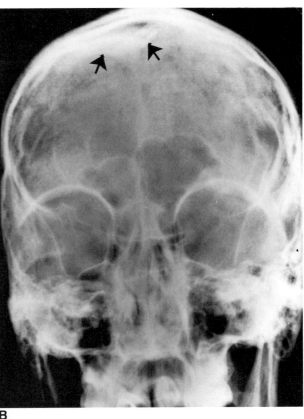

B

Fig. 2-3
Depressed skull fracture on radiography. AP (**A**) and lateral (**B**) cranial radiographs reveal depression of the frontal vertex region with visualization of both the inner and outer cortices displaced below the inner table of the skull (*arrows*). The location of the fracture should raise concern for superior sagittal sinus injury.

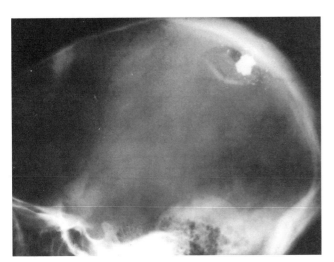

Fig. 2-4
Skull radiograph of bullet wound demonstrates a focal depression of parietal fragments at the impact site, requiring CT evaluation and probable surgical debridement.

Routine CT technique for traumatized patients should include noncontrast examination with 8- to 10-mm slice thickness, 8- to 10-mm slice interval, and 512^2 matrix reconstruction. In many institutions, slightly thinner sections (5 mm) are obtained through the posterior fossa, and thicker sections (10 mm) through the supratentorial region. Ideally, fast helical CT image acquisition, 2 seconds or less, is required to diminish artifacts from patient motion. Under selected clinical circumstances, thinner section CT images through selected areas, such as the posterior fossa, may be warranted (see below). As noted above, though CT is excellent for detecting most major intracranial pathology resulting from head trauma, some skull fractures may be undiagnosed. It is imperative that all CT scans of the head be reviewed with "bone windows" (center, 250 Hounsfield units [HU]; width, 3000 HU) to improve contrast discrimination between cancellous and cortical bone and optimize fracture detection. Unfortunately, even with ideal technique, small, linear, nondisplaced fractures can be missed because of volume averaging. In our experience, in the adult trauma population, such fractures alone are seldom of clinical significance; rather, it is the presence or absence of intracranial injury that is of greatest import. At the UMSTC, additional sets of CT images are also reviewed. These "subdural windows" (center, 60 HU; width, 120 HU) permit easier distinction of thin extraaxial collections of clotted blood from the adjacent bone of the inner table (Fig. 2-5).

In certain clinical situations, routine CT scanning protocols should be modified or augmented. In patients with suspected basilar skull fracture or cranial nerve deficits (especially the optic or facial nerve), high-resolution thin (0.5 mm to 1.5 mm) contiguous sections through the optic or facial nerve canal may prove beneficial to demonstrate bony impingement. Orbital sections may be improved with a true horizontal plane or a negative angulation to more closely parallel the orientation of the chiasm and optic nerves. In the presence of posterior fossa signs and symptoms, thinner (4 mm or 5 mm) contiguous sections, as well as a more true horizontal (parallel to Reid's baseline) scan orientation, are recommended to improve lesion detection in the posterior fossa.

Magnetic Resonance Imaging

Several studies suggest that MRI is not only more sensitive than CT at detecting many types of craniocerebral trauma but often demonstrates lesions earlier than CT when both modalities detect the same pathology.[3,7-9,14-18] However, this increase in sensitivity may not be necessary or even desired, especially in the acute trauma setting. Hartshorne[18] performed MRI acutely in head-injured patients and identified a large number of lesions not detected on acute CT examination. These injuries consisted primarily of areas of abnormal cortical hyperinten-

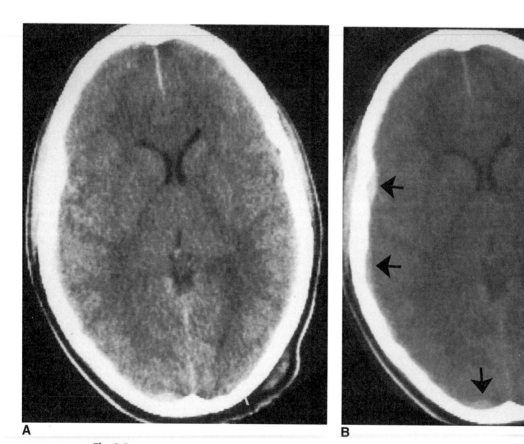

A   **B**

Fig. 2-5
"Subdural windows." **A,** Admission CT after blunt trauma shows no definite lesion. **B,** Photography in extended windows (center, 60 Hounsfield units (HU); width, 120 HU) shows a small right posterior frontoparietal SDH (*arrows*) that can be identified retrospectively in the routine windows used for brain parenchyma (center, 35 HU; width, 80 HU).

sity on T2-weighted images. Many of these lesions were found in patients without any detected neurologic abnormalities. In addition, serial follow-up studies in many of these patients who had abnormalities shown by MRI, but negative CT scan and clinically normal physical examination, demonstrated spontaneous resolutions of the cortical abnormalities. In the absence of a clinical or pathologic correlate for these abnormalities, their significance remains unclear. It continues to be true that use of MRI for the acutely head-injured patient should be limited to those instances where CT findings fail to explain the level of neurologic deficit, for patients suspected of having brainstem lesions, in evaluating patients with suspected vertex or infratemporal extraaxial hematomas (which may be difficult to discern by axial CT scanning), and in assessing the patency of the major dural sinuses[7-9] (Figs. 2-6 to 2-8). In our experience, the performance of MRI in the acute posttrauma setting has seldom resulted in a significant alteration in clinical management deci-

sions based on neurologic examination and CT observations, except when CT is unrevealing.

It has been firmly suggested by some authors that MRI be performed before discharge in all patients hospitalized for craniocerebral injuries.[15-17] Serial MRI may not be necessary, but complete documentation of the nature and full extent of injuries can best be acquired through MRI. Predischarge MRI could serve as a baseline for later follow-up MRI examinations. The true clinical value of routine predischarge cranial MRI studies is not well established in comparison with clinical evaluation that includes neuropsychiatric testing.[19-22]

MRI Techniques. The MR imaging protocol in acute head trauma consists of six sequences (Box 2-2). T1-weighted sagittal images are obtained primarily for localization of the remaining sequences that are all acquired in the axial plane. They also provide a detailed anatomic overview of the midline structures for a modest investment

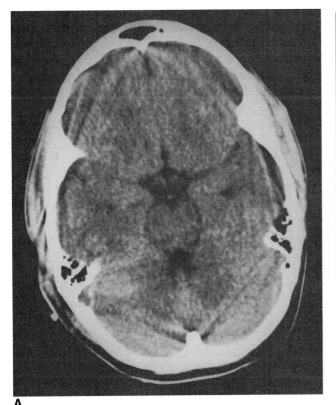

A

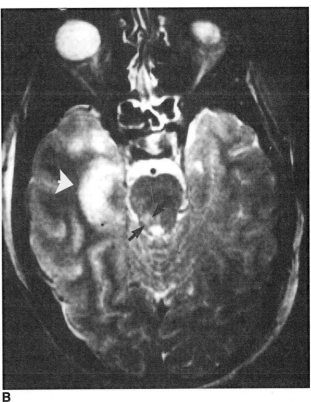

B

Fig. 2-6
Brainstem and temporal lobe contusion. **A,** Admission cranial CT study of a 15-year-old after a motor vehicle collision does not indicate evidence of injury, even though the patient is in a coma. **B,** T2-weighted MRI study shows increased signal (edema) in the right medial temporal lobe (*arrowhead*) and in the right side of the lateral and dorsal brainstem (*black arrows*), better explaining the patient's clinical condition.

Continued

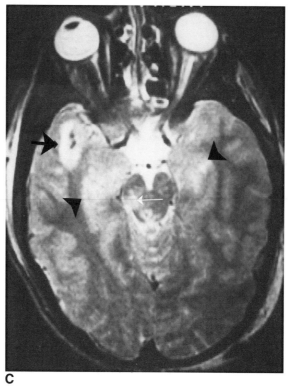

C

Fig. 2-6, cont'd
C, T2-weighted MRI obtained at a slightly different level demonstrates focal low signal centrally with surrounding high signal indicative of hemorrhage (*black arrow*) and bitemporal contusions (*arrowheads*). Again, a right lateral brainstem contusion is observed (*white arrow*).

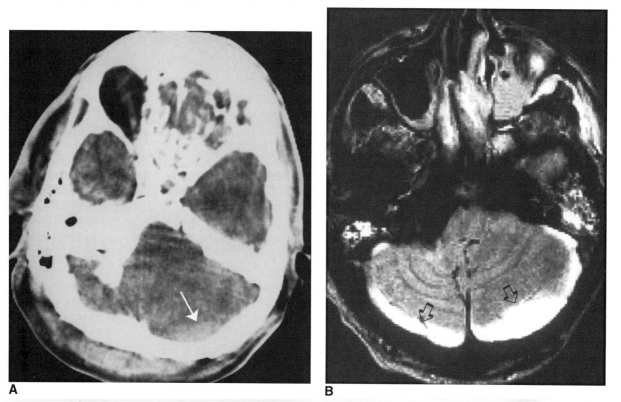

A   **B**

Fig. 2-7
CT and MRI of infratentorial SDH. **A,** CT image obtained after head trauma in a 53-year-old man initially interpreted as normal in infratentorial compartment. A small extraaxial hyperdensity is suggested on the left (*arrow*). **B,** Because of persistent neurologic symptoms an MRI study is performed and reveals bilateral infratentorial SDHs (*open arrows*). Left maxillary sinus fluid is incidentally observed.

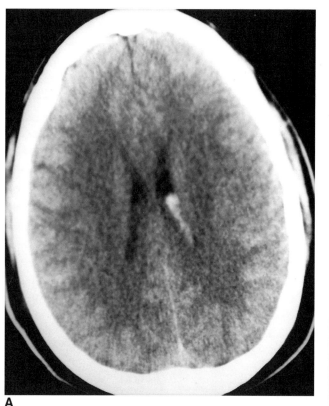

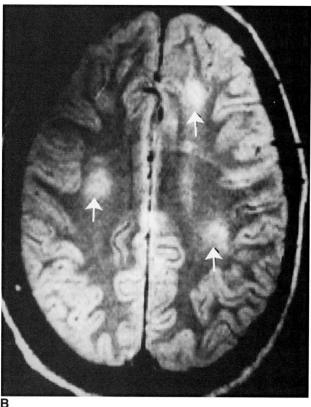

A **B**

Fig. 2-8
MRI of white matter contusions. **A**, CT image obtained in an obtunded middle-aged man after blunt head trauma reveals some blood in the left lateral ventricle, but no parenchymal lesion. **B**, T2-weighted MR image acquired at a slightly more rostral level shows three foci of increased signal representing white matter contusions (*arrows*) that are not detected by CT.

of time (approx. 1.25 minutes). The T1- and T2-weighted axial images provide morphologic characterization of brain anatomy that serves to identify fluid collections, shifts, local mass effect, and ventricular abnormalities.

Box 2-2
MRI Sequences Used in Craniocerebral Trauma

Core Sequences
  1. T1 sagittal
  2. T1 axial
  3. T2 axial
4a. FLAIR-conventional axial
5a. T2*-conventional axial
  6. DWI axial

Alternative Sequences
4b. FLAIR-interleaved axial (for subarachnoid hemorrhage)
5b. T2-echo planar axial (for speed; uncooperative patient)

Basic tissue characterization is also provided by these sequences and allows for identification of ischemic changes, edema, and gross hemorrhage.

Fluid attenuated inversion recovery (FLAIR) augments the T2-weighted acquisition by increasing sensitivity to the detection of tissue changes adjacent to CSF spaces, mainly in the cerebral cortex and in the periventricular zones. There are different versions of the FLAIR sequence, primarily distinguished by the thickness of the inversion slice that provides darkening of CSF. Depending on how this is performed, the homogeneity of CSF signal attenuation will determine the accuracy of this sequence in detecting hemorrhage in the subarachnoid spaces and ventricles. Because of the additional time required for more complete CSF signal elimination (4.5 min vs. 2.5 min for the base sequence), in most acute head trauma settings, the shorter sequence is used. In the event that the presence of blood in the subarachnoid compartment is of importance for clinical management, the interleaved version of the FLAIR sequence is used, permitting a doubling of the inversion slice thickness to better suppress CSF signal.

T2*-weighted axial images serve to identify parenchymal blood by virtue of its exquisite sensitivity to the magnetic susceptibility effect of most forms of hemoglobin. This causes pronounced decay of transverse magnetization and localized signal loss, a phenomenon accentuated by the use of gradient echoes rather than spin echoes in this sequence. Although acute blood containing pure oxyhemoglobin may theoretically be missed by this technique, in clinical practice sufficient deoxyhemoglobin is present even in the most acute presentations to permit detection. In addition, the magnetic susceptibility "artifact" produced by blood characteristically displays a focal round, curvilinear, or sometimes irregular focus of pronounced brightness near the edge of an otherwise hypointense hematoma, an occasionally helpful associated finding. There are two versions of the T2*-weighted sequence that may be considered for routine clinical use. The more rapid echo planar version requires only several seconds to obtain and is preferred when time is of the essence. Although this sequence has more exquisite sensitivity to blood, the more pronounced magnetic susceptibility that makes this possible also produces greater signal loss at bone-brain interfaces. Therefore peripherally located hypointense hemorrhage may be difficult to detect. The more conventional T2*-weighted sequence that acquires a single gradient echo per slice for each TR interval still exhibits considerable magnetic susceptibility sensitivity and much better spatial resolution. Overall, the accuracy for hemorrhage diagnosis by this sequence is slightly better than the echo-planar version, but the price is added scan time, requiring approximately 3 minutes.

Diffusion-weighted images round out the routine acute head trauma protocol. These images are highly sensitive to acute ischemia, a secondary effect of vascular injury or compression that may be seen in association with rotational deceleration and mass effect, respectively. Shear injury is also a by-product of these forces and can be manifested as diffusion hyperintensity at the outer margin of the corpus callosum and near gray-white matter interfaces. Such abnormalities are often accompanied by petechial hemorrhage that will be visible on the T2*-weighted images. Many implementations of diffusion-weighted imaging exist, and the available options are poised to grow considerably in the near future, ranging from higher "b values" for stronger diffusion sensitization, to increasing the number of directions for measuring diffusion. This latter development serves to better characterize the size and direction of the diffusion vector at each point and will likely improve depiction of white matter tract disruption in acute trauma. At the present time most high-performance scanners are capable of trace diffusion images, which represent a simple average of diffusion sensitization along the three major orthogonal axes.

Precautions for Craniocerebral Trauma Imaging

Ideally, all patients sent to the CT scanner for evaluation of craniocerebral injury will be hemodynamically and neurologically stable. In actuality these patients often have multisystem injury in association with head injury and may have ongoing neurologic deterioration. Initial resuscitation efforts to stabilize the patient hemodynamically must be performed before transfer to the CT suite, but critical-care monitoring and resuscitation equipment must be provided in the CT suite to adequately care for these patients after stabilization. It is *imperative* that adequately trained medical personnel accompany the patient to the CT area to monitor vital signs and look for evidence of systemic or neurologic deterioration. The CT scanning area should be in close proximity to the patient admitting area to minimize transport risks.

For the multitrauma patient, CT studies of many body areas are often requested simultaneously. Appropriate study prioritization before placing the patient on the CT bed is strongly advised (see Chapter 1). In general at most facilities, including the UMSTC, patients with CNS deficits undergo nonenhanced cranial CT before any other requested CT examination. Rapid scan and reconstruction times are important, and in most cases the cranial CT scan should be completed in less than 2 minutes. Rapid review of CT images is desirable to appropriately triage the patient to initial surgical or nonsurgical management. Radiology coverage should be available around the clock, either onsite or by telemedicine.

Extreme caution must be exercised in moving the patient's head into a CT head holder adaptor since, in many cases, the stability of the cervical spine may be unclear at the time of emergency cranial CT. In many such instances, a tabletop head CT can be performed with appropriate CT gantry angulation to avoid patient movement.

CRANIOCEREBRAL PATHOLOGY IN TRAUMA
Scalp Injuries

The skin and subcutaneous tissues are almost invariably damaged when contact injuries include the head. There may be bruising (contusion) in the scalp that increases the attenuation of the normally low-density fat. The galea aponeurotica, to which the scalp is attached, is separated from the skull and its periosteum by loose (areolar) connective tissue. This arrangement allows gliding of the scalp over the calvarium, which not only permits greater freedom of facial expression, but also provides a protective effect. The energy of an impact to the head may dissipate over a larger area of the head through the mechanism of scalp gliding. This action diffuses the energy of impact and lessens the severity of injury to the underlying skull and the intracranial content.[23]

The potential subgaleal space, between the galea and the periosteum, of the outer table fluid is not limited or bound by sutures. Hemorrhage or pus can accumulate within this space and is particularly likely to occur in children who sustain head injury. In children, hemorrhage into this space may become hemodynamically significant because of the relatively large size of the head in relation to the body (see section on pediatric TBI). The volume of the subgaleal potential space is a fraction of the total blood volume, and therefore bleeding into this space is of less consequence. Subgaleal hematomas and scalp contusions are useful in localizing the point of contact against the calvarium and thus in defining coup versus contrecoup injuries. Knowledge of the point of impact against the skull can indicate the vector of forces applied, help focus attention along the path of energy deposition in the cranium, and may help identify subtle injuries (Fig. 2-9). Documenting site impact against the calvarium may also be important for medical-legal reasons. Subgaleal blood can be a sign of both skull fracture and epidural hematoma (EDH). Because blood

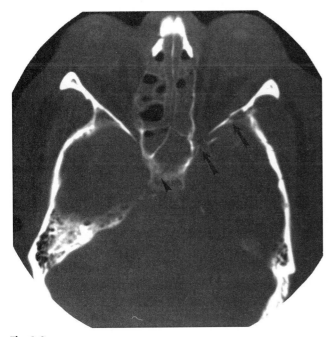

Fig. 2-9
Deep skull base fracture. This CT image of a male adolescent following a sports-related accident reveals a fracture of the left lateral orbital wall–greater sphenoid wing (*arrows*). The vector of force is directed posteriorly and medially. The fracture extends through the sphenoid sinus (opacified) and into the body of the sphenoid (*arrowhead*). The force vector crosses the left superior orbital fissure, damaging the cranial nerves at this site and producing a "superior orbital fissure syndrome" clinically. Analysis of the vector of force to the face and skull can be helpful in predicting associated injury. (From Corradino G, Wolf AL, Mirvis SE, Joslyn JN: *Neurosurgery* 27:592, 1990.)

from the epidural space can seep out through the skull fracture and into the loose connective tissue that separates the galea from the calvarium, a spontaneous decompression of an EDH into the subgaleal space can occur (Fig. 2-10).

Finally, hemorrhage can occur between the periosteum and the outer table of the calvarium, a cephalohematoma. Because the "pericranium" is firmly attached at the sutures, the sutures delimit the subperiosteal hematoma. A subperiosteal hemorrhage, a cephalohematoma, can stimulate ossification by elevating the periosteum and lead to alteration of the shape and thickness of the calvarium focally. Cephalohematomas may be seen with birth trauma and child abuse.

Skull Fractures

Skull fractures occur when forces applied to the bone exceed the ability of the bone to undergo elastic transformation. Fractures may be displaced or nondisplaced, depressed below the surrounding or nondepressed calvarium. The pattern of the fracture can be described as linear, stellate, eggshell, and so on. The fracture may involve only the cranial vault, the convex hemispheric bones—frontal, parietal, occipital, squamosal, temporal—or may involve the skull base, sphenoid, clivus, peduncle, orbitosphenoid, and so forth. If the dura remains intact, the fracture is closed, but if the dura is lacerated, the fracture is open, as in "open" head trauma.

The skull bones generally fracture in tension, rather than in compression. Thus, when a blow is struck to the head, the inner table under the impact zone will give way first, followed by fracture of the outer table. Impaction fractures of the skull bones are unusual. Fractures usually appear as radiolucent lines on radiography or CT (Figs. 2-11 to 2-13; see also Figs. 2-2 and 2-3). If, however, the fracture appears as a dense line, there is almost always overriding of the fragments, which invariably indicates a depressed skull fracture (Fig. 2-14; see also Fig. 2-3). Depressed skull fractures may or may not warrant surgical intervention.[24] In some less developed countries, nonsurgical management has been successful in the majority of cases, and less than 3% of patients so managed developed septic sequelae. At the UMSTC, the decision to elevate a depressed skull fracture is based on several factors. Closed depressed skull fractures are not elevated unless the fracture creates an unacceptable cosmetic deformity, because it does not decrease the incidence of late epilepsy.[25] All compound depressed fractures (open fractures) are debrided and elevated as soon as possible with a watertight dural closure to minimize the incidence of infection.

Basilar skull fractures usually occur when a linear skull fracture has a vertical or an oblique orientation and extends downward to involve the bones of the skull base.

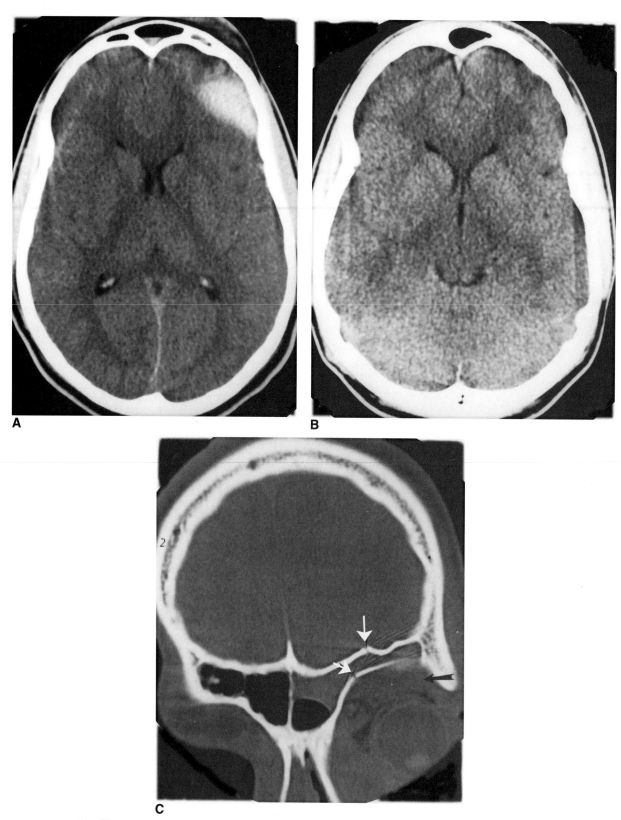

Fig. 2-10
Spontaneous evacuation of an epidural hematoma. **A,** Cranial CT obtained in a young man with a supraorbital impact site reveals frontal scalp contusion and an epidural hematoma (EDH) in the left frontal region. **B,** A follow-up CT the next day shows complete resolution of the hematoma. **C,** Coronal facial CT image, also obtained the day after admission, demonstrates fractures of the left orbital plate of the frontal bone and left orbit roof (*white arrows*). A hematoma (*black arrow*) in the superior left orbit displaces the globe inferiorly. It is speculated that the EDH spontaneously decompressed through the fractures into the adjacent frontal sinus and orbit.

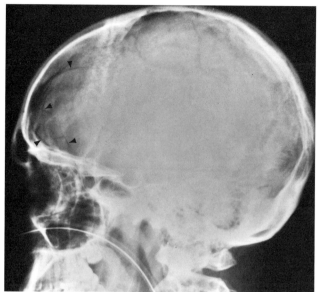

Fig. 2-11
Complex skull fracture on radiography. This lateral skull radiograph of a 16-year-old trauma victim shows a complex "eggshell" fracture of the frontal bone (*arrowheads*). There are several isolated bone fragments.

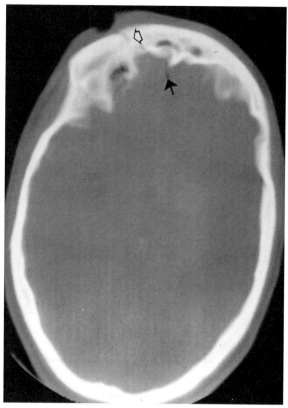

Fig. 2-13
Skull fracture. This image through the midventricular level shows a frontal skull fracture beneath a scalp laceration (*open arrow*). There is minimal pneumocephalus (*arrow*) indicating dural laceration and an open fracture.

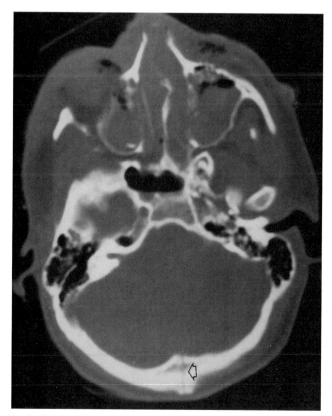

Fig. 2-12
Skull fracture. This image through the skull base reveals a focal lucency through the midline of the occipital bone (*arrow*), indicating a fracture. Complex midfacial fractures are noted.

Basilar skull fractures are of particular significance because of the long-term sequelae. Fractures of the skull base, commonly associated with severe head trauma, can lead to cranial nerve damage and vascular trauma (see below). The cranial nerves all exit through foramina at the skull base; at these openings they are tethered to both the dura and to the bone. A fracture may directly traumatize them, or a hematoma from the fracture can secondarily compress the exiting nerve (Fig. 2-15; see also Fig 2-9). Basilar fractures tend to crisscross the skull base, passing diagonally through the basiocciput, especially the clivus. This geometry of crossing the sphenoid can lead to fractures that lacerate the internal carotid arteries as they enter the skull, where they are "locked" in the cartilage of the foramen lacerum, or within the cavernous sinus (Fig. 2-16). The anatomy of this later situation may produce a carotid-cavernous fistula (see Fig. 2-15). Clinically, this leads to increased pressure in the orbital veins that become engorged and dilated. Capillary drainage is impaired, producing edema in the orbit, on the sclera (chemosis), and on the side of the face. Around the eye the arterial pressure is transmitted into the orbit

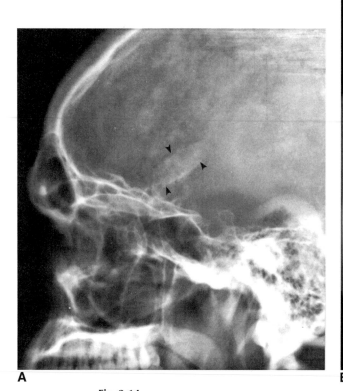

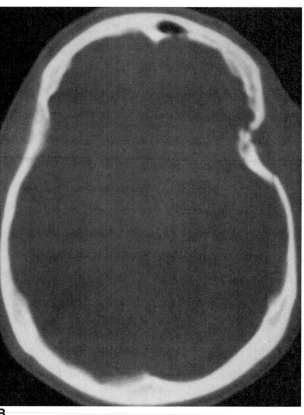

A **B**

Fig. 2-14
Depressed skull fracture increasing skull density. **A,** Lateral radiograph demonstrates an oval area of increased density in the posterior frontal region (*arrowheads*). **B,** Corresponding CT image reveals a depressed left posterior frontal calvarial fracture.

through the dilated veins, and the patient can develop pulsatile exophthalmos.

Other well-described clinical signs of basilar skull fracture include Battle's sign and "raccoon eyes" from subcutaneous ecchymoses. These occur when blood dissects from the trauma and fracture into the adjacent soft tissues of the scalp and orbit. Raccoon eyes (periorbital ecchymoses) are usually seen in association with fractures of the orbital roof when blood dissects in the extraconal space into the eyelids, and Battle's sign is due to petrotemporal fractures with blood dissecting into the retroauricular soft tissues, producing ecchymosis overlying the mastoid behind the ear.

Cranial Vault Fractures

Stellate Fracture. Stellate fractures are usually seen when the skull is impacted with relatively small-diameter objects, such as a bullet or a hammerhead. Stellate fractures resemble the appearance of a car windshield when struck by a rock. In the center, on the inside, is a pyrami-

dal-shaped bone defect, with the edge pointing outward and the base of the pyramid on the inner table aspect. A series of curvilinear fractures lead away from the central defect in a radial arrangement.

Linear Fracture. A linear or curvilinear skull fracture is usually the result of contact of the skull with an object that has one or two very large diameters. A cylindrical object, such as a baseball bat, typically produces a linear skull fracture. In this situation one diameter of the bat is long and the forces of impact are distributed over a large portion of the skull. In a more commonly encountered setting the skull impacts against a flat surface that distributes forces over a large area of the skull and leads to linear fracture, which is often not displaced at the time of radiologic evaluation (see Fig. 2-2).

Eggshell Fracture. The eggshell fracture (see Fig. 2-11) is rarely encountered in clinical practice, because the patient usually dies at the accident scene. This type of

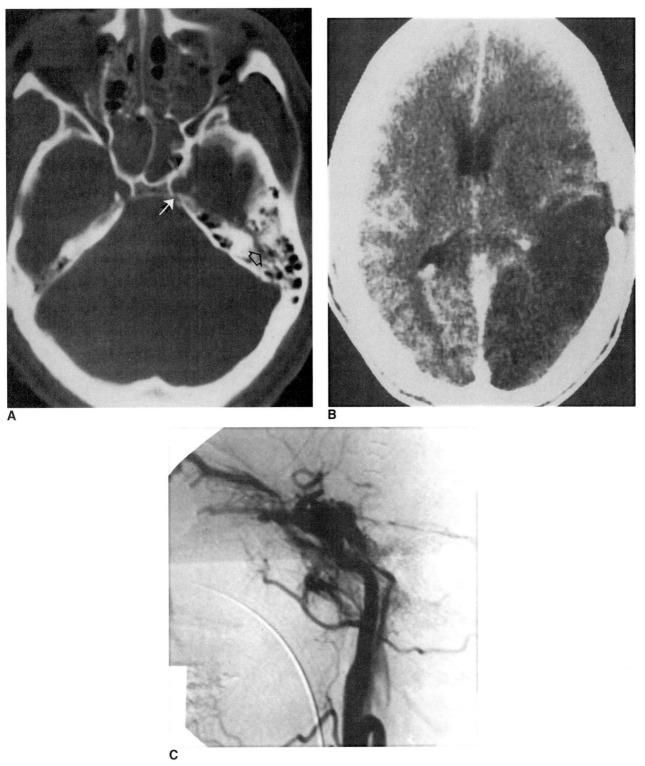

Fig. 2-15

Skull base fracture resulting in carotid artery injury. **A**, CT image of a 25-year-old man after a motor vehicle collision reveals a longitudinal left mastoid fracture (*open black arrow*) that extends across the precavernous carotid canal (*white arrow*). **B**, Contrast-enhanced CT study shows a left posterior middle cerebral and posterior cerebral distribution infarct. **C**, Left carotid intraarterial digital subtraction angiography (IA-DSA) (lateral projection) reveals complete occlusion of the left carotid artery at the cavernous portion and a carotid-cavernous fistula. (From Mirvis SE, Wolf AL, Numaguchi Y, et al: *AJNR* 11:355, 1990.)

fracture results from extensive injury that breaks the skull into multiple fragments, like tiles in a mosaic. The skull fragments are held together only by the scalp's soft tissue. The damage to the cranial contents is typically immediately fatal.

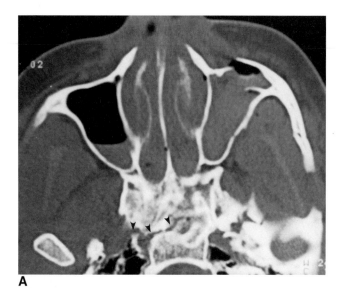

A

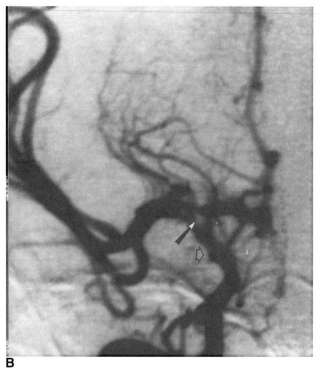

B

Fig. 2-16

Skull base fracture resulting in carotid artery injury. **A**, CT image of an 18-year-old woman after severe facial trauma demonstrates a fracture through the body of the sphenoid into the right carotid canal (*arrowheads*). **B**, The patient developed left-sided hemiplegia, and a right carotid angiogram was performed, demonstrating irregularity (*open arrow*) of the cavernous internal carotid and a thrombus in the proximal right middle cerebral artery (*solid arrow*).

Cranial Base Fractures

Frontal Bone. Frontal area (orbital roof, cribriform plate) basilar skull fractures may occur in discontinuous or contrecoup patterns.[26] This type of injury has been described in gunshot wounds, from the high velocity of a penetrating missile.[27] These discontinuous fractures occur because of hydraulic pressure waves similar to the mechanism of orbital blowout fractures. Fractures involving the frontal skull base most commonly result from direct impact to the naso-orbital-ethmoid region, or supraorbital frontal bone, and from lateral impact to the anterior face, producing transversely oriented fractures (Figs. 2-17 and 2-18) across the orbital roofs and greater and/or lesser sphenoid wings (see Chapter 5). In the setting of a possible frontal skull base fracture, intubation must be performed carefully. A nasogastric tube can pass directly through a cribriform plate fracture and enter the calvarium.

Petrous Bone. Whenever a fracture extends through the petrous portion of the temporal bone, the potential exists for damage to the cranial nerves, ossicular chain, otic capsule, vestibular system, and other related structures. High-resolution CT (i.e., slice thickness 1 to 2 mm, 512×512 matrix) has significant advantages over routine CT and radiography in diagnosing temporal bone fractures.[28] The acute or emergent CT can be performed with routine technique; serious sequelae of temporal bone trauma may warrant a repeat CT scan with high resolution. A laterally applied force may create a parietal fracture that can extend anteriorly, parallel to the long axis of the petrous pyramid (parallel to the petrous ridge) and produce a *longitudinal fracture* (Figs. 2-19 to 2-21). An occipital impact may fracture that bone and may continue anterolaterally and pass through the temporal bone perpendicular to its axis, creating a *transverse fracture* (see Fig. 2-21). This scheme seems useful in describing temporal fractures as either longitudinal or transverse. However, very commonly there is either a complex fracture or a combination of fractures.

When trauma disrupts the mechanics of the ossicular chain, the patient will experience immediate conductive hearing loss. If fluid accumulates within the middle ear, a conductive hearing loss will also occur, but this may be delayed if the fluid accumulates over time. Fractures of the bony otic capsule itself will produce an acute sensorineural hearing loss by disrupting the cochlea and/or its nerves. Longitudinally oriented fractures are the most common (10% to 90% of petrous bone fractures), have a high incidence of CSF otorrhea and rhinorrhea (via the eustachian tube), and cause conductive hearing loss, but affect the facial nerve in only 10% to 20% of cases.[29] The facial nerve deficit from a longitudinally oriented fracture is usually incomplete and may have delayed onset.[30] In contrast, the transversely oriented petrous fracture is less

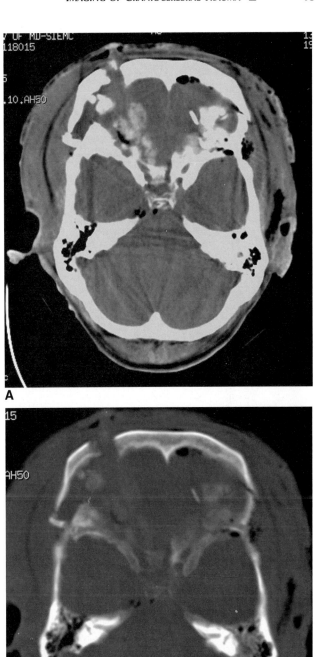

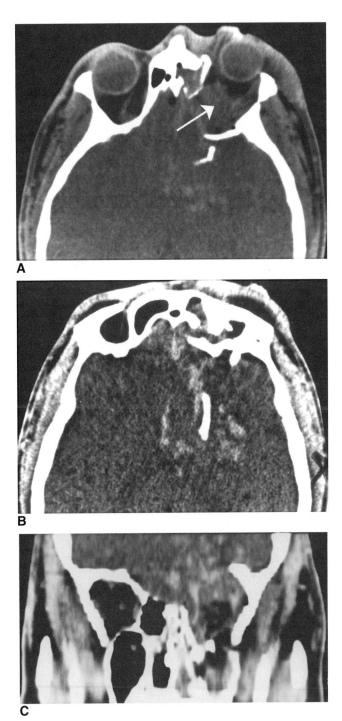

Fig. 2-17
CT of orbital blowout fracture. **A**, CT image of a young man who sustained severe left frontal impact reveals discontinuity of the left orbital roof and herniation of brain into the superior left orbit (*arrow*). **B**, A more rostral CT image shows the displaced orbital roof fragment imbedded within the left frontal lobe. **C**, Coronal CT-reformation also depicts displacement of the left orbit roof and a large left frontal contusion.

Fig. 2-18
CT of complex frontal bone and orbital roof fractures. **A**, CTs in brain parenchymal and **B**, bone windows, show a severe comminuted open fracture of the frontal bone and orbital plates with pneumocephalus after middle-aged man was struck in head by a light-rail train. Fluid in the left mastoid indicates probable oblique extension of a fracture across the skull base longitudinally into the left temporal bone.

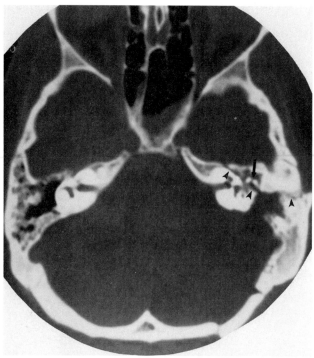

Fig. 2-19
Longitudinal petrous fracture. CT image through the skull base reveals a fracture extending (*arrowheads*) longitudinally across the petrous temporal bone. Fluid in the left middle ear and an abnormal orientation of the malleolus and incus indicate ossicular chain disruption (*arrow*).

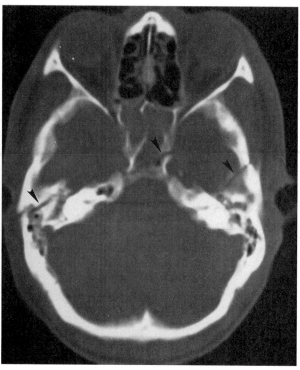

Fig. 2-21
Longitudinal and transverse petrous temporal fractures. CT image of a 16-year-old after a fall reveals a longitudinal fracture across the right petrous ridge and sphenoid sinus (filled with blood) with continuation transversely across the left petrous temporal bone (*arrowheads*). (From Corradino G, Wolf AL, Mirvis SE, Joslyn J: *Neurosurgery* 27:592, 1990.)

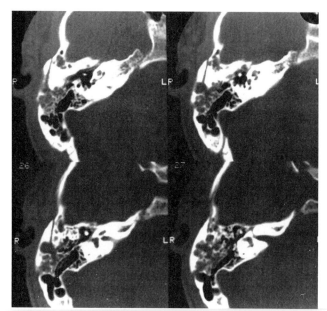

Fig. 2-20
Longitudinal petrous fracture. Sequential series of four CT images targeted on the right mastoid and petrous temporal bone reveal a fracture extending longitudinally through the bone. The patient has a conductive hearing loss.

common (10% to 30%), is complicated by extension through the labyrinth with sensorineural hearing loss and vestibular dysfunction, and commonly the damages involve the facial nerve (40% to 50%).[22] In this situation, facial nerve paralysis is usually immediate and complete.[30]

Clival Fracture. Clival fractures are extremely rare, most likely because of the centrally situated location of the clivus within the skull base. Nonetheless, high-impact injuries can be transmitted through the clivus. Fractures of the clivus have been divided into three categories, including longitudinal, transverse, and oblique.[29,31] Longitudinal fractures result from direct impact to the occipital midline, which transmits energy through the brainstem and into the clivus (Fig. 2-22). In the series of Corradino et al.,[32] the mortality of this type fracture was 67%, and extensive CNS injury occurred in survivors. In many cases it appears that the basilar or vertebral arteries are trapped within the diastatic clival fracture, leading to occlusion and brainstem infarction.[33] Transverse fractures most likely arise from a significant lateral impact and have a better prognosis, with 50% mortality. These fractures frequently extend to or from petrotemporal fractures and are associated with cranial nerve injuries

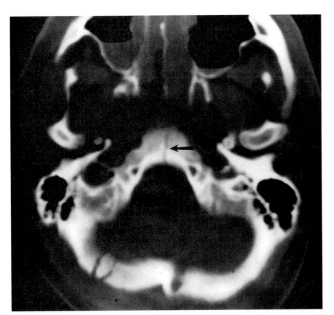

Fig. 2-22
Longitudinal fracture of the clivus. CT image through the skull base of a 12-year-old who struck his occiput on the ground after being hit by a car. Linear fractures through the right occipital bone are observed. A linear fracture line extends longitudinally through the clivus (*arrow*). Other images showed brainstem hemorrhage, and the patient died from this injury. (From Corradino G, Wolf AL, Mirvis SE, Joslyn J: *Neurosurgery* 27:592, 1990.)

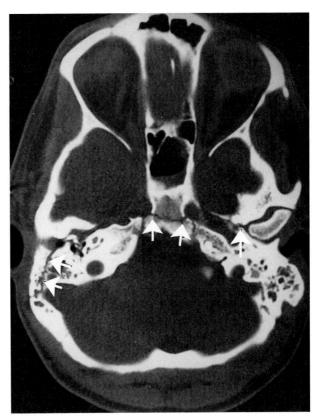

Fig. 2-23
Transverse clival fracture. CT demonstrates a fracture extending from the right petrous ridge, transversely across the clivus and foramen transversarium, and into the left condylar fossa (*arrows*).

(V to VII), and/or carotid artery injuries in survivors[29] (Figs. 2-23 and 2-24). In some cases, transverse fractures appear to follow the course of the developmental sphenoccipital synchondrosis, suggesting that this is an area of weakness within the bone.[31] Obliquely oriented clival fractures usually arise from impact to the lateral orbital walls or temporal mastoid regions. The petrous ridge and lateral orbital wall appear to act as buttresses that direct the impacting force into the clivus, producing an oblique fracture (Figs. 2-25 and 2-26). Of five patients with oblique clival fractures described by Corradino et al.,[32] only two (40%) survived; both had cranial nerve deficits, and one had a traumatic carotid-cavernous fistula.

Intracranial-Extraaxial Injury

Epidural Hematoma. EDHs are relatively uncommon injuries occurring from head trauma with a reported incidence of only 1% to 5%.[4,34] However, in the pre-CT era, the EDH was one of the most devastating of all consequences of craniocerebral trauma. The mortality rate varies from series to series, ranging from 7% to 32%,[4] and is surprisingly less than the mortality associated with *acute* subdural hematomas (SDHs). Patients with EDH have the following characteristics: 50 to 63% have no significant intradural injury; only 33% have a classic "lucid" interval; and mortality varies from 5 to 20%.[34] An

adult patient with an EDH almost always (>90%) has an associated skull fracture.[35] However, in children, it is well documented that blood may accumulate in the epidural space without evidence of a skull fracture, presumably because of the elasticity of the developing skull, which allows the dura and meningeal arteries to be torn without a fracture.[27] Thus, pediatric trauma is yet another situation where the skull series may be an adjunct to CT, but is a very ineffective screening tool when used alone.

Sources of Bleeding. The epidural space is only a potential space in the normal individual. The epidural space is created when the dura is forcibly stripped away from the inner table of the calvarium. With both layers of the dura mater stripped away, the EDH is actually a *subperiosteal hematoma* of the inner table of the calvarium. There are at least four potential sources for bleeding into the epidural space: the meningeal arteries, the meningeal veins, the dural vascular sinuses, and the vessels and sinusoids of the diploic bone marrow. On occasion, combined arterial and venous bleeding can occur and form a posttraumatic fistula. Fistula formation has been implicated as a cause for persistent epidural bleeding, which can cause delayed clinical deterioration. When a fracture line crosses a large

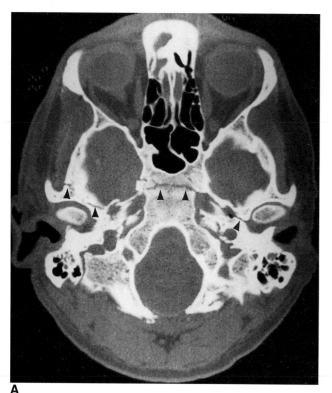

A

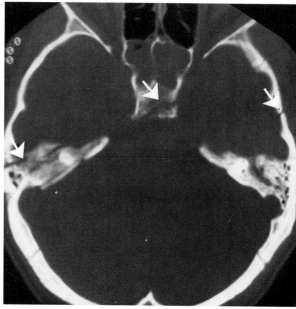

Fig. 2-25
Oblique transclival fracture. Image through the skull base demonstrates a longitudinal right petrous fracture extending obliquely across the clivus (*arrows*). A left temporal squamous fracture is noted. The sphenoid sinus is opacified by hemorrhage.

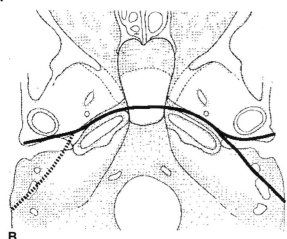

B

Fig. 2-24
Transverse clival fracture. **A,** CT image of a male patient who sustained a slow lateral crush injury of the skull shows a deep skull base fracture extending from the right middle cranial fossa, just anterior to the right condylar fossa along the right petrous ridge, transversely across the clivus, obliquely across the left middle cranial fossa, and into the left condylar fossa (*arrowheads*). The patient was awake and had bilateral deficits of the sixth and seventh cranial nerves and deficits of the second and third divisions of the trigeminal nerve on the right. **B,** This posterior transsphenoidal skull base fracture pattern that courses along the sphenopetrosal synchondrosis bilaterally represents a common injury pattern that follows a path of least resistance. The pattern is termed the posterior "U" based on its shape and orientation. (**A** from Corradino G, Wolf AL, Mirvis SE, Joslyn J: *Neurosurgery* 27:592, 1990.)

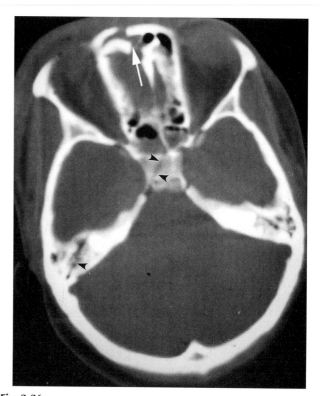

Fig. 2-26
Oblique transclival fracture. Image through the skull base reveals a longitudinal right petrous fracture and an oblique transclival fracture (*arrowheads*), as well as an open left frontal sinus fracture (*arrow*). The petrous ridges and lateral orbital walls appear to act as buttresses propagating energy into the deep skull base.

dural sinus, it may become lacerated. Although the sinuses are low-pressure systems, the flow volume is large enough to produce an expanding EDH. This type of EDH is most common in the occipital region and posterior fossa (Figs. 2-27 to 2-29) where the transverse and sigmoid sinus are torn, and can lead to an EDH tracking along the insertion of the tentorium (see Fig. 2-27).

Pathogenesis. One theory for the pathogenesis of the EDH makes the following assumptions: (1) a skull fracture exists; (2) the meningeal layer of the dura resists the laceration better than the periosteal layer; and (3) the fracture crosses the path of the meningeal vessels (and their vascular groove along the inner table of the calvarium). The two dural layers (meningeal and periosteal) are more firmly fixed to each other than to either the inner table or the underlying arachnoid. Step-by-step the following events occur in sequence. First is a blow to the head that transiently produces an inbending of the sku!l and the underlying dura. When the elastic limits of the skull are exceeded, the bone fractures, and at the instant of break, the dura (both layers) are mechanically separated from the bone. In addition to this initial mechanical stripping of the dura, the periosteal layer of the dura and the meningeal vessels between the two dural layers are also torn and lacerated. After these initial events, the bone may return to its original orientation, forming a nondisplaced fracture. However, whether the fracture is displaced or not, the lacerated meningeal vessels begin to bleed, and the blood begins to accumulate in the space between the periosteal layer of the dura and the naked inner table of the calvarium. Since the meningeal layer of the dura is intact, the hemorrhage cannot pass into the subdural or other intradural spaces, and the full thickness of the dura mater begins to be mechanically dissected from the bone by the force of the expanding hematoma. The force of the arterial blood, leading to expansion of the hematoma, is partially resisted by the adherence of the periosteal layer of the dura to the bone. Therefore the hematoma begins to form a lens-shaped (biconvex) mass. Even if the force of the expanding hematoma leads to the extension of the margins of the epidura, the attachment of the periosteal layer at the cranial sutures is almost never violated (Fig. 2-30). Therefore the EDH is a biconvex mass that does not cross the cranial sutures.[27,36,37] Most commonly, the skull fracture occurs in

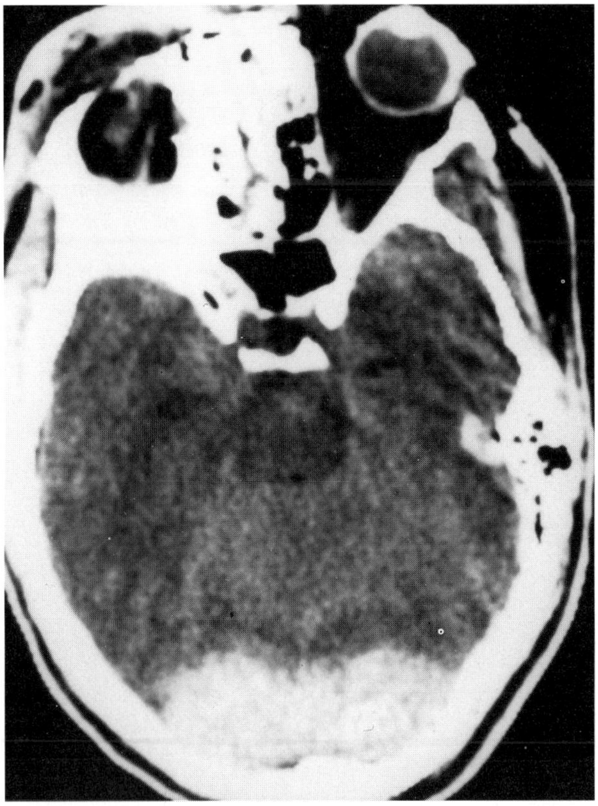

Fig. 2-27
Posterior fossa EDH. CT image reveals a high-density hematoma in the posterior fossa. There is compression of the posterior brainstem (shortened AP diameter) and fourth ventricle due to mass effect. The hematoma was limited laterally at the insertions of the lambdoid sutures, but extended above the tentorium into the supratentorial space (not shown).

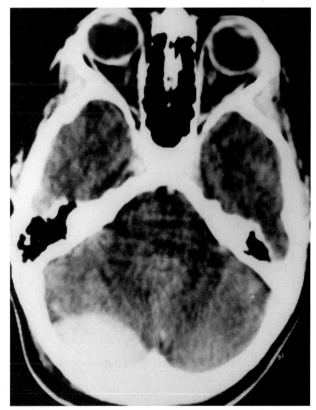

Fig. 2-28
Posterior fossa EDH. Image of an 18-year-old woman after a motor vehicle collision shows a focal right posterior fossa EDH compressing the fourth ventricle. The patient became increasingly obtunded on the CT table, and the scan was stopped after this image. The patient had complete recovery after emergency surgical drainage of the EDH.

the temporal bone, and the lacerated dura contains the branches of the middle meningeal artery (MMA), especially the anterior branch of the MMA, which lies just posterior to the coronal suture. Combining all these features, the classic EDH is an acute hematoma (and therefore of high-CT density attenuation) that forms a lenticular mass convex toward the brain, typically in the middle cranial fossa, displacing the temporal lobe medially (Fig. 2-31) and leading to medial and downward transtentorial herniation.[38] The EDH also causes direct compression of the adjacent cortical gyri (Figs. 2-32 and 2-33). Large EDHs can produce significant mass effects (Fig. 2-34).

CT Appearance. The CT appearance of the EDH recapitulates the gross pathology. On CT the EDH is typically seen as a biconvex or lens-shaped high-attenuation mass in the middle cranial fossa and lower lateral convexity, where the EDH is limited by the coronal suture anteriorly and lambdoidal suture posteriorly. The EDH usually has the high attenuation (60 to 90 HU) of clotted blood (see Figs. 2-27 to 2-34). On occasion, the EDH may be acute, in which case a blood clot is not completely formed and a heterogeneous lesion is observed (Figs. 2-35 and 2-36). Underlying anemia, or coagulation abnormalities, can also affect the density of the acute EDH. In some cases,

ongoing active bleeding may produce a "swirl sign" where fresh unclotted whole blood (40 HU) is seen as a spiral-shaped lucency within the hyperdense mass of previously clotted blood. Other causes of the swirl sign include extrusion of serum from the clot and intrusion of CSF (into an SDH).[39] The finding of mixed density clots in the epidural space has been associated with a more severe acute presentation and a reduced survival after surgery.[40]

On rare occasions, EDHs may be present in association with concurrent SDHs in which the separating dura remains intact (Fig. 2-37). This phenomenon may account for some cases of SDHs with convex centers (see below). EDHs can also present in the posterior fossa (see Figs. 2-27 to 2-29), where they are most often due to venous bleeding from laceration of the large dural sinuses. They may also appear over the vertex (Fig. 2-38) from fractures that cross the superior sagittal suture and sinus. Some EDHs have been observed to resolve spontaneously presumably by decompressing themselves through the fracture defect (see Fig. 2-10).[41] Last, the EDH has been reported to develop in a delayed fashion after an initially normal CT scan in almost 9% of patients.[42] This could be explained by initial hypotension, followed by resuscitation that produces more vigorous bleeding.

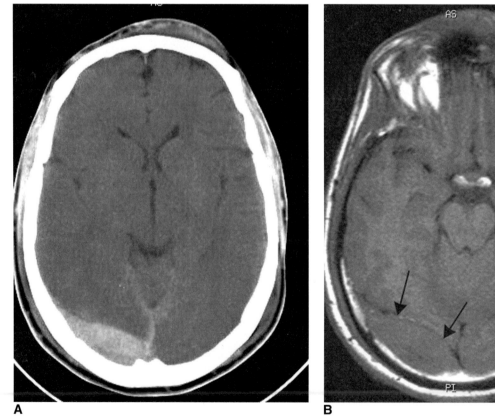

A　　　　　　　　　　　　　　　　　　B

Fig. 2-29
Posterior fossa EDH. **A,** CT shows an EDH arising in the right occipital epidural space and compressing the right occipital lobe. **B,** T1-weighted MRI shows an isointense signal EDH (*arrows*).

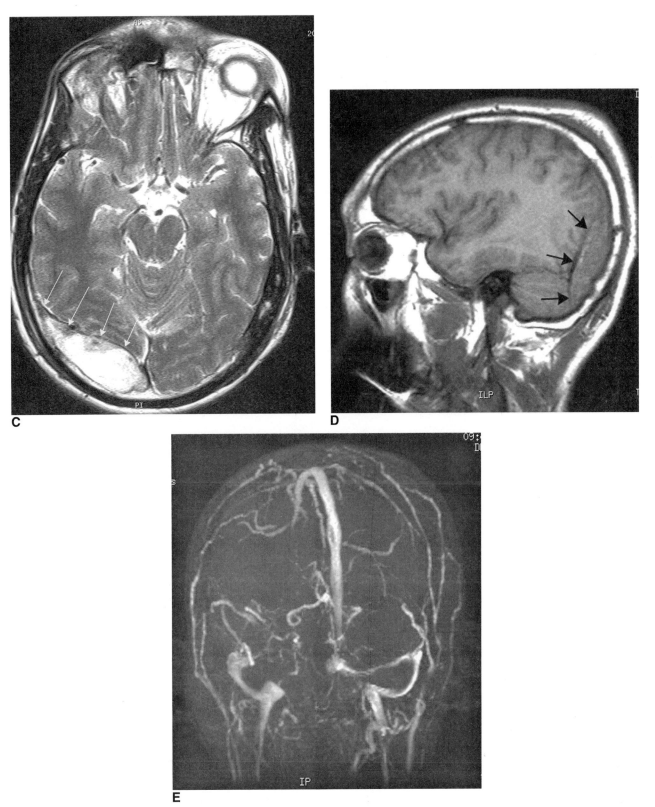

Fig. 2-29, cont'd
C, T2-weighted MRI shows the majority of the hematoma appears to lie between the meningeal layer (*arrows*) and periosteal layer (adjacent to bone) of the dura, and a small amount lies beneath both layers adjacent to the bone. **D**, A sagittal T1-weighted MR image shows that the EDH crosses the tentorium dividing the infra- and supratentorial spaces. **E**, An MR venogram shows occlusion of the right transverse sinus, indicating thrombosis.

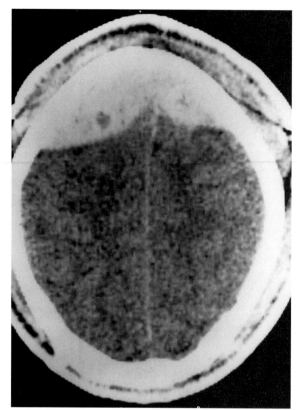

Fig. 2-30
Bifrontal EDH. CT image shows a bilateral frontal EDH. The bleeding crosses under the anterior falx, but is limited in spread at the coronal sutures. Marked frontal scalp contusion is noted.

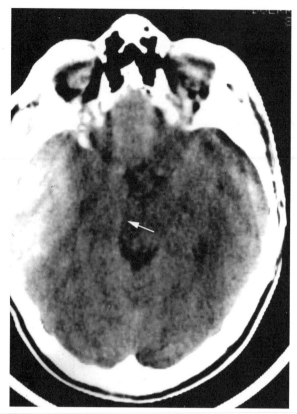

Fig. 2-31
Right temporal EDH. CT image demonstrates a right temporal EDH producing local medial herniation of the ipsilateral temporal lobe. There is effacement of the ipsilateral perimesencephalic cistern and brainstem distortion (*arrow*).

Subdural Hematoma. SDHs are considerably more complex than EDHs in terms of location, shape, composition, and clinical presentations. Isolated subdural collections are frequently seen in a subacute or chronic presentation. The SDH is also commonly seen in the acute posttrauma setting and in this situation is usually associated with cerebral injuries. SDH is rarely encountered in the acute setting without other evidence of intracranial pathology.

Source of Bleeding. The subdural space is a potential space, lying between the inner (meningeal) layer of the dura and the delicate arachnoid membrane. The subdural space is also called the "epiarachnoid space." Although the arachnoid is normally attached to the inner layer of the dura, a small collection of fluid may be in the subdural space. This fluid is not evenly distributed, but is concentrated in the vicinity of the large dural sinuses rather than over the convexities of the hemispheres. Several mechanisms produce hemorrhage into the subdural space. Penetrating injuries may lacerate blood vessels in the meninges, or a severe contusion may injure both cortical surface vessels and the arachnoid, allowing blood to reach the subdural space, and nontraumatic aneurysms may rupture into the "epiarachnoid space."

Classically, the SDH results from a tear in one or more bridging cortical veins. The bridging veins may tear when the brain and the skull (and its attached dura) move at different rates. The brain weighs between 1100 and 1500 gm.; however, suspended in a bath of CSF, the brain floats with an effective weight of only about 50 gm. When the head accelerates or decelerates, there may be a lag between movement of the skull and movement of the brain. This displacement leads to stretching of the bridging cortical veins and may tear these veins if the strain is sufficient. Since the surface of the brain is more compliant than the rigid dura, the veins usually tear where they enter the dural sinuses rather than at the surface of the brain. This mechanism for the production of isolated SDH has been confirmed by laboratory experiments using monkeys.[43] Hemorrhage that occurs at the site of insertion of bridging veins into the dural sinuses accumulates in the subdural space rather than in any other compartment.

Clinical Significance. Acute presentation with SDH occurs acutely in 10% to 30% of patients studied after severe head trauma. Patients with an acute SDH have a worse prognosis than those with EDH; the mortality rate varies from 30% to as high as 90%. In a report by Sahuquillo-Barris et al.,[44] the mortality from acute SDH was 31%, with 60% of the patients dying with evidence of concomitant diffuse axonal injury (DAI) (see below).

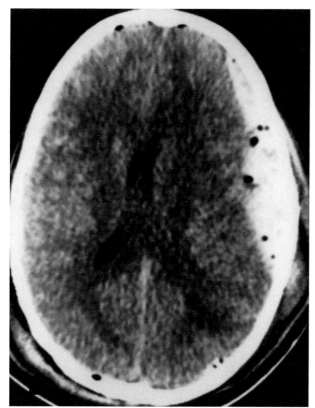

Fig. 2-32
Air mixed with EDH. CT image shows a large left frontoparietal EDH. Air from an adjacent open skull fracture has mixed with the epidural blood.

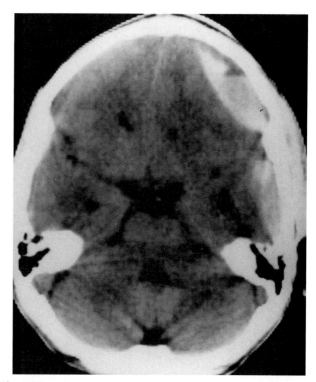

Fig. 2-33
EDHs with focal cortical mass effect. CT image reveals two small EDHs in the left frontotemporal region limited in extent at the coronal suture. The anterior bleed is incompletely clotted. Minimal mass effect exists on the left frontal horn and left temporal lobe.

These authors and others[45,46] have emphasized that the morbidity and mortality may not be related directly to the SDH itself, but, rather, to concurrent cerebral injury. The association of SDH with DAI should not be unexpected, since both can be produced by rapid acceleration-deceleration mechanism.[36] The mortality of the SDH relates directly to the promptness of diagnosis and surgical treatment. Patients with SDH who undergo surgery within four hours postinjury have a 30% mortality rate, whereas those who undergo surgery later than four hours postinjury have a 90% mortality rate,[46] another reason for rapid evacuation, diagnosis, and treatment.

Lesions Associated with Subdural Hematoma. In clinical practice, an SDH is typically not seen as an isolated finding, but as a component of a more complex and severe craniocerebral injury. Commonly, the SDH is only an associated finding with limited clinical significance in comparison with other lesions that are present, an "epiphenomenon" of some other injury.[44] Other significant lesions commonly occurring with acute SDH are focal or diffuse cerebral edema, diffuse axonal shearing, severe contusions, and EDH. Frequently, the SDH may be the most obvious lesion, whereas other injuries may be less apparent or even occult. The underlying injury may be less amenable to treatment than the obvious SDH. The

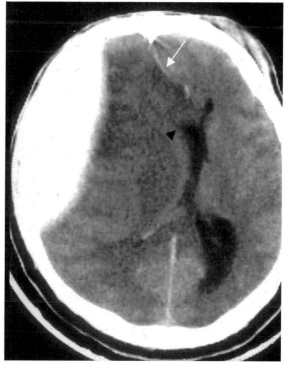

Fig. 2-34
Large right EDH producing subfalcine herniation. CT image reveals an extensive EDH in the right frontoparietal area, producing bowing of the anterior falx (*arrow*) and marked subfalcine herniation. The frontal horn of the right lateral ventricle appears partially amputated (*arrowhead*). (From Mirvis SE, Wolf AL, Numaguchi Y, et al: *AJNR* 11:355, 1990.)

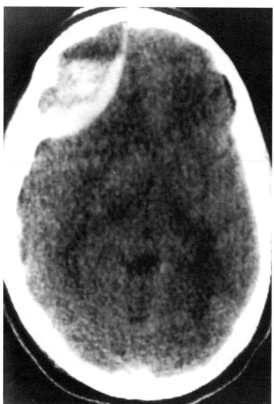

Fig. 2-35
Mixed attenuation EDH. A right frontal EDH displays a layered effect due to variation in blood clotting. Well-formed clot, highest attenuation, lies in the lowest position, with partially formed clot intermediate. Unclotted blood or serum occupies the upper position. Diffuse cerebral edema was also present, increasing compression of the ventricular system.

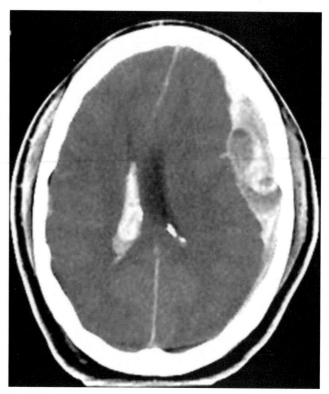

Fig. 2-36
Mixed attenuation EDH. Left EDH shows mixed attenuation. Lower density areas may represent nonclotted blood or active bleeding. Blood fills the right lateral ventricle.

common observation that the acute SDH produces more mass effect than can be accounted for by its size implies the presence of other injuries as hyperemic swelling, early contusions, or DAIs (Fig. 2-39). Yoshino et al.[47] reported that among a series of patients with SDH who died all exhibited "remarkable brain bulk enlargement" from edema or hyperemic swelling. The clinical history of immediate unconsciousness at the time of head trauma suggests diffuse axonal shearing as the major pathology rather than SDH.[44]

In cases where the acute SDH is the only lesion producing CNS symptoms and signs, the SDH is often unusually large or has accumulated with unusual rapidity. Several conditions may predispose a patient to the development of rapid or massive bleeding into the subdural space, including a hemorrhagic diathesis, chronic renal disease, and cerebral atrophy by increasing brain mobility.

CT Appearance. A SDH is usually crescentic and concave toward the brain—roughly paralleling the inner table of the skull. The typical CT features of acute SDH include high attenuation (in the range of 65 to 95 HU) (Figs. 2-40 to 2-42; see also Fig. 2-39), a swirl sign where

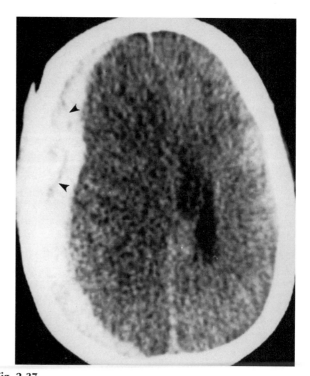

Fig. 2-37
Combined EDH and SDH. CT image demonstrates a large right convexity SDH with a central bulge. A smaller EDH was deep to the SDH. The lucent line separating them is the dura (*arrowheads*). A marked subfalcine herniation is to the left.

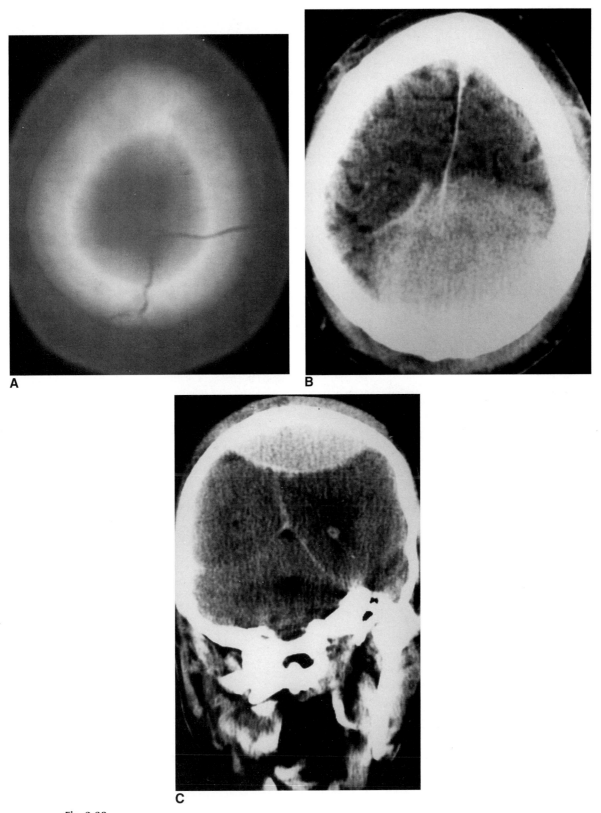

Fig. 2-38
Vertex EDH. **A,** CT image through the skull vertex photographed for bone shows a right parietal fracture and a midsagittal fracture. **B,** Image through the vertex reveals a large area of high-density clot over the cerebral vertex. **C,** Direct coronal CT confirms the epidural location of the hematoma with a classic biconvex configuration. The falx is displaced inferiorly and laterally. Presumably the hematoma arose from a laceration of the superior sagittal sinus.

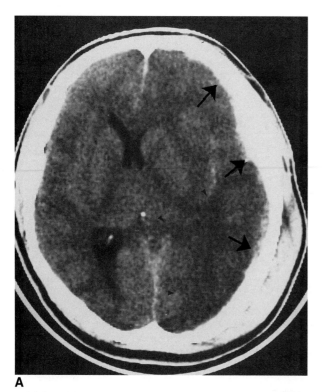

A

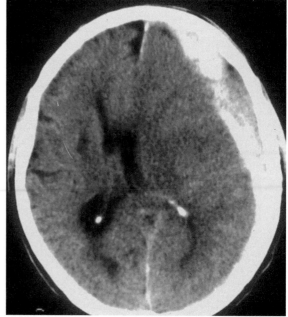

Fig. 2-40
SDH producing transfalcine herniation. CT image shows a left convexity SDH extending into the interhemispheric subdural space. Focal hemorrhage was observed in the centrum semiovale on the left. Marked transfalcine herniation is obliterating the left occipital horn. The left frontal horn is displaced posterior to "fit" under the rigid falx. Dilation of the right lateral ventricle indicates entrapment and developing unilateral hydrocephalus.

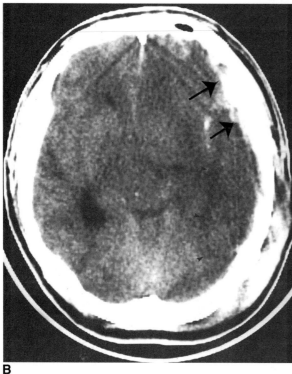

B

Fig. 2-39
Thin SDH associated with marked mass effect. **A** and **B**, CT images of a young man involved in a high-speed motor vehicle collision demonstrate a thin left frontal SDH (*arrows*). However, there was marked subfalcine herniation (note posterior displacement of the left frontal horn and obliteration of the left occipital horn). Low attenuation in the left occipital lobe is suggestive of ischemia or infarction. Presumably the mass effect from the left cerebral edema far outweighs the minimal mass effect attributable to the SDH alone.

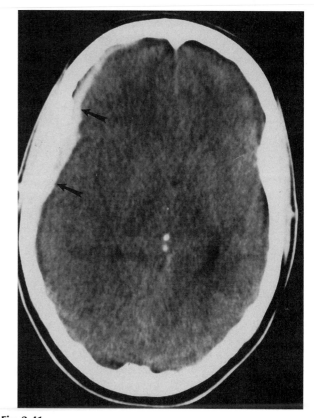

Fig. 2-41
SDH associated with severe intraparenchymal injury. CT image reveals a thin right frontoparietal SDH (*arrows*). Despite the small SDH there was severe diffuse cerebral edema with obliteration of the lateral ventricles. The patient underwent a lifesaving right deep temporal lobectomy with good neurologic recovery.

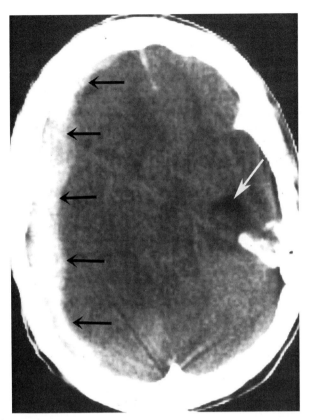

Fig. 2-42
SDH. CT image of a large right convexity SDH (*arrows*) producing both transfalcine and transtentorial herniation. The basal cisterns are obliterated and there is dilation of the contralateral temporal horn (*white arrow*).

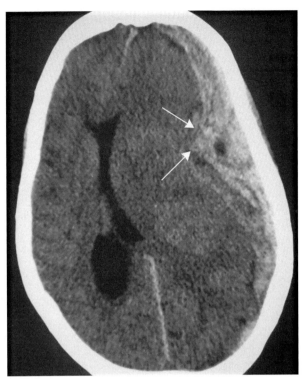

Fig. 2-43
SDH extending into the interhemispheric fissure. CT shows a left convexity SDH producing marked rightward subfalcine herniation. Note the convex bulge in the central portion of the subdural collection (*arrows*) mimicking an EDH, a feature not uncommon in large acute SDHs.

lower density unclotted whole blood swirls into a region of clotted blood that is hyperdense, extraaxial blood without a skull fracture, and an extraaxial collection of blood that crosses sutures but is limited by the falx and tentorium (Figs. 2-43 to 2-48). Rarely, even an acute SDH can be isointense with cerebral cortex if the patient is severely anemic (hemoglobin, 8 to 10 g/dl) or if there is a leakage of CSF (from an arachnoid tear) into the subdural space.[39,48] An acute SDH appears as a relatively thin collection that conforms to the surface of the brain and is therefore concave toward the brain. The SDH spreads more or less uniformly over the convexity and may fill the interhemispheric compartment or layer along the surface of the tentorium (see Figs. 2-43 to 2-48). The SDH is not related to skull fractures in a causal way and is not limited by the calvarial sutures in its extent. However, unlike the EDH, the SDH is limited in its spread by the rigid falx and tentorium. The CT density of the SDH is time dependent. In a patient with a normal hematocrit, the SDH is initially of high-CT attenuation. Over time, as the hemoglobin is digested and reabsorbed, the density of the collection gradually declines until eventually the fluid appears hypointense relative to the nonenhanced cerebral cortex. At some point, the fluid collection passes through the density range of normal brain attenuation, at

which point it may be difficult to separate these isodense components. Ancillary signs may be used to identify the isodense SDH. The mass effect of the subdural collection will produce focal effacement of the sulci at the cortical surface and the gray-white matter junction will appear medially displaced[49-51] (Figs. 2-49 to 2-52). The mass effect of a large SDH will produce distortion of the contour of the ipsilateral ventricle and may produce subfalcine herniation[49,52] (see Figs. 2-39, 2-40, 2-43, 2-49, and 2-52). This pattern occurs because the opening in the falx is centrally placed and is much smaller than both the hemispheres and the ventricles. Therefore when herniation is produced by a diffuse mass that is both anterior and posterior, the frontal horn of the ipsilateral lateral ventricle is "amputated" by the corpus callosum, as both are displaced posteriorly to clear the undersurface of the anterior falx. Simultaneously, the trigone of the lateral ventricle and its choroid plexus must move anteriorly to slip beneath the posterior edge of the falx opening. Thus, the frontal horn is displaced posteriorly, whereas the trigone and posterior horn are pushed anteriorly (see Figs. 2-39, 2-40, 2-43, and 2-52). This pattern is uncommon when the mass effect arises from a focal lesion or from an intraaxial process, such as an infarct or traumatic brain swelling, both of which may also appear isointense with brain tissue initially. Review of images with "subdural

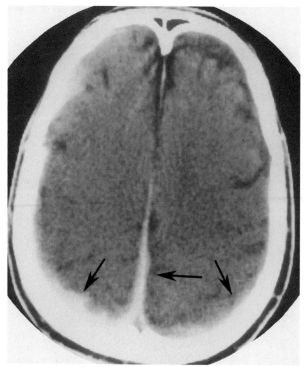

Fig. 2-44
Perifalx SDH. CT image demonstrates a smooth thickening of the posterior falx without high density in the cortical sulci. The appearance is diagnostic of a perifalx interhemispheric SDH. The SDH extends along the occipital subdural space bilaterally (*arrows*).

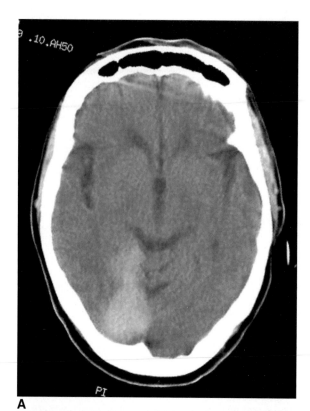

A

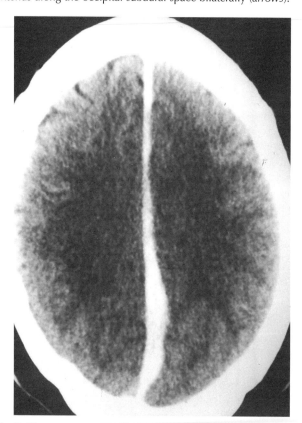

Fig. 2-45
Perifalx SDH. CT shows a diffuse apparent thickening of the falx due to layering of subdural blood along the left side of the falx. A convexity SDH was not observed. No blood interdigitates with the adjacent sulci to suggest a subarachnoid component.

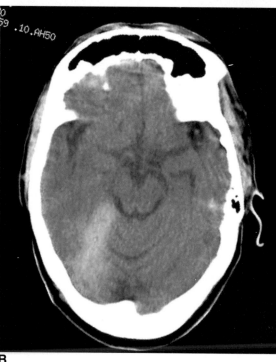

B

Fig. 2-46
Peritentorial SDH. **A** and **B**, CT demonstrates high-density blood bordering the right side of the tentorium with a sharp demarcation at the incisura consistent with a supratentorial SDH.

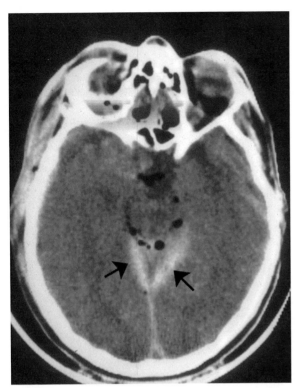

Fig. 2-47
Bilateral supratentorial SDH. CT image after blunt head impact reveals a V-shaped area of increased density along the margins of the tentorium (*arrows*). The blood is sharply marginated on the medial aspect and "fuzzy" on the lateral margins, indicating a supratentorial, peritentorial location. Pneumocephalus is also observed.

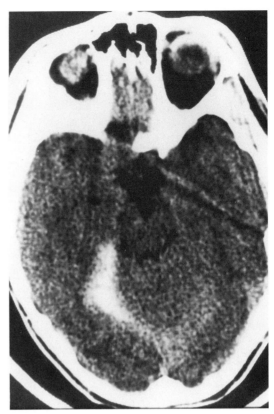

Fig. 2-48
Peritentorial SDH. Axial CT image through the posterior fossa reveals high-density blood along the right tentorium with a sharp medial demarcation and irregular lateral margin. This appearance suggests a supratentorial, peritentorial location of blood.

windows" should be used whenever trauma is suspected. In cases of a thin isodense SDH, a contrast-enhanced CT scan will increase the density of the cortical surface vessels and show them to be displaced from the inner table of the calvarium[50,51] (see Fig. 2-49). The increase in cortical density will increase the contrast between the brain and SDH. In addition, contrast may produce enhancement of neomembranes, encapsulating the subacute to chronic SDH, or may demonstrate dural enhancement. Delayed scanning after contrast injection may permit enough contrast to enter the subdural collection to increase its density above that of the adjacent brain.

As noted above, most subdural fluid collections are crescentic, concave towards the brain, and spread relatively thinly over a large area. On occasion, however, the acute SDH is strikingly limited in extent, very thick, and focally convex toward the brain[53] (Fig. 2-53). These atypical features of acute SDH often mimic the appearance of acute EDH.[39,53]

SDH layering along the tentorium may prove difficult to diagnose. The blood tends to increase the density and thickness of the tentorium on axial images. Typically, supratentorial subdural blood is sharply marginated on

its medial edge by the tentorial edge and has a fuzzy lateral border due to volume averaging along the angled tentorium. The supratentorial and peritentorial SDH often creates a V-shaped appearance of increased density along the falx (see Figs. 2-46 to 2-48). Infratentorial peritentorial subdural blood typically is sharply marginated laterally along the insertion of the tentorium into the inner table of the calvarium and is less sharply defined medially. In practice, we have found this distinction occasionally difficult and may resort to direct coronal CT images, when possible, to localize the site of the SDH if deemed clinically warranted. Alternatively, coronal reformations of thin-axial CT sections may be used. Infratentorial peritentorial SDH is quite uncommon as compared to a supratentorial location (Fig. 2-54).

SDH can commonly layer along the margin of the midline falx, producing a thickened, somewhat lobulated appearing pseudo-falx. Usually, clotted subdural blood can be seen to continue over the cerebral convexity or tentorium, confirming the diagnosis. On occasion, it is difficult to distinguish the normal falx from a thin parafalx SDH.[54,55] A calcified thickened falx can be dis-

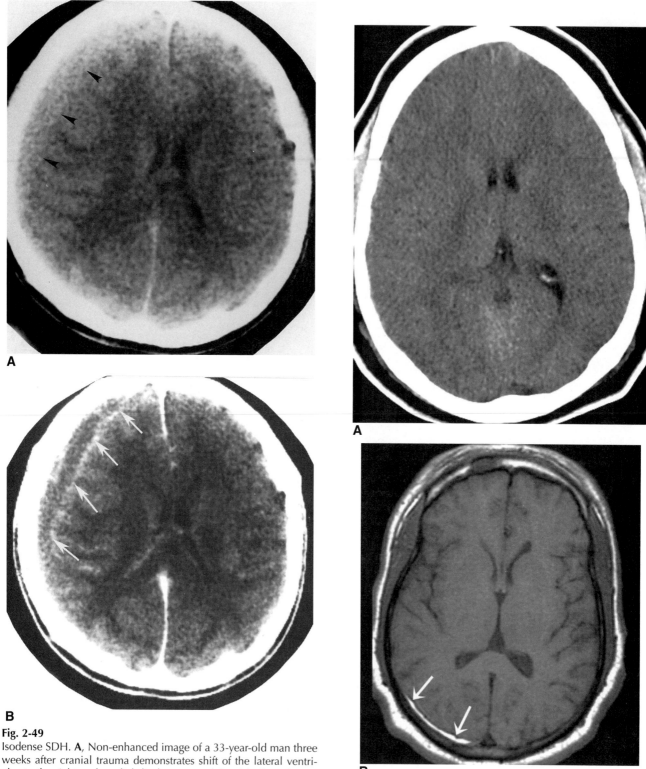

Fig. 2-49
Isodense SDH. **A**, Non-enhanced image of a 33-year-old man three weeks after cranial trauma demonstrates shift of the lateral ventricles to the right and medial displacement of the right frontal gray-white matter interface (*arrowheads*). In addition the cortical sulci over the right frontal-parietal region are obliterated by mass effect. **B**, Image acquired after intravenous contrast clearly demarcates the right convexity SDH (*arrows*).

Fig. 2-50
Subtle SDH revealed by MRI. **A**, CT of blunt head trauma patient shows no acute injury. **B**, MRI performed on the same patient clearly shows thin right occipital SDH (*arrows*).

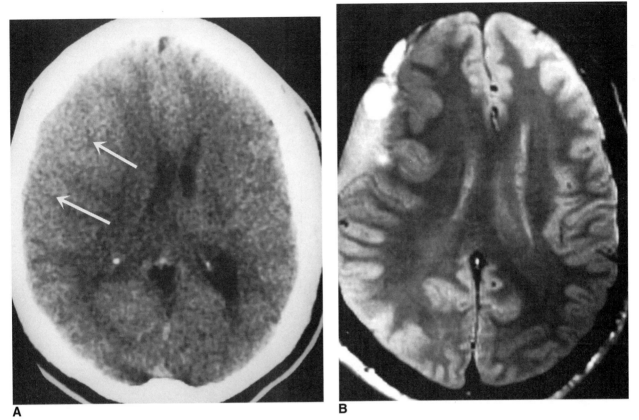

Fig. 2-51
Isodense SDH on CT and MRI. **A**, CT image of 31-year-old man 2 weeks after head trauma demonstrates an isointense collection producing mass effect and medial displacement of the gray-white matter interface (*arrows*). **B**, MRI reveals a collection of clotted blood (brighter areas) and proteinaceous fluid consistent with an evolving SDH.

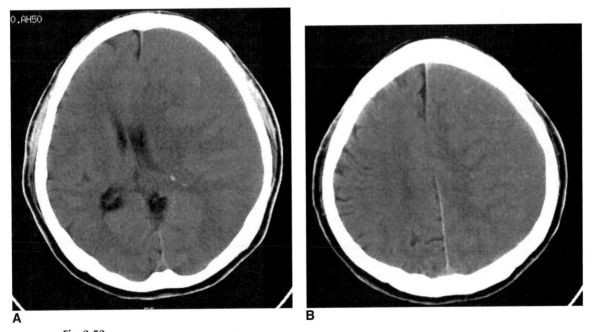

Fig. 2-52
Huge isodense SDH. **A** and **B**, CT images demonstrate a large left convexity SDH that is near isointense with gray matter. Significant mass effect displacing the ventricles to the right allows easy identification of this lesion.

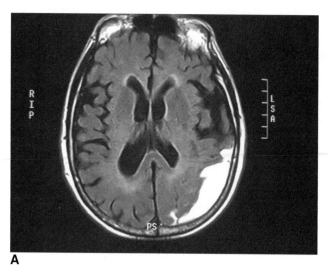

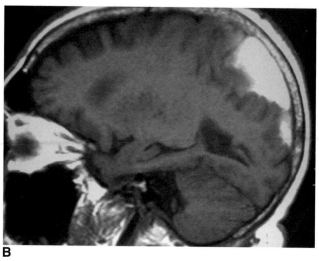

A

B

Fig. 2-53
SDH mimicking an EDH. **A,** Axial fluid attenuated inversion recovery (FLAIR) MR image shows a high signal collection in the left temporal-occipital region with a convex bulge toward the brain and sharply defined margins. **B,** A near midsagittal T1-weighted study shows a high-signal collection typical of hematoma with a convex bulge toward the brain. The hematoma was in the subdural space at surgery.

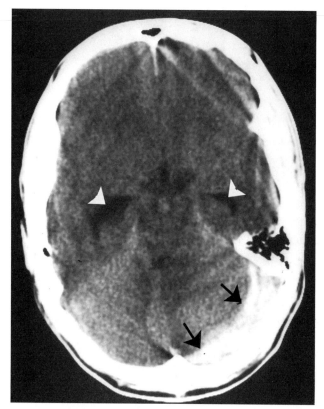

Fig. 2-54
Infratentorial SDH obstructing cerebral aqueduct. CT through the posterior fossa reveals a left SDH tracking along the insertion of the tentorium (*arrows*). Temporal tip distension (*arrowheads*) indicates cerebral aqueduct obstruction. Anterior focal midbrain hemorrhage is also observed.

tinguished from a parafalx SDH using bone windows in which dense calcification can still be seen, but hematoma blends with the adjacent brain.

Complications. In addition to the direct mass effect and secondary herniation effects of an acute SDH, other complications may occur, usually during the subacute or chronic phase. Neomembranes usually form from the outer (dural) border of the subdural collection and are often fully developed 2 to 3 weeks after the acute bleed. Subdural membranes are composed of proliferating capillaries and fibroblasts and enhance because the capillaries do not develop a blood-brain barrier. The neomembranes are fragile and are prone to spontaneous hemorrhage, leading to delayed acute rebleeding into a subacute or chronic SDH[56] (Figs. 2-55 and 2-56). Because of the potential for rebleeding, even a chronic SDH may present with high attenuation or blood-fluid levels. The neomembranes may form loculated collections in the subdural space in patients with multiple episodes of subdural hemorrhage.

With time, an SDH develops an expanded biconvex shape from its initial configuration, perhaps in part related to loculation by neomembranes. Repetitive hemorrhage, "osmotic effects of blood breakdown products," and an "active pump" from the membranes have all been suggested as possible factors in this transformation of size and shape. The end result is a symptomatic focal extraaxial compressive mass on the brain developing from a less innocuous concave collection.

Tension pneumocephalus may develop after surgical removal of an SDH, particularly in the subacute or chronic phase, when the deformed brain fails to return to its normal shape and the persistent void fills with air under tension[57,58] (Fig. 2-57). Tension pneumocephalus is readily recognized on CT by the abnormally large collection of air and the persistence of mass effect in the absence of fluid or blood. In practice, the authors have observed tension pneumocephalus on several occasions but have not seen significant clinical sequelae in the majority of these patients.

MRI Observations. The morphology, clinical evolution, and time course of SDHs can often be subtle and confusing. If CT fails to explain the clinical situation, MRI should be the next modality used. MRI is likely to be more sensitive than CT in detecting thin SDHs or those that may be misdiagnosed because of volume averaging with bone, such as at the vertex or subtemporal region. MRI will be more sensitive to thin isodense SDH since the bone signal will appear dark and the blood will appear bright on T1-weighted sequences from the paramagnetic effect of extracellular hemoglobin[59,60] (Fig. 2-58; see also Figs. 2-7, 2-50, and 2-51). The evolution of the MRI appearance of blood in the subdural space differs from that of intraparenchymal hematoma.[61] These differences include lack of hemosiderin deposition in chronic SDH (a hallmark of chronic parenchymal hematoma); absence of persistent hyperintensity, which is common in parenchymal hematomas; and a greater likelihood of rebleeding, which will produce complex signal patterns of mixed signal intensity due to differences in hematoma age. Fobben et al.[61] suggest that persistent high signal on short TR/TE images in the historically chronic SDH indicates rebleeding (Fig. 2-59). True CSF hygromas, which are likely the result of arachnoid tears with CSF entering the subdural space or abnormal CSF absorption into the venous sinuses, appear near isointense to CSF on different MRI sequences. Thus, MRI can better distinguish a chronic SDH from a subdural hygroma, which has a similar appearance by CT.

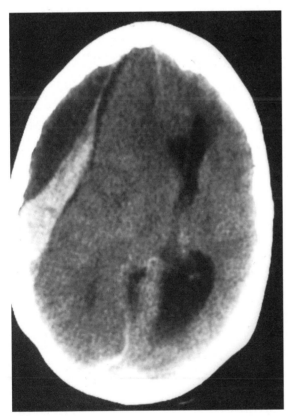

Fig. 2-55
Acute on chronic SDH. CT image shows a large right convexity SDH. A large low attenuation component was indicating a chronic SDH within a collection mixed with high-density fresh clot, suggesting an acute on chronic SDH. Marked right to left subfalcine herniation is present and left ventricular entrapment. The elderly female patient's history included an SDH.

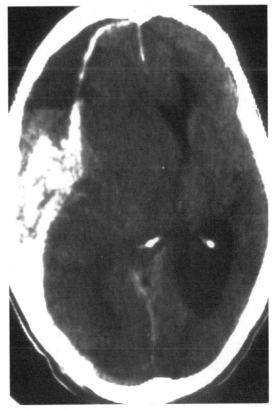

Fig. 2-56
Acute on chronic SDH. Another patient displays a large right convexity SDH containing a mixture of CT densities, suggestive of an acute on chronic SDH. Again, there is marked right to left transfalcine herniation with left lateral ventricular entrapment and dilation.

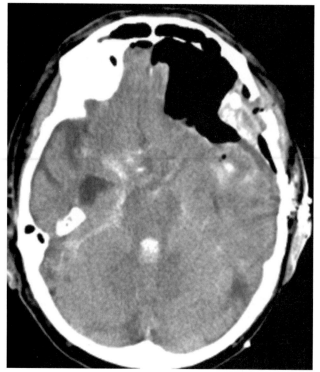

Fig. 2-57
Tension pneumocephalus. Following removal of a large left SDH, the postoperative CT reveals accumulation of air in the left frontal subdural space. A tension component is suggested by displacement of the left frontal lobe. Residual hemorrhage is present in the fourth ventricle, left temporal lobe, and subarachnoid space of the basal cisterns. The right temporal tip is dilated.

Subarachnoid Hemorrhage

Subarachnoid hemorrhage (SAH) is the most common type of bleeding after craniocerebral trauma, and trauma is the most common cause of SAH.[62] In our experience, however, isolated SAH visible on CT without other signs of craniocerebral injury is unusual after head trauma. If a clear-cut history of trauma is not available, the appearance of isolated SAH on CT should suggest the possibility of other etiologies such as an aneurysm rupture or a bleeding vascular malformation; less commonly an intraspinal process may bleed into the subarachnoid space. Acutely, traumatic SAH may be overshadowed by the presence of other more obvious and more significant gross injuries, such as EDH or SDH. The clinical manifestations of SAH, such as meningismus headache, and Kernig's sign are typically not well appreciated in the presence of more profound CNS dysfunction attributed to other lesions. Blood in the subarachnoid space from head trauma rarely forms the typical basilar clots seen from aneurysmal bleeding. SAH related to trauma may be seen in association with cortical contusions from blood leaking into the subarachnoid space, from extraaxial collections, as an SDH with a tear in the arachnoid membrane, from an intraparenchymal hematoma

with leakage of blood into the ventricular system, or from direct injury to the cortical (pial) vessels in the subarachnoid space itself (Figs. 2-60 and 2-61). The sequelae of traumatic SAH are similar to those resulting from a bleeding aneurysm: vasospasm with potential secondary infarction; chemical meningitis; and acute or delayed hydrocephalus either from obstruction of the cisterns or impaired CSF reabsorption due to occlusion of the arachnoid villi. However, vasospasm from traumatic SAH is less frequent than with aneurysms.[62]

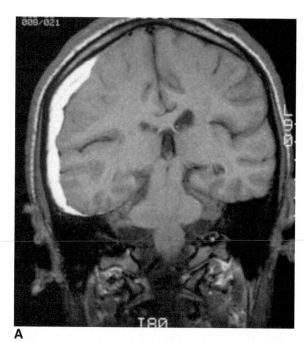

A

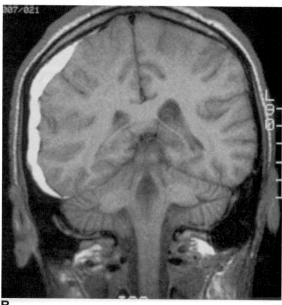

B

Fig. 2-58
MRI of SDH. **A** and **B**, Coronal CT images of trauma patient show bright signal of blood on T1-weighted sequence related to paramagnetic (T1 shortening effect) of extracellular methemoglobin.

Cerebral Contusion

Contusions are surface lesions that always involve the cortex, and may be limited entirely to the gray matter. They typically affect the crests or crowns of the gyri rather than the tissue at the base of a sulcus or fissure. A cerebral contusion (bruise) is a focal area of mixed hemorrhage,

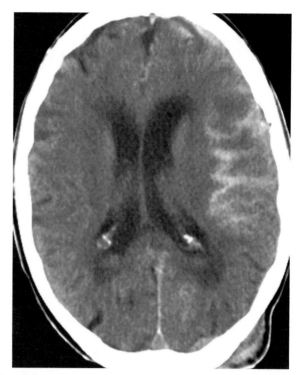

Fig. 2-60
Acute subarachnoid hemorrhage (SAH). CT image in acute head trauma victim shows linear collections of blood filling left-sided sulci. There is a thin left SDH. Mass effect with left shift is due to left cerebral edema.

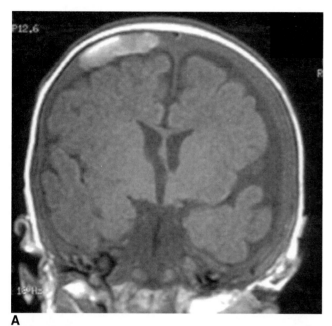

A

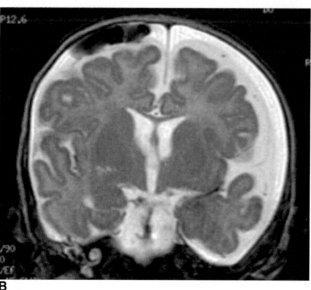

B

Fig. 2-59
MRI of acute on chronic SDH. **A,** Coronal T1-weighted study shows biconvex medium intensity collections of higher signal than cerebrospinal fluid (CSF). A focus of increased signal at the left vertex represents acute or subacute hemorrhage. **B,** Coronal image with T2-weighted sequence shows a bright subdural collection similar to the CSF with a dark region in the left vertex region presumably due to extracellular free methemoglobin and central areas of persistent intracellular deoxyhemoglobin or methemoglobin. The areas of altered signal indicate more recent hemorrhage into a chronic SDH.

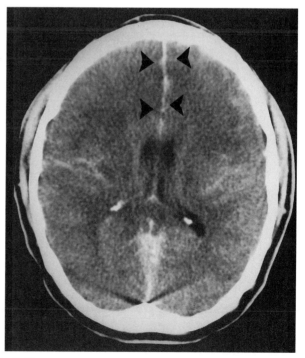

Fig. 2-61
SAH. CT shows bilateral linear density in the cerebral sulci indicating subarachnoid blood. SAH in the interhemispheric fissure interdigitates through the adjacent sulci (*arrowheads*), which would not occur with isolated perifalx subdural blood. There is also hemorrhage in the occipital horns.

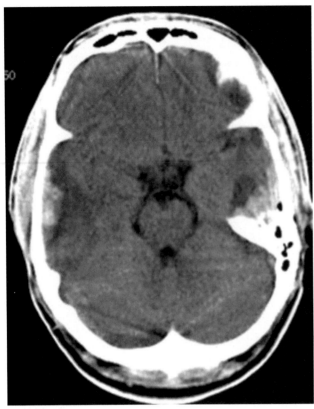

Fig. 2-62
Cerebral contusion. CT after right-sided temporal impact shows underlying right temporal coup contusion with contrecoup contusion of the left temporal lobe adjacent to calvarium.

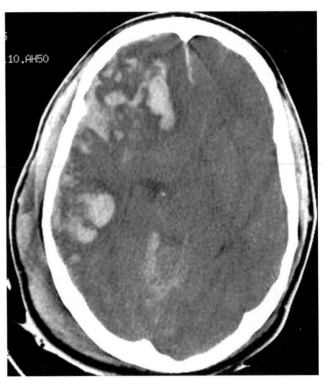

Fig. 2-63
Cerebral contusion. CT shows a large area of mixed hemorrhage and edema in the right frontal and temporal region. A large scalp contusion reflects the large impact site. There is marked right to left shift and compression of the ventricular system due to edema.

edema, and necrotic tissue, arising from mechanical forces transmitted to the brain (Figs. 2-62 to 2-64). These forces may be directly transmitted from a penetrating foreign body or displaced bone fragment. They may be transmitted through the calvarium to the underlying cortical surface, so-called "coup" contusions (see Figs. 2-62 and 2-63), or may result from impaction of the cerebrum against the rigid inner table at a point opposite to the site of the impacting force, a "contrecoup" contusion (see Fig. 2-64). In addition to the conventional coup and contrecoup contusions of the cerebral cortex, a third group, formerly called "intermediate" contusions, affects the deep central parts of the CNS, including the corpus callosum and the basal ganglia (Fig. 2-65). These deep injuries appear to arise from a different mechanism than the more superficial cortical contusions and most likely result from mechanical stresses—shearing injury—within the cerebral hemisphere (see below).

Regardless of the mechanism of injury, superficial contusions most frequently occur at the base of the anterior frontal lobes and in the anterior temporal lobes. It has been suggested that this localization is produced by the relatively irregular floor of the middle and anterior cranial fossae as compared with the smooth floor of the posterior fossa. Superficial or cortical contusions occur when sufficient force is applied to the tissue to mechanically disrupt the integrity of small vascular channels. Usually only capillaries and small venules are damaged, and they begin to ooze or leak small quantities of whole blood. The blood accumulates in the perivascular space around damaged vessels as multiple small petechial or "flame" hemorrhages. The bleeding is often self-limited and is frequently confined to the cortex (Fig. 2-66). However, if the total damage is significant, larger vessels may be disrupted, producing a confluent collection, such as a hematoma (see Fig. 2-63). The CT appearance of cerebral contusion will reflect the pleomorphic mixture of tissue densities, including focally dense blood clot, lower density cerebral edema, and mixtures intermediate between these two densities (see Figs. 2-62 to 2-64). The appearance of cerebral contusion may evolve dramatically over time from an initial region with undetectable bleeding to an area of frank cerebral hematoma representing gross ongoing bleeding into the parenchyma. During this time the mass effect attributable to the contusions may also increase substantially. In addition, edema associated with cerebral contusion may also increase for several days,

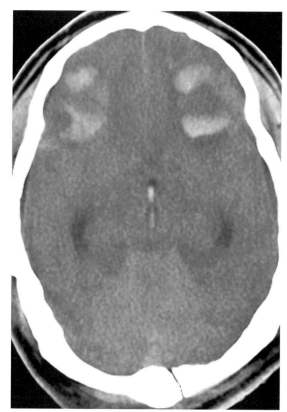

Fig. 2-64
Contrecoup contusion. CT image shows a midline occipital skull fracture that indicates the site of blunt impact. Areas of hemorrhage and edema are seen in the frontal lobe bases, reflecting impact into the frontal bone surfaces and effects of inertial forces.

usually reaching a peak between 3 and 5 days after injury. Edema may be increasing even as the hemorrhagic components are resolving on serial CT studies. Extensive cerebral contusions may cause enough mass effect to produce life-threatening herniation and require surgical resection of the damaged brain or extensive craniotomy to preserve life[63] (Fig. 2-67). Cerebral contusions that remain essentially "nonhemorrhagic" and produce limited mass effect may be too subtle to detect by CT and are better appreciated by MRI scanning[64,65] (see below).

Deep and/or Diffuse Cerebral Injuries

One group of cerebral injuries usually excludes the cortex and instead involves the deeper portions of the brain. These lesions tend to be diffuse and may be seen with or without an impact.[65] They are primary lesions and are variously called *shearing injury, diffuse white matter injury,* or *diffuse axonal injury* (DAI). These diffuse lesions are noted in up to 50% of severe head injuries, account for 30% of deaths from head injury, and are far more com-

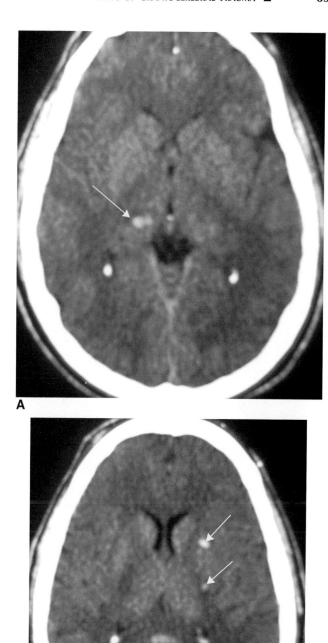

Fig. 2-65
Intermediate cerebral contusions. **A,** CT image of obtunded closed head trauma patient shows small focus of hemorrhage in the right thalamus (*arrow*). **B,** Another level shows foci of hemorrhage adjacent to the internal capsule. The findings are compatible with deep brain hemorrhages that can involve the basal ganglia and surrounding white matter from axonal shearing (*arrows*).

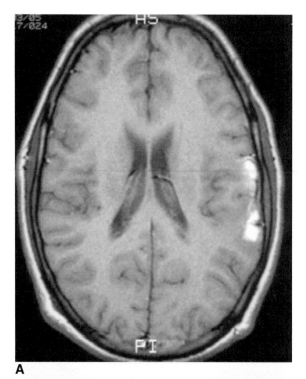

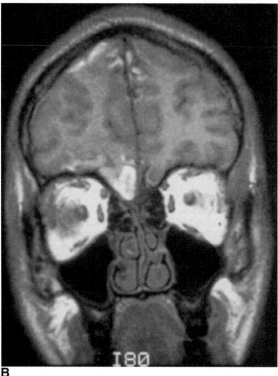

Fig. 2-66
Contusions confined to cortex on MRI. **A** and **B**, Axial and coronal T1-weighted MRI demonstrates hemorrhage that is principally confined to the cortex of the left parietal vertex, parietal lobe, and frontal base.

mon in patients presenting with a Glasgow Coma Scale (GCS) score of eight or less.[66] Three processes to be considered below include DAI, hyperemic brain swelling (HBS), and traumatic brain edema (TBE). These lesions

have numerous etiologic, clinical, and imaging similarities and are often confused with one another.

Diffuse Axonal Injury. DAI is thought to result from shearing strains applied to the brain and are frequently referred to as "shearing injuries."[66-71] Since the 1930s, pathologists have reported a series of abnormalities occurring in the deeper portions of the CNS that do not appear to be the result of a direct transmission of blunt forces. These were noted in patients who had survived head trauma, often of a severe nature, but who remained in a persistent vegetative state. Many of these patients had been rendered unconscious immediately at the moment of impact, consistent with a primary brain injury. Shearing forces do the most damage to the brain when applied in the coronal (lateral) plane, and especially when there is a component angle of acceleration.[67] Adams et al.,[68] in a study of 45 patients, concluded that DAI occurs at the time of injury and is not a secondary process that is the result of other pathology, such as edema, hypoxia, or herniation.

The pathologic characteristics of DAI include a "triad" of: (1) microscopic evidence of diffuse axonal damage (white matter lesions); (2) focal lesions of the corpus callosum; and, (3) focal lesions of the brainstem, especially in the dorsolateral quadrants of the upper brainstem.[66-70] Histologically the lesions include axon retraction balls, a sign of axonal transection. Long-term survivors may develop microglial clusters and later atrophy (Wallerian degeneration). Pathophysiologically, acceleration-deceleration forces transmitted through the brain cause disruption of axons perpendicular to the long axis of the axon. These injuries are typically found in regions of a high degree of parallel arrangement of axons, such as the corpus callosum, internal capsule, brainstem, basal ganglia, and subcortical white matter.[66-70] These lesions may be accompanied acutely by small hemorrhages from vessels in close proximity to the axon bundles. These hemorrhages may provide the major CT marker for these lesions. Deep parenchymal hematomas that occur without penetrating trauma are almost invariably the result of shearing force injury's disrupting small arterioles.[72-74] Clinically, patients sustaining DAI are usually reported to be unconscious from the time of impact and have a high incidence of primary cerebral death[66-71] or severe neurologic impairment. Diffuse posttraumatic cerebral atrophy frequently accompanies DAI as a result of Wallerian degeneration of nerve cells and axons (see below).

As noted above, CT scans cannot directly demonstrate the presence of axonal injuries, but can detect the multiple punctate hemorrhages that typically accompany DAI (Figs. 2-68 to 2-70; see also Fig. 2-65). Many authors insist that MRI is needed to exclude white matter shearing.[65] These foci of hemorrhage are appreciated at the gray-white matter junction, along the corpus callosum, in the basal ganglia, and in the rostral brainstem.[66-71]

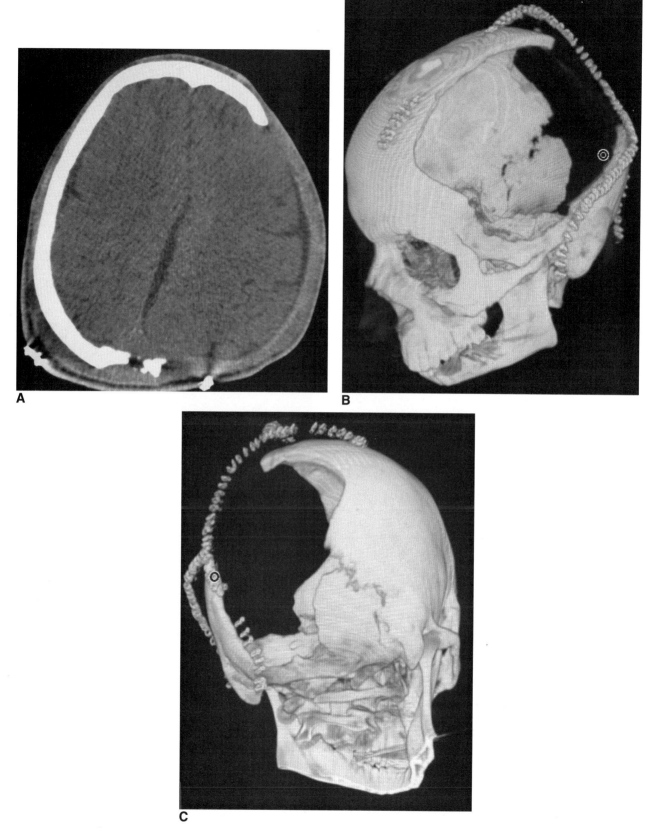

Fig. 2-67

Extensive craniectomy. **A**, Axial CT shows extensive left-sided craniectomy that was performed because of severe cerebral edema and increased intracranial pressure after blunt head trauma and a posterior fossa EDH. **B** and **C**, Extent of lifesaving craniectomy including large portion of temporal, parietal, and bilateral occipital bones is shown in three-dimensional display. The bone fragments are preserved in liquid carbon dioxide and replaced when brain swelling resolves completely.

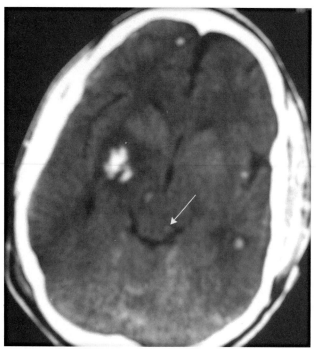

Fig. 2-68
Diffuse axonal injury (DAI). Typical pattern of punctate hemorrhage caused by shearing effects between connected tissues of different density. Note hemorrhages in gray-white junction, around the right basal ganglia, right subthalamic area, and dorsolateral brainstem (*arrow*).

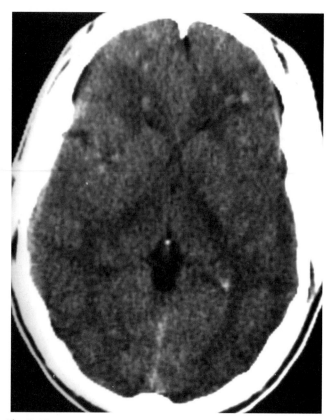

Fig. 2-69
CT of diffuse axonal shearing. Image at the midventricular level reveals numerous small foci of hemorrhage predominantly involving the gray-white matter junction, which is typical of diffuse axonal shearing.

Zimmerman et al.[69] postulated that disruption of small blood vessels, paralleling the axonal bundles, is also a result of the shear stress across the gray-white matter interface. The classic hypothesis is that these are produced by a difference in the physical density between the gray and white matter, leading to differential acceleration and deceleration as the mechanical stress is applied.

MRI is far more sensitive in identifying DAI than CT, and is frequently diagnostic when a corresponding CT scan appears normal[4,65] (Figs. 2-71 to 2-73). Furthermore, specialized MR studies are potentially more sensitive than conventional spin echo scans including FLAIR imaging, gradient recalled echo (GRE), diffusion-weighted imaging (DWI), apparent diffusion constant (ADC) mapping, magnetization transfer imaging (MTF), and MR spectroscopy (MRS).[75-81] Shearing lesions are usually defined as having the following characteristics: less than 15 mm in diameter; occurring in the hemispheric white matter, corpus callosum, and brainstem; and not significantly involving the cortex. GRE images are commonly abnormal when T2W SE images are "clean." Magnetization transfer studies are also more sensitive than standard MR pulse sequences. DWI may reveal characteristic lesions that are involving the corpus callosum, especially in the posterior body and splenium of the corpus callosum. Takayama et al.[80] reported a case where DWI was abnormal in a region of T2 hyperintensity, consistent with cytotoxic edema. Using special stains for amyloid precursor protein (APP), Leclercq et al.[73] have shown that axonal injury preferentially affects the caudal corpus callosum (posterior body and splenium). These areas of primary brain destruction in the splenium, and similar lesions in the pons, may have reduced NAA (N-acetyl aspartate) peaks on MRS and abnormal MTR (magnetization transfer ratio) even when they appear normal on conventional MR images.[78] White matter lesions in the body and splenium of the corpus callosum, especially involving the undersurface, are suggestive of DAI.[73,74] Research from Emory University involving a series of children with nonaccidental CNS trauma have suggested using DWI and ADC maps because of their inherently greater sensitivity than both CT and conventional MR studies, and better correlation with patient prognosis.[81] These authors recommend using DWI/ADC to "complement the routine MRI ... when child abuse is suspected."[81]

Posttraumatic Edema and Hyperemic Swelling.
Diffuse cerebral swelling after blunt head trauma can occur at any age, but is predominantly a lesion of infants and children. In fact, in 1981 Bruce et al.[82] reported that

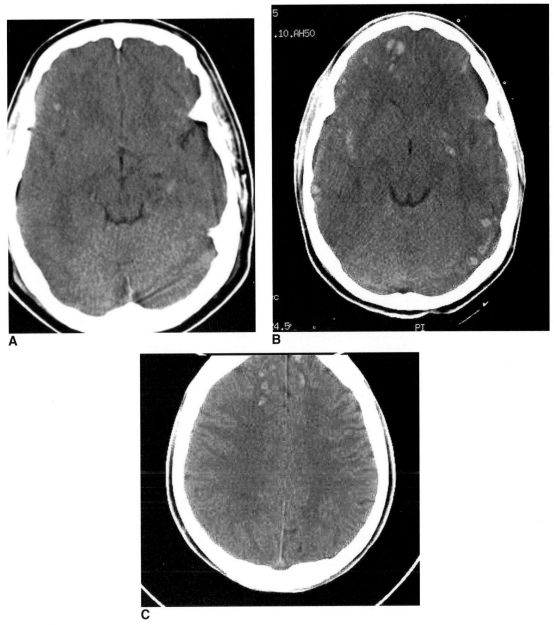

Fig. 2-70
Diffuse axonal shearing injury. **A** to **C**, CT of unconscious trauma patient at three levels shows multiple punctate hemorrhages involving the gray-white junction and the lateral basal ganglia.

bilateral cerebral swelling was the most common abnormality of head-injured children noted by CT. Excluding severe DAI, two different processes can lead to diffuse cerebral swelling: hyperemic swelling and true cerebral edema. Hyperemia may be related to a transient loss of autoregulation that leads to vasodilatation. That hyperemic brain swelling is due to vascular engorgement from a relative or absolute increase in cerebral blood flow has been confirmed directly by measurement of cerebral blood flow and indirectly by measurements of CT density and dynamic CT scanning.[82,83] The brain expands from hyperemia but remains constricted by the bony calvarium and dural folds. Consequently, a malignant elevation of intracranial pressure (ICP) occurs, leading to

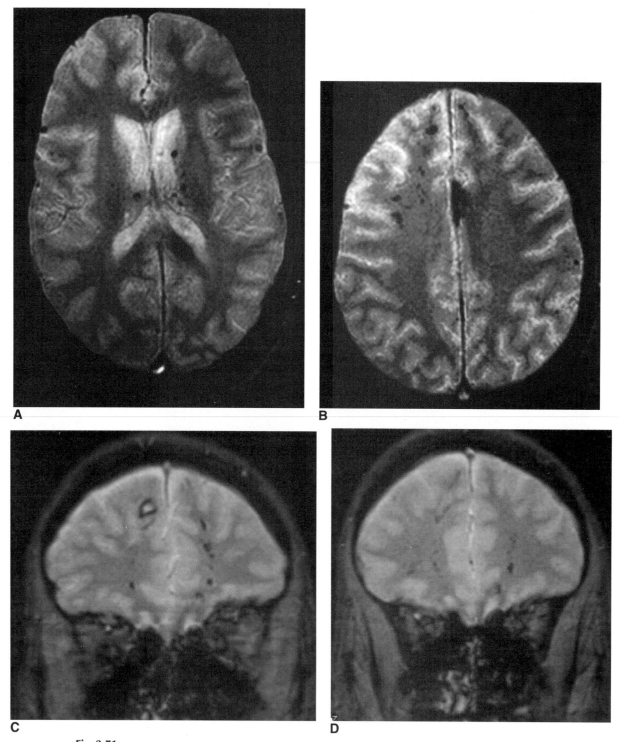

A

B

C

D

Fig. 2-71
Axonal shearing injury on MRI. Axial (**A** and **B**) and coronal (**C** and **D**) gradient echo images of head trauma patient show multiple diffuse low-signal foci of hemorrhage related to magnetic suscepti-bility effect of intracellular deoxy- and methemoglobin. Most lesions are confined to white matter bands or the gray-white matter junction.

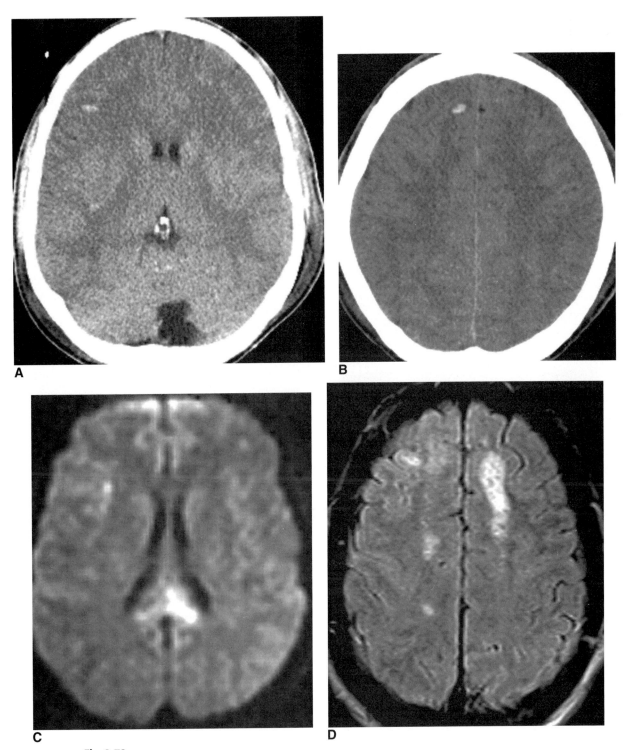

Fig. 2-72
Axonal shearing injury on CT and MRI. **A** and **B**, CT images obtained at two levels in an obtunded blunt trauma patient show a high right frontal punctate hemorrhage and possible hemorrhages (small) in the posterior right frontal and right deep temporal area. A diffusion-weighted (**C**) and FLAIR (**D**) MR sequence confirm the right posterior frontal and vertex lesions, but also demonstrate injury to the splenium and corona radiata bilaterally.

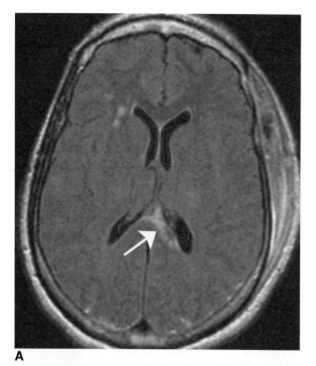

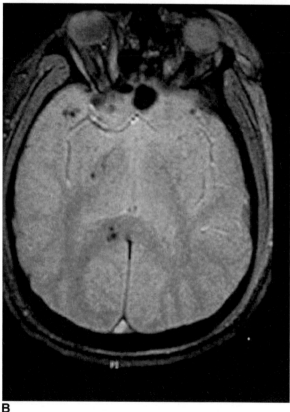

Fig. 2-73
Axonal shearing of brainstem and corpus callosum. **A**, FLAIR image of unconscious blunt trauma victim shows increased signal in the splenium of the corpus callosum (*arrow*), a typical location of deep shearing injury. Punctate injuries are also observed in the white matter lateral to the right caudate head. **B**, Gradient echo MRI of a different patient shows multiple punctate low-signal areas at the gray-white interface, right basal ganglia, and splenium, representing shearing injuries.

cerebral herniation. Elevation of ICP above 20 mm Hg impairs cerebral perfusion, producing secondary ischemia and necrosis.

Diffuse cerebral swelling is recognized on CT by obliteration of the CSF spaces of the sulci, loss of the basal cisterns, and, if severe, by compression and effacement of the lateral ventricles (Figs. 2-74 to 2-77; see also Figs. 2-35, 2-37, 2-41 and 2-42). In some patients the perimesencephalic cistern is also effaced, though this may be secondary to cerebral herniation rather than a direct result of swelling of the midbrain.

True brain edema can have a variety of causes, including blunt head trauma, and leads to an accumulation of interstitial water within the brain. The increased water content reduces the specific gravity of the cerebral tissue, leading to decreased CT attenuation. Typically, the edema collects within the white matter tracts and is caused by disruption of the blood-brain barrier associated with brain injury, that is, "vasogenic edema." Areas of white matter cerebral edema may be recognized as decreased attenuation of the white matter and local effacement of sulci (see Figs. 2-74 to 2-77).

Conversely, in hyperemic edema, CT attenuation values of brain increase, rather than decrease.[82,83] An increase would be anticipated if the brain contained more blood than normal. Bruce and coauthors[82] have suggested that this hyperemic swelling is the most common form of "malignant brain edema" and may be observed in more than 40% of children with major head injury. Bruce et al.[82] observed that patients with hyperemic edema have a higher mortality, a lower admission GCS, and a higher incidence of other associated brain injuries when compared with those without hyperemic edema.

Intraventricular Hemorrhage in Trauma

Posttraumatic intraventricular hemorrhage (IVH) is an uncommon phenomenon occurring in 3% to 8% of patients with major blunt head trauma, whether as an isolated process or in association with other lesions[84] (Fig. 2-78; see also Figs. 2-36 and 2-75). As an isolated process, IVH may occur from bleeding from the choroid plexus, a very vascular and somewhat friable structure. Inertial movements of the large mass of the choroid plexus glomus, within the open space of the ventricular trigone, may lead to small tears and intraventricular bleeding. Trigonal hemorrhage may layer in the dependent portions of the occipital (posterior) horns of the lateral ventricles. Intraventricular blood may accumulate from a parenchymal hematoma that decompresses itself through the ependyma and into the lumen (Fig. 2-79). This occurrence is most common in spontaneous basal ganglia and thalamic hemorrhages. Blood may also reflux into the ventricular system from the extraventricular

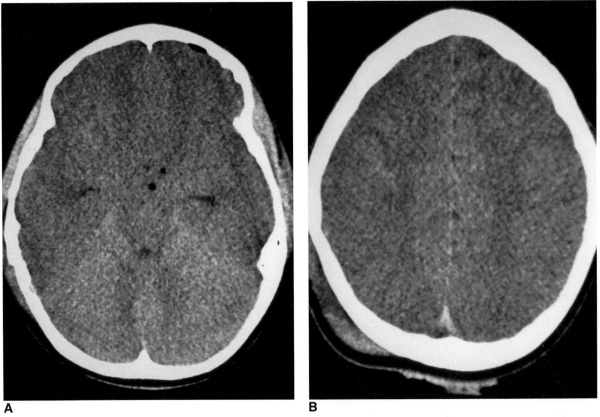

Fig. 2-74
Diffuse cerebral edema. **A**, CT of head trauma victim demonstrates diffuse loss of gray-white density difference and loss of the sulci and basal cisterns due to diffuse swelling. The tentorium appears slightly denser than usual because of the low attenuation of the adjacent brain. **B**, A more rostral image shows a scalp contusion over the right parietal region. The left-sided gray-white interface appears somewhat better preserved than the right, indicating more severe injury on the right.

subarachnoid space. Bleeding from a tear in the corpus callosum in patients with shearing injury may also produce IVH.

Brain Herniation—Diagnosis and Complications

Both CT and MRI are sensitive and specific in demonstrating brain herniation. Under the pressure of a mass lesion, the brain may herniate around the rigid dural folds that divide the cranial cavity, the cortex may herniate through a posttraumatic or postsurgical defect, or the medulla and cerebellar tonsils may herniate downward through the foramen magnum. The sequence of events occurring during herniation depends on the exact location of the mass and its resultant vector of force applied to the brain. Generally, in the context of trauma, most masses are supratentorial and produce lateral (subfalcine) and/or downward (transtentorial) herniation. Either type of herniation can result from either extraaxial

or intraaxial masses, and both these types of herniation may occur simultaneously.

Most well-known clinical sequelae of herniation occur in relation to medial temporal (uncal) herniation (see Figs. 2-31 and 2-33) and central downward (rostral-caudal) herniation (see Figs. 2-74, 2-75 and 2-77). The effects of herniation on the upper brainstem are often described as "lateral" when associated with uncal herniation and "central" when they occur without temporal lobe shift.[85] The ipsilateral third cranial nerve (oculomotor) and the posterior cerebral artery (PCA) may become compressed between the cerebral peduncle and the herniating uncus, producing dilatation of the ipsilateral pupil as a result of loss of parasympathetic innervation. Uncal herniation syndrome (lateral tentorial shift) may produce a sequence of neurologic events, such as ipsilateral paralysis of the oculomotor nerve, leading to ptosis, mydriasis, and ophthalmoplegia; altered consciousness; ipsilateral or bilateral long tract signs; and ultimately, decerebrate posturing.[85] If severe lateral displacement of

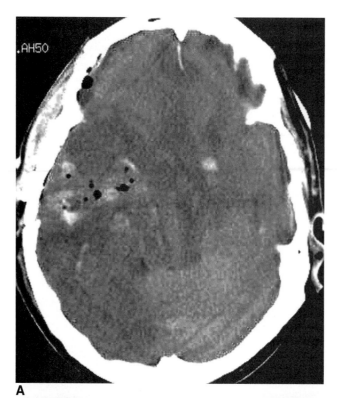

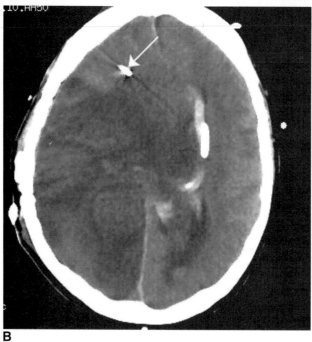

Fig. 2-75
Postsurgical cerebral edema. **A** and **B**, Follow-up of patient with right subdural and right temporal hematoma. Note marked edema of right hemisphere and upper brainstem, producing marked mass effect to the left. Intraventricular blood and enlargement of the left ventricle are due to entrapment. An intraparenchymal intracranial pressure monitor is placed on the right (*arrow*). Some of the edema may be due to infarction in the anterior and posterior cerebral artery territories from marked herniation and flow disruption.

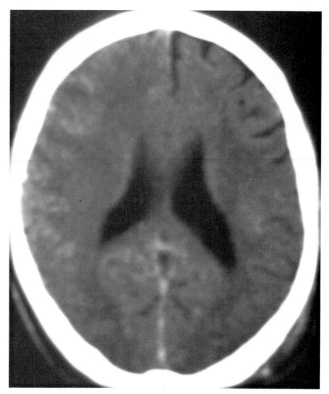

Fig. 2-76
Asymmetric vasogenic white matter edema. CT of blunt head trauma patient shows evidence of right-sided cerebral edema with loss of sulci and thickening of cortical gray matter band as compared with left side.

the midbrain occurs, the contralateral cerebral peduncle may become entrapped against the edge of the opposite leaf of the tentorium, producing corticospinal tract disruption above the level of decussation, and resulting in hemiplegia ipsilateral to both the pupillary dilation and the inciting mass lesion. Pathologically, the indentation of the contralateral cerebral peduncle against the tentorial edge produces an indentation in the lateral aspect of the contralateral midbrain (Kernohan's notch). In the central syndrome, stupor and Cheyne-Stokes respiration (without pupil dilatation) may precede a paralysis of upward and contralateral gaze, ultimately progressing to decerebrate or decorticate rigidity.[85]

The CT and MRI findings that are characteristic of herniation under the falx include slight arching of the falx and distortion of the ipsilateral lateral ventricle (Fig. 2-80; see also Figs. 2-34, 2-36, 2-37, 2-40, 2-43, 2-51, 2-52, 2-55, 2-56, 2-63, 2-75, 2-77, and 2-79). If the mass is anteriorly positioned, the frontal horn of the lateral ventricle may be amputated as it is pushed back by the corpus callosum. This situation occurs when both the frontal horn and ipsilateral corpus callosum are squeezed together through the narrow opening under the

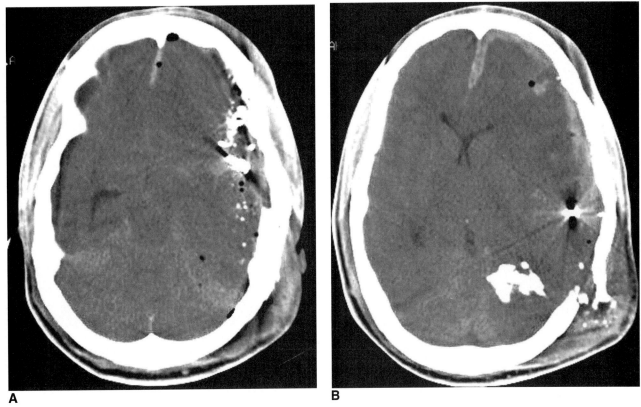

A   B

Fig. 2-77
Diffuse cerebral edema after gunshot to head. **A** and **B**, A bullet entered the left cerebral hemisphere from the left parietal region, causing displacement of calvarial fragments into the left occipital lobe. A SDH tracks along the left convexity into the perifalx subdural space. There is generalized loss of gray-white differentiation, cerebral sulci, and basal cisterns with compression of the lateral ventricles due to diffuse cerebral edema. The patient did not survive.

falx. Similarly, when the mass lesion is posterior and/or high, the trigone will be compressed and the glomus of the choroid will move anteriorly and medially as it squeezes around the posterior edge of the falx.

When the mass is extraaxial in the middle cranial fossa or in the temporal lobe itself, medial displacement of that lobe will displace the midbrain (and often the pons) laterally across the circummesencephalic cistern (see Fig. 2-31). This occurrence usually precedes the downward herniation of the uncus into the ambient or suprasellar cistern. Osborn[86] reported that the earliest CT sign of actual downward herniation was blunting of the ipsilateral suprasellar cistern as the herniating temporal lobe (uncus) is caudally displaced (see Fig. 2-33). However, depending on the location of the mass, lateral displacement of the hemisphere and brainstem may precede downward herniation, which can be recognized by widening of the perimesencephalic cistern *ipsilateral* to the mass lesion (see Fig. 2-80). Even in middle cranial fossa lesions, some degree of lateral herniation invari-

ably accompanies the caudal herniation of the temporal lobe, since the uncus must move medially to get over the ridge of the tentorium. More extensive mass effect may cause further lateral movement of the brainstem, which may enlarge the ipsilateral pontine cistern (see Fig. 2-80).

Displacement and distortion of the midbrain will kink or obstruct the cerebral aqueduct. CSF volume will then increase, dilating the third and the *contralateral* ventricle and adding to the supratentorial mass effect and increasing herniation. The ipsilateral ventricle is usually prevented from enlarging because it has already been effaced by pressure from the original mass lesion. With further herniation, the uncus and the hippocampus obliterate the interpeduncular and suprasellar cisterns and may cause anteroposterior elongation of the brainstem (Figs. 2-81 and 2-82). The PCA, which travels in the mesencephalic cistern, may be caught between the herniating brain tissue and the midbrain or compressed against the edge of the tentorium. This usually does not cause a

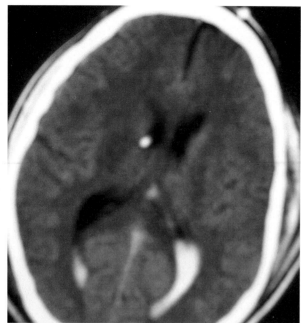

Fig. 2-78
Intraventricular hemorrhage. Blood layering dependently in the occipital horns following blunt trauma over left hemicranium. An intraventricular catheter terminates in the frontal horn of the right lateral ventricle.

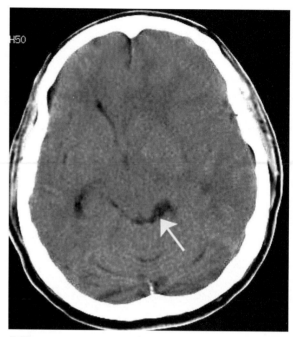

Fig. 2-80
Widened cistern ipsilateral to mass effect. Cerebral edema in the left hemisphere produces left to right shift of the brain. The movement of the brain also displaces the brainstem in the same direction, producing widening of the quadrigeminal cistern (*arrow*) ipsilateral to the displacing mass.

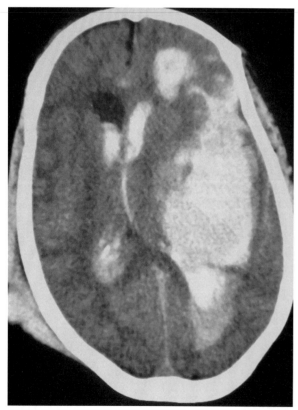

Fig. 2-79
Decompression of hematoma through lateral ventricle. A large post-traumatic intracerebral hematoma occurring after blunt trauma to the right hemicranium extends to and partially decompresses into the ventricular system. There is marked subfalcine herniation.

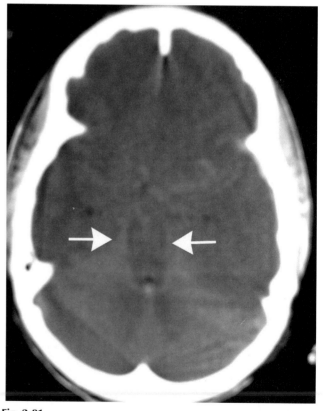

Fig. 2-81
Brainstem compression. Bilateral transtentorial herniation produces bilateral compression of the brainstem (*arrows*) with distortion of its shape and elongation in the anteroposterior direction.

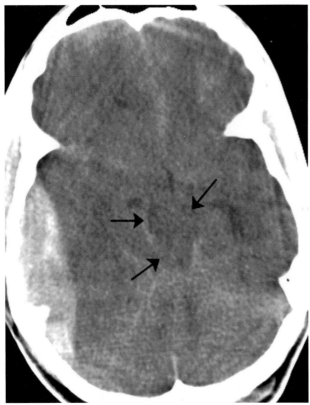

Fig. 2-82
Compression of the brainstem due to herniation. CT shows a right temporal EDH and diffuse edema, producing combined transtentorial and uncal herniation. The brainstem (*arrows*) is compressed bilaterally and elongated in the AP dimension.

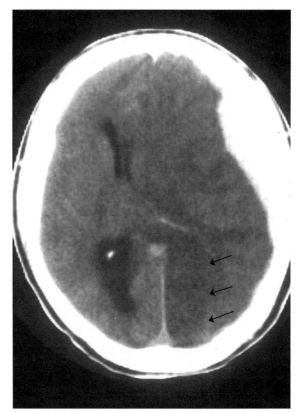

Fig. 2-83
Infarction resulting from transfalcine herniation. A large left SDH with central bulge produces marked left to right mass effect. Low attenuation in the left posterior cerebral artery distribution (*arrows*) indicates ischemia or infarction due to vascular supply compression.

complete occlusion, but it often limits flow sufficiently to produce ischemia and resultant infarction in the PCA distribution. PCA infarcts (see below) from herniation may be bilateral when severe herniation compresses both PCAs. The most common cause of hemorrhagic infarction in the occipital lobe is PCA compression from herniation (Fig. 2-83). Like hydrocephalus, swelling of the brain produced by the secondary infarction only serves to aggravate the process and produce further herniation. Rarely, hemorrhage into the posterior fossa can produce upward herniation of the brainstem, occluding the fourth ventricle (Fig. 2-84).

Traumatic Brainstem Hemorrhage/Contusion

Traumatic brainstem hemorrhage (TBH) after closed head trauma is an uncommon injury occurring in 0.75% to 3.6% of all patients admitted to emergency centers.[87-93] Clinically, TBH typically results in coma, decerebrate posturing, and autonomic nervous system dysfunction.[90] In general, TBH almost uniformly has been associated with a dismal clinical prognosis (31% to 45% of patients have concurrent supratentorial lesions) and a mortality rate of 83%; up to 50% of survivors remain in a persistent vegetative state.[90-92] Studies performed at the UMSTC indicate that the prognosis of TBH may not be as dismal as previously thought and often depends on the mechanism of the TBH[93] (see below).

Primary TBH is the result of direct mechanical distortion of the brainstem occurring during impact, whereas secondary TBH develops sometime after the initial injury and results from diffuse cerebral edema, hypoxia, posttraumatic vasospasm, and transtentorial herniation.[93-101] These secondary brainstem hemorrhages resulting from herniation may occur within 30 minutes of initial injury and thus may be difficult to distinguish from primary mechanical injury.[98]

A variety of mechanisms have been postulated to account for acute primary TBH, such as direct impact of the brainstem against the edge of the rigid tentorium, shear stresses created by rotational acceleration and deceleration associated with diffuse axonal disruption, tearing at the pontomedullary junction due to hyperdistraction, and avulsion of penetrating brainstem arteries due to craniocaudal displacement of the brainstem.[93,94,96-103]

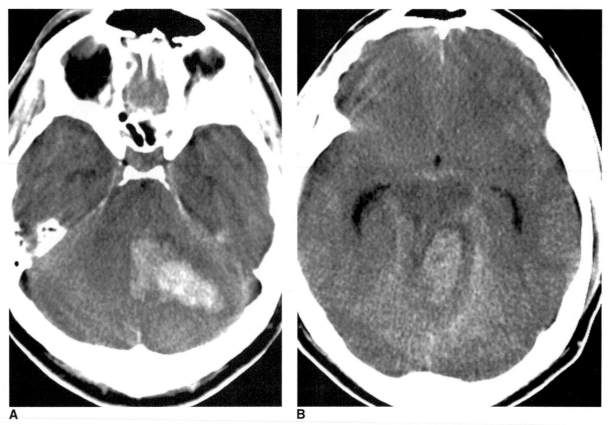

A   B

Fig. 2-84
Upward transtentorial herniation. **A,** CT of patient with cerebellar hematoma resulting from aneurysm rupture exerting mass effect on the brainstem. **B,** CT image at a rostral level showing lifting of brainstem through incisura and obliteration of mesencephalic cisterns. Obstructive hydrocephalus is indicated by temporal tip dilation.

Both CT and MRI are useful in the detection of both primary and secondary brainstem injuries.* On CT, brainstem lesions may appear as focal areas of decreased attenuation representing edema, as areas of focal high density representing hemorrhage, or as a mixture of both (Figs. 2-85 to 2-88). CT is principally hampered in the demonstration of brainstem lesions by the presence of artifacts arising from the osseous structures surrounding the brainstem. The thick (8 mm to 10 mm) axial sections acquired on the standard emergency cranial CT may miss these lesions because of volume averaging. Subtle areas of brainstem edema without significant hemorrhage may be below the contrast resolution of CT. If brainstem pathology is sought following head injury, 3 mm to 5 mm sections of the brainstem should be acquired with a field of view targeted to the brainstem. Alternatively, narrow collimation slices through the posterior fossa can be fused to improve the signal-to-noise ratio. Patient motion

contributes significantly to artifacts in the posterior fossa and should be limited as much as possible.

MRI has distinct advantages over CT for imaging the brainstem. MRI is not hampered by bone-creating artifact and has greater contrast resolution than CT, particularly for small and nonhemorrhagic lesions (Figs. 2-89 to 2-91). In our experience, and that of others, MRI is far more sensitive in detecting brainstem lesions than is CT, particularly in the subacute and chronic posttrauma setting.[14,15,17,104,106-108]

At the UMSTC, in a 5-year retrospective review of 45 patients with TBH,[93] patients were divided into different groups based on the location of their hemorrhage. Type I hemorrhage, occurring in the midline of the rostral brainstem posterior to the interpeduncular cistern, was the most common type of TBH, seen in 31 (69%) of the patients (see Figs. 2-85 and 2-86). Eight (18%) patients had type II hemorrhages, seen in a variety of locations within the brainstem, and six (13%) patients had type III brainstem hemorrhage associated with transtentorial herniation and brainstem compression (see Fig. 2-87).

---

*References 14, 15, 17, 87-89, 93, 99, 102-108.

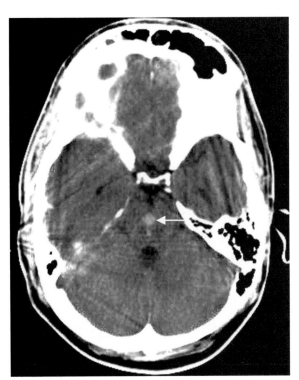

Fig. 2-85
Acute traumatic brainstem hemorrhage. CT image of an obtunded man after blunt head trauma shows a focal hemorrhage in the midline of the rostral brainstem posterior to the interpeduncular cistern (*arrow*).

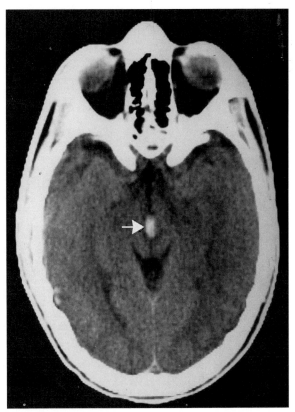

Fig. 2-86
Acute traumatic brainstem hemorrhage. CT in another patient also reveals linear midline hemorrhage in the rostral midbrain (*arrow*) posterior to the interpeduncular cistern. It is postulated that such hemorrhage occurs because of sudden caudal displacement of the brainstem and tearing of perforating anterior midbrain vessels that are tethered to the fixed carotid arteries.

Survival was 71% in type I injuries, 88% in type II, and 0% in type III. Patients with type I TBH frequently (77%) had CT evidence of either frontal or occipital impact sites. Experimental studies in canines have demonstrated that sudden craniocaudal displacement of the brain produces a hemorrhagic lesion in the same location as the type I injury seen in our patients.[93] Severing of the vascular connections between the carotid and basilar arteries in the canine model led to a statistically significant decrease in brainstem hemorrhage. Thus, it is postulated that the "tethering" of the basilar artery to the fixed carotid arteries produces stretching and distortion of the penetrating anterior brainstem vessels during cranial or caudal displacement of the brain[93, 101-103] (Fig. 2-92).

TBH can result from shearing injuries occurring during acceleration and deceleration. In the brainstem, these lesions are discrete, often hemorrhagic, and are typically demonstrated in the dorsolateral quadrant of the brainstem[87-89,104-108] (see Fig. 2-89). The vector of force required for TBH is somewhat distinct from the mechanism required to produce shearing injury. In the UMSTC experience only 22% of our patients with type I injuries (anterior rostral midbrain) had other CT evidence of diffuse axonal shearing.[93] Experimental studies in animal models suggest that animals subjected to a sagittal (cran-

iocaudal) inertial force had limited diffuse axonal shearing with good recovery, while those subjected to a coronal plane acceleration had typical DAI.[66] Recent studies have confirmed that ventral and superficial dorsal brainstem hemorrhages have a much better prognosis than deep dorsal bleeds.[103] Thus, TBH can occur without accompanying DAI, depending on the primary vector of force applied to the cranium.

Secondary TBH lesions (Duret hemorrhages) represent areas of hemorrhagic infarction due to compression, distortion, and disruption of the vascular supply to the caudal mesencephalon, and rostral pons due to devastating supratentorial injury and herniation with subsequent reperfusion.[94-97] Typically these lesions appear in the superior pontine or pontomesencephalic junction region and portend a dismal prognosis (see Fig. 2-87).

We have observed several patients with isolated contusions of the dorsal rostral brainstem by MRI without associated supratentorial injury and believe that these injuries may result from impaction of the dorsolateral

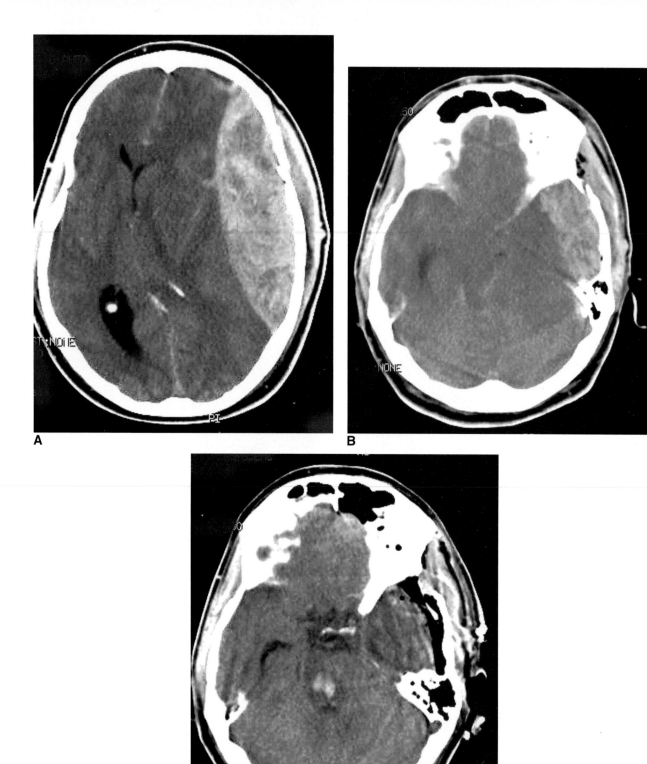

Fig. 2-87
Duret hemorrhage of the brainstem. **A**, Admission CT shows an extensive EDH with marked sub-falcine herniation. **B**, There is marked transtentorial herniation with obliteration of the bisal cisterns and distortion of the brainstem. **C**, Areas of hemorrhage are seen in the pontine portion of the brainstem. This appearance is usually seen in the late stage of transtentorial herniation and suggests non-survivability. The mechanism is debated and includes venous outflow obstruction from increased pressure on draining veins with subsequent parenchymal hemorrhage or reperfusion of arteries after initial occlusion and pontine infarction.

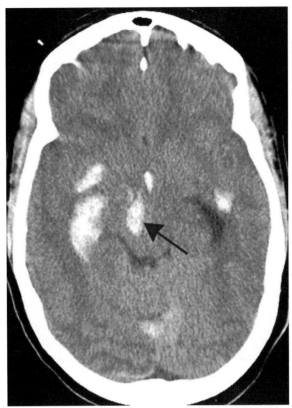

Fig. 2-88
CT of brainstem hemorrhage. Axial image shows focal hematoma of the right side of rostral midbrain (*arrow*) and deep medial temporal hematomas. Blood is also seen along the tentorium and in the third ventricle. Left temporal horn dilation indicates developing hydrocephalus.

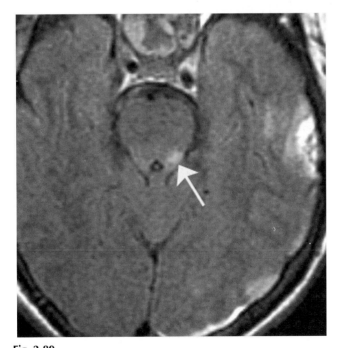

Fig. 2-89
MRI of brainstem contusion. T1-weighted sequence in trauma patient shows dorsal brainstem hemorrhage (*arrow*), left temporal cortical contusion, and thin occipital SDH.

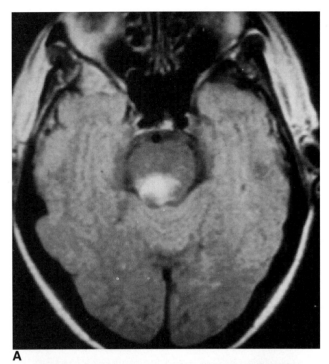

A

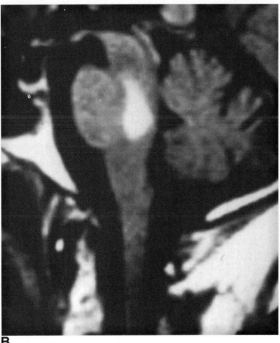

B

Fig. 2-90
MRI of brainstem hematoma. Axial (**A**) and sagittal (**B**) image of obtunded trauma patient reveals hematoma in the brainstem posterior to the pons.

brainstem against the tentorial edge created by inertial displacement of the brainstem.

Traumatic Pneumocephalus

Posttraumatic pneumocephalus is significant as an indicator of an abnormal communication between the

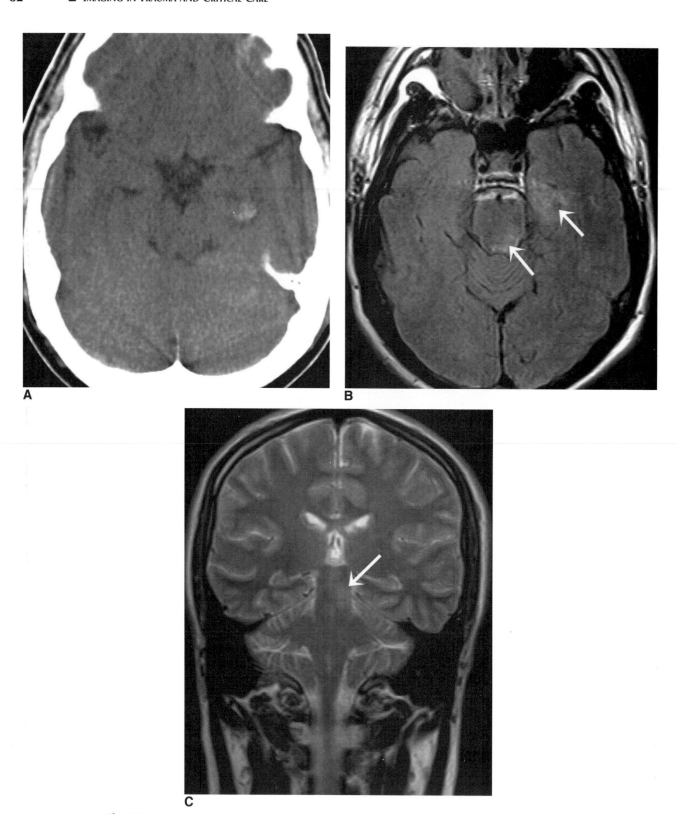

Fig. 2-91
MRI versus CT for brainstem contusion. **A,** CT shows deep left medial temporal contusion but no indication of brainstem injury. Axial FLAIR (**B**) and (**C**) coronal T2-weighted fast spin-echo sequences clearly demarcate abnormal increased signal (*arrows*) consistent with predominantly nonhemorrhagic contusion of dorsal and lateral left midbrain as well as left medial temporal contusion.

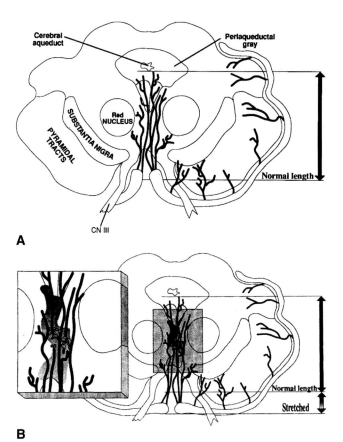

Fig. 2-92
Mechanism of brainstem hemorrhage. Proposed mechanism of midline anterior brainstem hemorrhage. **A,** Diagram demonstrates the normal anatomy of the rostral brainstem with penetrating vessels from the proximal posterior cerebral arteries supplying the brainstem. **B,** This diagram depicts stretching of the anterior brainstem perforating vessels as the brainstem is caudally displaced from frontal impact. The position of the basilar and posterior cerebral arteries is fixed by their attachment to the carotid arteries.

intracranial and extracranial spaces. Trauma to the head and face accounts for about 75% of cases of pneumocephalus after trauma, with the remainder due to postsurgical causes. The recognition of pneumocephalus by radiography or CT is important to indicate the presence of a basilar skull fracture and the potential complications of meningitis, cranial nerve injury, CSF otorrhea and rhinorrhea, or (rarely) tension aerocele (see below). CT is more sensitive in detection of pneumocephalus, with as little as 0.5 ml visualized, whereas skull radiographs detect as little as 2 ml.[5] Intracranial air has some predilection for localization in particular spaces, depending on the site of fracture. After fractures of the posterior ethmoid or sphenoid sinus roofs, air is likely to accumulate in the subarachnoid space of the basal cisterns because of the close apposition of the dura and arachnoid and the patency of the basal cisterns (Figs. 2-93 to 2-95). Fractures of the anterior ethmoidal and frontal sinuses

tend to introduce air into the subdural space because of the close adherence of the arachnoid to the brain over the frontal lobes and the thin dura, which is closely applied to the inner table (see Fig. 2-95).

After evacuation of an SDH, air frequently replaces the evacuated blood. On occasion, a larger volume of air than the original volume of blood replaced may be introduced, producing a component of mass effect (tension pneumocephalus)[58] (see Fig. 2-57). Ishiwata et al.[58] described five patients with subdural tension pneumocephalus after surgery for chronic SDH. They described posterior displacement of the frontal poles and widening of the anterior interhemispheric fissure as CT evidence of tension pneumocephalus ("Mt. Fuji sign"). In addition, they noted that numerous small air bubbles entered the basal cisterns, presumably because of a tear in the arachnoid and the high pressure of the subdural air collection. All five patients described by Ishiwata et al.[58] exhibited neurologic improvement after evacuation of the subdural air that produced the Mt. Fuji sign. In our experience, not all patients exhibiting this CT sign demonstrate evidence of neurologic sequelae; they may be followed without specific treatment if warranted by neurologic status. Goldmann[10] has reported the development of pneumocephalus as a consequence of barotrauma during scuba diving.

It is important to follow the quantity and duration of pneumocephalus on serial CT scans, particularly when associated with basilar skull fractures. Typically, pneumocephalus resolves over several days after injury. The persistence or recurrence of pneumocephalus after surgical repair of lacerated dura indicates a dural leak. Alternatively, the persistence of pneumocephalus after trauma may indicate development of posttraumatic brain infection[37] (see below). The presence of air within an extraaxial hematoma indicates an open skull fracture and is more typically seen with EDHs (Figs. 2-96 and 2-97; see also Fig. 2-32).

Role of MRI in Craniocerebral Trauma

Several studies have evaluated the role of MRI in the assessment of patients with craniocerebral trauma.[14-17,103,104,106-108] MRI has been shown to be more sensitive than CT, particularly in the subacute period, at demonstrating axonal shearing injuries, hemorrhagic and mainly nonhemorrhagic contusions, SDHs, and brainstem injuries.[14-17,103,104,106-108] The appearance of hemorrhage by MRI depends principally on the time after trauma at which the scan is performed and to some extent of the magnetic field strength. At a 1.5 Tesla field strength, acute hemorrhage (within 24 to 48 hours of injury) appears isointense to gray matter on T1-weighted sequences (short TR, short TE) and markedly hypointense on T2-weighted images (long TR, long TE)

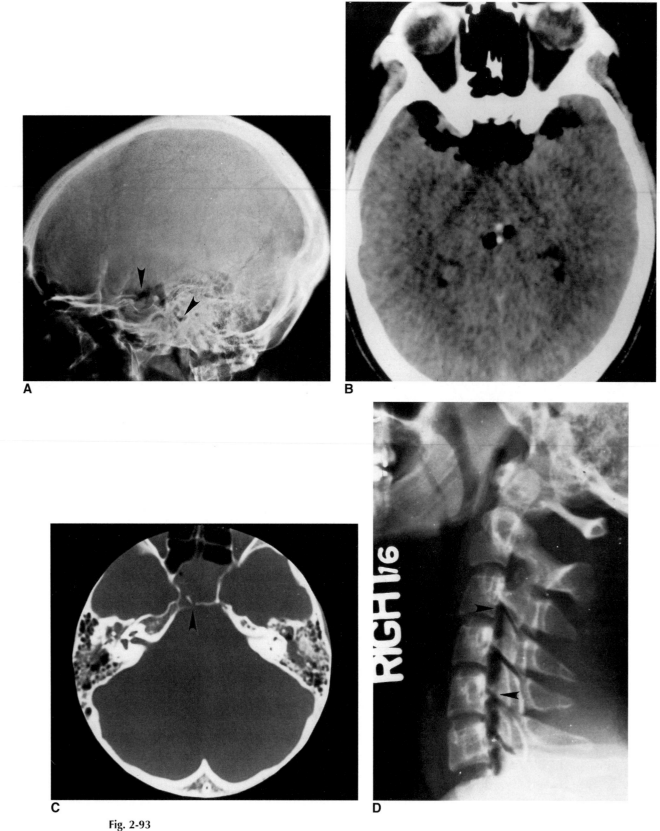

Fig. 2-93
Traumatic pneumocephalus. **A**, Lateral skull radiograph demonstrates air in the basal cisterns (*arrowheads*) around the pituitary fossa and clivus. **B**, Axial CT image of the same patient shows subarachnoid air in the basal cisterns (suprasellar). **C**, Image photographed in bone windows displays a fracture of the posterior sphenoid sinus (*arrowhead*) and blood in both mastoid sinuses (bilateral longitudinal petrous temporal fractures seen on other images). **D**, Horizontal lateral cervical radiograph demonstrates tracking of subarachnoid air into the cervical region (pneumorrhachis).

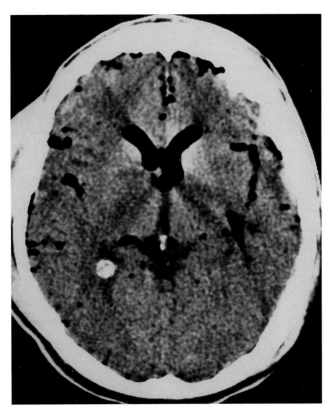

Fig. 2-94
Posttraumatic pneumocephalus. CT image of a 52-year-old man who sustained a skull base fracture reveals diffuse subarachnoid and intraventricular air.

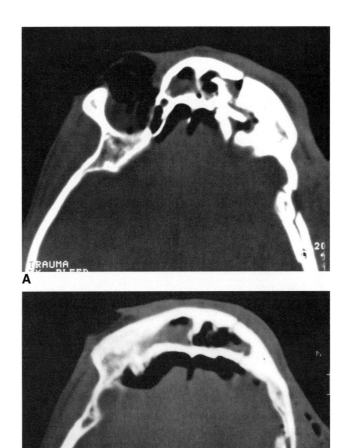

Fig. 2-95
Subdural pneumocephalus. **A** and **B**, CT images obtained after a frontal impact reveal fractures through the left anterior and posterior frontal sinus. Air has collected in the frontal subdural space, indicating a dural laceration.

due to increased magnetic susceptibility of intracellular deoxyhemoglobin.[59,60] In the subacute period, days to weeks after trauma, T1-weighted images are effective at demonstrating hemorrhage as regions of high signal intensity due to the combined effects of paramagnetic intracellular methemoglobin and cell lysis and watery dilution by resorption of free methemoglobin[59,60] (see Figs. 2-6, 2-7, 2-53, 2-58, 2-59, 2-66, and 2-89 to 2-91). T1-weighted hyperintensity appears earliest in the periphery of a hematoma and then gradually fills into the central portions of the hematoma. T2-weighted images show hemorrhage as regions of low- or high-signal intensity depending on the age and chemical state of hemoglobin (Fig. 2-98; see also Figs. 2-6 and 2-59). Edema appears as regions of increased signal strength on T2-weighted sequences, and hemosiderin deposits around subacute to chronic hematomas appear as regions of decreased signal intensity on T2-weighted images and due to selective T2 relaxation and also are low signal on gradient echo sequences due to increased magnetic susceptibility[59,60] (Figs. 2-99 and 2-100; see also Figs. 2-1, 2-6, 2-8, 2-71, 2-73, and 2-98).

Because of its higher contrast resolution, MRI can detect contusions, particularly when nonhemorrhagic,

better than CT[17] (see Figs. 2-6, 2-8 and 2-98). This attribute is particularly important in identifying white matter contusions that accompany axonal shearing and brainstem contusions (see Figs. 2-8, 2-71, 2-73, 2-89 and 2-91). The ability of MRI to image the head in any axis improves the sensitivity in localization of lesions (see Fig. 2-98). MRI has the advantage of not requiring contrast (which is also seldom used for CT in the acute posttrauma setting). MRI, however, has some significant disadvantages compared with CT in the acute setting. MRI examinations are contraindicated in clinically unstable patients with fluctuating vital signs, in patients who require intensive physiologic monitoring and support, and in patients who are combative and cannot be safely sedated. MRI scans have become much faster, particularly using gradient and fast spin echo sequences, allowing some types of examination to be completed in a few

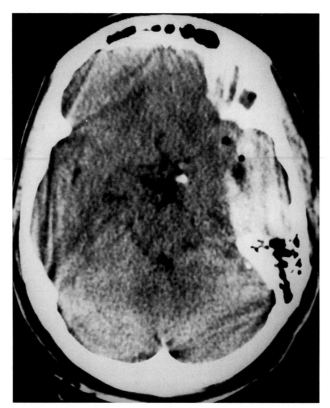

Fig. 2-96
EDH containing air. CT image shows a left temporal EDH containing air (*arrow*) indicating an open skull fracture.

minutes, but they are still more time-consuming than a helical cranial CT examination. CT is more accurate at detecting important findings such as pneumocephalus, SAH, and skull base fractures than is MRI. CT is better and more efficient for rapidly assessing the facial bones, spine, chest, abdomen, and pelvis for evidence of other systemic injury, particularly osseous.

At UMSTC, MRI is not used in the acute trauma setting in favor of rapid CT scanning. In patients whose CT findings do not explain their neurologic condition and in patients with equivocal CT findings, MRI is used selectively to search for brainstem injuries, shearing injuries, or thin extraaxial hematomas. We have not found that MRI findings significantly alter patient management but, more typically, that they confirm CT findings or detect subtle, nonsurgical lesions that better explain the clinical picture. MRI may be used selectively in the rehabilitation phase after head injury—again, when the evolving neurologic picture is not well explained by CT findings.

Cerebral Angiography in Trauma

Cerebral injury after blunt or penetrating trauma may be a consequence of damage to cerebral blood vessels (see section on vascular injury of the head and neck). Such damage may occur extracranially in the cervical region, along the intraosseous course of carotid artery within the skull base, along the course of the vertebral or basilar arteries, or to major intracerebral vessels (see Figs. 2-15, 2-83, and 2-110 to 2-112). Complications of vascular injury include intimal injury with or without thrombus formation and occlusion with cerebral or brainstem infarction (Figs. 2-101 to 2-104; see Figs. 2-16, 2-108, and 2-110 to 2-112), pseudoaneurysms (Figs. 2-105 and 2-106), embolization (see Fig. 2-108), and arteriovenous fistulas (see Figs. 2-15 and 2-109).

Severe hyperextension and rotation, producing intimal dissection and thrombosis, may injure the carotid vessels in the neck.[109,111] Missiles can injure the extracranial cerebral arteries through direct impact or close passage leading to occlusion, intimal injury, or pseudoaneurysm formation (see Figs. 2-105 and 2-106). The carotid arteries are prone to injury because of fractures that traverse their intraosseous course within the skull base[109-112] (see Figs. 2-15 and 2-16), leading to occlusion, intimal damage, and/or carotid-cavernous fistula formation. The vertebral arteries can similarly be injured within the transverse vertebral foramina of the cervical spine because of fracture-dislocations or mechanical overstretching from other blunt force (see Figs. 2-108 and 2-110 to 2-112). Rarely the basilar artery can be similarly injured or entrapped in a clival fracture leading to brainstem infarction[110] (see Fig. 2-101). Recurrent hematoma formation after penetrating injury to the cerebrum suggests pseudoaneurysm formation (Fig. 2-107).

Major cerebral vascular injury should be considered whenever the patient's neurologic deficit is not explained by initial CT evaluation, since ischemic changes may not be apparent by noncontrast CT studies obtained soon after the onset of cerebral ischemia or infarction. Injury to both intracranial and extracranial cerebral arteries should be sought. Patients presenting with ischemic symptoms after head injury should be considered for acute angiography. Therapy should be directed toward the management of ischemic complications because of the frequent occurrence of thrombosis and subsequent infarction.

Cerebral vascular injuries, including pseudoaneurysm formation and arteriovenous fistulas, may be managed surgically, if accessible, or by interventional angiographic techniques such as balloon occlusion[112] (Fig. 2-109). Intimal vascular injuries with thrombus formation and potential embolization may be managed by systemic anticoagulation when possible or by selective vascular interruption through surgical or interventional neuroradiologic techniques when adequate collateral blood flow is demonstrable angiographically.[112]

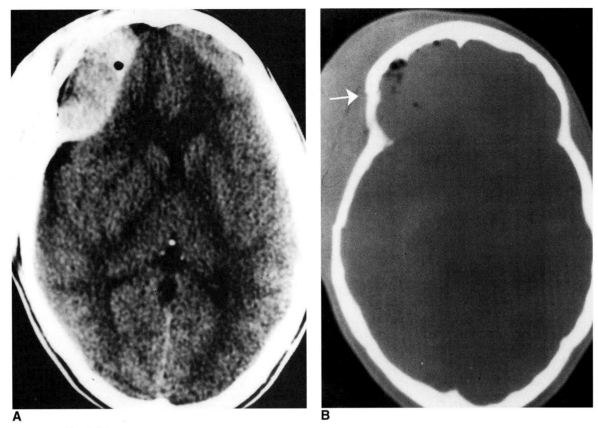

Fig. 2-97
EDH containing air. **A,** Axial CT reveals a right frontal EDH containing a small quantity of air. **B,** Bone windows show the pneumocephalus more readily and the open right frontal fracture (*arrow*).

Complications and Delayed Effects of Craniocerebral Trauma

Delayed Intracranial Hemorrhage. The appearance of delayed intracranial hemorrhage after initial evaluation is well known and can involve extracerebral[41,113-116] and intracerebral hematomas (ICHs).[117-122] The concept of a delayed intracranial bleed is a radiologic one and differs among various authors, but can include any significant new hemorrhage appearing on a subsequent CT/MRI examination that was not manifest on the initial CT/MRI study.[116] Most delayed intracranial hemorrhages are apparent within 2 weeks of injury,[113] with the majority diagnosed within 48 hours after injury.[117]

Reports of the incidence of delayed extracerebral hematoma (DECH) vary, depending on the definition applied, from approximately 5% to 10% of all cases[115] of extracerebral hematoma. Gudeman et al.[120] reported delayed intracerebral hematoma (DICH) in 7.5% of 162 patients with severe closed head injuries, whereas Diaz et al.[122] found posttraumatic DICH in 9 (1.3%) of 656 closed head trauma patients. Lipper et al.[121] reported 10 (8.4%) patients with DICH and 9 (7.5%) patients with DECH among 119 consecutive patients suffering severe head trauma.

A number of possible factors have been cited as contributors to the development of DICH: (1) loss of cerebrovascular autoregulation (vasoparalysis) possibly because of hypoxia and hypercapnia, permitting transmission of intraarterial pressure–damaged capillary beds; (2) loss of a mechanical tamponade effect on injured areas because of surgical, medical, or CSF leak decompression that reduces ICP; (3) vasospasm producing local ischemia and necrosis followed by hemorrhage; (4) posttraumatic hypotension followed by a return to normotensive blood pressure; (5) systemic intravascular coagulopathy and fibrinolysis; (6) venous congestion; (7) delayed rupture of a posttraumatic aneurysm; (8) hemorrhagic infarction; and (9) slow bleeding from a venous source, among others.[113-122]

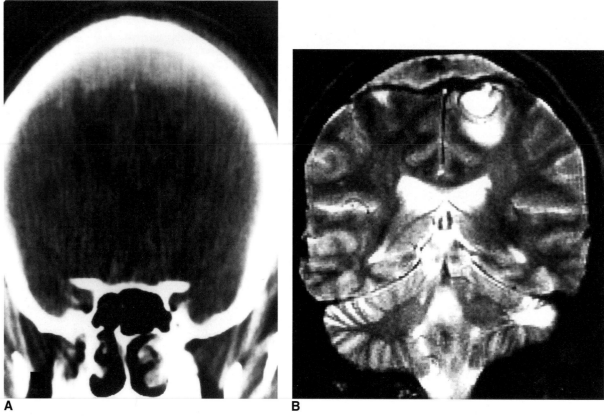

A   B

Fig. 2-98
Vertex EDH—CT and MRI. **A,** Coronal CT image demonstrates a high-density collection at the skull vertex, but its precise localization is unclear. **B,** Coronal T2-weighted MR image reveals the collection of blood to be extradural. The more intense outer rim indicates the paramagnetic effect of extracellular methemoglobin, while the central lower signal portion represents hemoglobin in intact red cells. A hematoma surrounded by a low-signal hemosiderin ring and adjacent cerebral edema was also observed in the left medial parietal lobe.

CT scanning is ideal for detection of DICH from a variety of mechanisms (Figs. 2-113 to 2-115). The appropriate use of delayed CT scanning in the follow-up evaluation of head trauma patients is not uniform. General indications for early repeat cranial CT include the following: (1) a patient undergoing maneuvers to lower ICP, including decompressive surgery, especially in the presence of a skull fracture, signs of bleeding adjacent to a skull fracture, or another cerebral hematoma not included in the original surgical site; (2) a patient who sustains an inexplicable increase in ICP, delayed neurologic deterioration, and/or who fails to improve neurologically or to maintain a persistently elevated ICP after decompressive surgery; (3) a patient who is intubated and paralyzed; and (4) a patient with hypotension after severe head injury, requiring vigorous fluid replacement.[113-122]

Because many DICHs after trauma do not produce immediate clinical deterioration, their development may often be heralded by subtle changes in neurologic status and/or ICP. Yet because prompt treatment often mitigates or remedies the pathologic effects of these delayed hemorrhages, their early recognition is crucial to optimize neurologic outcome.

Posttraumatic Cerebral Infarction. Posttraumatic cerebral infarction (PTCI) is a known complication of craniocerebral trauma and is a frequent form of "secondary injury." A variety of mechanisms may account for this complication, including cerebral vasospasm, direct vascular compression by mass effects, vascular injury, embolization, and systemic hypoperfusion.[123-136] Infarction of the occipital pole after compression of the PCA against the rigid edge of the tentorium by the herniating medial temporal lobe is the most recognized mechanism leading to cerebral infarction[123,125] (Figs. 2-116 and 2-117; see also Fig. 2-83).

A retrospective review of cranial CT scans of 1332 patients admitted over a 40-month period to the UMSTC with blunt-force craniocerebral trauma revealed 25 (1.9%) with PTCI.[136] Infarction was most common in

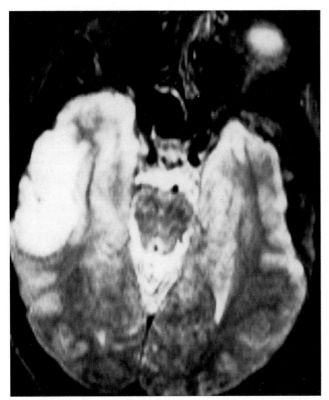

Fig. 2-99
MRI of cerebral contusion. This T2-weighted image shows increased signal in the right temporal lobe due principally to cerebral edema.

the PCA distribution, but infarcts were also relatively common in the anterior and middle cerebral, lenticulostriate/thalamoperforating, and anterior choroidal territories (Fig. 2-118; see also Figs. 2-83, 2-116, and 2-117). In 22 (88%) of 25 patients, infarction resulted from gross mechanical shift of the brain and herniation across the falx and/or tentorium. PTCI in the anterior cerebral artery (ACA) distribution was described by Rothfus et al.[124] They postulated that branches of the ipsilateral callosomarginal artery might be kinked against the free edge of the falx as the medial aspect of the hemisphere herniates across the midline. The extent of infarction would vary depending on how anteriorly the ACA was compressed. Downward displacement of the frontal lobes and impingement of the proximal ACA against the posterior ridge of the body and lesser wing of the sphenoid may produce both proximal and distal ACA infarction (see Fig. 2-117). The anterior choroidal artery may be compressed between the herniating medial temporal lobe and the cerebral peduncle.[123] Infarction due to anterior choroidal compression occurs in the posterior limb of the internal capsule (see Fig. 2-118).

Gross mass effects can produce stretching and attenuation of vessels, such as the fine lenticulostriate and thalamoperforators, and contribute to infarction in the basal

ganglia and thalamus (see Fig. 2-118). The role of vasospasm, which has been angiographically documented in 5% to 57% of patients with craniocerebral trauma[129-133] in producing PTCI, is unknown but can be assumed to be contributory.

Infarction of the cortex and subcortical region can also result from direct compression by overlying masses, such as an extraaxial hematoma.[126,136] Such infarcts extend beyond arterial vascular territories and may be hemorrhagic. These infarcts may result from direct pressure effects, leading to diminished distal arterial perfusion, or may be secondary to local venous drainage compression (Fig. 2-119). PTCI can also result from direct vascular injury involving the intracranial or extracranial cerebral blood supply (see above).

In the series by Mirvis et al.[136] the mortality of patients with craniocerebral trauma complicated by PTCI was 68%, reflecting the severity of injury usually associated with this complication. However, this mortality was not significantly different statistically from a population of patients with head trauma matched for admission GCS score without complicating PTCI, suggesting that aggressive management should not be abandoned even in the presence of PTCI.

Posttraumatic Cerebral Infection. Fortunately, posttraumatic cerebral infection is uncommon in our experience. The recognition of extraaxial empyema (Fig. 2-120), cerebral abscess formation (Fig. 2-121), or cerebritis (Fig. 2-122) is considerably complicated by the presence of similar CT changes associated with trauma and with surgical intervention.

Epidural empyemas are of relatively low CT attenuation, but greater than that of CSF. They typically assume a lentiform shape with focal mass effect and demonstrate enhancement of a thickened adjacent dura following intravenous contrast. Although uncommon in our experience, these collections may be expected to occur adjacent to open fractures, particularly entering the frontal or mastoid sinuses.

Subdural empyemas are crescentic or lentiform and display a CT density equal to or slightly greater than CSF. The medial aspect of the collection is well defined and enhances with intravenous contrast.[36] These collections may exert considerable mass effect and may extend into the interhemispheric fissure. Involvement of the adjacent parenchyma can cause thrombophlebitis with resultant infarction and/or abscess development.[36]

The distinction of cerebritis without cerebral abscess formation from cerebral contusion is difficult. Both lesions appear as regions of diminished CT density involving both gray and white matter; both may exhibit enhancement of the surrounding parenchyma or adjacent dura with intravenous contrast; and both exhibit variable amounts of mass effect. Both cerebral contusions

Text continued on p. 95.

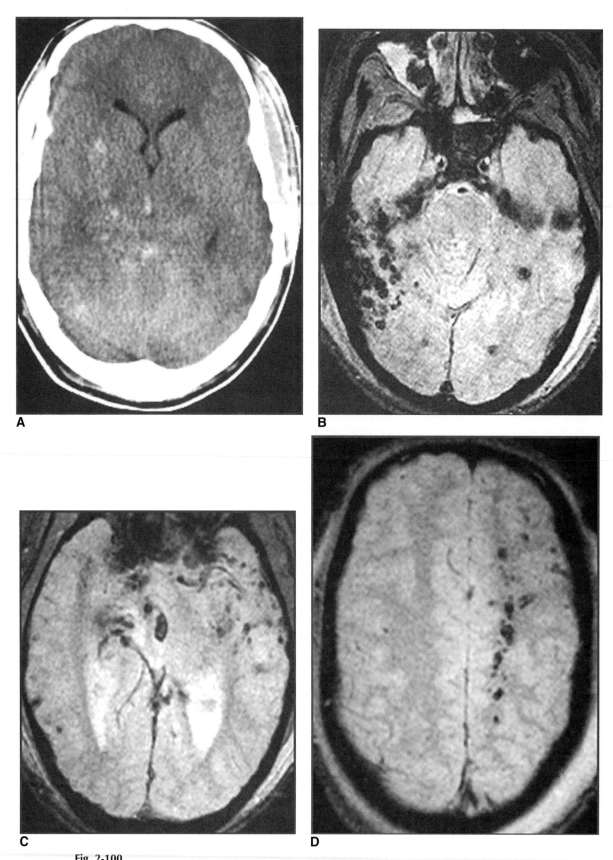

Fig. 2-100
MRI versus CT for DAI. **A**, CT of head trauma victim with Glasgow Coma Score of 3 shows multiple foci of hemorrhage around the right external capsule and basal ganglia in blood in the third ventricle. **B** to **D**, Gradient-echo images at three levels reveal innumerable discrete foci of hemorrhage indicative of axonal shearing. The GRE sequence is particularly sensitive to blood due to magnetic susceptibility effects of hemoglobin.

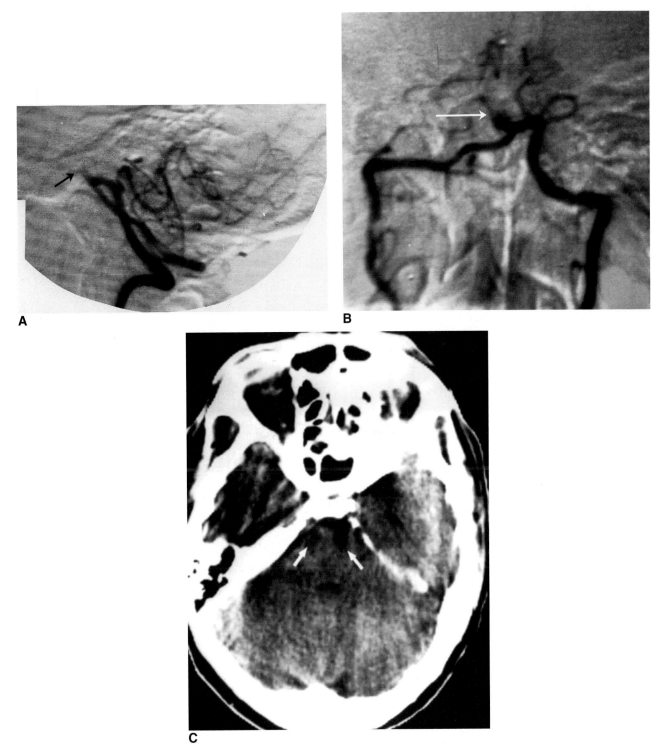

Fig. 2-101
Acute traumatic basilar artery thrombosis—CT and arteriography. Lateral (**A**) and AP (**B**) vertebral angiograms from a young woman with complete motor paralysis reveal occlusion of the proximal basilar artery (*arrow*). **C**, CT image shows bilateral foci of decreased density in the anterior pons (*arrows*), explaining the patient's "locked -in" neurologic picture.

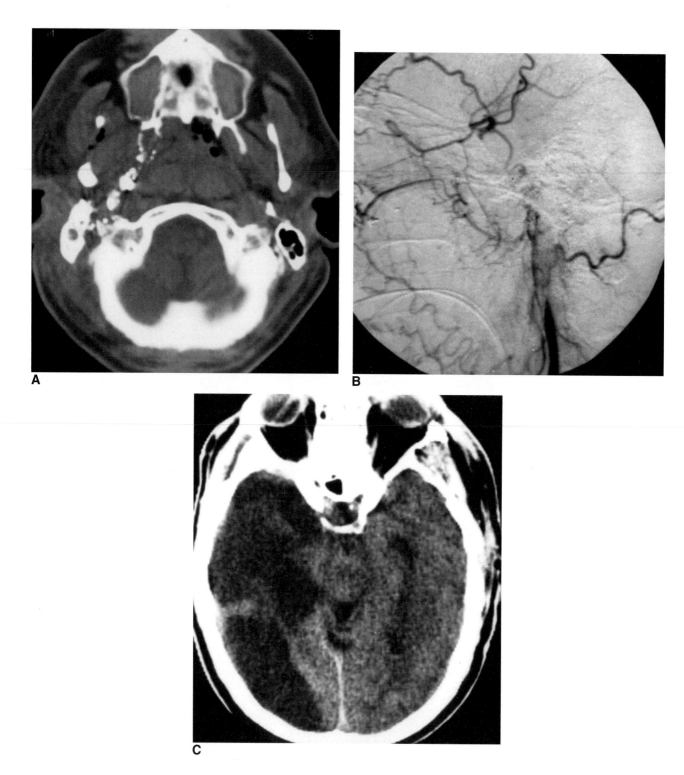

Fig. 2-102
Cervical ballistic injury leading to cerebral infarction. **A**, CT image shows a bullet path through the region of the right carotid sheath. **B**, Lateral cerebral arteriogram shows complete occlusion of the right common carotid artery. **C**, Subsequent cranial CT reveals extensive infarction in the right cerebral hemisphere.

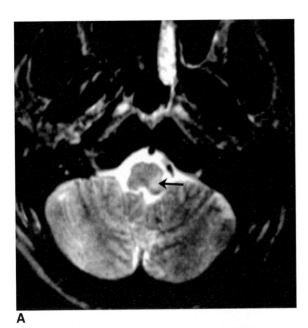

A

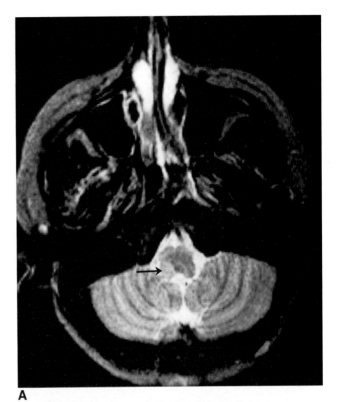

A

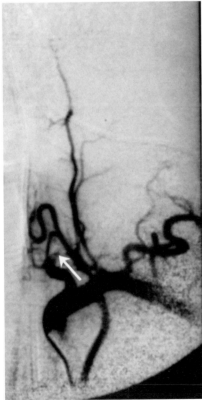

B

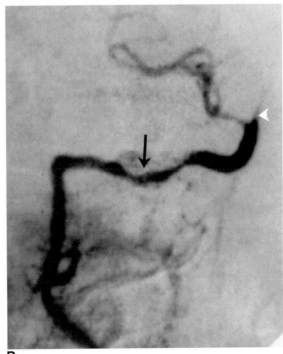

B

Fig. 2-103
Posttraumatic lateral medullary infarct—arteriography and MRI. **A**, T2-weighted image of a 34-year-old man after a motor vehicle collision reveals increased signal in the left lateral medulla (*arrow*) compatible with the clinical presentation of Wallenberg's syndrome. **B**, IA-DSA study shows a traumatic occlusion of the proximal left vertebral artery (*arrow*) producing the infarct.

Fig. 2-104
Posttraumatic brainstem infarction by MRI and arteriography. **A**, T2-weighted (2500/90) image of a 25-year-old woman who developed Wallenberg's syndrome (lateral medullary infarction) after a chiropractic manipulation reveals increased signal (edema) in the right lateral medulla (*arrow*). **B**, Right vertebral IA-DSA demonstrates an intimal dissection along the horizontal segment of the vertebral artery (*arrow*) and occlusion distally (*arrowhead*).

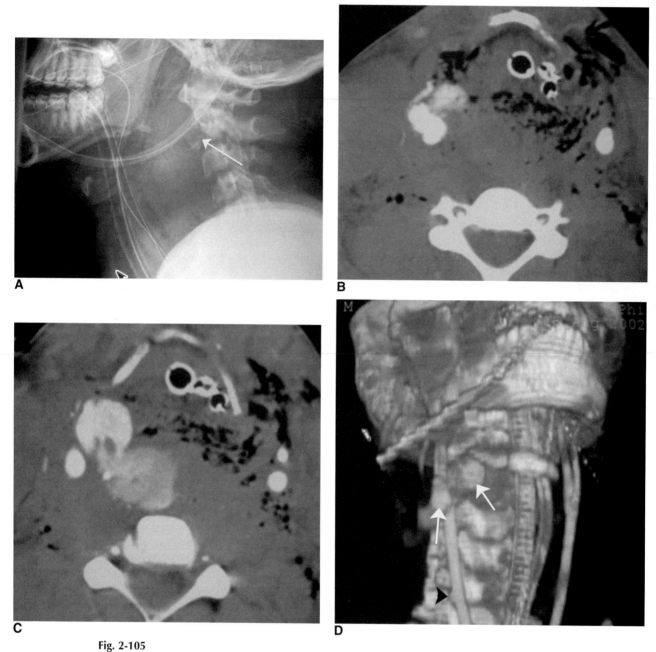

Fig. 2-105
Common carotid artery injury from gunshot wound. **A,** Lateral cervical radiograph of young man with gunshot wound (GSW) through the neck shows marked soft tissue swelling anterior to the vertebral column and a fracture of the anterior C2 body (*arrow*) secondary to ballistic impact. **B,** CT image at level of distal common carotid arteries shows extravasation of contrast from the right common carotid artery, marked surrounding soft tissue swelling (hemorrhage), and deep soft tissue air. **C,** CT image at a more rostral level shows extent of contrast leaking along ballistic tract toward C2 injury. **D,** Volume rendered 4D CT image from frontolateral perspective shows bilobed pseudoaneurysm (*white arrows*) arising from the distal right common carotid artery. A smaller more proximal vascular injury (*black arrowhead*) was confirmed at surgery.

Continued

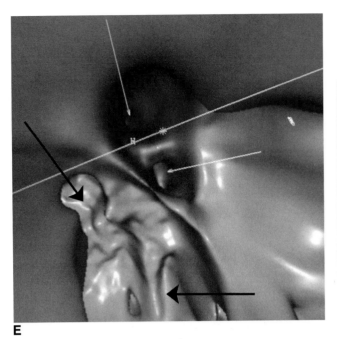

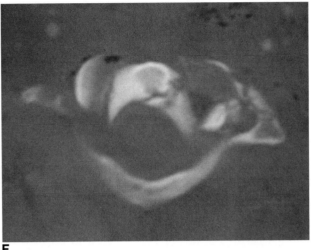

Fig. 2-105, cont'd
E, Endovascular view of injury looking up at the carotid bifurcation (*marked by white arrows*) shows irregular defect in the common carotid wall (*black arrows*). **F**, CT at lower C2 level shows comminuted C2 left body fracture from bullet impact. The left vertebral artery was partially occluded (not shown) and was embolized with coils proximally. The major common carotid lesion was repaired by interposition graft, but the patient suffered a right middle cerebral artery infarction 3 days after surgery.

and cerebritis exhibit the potential for increasing size and edema over a course of several days; however, we have noted a tendency for edema associated with cerebritis to persist and gradually increase after the initial 3 to 5 days after injury. Resolution of mass effect and edema without specific treatment of cerebral infection suggests noninfected contusion as the most likely pathology.

Cerebral abscesses classically are relatively low attenuation masses with a well-formed thick enhancing capsule and surrounding edema (see Fig. 2-121). With liberal use of parenteral antibiotics in the setting of multisystem trauma, this typical appearance seldom evolves completely. In addition, ICHs may lose their high-density blood component after initial trauma and develop enhancing capsules with surrounding edema, therefore mimicking the appearance of a cerebral abscess. We have noted, subjectively, that the cerebral enhancement surrounding a hematoma is less well formed and not as thick as that associated with cerebral abscess and that the edema and mass effect associated with a chronic ICH are less than that associated with an abscess. Serial evaluation of CT findings is useful diagnostically as infected collections tend to display increasing surrounding edema and

mass effect with time, unlike an evolving ICH. MRI may have advantages over CT in characterizing abscesses. In a population of 14 patients *without trauma*, Haimes et al.[137] found that MRI demonstrated concentric zones of varying signal intensity within the abscess cavity in seven patients and, in most, demonstrated a capsule of low signal intensity on long TR scans believed to be associated with paramagnetic T2 shortening caused by the presence of free radical products of phagocytosing macrophages. Use of these observations in distinguishing cerebral abscesses from hemorrhagic posttraumatic lesions, which also display hypointense capsules on T2-weighted sequences, has not been determined. Other CT or MRI findings that may indicate the presence of a cerebral abscess include adjacent satellite lesions and extension of the process into the ventricular system (ventriculitis) or adjacent CSF spaces.

Posttraumatic Cerebral Tension Aerocele. Posttraumatic cerebral tension aerocele is a rare complication of craniocerebral trauma (Fig. 2-123). After an open skull fracture (particularly involving the frontal sinus region), one-way communication may persist between the sinus and the cerebral parenchyma through a torn dura. This one-way

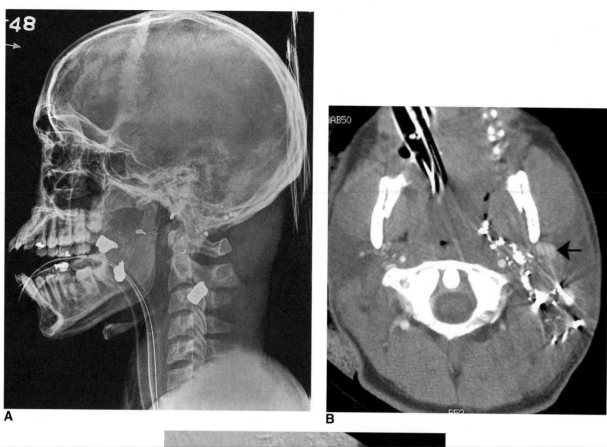

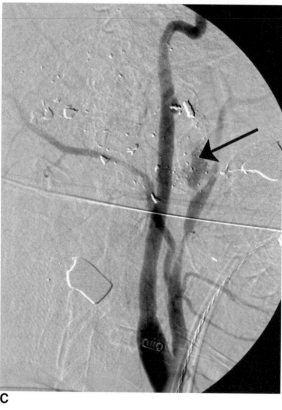

Fig. 2-106
Carotid injury from GSW to neck. **A**, Lateral radiograph of head, neck, and face of GSW victim shows multiple bullets projected over the posterior mandible and upper cervical spine. **B**, An axial CT image at the level of the oral pharynx shows a ballistic tract extending across the left anterior and posterior cervical triangles and crossing the carotid sheath. A blush of contrast extravasation (*arrow*) is seen posterior to the left mandibular angle. **C**, An arteriogram confirms extravasation from the left external carotid artery (*arrow*) and spasm in the proximal portion of the injured branch.

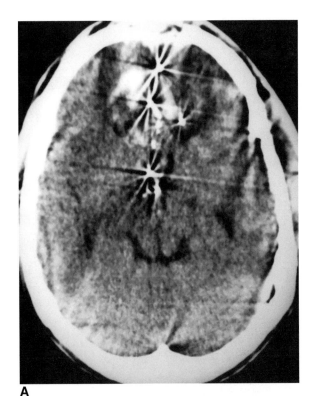

A

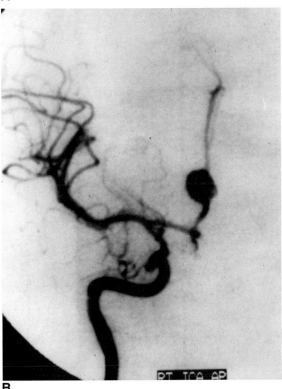

B

Fig. 2-107
Pseudoaneurysm following ballistic injury to the brain. **A,** CT image of a young man after a self-inflicted GSW to the head demonstrates ballistic fragments along the midline and punctate areas of hematoma in both frontal lobes. **B,** Because of persistent recurrence of frontal hemorrhage an arteriogram was performed that revealed a pseudoaneurysm of the anterior cerebral artery that was surgically clipped.

"valve" permits entrance of air from the sinus into the brain but no, or only limited, egress. In this manner, a cavity of air, under tension, develops at the site of communication. The cavity may decompress through the ventricular system and present as a large mass with an air-fluid level. This lesion is typically not seen acutely after trauma, but presents in a delayed fashion, usually weeks after the initial injury. This complication most often results from a complex open frontal sinus fracture with considerable comminution of bone and dural lacerations. To avoid this complication, attention must be paid to the presence of open frontal sinus fractures involving both anterior and posterior walls, complete surgical repair of the dura, and, when indicated, obliteration of the sinus.

Cerebrospinal Fluid Leaks. Acute CSF fistulas occur in 2% to 11.5% of all patients with closed head injury[138] and in 5% to 11% of patients with basilar skull fractures.[139] Rhinorrhea probably occurs after a dural tear and fracture of the ethmoid and/or sphenoid bone or the orbital plate of the frontal bone (Fig. 2-124). It is estimated that unilateral rhinorrhea will accurately predict the site of the dural tear and fracture more than 75% of the time.[140] On the other hand, bilateral rhinorrhea does not predict bilateral leaks. Anosmia accompanying a CSF leak suggests a fracture in the region of the ethmoid roof. Plain skull radiographs may demonstrate the presence of fluid or an air-fluid level within the paranasal sinuses, which may provide an important clue to the site of the fracture.

If the CSF fistula does not close after 72 hours of bed rest and an additional 72 hours of lumbar drainage, an indium[111]–DTPA scan is performed with introduction of the agent into the subarachnoid space.[141] Cotton pledgets are placed in the anterior and posterior roof of the nasal cavity, in the sphenoidal recess, and in the middle meatus in an attempt to localize the site of the leak to the anterior ethmoid and/or cribriform plate or from the posterior ethmoid or sphenoid sinus. Alternatively, CT cisternography using nonionic intrathecal contrast and high-resolution coronal CT can be used to attempt to directly visualize the fistula site.[142]

Otorrhea usually occurs secondary to a fracture in the temporal bone and may present with seventh or eighth nerve palsy. CSF leaks from temporal bone injury may initially appear as rhinorrhea or as both rhinorrhea and otorrhea, since the CSF travels through the eustachian canal into the back of the nasopharynx.[143]

Fractures of the petrous bone are classified in relationship to the long axis of the petrous pyramid (see above) as either longitudinal or transverse.[144] Both types are associated with a similar incidence of CSF otorrhea.[145] In experience at the UMSTC, both otorrhea and rhinorrhea cease spontaneously in the overwhelming majority of

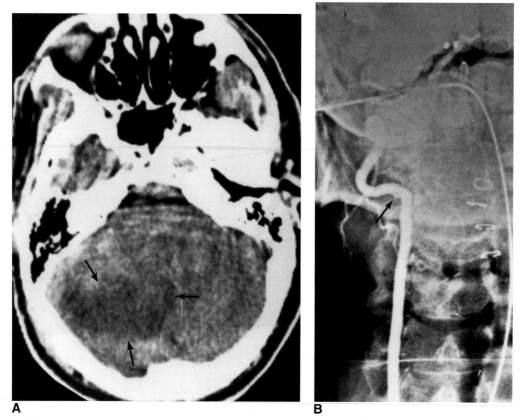

A   B

Fig. 2-108
Vertebral artery injury leading to infarction. **A,** CT study of a 35-year-old man who had sustained a
C2 hangman's fracture 2 days earlier reveals a large low-density area in the right cerebellar hemisphere (*arrows*) producing mass effect on the fourth ventricle. The lesion was believed to be an
acute infarction. **B,** Right vertebral angiogram performed after emergency decompressive suboc-
cipital craniotomy reveals an intimal injury in the vertebral artery (*arrow*) at the site where the vessel crosses the C2 transverse foramen. It was believed that this injury was a nidus for embolization.
(From Mirvis SE, Young JWR, Lim C, Greenberg J: *Radiology* 163:713-717, 1987.)

patients, with an incidence of required surgical repair or
meningitis of less than 1%.

Posttraumatic Cerebral Atrophy. Relatively little literature has been devoted to the development of diffuse
supratentorial cerebral atrophy as a result of blunt craniocerebral trauma. Over the past 6 years at the UMSTC,
approximately 60 patients have developed diffuse supratentorial cerebral atrophy patterns after blunt head
trauma. Such patients may have initial CT evidence of diffuse axonal shearing but, in the majority of cases, show
only focal contusions, hematomas, or no gross lesions
(Figs. 2-125 and 2-126). The patients tend to be young
adults who present with neurologic deficits greater than
predicted based on the extent of cerebral injury observed
by CT. The atrophic pattern is evident as early as 2 weeks
after injury, but is typically very obvious by 6 weeks after
injury. Since this injury is mainly observed in young
adults, it is extremely unlikely that the atrophic pattern

simply represents a return to the patient's baseline cerebral appearance. As expected, these patients are generally
vegetative or suffer severe cognitive deficits.

Other suggested etiologies for diffuse cerebral atrophy
include microscopic axonal disruption (i.e., below the
resolution of CT and perhaps MRI); the effects of
prolonged high pressure ventilatory support leading to
chronically elevated venous pressure, so-called "respirator-
brain"; or additive effects of global hypoxia combined
with parenchymal injury.

CONCLUSION

At this time, CT scanning provides the best initial diagnostic study of the cerebrum after trauma. CT provides a
rapid indication of the need for initial surgical management of injuries, provides a baseline evaluation that has
predictive value regarding prognosis, and can detect
delayed or secondary complications of the initial trauma.

Text continued on p. 108.

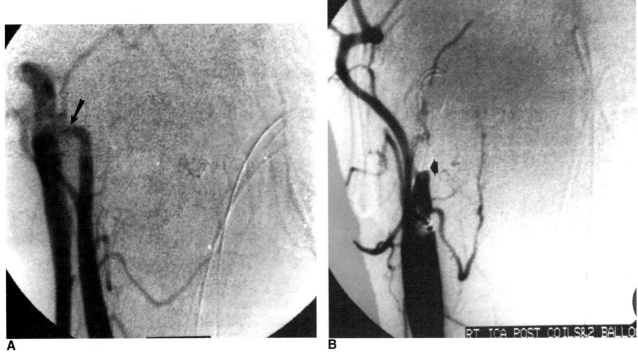

Fig. 2-109
Internal carotid-jugular fistula after penetrating trauma. **A,** Arteriogram of a 22-year-old man secondary to ballistic injury demonstrates a right internal carotid to jugular venous fistula (*arrow*). **B,** The internal carotid was occluded with coils and balloons after verifying adequate collateral circulation (*arrow*).

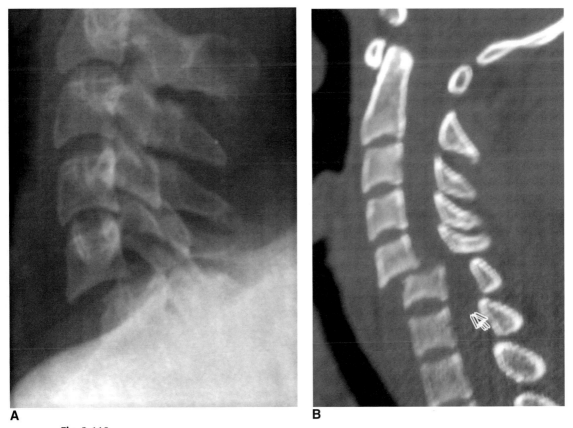

Fig. 2-110
Vertebral artery injury from cervical dislocation. **A,** Lateral radiograph of quadriplegic blunt trauma patient shows a bilateral facet dislocation at the C5-6 level. **B,** The finding is verified on the mid-sagittal CT reformation.

Continued

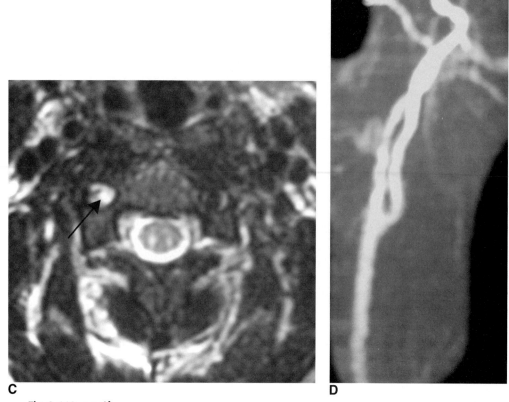

Fig. 2-110, cont'd
C, T2-weighted spin-echo sequence on axial MRI shows high signal in right vertebral artery (*arrow*) with absence of expected flow void (seen in the left vertebral artery). **D,** MRA shows normal right carotid system without flow in the right vertebral artery. The patient did not sustain a neurologic deficit related to this vertebral occlusion.

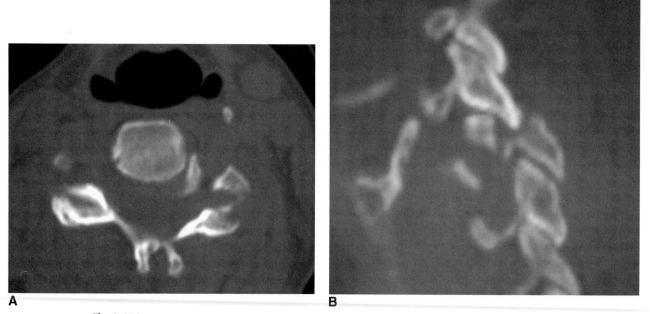

Fig. 2-111
Vertebral artery injury from cervical spine fracture-subluxation. **A,** Axial CT shows a cervical unilateral fracture-subluxation on the left side. Note uncovered posterior disc resulting from rotational subluxation of vertebral body. **B,** Parasagittal CT reformation confirms fracture of lower articular mass and forward displacement of adjacent (superior) articular pillar.

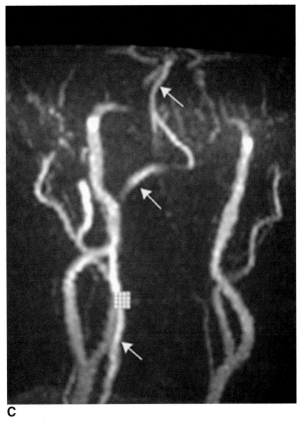

Fig. 2-111, cont'd
C, MRA shows an intact right vertebral artery signal (*arrows*), but no signal from the left vertebral artery, indicating occlusion.

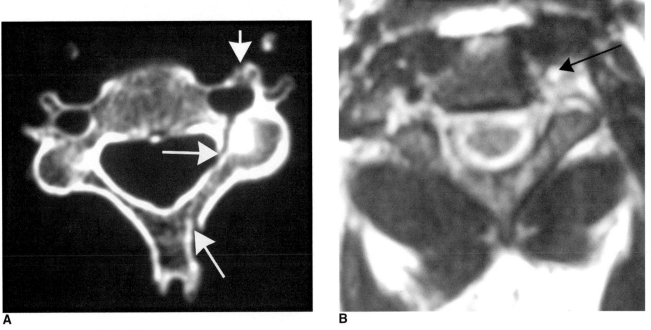

Fig. 2-112
Vertebral artery injury from fracture across foramen transversarium. **A**, Axial CT shows an isolated articular pillar or lamino-pedicular separation of the left with fractures in the lamina, pedicle, and across the left vertebral foramen (*arrows*). **B**, A T2-weighted axial MR image shows a high signal in the left vertebral foramen, indicating occlusion of the artery (*arrow*). Note normal right flow void.

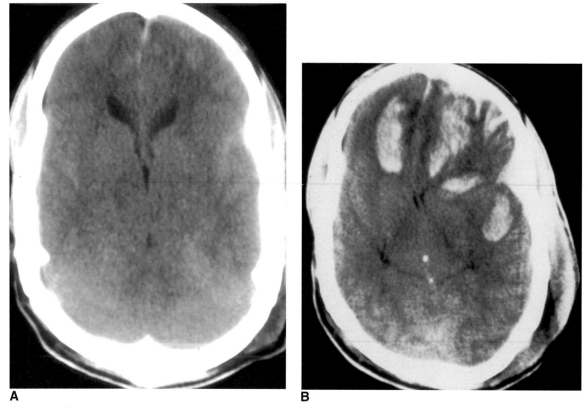

Fig. 2-113
Delayed intracerebral hemorrhage. **A**, Admission CT of blunt head trauma patient with impact to left parietal region shows faint small areas of hemorrhage in the frontal lobes, predominantly on the left. **B**, CT acquired 2 days after admission reveals new hemorrhages in both frontal lobes and left temporal lobe producing mass effect on the ventricles. Subdural blood probably tracks along the left frontal subdural space.

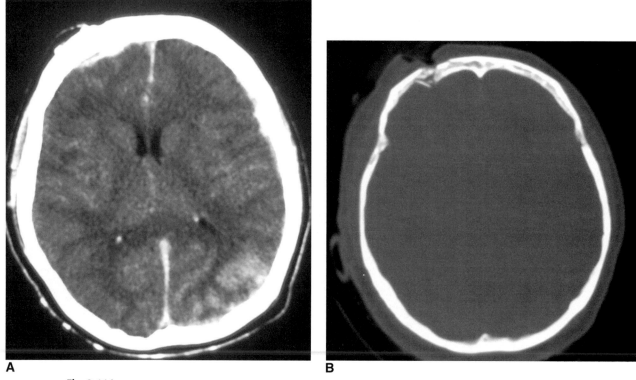

Fig. 2-114
Delayed intracerebral hemorrhage. **A**, Admission CT of blunt head trauma patient shows a right frontal skull fracture with a thin extraaxial hematoma (probable EDH), a thin left convexity extraaxial hematoma, and left occipital lobe contusion. **B**, Review of the CT on bone windows allows confirmation of a comminuted depressed right frontal bone fracture.

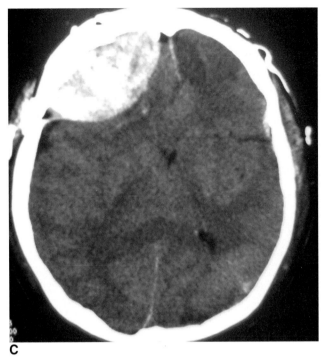

Fig. 2-114, cont'd
C, A follow-up CT scan 6 hours after the initial study shows a marked enlargement of a right frontal EDH and increasing cerebral edema with compression and displacement of the frontal horns.

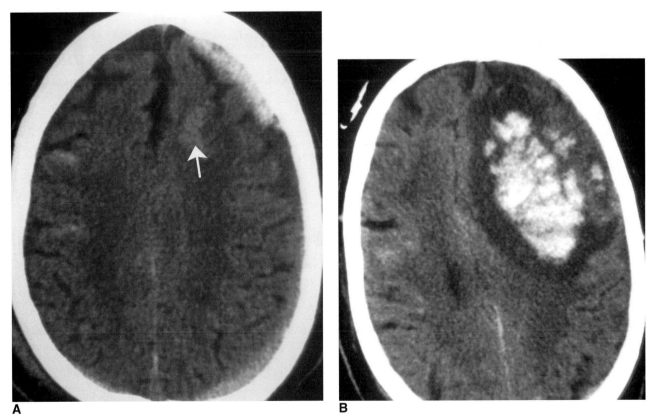

Fig. 2-115
Delayed intracerebral hematoma. **A**, Admission CT of 22-year-old assault victim shows thin left-sided SDH, a small anterior white matter hemorrhage on the left (*arrow*), and right-sided subarachnoid blood. **B**, Routine follow-up CT 6 hours after admission shows marked progression of left frontal and anterior parietal hematoma.

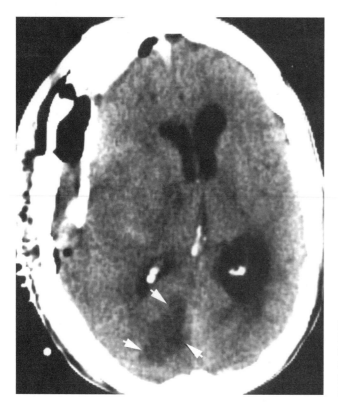

Fig. 2-116
Posterior cerebral infarct from mass displacement. This postoperative CT image obtained after evacuation of a large right SDH producing right to left subfalcine herniation reveals a focal low-density region in the right posterior cerebral territory, indicative of infarction (*arrowheads*).

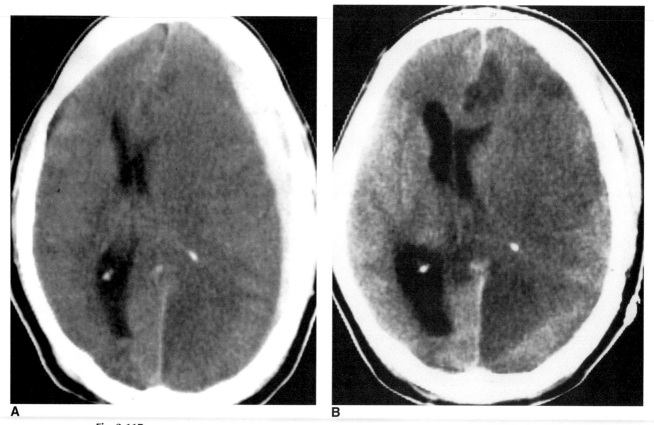

A

B

Fig. 2-117
Multifocal infarction following gross mass displacement. **A**, CT image reveals a large left convexity SDH markedly displacing the midline structures to the right. Low density adjacent to the posterior falx suggests early ischemic changes. **B**, Follow-up CT at the midventricular level after evacuation of the SDH reveals infarction in the left anterior and posterior cerebral and left thalamoperforating distributions. In addition, the left anterior middle cerebral territory is of low density, suggesting infarction or edema.

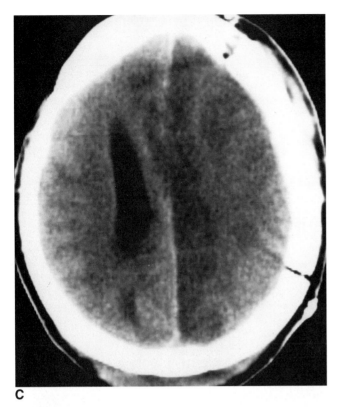

Fig. 2-117, cont'd
C, A high ventricular level image shows infarction in the anterior and posterior cerebral vascular distributions and low density in the left anterior middle cerebral territory. Some evidence of a distal right anterior cerebral artery infarct is also seen. (From Mirvis SE, Wolf AL, Numaguchi Y, et al: *AJNR* 11:355, 1990.)

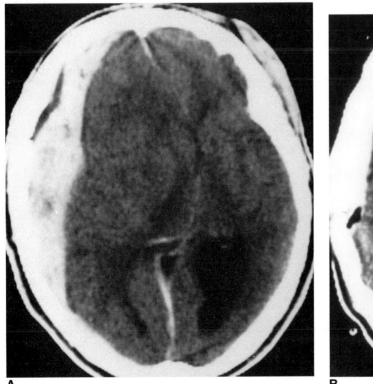

Fig. 2-118
Anterior choroidal infarction. **A**, CT image of an elderly woman after head trauma demonstrates a large right convexity SDH with marked subfalcine herniation. Subdural blood also tracks along the posterior and anterior falx. **B**, Follow-up CT study after surgical evacuation shows oval low density in the posterior limb of the internal capsule consistent with infarction in the distribution of the anterior choroidal artery (*arrows*). (From Mirvis SE, Wolf AL, Numaguchi Y, et al: *AJNR* 11:355, 1990.)

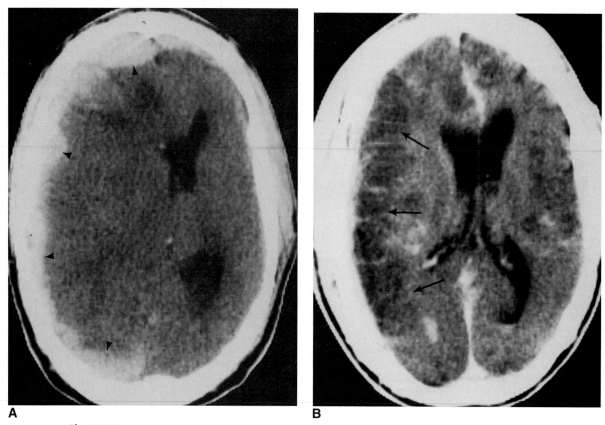

A   **B**

Fig. 2-119
Cortical cerebral infarction. **A,** CT image of an elderly man after head trauma reveals a large right
convexity SDH producing marked mass effect and subfalcine herniation. **B,** Enhanced CT obtained
after evacuation of the hematoma shows a large band *(arrows)* of low density along the middle
cerebral distribution involving the gray and subcortical white matter. The infarct is most likely due
to direct pressure effects of the overlying subdural mass limiting arterial inflow or venous outflow.
(From Mirvis SE, Wolf AL, Numaguchi Y, et al: *AJNR* 11:355, 1990.)

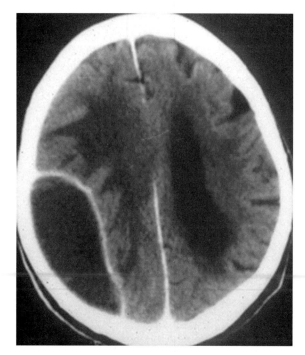

Fig. 2-120
Posttraumatic cerebral infection. Delayed contrast-enhanced CT
shows a low-attenuation fluid collection with convex bulge toward
the brain and sharp margins indicating an epidural location. The
collection is slightly higher density than CSF in the ventricles, and
the adjacent dura is thickened and enhanced. The collection proved
to be an epidural empyema arising from a previous open skull fracture at the site.

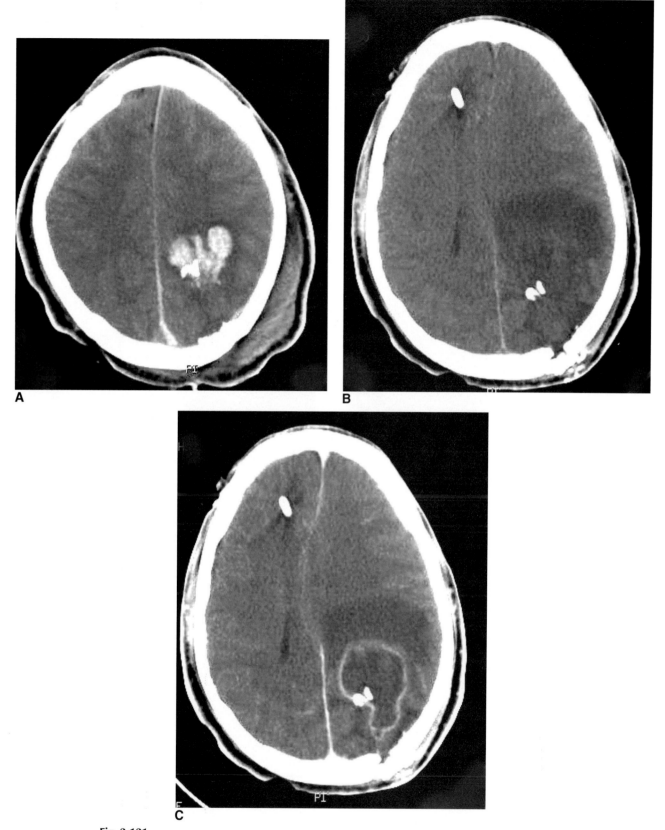

Fig. 2-121
Intracerebral abscess posttrauma. **A,** Admission CT following GSW to the left parietal region shows a hematoma and displaced bone fragments in the left parietal lobe. A thin SDH extends along the left posterior falx. A nonenhanced (**B**) and contrast-enhanced (**C**) CT obtained 3 weeks later show a ring-enhancing lesion at the site of the hematoma with persistent surrounding edema. An abscess was surgically drained.

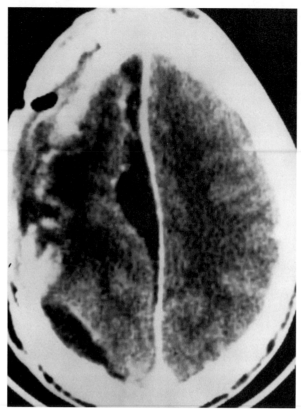

Fig. 2-122
Cerebritis. CT study was acquired 2 weeks after surgical evacuation of right intraparietal and subdural hematoma. Medially there is a subdural fluid collection in the interhemispheric fissure. Note the smooth inner margin and displacement of the cortical vessels (*white dots*). Laterally, a complex mixture of extraaxial fluid and air and a craniectomy site are present. The right parietal cortex is of low density, indicating edema. The patient proved to have cerebritis with loculated subdural empyema.

CT can readily be repeated to follow progression or resolution of injuries. State-of-the art CT scanners with laser cameras can provide complete studies, including a hard copy of the images, in less than 3 to 5 minutes.

MRI has been found to have application in improved detection of thin or isodense extraaxial hematomas, improved localization of lesions, improved sensitivity for predominantly nonhemorrhagic contusions in the brain and brainstem (such as occur in shearing injuries), and improved sensitivity in detecting traumatic cerebral vascular injury as compared with nonenhanced CT scan. The effect of information provided by MRI in *altering patient management* as compared with information derived from CT is not yet defined. The inability of MRI to easily demonstrate pneumocephalus and calvarial fractures is a significant limitation of the modality in acute head trauma imaging. The potential applications of MR angiography (MRA) in detecting intracranial or extracranial (cervical) vascular injury and the potential role of cerebral MRS to assess metabolic activity in injured brain parenchyma using phosphorus spectra remain as areas of investigation.

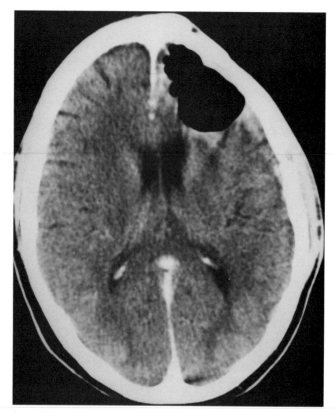

Fig. 2-123
Posttraumatic cerebral aerocele. CT obtained 2 weeks after discharge of a 40-year-old man who had sustained a complex frontal bone fracture shows an air collection in the left frontal region, but no significant mass effect.

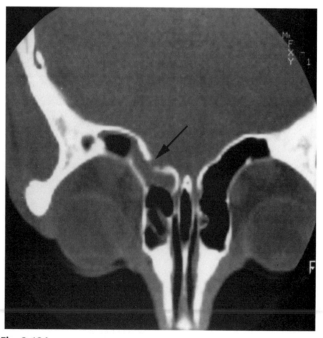

Fig. 2-124
CSF leaking from frontal extension of ethmoid sinus. CT image of a patient with CSF rhinorrhea reveals a fracture in the orbital plate of the frontal bone with fluid accumulation in the superior ethmoid air cells.

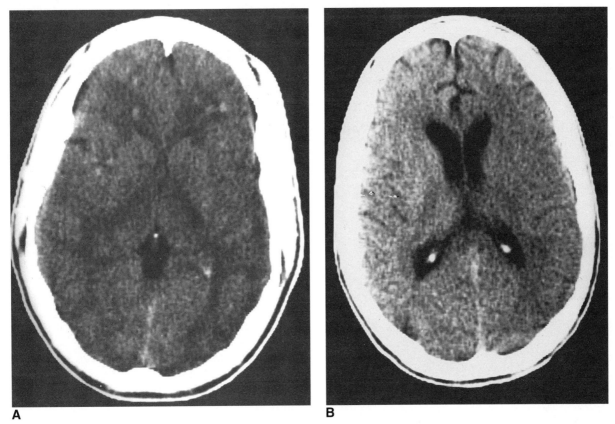

Fig. 2-125
Posttraumatic diffuse cerebral atrophy. **A**, Admission CT of a patient with diffuse axonal shearing injury.
B, Repeat CT several weeks later reveals generalized atrophy with sulcal and ventricular involvement.

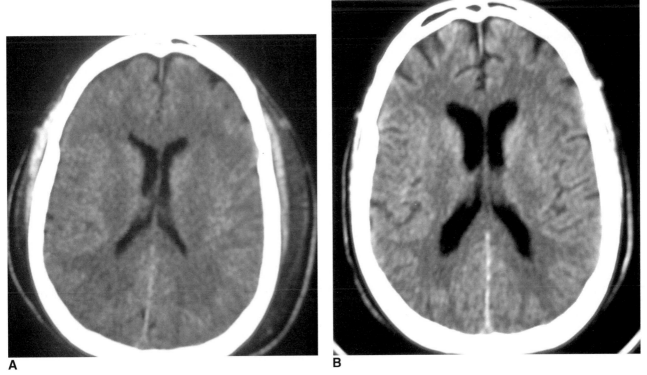

Fig. 2-126
Posttraumatic diffuse cerebral atrophy. **A**, Admission CT of a patient with no obvious cerebral injury
but diminished mental status. **B**, A 3-week follow-up cranial CT demonstrates both central and cortical atrophy compared with admission study.

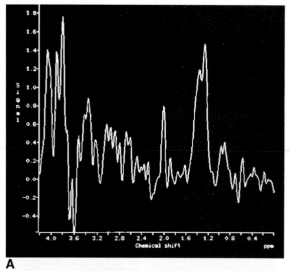

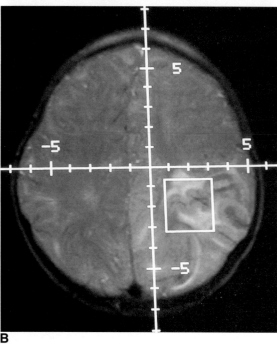

Fig. 2-127
MR spectroscopy (MRS) in closed head injury. **A,** Single voxel proton spectroscopy (STEAM, TE 270ms) shows markedly elevated lactate doublet (1.33 pm) with significant reduction in n-acetyl aspartate (2.01 ppm), choline (3.22 ppm) and creatine (3.02 ppm). **B,** Voxel position superimposed on axial FLAIR through a large cerebral contusion.

Pediatric Traumatic Brain Injury

Erin M. Simon and Robert A. Zimmerman

The imaging evaluation of the brain injured pediatric patient is directed at detecting the nature of the insults and the evolving pathologic process so that its rate and direction of progression can be determined. Once this is accomplished, measures can be instituted to protect the brain against still greater damage.

The direction and nature of the force that produced injury, the position of the head at the time of injury, and the protection afforded to the brain (i.e., by a helmet or the degree of ossification) at the time of injury are highly significant factors in determining the degree of intracranial trauma. The young infant, with open sutures and a thin flexible calvarium, can absorb traumatic forces better than the older child and the adult. The relative lack of myelination of the white matter affords additional impact absorption. However, this flexibility has inherent disadvantages, including allowing severe distortion between the skull, dura, and the cerebral vessels to occur.[146] This permits distraction between the brain and its meninges, which results in increased likelihood of tearing bridging veins and dural attachments (including the enclosed venous sinuses), producing interhemispheric SDHs and dural venous sinus rents, lesions less common in adults. With progressive development and maturation, the calvarium thickens, the sutures fuse, and myelination becomes complete. The patterns of brain injury in the adolescent are more typical of those seen in the adult.

As in adults, the optimal imaging evaluation of pediatric brain injury depends to a large extent on the probable nature of the injury and the clinical status of the patient. In most situations, evaluation of the intracranial structures is of paramount importance and necessitates CT scanning as the initial study. If there is a need to mobilize the patient for transport to the CT scanner, traumatic insults to the cervical spine must be considered and be excluded. Until this can be adequately done, the cervical spine must be immobilized. CT and MRI are currently the two highly accurate noninvasive modalities for showing the morphologic manifestations of the traumatic cerebral process at one point in time.[147] It is important to remember that the injured brain is in a dynamic state, with edema and hemorrhage evolving over time. CT delineates the changes that affect the brain parenchyma, subarachnoid spaces, ventricular system, and to some extent the cerebral vascular structures. Serial CT examinations can often document the morphologic manifestations of the posttraumatic process effectively.[148]

Unfortunately, the sensitivity of the CT evaluation to subtle brain injury can be poor. MRI can contribute greatly to visualization of the structural manifestations of cerebral injury and to understanding ongoing pathophysiologic processes. Unfortunately, MRI remains technically a more difficult study to achieve in the brain-injured patient than CT, because the acquisition times are longer and patient motion is more of a problem.[65] CT can be performed with individual slice scan times of less than 1 second and, with multi-detector spiral technique, the entire brain can be examined in less than 12 to 15 seconds. With MRI, most imaging sequences are on the order of several minutes, during which patient immobility is critical if the images are to be of diagnostic quality.

CT was reported to be superior to MRI in the setting of acute SAH, where CT depicts the increased density within the subarachnoid spaces, but this has been called into question in recent in vitro experiments.[150] It is possible that MRI may miss a small percentage of acute SAH, even with newer imaging techniques.[149] As in adults, CT is also better at depicting fractures.[151]

MRI examination for assessment of TBI generally includes: spin echo T1-weighted images (WI), turbo spin echo (fast spin echo) T2-WI, turbo FLAIR, T2-weighted gradient echo susceptibility sequence (GE T2*) and diffusion weighted imaging (DWI). The total imaging time can be less than 12 minutes. The application of these sequences in orthogonal planes, along with their ability to depict hyperacute, acute, subacute, and chronic hemorrhage, as well as cytotoxic and vasogenic edema, provides a fuller picture of the location and extent of injury.

Magnetic resonance spectroscopy (MRS) can depict and quantitate levels of certain metabolites within the brain.[152] Decreases in NAA, a neuronal marker, represent neuronal loss, whereas increases in lactate, a product of anaerobic glycolysis, can indicate necrosis and infarction of tissue (Fig. 2-127). DWI can depict acute cytotoxic cell swelling, which is thought to reduce extracellular water motion. MR perfusion imaging techniques can detect blood flow to and through the cerebral parenchyma.[153] Conventional MRI and MRA can demonstrate many vascular injuries, such as pseudoaneurysm, dissection, or occlusion.[154]

SKULL FRACTURES

In the pediatric population, the skull is often fractured without significant injury to the brain, but the fracture location or type may affect treatment. For example, a depressed fracture over the motor strip or a major dural venous sinus, or significant depression such that the outer table is forced deep to the inner table of the adjacent intact calvarium, may require surgical intervention. Additionally, a fracture that involves the paranasal sinuses or mastoid air cells, contains a foreign body, or is associated with an overlying laceration, can increase the risk of intracranial infection, particularly meningitis or empyema. Skull radiography may occasionally be complementary to CT in demonstrating depressed fractures and localizing foreign bodies, but CT remains the examination of choice for its depiction of the parenchymal and extraaxial spaces.

TRAUMATIC EXTRACEREBRAL INJURY
Subarachnoid Hemorrhage

In children traumatic SAH is usually focal, overlying sites of contusion, and/or found in the interhemispheric fissure paralleling the falx cerebri.[155] The normal falx and calcification of the falx in older children may be seen on CT and should not be falsely mistaken for SAH.[54] In general the incidence of SAH as seen on CT scanning increases with increased severity of brain injury. Subarachnoid blood loses its density over the ensuing days with the breakdown of the globin molecule. The high-density acute blood becomes isodense or hypodense within 7 days, making the blood more difficult to see.[54] Affected cisterns, fissures, and sulci may mistakenly appear obliterated by blood that is isodense to the surrounding tissues. This is a potential source of diagnostic error when the CT is at a delayed point after the brain trauma, or when no history of brain trauma is provided, as is often the case in the setting of nonaccidental trauma. As a complication of SAH, fibroblastic proliferation in the subarachnoid space and arachnoid villi may lead to the production of a communicating hydrocephalus. An in vitro model suggests that children with preexisting benign enlargement of the subarachnoid spaces (benign external hydrocephalus) may be more likely to develop extraaxial hemorrhage following minor head trauma.[156] FLAIR imaging has been reported to be more successful than CT in showing subacute SAH between 3 and 45 days after the injury[157] (Fig. 2-128).

Subdural Hematoma

Acute SDHs in children are similar in imaging characteristics to those seen in adults. They are nearly always

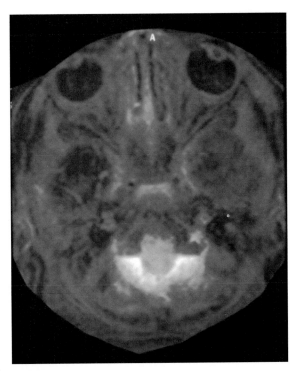

Fig. 2-128
Subacute SAH hemorrhage on FLAIR. Axial FLAIR through the foramen magnum shows dependently layering subacute SAH as hyperintense compared to CSF.

associated with underlying brain injury and, despite modern methods of treatment, carry significant morbidity and mortality risk.[147] SDH arising primarily within the interhemispheric fissure in infants is often due to "whiplash" or shaken-impact injury, which should raise the suspicion of nonaccidental trauma if accidental trauma is undocumented. In the normal infant, like the adult with significant volume loss, it is thought that the large subarachnoid spaces contribute to excessive mobility of the brain within the calvarium.[158] The infant's weak neck muscles and comparatively large head subject the brain to unconstrained anterior and posterior motion of a rapid nature. The brain moves at a different rate of speed than the calvarium and falx but is attached to them by bridging cortical veins. Violent shaking or whiplash-type motion results in stress on these veins, leading to their disruption and production of subdural bleeding, usually interhemispheric.[158] SDH that occurs in older children and adolescents is more often similar in location and appearance to that seen in adults.

Epidural Hematoma

The CT appearance of EDH depends on the source of bleeding (arterial or venous), the interval between injury and imaging, the hemorrhage severity, and the degree of clot organization or breakdown.[159] Overall, the appearance and typical locations are similar to those described in the nonpediatric population.

TRAUMATIC BRAIN INJURY
Shearing or Diffuse Axonal Injury

Rotational stress on the brain, such as occurs with rapid deceleration of one cerebral hemisphere relative to the other, can result in edematous and/or hemorrhagic injury to the pediatric brain and occurs at rather characteristic sites.[67-71] The splenium and posterior body of the corpus callosum, the gray-white matter junctions of the cerebral hemispheres, the axonal connections to the basal ganglia, and the dorsal upper brainstem, including the superior cerebral peduncles down into the middle cerebellar peduncles, are the usually affected sites[68,69] (Fig. 2-129). DAI is most commonly caused by high-speed collisions, such as motor vehicle accidents. There is evidence, however, that falls from heights and blows to the brain can produce DAI if they generate sufficient angular momentum. Clinically, severe DAI produces a comatose child who becomes vegetative and only occasionally recovers some function.

Detection of DAI by CT is generally limited to cases associated with focal hemorrhages. Bleeding into the lateral ventricles should alert the radiologist to the possibility of tears in the corpus callosum, particularly the

splenium. In most cases, the brain will not show significant mass effect from the injury, particularly on initial presentation. Thus, a comatose patient with small, scattered areas of hemorrhage at supratentorial gray-white matter junctions, a small amount of IVH, and perhaps basal ganglia or upper brainstem hemorrhage has CT-diagnosable DAI. The diagnostic difficulties arise when the hemorrhages are not visible with CT. Clearly, significant white matter injury can occur without associated hemorrhage, potentially resulting in a false-negative CT.

MRI, on the other hand, is highly sensitive to petechial hemorrhages and tiny foci of parenchymal insults. T2-weighted images, PD-weighted images, and FLAIR are sensitive to increased interstitial water at the site of torn axons.[88,160] Conventional spin echo T2-weighted images are more sensitive in demonstrating blood products than turbo/fast spin echo. However, GE T2* scans are even better for bringing out susceptibility effects due to blood products.[161] This is true whether the hemorrhage is acute or chronic. The combination of FLAIR and GE T2* can demonstrate characteristic lesions of DAI in the setting of a normal CT. Even when CT does detect abnormalities, MRI frequently demonstrates numerous additional areas of injury that were not visible on CT, allowing more accurate prediction of prognosis.[162] The routine application of DWI in the setting of TBI further improves sensitivity to DAI within the brain (Fig. 2-130). Newer imaging techniques, such as diffusion tensor imaging, hold the promise of even higher sensitivity to microscopic regions of parenchymal insult and may help in the development and assessment of neuroprotective agent in the acutely injured child.[75]

With DAI, the injured axons can produce relatively rapid changes of Wallerian degeneration. This will lead to parenchymal volume loss, which can produce striking ventricular and sulcal enlargement. The high signal intensity acutely present on FLAIR and T2-weighted images becomes less obvious or disappears with time.[163] However, the small hemorrhages will leave telltale hemosiderin deposition that can frequently be seen for many months to years after the injury, particularly with GE T2* sequences.

Cerebral Contusion

Petechial hemorrhages and torn capillaries, as well as evidence of mechanical damage to adjacent neurons, characterize the cerebral contusion. Apices of the cerebral convolutions are involved maximally, with progressively less involvement of the deeper portions of the brain. Crests of contiguous gyri are often involved, while portions of the intervening sulci are spared. The coup contusion results when an object impacts on the stationary brain, while the contrecoup contusion occurs at a

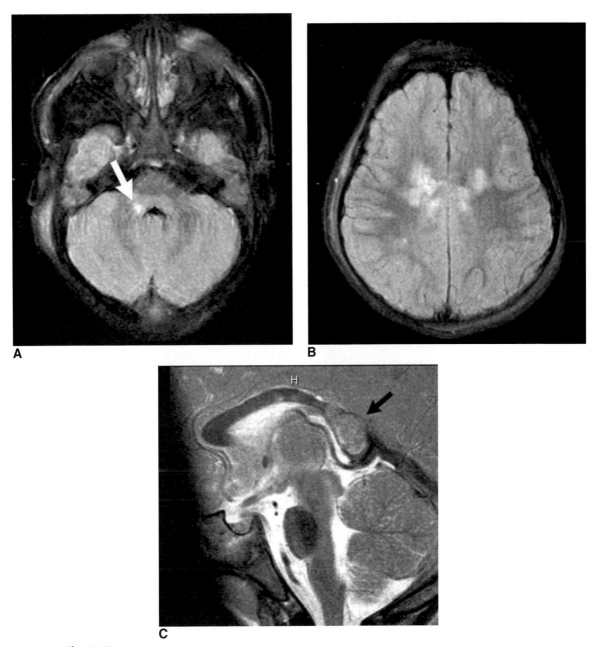

Fig. 2-129
DAI. **A**, Axial FLAIR through the level of the brainstem with a site of axonal injury in the dorsal pons (*arrow*). **B**, Extensive white matter injury within the centrum semiovale bilaterally on axial FLAIR. **C**, Axonal injury within the splenium of the corpus callosum (*arrow*) seen on sagittal T2-weighted imaging.

site remote from the point of impact, as seen in adults. Contusions are one of the most frequent manifestations of traumatic pediatric brain injury, are often multiple, and are frequently accompanied by other forms of traumatic injury, such as an acute SDH[147] (Fig. 2-131).

The presence of a contusion does not necessarily imply acute neurologic symptoms. Children with contu-

sions can present in a delayed fashion after the episode of trauma, because of the development of secondary effects, such as seizures from fibroglial scarring at the contusion site. In acute contusions the most frequent clinical manifestations are confusion, or focal cerebral dysfunction related to the site of injured cortex. Days after the injury, because of brain swelling around injured sites, increasing

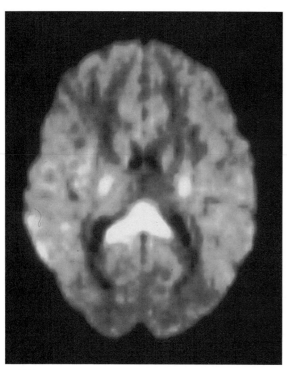

Fig. 2-130
Diffusion weighted imaging in diffuse axonal shearing. Reduced diffusion in the basal ganglia and splenium of the corpus callosum bilaterally from DAI seen on diffusion-weighted imaging.

mass effect can lead to cerebral herniation in the setting of large insults. Subsequent to resolution of the brain injury, in addition to seizures, personality changes or focal neurologic deficits may persist.

For the pediatric population, the CT and MRI appearance of parenchymal contusions, and the areas of encephalomalacia that develop in their wake, are similar to those seen in adults.

Intracerebral Hematomas

ICHs are a less frequent manifestation of brain trauma than are contusions, but occur in the same territorial distribution, that is, the frontal and temporal lobes and the basal ganglia (Fig. 2-132). They frequently arise in association with contusions, but are caused by disruption of larger vessels. Once the bleeding begins, blood dissects between the axons within the white matter and accumulates, leading to clot formation.[164] During the active phase of dissection of the clot through the white matter, the blood may rupture transependymally into the ventricular system.[147] This occurs in approximately one-third of the cases of ICH. While the incidence of ICH after trauma is low (4.5% to 6.3%), a higher incidence (20%) of bilat-

eral TBI is seen when a hematoma is present.[147,164] More than half of patients with IDH also will have other lesions, including SDH and EDH.[147] ICHs are much more frequent in adults than in children, by approximately a three to one margin.

A small percentage of posttraumatic ICH develops in a delayed fashion, appearing from 1 to 7 days after injury.[165-167] Delayed ICH occurs most often at sites of contusion or parenchymal ischemia. As with hemorrhagic contusions and acute-onset ICH, delayed ICH occurs most often in the frontotemporal regions. Whatever the etiology, such as removal of the tamponade effect of an extracerebral hematoma or lactic acidosis with ischemia of a vessel wall, recognition of delayed ICHs is crucial, since they can be associated with secondary deterioration of the patient, one that may require surgical intervention.

NONACCIDENTAL TRAUMA

Estimates are that at least 3000 deaths per year in the United States result from nonaccidental brain injury, and more than 10% of children with mental retardation and cerebral palsy are presumed to have been damaged by abuse.[168] Severe accidental brain trauma is relatively uncommon in children younger than 2 years old.[168] Within the subset of patients younger than 1 year old, accidental injury is 10 to 15 times more common than nonaccidental injury.[169] However, in patients younger than 2 years old, nonaccidental injury accounts for 80% or more of all deaths attributed to brain trauma.[170] Additionally, one large series found that abused children were more likely to suffer significant intracranial injury than those unintentionally injured (42% vs. 14%).[171] The same authors also found that children with nonaccidental blunt trauma were more likely to be admitted to intensive care units and to develop "extensive functional limitations" (9% vs. 3%). It has been reported that up to 50% of patients suffering from child abuse have skull fractures.[11,172]

The clinical history is often an important clue in recognizing abuse. A discrepancy between the report of how the injury occurred (i.e., fall from a standing height onto a rug) and the nature of the traumatic lesions seen with imaging (i.e., severe brain injury) should alert the clinician and radiologist to the possibility of nonaccidental trauma.[168,173,174] The presence of retinal hemorrhages, particularly when they are bilateral, is often presumptive evidence of abuse. Large hemorrhages can be seen with CT and MRI (Fig. 2-133). Retinal hemorrhages are rarely associated with accidental trauma or with cardiopulmonary resuscitation.[173,175] Idiopathic retinal hemorrhages may be found immediately after birth but disappear within the first few days of life.[176]

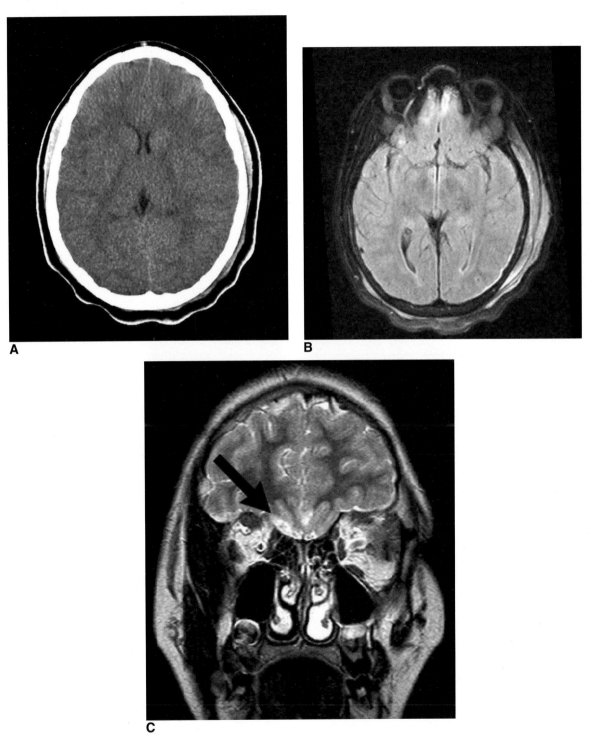

Fig. 2-131
Cerebral contusion. **A**, Axial unenhanced CT through the level of the basal ganglia shows mild asymmetry of the frontal horns of the lateral ventricles, but no appreciable abnormal parenchymal density. **B**, Contusions are evident bilaterally in the gyrus rectus on axial FLAIR. **C**, Coronal T2-weighted imaging confirms the intraaxial location of the contusion (*arrow*).

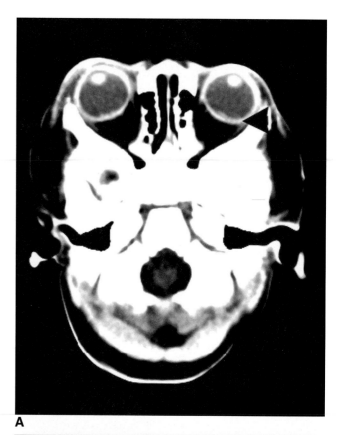

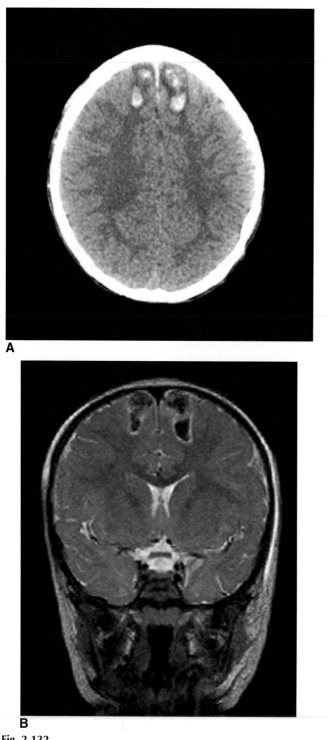

A

B

Fig. 2-132
Intracerebral hematomas. **A,** Bifrontal parasagittal hematomas with diffuse sulcal effacement on unenhanced CT. **B,** The contusions are seen as hypointense on coronal T2-weighted imaging, with no significant surrounding edema.

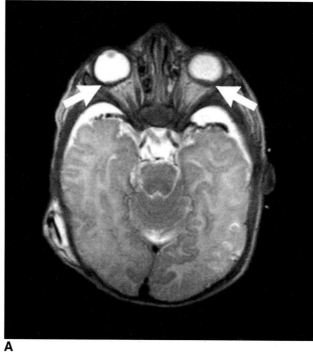

A

Fig. 2-133
Retinal hemorrhage from nonaccidental trauma. **A,** Axial CT reveals hyperdense hemorrhage along the posterior retina of the left globe (*arrowhead*). Hemorrhage in the right globe was questioned as well. **B,** Bilateral hemorrhages confirmed with axial T2-weighted imaging (*arrows*). Note also the contusions in the left posterior temporal lobe and the hypointense hemorrhage over the temporal poles bilaterally. The MR was performed following shunt placement.

Two primary mechanisms of abuse occur either singularly or in combination: battering and shaking. Skull fractures with overlying bruises are a sign of battering injury. Often the history is inconsistent with the imaging and clinical findings. A fall from a stroller onto a rug or a fall from a couch onto the floor will not produce a depressed calvarial fracture and brain injury in a normal child. Further evaluation of the long bones and ribs to search for other fractures, and careful physical examination for stigmata of prior abuse are indicated.

Brain injuries that result from acceleration/deceleration effects fall under the category of "whiplash," shaken injury or shaken-impact injury. The latter term is used in the setting of brain impact on a structure, such as a mattress.[177] These children do not usually have skull fractures or bruises but may have metaphyseal "corner" fractures of the long bones, where they are held while being shaken or thrown.

As previously detailed, the relatively large brain of the infant is not supported by the weak neck musculature, so when marked to-and-fro motion occurs, the skull and sagittal sinus move as a unit, while the brain moves within the subarachnoid space as a separate unit, yet is attached by the bridging veins to the sagittal sinus. Tearing of these bridging veins leads to interhemispheric SDH (Fig. 2-134). SDH over the convexities can develop as well.

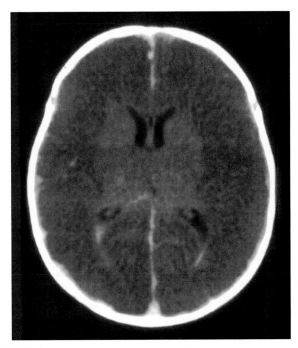

Fig. 2-134
Interhemispheric SDH from shaking injury. Hyperdense subdural blood is seen in the interhemispheric fissure both anteriorly and posteriorly. Note also the diffuse parenchymal hypodensity with relative sparing of the basal ganglia, from superimposed anoxic injury.

"Gliding" contusions result when the pial-covered surface of the outer cortex of the brain rubs against the inner table of the skull.[178,179] These are commonly seen in the gyrus rectus and the inferior temporal lobes. White matter shearing injuries occur more commonly in young children than in older children or adults, as the unmyelinated white matter is not strong. However, seeing these lesions on MRI or CT in the infant brain, with its high water content, can be difficult unless bleeding has occurred. DWI can be extremely helpful in this situation (Fig. 2-135).

One CNS effect of shaking an infant may be depression of central respiratory control, leading to apnea, hypoxia, and worsening cerebral edema.[180] Cerebral swelling may also occur because of cerebral hyperemia owing to loss of vasomotor control.

The injuries that come as a result of nonaccidental trauma otherwise have an identical appearance to lesions arising from accidental trauma. The CT and MRI appearances of intentionally inflicted cerebral contusions, DAI, and extraaxial hemorrhage are all as previously described. It is the constellation of findings and the clinical context that alerts the astute radiologist to the possibility of abuse in a patient of any age.

It is also important to realize that abuse does not always lead to immediate medical attention, but may present days to months after the event and may clinically mimic nontraumatic diseases. It is crucial to be alert to the presence of abnormally large extraaxial spaces around the brain of an infant or young child. This may represent benign enlargement of the subarachnoid spaces or may be due to volume loss from an underlying metabolic or cardiac disease. However, when on CT the density of the fluid is greater than that of CSF[169] or on FLAIR/PD the signal intensity is greater than that of CSF, chronic SDH should be suspected. The etiology should include the possibility of nonaccidental injury. When chronic SDH is seen with rehemorrhage, such as on CT where there is a hyperdense new area of blood products within the older chronic subdural collection, investigation into nonaccidental injury should be undertaken, particularly when coagulopathy and metabolic diseases (such as glutaric aciduria) have been excluded (Fig. 2-136).

CONCLUSION

The pediatric patient with TBI requires rapid and accurate diagnosis and intervention. By utilizing modern imaging techniques and recognizing the many variations of injury, the radiologist can assist the primary physicians in caring for these children. The astute radiologist may be the first to raise the "red flag," by familiarizing oneself with the patterns most commonly seen in the setting of nonaccidental trauma.

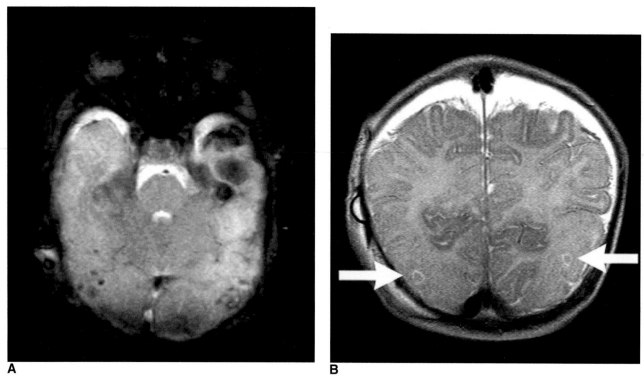

A   B

Fig. 2-135
Gliding contusions. **A**, Multiple bilateral temporal and occipital contusions are revealed with T2-weighted gradient-echo imaging. Hemorrhage over the temporal poles is also noted. **B**, Coronal T2-weighted imaging shows bilateral temporal contusions (*arrows*). Note also the subdural collections.

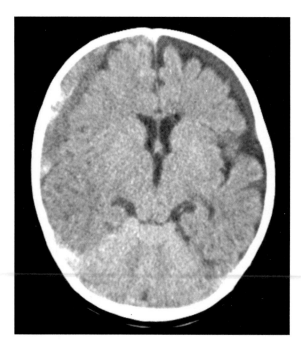

Fig. 2-136
SDH of varying stages due to nonaccidental trauma. Axial CT demonstrates SDH of at least three stages: more acute hyperdense blood along the periphery of the right convexity and right side of the tentorium; subacute, slightly hyperdense blood filling the majority of the right subdural space; and a chronic, hypodense SDH overlying the left hemisphere. The ventricular system is also enlarged from parenchymal volume loss.

Vascular Injury of the Head and Neck

M.J.B. Stallmeyer

TRAUMATIC INJURIES OF THE EXTRACRANIAL CAROTID AND VERTEBRAL ARTERIES

Traumatic injury to the extracranial carotid and vertebral arteries is a relatively uncommon but potentially devastating event. The mortality rate from posttraumatic carotid dissection ranges from 20% to 40% in reported series, and significant neurologic sequelae have been reported to occur in between 12.5% and 80% of survivors.[181-191] The corresponding mortality and neurologic morbidity rates for vertebral artery injury are 4% to 8% and 14% to 24%, respectively.[191,192] Traumatic injury of the carotid or vertebral arteries may be caused by penetrating (e.g., gunshot or stab wound) or blunt trauma. Mechanisms at high risk for producing blunt carotid and vertebral injury include direct blows to the neck, and hyperflexion-rotation or hyperextension-rotation injuries, with seat belt injury possibly playing a contributory role.[192] Basilar skull fractures that cross the petrous carotid canal can also produce carotid injury at this level. Motor vehicle collisions, falls, and assaults are the most common mechanisms.[184,191,193] Other etiologies of blunt injury to the extracranial carotid and vertebral artery include chiropractic manipulation,[194-198] athletic activity,[199-203] and rapid head turning or flexion-extension movements.[204,205] Several conditions have been reported as predisposing to "spontaneous" dissection, including Marfan's syndrome[206] and fibromuscular dysplasia.[207]

Recent literature suggests that the true incidence of blunt-force injury to the carotid and vertebral arteries is higher than initially described. Early studies described an incidence of carotid injury of 08% to 0.17% among patients admitted for blunt trauma.[184-187] However, centers performing aggressive screening of selected patients using cervico-cerebral arteriography have reported a higher incidence. Fabian et al.[208] identified 67 patients with 87 blunt carotid injuries over a period of 11 years, for a rate of 0.67% where motor vehicle collision was the mechanism of injury, and a rate of 0.33% for other blunt trauma. Before initiating an aggressive screening protocol, Biffl et al.[209] reported an incidence of carotid injury of 0.1% in patients admitted with blunt trauma; this increased to 0.86% when patients were routinely screened with angiography. Prall et al.[210] found an incidence of 3.5% when carotid arteriography was performed in patients undergoing aortogram for blunt traumatic injury. The corresponding incidence of vertebral artery injury in all patients with blunt trauma is somewhat smaller, at 0.53%.[191] However, where definite cervical spine injury is present (e.g., facet dislocation, fractures through the foramen transversarium, spinal cord injury), the reported incidence of vertebral artery injury ranges from 24% to 88%.[211-215] The true incidence of this type of injury likely is still underreported.

Traumatic Pathology

Dissection separates different layers of the arterial wall. Most commonly, the intimal layer is disrupted, allowing blood to track into the subintima, with subsequent formation of a false lumen. Hemorrhage may be confined to the subintimal layer or may extend through the media or adventitia. Subintimal hemorrhages tend to cause luminal narrowing, whereas subadventitial hemorrhages are more likely to result in pseudoaneurysm formation. This process may be self-limiting and asymptomatic, with healing within a few weeks. If the false lumen enlarges sufficiently, marked narrowing or occlusion of the vessel may occur, and clots forming in the true lumen because of vessel stenosis may then embolize distally. Hematomas forming in the false lumen may also result in thromboembolism and subsequent stroke.

Diagnosis: Clinical Presentation

Patients with carotid dissection most commonly complain of pain in the neck, face, or head ipsilateral to the side of dissection.[216] Pain alone is seen in about 15% of patients. Pain and headache may be mild or severe, sometimes resembling migraine, but more often is dull and nonthrobbing. Scalp tenderness has been reported in some. Pain may precede development of other symptoms by 1 to 2 days. Other presenting symptoms include pulsatile tinnitus, asymptomatic bruit, Horner's syndrome (40%) and cranial neuropathies.[217,218] The initial clinical symptoms of a vertebral artery dissection are most commonly a posterior unilateral headache with or without neck pain. Stroke or TIA is the next most common presenting symptom in both carotid and vertebral dissections.

Numerous authors have noted that neurologic symptoms secondary to traumatic injury to the extracranial carotid and vertebral arteries may be immediate or delayed.[182,183,191-193,219] About half of patients eventually developing a symptomatic dissection have a normal neurologic examination at presentation.[186] As described above, blunt carotid injury progresses to stroke in a significant number of patients. Cervico-cerebral arterial dissection, including "spontaneous" dissections and those occurring after minor trauma, is estimated to cause about 1% of all ischemic strokes and 5% of ischemic strokes in young adults. In the carotid artery distribution about 2.5% of all first strokes result from dissection. The patients are typically young (age 30 to 45).

External signs suggestive of possible carotid or vertebral arterial injury include epistaxis, hemorrhage from the mouth or ears, expanding cervical hematoma or pulsatile mass, cervical bruising or abrasions, and cervical bruit in a young patient.

Imaging Evaluation

The goal of imaging evaluation is to identify patients with blunt carotid injury before neurologically devastating or life-threatening complications can occur. While many patients develop neurologic complications at the time of the initial injury, various authors have reported delayed onset of neurologic sequelae more than 24 hours after trauma.[182,183,193] Therefore screening for vascular injury is indicated as soon as the patient is sufficiently stable to undergo imaging evaluation. The "gold standard" for diagnosis of traumatic carotid or vertebral injury is selective angiography. Although angiography is costly, invasive, and carries a risk of serious complications, it remains the definitive method for evaluation of extracranial cervico-cerebral arterial injury. Findings that should prompt consideration of angiographic screening for carotid or vertebral artery traumatic injury include closed head injury, especially DAI diagnosed on head CT; immediate or delayed neurologic deficits that cannot be accounted for by CT scan findings; displaced midface fractures; fractures through the petrous carotid canal; and cervical spine vertebral body fracture-dislocations, especially perched facet dislocations and foramen transversarium fractures.[195,196]

The most common finding in cervical internal carotid artery (ICA) injury is luminal narrowing.[220] Often this appears as an eccentric, tapered stenosis arising just distal to the carotid bulb, and extends cephalad toward the skull base. Pseudoaneurysms due to blunt trauma commonly occur just below the skull base, stopping where the carotid enters the petrous canal.[221-223] An associated dissection sometimes extends into the petrous carotid canal for a short distance. Extracranial cervical ICA dissections generally involve the medial layer.

Biffl et al.[224] have proposed a grading scale for the arteriographic appearance of cerebrovascular injuries (Fig. 2-137):

Grade I: Irregularity of the vessel wall, or a dissection or intramural hematoma with <25% luminal narrowing (Fig. 2-137, *A*)

Grade II: Intraluminal thrombus or raised intimal flap, or a dissection or intramural hematoma with >25% luminal stenosis (Fig. 2-137, *B*)

Grade III: Pseudoaneurysm (Fig. 2-137, *C*; see also Figs. 2-105 to 2-107)

Grade IV: Occlusion (Figs. 2-102, 2-137, *D*)

Grade V: Transection (Fig. 2-137, *E*)

Alimi et al.[192] proposed a three-grade classification of skull-base ICA dissections based on arteriographic findings:

Type I: wall involvement without significant stenosis or dilation

Type IIA: stenosis >70%

Type IIB: dilation >50%

Type III: ICA thrombosis (see Fig. 2-102)

Angiographic findings of vertebral artery dissection include decreased luminal diameter, and, less frequently, pseudoaneurysm or thrombosis (see Figs. 2-103, 2-104, 2-108, and 2-110 to 2-112). Most vertebral artery dissections are extracranial and occur above the C2 level.[225] Vertebral artery injuries extending intracranially may present with SAH.[226] The major disadvantage of angiography as a screening method for extracranial cerebrovascular injury is the attendant risk of serious complication of at least 0.33% to 4%[227-231] Moreover, in most reported series, screening angiography is negative in more than 50%, and often in more than 80% of cases.[209-211,213-215,219] This has led to the investigation and development of noninvasive methods for diagnosis of extracranial cervico-cerebral vascular injury.

Doppler ultrasound may show a luminal stenosis or a double lumen, or may show reduced or absent distal carotid artery flow at the level of the bifurcation.[189,232-234] Transcranial Doppler may help identify the subset of patients with carotid or vertebral arterial injury with increased risk for stroke due to thromboembolic phenomena.[235] Ultrasound, however, does not permit consistent visualization of lesions in the thorax and above the mandible.

MRA is effective in demonstrating flow signal abnormalities, pseudoaneurysms, dissection flaps, and intraluminal clot.[236-237] However, the use of MRA as an initial screening modality in the multiply injured patient may be limited by transport issues, availability in off-hours in many institutions, long scanning time, and the need for mechanical ventilation and external fixation devices. MRA has nevertheless been used successfully in screening for the presence of blunt carotid and vertebral injury[238] (see Figs. 2-110 and 2-111).

CT angiography (CTA), which may only add a few minutes to the time required for imaging workup of trauma patients, is a promising methodology for noninvasive screening for blunt carotid and vertebral arterial injury[239,240] (see Fig. 2-105). The latter authors, in a retrospective study, reported that following institution of a CTA protocol in patients sustaining blunt neck injury, patients with carotid arterial injury were more likely to be identified, were diagnosed more rapidly, and were treated more rapidly, with consequent decrease in neurologic morbidity.

Treatment

Many recent reports have stressed the importance of early diagnosis of carotid and vertebral arterial injury in order to start anticoagulation or antiplatelet therapy as soon as is possible.[191,208-209,241] These reports cited improved outcomes in patients who were treated with heparin, compared with patients who did not receive heparin therapy. For example, Fabian et al.[208] reported neurologic improvement in symptomatic patients treated with heparin, compared with untreated patients. Biffl et al.[209] identified 13 patients who were asymptomatic at the time of diagnosis. Ten of the 13 were placed on systemic heparin, with nine remaining free of neurologic complications. Miller et al.[190] were able to give heparin to 39 neurologically asymptomatic patients out of 50 patients with vertebral artery blunt trauma. In their series, treated patients had a stroke rate of 2.6%, versus 54% for untreated patients. Heparin therapy and antiplatelet therapy, however, remain controversial: Eachempati et al.[241] and Kerwin et al.[219] failed to show any statistically significant benefit for antiplatelet therapy or systemic heparin treatment in improving neurologic outcome.

In recent years, stenting has been used to treat traumatic dissections and pseudoaneurysms of the cervical carotid and vertebral arteries.[242-252] This has proven a particularly useful strategy in patients with symptomatic dissections in whom anticoagulation may be contraindicated because of concurrent injuries, patients who become symptomatic despite adequate anticoagulation, and patients with pseudoaneurysms, which are unlikely to heal even with anticoagulation.[224]

At the University of Maryland, patients are initially treated with heparin or antiplatelet therapy where feasible. Endovascular intervention with stenting is performed for progression of neurologic symptoms, worsening luminal compromise with impending occlusion, and enlarging or nonhealing pseudoaneurysms. Diagnostic angiography is performed, and the diameter of the artery to be stented is carefully measured in multiple planes. A suitable guide sheath (e.g., Shuttle, Cook Cardiology Inc., Bloomington, Ind.) is placed in the carotid artery or subclavian artery. Heparin is given to maintain activated clotting time of 200 to 250 seconds. Abciximab (ReoPro) (Eli Lilly and Company, Indianapolis) is given before traversing the injured segment. A soft tip microwire and microcatheter are then used to cross the dissected segment. The microwire is removed, and position in the true lumen is verified by hand injection of the microcatheter distal to the site of injury. Next an extra support 0.014 or 0.018 exchange length microwire is passed through the microcatheter, which is subsequently removed. The stent delivery system (e.g., S.M.A.R.T. Stent, Cordis Endovascular, Miami; WallStent, Boston Scientific, Minneapolis; S670 and S7, Medtronic AVE, Santa Rosa, Calif.) is then posi-

tioned across the injured segment, and the stent is deployed. Small pseudoaneurysms often resolve spontaneously as flow into the pseudoaneurysm sac is disrupted by the stent (Fig. 2-138). Alternatively, small pseudoaneurysms with well-defined necks can often be treated with coiling alone (Fig. 2-139). Larger pseudoaneurysms and those that do not resolve in time may require coil embolization, which can be performed by passing a microcatheter through the stent interstices and into the pseudoaneurysm sac (Fig. 2-140).

The severity of injury seen on initial angiography may be used as a guide to treatment options. Biffl et al.[224] found that two thirds of mild intimal injuries (grade I) were noted to heal, regardless of therapy. The majority (70%) of patients with grade II injuries (dissections or hematomas with luminal stenosis) progressed angiographically despite heparin therapy. Few (8%) pseudoaneurysms (grade III) healed with heparin treatment, but 89% resolved after endovascular stent placement. These authors further reported that in their series grade IV injuries (occlusions) did not recanalize in the early postinjury period and that grade V injuries (transections) were uniformly lethal. They recommended surgical treatment of accessible grade II-V lesions, and a course of anticoagulation for inaccessible grade II-IV injuries. They further noted that endovascular methods may offer the only feasible treatment for most grade V injuries, and may be helpful in the treatment of patients with pseudoaneurysms (grade III injury).

TRAUMATIC INJURIES OF THE INTRACRANIAL CEREBRAL ARTERIES

Traumatic injury to the intracranial arteries may occur in the setting of closed head injury, penetrating skull injury, or iatrogenic injury (e.g., during surgical or endovascular procedures). Although severe traumatic injury to the intracranial arteries is often obvious on the initial head CT, as with injuries of the cervical segments of the intracranial arteries, the nature of the injury and development of neurologic sequelae may not be immediately evident. Traumatic injuries of the large intracranial arteries fall into two main categories: (1) aneurysms and pseudoaneurysms and (2) arteriovenous fistulae.

Traumatic Aneurysms and Pseudoaneurysms

These involve partial or complete disruption of the arterial wall. In true aneurysms, the intima and adventitia are intact. In pseudoaneurysms, the artery is perforated, and the apparent wall of the aneurysm is contained within an extraluminal clot. It is often difficult to differentiate true aneurysms from pseudoaneurysms on the basis of cerebral angiography.

Aneurysms and pseudoaneurysms of the intracranial arteries result from penetrating trauma, such as stab wounds,[253] gunshot wounds,[254-257] nail-gun missile injuries[258] (see Fig. 2-107), and skull fracture with traumatic laceration or dissection of the artery.[259-261] They may also result from closed head injury[262-265] secondary to shear injury or impaction of arteries against fixed dural structures such as the falx cerebri.[264,266]

In the petrous and cavernous segments of the ICA, pseudoaneurysms are thought to be more common than true aneurysms. In these locations, a classic triad of presenting symptoms and signs is (1) skull base or orbital fracture, (2) visual deficits (e.g., unilateral blindness, blurred vision, extraocular muscle palsies), and (3) hemorrhage, such as bleeding into the middle ear cavity or epistaxis in cases where the bleeding site communicates with the sphenoid sinus.[261,267,268] Presentation of hemorrhagic symptoms and detection on angiography may be immediate or delayed.[261,262,268,269]

Pseudoaneurysms of arteries within the subarachnoid space can present as acute intracranial hemorrhage.[270] If a severe laceration is present, the injury is often immediately fatal. However, formation of a pseudoaneurysm may also be delayed, and hemorrhage or thromboembolic complications may not appear until weeks or even months after the traumatic episode.[255,256] Unless the managing physician suspects the injury enough to order angiographic workup, it may go undetected.

In general, traumatic pseudoaneurysms do not resolve spontaneously. Treatment alternatives include surgical clipping or arterial reconstruction, trapping of the aneurysm by surgical or endovascular means, occlusion of the parent vessel with detachable balloons or coils, and vascular bypass.[270,271]

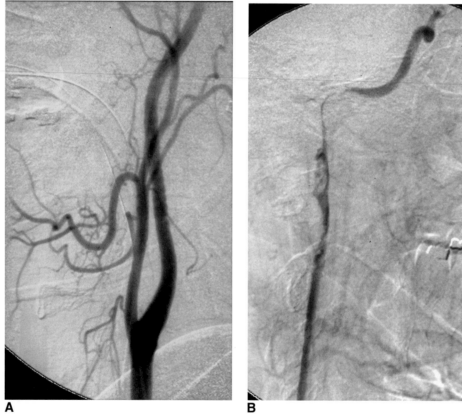

A **B**

Fig. 2-137
Vascular injury scale of Biffl.[224] **A**, Grade I: The hallmark of this injury is irregularity of the vessel wall. A dissection flap, without significant luminal compromise, may also be seen. **B**, Grade II: Intraluminal thrombus produces an irregular filling defect within the lumen. There is also luminal compromise secondary to a long segment dissection, extending from the cervical segment into the proximal petrous segment.

Continued

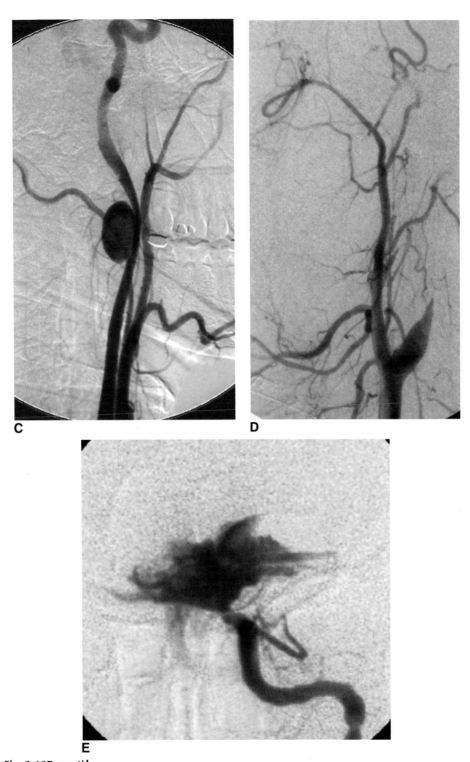

Fig. 2-137, cont'd
C, Grade III: Pseudoaneurysms appear as outpouchings of the vessel wall, most commonly occurring just below the skull base. **D**, Grade IV: The internal carotid artery (ICA) is occluded just beyond the carotid bulb. In some patients, this appearance may result from spasm in the affected vessel. On follow-up angiography, the artery may be patent. **E**, Grade V: Transection. Gross extravasation of contrast is seen. (**E** courtesy D. Coldwell, MD.)

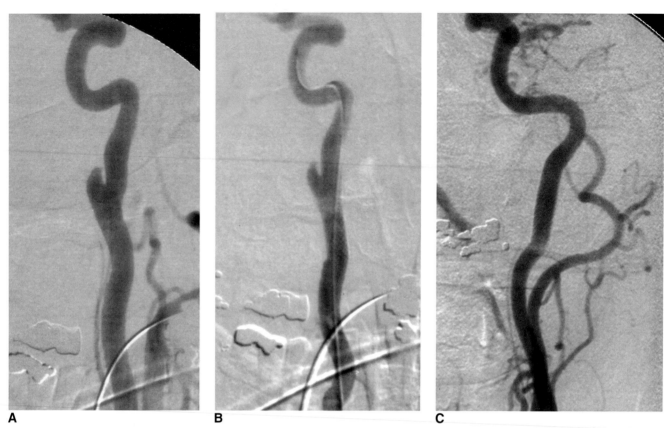

A **B** **C**

Fig. 2-138
Angiograms of left ICA pseudoaneurysm. Before treatment (**A**) immediately after treatment (**B**), and at follow-up 5 months after treatment with stent (**C**).

Intracerebral Arteriovenous Fistulas

Although intracerebral arteriovenous (AV) fistulas may occur after relatively minor trauma, they are more typically seen in the setting of more serious head trauma following a motor vehicle accident or assault injury. The majority of posttraumatic intracranial AV fistulas are carotid-cavernous fistulas (see Figs. 2-15 and 2-137). In these, the cavernous ICA or one of its small intracavernous branches is disrupted, resulting in a direct communication between the torn artery and the surrounding cavernous sinus. The mechanism of injury is thought to be due to laceration of the artery, either by spicules of bone associated with fracture or penetrating injury, or by rupture of the artery at points of dural attachment located between the foramen lacerum and the anterior clinoid process. In older patients, direct carotid-cavernous fistulas may result from rupture of a preexisting intracavernous aneurysm into the cavernous sinus, but this is less common. Posttraumatic direct arteriovenous fistulas have been reported in other locations [272,273] but are much less common. Dural arteriovenous malformations, in which meningeal arteries communicate with venous sinuses, have also been associated with a history of trauma.

Various classifications have been used to describe the spectrum of carotid-cavernous fistulas. The most commonly used classification[274] is as follows:

Intracavernous ICA to cavernous sinus

Dural branches of the ICA to cavernous sinus

Dural branches of the external carotid artery to cavernous sinus

Dural branches of both the internal and external carotid arteries to cavernous sinus

Patients with either direct carotid-cavernous fistulas or dural arteriovenous malformations of the cavernous sinus may present with headache, orbital or temporal bruit, chemosis, exophthalmos, cranial nerve deficits involving the extraocular muscles, visual disturbances, and venous infarcts. The timing and severity of presenting symptoms depend on a variety of factors, including the size of the arterial rent and the available routes of venous drainage.

The hallmark of angiographic findings in carotid-cavernous fistula is nearly instantaneous filling of the cavernous sinus. In most cases, the subcompartments of the ipsilateral cavernous sinus communicate freely with one another, and subsequently drainage occurs to the ipsilateral superior ophthalmic vein and inferior petrosal sinus. Drainage to the contralateral cavernous sinus via the intercavernous (circular) sinus is also common; in these patients, bilateral orbital symptoms may rarely result, as the arterialized cavernous sinuses drain to bilateral superior ophthalmic veins. Arterial-level pressures within the superior ophthalmic veins cause venous hypertension within the orbit, with resultant chemosis, proptosis, stretching of the optic nerve, and deterioration in vision. Infrequently, drainage is to cerebral cortical veins (most commonly the sphenoparietal sinus or uncal vein),[275] with cerebral venous hypertension and resulting cortical venous ischemia or infarct.[276]

Angiographic workup should include selective internal carotid and external carotid injections to distinguish direct fistulas from indirect ones, as well as vertebral injection to evaluate collateral flow in the Circle of Willis. High filming rates are essential in visualizing the fistula point. Extended filming during the venous phase is also useful to assess routes of venous drainage and to evaluate whether cerebral cortical venous hypertension is present.[277]

Indications for urgent treatment include (1) increased ICP or presence of cerebral cortical venous hypertension, (2) deterioration in vision, (3) increased intraocular pressure, and (4) worsening proptosis. Endovascular occlusion of carotid-cavernous fistulas with preservation of the parent artery is the current preferred treatment.[278-280] Direct carotid-cavernous fistulas are most commonly treated using a detachable balloon device (e.g., DSB Detachable Silicone Balloon, Boston Scientific Meditech

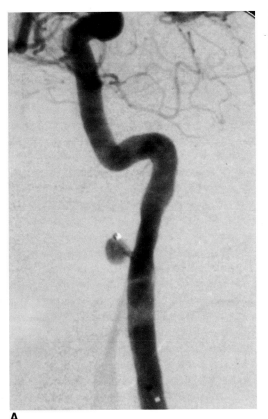 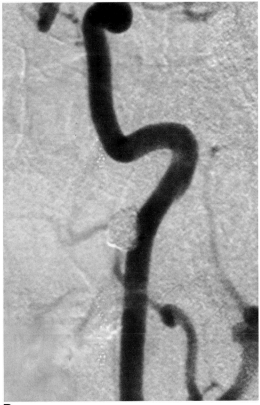

A **B**

Fig. 2-139
Angiography of small pseudoaneurysm of left ICA. **A**, before and **B**, after placement of Guglielmi Detachable Coils into the pseudoaneurysm sac.

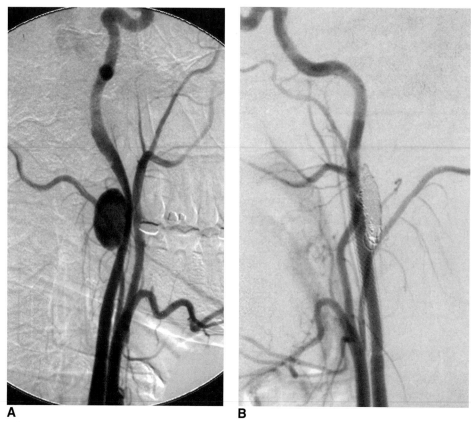

A   **B**

Fig. 2-140
Angiography of large pseudoaneurysm of left ICA. Before treatment (**A**) and after stent deployment (**B**) across the neck of the pseudoaneurysm and placement of Guglielmi Detachable Coils within the pseudoaneurysm sac.

Target, Fremont, Calif.; Coaxial Angiographic Catheter Set, Boston Scientific Meditech Target, Fremont, Calif.). The device is passed transarterially to the fistula point. With slight inflation of the balloon, the balloon is pulled through the fistula, into the cavernous sinus. Subsequent inflation of the balloon within the cavernous sinus will often tamponade the fistula point, without encroaching on the ICA.[278] Alternatively, coils may be placed within the cavernous sinus, either by transarterial or transvenous routes, to occlude the fistula.[278-282]

Facial Trauma and Epistaxis

Massive maxillofacial hemorrhage may be secondary to facial fractures[283-286] or penetrating trauma.[287,288] Clinical findings, such as obvious hemorrhage or expanding hematoma, may occur immediately or may be delayed.

Patients referred for potential endovascular treatment of severe facial bleeding and epistaxis following trauma often have multiple injuries and may be hemodynamically unstable. Appropriate triage to ensure that the most threatening injuries are treated first (e.g., treatment of craniofacial injury versus visceral or limb injury) is crucial. Intubation or tracheostomy to protect the airway is mandatory in severely injured patients. Even in a cooperative and conscious patient, prophylactic intubation before angiography is often prudent, as nasal and oral bleeding may recur during the procedure. Some patients may have had packing placed in the oropharynx or nasopharynx, and the site of bleeding may not be evident. It is thus important to review CT images and discuss with the referring physician clinical findings prior to packing in order to try to determine the most likely sources of bleeding.

Arch aortography or common carotid angiography, with the catheter positioned low in the artery, is usually a useful first step to evaluate for proximal injury and to evaluate the internal carotid circulation. If no internal carotid injury requiring immediate intervention is present, attention can then be directed to the external carotid artery. If no definite pseudoaneurysms or lacerations of the major external carotid branches are evident on common carotid angiography, selective injection of the external carotid artery should be performed.

Pseudoaneurysms or transections of major branches of the external carotid artery are often treated using coils. Because of the propensity of the external carotid branches to collateralize and reconstitute one another, it is important to deploy coils both distal and proximal to the injury wherever technically possible.

Where smaller branches are lacerated, or where a definitive site of bleeding is not identified, the goal of treatment is to decrease the pressure head to the region of injury. In this setting, superselective PVA embolization with particles in the 250 to 500 micron range is often effective.[289] For example, in LeFort fractures, superselective PVA embolization of bilateral internal maxillary arteries (and, where possible, descending palatine arteries) usually yields the desired result. PVA particles smaller than 250 microns should not be used, so as to avoid devascularization of the capillary bed and possible embolization to dangerous collaterals (e.g., ethmoidal branches of the ophthalmic artery). Following embolization, control angiography of both the ipsilateral and contralateral external carotid arteries should be performed to evaluate potential sources of collateral supply that may cause rehemorrhage.

REFERENCES

1. Frazee JG: Head trauma, Emerg Med Clin North Am 4:859, 1986.
2. Weller RO, Swash M, McLellan DL, Scholtz CL: Trauma to the central nervous system. In Clinical neuropathology, New York, 1983, Springer-Verlag.
3. Paterakis K, Karantanas AH, Komnos A, Volikas Z: Outcome of patients with diffuse axonal injury: the significance and prognostic value of MRI in the acute phase, J Trauma 49:1071, 2000.
4. Zimmerman RA, Bilaniuk LT, Gennarelli T, et al: Cranial computed tomography in the diagnosis and management of acute head trauma, AJR 131:27, 1978.
5. Masters SJ, McClean PM, Arcarese JS, et al: Skull X-ray examination after head trauma, N Engl J Med 316:84, 1987.
6. Heng RC, Bell KW: Interpreting urgent brain CT scans: does review by a radiology trainee make a difference in accuracy? Australas Radiol 45:134, 2001.
7. Bruce DA: Imaging after head trauma: why, when and which, Childs Nerv Syst 16:755, 2002.
8. Udstuen GJ, Claar JM: Imaging of acute head injury in the adult, Semin Ultrasound CT MR 22:135, 2001.
9. Woodcock RJ, Davis PC, Hopkins KL: Imaging of head trauma in infancy and childhood, Semin Ultrasound CT MR 22:162, 2001.
10. Goldmann RW: Pneumocephalus as a consequence of barotrauma, JAMA 255:3154, 1986.
11. Tsai FY, Zee CS, Apthorp JB, Dixon GH: Computed tomography in child abuse head trauma CT, J Comput Tomogr 4:277, 1980.
12. Saulsbury FT, Alford BA: Intracranial bleeding from child abuse: the value of skull radiographs, Pediatr Radiol 12:175, 1982.
13. Kleinman PK: Diagnostic imaging in infant abuse, AJR 155:703, 1990.
14. Gentry LR, Godersky JC, Thompson B, et al: Prospective comparative study of intermediate-field MR and CT in the evaluation of closed head trauma, AJNR 9:91, 1988.
15. Kelly AB, Zimmerman RD, Snow RB, et al: Head trauma: comparison of MR and CT—experience in 100 patients, AJNR 9:699, 1988.
16. Levin HS, Amparo E, Eisenberg HM, et al: Magnetic resonance imaging and computerized tomography in relation to the neurobe-havioral sequelae of mild to moderate head injuries, J Neurosurg 66:706, 1987.
17. Hesselink JR, Dowd CF, Healy ME, et al: MR imaging of brain contusions: a comparative study with CT, AJNR 9:269, 1988.
18. Hartshorne MF: Clinical experience with ultra-low field MRI: presented at "Present Concepts in Diagnostic Radiology," San Antonio, Tex, April 24-26, 1989.
19. NIH Consensus Development Panel: Rehabilitation of persons with traumatic brain injury, JAMA 282:974, 1999.
20. Parizel PM, Ozsarlak O, VanGoethem JW, et al: Imaging findings in diffuse axonal injury after closed head trauma, Eur Radiol 8:960, 1998.
21. Wallesch CW, Curio N, Galazky I, Jost, S, Synowitz H: The neuropsychology of blunt head injury in the early postacute stage: effects of focal lesions and diffuse axonal injury, J Neurotrauma 18:11, 2001.
22. Parizel PM: Outcome after mild-to-moderate blunt head injury: effects of focal lesions and diffuse axonal injury, Brain Inj 15:401, 2001.
23. Guardjian ES: Recent advances in the study of the mechanism of impact injury of the head—summary, Clin Neurosurg 19:1, 1972.
24. Heever CM, Merwe DJ: Management of depressed skull fractures, Neurosurgery 71:186, 1989.
25. Jenett B, Miller SO, Braakman R: Epilepsy after nonmissile depressed skull fracture, J Neurosurg 41:208, 1974.
26. Meservy CH, Towbin R, McLaurin PL, Myers PA, Ball W: Radiographic characteristics of skull fractures resulting from child abuse, AJNR 8:455, 1987.
27. Tedeschi CG: Injury to the central nervous system by physical agents. In Tedeschi CG, ed: Neuropathology: methods and diagnosis, Boston, 1970, Little, Brown.
28. Lindenberg R: Pathology of craniocerebral injuries. In Newton TH, Potts DG, eds: Radiology of the skull and brain, St Louis, 1977, Mosby.
29. Holland BA, Brant-Zawadski M: High-resolution CT of temporal bone trauma, AJR 143:391, 1984.
30. Dolan KD: Temporal bone fractures, Semin Ultrasound CT MR 10:262,1989.
31. Joslyn JN, Mirvis SE, Markowitz B: Complex fractures of the clivus: diagnosis with CT and clinical outcome in 11 patients, Radiology 166:817, 1988.
32. Corradino G, Wolf AL, Mirvis SE, Joslyn J: Fractures of the clivus: classification and clinical features, Neurosurgery 24:592, 1990.
33. Anthony DC, Atwater SK, Rozear MP, Burger PC: Occlusion of the basilar artery within a fracture of the clivus, J Neurosurg 66:929, 1987.
34. El Gindi S, Salma M, Tqwfik E, Nasr HA, El Nadi F: A review of 2,000 patients with craniocerebral injuries with regard to intracranial hematomas and other vascular complications, Acta Neurochir (Wien) 28:237,1979.
35. Cooper PB: Post-traumatic intracranial mass lesions. In Cooper PB, ed: Head injury, Baltimore, 1978, Williams & Wilkins.
36. Hardman JM: The pathology of traumatic brain injuries. In Thompson RA, Green JR, eds: Advances in neurology, vol 22, New York, 1979, Raven Press.
37. Zimmerman RA, Bilaniuk LT: Head trauma. In Rosenberg RN, ed: Neuroradiology, vol 4, Clinical neurosciences, New York, 1984, Churchill Livingstone.
38. Voris HC: Craniocerebral trauma. In Baker AB, Baker LH, eds: Clinical neurology, New York, 1982, Harper & Row.
39. Reed D, Robertson WD, Graeb D, et al: Acute subdural hematomas: atypical CT findings, AJNR 7:417, 1986.
40. Lobato RD, Rivas JJ, Cordobes F, et al: Acute epidural hematoma: an analysis of factors influencing the outcome of patients undergoing surgery in coma, J Neurosurg 68:417, 1988.
41. Aoki N: Rapid resolution of acute epidural hematoma: report of two cases, J Neurosurg 68:149, 1988.

42. Borovich B: Delayed onset of traumatic extradural hematoma, *J Neurosurg* 63:30, 1985.

43. Gennarelli TA, Thibault LE: Biomechanics of acute subdural hematoma, *J Trauma* 22:680, 1982.

44. Sahuquillo-Barris J, Lamarca-Ciuro J, Vilata-Castan J, et al: Acute subdural hematoma and diffuse axonal injury after severe head trauma, *J Neurosurg* 68:894, 1988.

45. Zimmerman RA, Bilaniuk LT, Bruce D, et al: Interhemispheric acute subdural hematoma: a computed tomographic manifestation of child abuse by shaking, *Neuroradiology* 16:39, 1978.

46. Seelig JM, Becker DP, Miller JD, et al: Traumatic acute subdural hematoma, *N Engl J Med* 304:1511, 1981.

47. Yoshino E, Yamaki T, Higuchi T, Horikawa K: Acute brain edema in fatal head injury: analysis by dynamic CT scanning, *J Neurosurg* 63:830, 1985.

48. Smith WP, Batnitzky S, Rengachary SS: Acute subdural hematomas: a problem in anemic patients, *AJNR* 2:37, 1981.

49. Mancu H, Becker H: Computed tomography of isodense chronic subdural hematomas, *Radiology* 14:81, 1977.

50. Kim KS, Hemmati M, Weinberg PE: Computed tomography in isodense subdural hematoma, *Radiology* 128:71, 1978.

51. Hayman LA, Evans RA, Hinck VC: Rapid high-dose contrast computed tomography of isodense subdural hematoma and cerebral swelling, *Radiology* 131:381, 1978.

52. Moller A, Erickson K: Computed tomography of isoattenuating subdural hematomas, *Radiology* 130:149, 1979.

53. Braun J, Borovich B, Guilburd JN, et al: Acute subdural hematoma mimicking epidural hematoma on CT, *AJNR* 8:171, 1987.

54. Osborn AG, Anderson RE, Wing SD: The false falx sign, *Radiology* 134:421, 1980.

55. Zimmerman RD, Russel EJ, Yurberg E, Leeds NE: Falx and interhemispheric fissure on axial CT. II. recognition and differentiation of interhemispheric subarachnoid and subdural hemorrhage, *AJNR* 3:635, 1982.

56. Friede RL, Schachnmayr W: The origin of subdural neomembranes, *Am J Pathol* 92:69, 1978.

57. Lundsford LD, Maroon JC, Sheptek PE, Albin MS: Subdural tension pneumocephalus, *J Neurosurg* 50:525, 1979.

58. Ishiwata Y, Fugitsu K, Sekino T, et al: Subdural tension pneumocephalus following surgery for chronic subdural hematoma, *J Neurosurg* 68:58, 1988.

59. Gomori JM, Grossman RI, Goldberg HI, et al: Intracranial hematomas: imaging by high-field MR, *Radiology* 157:87, 1985.

60. Gomori JM, Grossman RI, Hackney DB, et al: Variable appearance of subacute intracranial hematomas on high-field spin-echo MR, *AJR* 150:171, 1988.

61. Fobben ES, Grossman RI, Atlas SW, et al: MR characteristics of subdural hematomas and hygromas at 1.5T, *AJNR* 10:587, 1989.

62. Fukuda T, Hasue M, Ito H: Does traumatic subarachnoid hemorrhage caused by diffuse brain injury cause delayed ischemic brain damage? Comparison with subarachnoid hemorrhage caused by ruptured intracranial aneurysms, *Neurosurgery* 43:1040, 1998.

63. Nussbaum ES, Wolf Al, Sebring L, Mirvis SE: Surgical resuscitation of transtentorial herniation by complete temporal lobectomy in unilateral hemispheric swelling, *Neurosurgery* 29:62, 1991.

64. Orrison WW, Gentry LR, Stimac GK, et al: Blinded comparison of cranial CT and MR in closed head injury evaluation, *AJNR* 15:351, 1994.

65. Zimmerman RA, Bilaniuk LT, Hackney DB, et al: Head injury: early results of comparing CT and high-field MR, *AJR* 147:1215, 1986.

66. Clifton GL, Grossman RG, Makela ME, et al: Neurologic course and correlated computerized tomography findings after severe closed head injury, *J Neurosurg* 52:611, 1980.

67. Gennarelli TA, Thibault LE, Adams JH, et al: Diffuse axonal injury and traumatic coma in the primate, *Ann Neurol* 12:564, 1982.

68. Adams JH, Graham DI, Murray LS, Scott G: Diffuse axonal injury due to nonmissile head injury in humans: an analysis of 45 cases, *Ann Neurol* 12:557, 1982.

69. Zimmerman RA, Bilaniuk LT, Gennarelli T: Computed tomography of shearing injuries of the cerebral white matter, *Radiology* 127:393, 1978.

70. Sahuquillo J, Vilalta J, Lamarca J, et al: Diffuse axonal injury after severe head trauma, *Acta Neurochir (Wien)* 101:149, 1989.

71. Cardobes F, Lobato RD, Rivas JJ, et al: Posttraumatic diffuse axonal injury: analysis of 78 patients studied with computed tomography, *Acta Neurochir (Wien)* 81:27, 1986.

72. Maki Y, Akimoto H, Encomoto T: Injuries of basal ganglia following head trauma in children, *Childs Brain* 7:113, 1980.

73. Leclercq PD, McKenzie JD, Graham DK, Gentleman SM: Axonal injury is accentuated in the caudal corpus callosum of head-injured patients, *J Neurotrauma* 13:1, 2001.

74. Friese SA, Bitzer M, Freudenstein D, et al: Classification of acquired lesions of the corpus callosum with MRI, *Neuroradiology* 42:795, 2000.

75. Rugg-Gunn FJ, Symms MR, Barker GJ, et al: Diffusion imaging shows abnormalities after blunt head trauma when conventional magnetic resonance imaging is normal, *J Neurol Neurosurg Psychiatry* 70:530, 2001.

76. Nakahara M, Erickson K, Bellander BM: Diffusion-weighted MR and apparent diffusion coefficient in the evaluation of severe brain injury, *Acta Radiol* 42:365, 2001.

77. Bagley LJ, McGowan JC, Grossman RI, et al: Magnetization transfer imaging of traumatic brain injury, *J Magn Reson Imaging* 11:1, 2000.

78. Sinson G, Bagley LJ, Cecil KM, et al: Magnetization transfer imaging and proton MR spectroscopy in the evaluation of axonal injury: correlation with clinical outcome after traumatic brain injury, *Am J Neurosurgery* 22:14, 2001.

79. Brooks WM, Friedman SD, Gasparov C: Magnetic resonance spectroscopy in traumatic brain injury, *J Head Trauma Rehabil* 16:149, 2001.

80. Takayama H, Kobayashi M, Sugishita M, Mihara B: Diffusion-weighted imaging demonstrates transient cytotoxic edema involving the corpus callosum in a patient with diffuse brain injury, *Clin Neurol Neurosurg* 102:135, 2000.

81. Suh DY, Davis, PC, Hopkins KL, et al: Nonaccidental pediatric head injury: diffusion-weighted imaging findings, *Neurosurgery* 49:309, 2001.

82. Bruce DA, Alavi A, Bilaniuk L, et al: Diffuse cerebral swelling following head injuries in children: the syndrome of "malignant cerebral edema," *J Neurosurg* 54:170, 1981.

83. Bullock R, Smith R, Favier J, et al: Brain specific gravity and CT scan density measurement after human head injury, *J Neurosurg* 63:64, 1985.

84. Oliff M, Fried AM, Young AB: Intraventricular hemorrhage in blunt head trauma, *J Comput Assist Tomogr* 2:625, 1978.

85. Adams RD, Victor M: Intracranial neoplasms. In Adams RD, Victor M, eds: *Principles of neurology*, New York, 1977, McGraw-Hill.

86. Osborn AG: Diagnosis of descending transtentorial herniation by cranial computed tomography, *Radiology* 123:93, 1977.

87. Tsai FY, Teal JS, Quinn MF, et al: CT of brainstem injury, *AJR* 134:717, 1980.

88. Gentry LR, Godersky JC, Thompson B: MR imaging of head trauma: review of the distribution and radiopathologic features of traumatic lesions, *AJR* 150:663, 1988.

89. Zuccarello M, Fiore DL, Trincia G, et al: Traumatic primary brainstem hemorrhage: a clinical and experimental study, *Acta Neurochir (Wien)* 67:103, 1983.

90. Adams JH, Mitchell DE, Graham DI, Doyle D: Diffuse brain damage of immediate impact type, *Brain* 100:489, 1977.

91. Espersen JO, Petersen OF: Computerized tomography in patients with head injuries. *Acta Neurochir (Wien)* 56:201, 1981.

92. French BN, Dublin AB: The value of computerized tomography in the management of 1000 consecutive head injuries, *Surg Neurol* 7:171, 1977.

93. Meyer CA, Mirvis SE, Wolf AL, Thompson RK: CT of acute traumatic midbrain hemorrhage: experimental and clinical observations, *Radiology* 179:813, 1991.

94. Friede TL, Roessmann U: The pathogenesis of secondary midbrain hemorrhages, *Neurology* 16:1210, 1966.

95. Galyon DD, Winfield JA: An unusual syndrome of pediatric brainstem trauma, *Pediatr Neurosci* 14:272, 1988.

96. Klintworth GK: The pathogenesis of secondary brainstem hemorrhages as studied in an experimental model, *Am J Pathol* 47:525, 1965.

97. Lindenberg R: Compression of brain arteries as pathogenetic factor for tissue necrosis and their areas of predilection, *J Neuropathol Exp Neurol* 14:223, 1955.

98. Freytag E: Autopsy findings in head injuries from blunt forces, *Arch Pathol* 75:402, 1963.

99. Lindenberg R: Significance of the tentorium in head injuries from blunt forces, *Clin Neurosurg* 12:129, 1966.

100. Cooper PR, Maravilla K, Kirkpatrick J, et al: Traumatically induced brainstem hemorrhage and the computerized tomographic scan: clinical, pathological and experimental observations, *Neurosurgery* 4:115, 1979.

101. Thompson RK, Salcman M: Dynamic axial brainstem distortion as a mechanism in the production of brainstem hemorrhages: role of the carotid arteries, *Neurosurgery* 22:629, 1988.

102. Weintraub CM: Bruising of the third cranial nerve and the pathogenesis of midbrain hemorrhage, *Br J Surg* 48:62, 1960.

103. Shibata Y, Matsumura A, Meguro K, Narushima K: Differentiation of mechanism and prognosis of traumatic brainstem lesions detected by magnetic resonance imaging in the acute stage, *Clin Neurol Neurosurg* 102:124, 2000.

104. Gentry LR, Godersky JC, Thompson BH: Traumatic brainstem injury: MR imaging, *Radiology* 171:177, 1989.

105. Jacobs L, Kinkel WR, Heffner RR: Autopsy correlation of computerized tomography: experience with 6,000 CT scans, *Neurology* 26:1111, 1976.

106. Komiyama M, Bab M, Hakuba A, et al: MR imaging of brainstem hemorrhage, *AJNR* 9:261, 1988.

107. Han JS, Kaufman B, Alfidi RJ, et al: Head trauma evaluated by magnetic resonance and computed tomography, *Radiology* 150:71, 1984.

108. Wilberger JE, Deeb Z, Rothfus W: Magnetic resonance imaging in cases of severe head injury, *Neurosurgery* 20:571, 1987.

109. Pozzati E, Giuliano G, Poppi M, Faenza A: Blunt traumatic carotid dissection with delayed symptoms, *Stroke* 20:412, 1989.

110. Shaw CM, Alvord EC: Injury of the basilar artery associated with closed head trauma, *J Neurol Neurosurg Psychiatry* 35:247, 1972.

111. Fakhry SM, Jaques PF, Proctor HJ: Cervical vessel injury after blunt trauma, *J Vasc Surg* 8:501, 1988.

112. Fry WJ, Fry RE: Management of carotid artery injury. In Bergan JJ, Yao JST, eds: *Vascular surgical emergencies*, Orlando, 1987, Grune & Stratton.

113. Nelson AT, Kishore PRS, Lee SH: Development of delayed epidural hematoma, *AJNR* 3:583, 1982.

114. Bucci MN, Phillips TW, McGillicuddy JF: Delayed epidural hemorrhage in hypotensive multiple trauma patients, *Neurosurgery* 19:65, 1986.

115. Milo R, Razon N, Schiffer J. Delayed epidural hematoma, *Acta Neurochir (Wien)* 84:13, 1987.

116. Piepmeier JM, Wagner FC: Delayed posttraumatic extracerebral hematomas, *J Trauma* 22:455, 1982.

117. Fukamachi A, Kohno K, Nagaseki Y, et al: The incidence of delayed traumatic intracerebral hematoma with extradural hemorrhages, *J Trauma* 25:145, 1985.

118. Hirsch LF: Delayed traumatic intracerebral hematomas after surgical decompression, *Neurosurgery* 5:653, 1979.

119. Brunetti J, Zingesser L, Dunn J, Rovit RL: Delayed intracerebral hemorrhage as demonstrated by CT scanning, *Neuroradiology* 18:43, 1979.

120. Gudeman SK, Kishore PRS, Miller JD, et al: The genesis and significance of delayed traumatic intracerebral hematoma, *Neurosurgery* 5:309, 1979.

121. Lipper MH, Rad FF, Kishore RS, et al: Delayed intracranial hematoma in patients with severe head injury, *Radiology* 133:645, 1979.

122. Diaz FG, Yock DH, Larson D, Rockswold GL: Early diagnosis of delayed posttraumatic intracerebral hematoma, *J Neurosurg* 50:217, 1979.

123. Sato M, Tanaka S, Kohama A, Fugi C: Occipital lobe infarction caused by tentorial herniation, *Neurosurgery* 18:300, 1986.

124. Rothfus WE, Goldberg AL, Tabes JH, Deeb ZL: Callosomarginal infarction secondary to transfalcine herniation, *AJNR* 8:1073, 1987.

125. Kearne JR: Blindness following tentorial herniation, *Ann Neurol* 8:186, 1986.

126. Mauskop A, Wolintz AH, Valderrama R: Cerebral infarction and subdural hematoma, *J Clin Neuroophthalmol* 4:251, 1984.

127. Suwanwela C, Suwanwela N: Intracranial arterial narrowing and spasm in acute head injury, *J Neurosurg* 36:314, 1972.

128. Mooney RP, Bessen HA: Delayed hemiparesis following nonpenetrating carotid artery trauma, *Am J Emerg Med* 6:341, 1988.

129. Marshall LF, Bruce DA, Bruno L, Langfitt TW: Vertebrobasilar spasm: a significant cause of neurologic deficit in head injury, *J Neurosurg* 48:560, 1978.

130. Pasqualin A, Vivenza C, Licata C, et al: Cerebral vasospasm after head injury, *Neurosurgery* 15:855, 1984.

131. Wilkens RH, Odom GL: Intracranial arterial spasm associated with craniocerebral trauma, *J Neurosurg* 32:626, 1970.

132. Weisberg LA: CT and acute head trauma, *Comput Radiol* 3:15, 1979.

133. MacPherson P, Graham DI: Arterial spasm and slowing of the cerebral circulation in the ischemia of head injury, *J Neurol Neurosurg Psychiatry* 36:1069, 1973.

134. Tsai FY, Teal JS, Heishima GB: *Neuroradiology of head trauma*, Baltimore, 1984, University Park.

135. Mears GD, Leonard RB: Blunt carotid artery trauma: a case report, *Am J Emerg Med* 6:281, 1988.

136. Mirvis SE, Wolf AL, Numaguchi Y, et al: Posttraumatic cerebral infarction diagnosed by CT: prevalence, origin, and outcome, *AJNR* 11:355, 1990.

137. Haimes AB, Zimmerman RD, Morgello S, et al: MR imaging of brain abscesses, *AJNR* 10:279, 1989.

138. Eljamel MS, Foy PM: Acute traumatic CSF fistulae: the risk of intracranial infection, *Br J Neurosurg* 4:381, 1990.

139. Calcaterra TC: Extracranial surgical repair of cerebrospinal fluid rhinorrhea, *Ann Otol Rhinol Laryngol* 89:103, 1980.

140. Lewin W: Cerebrospinal fluid rhinorrhea in closed head injuries, *Br J Surg* 42:1, 1954.

141. Glaubitt D, Haubrich J, Cordoni-Voutsas M: Detection and quantification of intermittent CSF rhinorrhea during prolonged cisternography with ^{111}In-DTPA, *AJNR* 4:560, 1983.

142. Manelfe C, Cellerier P, Sobel D, et al: Cerebrospinal fluid rhinorrhea: evaluation with metrizamide cisternography, *AJR* 138:471, 1982.

143. Gardner T, Gage R: Cerebrospinal otorrhea, *Arch Otolaryngol* 1:19, 1970.

144. Henry RC, Taylor PH: Cerebrospinal fluid otorrhea and rhinorrhea following closed head injury, *J Laryngol Otol* 92:743, 1978.

145. Hicks GW, Wright JR Jr, Wright JW III: Cerebrospinal fluid otorrhea., *Laryngoscope* 90:1, 1980.

146. Zimmerman RA, Bilaniuk LT: Computed tomography in pediatric brain trauma, *J Neuroradiol* 8:257, 1981.

147. Zimmerman RA, Bilaniuk LT, Gennarelli T, et al: Cranial computed tomography in diagnosis and management of acute brain trauma, *AJR* 1311:27, 1978.

148. Zimmerman RA, Bilaniuk LT, Bruce D, et al: Computed tomography of pediatric brain trauma: acute general cerebral swelling, *Radiology* 126:403, 1978.

149. Noguchi K, Seto H, Kamisaki Y, et al: Comparison of fluid-attenuated inversion-recovery MR imaging with CT in a simulated model of acute subarachnoid hemorrhage, *AJNR* 21:923, 2000.

150. Mitchell P, Wilkinson ID, Hoggard N, et al: Detection of subarachnoid hemorrhage with magnetic resonance imaging, *J Neurol Neurosurg Psychiatry* 70:205, 2001.

151. Zimmerman RA, Bilaniuk LT, Hackney DB, et al: Magnetic resonance imaging in temporal bone fracture, *Neuroradiology* 29:246, 1987.

152. Sutton LN, Wehrli SL, Genarelli L, et al: High-resolution 1H magnetic resonance spectroscopy of pediatric posterior fossa brain tumors, *Neurosurgery* 81:443, 1994.

153. Zimmerman RA, Haselgrove JC, Wang Z: Advances in pediatric neuroimaging. *Brain Dev* 20:275, 1998.

154. Zimmerman RA, Naidich TP: Magnetic resonance angiography. In Salcman M, ed: *Current techniques in neurosurgery*, Philadelphia, 1993.

155. Dolinskas C, Zimmerman RA, Bilaniuk LT: A sign of subarachnoid bleeding on cranial computed tomograms of pediatric brain trauma patients, *Radiology* 126:409, 1978.

156. Papasian NC, Frim DM. A theoretical model of benign external hydrocephalus that predicts a predisposition towards extra-axial hemorrhage after minor head trauma, *Pediatr Neurosurg* 33:188, 2000.

157. Noguchi K, Ogawa T, Seto H, et al: Subacute and chronic subarachnoid hemorrhage: diagnosis with fluid-attenuated inversion-recovery imaging, *Radiology* 203:257, 1997.

158. Zimmerman RA, Bilaniuk LT, Bruce D, et al: Computed tomography of craniocerebral injury in the abused child, *Radiology* 10:687, 1979.

159. Greenberg J, Cohen WA, Cooper PR: The "hyperacute" extra-axial intracranial hematoma: computed tomographic findings and clinical significance, *Neurosurgery* 17:48, 1985.

160. Gentry LR, Thompson B, Godersky JC: Trauma to the corpus callosum: MR features, *AJNR* 9:1129, 1988.

161. Seidenwurm D, Tze-Kong M, Kowalski K, et al: Intracranial hemorrhagic lesions evaluated with spin-echo and gradient-refocused MR images at 0.5 and 1.5 T, *Radiology* 172:189, 1989.

162. Groswasser Z, Reider-Groswasser I, Soroker N, Machtey Y: Magnetic resonance imaging in brain injury patients with normal late computed tomography scans, *Surg Neurol* 27:331, 1987.

163. Levin HS, Williams DH, Valestro M, et al: Corpus callosal atrophy following closed brain injury: detection with MR, *J Neurosurg* 73:77, 1990.

164. Soloniuk D, Pitts LH, Lovely M, Bartowski H: Traumatic intracerebral hematomas: timing of appearance and indications for operative removal, *J Trauma* 26:787, 1986.

165. Koo AH, LaRoque RL: Evaluation of brain trauma by computed tomography, *Radiology* 123:345, 1977,

166. Young HA, Gleave JRW, Schmidek HH, Gregory S: Delayed traumatic intracerebral hematomas: report of 15 cases operatively treated, *Neurosurgery* 14:22, 1984.

167. Ninchoji T, Nemura K, Shimoyama I, et al: Traumatic intracerebral haematomas of delayed onset, *Acta Neurochir (Wien)* 71:69, 1984.

168. Radkowski MA, Merten DR, Leonidas JC: The abused child: criteria for the radiological diagnosis, *Radiographics* 3:262, 1983.

169. Bruce DA, Zimmerman RA: Shaken impact syndrome, *Pediatr Ann* 18:482, 1989.

170. Rivera FP, Kamitsuka MD, Quan L: Injuries to children younger than one year of age, *Pediatrics* 81:93, 1988.

171. DiScala C, Sege R, Li G, Reece RM. Child abuse and unintentional injuries: a 10-year retrospective, *Arch Pediatr Adolesc Med* 154:16, 2000.

172. Merten DF, Osborne DRS, Radkowski MA, et al: Craniocerebral trauma in the child abuse syndrome: radiological observations, *Pediatr Radiol* 14:272, 1984.

173. Billmire ME, Myers PA: Serious brain injury in infants: accident or abuse? *Pediatrics* 75:340, 1985.

174. Harwood-Nash DC: Abuse to the pediatric central nervous system, *AJNR* 13:569, 1992.

175. Kanter RK: Retinal hemorrhage after cardiopulmonary resuscitation or child abuse, *J Pediatr* 108:430, 1986.

176. Planten JT, Schaaf PC: Retinal hemorrhages in the newborn, *Ophthalmologica* 162:213, 1971.

177. Duhaime AC, Gennarelli TA, Thibault LE, et al: The shaken baby syndrome: a clinical, pathological, and biochemical study, *J Neurosurg* 66:409, 1987.

178. Calder IM, Hill I, Scholtz CL: Primary brain trauma in non-accidental injury, *J Clin Pathol* 37:1095, 1984.

179. Lindenberg R, Freytag E: Morphology of brain lesions from blunt trauma in early infancy, *Arch Pathol* 87:298, 1969.

180. Bird CR, McMahan JR, Gilles FH, et al: Strangulation in child abuse: CT diagnosis, *Radiology* 163:373, 1987.

181. Yamada S, Kindt GW, Youmans JR: Carotid artery occlusion due to nonpenetrating injury, *J Trauma* 7:333, 1967.

182. Krajewski LP, Hertzer NR: Blunt carotid artery trauma: report of two cases and review of the literature, *Ann Surg* 191:341, 1980.

183. Perry MO, Snyder WH, Thal ER: Carotid artery injuries caused by blunt trauma, *Ann Surg* 192:74, 1980.

184. Davis JW, Holbrook TL, Hoyt DB, et al: Blunt carotid artery dissection: incidence, associated injuries, screening, and treatment, *J Trauma* 30:1514, 1990.

185. Martin RF, Eldrup-Jorgensen J, Clark DE, et al: Blunt trauma to the carotid arteries, *J Vasc Surg* 14(6):789, 1991.

186. Cogbill TH, Moore EE, Meissner M, et al: The spectrum of blunt injury to the carotid artery: a multicenter perspective, *J Trauma* 37:473, 1994.

187. Ramadan F, Rutledge R, Oller D, et al: Carotid artery trauma: a review of contemporary trauma center experiences, *J Vasc Surg* 21:46, 1995.

188. Carrillo EH, Osborne DL, Spain DA, et al: Blunt carotid artery injuries: difficulties with the diagnosis prior to neurologic event, *J Trauma* 46:1120, 1999.

189. Kraus RR, Bergstein JM, DeBord JR: Diagnosis, treatment, and outcome of blunt carotid arterial injuries, *Am J Surg* 178:190, 1999.

190. Miller PR, Fabian TC, Bee TK, et al: Blunt cerebrovascular injuries: diagnosis and treatment, *J Trauma* 51:279, 2001.

191. Biffl WL, Moore EE, Elliott JP, et al: The devastating potential of blunt vertebral arterial injuries, *Ann Surg* 231:672, 2000.

192. Alimi Y, Di Mauro P, Tomachot L, et al: Bilateral dissection of the internal carotid artery at the base of the skull due to blunt trauma: incidence and severity, *Ann Vasc Surg* 12:557, 1998.

193. Fabian TC, George SM, Jr., Croce MA, et al: Carotid artery trauma: management based on mechanism of injury, *J Trauma* 30:953, 1990.

194. Lee KP, Carlini WG, McCormick GF, et al: Neurologic complications following chiropractic manipulation: a survey of California neurologists, *Neurology* 45:1213, 1995.

195. Peters M, Bohl J, Thomke F, et al: Dissection of the internal carotid artery after chiropractic manipulation of the neck, *Neurology* 45:2284, 1995.

196. Hufnagel A, Hammers A, Schonle PW: Stroke following chiropractic manipulation of the cervical spine, *J Neurol* 246:683, 1999.

197. Parenti G, Orlandi G, Bianchi M, et al: Vertebral and carotid artery dissection following chiropractic cervical manipulation, *Neurosurg Rev* 22:127, 1999.

198. Parwar BL, Fawzi AA, Arnold AC, et al: Horner's syndrome and dissection of the internal carotid artery after chiropractic manipulation of the neck, *Am J Ophthalmol* 131:523, 2001.

199. Rogers L, Sweeney PJ: Stroke: a neurologic complication of wrestling: a case of brainstem stroke in a 17-year-old athlete, *Am J Sports Med* 17:352, 1979.

200. Tramo MJ, Hainline B, Petito F, et al: Vertebral artery injury and cerebellar stroke while swimming: case report, *Stroke* 16:1039, 1985.

201. Lannuzel A, Moulin T, Amsallem D, et al: Vertebral-artery dissection following a judo session: a case report, *Neuropediatrics* 25:106, 1994.

202. Schievink WI, Atkinson JL, Bartleson JD, et al: Traumatic internal carotid artery dissections caused by blunt softball injuries, *Am J Emerg Med* 16:179, 1998.

203. McCrory P: Vertebral artery dissection causing stroke in sport, *J Clin Neurosci* 7:298, 2000.

204. Traflet RF, Babaria AR, Bell RD, et al: Vertebral artery dissection after rapid head turning, *AJNR* 10:650, 1989.

205. Egnor MR, Page LK, David C: Vertebral artery aneurysm—a unique hazard of head banging by heavy metal rockers: case report, *Pediatr Neurosurg* 17:135, 1991.

206. Schievink WI, Bjornsson J, Piepgras DG: Coexistence of fibromuscular dysplasia and cystic medial necrosis in a patient with Marfan's syndrome and bilateral carotid artery dissections, *Stroke* 25:2492, 1994.

207. Duncan MA, Dowd N, Rawluk D, et al: Traumatic bilateral internal carotid artery dissection following airbag deployment in a patient with fibromuscular dysplasia, *Br J Anaesth* 85:476, 2000.

208. Fabian TC, Patton JH, Jr, Croce MA, et al: Blunt carotid injury: importance of early diagnosis and anticoagulant therapy, *Ann Surg* 223:513, 1996.

209. Biffl WL, Moore EE, Ryu RK, et al: The unrecognized epidemic of blunt carotid arterial injuries: early diagnosis improves neurologic outcome, *Ann Surg* 228:462, 1998.

210. Prall JA, Brega KE, Coldwell DM, et al: Incidence of unsuspected blunt carotid artery injury, *Neurosurgery* 42:495, 1998.

211. Louw JA, Mafoyane NA, Small B, et al: Occlusion of the vertebral artery in cervical spine dislocations, *J Bone Joint Surg Br* 72:679, 1990.

212. Woodring JH, Lee C, Duncan V: Transverse process fractures of the cervical vertebrae: are they insignificant? *J Trauma* 34:797, 1993.

213. Willis BK, Greiner F, Orrison WW, et al: The incidence of vertebral artery injury after midcervical spine fracture or subluxation, *Neurosurgery* 134:435, 1994.

214. Friedman D, Flanders A, Thomas C, et al: Vertebral artery injury after acute cervical spine trauma: rate of occurrence as detected by MR angiography and assessment of clinical consequences, *AJR* 164:443, 1995.

215. Weller SJ, Rossitch E Jr, Malek AM: Detection of vertebral artery injury after cervical spine trauma using magnetic resonance angiography, *J Trauma* 46:660, 1999.

216. Mokri B, Sundt TM Jr, Houser OW, et al: Spontaneous dissection of the cervical internal carotid artery, *Ann Neurol* 19:126, 1986.

217. Mokri B, Schievink WI, Olsen KD, et al: Spontaneous dissection of the cervical internal carotid artery: presentation with lower cranial nerve palsies, *Arch Otolaryngol Head Neck Surg* 118:431, 1992.

218. Schievink WI, Mokri B, Garrity JA, et al: Ocular motor nerve palsies in spontaneous dissections of the cervical internal carotid artery, *Neurology* 43:1938, 1993.

219. Kerwin AJ, Bynoe RP, Murray J, et al: Liberalized screening for blunt carotid and vertebral artery injuries is justified, *J Trauma* 51:308, 2001.

220. Houser OW, Mokri B, Sundt TM Jr, et al: Spontaneous cervical cephalic arterial dissection and its residuum: angiographic spectrum, *AJNR* 5:27, 1984.

221. Blankenship BA, Baxter AB, McKann GM II: Delayed cerebral artery pseudoaneurysm after nail gun injury, *AJR* 172:541, 1999.

222. Bavinski G, Killer M, Knosp E, et al: False aneurysms of the intracavernous carotid artery—report of 7 cases, *Acta Neurochir (Wien)* 139:37,1997.

223. Uzan M, Cantasdemir M, Seckin MS, et al: Traumatic intracranial carotid tree aneurysms, *Neurosurgery* 43:1314, 1984.

224. Biffl WL, Moore EE, Offner PJ, et al: Blunt carotid arterial injuries: implications of a new grading scale, *J Trauma* 47:845, 1999.

225. O'Sullivan RM, Graeb DA, Nugent RA, et al: Carotid and vertebral artery trauma: clinical and angiographic features, *Australas Radiol* 35:47, 1991.

226. Conforto AB, Yamamoto F, Evaristo EF, et al: Intracranial vertebral artery dissection presenting as subarachnoid hemorrhage: successful endovascular treatment, *Acta Neurol Scand* 103:64, 2001.

227. Mani RL, Eisenberg RL, McDonald EJ Jr, et al: Complications of catheter cerebral arteriography: analysis of 5,000 procedures. I. Criteria and incidence, *AJR* 131:861, 1978.

228. Mani RL, Eisenberg RL: Complications of catheter cerebral arteriography: analysis of 5,000 procedures. II. Relation of complication rates to clinical and arteriographic diagnoses, *AJR* 131:867, 1978.

229. Mani RL, Eisenberg RL: Complications of catheter cerebral arteriography: analysis of 5,000 procedures. III. Assessment of arteries injected, contrast medium used, duration of procedure, and age of patient, *AJR* 131:871, 1978.

230. Dion JE, Gates PC, Fox AJ, et al: Clinical events following neuroangiography: a prospective study, *Stroke* 18:997, 1987.

231. Warnock NG, Gandhi MR, Bergvall U, et al: Complications of intraarterial digital subtraction angiography in patients investigated for cerebral vascular disease, *Br J Radiol* 66:855, 1993.

232. Executive Committee for the Asymptomatic Carotid Atherosclerosis Study: Endarterectomy for asymptomatic carotid artery stenosis, *JAMA* 273:1421, 1995.

233. Steinke W, Rautenberg W, Schwartz A, et al: Noninvasive monitoring of internal carotid artery dissection, *Stroke* 25:998, 1995.

234. Rommel O, Niedeggen A, Tegenthoff M, et al: Carotid and vertebral artery injury following severe head or cervical spine trauma, *Cerebrovasc Dis* 9:202, 1999.

235. Srinivasan J, Newell DW, Sturzenegger M, et al: Transcranial doppler in the evaluation of internal carotid artery dissection, *Stroke* 27:1226, 1996.

236. Sue DE, Brant-Zawadzki MN, Chance J: Dissection of cranial arteries in the neck: correlation of MRI and arteriography, *Neuroradiology* 34:273, 1992.

237. Klufas RA, Hsu L, Barnes PD, et al: Dissection of the carotid and vertebral arteries: imaging with MR angiography, *AJR* 164:673, 1995.

238. Bok AP, Peter JC: Carotid and vertebral artery occlusion after blunt cervical injury: the role of MR angiography in early diagnosis, *J Trauma* 40:968, 1996.

239. Rogers FB, Baker EF, Osler TM, et al: Computed tomographic angiography as a screening modality for blunt cervical arterial injuries: preliminary results, *J Trauma* 46:380, 1999.

240. Ofer A, Nitecki SS, Braun J, et al: CT angiography of the carotid arteries in trauma to the neck, *Eur J Vasc Endovasc Surg* 21:401, 2001.

241. Eachempati SR, Vaslef SN, Sebastian MW, et al: Blunt vascular injuries of the head and neck: is heparinization necessary? *J Trauma* 45:997, 1998.

242. Miyachi S, Ishiguchi T, Taniguchi K, et al: Endovascular stenting of a traumatic dissecting aneurysm of the extracranial internal carotid artery: case report. *Neurol Med Chir (Tokyo)* 37:270, 1997.

243. Yamashita K, Okamoto S, Kim C, et al: Emergent treatment of iatrogenic dissection of the internal carotid artery with the Palmaz-Schatz stent: case report, *Neurol Med Chir (Tokyo)* 37:336, 1997.

244. Duke BJ, Ryu RK, Coldwell DM, et al: Treatment of blunt injury to the carotid artery by using endovascular stents: an early experience, *J Neurosurg* 87:825, 1997.

245. Klein GE, Szolar DH, Raith J, et al: Posttraumatic extracranial aneurysm of the internal carotid artery: combined endovascular treatment with coils and stents, *AJNR* 18:1261, 1997

246. DeOcampo J, Brillman J, Levy DI: Stenting: a new approach to carotid dissection, *J Neuroimaging* 7:187, 1997.

247. Dorros G, Cohn JM, Palmer LE: Stent deployment resolves a petrous carotid artery angioplasty dissection, *AJNR* 19:392, 1998.

248. Coric D, Wilson JA, Regan JD, et al: Primary stenting of the extracranial internal carotid artery in a patient with multiple cervical dissections: technical case report, *Neurosurgery* 43:956, 1998

249. Price RF, Sellar R, Leung C, et al: Traumatic vertebral arterial dissection and vertebrobasilar arterial thrombosis successfully treated with endovascular thrombolysis and stenting, *AJNR* 19:1677, 1998.

250. Coldwell DM, Novak Z, Ryu RK, et al: Treatment of posttraumatic internal carotid arterial pseudoaneurysms with endovascular stents, *J Trauma* 48:470, 2000.

251. Bush RL, Lin PH, Dodson TF, et al: Endoluminal stent placement and coil embolization for the management of carotid artery pseudoaneurysms, *J Endovasc Ther* 8:53, 2001.

252. Redekop G, Marotta T, Weill A: Treatment of traumatic aneurysms and arteriovenous fistulas of the skull base by using endovascular stents, *J Neurosurg* 95:412, 2001.

253. Kieck CF, deVilliers JC: Vascular lesions due to transcranial stab wounds, *J Neurosurg* 60:42, 1984.

254. Ferry DJ J., Kempe LG: False aneurysm secondary to penetration of the brain through orbitofacial wounds: report of two cases, *J Neurosurg* 36:503, 1972.

255. Aarabi B: Traumatic aneurysms of brain due to high velocity missile head wounds, *Neurosurgery* 22:1056, 1988.

256. Aarabi B: Management of traumatic aneurysms caused by high-velocity missile head wounds, *Neurosurg Clin N Am* 6:775, 1995.

257. Amirjamshidi A, Rahmat H, Abbassioun K: Traumatic aneurysms and arteriovenous fistulas of intracranial vessels associated with penetrating head injuries occurring during war: principles and pitfalls in diagnosis and management: a survey of 31 cases and review of the literature, *J Neurosurg* 84:769, 1996.

258. Rezai AR, Lee M, Kite C, Smyth D, Jafar JJ: Traumatic posterior cerebral artery aneurysm secondary to an intracranial nail: case report, *Surg Neurol* 42:312, 1994.

259. Lee JP, Wang AD: Epistaxis due to traumatic intracavernous aneurysm: case report, *J Trauma* 30:619, 1990.

260. Quintana F, Diez C, Gutierrez A, et al: Traumatic aneurysm of the basilar artery, *AJNR* 17:283, 1996.

261. Proust F, Callonec F, Bellow F, et al: Tentorial edge traumatic aneurysm of the superior cerebellar artery: case report, *J Neurosurg* 87:950, 1997.

262. Ohta M, Matsuno H: Proximal M2 false aneurysm after head trauma: case report, *Neurol Med Chir (Tokyo)* 41:131, 2001.

263. Nakstad P, Nornes H, Hauge HN: Traumatic aneurysms of the pericallosal arteries, *Neuroradiology* 28:335, 1986.

264. Banfield GK, Brasher PF, Deans JA, et al: Intrapetrous carotid artery aneurysm presenting as epistaxis and otalgia, *J Laryngol Otol* 109:865, 1995.

265. Chen D, Concus AP, Halbach VV, Cheung SW: Epistaxis originating from traumatic pseudoaneurysm of the internal carotid artery: diagnosis and endovascular therapy, *Laryngoscope* 103:326, 1998.

266. Hern JD, Coley SC, Hollis LJ, Jayaraj SM: Delayed massive epistaxis due to traumatic intracavernous carotid artery pseudoaneurysm, *J Laryngol Otol* 112:396, 1998.

267. Hemphill JC 3rd, Gress DR, Halbach VV: Endovascular therapy of traumatic injuries of the intracranial cerebral arteries, *Crit Care Clin* 15:811, 1999.

268. Holmes B, Harbaugh RE: Traumatic intracranial aneurysms: a contemporary review, *J Trauma* 35:855, 1993.

269. Higashida RT, Halbach VV, Tsai FY, et al: Interventional neurovascular treatment of traumatic carotid and vertebral artery lesions: results in 234 cases, *AJR* 153:577, 1989

270. Teitelbaum GP, Bernstein K, Choi S, Giannotta SL: Endovascular coil occlusion of a traumatic basilar-cavernous fistula: technical report, *Neurosurgery* 42:1394, discussion, p 1397, 1998.

271. Barrow DL, Spector RH, Braun IF, et al: Classification and treatment of spontaneous carotid-cavernous sinus fistulas, *J Neurosurg* 62:248, 1985.

272. Halbach VV, Higashida RT, Heishima GB, et al: Transvenous embolization of direct carotid cavernous fistulas, *AJNR* 9:741, 1988.

273. Lin TK, Chang CN, Wai YY: Spontaneous intracerebral hematoma from occult carotid cavernous fistula during pregnancy and puerperium, *J Neurosurg* 76:714, 1992.

274. Morris PP: *Practical neuroangiography*, Baltimore, 1997, Williams & Wilkins.

275. Higashida RT, Halbach VV, Barnwell SL, et al: Treatment of intracranial aneurysms with preservation of the parent vessel: results of percutaneous balloon embolization in 84 patients, *AJNR* 11:633, 1990.

276. Wadlington VR, Terry JB: Endovascular therapy of traumatic carotid-cavernous fistulas, *Crit Care Clin* 15:831, 1999.

277. Phatourous CC, Meyers PM, Dowd CF, et al: Carotid artery cavernous fistulas, *Neurosurg Clin N Am* 11:67, 2000.

278. Halbach VV, Higashida RT, Barnwell SL, et al: Transarterial platinum coil embolization of carotid-cavernous fistulas, *AJNR* 12:429, 1991.

279. Roy D, Raymond J: The role of transvenous embolization in the treatment of intracranial dural arteriovenous fistulas, *Neurosurgery* 40:1133; discussion, p 1141, 1997.

280. Bavinzski G, Killer M, Gruber A, Richling B: Treatment of posttraumatic carotico-cavernous fistulae using electrolytically detachable coils: technical aspects and preliminary experience, *Neuroradiology* 39:81, 1997.

281. Kanner AA, Maimon S, Rappaport ZH: Treatment of spontaneous carotid-cavernous fistula in Ehlers-Danlos syndrome by transvenous occlusion with Guglielmi detachable coils: case report and review of the literature, *J Neurosurg* 93:689, 2000.

282. Wilms G, Demaerel L, Lagae L, et al: Direct caroticocavernous fistula and traumatic dissection of the ipsilateral internal carotid artery: endovascular treatment, *Neuroradiology* 42:62, 2000.

283. Rogers SN, Patel M, Beirne JC, Nixon TE: Traumatic aneurysm of the maxillary artery: the role of interventional radiology: a report of two cases, *Int J Oral Maxillofac Surg* 24:336, 1995.

284. Borden NM, Dungan D, Dean BL, Flom RA: Posttraumatic epistaxis from injury to the pterygovaginal artery, *AJNR* 17:1148, 1996.

285. Mehrotra ON, Brown GE, Widdowson WP, Wilson JP: Arteriography and selective embolisation in the control of life-threatening hemorrhage following facial fractures, *Br J Plast Surg* 37:482, 1984.

286. Murakami R, Kumazaki T, Tajima H, et al: Transcatheter arterial embolization as treatment for life-threatening maxillofacial injury, *Radiat Med* 14:197, 1996.

287. Demetriades D, Chahwan S, Gomez H, et al: Initial evaluation and management of gunshot wounds to the face, *J Trauma* 45:39, 1998.

288. Borsa JJ, Fontaine AB, Eskridge JM, et al: Transcatheter arterial embolization for intractable epistaxis secondary to gunshot wounds, *J Vasc Interv Radiol* 10:297, 1999.

289. Kurata A, Kitahara T, Miyasaka Y, et al: Superselective embolization for severe traumatic epistaxis caused by fracture of the skull base, *AJNR* 14:343, 1993.

3

Computed Tomography of Maxillofacial Trauma: Patterns of Osseous Injury and Associated Soft Tissue Involvement

Jay Cinnamon, K. Shanmuganathan, and Bradley C. Robertson

Craniofacial trauma represents a common clinical indication for the radiologic evaluation of the face and skull base in the twenty-first century. Motor vehicle accidents and assaults are the leading causes of craniofacial trauma.[1-4] The combined use of airbags and seat belts has been shown to reduce the incidence considerably.[5] Since aggressive, early surgical intervention for severe injuries is frequently desired,[6-11] the challenges exist for the imaging community to provide diagnostic insight into the full scope of the injuries as quickly and efficiently as possible, often even before the severely injured trauma patient has been stabilized. Advances in the imaging technology armamentarium, particularly with regard to the introduction of multislice spiral CT and advanced postprocessing techniques, can enable the radiologist to provide all the critical anatomical detail with the required efficiency. The challenge for the radiologist, then, is to understand the disease—i.e., the patterns of osseous and soft tissue injuries—and then couple that to a thorough working understanding of the imaging technologies to generate a comprehensive imaging study that will not only *detect* the injuries but also *demonstrate* these injuries for the clinicians who need to repair them in a meaningful manner.

This chapter reviews craniofacial anatomy and presents a functional classification of facial injuries. Every diagnostic imaging study (and report) must address the major clinical considerations of the treating physicians. It is therefore incumbent on the interpreting radiologist to possess an adequate understanding of these issues—i.e., to understand what it is that the clinician needs to know. These concepts are covered herein as well. This chapter covers the basic concepts of optimizing multislice spiral CT imaging protocols, as well as the value of three-dimensional imaging, in the evaluation of craniofacial trauma.

CRANIOFACIAL ANATOMY

There are three dimensions to understanding craniofacial anatomy. The first, and most direct dimension, is to recognize the numerous bones that actually compose the facial skeleton, as well as the relationships they have to one another. The second is the functional dimension, to appreciate the structures in terms of the struts and buttresses that provide support and stability.[12] Finally, one must understand the general relationship between the face and the skull base and the specific points where the anterior and central skull base join the facial skeleton.

Osseous Anatomy

The facial skeleton can be divided, from superior to inferior, into the supraorbital, orbital, and midface regions and the mandible. The temporomandibular joints and temporal bones, although technically skull base structures, are common associated sites of injury in cases of significant facial trauma.

The supraorbital region is mainly composed of the frontal calvarium as it curves down to meet the facial skeleton (Fig. 3-1). Rudimentary development of the frontal sinuses can be noted as early as the age of 12 months, but these sinuses typically remain difficult to identify as discrete structures until they extend above the superior orbital rims several years later.[13] In young children, a suture separates the two halves of the frontal bone; fusion typically occurs between the ages of 6 and 10. When the suture persists, it is identified as the metopic suture.[14] The frontal sinuses are formed from anterior and posterior tables (Fig. 3-2). In evaluating frontal sinus fractures, identifying involvement of the posterior table can often be a critical point, since a fracture through this structure provides communication between the sinonasal cavity and the intracranial compartment.

As the frontal sinuses extend medially along the superior orbital rims, they come to a critical anatomic point known as the nasoethmoidal-orbital (NEO) region. This represents the junction point at which the frontal sinuses and calvarium meet the nasal bridge anteriorly, in turn joining with the cribriform plate and ethmoid labyrinths posteriorly[15] (Fig. 3-3). Fractures in this location take on an added clinical significance, since the region represents the union of the upper facial skeleton with the anterior skull base.

Seven separate bones join to form the walls of the orbit (Fig. 3-4). The orbital roof is formed almost exclusively by the posterior reflection of the frontal bone, known as the orbital plate. The orbital plates serve as the largest individual components of the floor of the anterior cranial fossa. The orbital surfaces of the orbital plates, as viewed from within the orbit, are smooth, whereas the intracranial surfaces are somewhat irregular and rough. This is one reason why the inferior frontal lobes are among the most common sites of contusion in the setting of head trauma. The supraorbital notch is located along the superior orbital rim, just medial to the midline point between the lateral and medial walls of the orbit. This notch carries the supraorbital branch of the trigeminal nerve, which provides sensory innervation to the upper eyelid, forehead, and scalp.[16] The medial margins of the orbital plates join the cribriform plate. Most of the orbital roof is formed from the orbital plate of the frontal

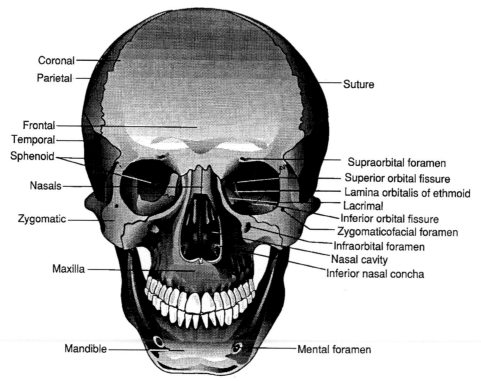

Fig. 3-1
Frontal view of skull with anatomic landmarks labeled.

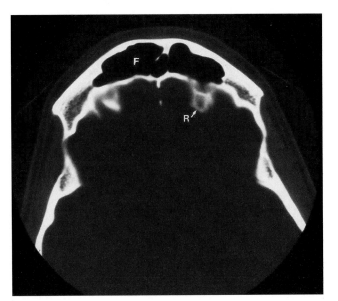

Fig. 3-2
Axial CT showing anterior and posterior walls of frontal sinus (*F*) and superior-most orbital roof (*R*).

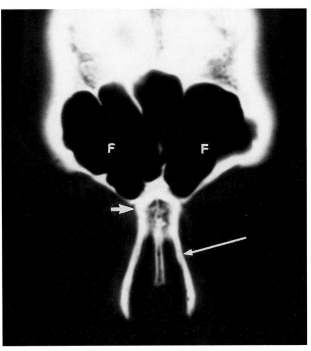

Fig. 3-3
Normal coronal view of face at level of the frontal sinuses (*F*), showing frontal process of the maxilla (*short arrow*) and nasal bones (*long arrow*).

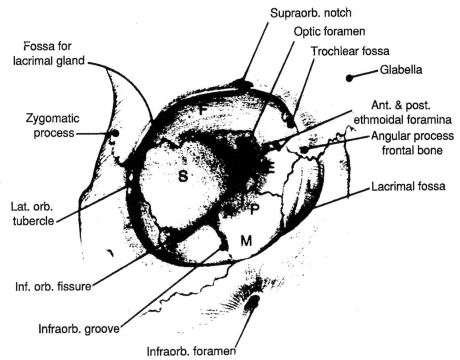

Fig. 3-4
Right orbit viewed along its axis. The rims and walls can be best visualized in this orientation. *F,* Frontal. *E,* ethmoid. *L,* lacrimal. *M,* maxilla. *P,* palatine. *Z,* zygoma. *S,* sphenoid (greater wing). (Illustration by Elizabeth Roselius, 1987; from Foster CA, Sherman JE: *Surgery of facial bone fractures,* New York, 1987, Churchill Livingstone.)

bone, but the most posterior extent of the roof is actually formed from the lesser wing of the sphenoid.

Four bones form the medial wall of the orbit. The most anterior portion of the medial wall is formed from the frontal process of the maxilla, a thin slit of bone that sweeps up from the maxilla to reside between the nasal bones anteriorly and the lacrimal bone posteriorly. Posterior to the lacrimal bone is the largest individual component of the medial orbital wall, the orbital plate of the ethmoid, also known as the lamina papyracea for its paper-thin composition (Figs. 3-1, 3-4, and 3-5). The sphenoid bone contributes the most posterior portion of the medial wall in the vicinity of the orbital apex (Figs. 3-1, 3-4, and 3-5).

The lateral wall of the orbit is formed posteriorly by the greater wing of the sphenoid and anteriorly by the zygoma. The zygoma, known to the general population as the cheekbone, also wraps around inferiorly to contribute to the floor of the orbit, although the majority of the floor is formed by the orbital surface of the maxilla[14] (Figs. 3-1, 3-4, and 3-5). A groove in the floor of the orbit carrying the infraorbital nerve and vessels terminates as the infraorbital foramen just below the inferior orbital rim.

When one peers into the orbit from the front, one can identify three outlets—the inferior orbital fissure, the superior orbital fissure, and the optic canal. The superior orbital fissure and the optic canal connect the orbit to the intracranial compartment, whereas the inferior orbital fissure represents a communication between the orbit and the infratemporal fossa, not the intracranial space. As one moves from the floor of the orbit superiorly, these channels of communication move medially. Thus the inferior-most opening, the inferior orbital fissure, is also the most laterally oriented; the optic canal is the most superiorly and medially located; and the superior orbital fissure lies in between (Figs. 3-4 to 3-7).

The midface comprises the maxillae, the nasal bones and bony architecture of the nasal cavity, and the zygomas. The latter is included in this category not only because of the frequency with which the zygoma is fractured in association with maxillary fractures but also because one of the keys to successful operative fixation of midface fractures is the reestablishment of the normal dimensions and contours of the zygomatic arches and zygoma bodies.[6,7,9,17] The inferior margin of the midface is the maxillary alveolar ridge and maxillary teeth along the periphery and the hard palate central. The hard palate can also be considered the floor of the nasal cavity (Fig. 3-8). The midface skeleton is primarily affected in Le Fort and zygomaticomaxillary (ZMC) fractures, which are described in detail later.

The mandible is a three-dimensional structure whose only articulation with the skull base is at the temporomandibular joints (Fig. 3-8). The symphysis represents the anterior midline prominence that forms the bony architecture of the chin. From this point, the mandibular bodies extend posteriorly to the mandibular angles. The ramus on each side continues superiorly from the angle and then splits into the anterior coronoid process and posterior condyle. The latter sits within the glenoid fossa of each temporal bone. The mandible is composed of a combination of strong cortical and cancellous bone, giving it the strength and stability to withstand a lifelong course of mastication. However, there are several relative weaknesses within the structure. Vulnerable points include the condylar neck, angle of the mandible, mental foramen, and sites of impacted teeth.[18-20] In addition, various portions of the mandible may be weakened by the presence of underlying lesions of either odontogenic or nonodontogenic etiology.[18]

Struts and Buttresses

The facial skeleton can be conceptually viewed as a network of vertically and horizontally oriented struts or buttresses that provide its stability (Fig. 3-9). First described by Gentry in 1983,[12] these interconnected struts actually run in all three planes—axial, coronal, and sagittal. There are three horizontal or axial struts that run from one side of the face to the other. The superior horizontal strut runs across from one orbital roof, through the cribriform plate, to the other roof; the middle horizontal strut is formed from the orbital floors and zygomatic arches; and the inferior horizontal strut comprises the hard palate.

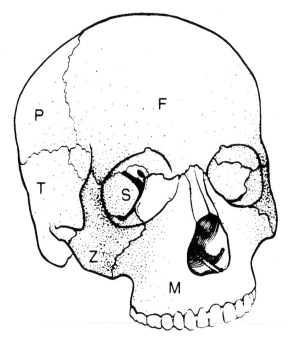

Fig. 3-5
Anterolateral view of the facial bones, emphasizing position of sphenoid bone as component of orbit. *F,* Frontal; *S,* sphenoid; *P,* parietal; *T,* temporal; *Z,* zygoma; *M,* maxillary.

Five vertical struts run in the sagittal plane. There is a single midline strut that is represented by the nasal septum. Two paramedian struts are formed from the medial walls of the orbits and maxillary sinuses and the pterygoid plates. The lateral walls of the orbits and maxillary sinuses compose the lateral struts, one on each side of the face.

There are two vertically oriented struts that run in the coronal plane. The anterior strut runs along the anterior surface of the facial skeleton, whereas the posterior coronal strut is formed from the posterior walls of the maxillary sinuses and the pterygoid plates.

Sites of Union Between the Facial Skeleton and Skull Base

The face is anchored to the skull base in several locations (Figs. 3-10 and 3-11). One site is the roof of the orbit, which is also the floor of the anterior skull base, as previously described. Conceptually, the midface is anchored in several locations. The frontal process of the zygoma, which forms a portion of the lateral wall of the orbit, is attached to the frontal calvarium as it descends laterally (Fig. 3-11). The temporal process of

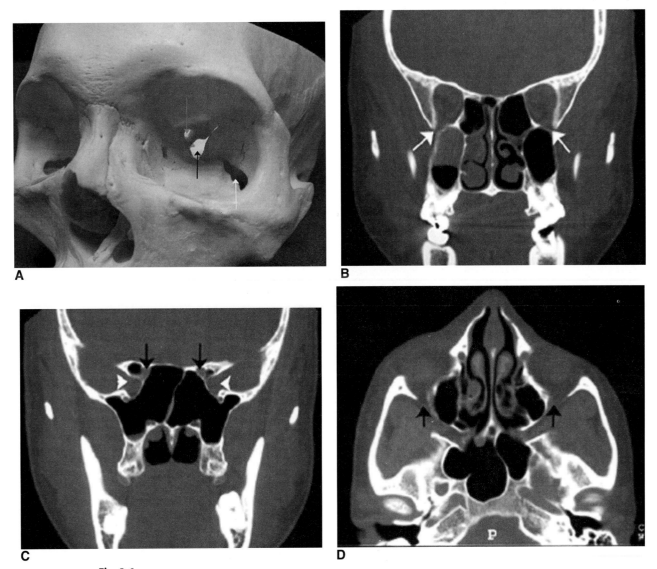

Fig. 3-6

Orbital anatomy. **A,**Three orbital outlets are the inferior orbital fissure (*right arrow*), which is the most inferior and lateral of the outlets and connects the orbit with the masticator space; the superior orbital fissure (*black arrow*); and the optic canal (*left arrow*). The optic canal is the most superior and medial of the outlets. **B,** Coronal CT image demonstrating the inferior orbital fissure (*arrows*). **C,** Coronal CT image demonstrating the superior orbital fissure (*arrowheads*) and optic canal (*arrows*). **D,** Axial image demonstrating the laterally oriented inferior orbital fissure (*arrows*), offering communication between the orbit and the masticator space (infratemporal fossa).

Continued

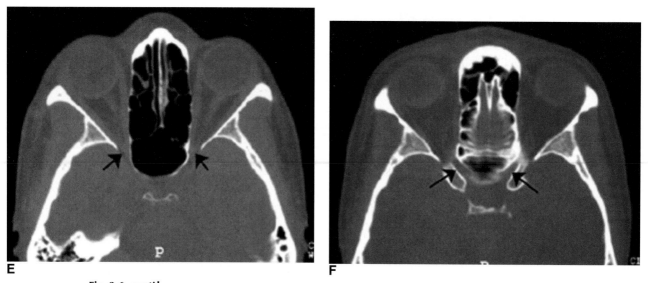

E   **F**

Fig. 3-6, cont'd
E, Axial image more superiorly demonstrates the superior orbital fissure. **F,** More superiorly, the optic canal is also noted to be the most medially oriented of the orbital outlets (*arrows*).

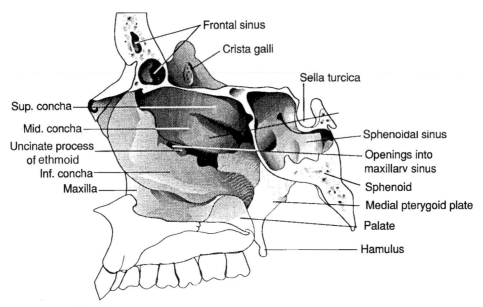

Sup. concha —
Mid. concha —
Uncinate process of ethmoid —
Inf. concha —
Maxilla —

— Frontal sinus
— Crista galli
— Sella turcica
— Sphenoidal sinus
— Openings into maxillary sinus
— Sphenoid
— Medial pterygoid plate
— Palate
— Hamulus

Fig. 3-7
Normal sagittal midline facial anatomy with nasal septum removed.

the zygoma runs posteriorly to meet the zygomatic process of the temporal bone to create the zygomatic arch, another anchoring structure (Fig. 3-11). Perhaps the most interesting site of union between the facial bones and the skull base, however, is in an area that cannot be clearly visualized when inspecting the facial skeleton from the outside, and that is in the vicinity of the pterygopalatine fossa. With the mandible disarticulated, the side view of the facial skeleton reveals that the pterygoid plates fuse to the posterior walls of the maxil-

lary sinuses, just above the maxillary ridge and just below the pterygopalatine fossa (Fig. 3-12). The pterygoid plates are outgrowths from the sphenoid bone, the main osseous structure of the central skull base. The maxillae are facial structures. The fusion of these structures therefore represents the deepest of the anchors of the face. It is this union that is severed in each of the Le Fort fractures, and it is for this reason that the main concept common to all Le Fort fractures is some degree of craniofacial separation.

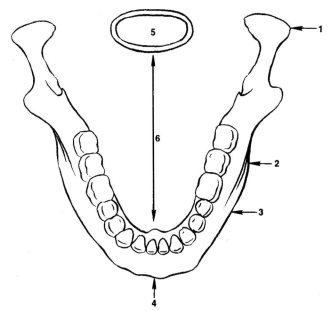

Fig. 3-8
Submental view of the normal mandible. The contour of the mandible is formed from the condyles (*1*), angles (*2*), bodies (*3*), and symphysis (*4*). With the normal mandibular contour, the muscles of the tongue and floor of the mouth are firmly supported, preventing obstruction of the oropharynx (*5*). The arrow (*6*) shows the distance between the mandibular symphysis and the oropharynx. (From Gerlock AJ: *Clinical and radiographic interpretation of facial fractures,* Boston, 1981, Little, Brown.)

FRACTURE CLASSIFICATION

Classification systems for facial fractures can be based on numerous factors, including mechanism of injury, severity of injury, pattern of involved structures, and ramification of therapeutic options.[12,15,21,22] One practical approach to such a classification relates specifically to two of the concepts previously discussed. By integrating the strut/buttress analysis with an understanding of the relationship between the facial skeleton and skull base, a classification system that stratifies most facial fractures into one of three main categories emerges (Box 3-1). In addition to serving as a functional framework for the conceptualization of the injuries, this system also correlates fairly well with therapeutic decision making. Solitary strut injuries are simple fractures that involve a single bony wall and often do not require open reduction. The relationship between the facial skeleton and the skull base is intact. Complex strut fractures are of higher severity, typically requiring open fixation to address what would otherwise result in a significant cosmetic deformity. The most common injury in this category is the zygomaticomaxillary complex fracture (Fig. 3-12). With this type of injury, the relationship between the facial skeleton and the skull base is partially severed, superficially and unilaterally. In this situation, most of the facial skeleton is still firmly anchored to the skull base; how-

ever, the zygoma, a prominent facial bone, has become detached from the skull base because of the fractures through the lateral orbital wall and the zygomatic arch. The most severe injuries are the transfacial fracture complexes, comprising markedly comminuted bilateral fractures. These fractures sever the union to the skull base and require extensive reconstructive surgery.

SOLITARY STRUT FRACTURES
Blowout Fractures of the Orbit

Orbital blowout fractures are among the most common facial injuries encountered in trauma centers. Blunt trauma to the orbit results in an acute rise in intraorbital pressures, leading to the generation of the fracture. Thus "pure" orbital blowout fractures (Figs. 3-13 to 3-16), which typically involve either the orbital floor, the medial orbital wall, or the combination of the medial aspect of the orbital floor and the inferior aspect of the medial orbital wall, result from a direct, blunt blow to the globe and anterior orbital soft tissue structures.[6,17,23-25] These fractures represent a route of decompression of the increased intraorbital pressures and can almost be considered a protective measure to maintain the integrity of the globe, which would otherwise bear the brunt of the pressure changes. On the other hand, "impure" orbital blowout fractures (Fig. 3-17) are typically associated with other facial fractures, such as the orbital rim, zygoma, and transfacial fractures. In these circumstances, the orbital blowout components of these more complex fractures are secondary to direct and intense blunt trauma, generating powerful lines of force applied to the facial skeleton that then traverse the orbital walls in their trajectories, thus differing from acute rises in intraorbital pressures that are associated with the simple "pure" blowout fractures.

The orbital floor is involved in the majority of blowout fractures. Typically, the medial aspect of the orbital floor is the actual site of fracture.[6,18] This may be the only site of fracture, although often these injuries are accompanied by a fracture of the inferior aspect of the medial wall.[6,15,26] Together, these sites represent the weakest points in the orbital skeleton. The medial wall of the orbit may also be the sole site of fracture; however, this is less common (Figs. 3-18 to 3-20), assumedly because of the intricate architecture of the ethmoid bone, with its numerous septa between the air cells serving as scaffolding that adds strength and stability to the lamina papyracea.[15]

Clinical examination of patients who have sustained orbital floor fractures typically demonstrates signs and symptoms associated with injury to the infraorbital nerve. Facial numbness in this distribution is one of the most sensitive clinical findings in this condition.[6] The infraorbital nerve courses obliquely along the floor of

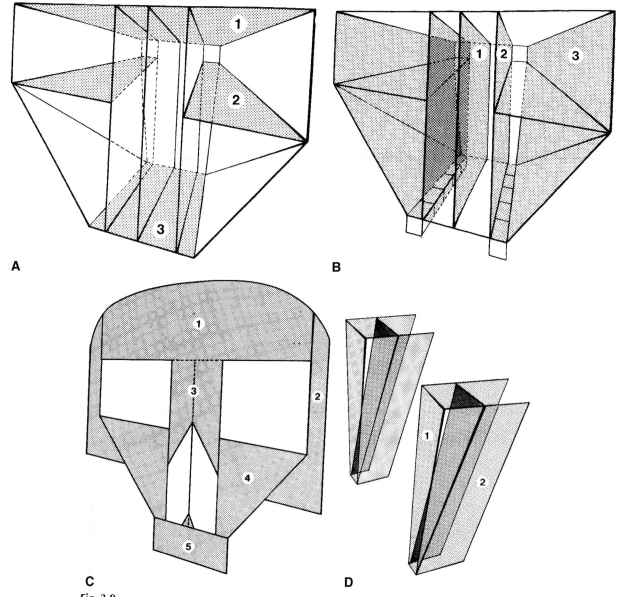

Fig. 3-9
Geometric representation of the triplanar facial struts. **A,** Horizontal struts consisting of superior-fovea ethmoidalis/cribriform plate (*1*), middle-zygomatic arch/orbital floor (*2*), and inferior-hard palate (*3*). **B,** The sagittal struts consist of the median-nasal septum (*1*), paramedian-medial maxillary sinus wall/medial orbital wall (*2*), and lateral-lateral alveolar ridge/lateral maxillary sinus wall/lateral orbital wall (*3*). **C,** The anterior coronal strut consists of frontal bone (*1*), zygomaticofrontal suture (*2*), nasofrontal (*3*), anterior maxillary wall (*4*), alveolar ridge (*5*). **D,** The posterior coronal strut consists of the posterior maxillary sinus walls (*1*) and the pterygoid plates (*2*). (From Gentry LR, Manor WF, Turski PA, Strother CM: *AJR* 140:523, 1983.)

the orbit. Anteriorly, its branches receive sensory stimulation from the cheek, upper lip, and anterior maxillary teeth. The branches merge into the nerve proper as the latter enters the infraorbital foramen, just below the inferior orbital rim near the midline. The nerve continues posteriorly in the canal that is embedded within the orbital floor for a short distance and then emerges from

the canal to continue posteriorly in the infraorbital notch along the floor. As it courses posteriorly, it also migrates laterally as it makes its way to the inferior orbital fissure.

Diplopia is another common finding associated with blowout fractures, although it may result from a variety of mechanisms.[6,15,22,27] Distinguishing among these possible etiologies may be of great clinical significance, since

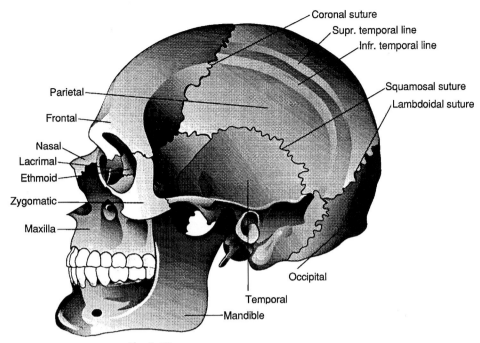

Fig. 3-10
Lateral view of normal skull and facial anatomy.

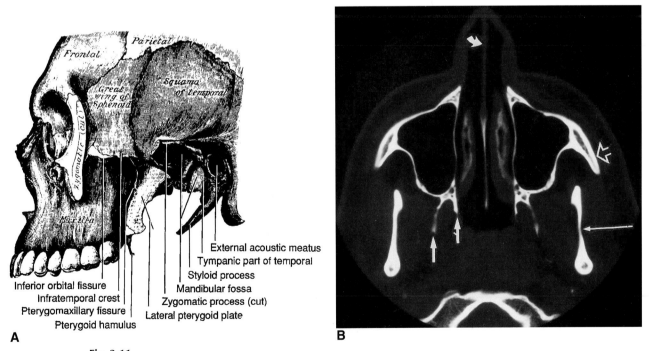

Fig. 3-11
A, Lateral view of the face, with the zygomatic arch removed. **B**, Axial CT view at the level of the midmaxillary sinuses shows medial and lateral pterygoid plates (*short arrows*), the temporal process of the zygoma (*open arrow*), the ramus of the mandible (*long arrow*), and the cartilaginous nasal septum (*curved arrow*). (**A** from Williams PL, Warwick R: *Gray's anatomy*, ed 36, Philadelphia, 1985, WB Saunders.)

the orbital floor defect with a distorted appearance that suggests incarceration. This is most likely to be associated with small fractures rather than larger fracture fragments, as the latter results in a defect large enough that actual entrapment of the muscle does not commonly occur. Thus descent of the muscle through the plane of the orbital floor fracture does not indicate with certainty that there is clinical entrapment. One needs to analyze the overall radiographic picture and integrate it into the clinical examination before the diagnosis of true entrapment can be established. Once it is established, emergency decompression is often considered.[8,11,28] However, true entrapment can also be present even when the muscle remains above the plane of the orbital floor. Herniation of fat alone, which may be tethered to the muscle by thin ligaments, can result in the same clinical impairment. A small branch of the oculomotor nerve (CN III) that innervates the inferior oblique muscle runs along the orbital floor and may also be injured in orbital floor trauma, leading to another cause of diplopia.[27] The most common cause of diplopia, however, is trauma to the inferior rectus muscle itself, leading to impairment of contractility.[6]

In cases of trauma to the inferior rectus muscle, the most common radiographic finding is enlargement of the belly of the affected muscle, which also often demonstrates shaggy margins indicative of the hematoma or edema within the muscle. As one would expect, this effect

they imply different lines of therapeutic action. Entrapment of the inferior rectus muscle in an orbital floor fracture is one of the better-known complications of such fractures, although true entrapment of the muscle itself is actually an uncommon development. Radiographic evaluation utilizing coronal imaging through the orbits demonstrates descent of the inferior rectus muscle through

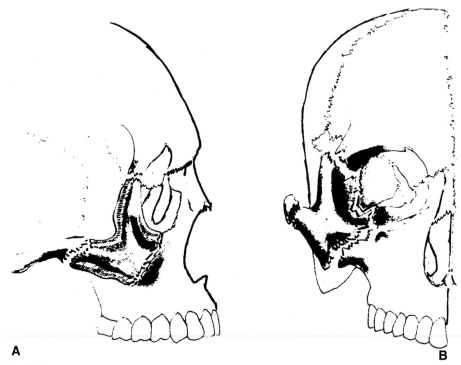

Fig. 3-12
A, Lateral view of zygoma fracture. **B**, Frontal view of zygoma fracture. (From Alling CM, Osbon DB: *Maxillofacial trauma*, Philadelphia, 1988, Lea & Febiger.)

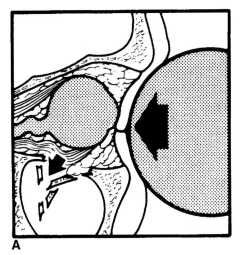
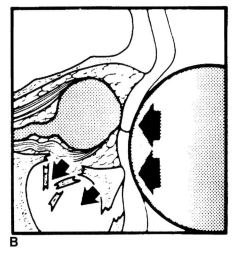

Fig. 3-13
A, Diagram of a pure blowout fracture. **B**, Diagram of an impure blowout fracture, showing involvement of the anterior maxillary sinus. (Illustration by Elizabeth Roselius, 1987; from Foster CA, Sherman, JE: *Surgery of facial bone fractures*, New York, 1987, Churchill Livingstone.)

is also best appreciated on coronal imaging. From a clinical point, it may not be easy to distinguish these various causes of diplopia from one another. Many of these causes of double vision will be transient and self-resolving over the few days following the trauma. A short course of steroids may help as well. Recognizing true entrapment therefore requires a thorough clinical evaluation with forced duction, integrated into a detailed coronal imaging study. Even in this circumstance, some surgeons advocate a trial observation period of 1 to 2 weeks before embarking on surgical exploration.[6]

As with orbital floor fractures, medial wall fractures can lead to impaired oculomotor motility by injuring the medial rectus muscle. In this situation, swelling of that muscle will be easily identified on axial imaging (Figs. 3-18 to 3-20). Acute medial wall fractures are virtually always associated with opacification of the adjacent ethmoid air cells. Deformity without such opacification is therefore reflective of a subacute or older injury.

Orbital roof and lateral orbital wall blowout fractures are much less common than floor and medial wall fractures[23,29] (Figs. 3-21 to 3-26). Orbital roof fractures are

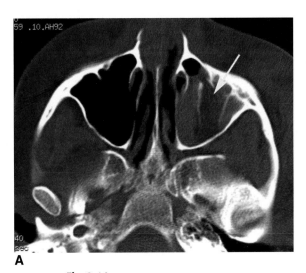
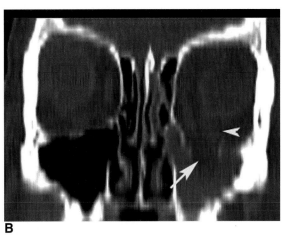

Fig. 3-14
Orbital floor fracture with fat herniation in a 31-year-old man admitted following blunt trauma to the face. **A**, Axial CT in bone window shows bone fragments from left orbital floor blown down into the superior maxillary sinus, with herniation orbital fat (*arrow*) between fragments. **B**, A coronal view shows the same findings. The bone fragments resemble the opened doors of a bomber; thus the appearance may be referred to as the "bomb bay door" sign. Orbital fat is herniated (*arrow*), but the inferior rectus muscle projects above the plane of the fracture (*arrowhead*).

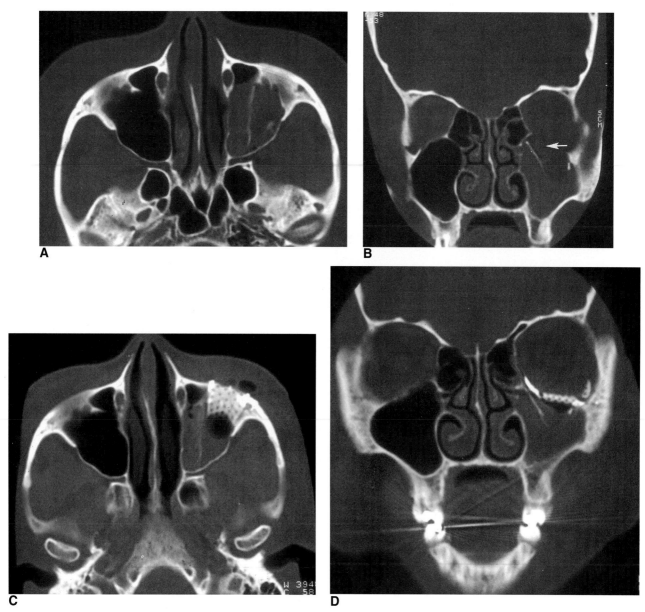

Fig. 3-15
Pure orbital blowout fracture. **A**, Axial spiral CT image shows a left orbital floor fracture with displaced bone fragments, maxillary sinus hemorrhage, and herniated orbital fat between bone fragments. **B**, Direct coronal image shows orbital fat herniating through orbital floor defect. The swollen inferior rectus muscle (*arrow*) is herniated below the level of the normal orbital floor but not entrapped. **C** and **D**, Axial and coronal views obtained after surgical repair show titanium miniplate and screws establishing near anatomic restoration of the orbital floor.

typically seen in association with fractures in the supra-orbital region involving the frontal sinuses and frontal calvarium (Figs. 3-21 and 3-22) that have extended into the floor of the anterior cranial fossa/orbital roof. Dural tears and frontal lobe contusions are commonly identified in this setting (Figs. 3-21 to 3-25). Lateral orbital wall fractures are also rarely solitary injuries and are more

commonly seen as part of the injured zygomaticomaxillary complex, which is described later.

In the acute setting, the patient who has sustained an orbital blowout fracture presents with periorbital soft tissue swelling associated with palpebral and subconjunctival hematomas.[6] As the swelling and hematomas resolve over time, enophthalmos may develop. Increased orbital

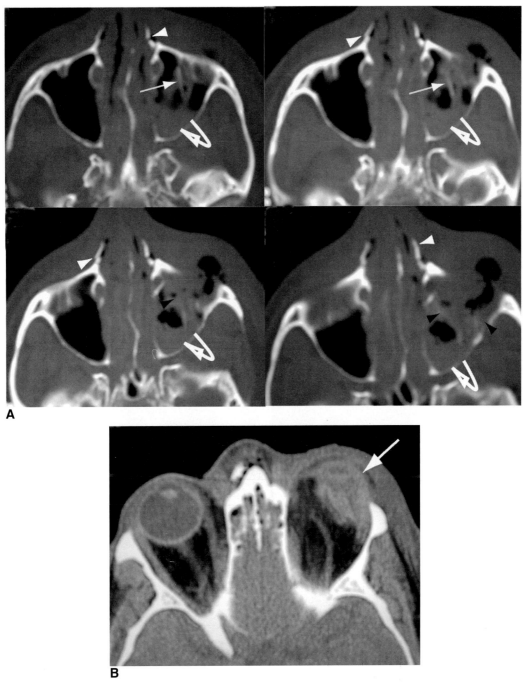

Fig. 3-16
Orbital floor fracture with rupture of globe. **A**, Contiguous spiral CT images of orbits show a defect in orbital floor (*black arrowheads*) with a floating bone fragment (*arrows*) within the left maxillary sinus arising from left orbital floor. A minimally displaced nasal fracture (*white arrowheads*) and blood (*curved arrow*) within the left maxillary sinus are also seen. **B**, CT image obtained in soft tissue window and level shows soft tissue swelling and a ruptured left globe (*arrow*), which is deformed.

volume secondary to the fracture(s) results in displacement of orbital soft tissue volume into the maxillary sinus or ethmoid air cells (depending on the site of fracture). Atrophy of the orbital fat and scarring within the fat causes retraction and displacement of the globe posteriorly. It has been determined that fracture fragments

that have an area greater than 2 cm^2 and that are displaced greater than 3 cm are generally expected to lead to enophthalmos and are considered a potential surgical indication.[6,22,30]

There are direct and indirect imaging signs of orbital blowout fractures. Although the diagnosis of an orbital

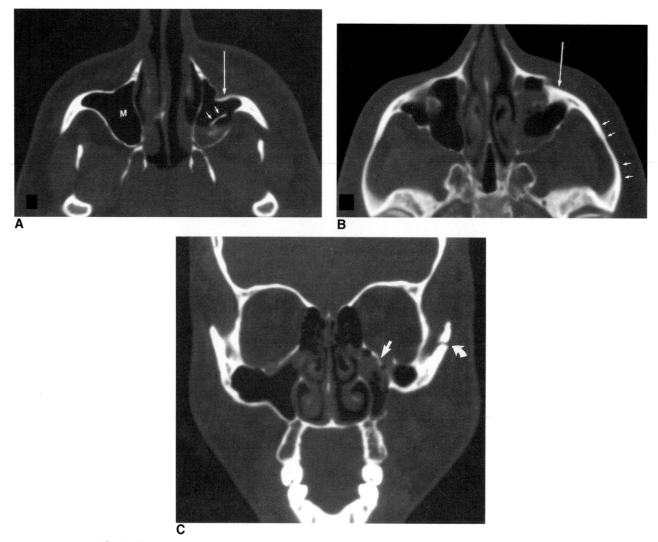

Fig. 3-17
Impure orbital blowout fracture. **A**, CT image shows displaced fracture of the anterior maxillary sinus wall (*long arrow*), extending to the anterior orbital rim, with displaced bone fragments from the orbital floor (*short arrows*). **B**, More cephalad view shows posterior displacement of the zygomatic recess of the left maxillary sinus (*long arrow*). The left zygomatic arch appears intact (*short arrows*) in this view. **C**, Coronal CT image through the orbits demonstrates a depressed fracture of the orbital floor (*straight arrow*) and a zygomatic fracture (*curved arrow*).

floor fracture can be made or suspected based on axial imaging alone, it is the coronal imaging that is necessary for proper fracture characterization. In the axial plane, the orbital floor is suboptimally visualized, since it courses in a plane that is tangential to the transverse plane of the image acquisition. As the axial images through the facial bones proceed superiorly from the level of the maxillary sinuses to the orbits, the orbital floors move from being an anterior structure to a posterior structure but are always identifiable as the piece of bone that separates the maxillary sinus from the orbital

soft tissues. In this plane, the structure typically appears curvilinear. Therefore one must develop a strong appreciation of this normal curvature before fracture irregularities can be identified as such.

Orbital blowout fractures are typically associated with other indirect imaging findings, such as air-fluid levels in the adjacent sinuses and orbital emphysema. In rare circumstances, an orbital floor fracture will not lead to fluid accumulation in the maxillary sinus but rather to a focal hematoma or fat density that extends through the orbital floor fracture into the superior portion of the sinus.

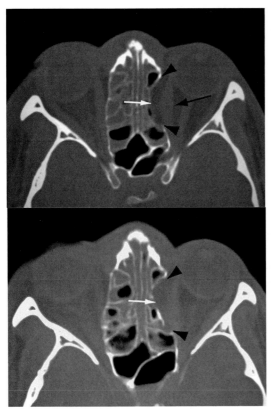

Fig. 3-18
Medial wall fracture with fat herniation into ethmoid sinus in blunt trauma patient. Multislice CT images show a large medial wall fracture (*arrowheads*) with orbital fat (*white arrows*) herniating into the left ethmoid sinus. The belly of the left medial rectus muscle (*black arrow*) is enlarged from contusion. Opacification of ethmoid air cells is also seen.

Isolated Zygomatic Arch Fractures

Only a small percentage of zygoma fractures are limited to the arch, with the majority involving additional components. Arch fractures typically result from a very focused blow to the side of the face. The fracture fragments may be nondisplaced or displaced inward or outward (Figs. 3-27 and 3-28). When ZMC fractures are inwardly displaced, they may impinge on the coronoid process of the mandible and limit the range of mandibular motion.[6] Even in the absence of functional impairment, displaced zygomatic arch fractures are usually repaired operatively to address the cosmetic deformity that would otherwise result.

Isolated Frontal or Maxillary Sinus Wall Fractures

Isolated fractures of the frontal sinus walls can result from a direct blow to the supraorbital region, although commonly such fractures are encountered as part of severe craniofacial trauma that results in injuries to other facial bone and anterior skull base structures. Fractures

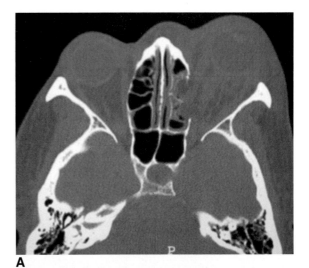

A

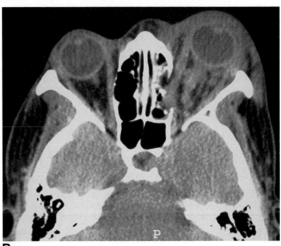

B

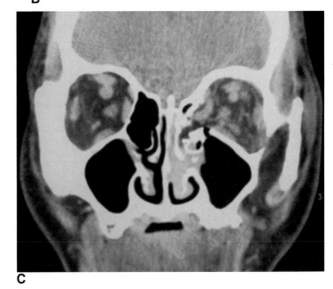

C

Fig. 3-19
Medial orbital wall fracture. **A**, CT image across orbit shows disruption of the medial wall, with fat and muscle herniation into the ethmoid sinus. There is adjacent orbital hemorrhage. **B**, Same findings seen in soft tissue settings. **C**, Coronal view shows herniation of swollen medial rectus herniated into ethmoid sinus.

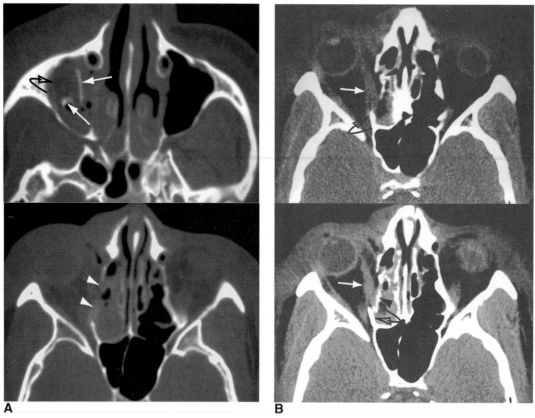

Fig. 3-20
Medial and floor fracture in a 48-year-old man admitted following assault to face. **A**, Multislice CT images show orbital floor bone fragments (*arrows*) and intraorbital fat (*curved arrow*) in right antrum secondary to orbital floor fracture. There is a concurrent medial wall fracture (*arrowheads*) with opacification of right ethmoid air cells. **B**, More cephalad CT images through the orbit show the right medial rectus muscle (*arrows*) is deformed and impaled by a bone fragment (*curved arrow*) arising from posterior aspect of the medial wall. A displaced medial wall bone fragment (*arrowheads*) is seen within the right ethmoid sinus.

that involve the frontal sinuses can involve the anterior table or both the anterior and posterior tables[6,17,31] (Figs. 3-29 to 3-31). Identifying involvement of the posterior table is important, since this represents a pathologic connection between the sinonasal cavity and the intracranial compartment and is therefore a potential source of infection from the sinonasal flora. In addition, posterior table fractures are associated with an increased incidence of dural tears along the anterior skull base, frontal lobe contusions, and other intracranial injuries.

Isolated anterior and lateral maxillary wall fractures are uncommon injuries and may respond to conservative measures (Figs. 3-32 and 3-33). Severely depressed anterior fractures may require surgical fixation for cosmetic purposes. Sensory changes in the distribution of the infraorbital nerve can result if the fracture extends up toward the inferior orbital rim.

Nasal Fractures

The architecture of the nose can be divided into the surface anatomy (or *pyramid*) and the internal nasal septum, both of which are composed of osseous and cartilaginous components (Fig. 3-34). The bony surface anatomy is made up of four bony structures—one nasal bone and the frontal process of the maxilla on each side, with the upper and lower nasal cartilages on each side filling out the remainder of the surface architecture. The internal nasal septum comprises the perpendicular plate of the ethmoid, the vomer that rises up from the hard palate, and the more anteriorly located septal cartilage; all three articulate with each other.

Trauma to the nasal region can result in isolated fractures of the nasal pyramid (surface architecture) or may involve the nasal septum as well (Figs. 3-35

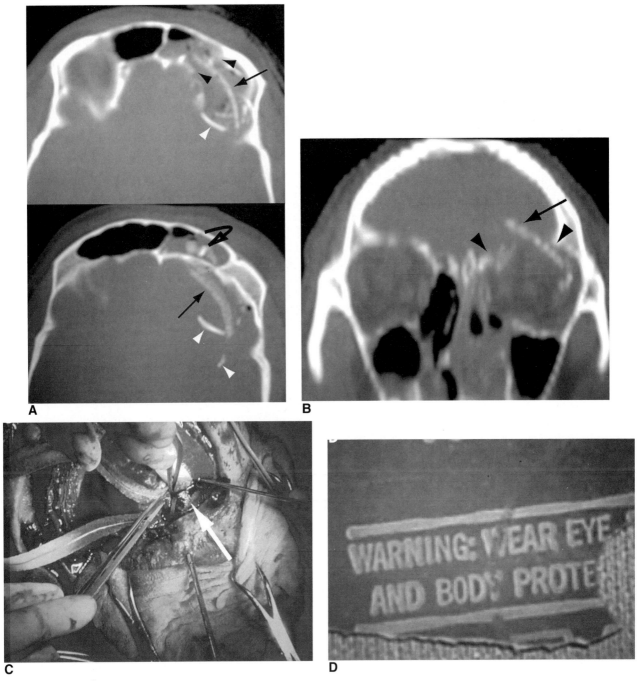

Fig. 3-21
Blowout fracture of orbital roof in a patient admitted following an industrial accident. **A**, Spiral CT images show a radio-opaque foreign body (*arrows*) entering the left anterior cranial fossa through the orbital roof. The orbital roof is fractured, with bone fragments (*white arrowheads*) displaced superiorly into the brain parenchyma. There is direct communication between the left frontal sinus and the superior aspect of the left orbit through a defect (*black arrowheads*). Bone fragments (*curved arrow*) are seen floating within the left frontal sinus blood. **B**, Coronal reformatted image shows herniation of a foreign body (*arrow*) through a large defect (*arrowheads*) in the orbital roof into the left frontal lobe. **C**, Intraoperative picture shows a foreign body (*arrow*) within anterior cranial fossa. **D**, Picture shows foreign body that entered left anterior cranial fossa through left orbit from electric sander.

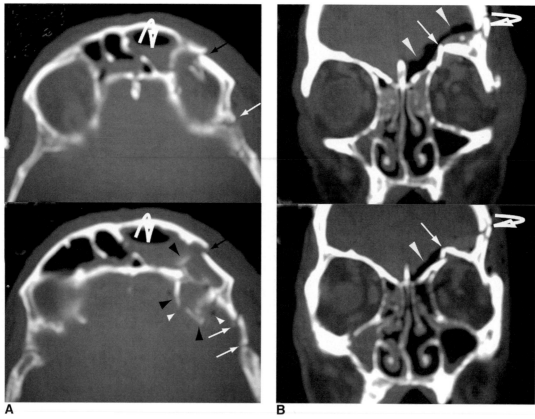

Fig. 3-22
Blowout and frontal sinus fracture in a man admitted following blunt trauma. **A,** CT images show orbital roof fragments (*black arrowheads*) displaced into brain parenchyma and left frontal sinus. Fractures of anterior wall of the left frontal sinus (*black arrows*), comminuted frontal bone fractures (*white arrows*), pneumocephalus (*white arrowheads*), and air-fluid levels (*curved arrows*) in frontal sinus are also seen. **B,** Coronal CT images show bone fragments (*arrows*) from left orbital roof displacement into frontal lobe. Pneumocephalus (*white arrowheads*) and a comminuted left frontal bone fracture (*curved arrows*) are also seen.

to 3-38). The fractures may be isolated injuries or associated with other facial fractures, depending on the nature, amount, and direction of force applied to the facial skeleton. Fractures may be nondisplaced, displaced, or depressed; solitary or comminuted; or restricted to the nasal bones or more extensive, leading to the nasofrontal, nasomaxillary, or nasoethmoidal fracture complexes that are discussed in greater detail later.

Nasal fractures are among the most common facial injuries, representing approximately 50% of facial fractures.[6,15,17] When a nasal fracture is identified clinically, much of the emphasis in the imaging evaluation is placed on the search for other associated injuries. Nonetheless, characterizing the degree of comminution and displacement of the fracture fragments can be helpful to the surgeon who is planning an operative fixation. CT imaging can identify the full extent of injury, and three-dimensional postprocessing can assist in surgical planning and in patient education.[32]

The nasal mucosa and nasal septum are richly vascularized. Bleeding into the nasal cavity in the setting of trauma can lead to respiratory compromise. Septal fractures (Fig. 3-38) can lead to the development of septal hematomas that can interfere with the cartilaginous blood supply and result in necrosis, leading to a saddle nose deformity.[15] Septal abscesses can develop when the hematomas become infected. Septal insults such as these can ultimately lead to the development of thick granulation tissue that can impede smooth airflow through the nasal cavity.[15] Septal fractures are often reduced by forceps manipulation of bone fragments. Antibiotic impregnated packing is then often placed within each nostril for support.[6]

In the setting of nasal bone fractures, the rich blood supply of the nasal mucosa can also lead to the accumulation of blood within one or both of the maxillary sinuses. Plain films in this context can be misleading, suggesting the presence of additional maxillary fractures. CT imaging can accurately differentiate between these two possibilities.[33]

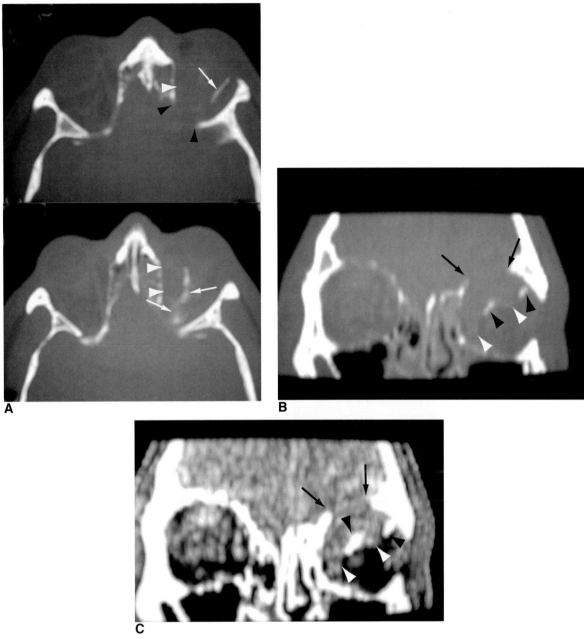

Fig. 3-23
Blow-in fracture of the orbital roof with an encephalocele. **A,** Single-slice helical CT images show bone fragments (*arrows*) arising from left orbital roof displaced inferiorly into extraconal space. A defect (*black arrowheads*) is seen in left orbital roof with a large extraconal soft tissue mass (*white arrowheads*) similar in attenuation as brain parenchyma. Coronal reformatted images of bone (**B**) and soft tissue (**C**) windows show a defect (*arrows*) in left orbital roof, with brain parenchyma (*white arrowheads*) herniating into orbit. Orbital roof bone fragments (*black arrowheads*) have been displaced inferiorly.

COMPLEX STRUT FRACTURES
Nasoethmoidal-Orbital and Nasomaxillary Fractures

The anatomic point on the face located just superior to the nasal bridge and between the eyebrows represents a point of junction of several key facial bone structures. Along the superficial contour of the face, this is the point at which the nasal bones meet the bones forming the anterior portion of the medial orbital walls (i.e., frontal process of the maxilla, lacrimal bone, and anterior lamina papyracea) and the inferomedial extensions of the frontal bones. Deep to this anatomic region is the cribriform plate and crista galli. As a result of these complex anatomic relationships, powerful injuries to this region result in complex strut fractures that mandate surgical

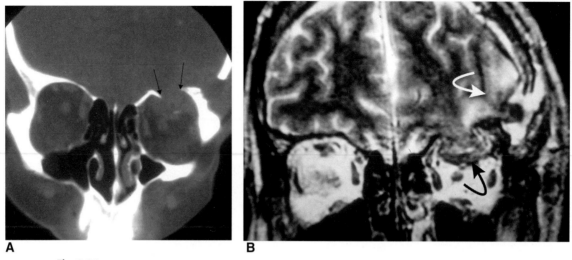

Fig. 3-24
Chronic blow-in fracture of orbital roof with an encephalocele. Coronal CT **(A)** and MR image **(B)** show an orbital roof defect (*black arrows*) in left orbit, with brain parenchyma herniating into left orbit (*black curved arrow*). A bone fragment rising from the orbital roof has been displaced inferiorly into orbit on CT. Encephalomalacia (*white curved arrow*) is seen in the frontal lobe.

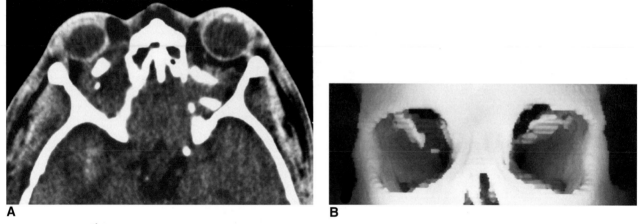

Fig. 3-25
Blow-in orbital roof fractures with encephaloceles. **A**, CT image through the superior orbits shows bone fragments displaced inferiorly into the orbits and soft tissue density in the superior medial orbits compatible with herniated anterior frontal lobe parenchyma. **B**, Three-dimensional surface contour rendering from single-slice nonhelical scanner shows both orbital roof fragments displaced into the superior orbits.

fixation that is typically much more intricate than is required for simple strut fractures.

There are four distinct facial struts that converge in this small anatomic region (see Fig. 3-9). Three of the five vertical facial struts are present here—the single midline strut that runs along the course of the nasal septum and the two paramedian struts formed by the medial walls of the orbits and maxillary sinuses. The fourth strut is the superior horizontal strut that runs from one orbital roof, across the cribriform plate, to the opposite orbital roof. The interrelationship of these struts gives insight into the

complexity of injuries to this region and also serves to explain the conceptual basis of the classification of injuries to this region. Specifically, the various subtypes of nasoethmoidal-orbital and nasomaxillary fractures all share the following two features: the fractures are always comminuted, and they always involve at least two of the four struts that cross this region.

The essence of these fractures is involvement of the nasal bones and involvement of the frontal process of the maxilla. Approximately half of these injuries are unilateral.[6] In addition, in about one half of cases, the injury is

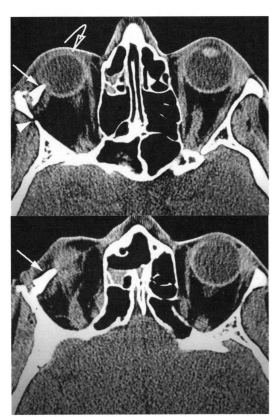

Fig. 3-26
Displaced superior orbital rim fracture in patient admitted following a blow to right orbit and head. Conventional CT images show a displaced fracture of the lateral superior orbital rim (*arrows*) and a nondisplaced fracture (*arrowhead*) of the right lateral orbital wall. The depressed superior orbital rim bone fragment impinges on the globe (*curved arrow*).

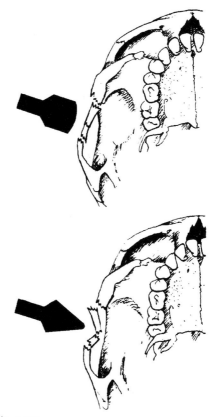

Fig. 3-27
Examples of isolated zygomatic arch fractures. (From Alling CM, Osbon DB: *Maxillofacial trauma*, Philadelphia, 1988, Lea & Febiger.)

limited to this region, while in the other half, the injury is more severe and the fractures extend to other facial bone structures.[6] The classic clinical finding is nasal bone fractures associated with free movement of the frontal process of the maxilla on one side or both sides, the latter facilitated by an accompanying fracture through the inferior orbital rim.

These fractures are comminuted and complex. The fracture fragments may be displaced posteriorly, laterally, or in both dimensions simultaneously (Figs. 3-39 to 3-41). Because the cribriform plate is located immediately posterior to these structures, injury to this structure is common, thereby explaining the relative high incidence of associated dural tears, intracranial hemorrhage, and pneumocephalus. Cerebrospinal fluid rhinorrhea may result in as many as 40% of these patients, and in rare circumstances even nasal encephaloceles or intracranial infection may develop.[34] When lateral displacement is the dominant result, there is a 20% incidence of associated injury to the nasolacrimal and nasofrontal ducts and a 30% incidence of ocular injury resulting in visual impairment.[34] With much of the force being displaced

laterally, postseptal hemorrhage within the orbits often ensues. Injury to the medial canthal ligaments may occur, resulting in telecanthism[6,33] (Fig. 3-42).

These injuries virtually always require open reduction and fixation, using the combination of interfragmentary wiring and hardware fixation.[6,7,17,22] Even with a prompt and aggressive surgical approach, this injury often leads to a significant posttraumatic deformity. CT imaging can demonstrate the full extent of the fractures in the acute setting and, together with three-dimensional imaging, can help define the full extent of deformity in the chronic setting as cosmetic reconstructive surgery is planned.[32] Radionuclide cisternography can help to provide objective evidence of a CSF leak, although it lacks the spatial resolution necessary to map out the full anatomic detail necessary before surgical fixation. High-resolution CT imaging in association with contrast cisternography is the study of choice.

Zygomaticomaxillary Fractures

If the maxilla is the bone that is recognized by the general population as the structure beneath the *cheek*, it is the zygoma that represents the *cheekbone*. In fact, the high

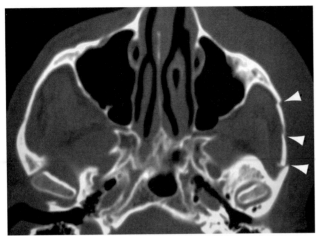

Fig. 3-28
Isolated zygomatic arch fracture in a man admitted following an assault. Multislice CT images show a comminuted minimally depressed left zygomatic arch fracture (*arrowheads*).

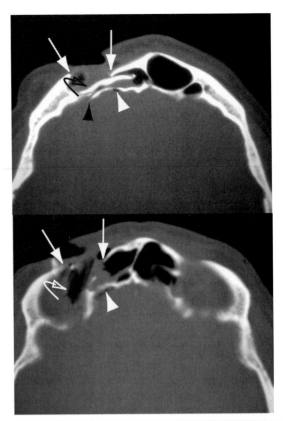

Fig. 3-30
Open frontal sinus fracture in a 51-year-old man who struck his face while falling on wood. Helical CT images show a defect in the anterior wall of the right frontal sinus (*arrows*), with a floating bone fragment (*black curved arrow*) within the right frontal sinus. A subtle fracture (*black arrowhead*) of the posterior wall of the right frontal sinus and pneumocephalus (*white arrowheads*) indicate an open frontal sinus fracture. Wood (*white curved arrow*) is also seen within the right orbit and frontal sinus.

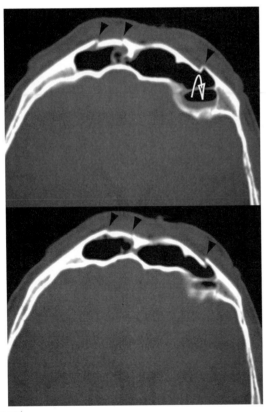

Fig. 3-29
Isolated anterior table fracture of frontal sinus in a 54-year-old man who fell onto his face. Multislice spiral CT images show a comminuted fracture (*arrowheads*) of the anterior table of both the right and left frontal sinuses. Soft tissue swelling is seen anterior to the fractures, with an air-fluid level (*curved arrow*) in the left frontal sinus.

cheekbone feature so admired in fashion models is a direct reference to the relationship between the zygoma and the remainder of the facial skeleton. The zygoma delin-

eates the inferolateral margin of the orbit, representing a cornerstone between various facial structures and a point of intersection between the lateral sagittal, middle horizontal, and anterior coronal struts of the face (see Fig. 3-9). Specifically, the structure articulates superiorly with the zygomatic process of the frontal bone, where it completes the lateral orbital rim; posteriorly, within the orbit, with the greater wing of the sphenoid bone, where it contributes to the lateral wall of the orbit; medially and inferiorly with the maxilla, where it contributes to the orbital floor and inferior orbital rim and leads to the slope of the cheek; and posterolaterally with the zygomatic process of the temporal bone, thereby completing the zygomatic arch (see Figs. 3-1, 3-4, 3-5, and 3-10).

Studies have shown that fractures of the zygoma account for more than half of midface injuries.[15] In one study of midface fractures, the zygoma was involved in 69% of cases.[35] These injuries fall along a spectrum, from simple fractures of the zygomatic arch to the more extensive zygomaticomaxillary complex fractures (Figs. 3-12

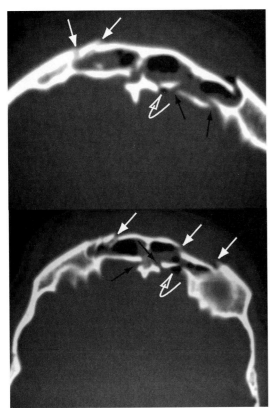

Fig. 3-31
Open frontal sinus fracture. Multislice spiral CT images show displaced comminuted fractures of both the anterior (*white arrows*) and posterior tables (*black arrows*) of the right and left frontal sinuses. Pneumocephalus (*curved arrows*) is also present. Frontal sinus exoneration and repair of a dural tear was performed.

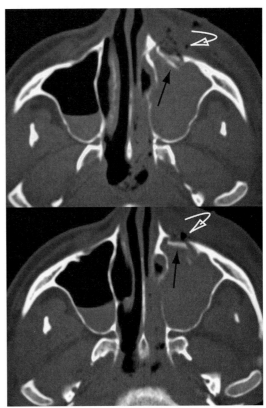

Fig. 3-32
Isolated anterior wall fracture of maxillary sinus in a 42-year-old man struck in the face by a hockey puck. Multislice spiral CT images show a comminuted anterior wall fracture (*arrows*) of the left maxillary sinus with subcutaneous emphysema (*curved arrows*). Complete opacification of the left maxillary sinus and an air-fluid level in the right maxillary sinus can also be seen.

and 3-43 to 3-46). The latter were previously referred to as "tripod" fractures, but that term has been largely abandoned, since it failed to reflect the complexity and severity of fractures associated with this injury. In actuality, the ZMC complex often does not involve the zygoma itself as much as the abutting weaker bones to which it is attached. In the simplest conceptualization, the ZMC injury represents a disjunction of the zygoma from its adjacent osseous connections so that the cheekbone becomes a freely moveable piece of bone. Thus there is a fracture through the lateral orbital rim in the vicinity of the zygomaticofrontal suture (Fig. 3-47), a fracture through the lateral wall of the orbit near the zygomaticosphenoid suture, a fracture through the inferior orbital rim (and typically orbital floor as well), and a fracture through the zygomatic arch, severing the connection to the temporal bone. Typically, there are additional fractures through the anterior and posterior walls of the maxillary sinus, thereby releasing the zygoma (Figs. 3-12 and 3-43 to 3-46). Rarely, incomplete ZMC fractures result when one of the osseous connections remains intact, as is discussed later.

Numerous classification systems have been devised to categorize the various types of ZMC injuries. Some of these have been based on the mechanism and force of injury, the fracture patterns, and therapeutic decision making.[15,35-37] From a purely anatomic point of view, ZMC fractures can be subdivided into those that are nondisplaced, displaced without rotation, and displaced with rotation. This classification system offers value beyond the conceptualization of injuries, since it relates directly to numerous other dimensions of the injury, including extent of bony injury, associated soft tissue injury, clinical presentation and sequelae, and surgical planning.

Nondisplaced ZMC fractures are often secondary to incomplete fracturing of one or more of the buttresses, often at the zygomaticofrontal suture. Such fractures may lend themselves to closed reduction, since the zygoma has not been completely severed from its adjacent bony attachments.

Rotated and displaced fractures present more of a challenge to repair (Figs. 3-45 to 3-47). The intact lateral facial buttress is the stabilizing strut for the force of the

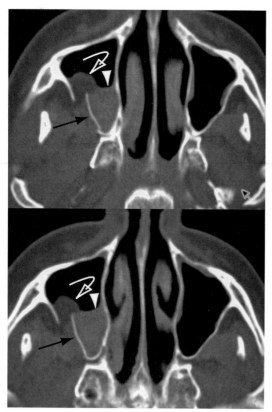

Fig. 3-33
Isolated lateral wall fracture of maxillary sinus with fat herniation. Multislice CT images show a medially displaced isolated comminuted lateral wall fracture (*arrows*) of the right maxillary antrum. Fat (*curved arrows*) from the infratemporal fossa herniates into the antrum through the lateral wall defect. An air-fluid level (*arrowheads*) is also seen in the right maxillary antrum.

contraction of the masseter muscle, which has a broad attachment against the body and arch of the zygoma.[15] Accordingly, fractures of this buttress serve as one of the key factors, along with the magnitude and direction of the traumatic force, that allows for displacement and rotation of the zygoma. The zygoma can be displaced inferiorly, laterally, or posteriorly (Figs. 3-45 and 3-47). Rotation of the main corpus of the zygoma can also be multidirectional. When viewing the facial skeleton in a frontal projection, one can see that the left zygoma, for example, can be rotated medially or laterally. Lateral rotation of the left zygoma implies a clockwise rotation as viewed when facing the patient, and medial rotation refers to counterclockwise rotation. Rotation can also occur along the vertical (craniocaudal) axis. Thus when viewing the fracture on axial CT imaging, one can assess whether the zygoma is rotated medially or laterally in this dimension (Figs. 3-44 to 3-46).

Rotation and displacement of the zygoma can result in enophthalmos or exophthalmos if it influences the orbital volume, and such fractures are also at risk for increased instability.[38] In fact, displacement at the zygomaticofrontal suture alone is an indication for open reduction.[6] Furthermore, inferior displacement leads to distortion of the lateral canthus and other cosmetic deformities. The involvement of the inferior orbital rim and orbital floor accounts for the high prevalence of injury to the infraorbital nerve. However, entrapment of the inferior rectus muscle is encountered less frequently in ZMC fractures than in orbital blowout fractures because the orbital floor involvement in ZMC injuries is

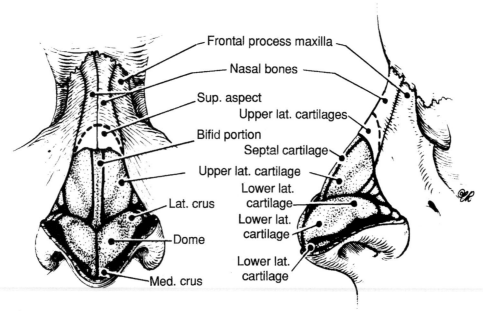

Fig. 3-34
Bony and cartilaginous nasal septum. Note that in the sagittal section, the nasal bone has a thick upper portion and thinner lower portion. (Illustration by Elizabeth Roselius, 1987; from Foster CA, Sherman, JE: *Surgery of facial bone fractures*, New York, 1987, Churchill Livingstone.)

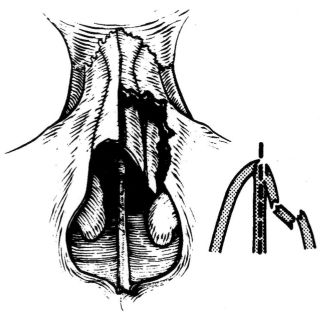

Fig. 3-35
Frontal and axial cross-section illustrations of a unilateral depressed fracture of the nasal bone and frontal process of the maxilla. (Illustration by Elizabeth Roselius, 1987; from Foster CA, Sherman, JE: *Surgery of facial bone fractures*, New York, 1987, Churchill Livingstone.)

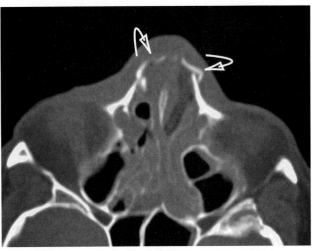

Fig. 3-37
Displaced fracture of nasal bone in a man punched in the nose. Bilateral displaced nasal bone fractures (*curved arrows*) are seen. Soft tissue swelling over the nose is also present.

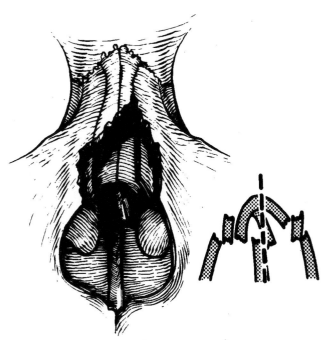

Fig. 3-36
Frontal and axial cross-section illustrations of depressed fracture of both nasal bones, frontal processes of the maxilla, and nasal septum. (Illustration by Elizabeth Roselius, 1987; from Foster CA, Sherman, JE: *Surgery of facial bone fractures*, New York, 1987, Churchill Livingstone.)

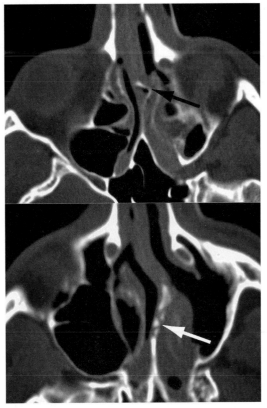

Fig. 3-38
Nasal septum fracture. Multislice spiral CT images show nasal septum is deformed (*black arrow*) and fragmented (*white arrow*), indicating a comminuted fracture.

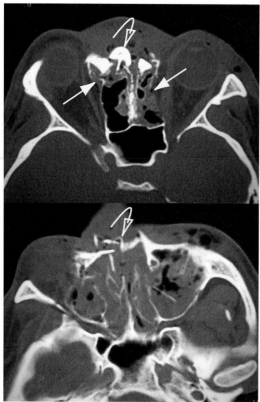

Fig. 3-39
Nasoorbital-ethmoid complex fracture. Conventional CT images show nasal bones (*curved arrow*) are driven posteriorly into the ethmoid sinuses, with fractures (*arrows*) of medial walls of both orbits. The anteromedial walls of both orbits are displaced laterally by posterior displacement of nasal bones.

typically more laterally oriented, beyond the course of the inferior rectus muscle, than in the more classic blowout fracture. Finally, in addition to the orbital consequences of ZMC injuries, such injuries also often lead to impingement on the coronoid process of the mandible or the temporomandibular joint itself or impairment of temporalis muscle function, all of which can lead to restricted range of mandibular motion and excursion and impaired mastication.

TRANSFACIAL FRACTURES

Le Fort Fractures

Complex midface fractures were classified by Rene Le Fort during the early 1900s in an attempt to provide a general conceptual approach to the various injury patterns that can occur in the midface in the setting of severe trauma. The greatest value of this system was in the pre-CT era, when plain film analysis could provide valuable but limited anatomic detail of facial fractures to supplement the physical examination findings and aid in surgical plan-

ning. In actuality, however, severe midface trauma usually results in a constellation of fractures that typically do not fit neatly into the Le Fort classification system, often demonstrating mixed or incomplete Le Fort patterns or additional fractures that are not part of the Le Fort system at all. With the advent of routine CT imaging for the evaluation of craniofacial trauma, the anatomic information that can now be attained is so detailed that to simply assign a Le Fort typing to a set of fractures may at times be an oversimplification. Great advances in craniofacial reconstructive techniques make it imperative that the full extent of injury be identified on high-resolution imaging.

Common to all of the Le Fort fractures are a number of anatomical and conceptual points. All are complex fractures that involve multiple struts and require open reduction and fixation. They all have the potential to result in considerable facial deformity and functional impairment. But perhaps the most important point is that they all represent some degree of disconnection between the facial skeleton and the skull base. The single most characteristic feature of all Le Fort fractures is involvement of the pterygoid plates. Noting again that these bony structures are osseous extensions from the sphenoid bone, the main bone of the central skull base, and that they are fused to the posterior surface of the maxillae, it becomes apparent how fractures that involve the pterygoid plates serve to sever one of the sites of facial-skull base union.

The Le Fort I fracture pattern is a horizontally oriented fracture line that involves the inferior portion of the midface (Figs. 3-48 to 3-50). Classically, the fracture line extends across the inferior portions of both maxillary antra, involving all of the walls of the maxillae, as well as the inferior nasal cavity. Extension posteriorly through the pterygoid plates completes the pattern, leading to the "floating palate." The palate, along with the maxillary ridge and alveolus of the maxillae, becomes a free fragment, separated from the upper portion of the midface skeleton. The palate itself may or may not be fractured as well. Although delineation of the full extent of injury was at times challenged by early CT imaging techniques because of the in-plane nature of some of the fractures, current high-resolution multislice CT imaging provides a thorough evaluation, especially when employing multiplanar reformatting techniques for the generation of high-quality coronal, sagittal, and oblique images.

As one would expect, the most dominant clinical finding on physical examination in a patient with a Le Fort I fracture is mobility of the maxillary dental arch.[6] Such mobility may be hindered if the fracture is impacted or incomplete. Midface swelling and ecchymosis are extensive, and nasopharyngeal bleeding is profuse.

The Le Fort II fracture complex represents a more extensive injury. It is also the most commonly encountered pattern of the various Le Fort fractures. Whereas the

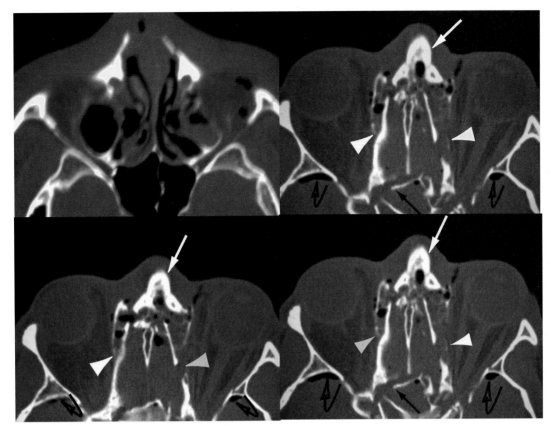

Fig. 3-40
Nasoorbital-ethmoid fracture in a 23-year-old tree surgeon who fell 20 feet from a tree onto his face. Multislice CT images show posterior displacement of nasal bones (*white arrows*) into the orbits and ethmoid sinuses bilaterally. Both medial orbital walls are fractured (*arrowheads*) and displaced laterally. A skull base fracture (*black arrows*) and pneumocephalus (*curved arrows*) are also seen.

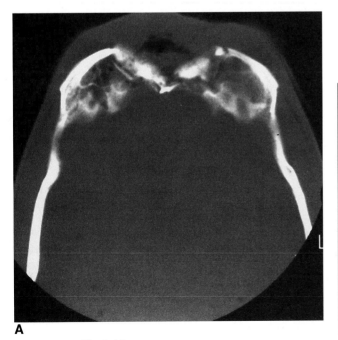

A

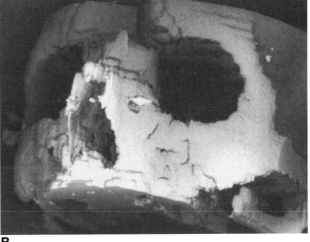

B

Fig. 3-41
Nasoorbital-ethmoid fracture. **A**, CT image through the orbital plates of the frontal bones demonstrates a severely comminuted and posteriorly displaced fracture of the nasal bridge and inferior frontal bone. **B**, Three-dimensional surface contour image of the injury from a frontolateral perspective.

Disrupted MCL

Lacrimal
sac injury

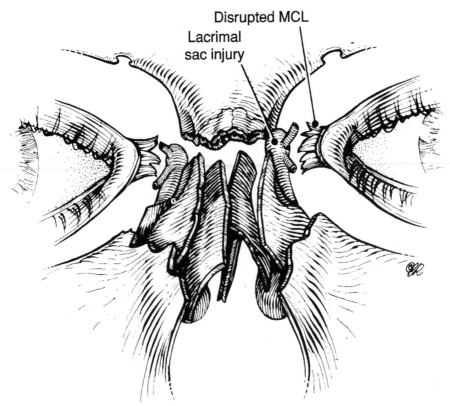

Fig. 3-42
Diagram of nasoorbital-ethmoid fracture, illustrating concurrent injury to the medial canthal ligament (*MCL*) and lacrimal sac. (Illustration by Elizabeth Roselius, 1987; from Foster CA, Sherman, JE: *Surgery of facial bone fractures*, New York, 1987, Churchill Livingstone.)

Le Fort I pattern releases the palate and maxillary ridge from its other skull base and facial skeletal attachments but leaves the orbits and upper nasal cavity structures intact, the Le Fort II involves these structures, leading to the pyramidal shape of disconnected facial structures that gives it its other name (Figs. 3-51 and 3-52). Thus the fracture lines, when viewed in the frontal view, assume a three-dimensional triangular configuration, with the apex of the pyramid centered at the nasal bridge and frontonasoethmoid complex. As the sides of the triangle descend from its apex, the fractures involve the medial orbital walls (lacrimal bone and lamina papyracea) and the orbital floors in the region of the infraorbital canals and then continue in an inferolateral course to involve the anterior and posterolateral walls of the maxillary sinuses, ultimately terminating in the pterygoid plates. In the classic Le Fort II fracture, the central pyramidal unit of the midface skeleton stays united, although typically displaced posteriorly, giving rise to the characteristic "dish face" deformity. The medial walls of the maxillary sinuses remain intact, as does the inferior nasal septum. The hard palate does not "float" as in the Le Fort I but rather serves as the base of the detached pyramidal midface unit. Furthermore, there is no involvement of the lateral orbital walls or zygomatic arches. These structures remain

anchored to their skull base attachments, thereby distinguishing the Le Fort II from the Le Fort III, which is discussed later.

Complications of Le Fort II injuries include severe cosmetic deformity associated with the "dish face" depression, malocclusion, and sensory impairment secondary to injury of the infraorbital nerves. The latter has been reported to occur in almost 80% of patients.[15]

The Le Fort III fracture represents the most dramatic and severe injury among the Le Fort midface fracture patterns. This fracture involves complete disconnection of the facial skeleton from the skull base structures. In this injury, also known as craniofacial dysjunction (Figs. 3-53 to 3-55), the lateral midface structures, including the lateral orbital walls and zygomatic arches, are fractured, along with the central upper midface structures that form the apex of the pyramid in the Le Fort II injury. Thus the fracture lines extend right across the upper facial skeleton from side to side. At their lateral margins, the fractures then extend down through the zygomatic arches. Once the upper facial skeleton is separated from the anterior skull base and the zygomas are separated from their points of junction to the temporal bones on each side, the only remaining site of junction between the facial skeleton and skull base is at the pterygoid plates/maxil-

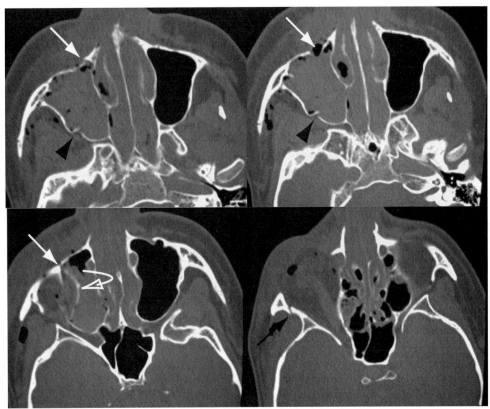

Fig. 3-43
Nondisplaced zygomaticomaxillary complex injury in a 16-year-old admitted with facial hematoma following a motor vehicle collision. Multislice spiral CT images through the face and orbit show fractures of the lateral (*arrowheads*) and anterior walls (*white arrows*) of the right maxillary sinus, lateral orbital wall (*black arrow*), and orbital floor (*curved arrow*).

lae. As the fractures continue to extend inferiorly and involve these structures, the end result is complete detachment of the facial skeleton from the skull base. In its purest form, the midface remains a solitary unit, as the anterior and lateral maxillary sinus walls are left intact.

Smash Fractures

High-energy injuries that result in severe comminution of the facial skeleton and that reflect multiple fracture planes and patterns are considered smash fractures (Fig. 3-56). These injuries are typically more serious than the other midface fractures previously discussed and are typically associated with other life-threatening injuries, including intracranial hemorrhage, temporal bone fractures, and cervical spine injuries.

MANDIBULAR FRACTURES

Mandibular fractures can occur as isolated injuries or in association with other facial fractures (Fig. 3-57). In approximately 50% of the cases, there is a solitary fracture within the mandible, whereas in the other half of the cases, the mandible is fractured in multiple sites.[25,39,40]

The fractures are generally characterized based on severity and location.[18] *Simple* fractures are those in which there is a single fracture line and no communication between the fracture and the oral cavity or extension through the overlying skin, as opposed to *compound* fractures, which result in one or both of these connections. Mandibular fractures may also be considered *comminuted* when there are multiple fracture fragments and *impacted* when there is foreshortening and restricted movement of the fragments. *Greenstick* fractures involve only one side of the cortex, while the other side is bent; these rare fractures are most commonly encountered in children and occur in the subcondylar region. Finally, fractures may be considered *pathologic* if they occur at a site of underlying osseous disease.

The most frequently fractured portion of the mandible is the condylar/subcondylar region[18,39,41] (Figs. 3-58 to 3-60). Since this portion of the mandible is protected from direct impact by the overlying zygomatic arch, these fractures are typically due to an impact elsewhere, such as the symphysis or body (Fig. 3-61; see Fig. 3-60). The fractures are often angulated or displaced and not infrequently associated with condylar subluxation out of the glenoid fossa.[42] These fractures may be further subcategorized

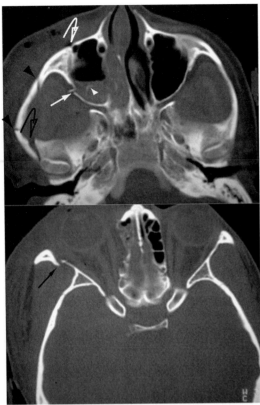

Fig. 3-44
Zygomaticomaxillary complex fracture with involvement of the temporomandibular joint. Axial images show a displaced comminuted fracture of the right zygoma (*black arrowheads*), with a fracture of the posterior zygomatic arch extending into the anterior wall of the temporomandibular joint (*black curved arrows*). Fractures of the right orbital floor (*white arrowhead*), lateral wall of the orbit (*black arrow*), and anterior (*white curved arrow*) and lateral walls (*white arrow*) of the maxillary sinus are also seen.

into intracapsular and extracapsular. The intracapsular fractures are the less common of the two forms (Figs. 3-58 and 3-59) and occur most frequently in children.[18] Because intracapsular fractures extend to the articular surface of the condyle, they may ultimately lead to the development of debilitating secondary arthritic changes. As one would expect, these very superior fractures often elude detection on plain films and require CT imaging for their identification and characterization.[43] Extracapsular fractures involve the subcondylar region and are more frequently unilateral than bilateral, although the unilateral fractures are often associated with contralateral mandibular angle fractures[18] (Fig. 3-62). In rare circumstances, the force of the impact of the condyle in the glenoid fossa will be transmitted into the temporal bone and specifically into the adjacent carotid canal, resulting in traumatic injury to the internal carotid artery.

Fractures involving the mandibular angles, bodies, and symphysis/parasymphyseal region occur with similar frequencies, although solitary fractures most commonly

involve the angle.[18] Coronoid process and ramus fractures occur much less frequently, owing to the protection afforded these structures by the overlying musculature and zygoma. In all sites, the direction and displacement of the fracture fragments will vary, depending on the magnitude and direction of the injuring force.

In a minority of cases, mandibular fractures can lead to mechanical airway obstruction. This can result from associated hematoma or posterior displacement of the tongue. Thus in the hyperacute setting, the evaluation should include specific attention being paid to the airway. In addition, the identification of loose teeth should be noted because of the risk they pose if they break free and are aspirated.

CT imaging is the modality of choice for the evaluation of mandibular fractures. High-resolution spiral imaging with the generation of 1-mm axial images is ideal for both identifying the extent of injury in the transverse plane and generating multiplanar reformatted images. Sagittal oblique images are particularly useful to demonstrate fracture lines that involve the mandibular body and ramus. Curved reformatted images simulate Panorex films and offer clear depiction of the symphysis/parasymphyseal region as well as the mandibular condyles (Fig. 3-63). Three-dimensional imaging with multitissue displays can be of additional value in surgical planning (Fig. 3-63), which is addressed later.

RADIOLOGIC EVALUATION AND INTERPRETATION

Overview

The armamentarium available to the radiologist evaluating the craniofacial trauma patient and the clinician charged with the mandate to treat that individual has evolved quite significantly over the past 25 years. Plain films, comprising multiple standard views (Waters, Caldwell, Towne, and lateral) and supplemented by specialized views (submental vertex, lateral nasal, and mandibular) when indicated, represented the earliest method of evaluating such patients.

The introduction of CT in the 1970s brought a new method of achieving highly detailed imaging that quickly demonstrated its superiority over plain films.[44,45] Axial imaging with 2.5- to 3-mm sections provided detail regarding fracture delineation, comminution, and displacement that simply could not be ascertained with plain films. Direct coronal imaging proved invaluable for investigating those bony structures that course in the transverse plane, parallel to the axial plane, such as the orbital roof and floor, cribriform plate and planum sphenoidale, hard palate, and floor of the middle cranial fossa. Furthermore, evaluation of the soft tissues of the

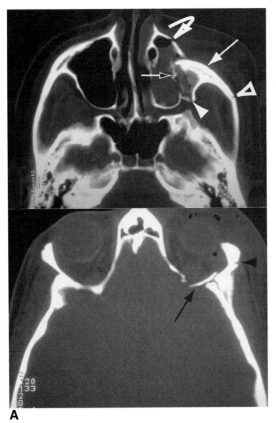

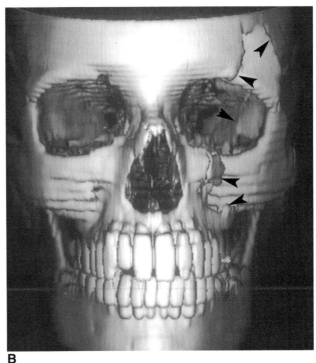

Fig. 3-45
Displaced atypical left zygomaticomaxillary complex (ZMC) fracture. **A,** Axial conventional CT images show posterior inferior displacement of the body of the left zygoma (*white arrow*). Fractures of the orbital roof (*black arrow*), zygomatic arch (*open arrowhead*), lateral wall of the orbit (*black arrowhead*), orbital floor (*black and white arrow*), and anterior (*curved arrow*) and lateral (*white arrowhead*) walls of the maxilla are also seen. **B,** Three-dimensional surface contour image from the frontal perspective shows these fractures (*arrowheads*) and displacement of the zygoma posteroinferiorly. Involvement of the frontal bone is atypical with this fracture pattern.

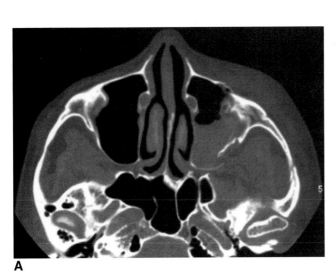

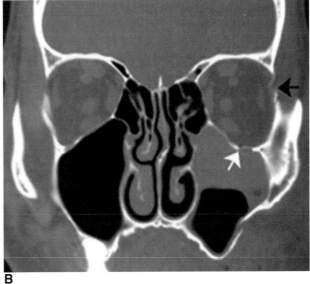

Fig. 3-46
ZMC fracture. **A,** CT image shows fractures of anterior and posterolateral wall of left maxillary sinus and midzygomatic arch consistent with ZMC pattern. **B,** Coronal view shows minimally displaced orbital floor (*white arrow*) and lateral orbital wall (*black arrow*) fractures and hemorrhage layers in the maxillary sinus.

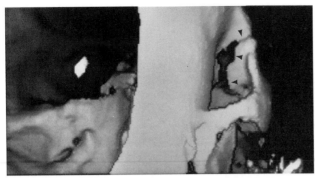

Fig. 3-47
Lateral orbital wall fracture. This 3-D-rendered posterior view of the lateral orbital wall in a patient with a ZMC injury shows a typical fracture pattern involved in this injury as well as the Le Fort fractures (see Fig. 3-48). The fracture begins as a frontozygomatic suture separation and continues inferiorly through a suture between the orbital process of the greater sphenoid wing posteriorly and the orbital process of the zygoma anteriorly (*arrowheads*). These sutures are a natural line of weakness in the lateral orbital wall.

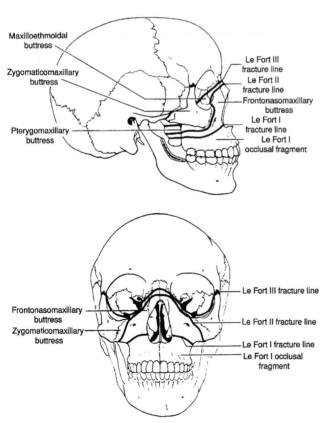

Fig. 3-48
Lateral and frontal views of the facial anatomy show classic Le Fort fracture patterns representing lines of anatomic weakness and major supporting buttresses. (From Federle MP, Brant-Zawadski M: *Computed tomography in the evaluation of trauma*, ed 2, Baltimore, 1986, Williams & Wilkins.)

face and orbits was now standard. Ruptured globes, retinal hemorrhage, intraorbital and intraocular foreign bodies, as well as edematous and entrapped extraocular muscles could now be readily identified, not to mention the threatened oropharyngeal airway and associated intracranial injury (Figs. 3-64 to 3-71). Computed tomography became the study of choice to delineate the extent of injury.

During this time, plain films remained a reasonable diagnostic tool, primarily because of the limited availability of CT scanners and the apprehension to jump immediately from the emergency room to CT without first obtaining a study that served to at least confirm the clinical suspicion of facial fractures. Furthermore, the CT examination itself was time-consuming, and direct coronal positioning in either the prone or supine position was challenging even for cooperative, healthy patients, not to mention the challenge it presented to the acute trauma patient, who was often either not stable enough to tolerate this positioning or not yet deemed stable because the cervical spine had not been cleared. Thus the plain film examination still maintained a role.

With the development of the spiral CT technology in the late 1980s and, more recently, with the introduction of the multislice or multidetector spiral CT technology in the 1990s, there has been clear movement toward a paradigm shift in the evaluation of acute trauma patients.[24,25,46-49] This advanced technology offers the benefits of high-resolution imaging that can be completed in a matter of seconds. The multislice spiral technology, in particular, allows for the generation of cross-sectional images that not only possess high spatial resolution and image detail but also serve as the substrate for the generation of high-quality computer-generated reformatted images. Coupled with advances in computer postprocessing hardware and software, the finished imaging product may now consist of an array of cross-sectional axial images; coronal, sagittal, and curved two-dimensional reformatted images; and three-dimensional images that may display either a single tissue (e.g., bone) or multiple tissues (e.g., bone, fat, or muscle) in the same image. Furthermore, the increasing availability of this technology around the clock, especially in the high-volume trauma centers, has led to much greater accessibility. Many trauma centers have a CT unit in the emergency radiology department in proximity to the patient care areas. Many of these patients are polytrauma patients and will already undergo CT imaging of the head, abdomen, pelvis, and perhaps other body parts as well. Adding a high-resolution CT study of the facial bones when facial fractures are suspected is then relatively easy to do, efficient, and comprehensive. All this, however, is not to say that there is no longer a role for plain films even when such powerful CT technology is readily available. One recent study identified the poten-

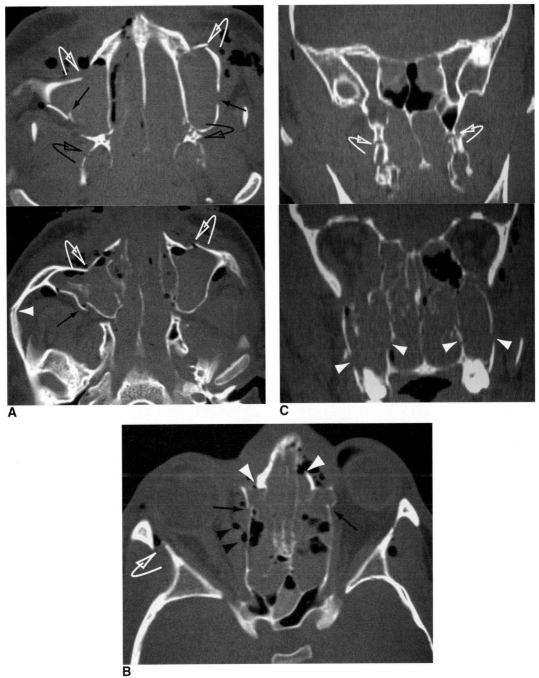

Fig. 3-49
Asymmetric Le Fort fractures in man injured in a motor vehicle collision. **A**, Multislice CT images show bilateral pterygoid plate fractures (*black curved arrows*) and fractures of the anterior (*white curved arrows*) and lateral walls (*arrows*) of both maxillary sinuses. These fractures extend to the lower aspect of the maxillary sinuses. Fractures on the right side are more displaced than those on the left. A laterally displaced fracture (*arrowhead*) of the right zygoma is also seen. **B**, Image through orbits shows fractures (*white arrowheads*) of both nasal bones, medial walls of the orbits (*arrows*), and the lateral wall of the right orbit (*curved arrow*). Within a right extraconal hematoma, orbital emphysema (*black arrowheads*) is seen. These fractures indicate a bilateral Le Fort I and II fracture, with a Le Fort III fracture on the right side. **C**, Multiplanar reformatted images in the coronal plane better reveal the bilateral Le Fort I (*arrowheads*) with pterygoid plate fractures (*curved arrows*).

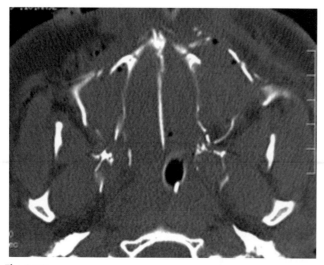

Fig. 3-50
Le Fort I pattern. All three walls of both maxillary sinuses are fractured just above the hard palate. Fractures are present in both pterygoid plates and in the bony nasal septum.

tial economic benefits of screening for facial fractures using a single occipitomental 15-degree plain film.[50] This certainly merits consideration at a time when health care resources are limited, yet such technology is designed to address a screening goal, which is considerably different from the highly detailed diagnostic study required by clinicians to determine and plan a surgical approach.

Imaging Goals

The advent of robust CT imaging and postprocessing tools that now supplement the more basic and established utility of plain films brings to light new challenges. When the only diagnostic tool was the plain film series, there were few difficult decisions to be made. Deviation from the standard series was uncommon and typically unnecessary. Now, however, there are many decisions to be made. Indeed, after the choice to evaluate with CT rather than plain films is made, the questions just begin.

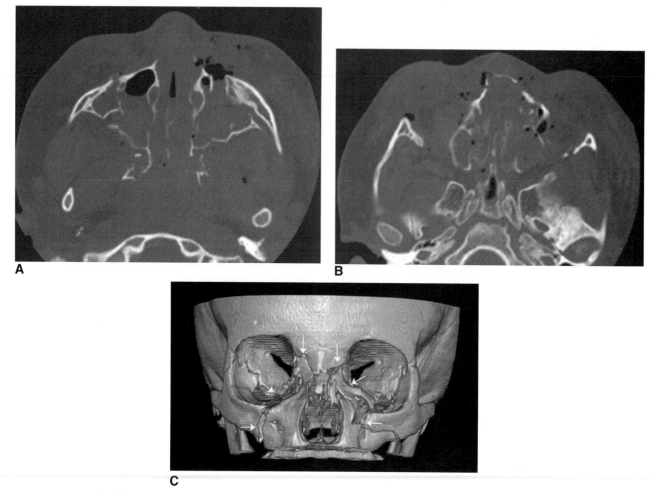

Fig. 3-51
Le Fort II fracture pattern. **A**, CT image showing marked comminuted fractures of the walls of the maxillary sinuses, pterygoid plates, and left frontal process of the maxilla. **B**, CT through a higher level shows comminuted bilateral nasal bone fractures. Zygomatic arches are intact. **C**, Three-dimensional volumetric surface contour image nicely depicts the pyramidal nature of the Le Fort II pattern (*arrows*).

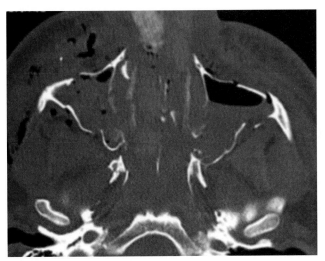

Fig. 3-52
CT of Le Fort II pattern. Image at the level of the frontal processes of the maxilla shows fractures of all walls of the maxillary sinuses and bony nasal septum. There is nasal packing in place. Fractures of the right pterygoid plates are evident, but left pterygoid fractures were noted at adjacent levels (not shown).

How should the CT study be done? What technique factors should be used? How, if at all, should the postprocessing be done? Now, more than ever before, there has to be a clear definition of one's imaging goals. Studies can now be sharply tailored to meet the needs of the patient and the referring clinician but only if the radiologist recognizes those needs.

Defining one's imaging goals must be done in two realms. In the first realm, one must deal with certain abstract concepts, even though they ultimately lead to concrete protocol design issues. Thus, in this realm, one must consider whether the imaging study is being carried out to *screen* for injury, to *detect* the injury, or to *depict* the injury.

To *screen* for facial skeletal injury, one could argue that plain films are an inexpensive yet effective way to accomplish this.[50] On the other hand, one could utilize intermediate to thick section (e.g., 3 to 5 mm) CT imaging to achieve the same goal. If the trauma patient is already destined to undergo CT imaging of another body part, one could easily see the benefits, in terms of disposition

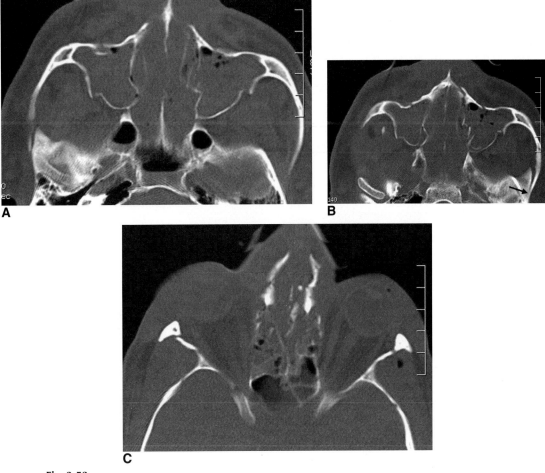

Fig. 3-53
CT of Le Fort III pattern. **A**, CT at level of the midmaxillary sinuses shows fractures of the anterior and posterolateral sinus walls, bony nasal septum (*arrowhead*), and right posterior zygomatic arch. **B**, More cephalad image shows fracture involving left zygomatic arch as well (*arrow*). **C**, Image at midorbit level shows bilateral lateral and medial wall orbit fractures with associated zygomatic arch fractures as part of Le Fort III pattern.

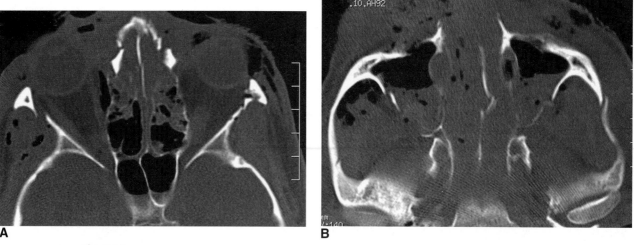

Fig. 3-54
CT of Le Fort III pattern. **A**, CT at midorbit level shows bilateral medial and lateral orbit wall fractures with associated comminuted nasal bone fractures. **B**, CT at midmaxillary sinus level shows fractures of zygomatic arches, all six maxillary sinus walls, midline nasal septum, and frontal processes of the maxilla. Pterygoid plate fractures were seen at other levels.

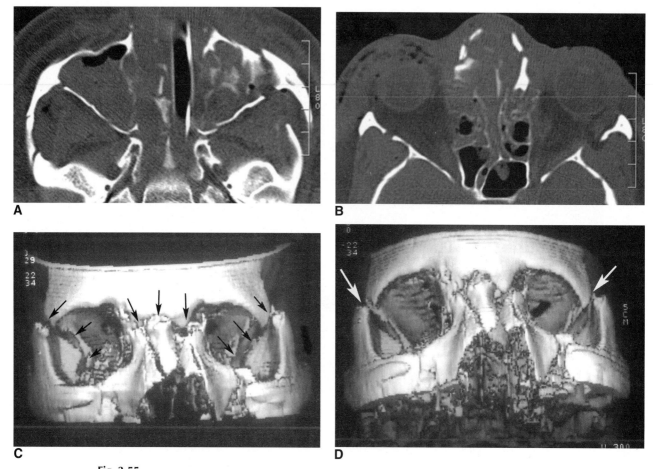

Fig. 3-55
CT of Le Fort III pattern. **A**, CT image at midmaxillary sinus level shows bilateral zygomatic arch fractures, left anterior and bilateral posterolateral maxillary wall fractures, and a nasal septal fracture. **B**, CT at midorbit level shows displaced lateral and medial wall fractures and comminuted nasal fractures. **C** and **D**, Surface contour images in frontal and inferior frontal views show W-shaped Le Fort fracture as it courses from the lateral orbital wall to the medial orbital wall and across the midline (*black arrows*). The frontozygomatic sutures (*white arrows*) and lateral orbital sutures are split, and there is a nasoorbital-ethmoid fracture pattern.

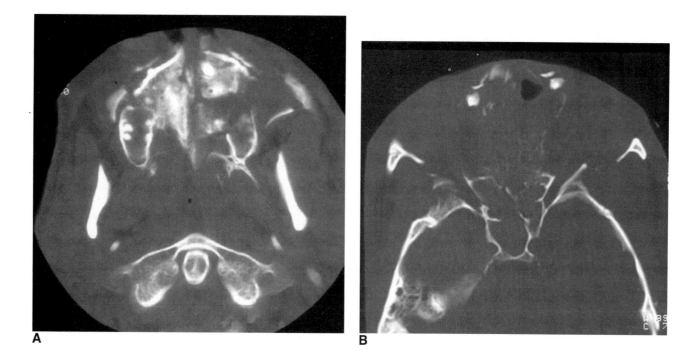

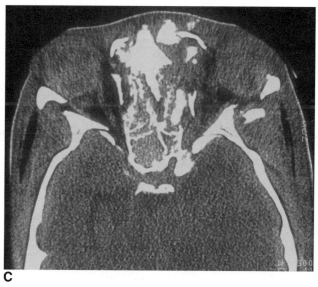

Fig. 3-56
CT of "facial smash." **A** to **C**, CT images through face in blunt trauma patient show features of combined Lefort I, II, and III patterns with comminuted fractures. There is a concurrent NOE injury pattern with posterior displacement of the nasal bridge and lateral displacement of the nasal bones. There is severe comminution of the hard palate and orbital walls with bilateral hemorrhagic globes.

time and accuracy of diagnosis, of adding this study on while the patient is on the CT table. Indeed, one could argue that if it has already been determined that the patient is to undergo CT imaging of the brain, one could simply modify the angulation of the slice acquisition to include visualization of the facial skeleton; even with standard 5-mm axial imaging, one will likely be left with

an adequate screening study of the facial bones. Since the multislice CT manufacturers offer various software programs for image splitting and image fusion, it might even be possible to achieve thinner sections through the facial bones while maintaining 5-mm thick sections through the brain and accomplish this all in a single acquisition.

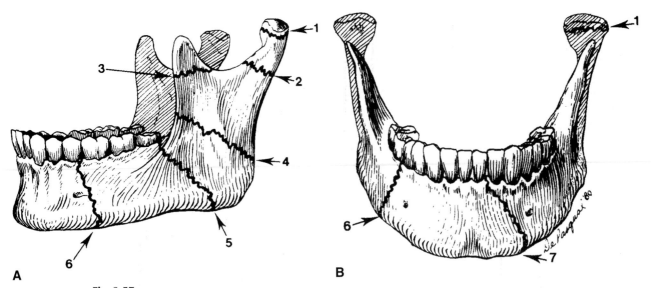

A

B

Fig. 3-57
A and **B**, Locations of mandibular fractures. *1,* Condylar; *2,* subcondylar. *3,* coronoid; *4,* ramus; *5,* angle; *6,* body; *7,* parasymphyseal. (Illustration by DePasqual JA. Reprinted with permission from Gerlock AJ: *Clinical and radiographic interpretation of facial fractures,* Boston, 1981, Little, Brown.)

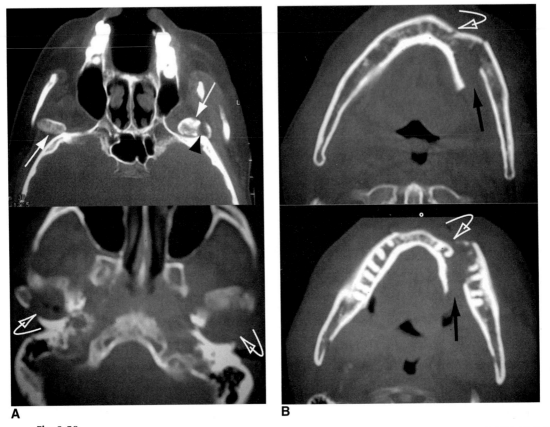

A

B

Fig. 3-58
Condylar head fracture in a man complaining of malocclusion after a fall. **A**, Single-slice spiral CT images show anteroinferior dislocation of the mandibular condyles (*arrows*) from the glenoid fossae (*curved arrows*). A fracture of the left condylar head is also seen (*arrowhead*). **B**, A fracture of the contralateral body (*curved arrow*) with bicortical involvement and moderate displacement (*straight arrow*).

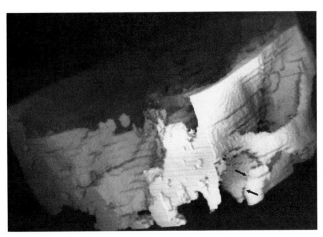

Fig. 3-59
Surface contour CT of a minimally displaced oblique intracapsular fracture (*arrows*) of the mandibular condyle from a posterior lateral perspective.

Detecting and *diagnosing* the extent of facial fractures is a significantly different goal from screening for them. In this context, the generation of high-quality axial and coronal images is the primary goal. In the early CT days, this was done with direct imaging in both planes. Now this can be done either the same way or with high-resolution imaging in the axial plane and then the generation of high-quality coronal reformatted images. The latter technique is of particular benefit in the acute trauma patient for the various reasons discussed earlier. The multislice technology has had a powerful impact on this imaging approach and is discussed in greater detail later.

Fracture *depiction* is still another abstract imaging goal. It is one thing to identify the full extent of craniofacial injury that a patient may have sustained. High-quality axial and coronal images are quite valuable in this regard. However, to be able to *depict* the fractures in a way that is particularly meaningful to the surgeon who needs to address them is quite another goal. Radiologists are trained to examine a series of two-dimensional images and construct a three-dimensional model in their minds. Clinicians have been forced to do this as well because the fundamental product of the CT acquisition has, until recently, been the two-dimensional images. In truth, the value of three-dimensional reformatted images for craniofacial trauma has been documented in numerous studies,[32,51-55] although not without some controversy. It has been debated whether three-dimensional images add true diagnostic value to that provided by the two-dimensional images, with a minority of authors arguing that they do. On the other hand, it has been stated fairly unanimously that three-dimensional images aid in surgical planning and in patient education. Nevertheless, three-dimensional imaging has come a long way since many of these studies were conducted. Advances in computer hardware and software make the generation of such images an easy task. Indeed, more advanced three-dimensional postprocessing is readily available and may prove even more valuable to the clinicians than they currently realize. Volumetric assessments and advanced volume-rendering techniques are already available; other sophisticated applications, such as virtual surgery, may be coming soon. It may even turn out that the *primary* imaging goals for craniofacial trauma patients (and other CT patients) may not be the two-dimensional image sets but rather three-dimensional portrayals of the anatomy and pathology.

The first realm of goal definition is the abstract—screening, detection, or depiction. The second realm relates to the quality and depth of the concrete knowledge ascertained from the CT study. To illustrate this, one could consider the example of a patient with a ZMC fracture. The first and most basic information to acquire from the CT study is which bones are in fact fractured. This allows the radiologist and clinician to correctly classify that patient's injury into the ZMC category. The next order of information is to identify fundamental issues that relate to treatment, such as whether there is displacement or rotation of the zygoma or entrapment of the extraocular muscles. The third and highest order of information is to assess other issues that are more complex but that may nonetheless impact significantly on management, such as orbital volumes.[30,56,57] Since this is a critical determinant as to whether the patient will develop enophthalmos or exophthalmos, identifying a significant discrepancy in orbital volumes between the injured orbit and the contralateral normal orbit may emerge as an important diagnostic focal point that influences management.

Multislice Spiral CT: Technologic Advances

A comprehensive discussion of the technologic advances of multislice spiral CT is beyond the scope of this text. In broad, general concepts, the introduction of this technology has led to the ability to carry out imaging studies of higher resolution and with greater speed and more extensive volumetric coverage than that which was possible with the single-slice spiral technology. The advantages are even more magnified when compared with the nonspiral step-and-shoot technology that predated the single-slice equipment. Thus the entire facial skeleton can now be covered with volumetric scanning in less than a minute, leading to the generation of 1 to 1.5-mm overlapping images. Some manufacturers even offer the ability to generate images with submillimeter slice thicknesses. These axial image data sets serve as the substrate for the generation of high-quality 2-D and 3-D reformatted images, which is discussed in greater detail later. The benefits of high-speed, high-resolution, and high-volume coverage

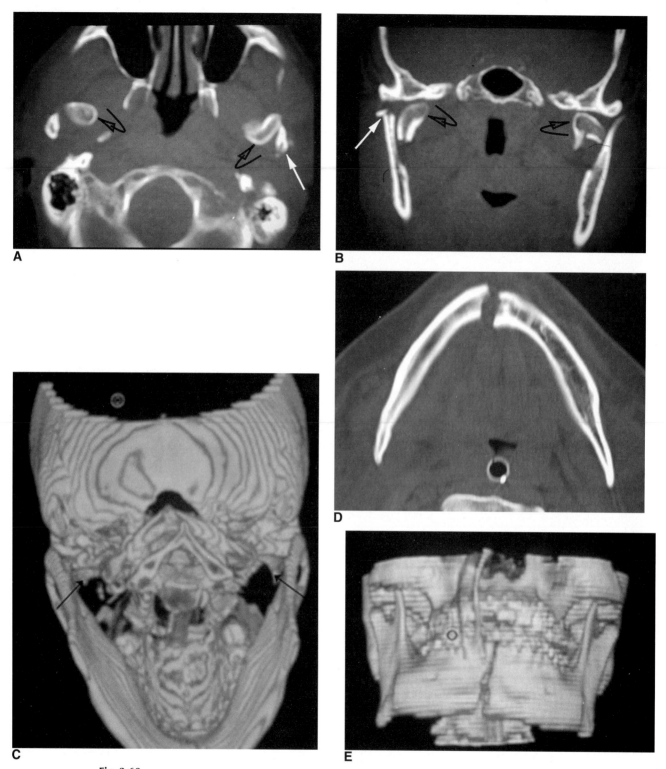

Fig. 3-60
Bilateral mandibular subcondylar fractures. **A**, CT shows bilateral subcondylar fractures (*arrows*) with inferomedial displacement of condyle heads (*curved arrows*). **B**, Same injury viewed as a coronal MPR. **C**, Same injury as a volume-rendered view from posteroinferior perspective, with medially displaced condylar heads with subcondylar fractures (*arrows*). **D**, CT shows fracture of the mandibular symphysis, which often leads to bilateral condyle fractures due to transmission of impacting force into both condyles or neck. **E**, Volumetric appearance in frontal view of same injury.

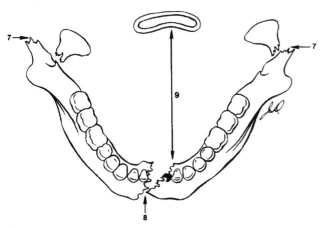

Fig. 3-61
Mechanism that allows lateral flaring of the mandibular angles and bodies. The arrow (9) represents the shortened distance between the symphysis and the oropharynx as a result of the disruption in the normal mandibular contour. The muscles of the tongue can obstruct the oropharynx. Subcondyle fractures (7) and a mental symphysis fracture (8) are also indicated.

have direct application in trauma patients who are typically agitated and also unable to undergo direct coronal imaging.

Multislice Spiral CT: Image Quality

Image quality in CT imaging can be broken down, conceptually and pragmatically, into three areas: spatial, contrast, and temporal resolution. A successful imaging study, possessing inherent high diagnostic yield, will strike the correct balance between these parameters. Thus it becomes imperative for the radiologist to have a working understanding of these concepts in order to design the correct CT sequence.

In its most basic form, *spatial resolution* relates to the ability of an image to accurately portray two discrete structures that are very close to each other as being in fact separate entities. For example, if a CT image correctly displays two 3-mm lung nodules that are located within millimeters of each other as two separate nodules, the image

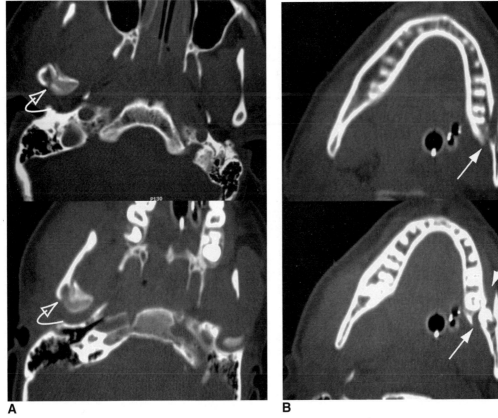

A   **B**

Fig. 3-62
Extracapsular fracture of neck of mandible. Multislice CT images show an extracapsular fracture (*curved arrows*) of the right neck of the mandible (**A**) and a displaced contralateral fracture (*arrows*) of the left angle of the mandible (**B**).

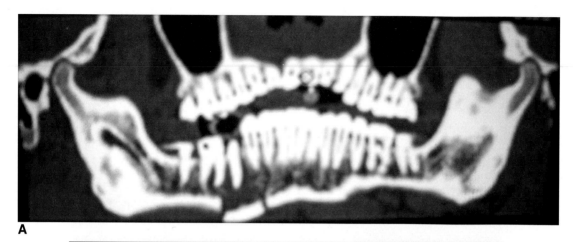

A

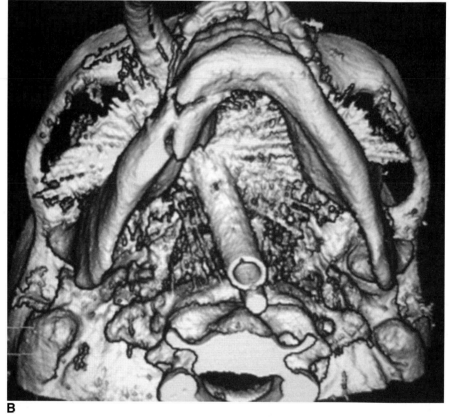

B

Fig. 3-63
Various techniques for demonstrating mandibular body fracture. **A,** Curved multiplanar reformation (pseudo-Panorex). **B,** Surface contour 3-D from inferior perspective.

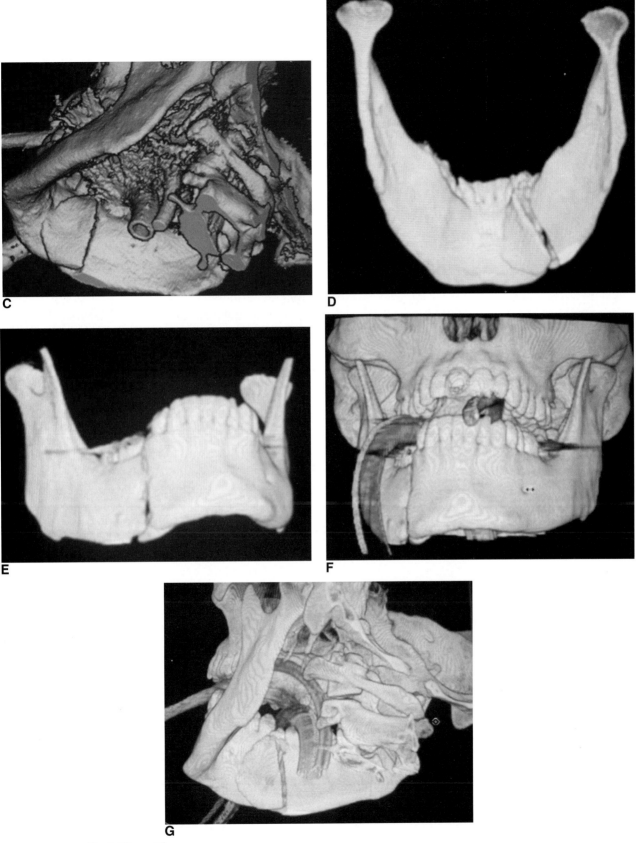

Fig. 3-63, cont'd
C, Surface contour 3-D from inferior oblique perspective. **D,** Disarticulated mandible body fracture from posterior perspective. **E,** Disarticulated mandible from anterior oblique view. **F,** Volume (4-D) anterior view. **G,** Volume (4-D) from posteroinferior and oblique view.

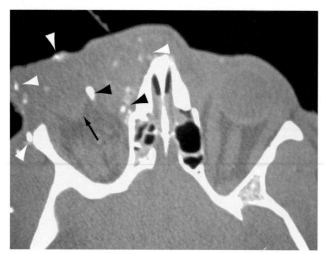

Fig. 3-64
Ruptured globe and intraorbital foreign bodies in a patient involved in a motor vehicle collision. The CT image of the orbit shows a ruptured right globe (*arrow*). Multiple intraorbital (*black arrowheads*) and soft tissue (*white arrowheads*) foreign bodies are seen in the right side of the face.

possesses higher spatial resolution than the CT image that blends these two lesions into one larger one. In essence, spatial resolution relates to spatial detail. Partial volume averaging is an imaging artifact that detracts from high spatial resolution. These basic concepts of spatial resolution relate to image quality not only in the directly acquired CT image (e.g., axial image) but also in computer-generated reformatted images.

Contrast resolution relates to the ability of an image to demonstrate different tissues based on their differences in density or X-ray attenuation. In its fundamental nature, contrast resolution has little to do with the size or spatial relationship between two tissues or lesions. For example, the ability to identify a soft tissue abnormality against background normal soft tissue (as in a case of liver lesion or retinal hemorrhage) is a reflection of the contrast resolution inherent in that image. Several factors affect the contrast-resolving abilities of an image. These factors include the mAs, slice thickness, and reconstruction algorithm utilized in image reconstruction. Strong contrast resolution is particularly important in evaluating soft tissue abnormalities. Osseous abnormalities, such as facial fractures, are less dependent on *image* contrast resolution, since they possess high *subject* contrast because they are positioned adjacent to soft tissues.

Quantum mottle image noise is a degrading influence on contrast resolution. Quantum mottle is a statistical phenomenon that is ultimately due to the photon concentration utilized in the generation of an image. Thus quantum mottle will be reduced in thicker images compared with thinner images. Assuming all other imaging parameters are kept constant, this means that, in general, thicker images possess greater contrast resolution, but less spatial resolution, than thinner images. Hence one can observe the relative inverse relationship between these two image quality parameters.

Temporal resolution relates to the various time issues in a CT sequence. On the most basic level, temporal resolution has to do with the amount of time required to complete

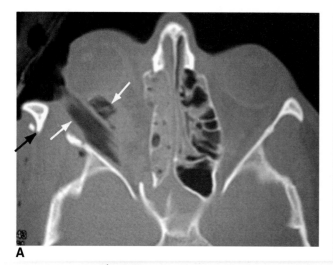

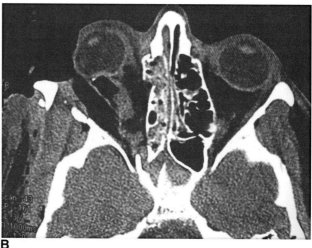

A   B

Fig. 3-65
Intraorbital wood in patient admitted following a fall. CT images in bone windows and levels show intraorbital wood (*white arrows*) and a displaced right lateral orbital wall fracture (*black arrow*) **(A)**. Note that by using the same soft tissue windows and levels, the intraorbital wood can easily be misdiagnosed as intraorbital air **(B)**.

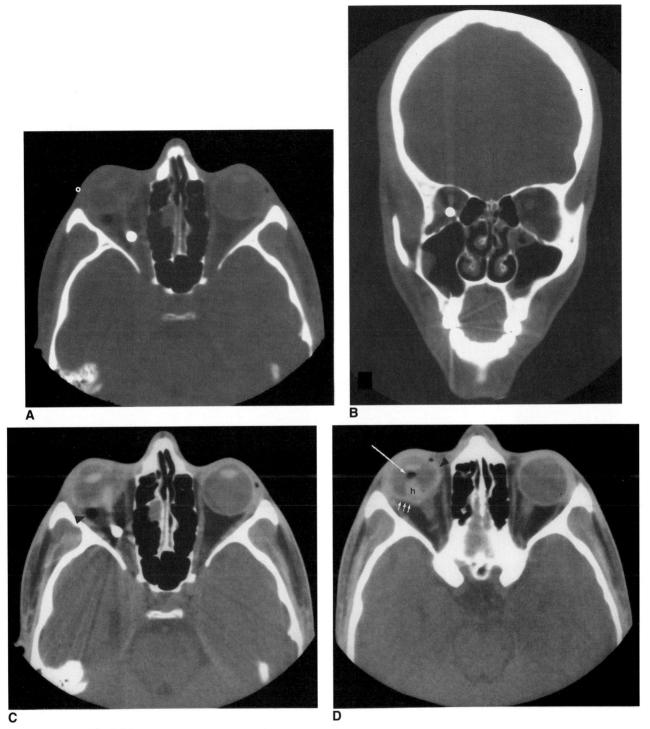

Fig. 3-66
Foreign body of the right orbit. Axial **(A)** and coronal **(B)** bone window CT images of orbits precisely demonstrate the location of a foreign body in the posterior orbit of a patient shot with a BB gun. The bony orbital walls are intact. **C**, Soft tissue window of **A** shows right orbital emphysema (*arrowhead*). **D**, Soft tissue image slightly superior to **C** shows "flat tire" (*small arrows*), hemorrhage in posterior chamber (*h*), scleral thickening (*arrowhead*) with respect to normal sclera on left, and posterior chamber air (*long arrow*). All of these are signs of scleral laceration. Note the lens just anterior to the posterior chamber air collection.

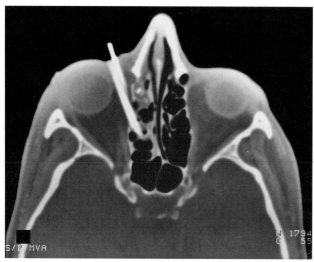

Fig. 3-67
Axial CT shows a large shard of glass penetrating the medial right orbit and right ethmoid sinus. The medial canthal ligament was severed.

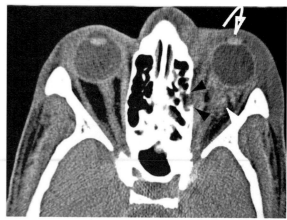

Fig. 3-69
CT of ectopic lens. Posttrauma patient shows dislocation of lens into anterior chamber of left globe (*curved white arrow*). Optic nerve is swollen and irregular in contour, suggesting laceration (*white arrowhead*). There is a small fracture of the left medial orbital wall (*black arrowheads*), and left medial rectus muscle appears contused.

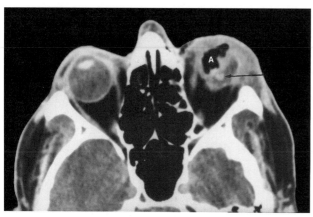

Fig. 3-68
Left scleral laceration from penetrating injury from a tree branch. There is extensive air (*A*) in the left globe. The lens (*arrow*) is dislocated into the posterior globe. There is a marked loss of volume to the left globe that appears flattened ("flat tire" sign), indicating scleral rupture.

an imaging study. Imaging of the facial skeleton in the nonspiral step-and-shoot CT era required as much as 30 to 40 minutes for completion of a comprehensive evaluation in axial and coronal planes. Spiral technology shortened these scan times by an order of magnitude. Decreased overall scan times impact not only on patient throughput but also on the quality of the studies themselves by reducing the opportunity for motion artifact to degrade image quality and by the facilitation of breathhold studies. Spiral technology also opened the door for new clinical applications, such as CT angiography and organ perfusion imaging.

Spiral CT: Technique Factors

Numerous technical factors associated with the spiral CT sequence influence image quality. These include the slice thickness, slice reconstruction increment or interval, mAs, and reconstruction algorithm.

Slice thickness is the resultant thickness of the individual images that are generated from the volumetric data set once the spiral acquisition has been completed. Most spiral CT sequences are carried out along the longitudinal (z-) axis of the patient, and the resultant images are then portrayed in the axial or transverse plane. Slice thickness is a key factor in determining the spatial and contrast resolution properties of a study and provides the substrate for multiplanar and 3-D reformatted images.

Once the volumetric data is acquired through the spiral acquisition, images can be reconstructed at any point along the path of data acquisition. *Slice reconstruction increment* represents the gap between adjacent slices in an image set. If the slice reconstruction increment is less than the slice thickness, then there will be image overlap. For example, if 3-mm images are to be reconstructed every 2 mm, then there will be a 50% overlap between the sequential images that are generated from the data. The advantage of image overlap rests in the improved multiplanar and 3-D image quality that results when overlapping images are used in their creation. In actuality, this type of imaging was used even before the spiral technology was introduced; however, with the step-and-shoot technology, the creation of overlapping images required overlapping irradiation (i.e., beam thickness of 3 mm with the patient advanced 2 mm after each beam rotation).

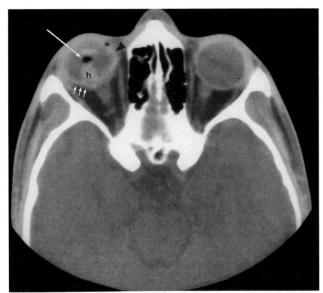

Fig. 3-70
CT of ruptured globe. A right globe injury in trauma shows air within the sclera and posterior chamber (*long white arrow*), indicating loss of scleral integrity (perforation). There is focal vitreous hemorrhage (*h*) and high density in the sclera, indicating hemorrhage (*arrowhead*). There is some flattening of the lateral contour of the globe (*small white arrows*), indicating loss of volume.

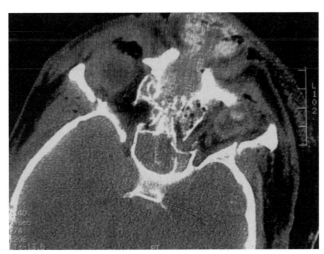

Fig. 3-71
"Flat tire" sign. The CT shows severe Le Fort III and nasoorbital-ethmoid facial fractures with marked loss of the left globe volume, indicating rupture.

The *mAs* is a reflection of the photon density of the X-ray beam used in an imaging study and influences the contrast resolution of the resultant images. For body parts that possess high inherent subject contrast, such as bones and lungs, low mAs techniques are usually adequate. Since the mAs of a study relates directly to the radiation dose delivered, it becomes imperative to understand and implement these concepts in order to minimize patient dose.

The *reconstruction algorithm* is the data processing formula used to take the raw data from the CT acquisition and convert it to a set of interpretable images. Each CT manufacturer typically offers various soft tissue and bone algorithms from which to choose. Variations in image detail, image noise, and edge enhancement are characteristics of each algorithm.

Image Postprocessing

The spiral CT technology and the accompanying advances in computer postprocessing technology have had a substantial impact on the evaluation of the acutely injured patient. For the patient who has sustained significant facial trauma, the imaging goals are often along the lines of both *detection* and *depiction* of the extent of injury. For the detection of facial fractures, axial, coronal and, at times, oblique imaging is necessary. The axial images are generated directly from the spiral acquisition, while the coronal and oblique images can be generated from the axial images using sophisticated multiplanar (MPR) postprocessing programs. The critical point is that the axial image set must be of sufficient quality to serve as the effective substrate for the MPR program. As mentioned before, there are two CT technique factors that impact directly on the quality of the multiplanar reformatted images—slice thickness and slice reconstruction increment (slice overlap). Thinner slice thicknesses and the generation of overlapping images are both benefits of the spiral CT technology; however, it is worth emphasizing that the quality of reformatted images is influenced much more by the slice *thickness* of the axial images used in their generation than by the amount of overlap between the axial images in the set. Thus 1-mm nonoverlapping axial images will lead to the generation of much higher-quality reformatted images than will 3-mm axial images that are reconstructed with 50% overlap. In the latter, stairstep artifact will typically degrade the quality of the reformatted images and make evaluation of structures like the orbital floor and roof somewhat challenging. When thinner (1-mm or submillimeter) axial images are used, the quality of the coronal reformatted images is often as good as or even better than that of directly acquired coronal images because the latter are often degraded by motion artifact as well as artifact from dental amalgam, both of which are typically absent in the reformatted images. Considering the additional point that most acute trauma patients cannot undergo direct coronal imaging, it becomes even more apparent how this technology offers robust solutions to a variety of imaging challenges that are present with these patients.

Issues such as spatial and contrast resolution apply to multiplanar reformatted images in much the same way as to the axial images. It therefore becomes imperative to identify the optimal slice thickness and spacing of the reformatted images in order to achieve the desired imaging goals. Thinner reformatted images will possess greater spatial resolution, but less contrast resolution, than thicker reformats. The sacrifice made in contrast resolution may well be worth it, since the primary goal of the reformatted images is the identification of osseous abnormalities (i.e., fractures) that may be difficult to identify in the axial plane. In one study, coronal reformatted images of submillimeter (0.4-mm) thickness and spaced at 1-mm intervals were found to be most effective.[49] On the other hand, image fusion, which can often be accomplished on the CT operator's console or on the postprocessing workstation, may prove to be a valuable tool, since it allows the generation of fused (thicker) axial images that possess higher contrast resolution than the original thin axial images.

In addition to standard coronal reformatted images, other planar orientations may be beneficial in the depiction of various injuries. Sagittal oblique images may prove valuable for both orbital floor and mandibular injuries. Curved reformatted projections allow simulation of the Panorex image of the mandible but often offer superior visualization of the mandibular condyles and coronoid processes than that provided on the Panorex. As previously discussed, 3-D images and multitissue displays are additional methods of lesion depiction that may aid in surgical planning and patient education.

New Horizons

Technologic advances continue to be made in the areas of spiral CT technology, image postprocessing, and surgical technique, all of which will influence the role of imaging in the setting of craniofacial trauma. Intraoperative CT has shown benefits in the management of patients with significant facial trauma.[58] Three-dimensional imaging will in all likelihood assume an even greater role in the evaluation of facial trauma patients as postprocessing becomes more thoroughly integrated into the primary CT process. Volumetric CT data collection may proceed straight to 3-D image displays to parallel the increasing demands of clinicians for more meaningful depictions of the pathology than that afforded by two-dimensional axial or coronal images. New stabilization and fixation materials, many of which are nonmetallic and resorbable, are being introduced continually, thereby leading to postoperative imaging studies that are of higher quality and more informative.

FACIAL TRAUMA: A SURGEON'S PERSPECTIVE

The introduction of CT in the early 1980s dramatically changed the diagnostic process and management of craniofacial trauma. Up to this point, radiographs were the standard, and their acquisition was all too often limited by problems with positioning, resulting in inadequate visualization of skeletal structures and/or inaccuracies leading to improper interpretation. CT added a third dimension to aid in craniofacial trauma analysis, and the era of CT-guided surgery was born.

For the first time, surgeons were able to accurately assess and define the subtleties and/or complexities of craniofacial fractures and correlate the displacement of skeletal buttresses with the clinical findings of soft tissue disruption. Accurate visualization of the fracture, its comminuted parts, and direction of displacement has allowed surgeons to understand and link the mechanism (vector and force) of injury with the pattern of fracture and the associated soft tissue damage. Fractures are now not only categorized (e.g., Le Fort pattern) but also designated as low-, mid-, or high-velocity. CT now directs surgical approach, such that as the velocity of injury increases, the requirement for wider exposure and greater fixation increases. For example, in a low-velocity fracture where there is minimal inward displacement of the malar eminence, only anterior approaches are necessary to stabilize the supportive buttresses, but in a high-velocity fracture with lateral displacement of buttresses and increased soft tissue disruption, wide exposure and greater rigid fixation is needed for fracture stabilization.

Today, acquisition of axial and coronal CT images—either as true coronal images or reformations via a multislice spiral CT—and advanced processing techniques have become standard procedure. The value of these images is critical in understanding the relationship of fracture segments and adjacent vital soft tissue structures. It is paramount to disclose the precise three-dimensional relationship of periorbital fractures to the optic nerve and/or extraocular eye muscles; surgical indications and outcomes are determined by comparing the CT images with clinical findings. Assessment of altered orbital volumes and the potential for primary and/or secondary enophthalmos is determined by similar comparisons. CT is essential for the analysis of mandibular condyle fractures and for relating the position of the condyle to the glenoid fossa. A subtle temporomandibular effusion or hemarthrosis as the etiology for a subtle malocclusion will not be diagnosed on plain radiography but will be observed on axial and coronal scans as a widened joint space. The position of a foreign body and the relationship to critical structures is markedly improved with utilization of axial and coronal CT. It is critical with severely comminuted fractures that the surgeon understands the structural relationship of the components to allow accurate reconstruction.

CT alone has been criticized for missing minimally or nondisplaced fractures of the midface and/or mandible when the fracture line is parallel to the plane of scanning. However, with experience using axial images and the addition of coronal views, injury documentation is rarely a problem. This becomes even less likely as slice profiles get thinner and volume averaging decreases. Acquisition of true coronal views is contraindicated in patients who are intubated and/or have potential cervical injuries. Since the introduction of multislice CT, this problem has been essentially overcome. The newest scanners provide coronal reformations that are nearly indistinguishable from direct coronal imaging.

CT has, in almost all instances, replaced radiography for management of both simple and complex craniofacial injuries; its role in diagnosis as well as in planning the surgical approach is unsurpassed. However, there still remains a role for radiography. Specifically, radiographs should be obtained in all midface and/or mandibular fractures where the fracture is in proximity to the dentition. Only a plain radiograph will identify the subtleties of the fracture as it relates to the teeth, roots, and related structures. The plain radiograph will permit identification of a root-tip fracture not seen on CT. The potential accuracy of dedicated dental CT software in this application is

not well known. CT assessment of periapical pathology often associated with periodontal and/or dental pulp disease will be inadequate (see Fig. 3-10). Plain radiographs best define a general overview of the relationship of the fracture to the dentition, and the gold standard for fractures of the maxillary dental alveolar process and/or mandible is a Panorex radiograph (Figs. 3-72 and 3-73). Additionally, plain radiographs in craniofacial trauma should be obtained in the immediate postoperative phase to document the placement of fracture stabilization hardware and the overall craniofacial skeletal reduction (Fig. 3-12). These films can then be used for future reference as a baseline from which comparisons can be made and more sophisticated CT requested should complications arise during the convalescent phase of healing.

CONCLUSION

Craniofacial trauma remains a prevalent condition that typically requires intense and immediate clinical decision making that is largely dependent on the radiologic *detection* and *depiction* of injuries. Recent advances in the spiral CT and computer postprocessing technologies have had an impressive impact on the ability to evaluate craniofacial trauma patients thoroughly and efficiently; the increasing front-line availability of this technology in trauma centers solidifies its role in becoming the imaging modality of choice for these conditions.

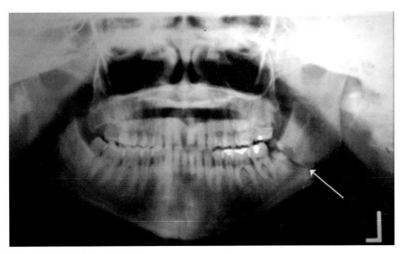

Fig. 3-72
Panorex showing angle fracture (*arrow*) extending through retained third molar root tips with periapical radiolucent pathology. This type of injury is often missed on CT.

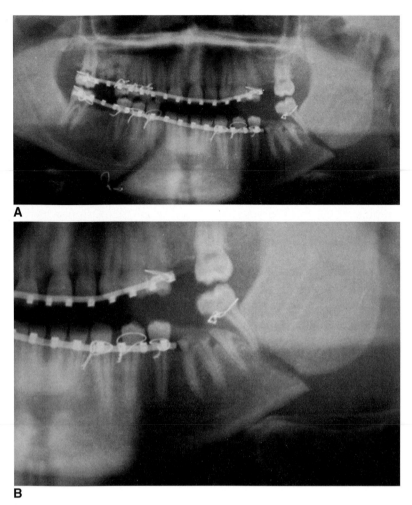

Fig. 3-73
A, Panorex showing bilateral mandibular fractures and relationship to adjacent tooth structures. **B**, Close-up view shows the fracture extending through the mesial root of the last molar. This finding was not reported on the original mandibular CT (not shown).

REFERENCES

1. Rogers LF: *Radiology of skeletal trauma*, ed 2, New York, 1992, Churchill Livingstone.
2. Iida S, Kogo M, Sugiura T, et al: Retrospective analysis of 1502 patients with facial fractures, *Int J Oral Maxillofacial Surg* 30:286, 2001.
3. Huang V, Moore C, Bohrer P, et al: Maxillofacial injuries in women, *Ann Plastic Surg* 41:482, 1998.
4. Amrith S, Saw SM, Lim TC, et al: Ophthalmic involvement in craniofacial trauma, *J Cranio-Maxillo-Fac Surg* 28:140, 2000.
5. Mouzakes J, Koltai PJ, Kuhar S, et al: The impact of airbags and seatbelts on the incidence and severity of maxillofacial injuries in automobile accidents in New York state, *Arch Otolaryngol Head Neck Surg* 127:1189, 2001.
6. Manson PN: Facial fractures. In Aston SJ, Beasley RW, Thorne CHM, eds: *Grabb and Smith's plastic surgery*, ed 5, Philadelphia, 1997, Lippincott-Raven.

7. Gruss JS, Kassel EE, Bubak P: Clinical, surgical, and treatment perspectives in the management of craniomaxillofacial trauma, *Neuroimaging Clin N Am* 1:341, 1991.
8. Jordan DR, Allen LH, White J, et al: Intervention within days for some orbital floor fractures: the white-eyed blowout, *Ophth Plas Reconstruc Surg* 14:379, 1998.
9. Laskin DM, Best AM: Current trends in the treatment of maxillofacial injuries in the United States, *J Oral Maxillofac Surg* 58:207, 2000.
10. Ochs MW, Beatty RL: Complex fractures in the periorbital region, *Sem Ophthal* 9:218, 1994.
11. Courtney DJ, Thomas S, Whitfield PH: Isolated orbital blowout fractures: survey and review, *Br J Oral Maxillofac Surg* 38:496, 2000.
12. Gentry LR, Manor WF, Turski PA, et al: High-resolution CT analysis of facial struts in trauma. 1. Normal anatomy, *AJR* 140:523, 1983.
13. Robertson RL, Ball WS Jr, Barnes PD: Skull and Brain. In Kirks DR, Griscom NT, eds: *Practical pediatric imaging: diagnostic*

radiology of infants and children, ed 3, Philadelphia, 1998, Lippincott-Raven.

14. Netter FH: Bone coverings of brain and spinal cord. In Brass A, Dingle RV, eds: *The CIBA collection of medical illustrations*, vol 1, *Nervous system*, ed 2, West Caldwell, NJ, 1986, CIBA Pharmaceutical.

15. Kassel EE, Gruss JS: Imaging of midfacial fractures, *Neuroimaging Clin N Am* 1:259, 1991.

16. Pansky B: *Review of gross anatomy*, ed 4, New York, 1979, Macmillan.

17. Crawley WA, Vasconez HC: Midface, upper face, and panfacial fractures. In Ferraro JW, ed: *Fundamentals of maxillofacial surgery*, New York, 1997, Springer-Verlag.

18. DelBalso AM, Hall RE: Mandibular and dentoalveolar fractures, *Neuroimaging Clin N Am* 1:285, 1991.

19. Hodgson VR: Tolerance of facial bones to impact, *Am J Anat* 120:113, 1967.

20. Huelke DF: Study of mandibular fractures, stress coat, *J Dent Res* 40:1042, 1961.

21. Haug RH, Greenberg AM: Etiology, distribution, and classification of fractures. In Greenberg AM, ed: *Craniomaxillofacial fractures*, New York, 1993, Springer-Verlag.

22. Lew D, Sinn DP: Diagnosis and treatment of midface fractures. In Fonseca RJ, Walker RV, eds: *Oral and maxillofacial trauma*, ed 2, Philadelphia, 1997, WB Saunders.

23. Weinstein JM, Lissner GS: Trauma to the orbit, neurovisual system, and oculomotor apparatus, *Neuroimaging Clin N Am* 1:357, 1991.

24. Mauriello JA, Lee HJ, Nguyen L: CT of soft tissue injury and orbital fractures, *Radiol Clin North Am* 37:241, 1999.

25. Rhea JT, Rao PM, Novelline RA: Helical CT and three-dimensional CT of facial and orbital injury, *Radiol Clin North Am* 37:489, 1999.

26. Dodick JM, Galin MA, Littleton JT, et al: Concomitant medial wall fracture and blowout fracture of the orbit, *Arch Ophthalmol* 85:273, 1971.

27. Manson PN, Hiff N: Management of blowout fractures of the orbital floor, *Surg Ophthal* 35:280, 1991.

28. Brady SM, McMann MA, Mazzoli RA, et al: The diagnosis and management of orbital blowout fractures: update 2001, *Am J Emerg Med* 19:147, 2001.

29. Rothman MI, Simon EM, Zoarski GH, et al: Superior blowout fracture of the orbit: the blowup fracture, *Am J Neuroradiol* 19:1448, 1998.

30. Jin HR, Shin SO, Choo MJ, et al: Relationship between the extent of fracture and the degree of enophthalmos in isolated blowout fractures of the medial orbital wall, *J Oral Maxillofac Surg* 58:617, 2000.

31. Graham SM, Hoffman HT: Traumatic injuries to the frontal sinus. In Fonseca RJ, Walker RV, eds: *Oral and maxillofacial trauma*, ed 2, Philadelphia, 1997, WB Saunders.

32. Remmler D, Denny A, Gosain A, et al: Role of three-dimensional computed tomography in the assessment of nasoorbitoethmoidal fractures, *Ann Plast Surg* 46:191, 2001.

33. Lawrason JN, Novelline RA: Diagnostic imaging of facial trauma. In Mirvis SE, Young JWR, eds: *Diagnostic imaging in trauma and critical care*, ed 1, Baltimore, 1992, Williams & Wilkins.

34. Cruse CW, Blevins PK, Luce EA: Naso-ethmoid-orbital fractures, *J Trauma* 20:551, 1980.

35. Yangisawa E: Pitfalls in management of zygomatic fractures, *Laryngoscope* 83:527, 1973.

36. Som PM, Brandwein M: Sinonasal cavities: inflammatory diseases, tumors, fractures, and post-operative findings. In Som PM, Curtin HD, eds: *Head and neck imaging*, ed 3, St Louis, 1996, Mosby.

37. Gruss JS, VanWick L, Phillips JH, et al: The importance of the zygomatic arch in complex midfacial fracture repair and correction of

post traumatic orbitozygomatic deformities, *Plast Reconstruct Surg* 85:878, 1990.

38. Jackson IT: Classification and treatment of orbitozygomatic and orbito-ethmoid fractures, *Clin Plast Surg* 16:77, 1989.

39. Barber HD, Woodbury HC, Silverstein KE, et al: Mandibular fractures. In Fonseca RJ, Walker RV, eds: *Oral and maxillofacial trauma*, ed 2, Philadelphia, 1997, WB Saunders.

40. Crawley WA, Sandel AJ: Fractures of the mandible. In Ferraro JW, ed: *Fundamentals of maxillofacial surgery*, New York, 1997, Springer-Verlag.

41. Olsen RA: Fractures of the mandible: review of 580 cases, *J Oral Maxillofac Surg* 40:23, 1982.

42. Raustia AM, Pyhtinen J, Oikarinen KS, et al: Conventional radiographic and computed tomographic findings in cases of fracture of the mandibular condylar process, *J Oral Maxillofac Surg* 48:1258, 1990.

43. Yamaoka M, Furusawa K, Iguchi K: The assessment of fracture of the mandibular condyle by use of computerized tomography: incidence of sagittal split fracture, *Br J Oral Maxillofac Surg* 32:77, 1994.

44. Hammerschlag SB, Hughes S, O'Reilly GV, et al: Blow-out fractures of the orbit: a comparison of computed tomography and conventional radiography with anatomical correlation, *Radiology* 143:487, 1982.

45. Zilkha A: Computed tomography in facial trauma, *Radiology* 144:545, 1982.

46. Venema HW, Phoa SS, Mirck PGB, et al: Petrosal bone: coronal reconstructions from axial spiral CT data obtained with 0.5mm collimation can replace direct coronal sequential CT scans, *Radiology* 213:375, 1999.

47. Klevansky A: The efficacy of multiplanar reconstructions of helical CT of the paranasal sinuses, *AJR* 173:493, 1999.

48. Rosenthal EL, Quint D, Johns M, et al: Diagnostic maxillofacial coronal images reformatted from helically acquired thin-section CT data, *AJR* 175:1177, 2000.

49. Hoeffner EG, Quint DJ, Peterson B, et al: Development of a protocol for coronal reconstruction of the maxillofacial region from axial helical CT data, *Br J Radiol* 74:323, 2001.

50. Sidebottom AJ, Lord TC: Single view radiographic screening of midfacial trauma, *Int J Oral Maxillofac Surg* 27:356, 1998.

51. Broumand SR, Labs JD, Novelline RA, et al: The role of three-dimensional computed tomography in the evaluation of acute craniofacial trauma, *Ann Plast Surg* 31:488, 1993.

52. Tello R, Suojanen J, Costello P, et al: Comparison of spiral CT and conventional CT in 3D visualization of facial trauma: work in progress, *Comput Med Imaging Graph* 18:423, 1994.

53. Luka B, Brechtelsbauer D, Geltrich NC, et al: 2D and 3D CT reconstructions of the facial skeleton: an unnecessary option or a diagnostic pearl? *Int J Oral Maxillofac Surg* 24:76, 1995.

54. Girod S, Keeve E, Girod B: Advances in interactive craniofacial surgery planning by 3D simulation and visualization, *Int J Oral Maxillofac Surg* 24:120, 1995.

55. Fox LA, Vannier MW, West OC, et al: Diagnostic performance of CT, MPR, and 3DCT imaging in maxillofacial trauma, *Comput Med Imaging Graph* 19:385, 1996.

56. Ramieri G, Spada MC, Bianchi SD, et al: Dimensions and volumes of the orbits and orbital fat in posttraumatic enophthalmos, *Dento-Maxillo-Facial Radiology* 29:302, 2000.

57. Schuknecht B, Carls F, Valvanis A, et al: CT assessment of orbital volume in late post-traumatic enophthalmos, *Neuroradiology* 38:470, 1996.

58. Stanley RB: Use of intraoperative computed tomography during repair of orbitozygomatic fractures, *Arch Facial Plast Surg* 1:25, 1999.

4 Imaging of Cervical Spinal Trauma

Stuart E. Mirvis

Cervical spine imaging must be considered within the context of the overall clinical picture of the patient, which dictates management priorities and the type and sequence of diagnostic evaluations. All trauma patients with clinical signs of spine or spinal cord injury and all uncommunicative or unreliable patients in whom the available information on the mechanism of injury is consistent with spine or spinal cord injury must undergo at least frontal (anteroposterior [AP]) and horizontal beam lateral cervical radiography during initial evaluation. If the cervical spine cannot be "cleared" (i.e., declared negative for injury) by combined limited clinical and radiologic studies, or if the patient's condition requires immediate surgical intervention or more complex imaging procedures of other organ systems, the spine must be immobilized to protect the cord. Immobilization must be maintained until the patient has been stabilized sufficiently to complete definitive imaging examinations.

Diagnostic imaging of the spine is the definitive method for determining the presence, location, extent, and nature of injury to the cord and vertebral column. Spinal imaging is, therefore, essential to the accurate assessment, evaluation, and management of cervical spinal injury. Efficient and economic application of diagnostic imaging for spinal trauma requires a thorough knowledge of the indications for and limitations of various imaging techniques available and the sequence in which they should be applied.

The first part of this chapter considers available imaging modalities for evaluating potential acute cervical spinal injury, beginning with the plain radiographic study, and includes illustrations of normal anatomy with examples of common injuries as they relate to the imaging concepts discussed. This section also reviews the strengths and weaknesses of each major imaging modality used in assessing spinal injury. The following section describes approaches to the imaging evaluation of potential acute cervical spine injury using various clinical features and considers many of the controversies that surround this subject. The diagnostic approach presented reflects experience in the imaging evaluation of acute cervical spinal injuries within the environment of a level I trauma center, but it is applicable to spinal injuries seen in any setting. The final section reviews specific cervical spine injury patterns, their proposed mechanism(s), and imaging features. The last section also considers imaging the traumatized cervical spines of patients with preexisting conditions which may alter significantly the appearance of the cervical spine.

DIAGNOSTIC MODALITIES IN IMAGING CERVICAL SPINAL TRAUMA: AN OVERVIEW

The diagnostic imaging modalities useful in the evaluation of spinal trauma include plain film radiography, computed tomography (CT), including two-dimensional (2D) and three-dimensional (3D) data reformation, CT myelography (CTM), magnetic resonance imaging (MRI), and nuclear scintigraphy. Cervical vascular injury, with the potential for devastating neurologic consequences, is associated not uncommonly with cervical spine trauma. These potential vascular injuries may be recognized by CT using intravenous contrast or with routine MRI but are diagnosed definitively by magnetic resonance angiography (MRA), Doppler sonography, CT angiography, and catheter angiography. The development and increasing availability of ultrafast, multirow-detector CT will make screening cervical CT angiography practical for selected trauma patients at high risk for injury to the carotid and vertebral arteries.

Plain Film Radiography of the Cervical Spine

All imaging examinations of spinal trauma begin with plain radiographic studies. Plain film radiography is readily available in all emergency centers; it is a reliable and quick method and can be performed with portable or fixed equipment. Radiography provides an excellent overview of the extent and magnitude of injury and makes a definitive and specific diagnosis possible in certain spinal injuries. The flexibility of the x-ray tube–film geometry provides the positioning latitude necessary for obtaining a comprehensive examination without patient motion, which is essential for patients suspected of having a spinal injury.

The quality of the plain radiographic study is of paramount importance to the identification of cervical spine injury. A properly exposed radiograph must display both the skeleton and the soft tissues and must be free of motion or grid artifacts that could obscure or mimic fractures. Prevention of artifact is of primary importance in detecting subtle, minimally displaced osseous injuries. A properly collimated plain film study effectively limits patient radiation, and the examination is relatively inexpensive.

Lateral View. Evaluation of the initial screening lateral radiograph should be done methodically. An adequate study must include the cervicothoracic junction (to include the top of T1), and the patient should be positioned without rotation or tilting of the head. Every reasonable effort must be made to visualize the cervicothoracic junction on the initial plain radiographic examination. If the C7-T1 level is not visualized adequately on the lateral radiograph, the cervical spine cannot be cleared, and other plain film studies (see later discussion) or CT must be performed.

The cross-table lateral radiograph is at least 74% to 86% sensitive for detection of cervical spine injuries, depending to a large extent on the expertise and experience of the examiner.[1-4] Missed injuries may result from

the following: (1) overlapping of bone, particularly involving the cervicocranial junction, the articular masses, and the laminae, (2) nondisplaced or minimally displaced fractures, particularly involving the atlas and axis, and (3) ligament injuries that may not be manifested when the radiograph is taken with the patient in a supine position, with the neck in extension and stabilized by a cervical collar (i.e., no stress applied). Some cervical spine subluxations or dislocations can reduce spontaneously or be reduced with placement in a cervical collar prior to imaging evaluation, making their detection more difficult. Obviously, poor imaging technique related to positioning, exposure, or motion can significantly impair diagnostic accuracy.

Review of the lateral cervical radiograph involves assessment of anatomic lines, including the anterior and posterior vertebral margins, alignment of the articular masses, and alignment of the spinolaminar junctions[5] (Fig. 4-1). It is important to recognize minimal degrees of anterior and posterior intervertebral subluxation which occur normally with physiologic cervical flexion and extension (Fig. 4-2). Such physiologic displacement typically occurs at multiple contiguous levels and usually does not exceed 3 mm.[6] The spacing between the laminae, articular facets, and spinous processes should be similar at contiguous levels. The intervertebral disc spaces should appear nearly uniform in height across the disc space. The orientation of each vertebra should be assessed for any rotational abnormalities. On a true lateral radiograph, the articular masses should be superimposed, whereas abrupt offset of the masses indicates a rotational injury such as a unilateral facet dislocation (Fig. 4-3). Similarly, an abrupt change in the distance from the posterior margin of the articular pillar to the spinolaminar line (the laminar space) also indicates a rotational injury[7] (Fig. 4-4). Focal prevertebral or retropharyngeal soft tissue edema or hematoma sometimes can indicate an otherwise radiographically occult injury (Fig. 4-5). However, absolute measurements of the prevertebral soft tissues are not particularly accurate indications of injury and can vary with head position, body habitus, and phase of inspiration, among other factors.[8,9] Herr et al.[8] evaluated prevertebral soft tissue measurements at the C3 level in 212 blunt trauma patients using a 4-mm upper limit of normal. They found that a measurement greater than 4 mm was only 64% sensitive for detecting cervical spine fractures involving the anterior, posterior, upper, or lower cervical spine.[8] Precervical soft tissue prominence from the skull base to the axis is particularly important to recognize, because injuries at the craniocervical junction are often not apparent on the lateral radiograph. Harris[10] has shown that the contour of the craniocervial prevertebral soft tissues can be particularly useful in detecting subtle upper cervical spine injuries (see Fig. 4-5).

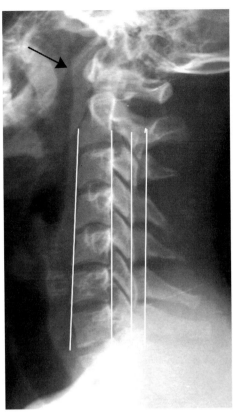

Fig. 4-1
Normal lateral radiograph. Admission study obtained in a cervical collar in cross-table projection often creates loss of cervical lordosis, as may also occur from a tucked chin position (or military posture). The lines connecting the anterior vertebral body, posterior vertebral body, posterior margins of the articular pillars, and spinolaminar junctions are straight (*white lines*). The prevertebral soft tissue is normal in thickness and contour, with a slight convex bulge anterior to C1 (*black arrow*) (see below). The C7-T1 region is not well exposed and would require further evaluation to assess adequately.

Assessment of the axis is aided by identification of the Harris ring,[11] a composite shadow of cortical bone along the margins of the neurocentral synchondrosis (Fig. 4-6). In a true lateral projection, the Harris rings from both sides of C2 are superimposed, whereas two parallel Harris rings result from an oblique (off-lateral) projection. Also in the lateral projection, the ring of cortical bone is interrupted in its posteroinferior aspect by the smaller ring of the foramen transversarium (Fig. 4-7). The Harris ring is particularly helpful in detecting atypical cases of traumatic spondylolisthesis[12] (hangman's fracture) (Fig. 4-8) and the classic type III or low odontoid fracture[13] (Fig. 4-9).

Radiologic identification of subluxation at the atlantooccipital articulation can be difficult. Previously the Powers ratio[14-16] was emphasized to assess this alignment. However, the anatomic landmarks required for this measurement are often difficult to visualize.[14,15]

Alignment at this articulation can be assessed by reference to three anatomic landmarks in the neutral position. First, the occipital condyle should lie within the condylar fossae of the atlas ring, with no gap between them in the adult patient. Second, a line drawn along the posterior surface of the clivus should intercept the superior aspect of the odontoid process. Third, a line drawn along the C1 spinolaminar line should intercept the posterior margin of the foramen magnum (Fig. 4-10). A more precise assessment of this anatomic relationship can be determined by direct measurement, regardless of the degree of cervical flexion and extension. The tip of the odontoid process should lie within 12 mm of the basion (inferior tip of the clivus), and a vertical line drawn along the posterior cortex of C2 (posterior axial line) should lie within 12 mm of the basion[14,15] (Fig. 4-11). Cranial distraction and anterior displacement are indicated by measurements of greater than 12 mm. The C1-2 articulation should be evaluated for the anterior atlantodental interval, normally less than 3 mm in the adult.[17] A larger anterior atlantodental interval associated with a cervicocranial hematoma indicates acute transverse atlantal ligament injury and instability of the articulation.

Anteroposterior View. The AP radiograph of the cervical spine supplements information provided on the lateral cervical radiograph and can identify additional injuries.[3,5,18,19] On the normal AP view, the spinous processes are aligned vertically, the lateral masses form smoothly undulating margins without abrupt interruption, the disc spaces are uniform in height from anterior to posterior, and the alignment of the vertebral bodies is assessed easily (Fig. 4-12). Typically, the craniocervical junction region and the odontoid process are not visible, being obscured by the face, mandible, and occipital skull. Lateral translation (displacement) of the vertebral bodies is best appreciated in this view. Similarly, lateral flexion injuries compressing a lateral mass or the lateral portion of a vertebral body are demonstrated to advantage, also. Rotational injuries are indicated by an abrupt offset of spinous process alignment, as occurs with unilateral facet dislocation (Fig. 4-13). Fractures of the vertebral body in the sagittal plane are often evident on the AP view (Fig. 4-14). Facet and articular mass fractures sometimes can be visualized, as well. Laminopedicular separation (fracture separation of the articular mass) may occur with hyperflexion-rotation injuries[20] or, rarely, hyperextension[21] and produces a horizontal orientation of the articular mass, leading to an open-appearing facet joint (Fig. 4-15). Normally these joints are not seen in tangent on the AP view because of their 35-degree inclination from the horizontal plane.[20] Some studies suggest that the AP view contributes no significant additional diagnostic information to that available from the lateral and open-mouth projection.[22] West et al.[23] have shown that, for

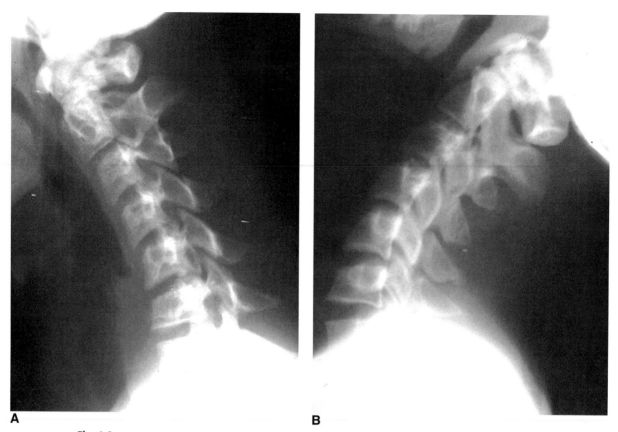

A   **B**

Fig. 4-2
Flexion-extension views. The flexion (**A**) and extension (**B**) stress views show physiologic motion without increased movement at a single level, as compared with others. Facet coverage is relatively uniform throughout. The interspinous and interlaminar distances are similar at each level, and the disc space heights remain uniform anteriorly to posteriorly, except for slight changes associated with the movement. The prevertebral soft tissue is normal. The amount of flexion and extension is only moderate. The study is inadequate in that C6-7 and C7-T1 are not shown adequately or at all.

experienced interpreters, a single lateral cervical spine radiograph is as sensitive for injury diagnosis as the standard three-view series.

Open-Mouth Odontoid View. The open-mouth odontoid (OMO) or atlantoaxial view requires patient cooperation for optimal studies. Ideally, the skull base (occiput), atlas, and axis are well displayed without overlap from the mandible or dentition (Fig. 4-16). The normal OMO view demonstrates the lateral margins of the C1 ring aligned within 1 or 2 mm of the articular masses of the axis. The articular masses of C2 should appear symmetric, as should the joint spaces between the articular masses of C1 and C2, as long as there is no rotation of the head. The measured distance between the odontoid and the C1 medial border (i.e., the lateral atlantodental space [LADS]) should be equal, but a discrepancy of 3 mm or greater is seen often in patients without pathology.[24] Finally, a vertical line bisecting the odontoid process should form a 90-degree angle with a line placed horizontally across the superior aspect of the C2 articular masses.[25] Rotation of the head will cause the C1 lateral masses to appear to change in size and shape, the disc space height to differ, and the apparent distance from the medial aspect of the lateral mass to the dens to change. The lateral mass moving anteriorly will appear larger, closer to the dens, and have a wider disc space with C2 (Fig. 4-17). Voluntary rotation, head tilting, or torticollis can be difficult to distinguish from atlantoaxial rotatory subluxation based on radiography alone. Dynamic CT studies can be useful in differentiating a locked atlantoaxial dislocation from subluxation without locking.[26] Injuries that are best seen on the OMO view include the C1 burst fracture (Jefferson fracture) (Fig. 4-18), odontoid fractures (Fig. 4-19), and lateral flexion fractures of the axis (Fig. 4-20). Lateral spreading of the C1 lateral masses of greater than 6 to 7 mm in the Jefferson burst fracture suggests coexisting disruption of the transverse portion of the cruciate ligament, producing an unstable "atypical" Jefferson fracture.[27] This pattern usually creates two fractures on one side of the C1 ring and probably results from asymmetric axial loading or bending forces (Fig. 4-21).

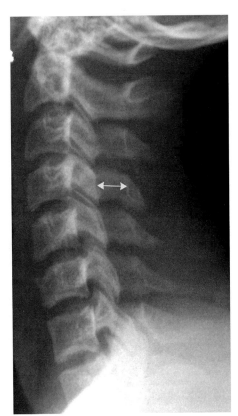

Fig. 4-3
Normal lateral cervical spine. The spacing between vertebral bodies, articular pillars, and spinous processes is uniform. When a true lateral view is obtained, the articular pillars are superimposed and the laminar space (distance from the posterior aspect of the articular pillar to the spinolaminar line—*two-headed arrow*) is uniform.

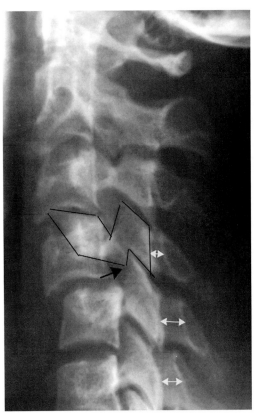

Fig. 4-4
Laminar space sign. The lateral cervical radiograph reveals a unilateral facet dislocation at C4-5 (*black arrow*). Note the abrupt decrease (or increase in some cases) in the distance from the back of the articular pillar to the spinolaminar line (*two-headed white arrows*—the laminar space) at the injury level as a result of rotation between the two sections of the spine. The "bow-tie" sign of the profile of the locked articular processes is outlined in black.

Supine Oblique or Trauma Oblique View. The supine oblique, or "trauma" oblique, projection is obtained with the patient maintained in collar stabilization in the supine and neutral position. The film-screen cassette is placed next to the patient's neck, and the x-ray tube is angled 45 degrees from the vertical.[5] The normal oblique view shows the neural foramina on one side and the pedicles of the contralateral side. The laminae are normally aligned like shingles on a roof (Fig. 4-22). This projection can be used to improve visualization of the cervicothoracic junction when the lateral view is insufficient and often is utilized to clear the cervicothoracic junction.[28] Subluxation or dislocation of the articular masses and laminae that may not be seen on other standard views may be shown to advantage in this projection. If the cervicothoracic junction cannot be visualized adequately on the neutral lateral view, clinicians at most institutions perform a swimmer's lateral radiograph (89%), as opposed to bilateral supine oblique (11%), as the next imaging study.[29] The supine oblique view is more cost effective than CT scanning to selectively clear the cervicothoracic junction.[29]

Swimmer's Lateral Projection. This view often is acquired to visualize the cervicothoracic junction when it is obscured by the density of shadows produced by the shoulders in the true lateral projection. Optimal positioning requires that one of the patient's arms be abducted 180 degrees and extended above the head—which may be difficult or impossible in patients with arm and shoulder injuries—while the opposite shoulder is extended posteriorly to decrease overlapping of skeletal structures (Fig. 4-23).[5] The projection further requires that the patient be rotated slightly off the true lateral. Position changes required to obtain the swimmer's view are contraindicated for patients who are unconscious or who have cervical cord injuries. The swimmer's view results in a somewhat distorted oblique projection of the cervicocranial junction, with the vertebrae obscured by portions of the shoulder girdle or the ribs, or both. However, even with its limitations, this view is generally suitable to assess alignment and detect gross injuries. A modification of the swimmer's projection[30] is designed to improve the quality of the image by producing a truer lateral projection.

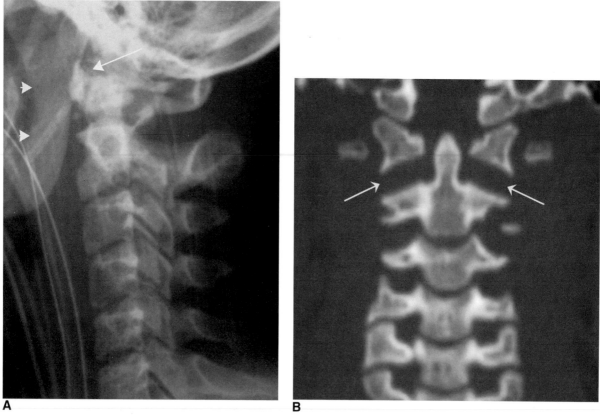

A   B

Fig. 4-5
Prevertebral soft tissue swelling. Both the contour and width of the prevertebral soft tissues are important to observe. Although absolute measurements are quite frequently falsely positive or negative, significant thickening (>10 mm) or a clearly abnormal contour should mandate careful inspection of the radiographs and the performance of CT in unresponsive patients and those with cervical spine symptoms. An endotracheal tube and nasogastric tube further confound this determination. **A,** In this case, the lateral radiograph in an unresponsive, intubated patient shows definite soft tissue swelling (*arrowheads*) above the level of the indwelling tubes. A careful review also shows tilting of the axis ring and elevation of the anterior atlas ring above the top of the dens (*arrow*). **B,** Coronal CT multiplanar reformation shows a clear atlantoaxial dissociation injury (*arrows*).

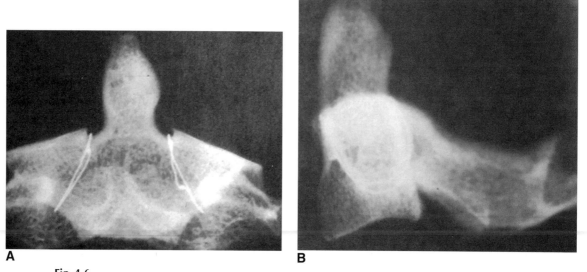

A   B

Fig. 4-6
Harris composite ring shadow. Lateral (**A**) and anteroposterior (**B**) views of axis vertebral body specimen showing wire around cortical bone that contributes to the Harris ring in the lateral cervical spine radiograph. (From Harris JH, Burke JT, Ray RD, et al: *Radiology* 153:353, 1984.)

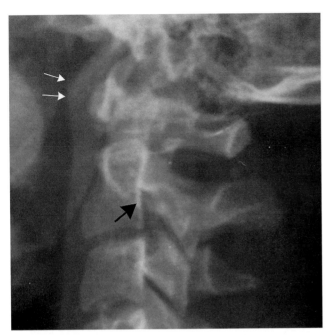

Fig. 4-7
Normal Harris composite shadow. Lateral view of upper cervical spine shows a well-defined Harris ring, with interruption only at the inferior aspect (*black arrow*) due to foramen transversarium. A normal soft tissue convex bulge anterior to the atlas is seen (*white arrows*).

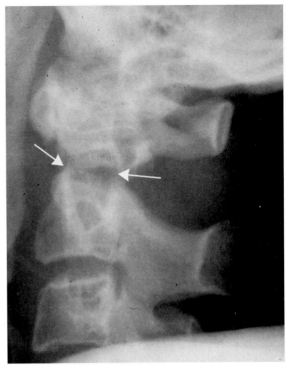

Fig. 4-9
Disruption of Harris axis ring shadow. Coned-down lateral view of upper cervical spine shows two breaks (*arrows*) in the upper Harris ring corresponding to the type III or low odontoid fracture. The odontoid process is tilted anteriorly.

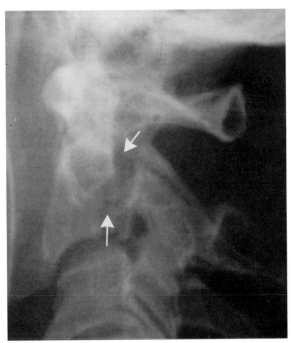

Fig. 4-8
Disruption of the Harris ring. Coned-down lateral cervical spine view shows a fracture of the C2 body that causes disruption of the Harris composite ring shadow at two sites (*arrows*). This is an atypical type I hangman's fracture that extends into the posterior C2 body, disrupting the cortex.

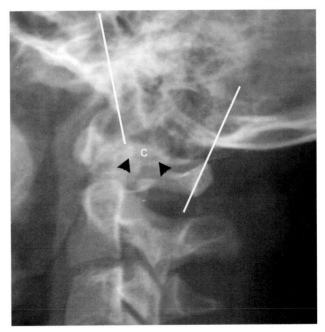

Fig. 4-10
Anatomic relationships of the normal atlantooccipital junction. A line drawn along the posterior margin of the clivus should intercept the posterior tip of the odontoid process, and a line drawn through the C1 spinolaminar line should intercept the opisthion (posterior midline of the foramen magnum) where the inner and outer tables of the skull join. The occipital condyles (*C*) should lie within the C1 condylar fossae (*arrowheads*) without intervening space.

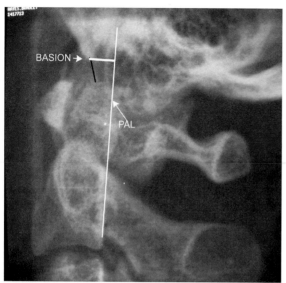

Fig. 4-11
Normal atlantooccipital alignment. Using the method of Harris et al., the distance between the basion (tip of the clivus) should lie within 12 mm of the top of the odontoid process (*black line*). A line extended along the posterior cortex of the axis (PAL) (*white line*) should lie within 12 mm of the basion (*thicker white line* perpendicular to the PAL).

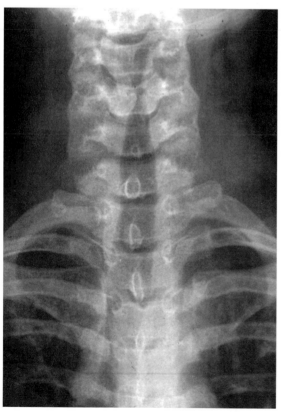

Fig. 4-12
Normal anteroposterior projection. The lateral margins of the spine should appear smoothly undulating without sudden disruptions, and the spinous processes should be aligned or gradually offset due to head turning.

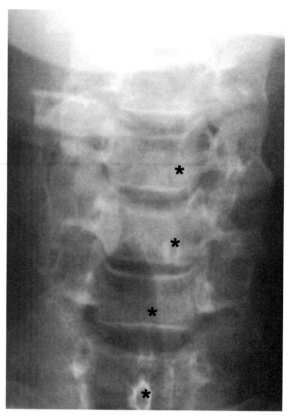

Fig. 4-13
Offset of spinous process due to unilateral facet dislocation. Anteroposterior projection of the cervical spine shows offset of the spinous processes of C4 and C5 compared with C6 and C7 (*asterisks*). This sudden change in orientation of the spinous processes is due to rotational injury at the C5-6 level.

Pillar View. The pillar view (Fig. 4-24) is designed specifically to visualize the cervical articular masses directly in the frontal projection. Weir[31] contends that the pillar view should be included in all acute cervical injuries. It is generally agreed, however, that this view should be reserved for those neurologically intact patients who are radiographically suspected of having articular pillar fractures. The pillar view is obtained by rotating the patient's head in one direction, positioning the x-ray tube off-center approximately 2 cm from the midline in the opposite direction, and angling the central x-ray beam approximately 30 degrees caudally, centered at the level of the superior margin of the thyroid cartilage.[5] The caudally angled central beam is tangential only to the plane of the facet joints in the middle and lower cervical spine because of normal cervical lordosis. Rotation of the head is essential, to eliminate superimposition of the mandible on the lateral masses. Therefore, the patient must be able to rotate the head on command, and an upper cervical injury must have been

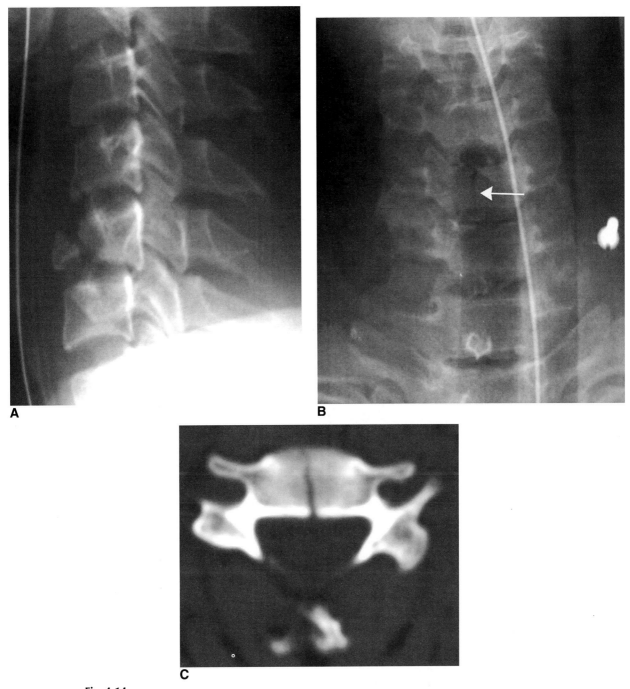

Fig. 4-14
Sagittal plane fracture of vertebral body. **A,** Lateral cervical radiograph shows a flexion tear drop fracture of C5, with posterior displacement of the body and an anteriorly displaced triangular bone fragment. **B,** The anteroposterior view shows a vertical midsagittal fracture of the C5 body typical of this pattern (*arrow*). **C,** Axial CT confirms the midsagittal fracture, as well as a minimally displaced right lamina fracture.

excluded previously on the initial plain radiographic evaluation. Articular pillar and pedicle fractures often occur with rotational injuries,[20] so further rotation is contraindicated when assessing these injuries. If injuries to the lateral cervical pillars are suspected based upon the initial plain film screening, they are further assessed best by CT.

Flexion-Extension Stress Views. Demonstration of ligament injury may require placing stress on the cervical

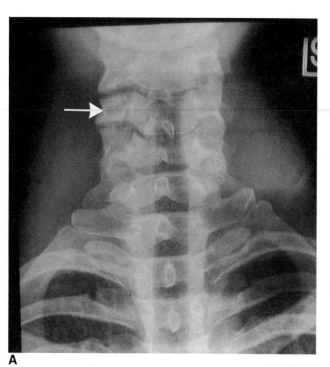

A

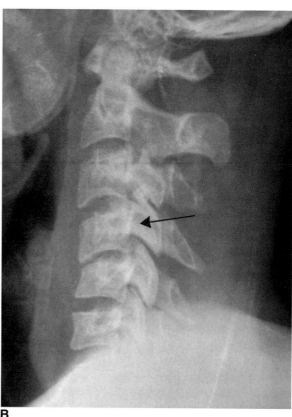

B

Fig. 4-15
Isolated articular pillar. **A**, This anteroposterior radiograph shows an abnormal orientation of the right C5 articular pillar (*arrow*) as compared with other levels. The facet joints are visualized directly due to rotation into a horizontal plane rather than the usual 35-degree tilt. Both the lamina and ipsilateral pedicle must be fractured to permit this motion. **B**, Lateral view of another patient with a similar injury shows rotation of an articular pillar at C4 into a more horizontal orientation (*arrow*).

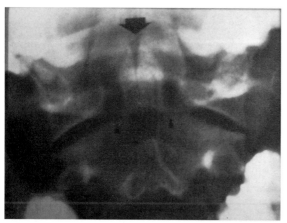

Fig. 4-16
Normal open-mouth odontoid view. The image shows that the lateral masses of the atlas align with the lateral margins of the axis. The joint spaces and lateral atlantodental spaces are nearly symmetric. A lucent line at the base of the odontoid process is a pseudofracture created by the bottom surface of the atlas (*arrowheads*). Note the lucent line extends beyond the lateral margins of the odontoid. A vertical lucent line (*arrow*) is created by the air gap between the incisors.

ligaments. It is imperative that cervical flexion and extension views are obtained only in alert, cooperative, and neurologically intact patients who can describe pain or early onset of any subjective neurologic symptoms. During the evaluation of acute injuries, active flexion-extension radiographs should be physician supervised, preferably by a clinical physician. Fluoroscopically guided passive flexion-extension cervical spine assessment will be discussed in detail in the following section on imaging approaches. Although in most patients evidence of cervical instability will be apparent on the neutral lateral radiograph, some injuries can be reduced effectively to an anatomic position with the patient in a cervical collar and may be completely invisible in the stabilized neutral position. Normally flexion and extension will produce minimal physiologic motion of adjacent vertebrae and anterior or posterior sliding movement across the articular facets. An abrupt change in facet coverage at one level indicates injury to the ligament support (Fig. 4-25). Finally, degenerative disease (cervical spondylosis) of the facet articulations with loss of the

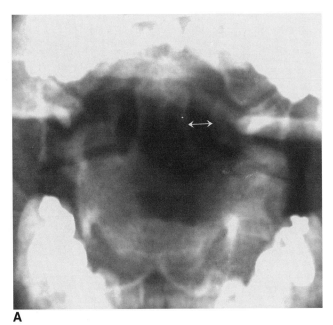

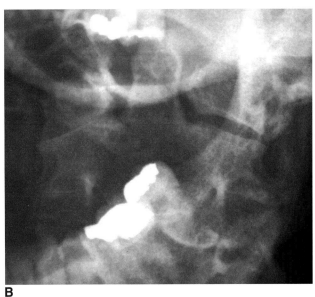

A

B

Fig. 4-17
Change in appearance of C1-2 with rotation on the open-mouth radiograph. **A**, In the neutral position, the lateral masses of the atlas are similar in size and shape, the joint space between the lateral masses and C2 facets appears equal, and the lateral atlantodental spaces (*two-headed arrow*) are nearly equal. **B**, With head rotation to the right of about 30 degrees, note the change in apparent size and shape of the lateral masses of the atlas, the apparent difference in width of the joint spaces, and the change in the lateral atlantodental distance from side to side.

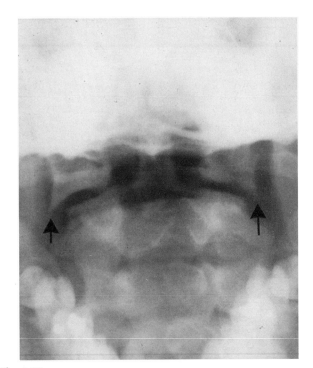

interarticular fibrocartilage may allow excessive anterior translation at one or more levels that can mimic pathologic movement owing to acute injury (Fig. 4-26). In degenerative slippage, the shape of the articular facet and width of the facet joint spaces may be normal; however, in most cases the articular facet has become "ground down," the facet joints are narrowed, and the articular

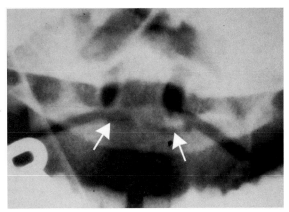

Fig. 4-18
Open-mouth odontoid (OMO) view of Jefferson burst fracture. OMO view shows lateral displacement of the lateral masses of the atlas relative to the lateral borders of the axis (*arrows*).

Fig. 4-19
Open-mouth view of type III (low) odontoid fracture (*arrows*). Same patient shown in Fig. 4-9.

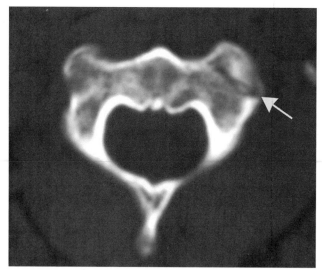

Fig. 4-20
Axial CT shows isolated lateral fracture of the axis (*arrow*) that most likely results from lateral bending with axial loading.

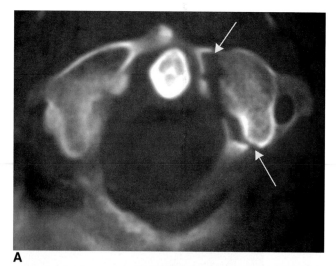

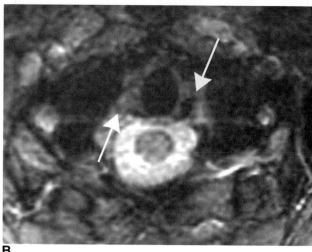

Fig. 4-21
Atypical Jefferson fracture. **A**, Axial CT shows two fractures of C1 ring on the left side (*arrows*). **B**, Gradient echo MR image shows tears at both ends of the transverse atlantal ligament (*arrows*) rendering the injury unstable.

processes are thinned. In traumatic subluxation, the articular facets will be either normally shaped or fractured, and the joint spaces will be widened.[32] In a national survey of 165 trauma centers, Grossman et al.[33] found that flexion-extension views were more likely to be performed as part of the cervical spine imaging evaluation in level 1 than in level 2 of lower level trauma centers. Brady et al.[34] evaluated use of dynamic flexion-extension views in 451 patients with blunt trauma who manifested neck pain, midline tenderness, or an abnormal spinal contour on static cervical radiographs. Patients with abnormal cervical static radiographic findings were statistically more likely to have abnormal active flexion-extension study results than those with normal static study results and were more likely to require invasive fixation.

Criteria for performing cervical spine flexion-extension stress series are not clearly established. Based on a study of normal volunteers, Knopp et al.[35] recommended that subluxation of greater than 2 mm on neutral radiographs was an appropriate indication. Wang et al.[36] have challenged the utility of flexion-extension views, citing the high frequency of inadequate studies due to limited amounts of applied stress due to spasm and neck pain. Dwek and Chung[37] have found little utility for these stress views for pediatric cervical trauma victims with normal static radiographs.

Computed Tomography of the Cervical Spine

CT allows images to be obtained in any plane determined by the radiologist to demonstrate the pathology in question to maximal advantage. Multiplanar computed tomography (MPCT) is CT with routinely obtained sagittal and coronal reformatted images. The

role of MPCT in the evaluation of injuries of the axial skeleton has been well established.[38-48] Simply put, MPCT (including 3D CT) is the imaging technique of choice for spinal injury. The principal value of CT is in the axial image, which demonstrates the neural canal and the relationship of fracture fragments to the canal. Axial data obtained in the supine patient is converted into images displayed in the sagittal and coronal planes, without requiring movement of the injured patient. The development of multislice CT technology with 0.5-sec gantry rotation allows up to eight axial images to be acquired per second on a four-detector row CT and is continuing to expand to more images per second. The speed of data acquisition decreases patient motion and permits thinner section images to be obtained routinely

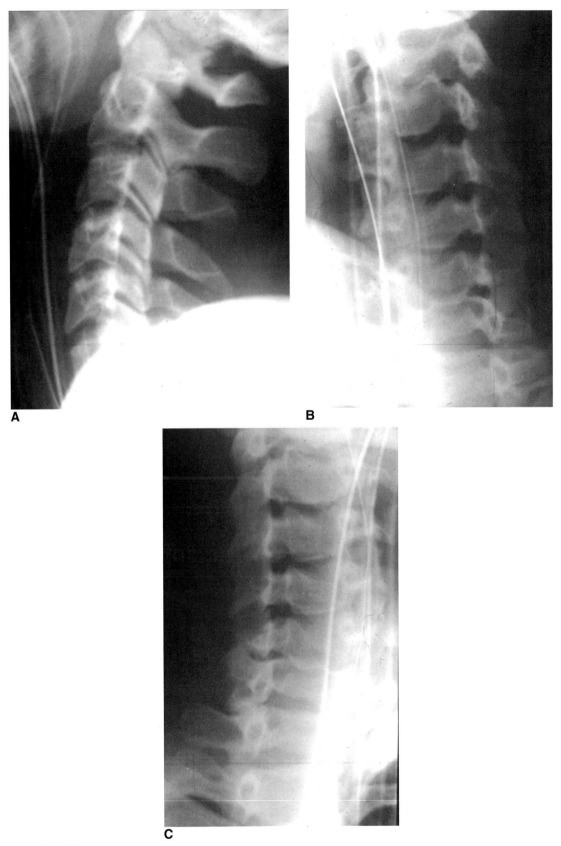

Fig. 4-22
Supine oblique projection. **A,** The lateral projection of this trauma patient includes only to the top of C6 and is inadequate to assess fully the cervical spine. **B** and **C,** The supine oblique projection well demonstrates the cervicothoracic junction, allowing the spine to be declared free of injury.

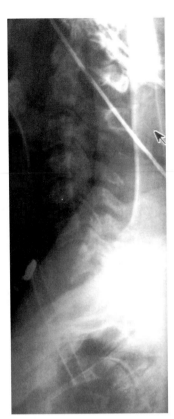

Fig. 4-23
Swimmer's view. Lateral view using increased exposure, with the shoulders offset above and below the cervicothoracic junction, helps to penetrate the soft tissues of lower neck and shoulders and visualize the area.

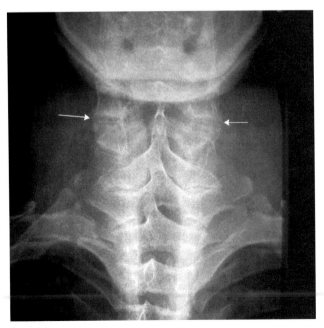

Fig. 4-24
Pillar view. Angled projection along the axis of the articular facets allows visualization of facet joints (*arrows*) and articular mass contour to detect injuries.

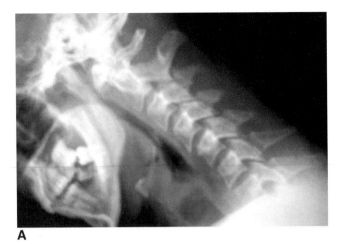

A

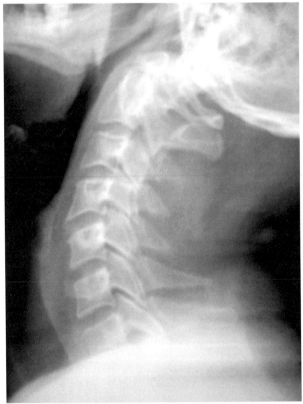

B

Fig. 4-25
Flexion-extension views. Flexion (**A**) and extension (**B**) lateral cervical radiographs must exhibit a significant degree of stress movement in both positions and include C7 through the top of T1 to be considered acceptable. Many studies fail in these respects and are, therefore, inadequate.

than single-slice spiral CT. These factors contribute to a major improvement in the quality of reformatted 2D and 3D images. The volume elements obtained (voxels) with multislice spiral scanning can be made equivalent in size in all three orthogonal axes (isotropic), permitting image quality that is equivalent to axial images in any orientation. The addition of more detector arrays

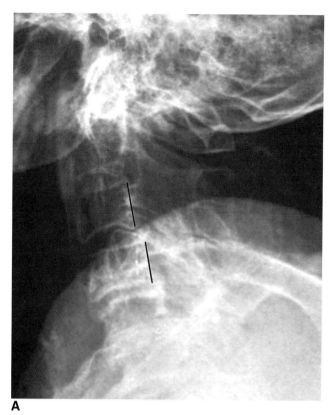

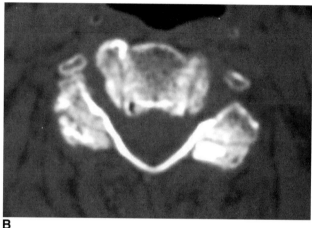

A   **B**

Fig. 4-26
Pseudosubluxation due to facet joint degeneration. **A**, A lateral cervical radiograph in an elderly woman with osteoporosis shows mild anterolisthesis of C3 on C4. **B**, Axial CT through this level shows loss of articular cartilage and sclerosis of the articular processes. Loss of cartilage allows closer apposition of the articular (facet) surfaces, permitting forward movement of the superior vertebral body in response to altered anatomy. The uncovertebral joints are similarly narrowed with periarticular bony hypertrophy.

increases the speed of image acquisition and further improves image quality.

Spinal CT imaging without intrathecal contrast is performed to (1) evaluate uncertain radiographic findings, (2) provide details of osseous injury as an aid to surgical planning, (3) assess focal or diffuse spine pain when no radiographic abnormalities are demonstrated, (4) clear the lower cervicothoracic region in symptomatic patients in whom cervical radiography provides inadequate visualization, (5) assess the adequacy of internal fixation and detect postoperative complications, and (6) localize foreign bodies and bone fragments in relation to neural elements.

CT imaging is not indicated for some spinal injuries identified radiographically. These include simple wedge compression fracture, clay shoveler's fracture, anterior subluxation (AS), hyperextension–tear drop fracture,[49] typical hangman's fractures, and typical odontoid fractures. CT often shows additional injuries not suspected on review of plain radiographic views.[50] CT is particularly useful in identifying fractures of the occipital condyles[51] (Fig. 4-27), articular masses, and laminae that may occur in association with hyperflexion facet dislocations[20] (Fig. 4-28), hyperextension fracture-dislocations, hyperflexion

tear drop fractures (Fig. 4-29), axial loading fractures of C1 (Jefferson fracture) (Fig. 4-30), and vertebral body burst fractures (Fig. 4-31).

Assessment of subluxation and dislocation is aided by 2D multiplanar as well as 3D surface contour or 4D volume-rendered image reformations (Fig. 4-32). The quality of both 2D reformations and 3D surface contour images is improved by the use of thinner axial CT slice thickness and by overlapping axial CT images. Axial CT slice thickness should be no greater than 3 mm in the cervical spine, preferably with slice overlap. Spiral CT scanners allow reconstruction of images at any slice thickness down to 0.5 mm and, therefore, generally provide higher quality reformatted images. Use of such thin-section scans with slice overlap assists in detection of fractures that are oriented in the plane of scanning (axial), such as the type II or high odontoid fracture, as well as for any minimally displaced fracture (Fig. 4-33). Multidetector CT can routinely perform 1-mm-slice thickness studies of the entire cervical spine, permitting superb 2D reformations (Fig. 4-34).

Potential limitations of axial CT include "volume averaging," accentuated by use of thick and axial images

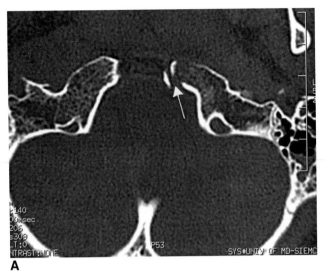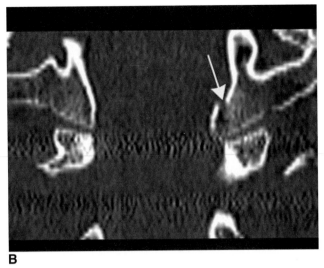

Fig. 4-27
CT of type I occipital condyle fracture. **A,** A small bone fragment arises from the medial aspect of the left occipital condyle (*arrow*). **B,** Coronal multiplanar reformation shows fracture line with minimal medial displacement. Upper neck pain was the patient's only symptom.

that do not overlap and may simulate or obscure a fracture (particularly those oriented along the axial imaging plane), radiation exposure, and time constraints. Minimally displaced fractures may be difficult to identify on reformatted sagittal and coronal images because of degradation in spatial resolution inherent in these images. CT quality also is adversely affected by patient motion. As described above, multidetector spiral CT with 0.5-sec tube rotation will diminish significantly these CT limitations.

Computed Tomography with Intrathecal Contrast.
CTM is MPCT performed following the intrathecal introduction of nonionic water-soluble contrast medium. Depending on the patient's condition and level of suspected cord involvement, the contrast can be introduced in the usual myelographic fashion or, more often, laterally at the C1-2 level with the patient supine.[44] Because it is not viscid, nonionic contrast can be introduced through a 22-gauge needle, which can then be removed, with the contrast absorbed through the meninges and subarachnoid villi. The water-soluble contrast diffuses through the cerebrospinal fluid, thereby requiring less patient movement to visualize the clinically indicated areas of the spine.[44] Typically, the area of interest is examined fluoroscopically with spot and overhead radiography. If desired, CTM can be performed immediately after introduction of nonionic contrast, because CT scanners can easily produce good quality images despite the high density of the contrast material.[52-55]

CTM provides direct visualization of the spinal cord, cauda equina, and nerve roots, thereby permitting distinction between extramedullary and intramedullary cord or root injury, localization of cord compression by frac-

ture fragments or herniated disc, or identification of root avulsion,[56] partial or complete "block" of cerebrospinal fluid,[46] dural tear,[57] or posttraumatic syringomyelia.[58] Contrast material in the cord itself indicates a penetrating injury, such as might be caused by a fracture fragment displaced into the canal.[59]

MRI has replaced most of the applications of CTM for evaluation of spinal cord injury. In those institutions in which magnetic field–compatible patient immobilization, support, and monitoring systems are available, MRI of the spinal cord should be performed as soon as clinically feasible in all patients with myelopathy. If MRI is not available, the traditional indications for CTM remain valid. CTM, however, continues as the imaging technique of choice for demonstrating the presence and extent of dural tears, nerve root herniation, and root avulsion[59] (Fig. 4-35).

Computed Tomography with 3D Display. 3D CT is the logical extension of the concept of sagittal and coronal reformation of axial image data. In essence, 3D CT software programs transform axial CT data into a 3D optical illusion of the portion of the spinal skeleton being examined. The 3D images are derived from the data of the axial CT scan.[60,61] Thus, 3D display increases neither examination time nor patient radiation dosage. In more contemporary CT systems, the CT data are transferred immediately upon acquisition to independent workstations dedicated to large image data set manipulation. Some workstations can be programmed to present "instant" preselected 3D renderings of the spine, with or without adding surrounding soft tissues. Tissues of different density are assigned different colors and degrees of

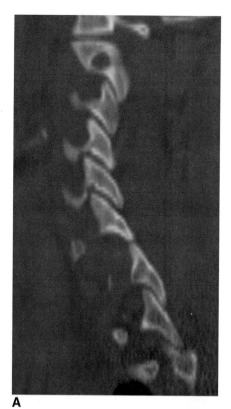

A

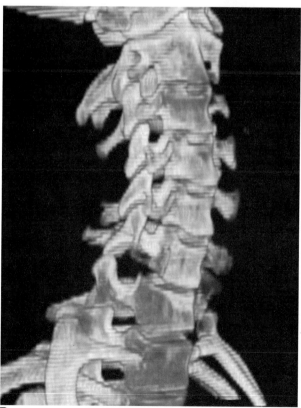

B

Fig. 4-28
Hyperflexion "perch." **A**, CT multiplanar reformation shows complete dislocation of the facet surfaces from a flexion force, resulting in perching of the tips of the articular processes. **B**, Volumetric rendering of the injury.

transparency to enhance distinction. The 3D volume images can then be manipulated in real time to find the preferred angle of viewing or perspective to enhance appreciation of pathology. The spine can be cut electronically along any axis to view the neural canal from within or to delete anatomic structures that might obscure the skeletal pathology. The surface contour–rendered 3D image clearly defines, and reduces or eliminates, ambiguity of complex fractures and fracture-dislocations (Fig. 4-36).

Magnetic Resonance Imaging of the Cervical Spine

Simplistically, MRI scans are derived from the energy released by the hydrogen protons of the body. When placed in a magnetic field, these protons change their orientation and energy state because of an additional radiofrequency current introduced into the static uniform external magnetic field. Only tissues within a specific slice within the body will have protons "precessing" at the correct frequency to absorb the radiofrequency energy. Release of this excess applied radiofrequency energy (relaxation) accompanies reorientation of hydrogen protons with the external magnetic field. A map is created of the location and energy intensity at each point in a slice that reflects the magnetic properties of the particular tissues within the slice. MR images also are influenced by the number of protons within a tissue relative to other tissues, the bulk and microscopic movement of protons, and the chemical state of some tissues such as hemoglobin. Contrast agents such as gadolinium chelates can be used to manipulate tissue relaxation properties and increase or decrease signal and, therefore, intensity.

The intrinsic advantages of MRI have made it the imaging technique of choice for the central nervous system, including the spinal cord, its meninges, and its roots.[62-69] These advantages include the following:

1. Direct imaging of the spinal canal in any orientation
2. Superior contrast resolution, when compared with other techniques, in the detection of soft tissue injury, including ligamentous, with greater sensitivity
3. Creation of myelography-equivalent images to assess the epidural space for evidence of hematoma, bone fragments, herniated disc material, and osteophytes, without use of instilled intrathecal contrast
4. Direct imaging of the spinal cord to detect evidence of contusion, hematoma, or laceration
5. Provision of prognostic information regarding the potential for recovery of function based on the MRI appearance of cord injuries

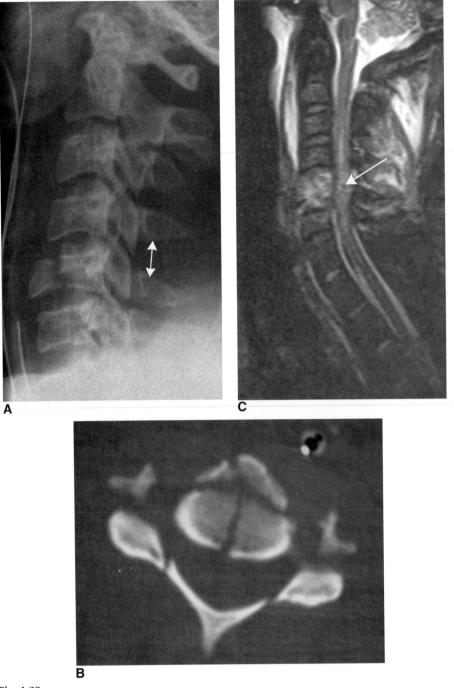

Fig. 4-29

Hyperflexion tear drop fracture pattern. **A**, Lateral cervical radiograph shows a tear drop–shaped anterior fragment arising from the C5 body, with retropulsion of the posterior body. There is also widening of the spinous processes between C4 and C5 (*two-headed arrow*). Fractures of the posterior elements are not seen. **B**, Axial CT image shows the anterior fracture fragment that composes the tear drop and a sagittal split in the body, typical of this pattern. Also seen are bilateral laminar fractures, again typical of the pattern. **C**, A T2-weighted spin-echo sagittal MR image shows a large, high-signal contusion extending from inferior C3 to the top of C7. There is apparent disruption of the ligamentum flavum at C4-5. A focus of low signal in the center of the cord at C5 indicates hemorrhage (*arrow*).

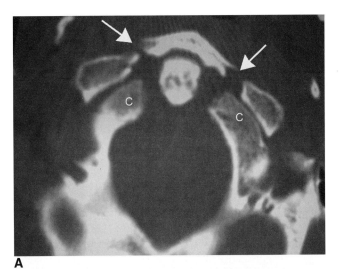

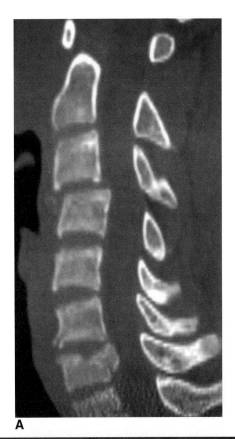

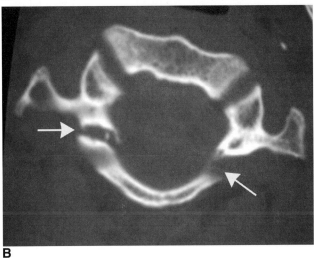

Fig. 4-30
CT of a Jefferson burst fracture. **A** and **B**, Two axial images demonstrate four fractures involving the atlas at the anterolateral and posterolateral margins. Note that the occipital condyles (*C* in **A**) lie medial to the C1 lateral masses.

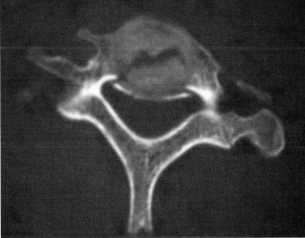

Fig. 4-31
Vertebral body burst fracture. **A**, Lateral cervical spine image of trauma patient shows a hyperflexion subluxation at C3 on C4 and a burst fracture of C7. Note loss of height of both the anterior and posterior cortex and retropulsion of the posterior body. A fracture of the C6 inferior endplate is also seen. **B**, Axial image at C7 shows retropulsed posterior body.

6. Visualization of flowing blood—which appears dark or bright, depending on the imaging sequence used—for assessment of major blood vessels, such as the vertebral arteries, without the necessity for intravascular contrast enhancement

7. No requirement for intravenous contrast or ionizing radiation

Several imaging sequences are performed routinely to emphasize various aspects of normal and pathologic anatomy. In general, most centers employ the following sequences:

1. Sagittal T1-weighted spin echo to define basic anatomy (Fig. 4-37, *A*)

2. Sagittal proton and T2-weighted spin-echo sequence to emphasize pathologic processes and ligamentous structures (see Fig. 4-37, *B* and *C*)

3. Sagittal gradient-echo sequence to optimize detection of hemorrhage and distinguish osteophytes from disc material
4. Axial T1-weighted fast spin echo to assess the epidural space, spinal cord, and neural foramen through areas of interest seen on sagittal sequences (see Fig. 4-37, *D*)
5. Axial gradient-echo sequences to visualize gray–white matter delineation and exiting nerve roots and neural foramen (see Fig. 4-37, *E*)
6. Optional MRA sequence to assess cervical arteries, depending on the type of spinal injury (see Fig. 4-37, *F*)

A variety of other, more recently developed, sequences are available, which may improve detection of certain types of spinal pathology. The use of a particular sequence (short tau inversion recovery) can improve detection of subtle spinal cord contusions compared with other standard imaging sequences[70] (Fig. 4-38).

The limitations of MRI are few but should be mentioned. Because cortical bone contains essentially no hydrogen atoms, it is not well visualized by MRI. The proton signal of blood and fat in its medullary portion is used to identify bone. Consequently, MRI reveals only major osseous injuries and cannot be depended upon to diagnose subtle bone injury, particularly that involving the posterior spinal elements.[71] Comprehensive MRI examinations of the spine require more time than comparable CT studies because of the longer data acquisition. New imaging acquisition sequences potentially can make MRI as fast as or faster than CT scanning. Hemodynamically unstable patients should not be studied by MRI, because acute cardiopulmonary resuscitation is not performed easily or safely in the MRI environment. The need for sophisticated physiologic monitoring and support requires MRI-compatible systems that can function reliably with the fringe magnetic field around the MRI device and that will not create radiofrequency noise in the image acquisition process. The development of such systems has made the application of MRI to patients with acute spinal injury possible.[72-75] However, patients with ferromagnetic intracranial aneurysm clips and pacemakers are excluded from the MRI environment, because some aneurysm clips undergo torque when moved through the external magnetic field, and pacemakers can malfunction.[76] Also, patients with metal in close proxim-

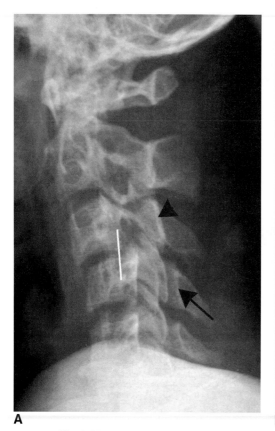

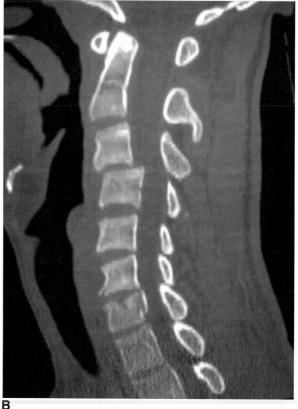

A   **B**

Fig. 4-32
Unilateral facet fracture-dislocation. Multiple display modes. **A,** Lateral radiograph shows the anterior displacement of C3 on C4 (*white line* marks posterior cortex of C3). The laminar space is wider at C4 (*arrow*) than C3 (*arrowhead*) due to rotation (see below). **B,** Midsagittal CT reformation confirms anterior displacement of C3.

Continued

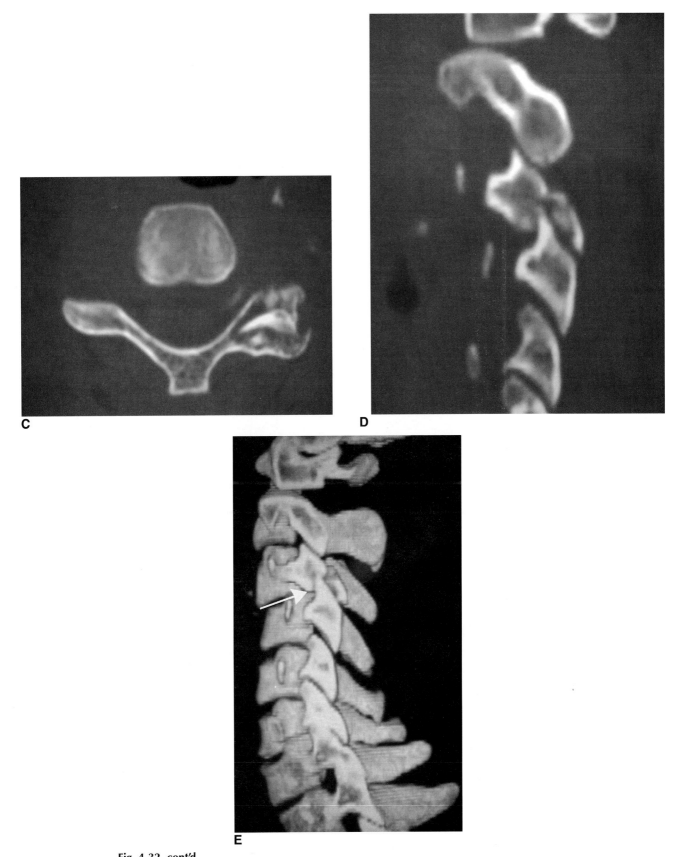

Fig. 4-32, cont'd
C and **D**, Axial CT with parasagittal reformation through the left articular pillars shows the superior articular process of C4 embedded in and fracturing the C3 articular mass. **E**, Volume-rendered view of same injury from lateral perspective nicely illustrates mechanism of C3 articular pillar fracture (*arrow*).

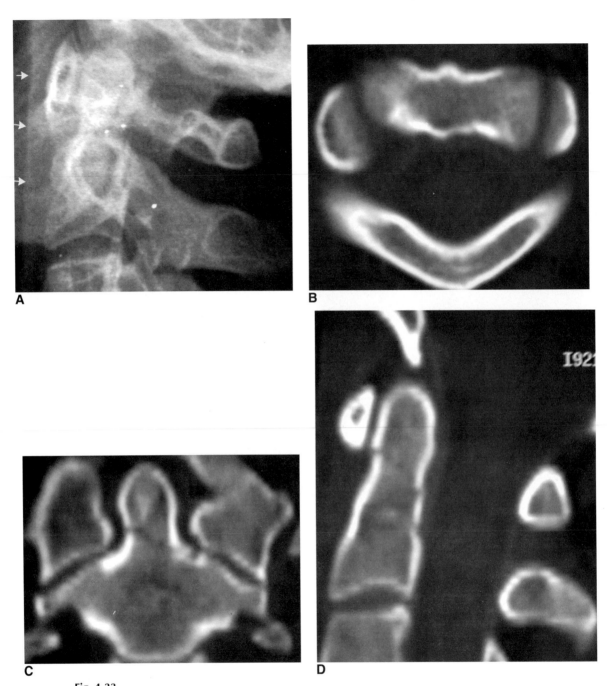

Fig. 4-33
Nondisplaced type II (high) odontoid fracture. **A,** The coned down lateral radiographic view was believed unremarkable. Note straightening of prevertebral soft tissues anterior to the axis from edema (*arrows*). **B,** Thin axial CT images (1 mm) through the odontoid were nondiagnostic—representative image shown. **C** and **D,** Coronal and sagittal multiplanar reformation images reveal the nondisplaced fracture with certainty.

ity to vital soft tissue structures such as the spinal cord, nerve roots, or orbit are at increased risk for further tissue injury when positioned in the magnet, particularly when metal foreign body penetration is acute. Patients in whom a history of possible exposure to metal fragments cannot be obtained (e.g., welders who are unconscious)

must be screened radiographically for metal foreign bodies.

MRI is indicated in the evaluation of all patients with incomplete or progressive neurologic deficit after cervical spinal injury, when permitted by the patient's overall clinical status and absence of direct contraindications to

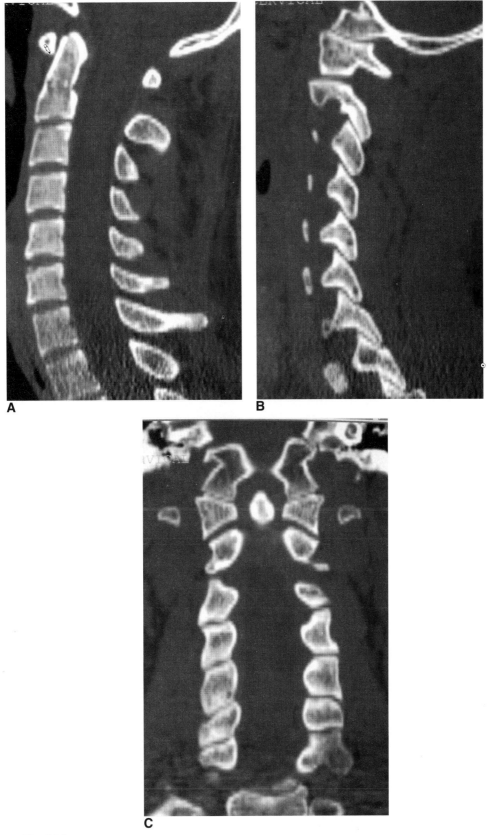

Fig. 4-34
Routine sagittal and coronal multiplanar reformations using quad-multidetector (Philips MX8000, Best, Netherlands). Scan protocol: 1.3-mm slice thickness, increment 1.3 mm, pitch 0.875, scan rotation time 0.75 to 1.0 sec, FOV 18 cm², reformat coronal and sagittal using 1.3-mm slices every 3 mm (kVp 140, mA 200 to 250). **A**, Midsagittal. **B**, Parasagittal plane through articular pillars. **C**, Coronal plane to assess articular pillars.

MRI. Patients with complete deficits should also undergo MRI assessment to demonstrate any cord-compressing lesions (e.g., herniated disc material, epidural hematoma [EDH], or bone fragments), the removal of which may allow some neurologic improvement. Other patients for whom spinal MRI is indicated include those with myelopathy or radiculopathy after spinal trauma, but with radiographic or CT studies with negative findings or results that fail to account for the deficit. Another strong indication is when the level of the deficit does not correlate with the injury location depicted by radiography or CT.[3,50,66] Finally, MRI can demonstrate the level and extent of ligament disruption and intervertebral disc herniation. This information helps determine the need for and the type of internal fixation required to restore a patent spinal canal and ensure mechanical stability.[77] MRI is particularly helpful in determining the extent of ligament injury and instability that typically accompanies injuries occurring in the fused spine, such as ankylosing spondylitis and diffuse idiopathic skeletal hyperostosis (see below).

Magnetic Resonance Imaging of Specific Acute Spinal Injuries

Parenchymal Lesions. MRI is unique in its ability to detect acute injury to the spinal cord, including edema, hemorrhage, and laceration. Cord edema appears isointense or slightly hypointense in relation to the normal cord on T1-weighted spin-echo images but becomes brighter in signal than the normal cord on T2-weighted image sequences (Fig. 4-39). When hemorrhage is present within the cord, its MRI appearance depends on a complex relationship between the chemical state of the blood, the field strength of the magnet, and the imaging sequence used.[78] During the acute to subacute period after injury (1 to 7 days), blood generally appears dark (low intensity signal) on T2-weighted sequences, whereas edema has a bright signal (Fig. 4-40). After about 7 days, as red blood cells are lysed, blood acquires a high-intensity signal on both T1- and T2-weighted studies.

Kulkarni and colleagues[64] were the first to describe a relation between the characteristics of the MRI cord signal and patient outcome, suggesting that MRI cord signal characteristics reflect the type of cord histopathology—that is, hemorrhage (type I), edema (type II), and mixed edema and hemorrhage (type III). The prognostic information provided by MRI regarding potential recovery of function has been verified by several other studies.[65,69,79-82] The ability of the MRI signals to identify the histopathology of acute cord injury has been confirmed by direct comparison of the MRI signal with histologic findings in experimentally induced spinal cord injuries.[79,83,84]

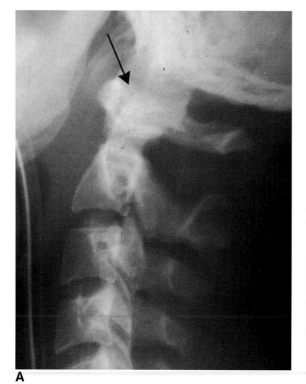

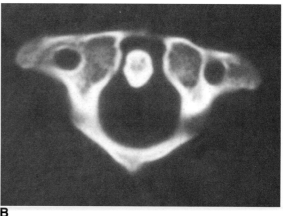

A **B**

Fig. 4-35
Use of CT myelography in trauma. **A**, Admission lateral cervical radiograph in trauma patient shows prevertebral soft tissue swelling anterior to the upper cervical spine and slight widening of the atlantodental space (*arrow*). **B**, Axial CT confirms a widened atlantodental space indicating injury to the transverse atlantal ligament.

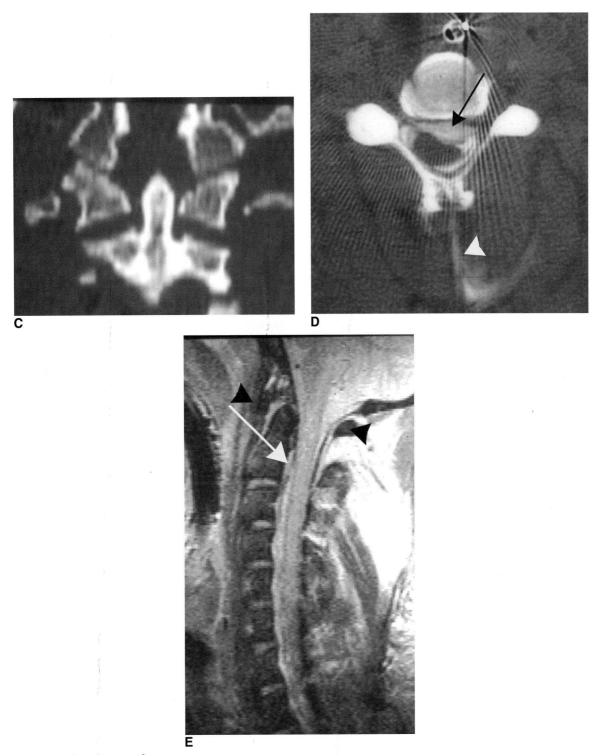

Fig. 4-35, cont'd
C, A coronal multiplanar reformation shows symmetric widening of the atlantoaxial joints indicating distracting injury. **D**, CT myelogram shows an epidural hematoma compressing the left anterior thecal scan and cord (*arrow*), as well as contrast leak from a torn dura (*arrowhead*). **E**, MRI confirms the small epidural hematoma anteriorly (*arrow*), the widened atlantodental space, and elevation of the atlas ring (*arrowheads*).

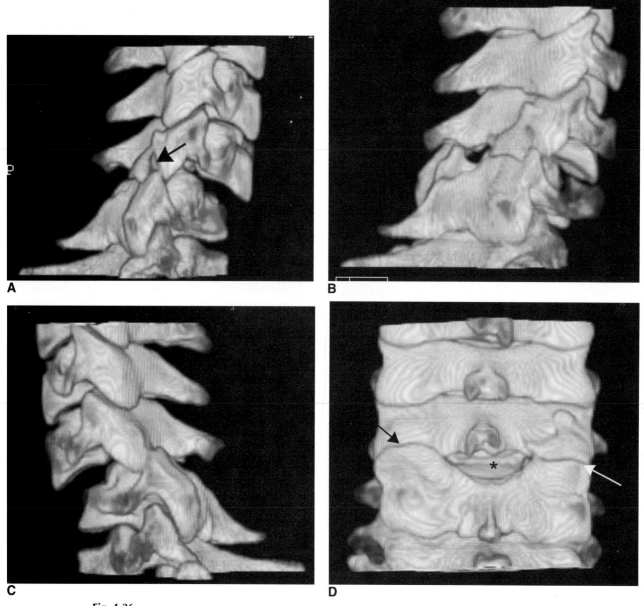

Fig. 4-36
Volume-rendered imaging of complex fracture-dislocation. **A**, Lateral perspective shows a fracture-dislocation of the articular facets at C5-6. Note how the superior articular process of C5 has impaled the C4 articular pillar separating off a fragment (*arrow*). **B**, The same injury from a posterolateral view. **C**, The contralateral side shows a facet dislocation without fracture. **D**, The injury as seen from the posterior view shows the fracture-dislocation on the left (*white arrow*) and the pure dislocation on the right (*black arrow*). Note the widening of the interlaminar and interspinous space (*asterisk*) created by the injury so that the posterior vertebral bodies are seen. Also, note the offset of the spinous processes created by a rotational component.

Ligament Injury. Ligament injury sustained from acute spinal trauma is inferred from the mechanism of injury, the ultimate fracture pattern, and the alignment of the spine after injury. However, even significant ligament injury leading to spinal mechanical instability may not be apparent when the spine is studied radiographically in the neutral position, particularly hyperflexion and hyperextension sprains without concurrent fractures. Furthermore, the spinal alignment demonstrated by plain radiographs may serve to reveal the site of major or

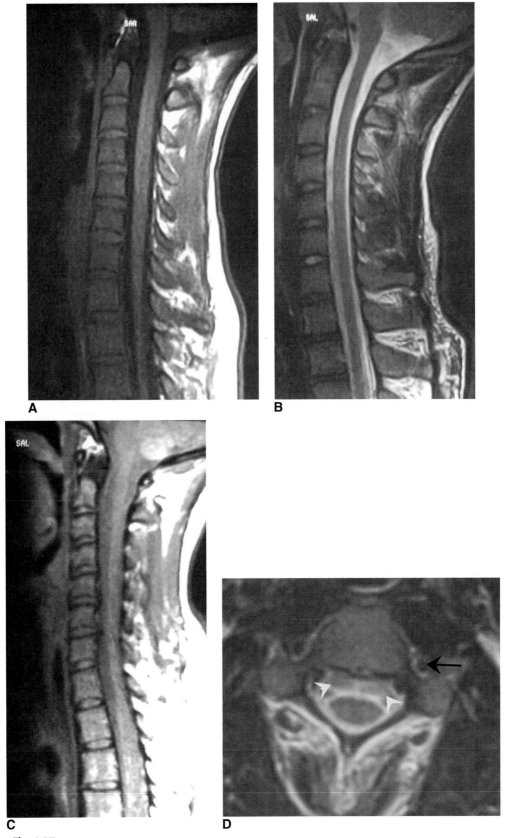

Fig. 4-37
Normal MRI/MRA sequences. **A**, Sagittal T1-weighted. **B**, Sagittal T2-weighted. **C**, Proton-weighted. **D**, Axial fast T2-weighted spin echo. Signal voids noted in vertebral arteries (*arrow*). CSF motions induced flow voids (*arrowheads*).

Continued

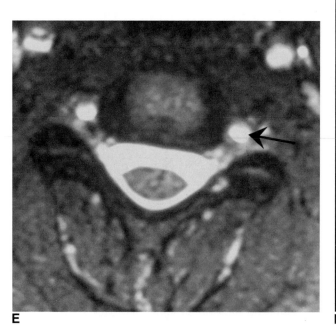

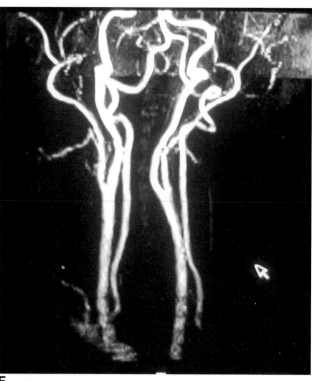

Fig. 4-37, cont'd
E, Axial gradient echo. **F,** MR time-of-flight angiogram.

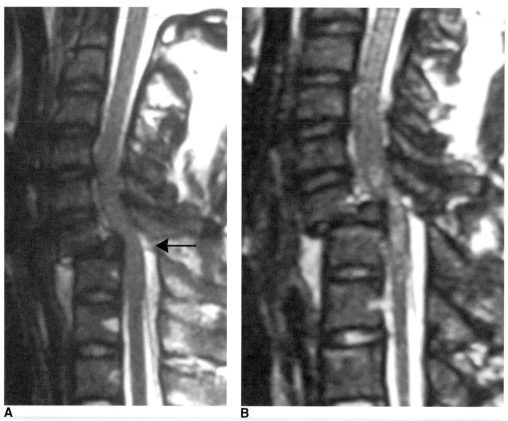

Fig. 4-38
MRI using short tau inversion recovery. **A,** Lateral T2-weighted MR image of patient with acute bilateral facet dislocation sustained in jump from a moving car shows stripping of anterior and posterior longitudinal ligaments and disruption of ligamentum flavum low signal (*arrow*). A slight increase in cord signal is seen around the injury site. **B,** Although the image is noisier, an inversion recovery sequence better demonstrates the high signal cord edema.

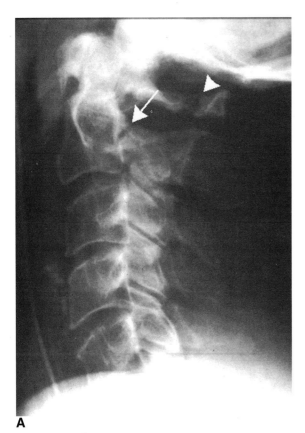
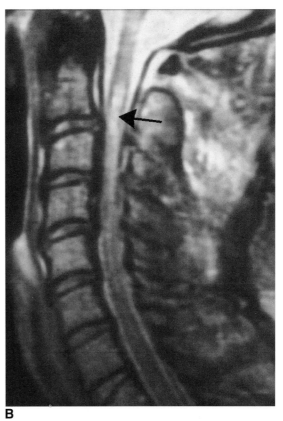

Fig. 4-39
MRI of cord contusion. **A**, Lateral cervical radiograph following blunt trauma demonstrates a type I hangman's fracture (*arrow*) and a posterior arch fracture of the atlas (*arrowhead*). **B**, A T2-weighted sequence shows increased cord signal at the C2 and C3 levels indicating edema (*arrow*). The T1-weighted sequence (not shown) appeared normal for the cord.

principal mechanical instability but may not demonstrate all major ligament injuries and other potential sites of immediate or delayed instability.

MRI depicts normal ligaments as regions of low signal intensity owing to lack of mobile hydrogen. Disruption of the ligament will be seen on MRI scans as an abrupt interruption of the low signal, ligament attenuation or stretching of the ligament, or association of a torn ligament with an attached avulsed bone fragment (Fig. 4-41). Determination of the status of the major support ligaments of the spine as revealed by MRI has a definite bearing on management approaches.[18,85-88] MRI can demonstrate unsuspected ligament injury or injury that is greater than anticipated based on the results of other available imaging modalities.[19]

Intervertebral Disc Herniation. Acute intervertebral disc herniation may accompany fractures or dislocations or may occur as an isolated lesion. If the disc impacts the spinal cord or roots, a neurologic injury may result. MRI demonstration of a single-level acute intervertebral disc herniation that impinges on the spinal cord is crucial in surgical management of spinal trauma to optimize neurologic recovery. MRI clearly depicts disc material herniation on essentially all imaging sequences (Fig. 4-42) but best separates disc material from posterior osteophyte on the gradient-echo sequence, which creates relatively bright disc material against a dark background of bone. The advantage of MRI over CT myelography in detecting acute traumatic disc herniation was shown clearly by Flanders et al.[80] In their study, 40% of acute disc herniations producing neurologic deficits were demonstrated by MRI but not by CTM. Rizzolo and colleagues[88a] found a 42% incidence of herniated nucleus pulposus in 53 patients studied by 1.5-T MRI within 72 hours of injury. The highest incidence occurred among patients with bilateral facet dislocations (80%) and anterior cord syndromes (100%). Doran et al.[89] described a high incidence of traumatic disc herniation among patients with both unilateral and bilateral facet dislocations. Patients with traumatically herniated intervertebral discs may sustain a neurologic deterioration when the cervical spine is reduced, because the disc may then compress neural tissue.[89-92] However, this point is controversial, because

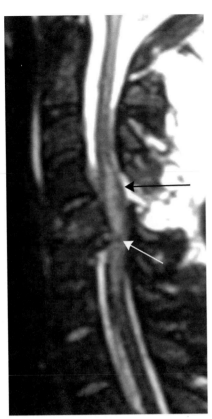

Fig. 4-40
MRI of cord contusion. Midsagittal T2-weighted sequence of patient with flexion tear drop pattern shows increased signal spanning cord from C3-4 to C7. Within the center of the area of edema adjacent to the point of bone impact into the cord, there is a focus of low signal due to hemorrhage (*white arrow*). Interruption of the ligamentum flavum is well delineated at C4-5 (*black arrow*).

others find no evidence of neurologic deterioration when closed reduction is performed for patients with disc herniation or disruption.[93]

Epidural Hematoma. EDHs are an uncommon sequela of spinal trauma and occur in 1% to 2% of cervical spine injuries.[94] The cervical spine is the most common location of EDHs of traumatic origin.[94] EDH most commonly occurs in the dorsal epidural space as a result of close adherence of the ventral dura to the posterior longitudinal ligament.[94] Bleeding most likely arises from sudden increases in pressure in the rich epidural venous plexus, which comprises valveless veins.[94,95] EDHs may develop acutely after trauma, in a delayed fashion, or after open or closed spinal column reduction. Up to 50% of posttraumatic EDHs may occur among patients without overt cervical spine injuries.[94] For this reason, myelopathy without an injury demonstrated by radiography or CT without intrathecal contrast should suggest an EDH. Garza-Mercado[94] described an increased likelihood of cervical spine EDH in younger trauma victims owing to increased elasticity of the vertebral column and among patients with

fused cervical spines, including those with ankylosing spondylitis and diffuse idiopathic skeletal hyperostosis. The onset of cord compression from an expanding EDH may be heralded by progressive, unexplained neurologic deterioration among patients sustaining spinal trauma.

Again, the MRI appearance of EDH depends on the age of the blood, magnetic field strength, and imaging sequence used. During the acute phase of trauma (1 to 3 days after injury), blood appears isointense (bright) relative to the spinal cord on the T1-weighted sequence (Fig. 4-43) and hypointense (dark) relative to the spinal cord on T2-weighted sequences. At 3 to 7 days after injury, the central portion of the hematoma, which contains intact red blood cells, has low signal intensity on T2-weighted sequences, whereas the periphery, composed of lysed red blood cells, shows increased signal strength on both T1- and T2-weighted sequences.[78]

Congenital or Acquired Spinal Stenosis. Spinal cord injury may be caused by impaction of posteriorly projecting osteophytes or hypertrophied, calcified, or ossified ligaments on the anterior surface of the cord during traumatic deformation of the cervical spine. Posterior spinal cord injury can result from buckling of hypertrophied ligamentum flavum during hyperextension.[96] Patients with congenital spinal stenosis or spinal stenosis acquired from degenerative changes (spondylosis) have an increased likelihood of injury from cervical spine trauma or even physiologic cervical spine motion. Posttraumatic myelopathy without radiographic evidence of acute injury among older patients with posterior spinal osteophytes, ossification of the posterior longitudinal ligament, or congenital spinal stenosis suggests that these conditions are likely to be etiologic.[97,98] Cervical spinal cord impaction by posterior cervical osteophytes typically produces a central cord syndrome.[99]

In the sagittal and axial orientation, MRI depicts spinal canal compromise produced by degenerative processes (Fig. 4-44). Comparison of T2-weighted spin-echo and T2-weighted gradient-echo sequences can be helpful in differentiating acutely herniated soft disc material from osteophytes surrounding chronic disc herniations. Both sequences produce a myelographic appearance that demonstrates the relationship of osteophytes and intervertebral discs to the spinal cord. However, gradient-echo sequences produce very dark–appearing osteophytes and increased contrast, with brighter signal disc material when compared with these features on T2-weighted spin-echo sequences. MRI is crucial in planning the extent of posterior surgical decompression by showing the points at which the thecal sac and direct spinal cord compression occur. It should be noted that the gradient-echo pulse sequence tends to make bone appear larger then in actuality (blooming), and this may accentuate the apparent degree of spinal canal encroachment.

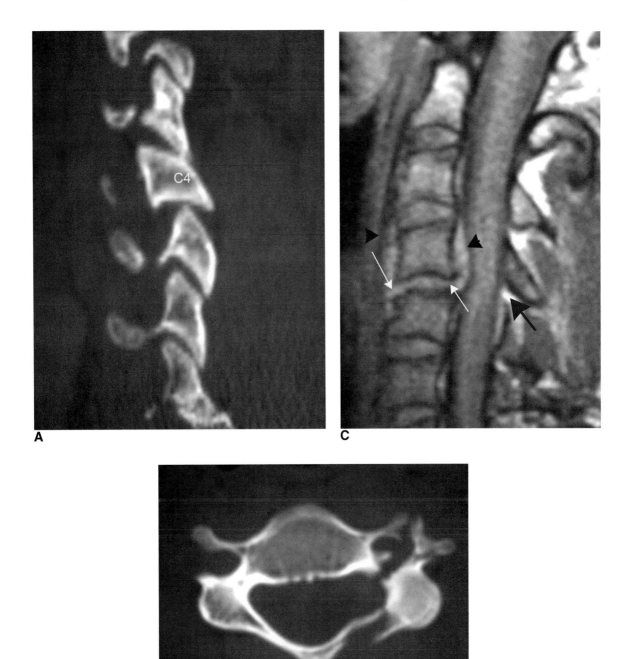

Fig. 4-41
MRI of ligament is associated with isolated articular pillar. **A**, Parasagittal CT multiplanar reformation shows rotation of the C4 articular pillar. **B**, Axial CT through the injured level shows fractures of the pedicle and ipsilateral lamina. The fracture crosses the left transverse process and foramen transversarium. **C**, Proton-density MR image shows disruption of both anterior and posterior annulus fibers at C4-5 (*white arrows*) and tearing of the ligamentum flavum at this level (*black arrow*). Disc material has herniated under the longitudinal ligaments. The appearance indicates bowing and stretching of the longitudinal ligaments (*arrowheads*). There is also a C5 anterior compression fracture.

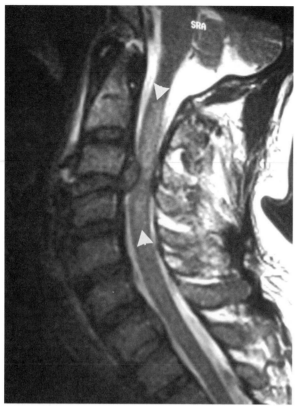

Fig. 4-42
MRI of acute disc herniation. Midsagittal T2-weighted MR image in a patient with a hyperextension injury at C3-4 shows an acute disc herniation at this level leading to cord impact. Higher signal intensity in the cord represents contusion (*between arrowheads*).

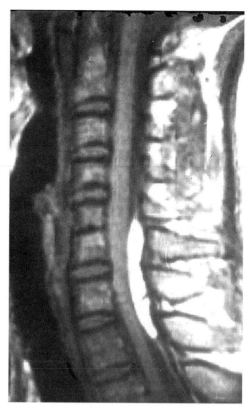

Fig. 4-43
MRI of epidural hematoma. T1-weighted sequence in trauma patient shows a high signal mass in the lower dorsal cervical spinal canal that is convex toward the canal and consistent with epidural hematoma.

Magnetic Resonance Imaging of Chronic and Postoperative Spinal Injuries. It has been well documented that MRI is superior to myelography, CT, and CTM in evaluation of chronic injuries of the spinal cord, particularly for the differentiation of myelomalacia and post-traumatic spinal cord cyst.[100-102] Myelomalacia typically appears as a focal low-signal area on T1-weighted sequences and as a high-signal area on T2-weighted sequences in a cord of normal or decreased caliber.[103] Syringomyelia has a similar appearance but is more sharply delineated and typically occurs in an expanded cord. Flow-sensitive imaging sequences may help to demonstrate a syrinx by demonstrating cerebrospinal fluid movement within the cavity.[103] Postoperative MRI studies performed in patients with internal fixation devices are improved when titanium fixation devices are used.[104] These produce far less magnetic susceptibility artifact than do stainless steel fixation devices and permit visualization of the cord and surrounding epidural space without artifact[104,105] (Fig. 4-45).

Magnetic Resonance Angiography. MRA is used as a screening assessment of the vertebral arteries. The exact incidence of vertebral artery injury occurring after cervical spine fracture-dislocation is unknown, but the injury is being reported with increasing frequency.[106-117] Vertebral artery injuries from cervical spine trauma generally involve the second portion of the artery extending from C6 to C2. Fixation of the artery within the confines of the transverse foramina predisposes this vessel to injury from cervical dislocations. Although a variety of cervical spine injuries have been associated with vertebral artery injury, unilateral and bilateral dislocations are most commonly implicated.[111,112,114] Vertebral artery injury can occur from fractures extending across the foramen transversarium and has been reported with lateral cervical dislocations.[111,115,116]

MRA screening of the vertebral arteries should be considered for all patients with blunt cervical spine trauma with significant degrees (>1 cm) of dislocation or subluxation or fracture of the foramen transversarium or with neurologic deficits consistent with vertebral vessel insufficiency.[109,115-117] Routine assessment of the cervical spine by MRI should include axial T1-weighted images. On these sequences, flowing blood creates a signal void (dark image). Conversely, on gradient-echo sequences,

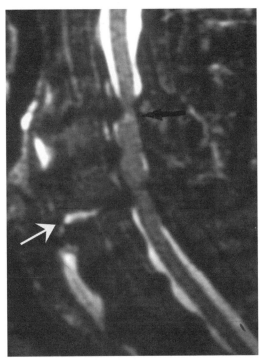

Fig. 4-44
MRI of contusion with spinal stenosis. Midsagittal T2-weighted MR image shows multiple areas of spinal stenosis secondary to osteophytes. There is a focal spinal cord contusion (*black arrow*) from impact against the osteophyte and a hyperextension injury with widening of the anterior C5-6 disc space (*white arrow*).

penetrating trauma. The role of CT angiography for penetrating injury to the neck remains to be investigated (Fig. 4-48). Although the incidence of vertebral artery injury from blunt trauma to the cervical spine appears to be higher than previously suspected, the injury usually results in complete thrombosis without producing a neurologic deficit,[107,109,111,112,116] although this point is controversial.[117] It also appears that thrombosed vessels remain occluded on long-term follow-up, obviating the need to perform endovascular occlusion.[112] Vertebral arteries which are injured but patent can lead to formation of clot and embolization with infarction.[117] These injuries, when identified, require management to prevent or minimize the chance for embolization, using antiplatelet or anticoagulant agents, as permitted by the patient's condition, or open surgical or endovascular techniques.[118]

Catheter Angiography

Conventional angiography (see Chapter 2) is used to detect or confirm vertebral artery injury resulting from cervical spine trauma. Although associated with higher procedure-related morbidity than MRA, the technique offers greater spatial resolution for detection and characterization of vascular injuries. As stated earlier, conventional angiography is the study of choice for assessment of potential vertebral artery injury resulting from penetrating injury to the cervical spine. In addition, angiography can provide the potential for intravascular thrombolysis and endovascular stent management of selected vertebral injuries.[118]

Radionuclide Bone Imaging

Radionuclide bone imaging (RNBI) (see Chapter 12) has been used in the assessment of spinal trauma, primarily to determine whether a radiographic abnormality represents an acute process that is potentially responsible for the patient's pain or to exclude an osseous abnormality as a source of spine pain when radiograph findings are normal. In the cervical spine, image resolution is improved by placing the patient's neck directly on the collimator surface, decreasing distance from the nuclide activity. Slightly posterior oblique images of the cervical spine also can assist diagnostically. Reports[119,120] and anecdotal experience indicate that an acute, nondisplaced cervical fracture cannot be excluded entirely, even when the initial RNBI scan results are normal. RNBI has been assessed in patients with whiplash,[121,122] and no correlation was found between symptoms and signs of injury and scintigraphic findings. However, one retrospective study of 35 cases[121] found that a negative bone scan excluded a skeletal injury, and in another prospective study of 20 patients[122] with whiplash injuries, no

flowing blood creates a bright image. Inspection of the major cervical arteries for the anticipated signal characteristics should be performed as part of overall assessment of the MRI study. Absence or irregularity of the expected flow signal should raise a question of vascular injury (Figs. 4-46 and 4-47). Injuries identifiable by MRA include intimal flaps, intramural dissection or hematoma, pseudoaneurysm, and thrombosis. Care must be taken to distinguish an injury from flow-related artifact, vessel hypoplasia or atherosclerotic disease. Positive MRA findings of vessel injury are confirmed and better characterized by direct contrast angiography, which offers greater spatial resolution than that possible with MRA. CT angiography also is expected to play a role in determining the status of the vertebral and carotid arteries, particularly with the increasing use of multidetector systems.

Penetrating injury accounts for most cervical vertebral injuries from trauma. Retained metal fragments from ballistic injury precludes vascular MRA assessment because of artifacts created by close proximity of metal. In addition, because MRA is less sensitive for detection of subtle intimal injuries or mural hematoma, conventional arteriography generally is recommended for evaluation of suspected vertebral artery injury from

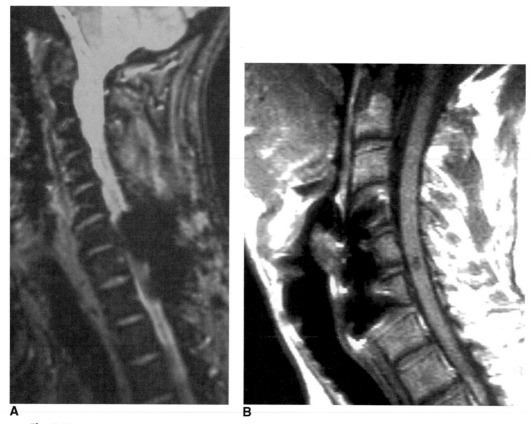

A   B

Fig. 4-45
Limited magnetic susceptibility of titanium fixation. **A**, T2-weighted sagittal MR image shows severe low loss of field homogeneity and signal drop-out related to ferromagnetic posterior fixation wires that obscure cord signal. **B**, T1-weighted sagittal image of a patient with previously placed internal fixation from C4 to C6 by anterior titanium plate and screws for C5 tear drop fracture. Artifact is in close proximity to the metal allowing assessment of the cord, which demonstrates a focal low-signal area of myelomalacia or cyst formation at C5-6. (From Mirvis SE, Harris JH Jr: Spinal imaging. In Browner BD, Jupiter JB, Levine AM, Trafton PG, eds: *Skeletal trauma*, ed 2, vol 1, Philadelphia, 1998, WB Saunders.)

patients had bone scan findings suggestive of fracture, and none was diagnosed subsequently with fracture. Increased activity within the cervical spine on delayed bone imaging includes a differential diagnosis of nonspecific stress response, degenerative arthritis, or healing fracture. Single photon emission computed tomography could increase the diagnostic accuracy of bone imaging for acute spinal trauma.

RNBI in the thoracic and lumbar spine is technically easier than in the cervical spine. Acute fractures can be detected on both blood pool and delayed images. Increased linear activity at the superior endplate is characteristic of traumatic fracture. RNBI may be particularly helpful in detecting acute compression fractures among patients with severe osteoporosis that may be quite subtle radiographically. Increased lateral activity on the concave side of a scoliotic spine that is not sharply marginated most likely represents stress-related or degenerative change. In patients with nonlocalized

lower back pain after trauma and normal lumbar radiographic findings, large field-of-view RNBI can screen for small laminar, transverse process, or articular process fractures that might otherwise require multilevel CT scanning to detect.

IMAGING APPROACH TO THE POTENTIALLY INJURED CERVICAL SPINE
Spinal Imaging of the Polytraumatized Patient: an Overview

Acute injuries of the cervical spine range in significance from clinically trivial to permanent paralysis. Therefore, the evaluation of cervical spinal injury must begin with clinical examination of the patient by an experienced physician who can appraise the location, extent, and magnitude of the spinal injury. Unconscious, intoxicated, or elderly patients with a history of trauma must be considered to have a cervical spinal injury until proven otherwise.

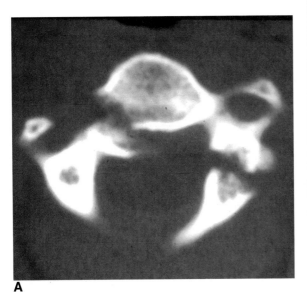

A

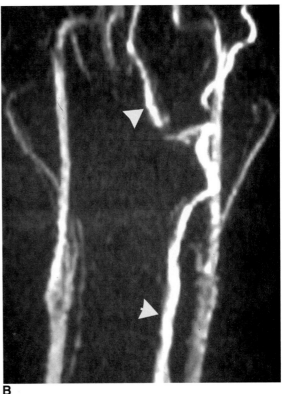

B

Fig. 4-46
Vertebral occlusion associated with hangman's fracture. **A,** Axial CT shows an asymmetric hangman's fracture with the right-sided injury crossing into the right vertebral foramen. **B,** MR angiogram shows occlusion of right vertebral artery and a patent left vertebral artery (*arrowheads*).

The type and extent of imaging evaluation are governed by the patient's neurologic status and overall condition, particularly the hemodynamic status. In all patients with spinal injury, however, the following guidelines should be observed:

1. The spine must remain immobilized to protect it and the cord during the initial examination and until the spine has been declared negative for injury.
2. The radiologic evaluation begins with plain radiographs.
3. The initial examination must be monitored by a radiologist or other qualified physician to establish the radiologic diagnosis as accurately and quickly as possible and to determine whether additional examinations are indicated. If so, the most efficient sequence of studies for optimal patient care must be established.

In the absence of neurologic findings and with the spine immobilized, other injuries, if any, can be managed initially. Alternatively, it may be clinically appropriate to clarify the status of the spine prior to managing a coexistent injury. In any case, the examination of the spine must be personally supervised and sequentially monitored by a radiologist or other qualified physician until either the spine study findings have been declared negative or a definitive diagnosis has been established.

Recommended Imaging Approach for Potential Cervical Spinal Trauma Based on Clinical Picture

Trauma Patient with a Neurologic Deficit Referable to the Cervical Spinal Cord. The optimal radiologic approach to the trauma patient with spinal injury and signs of cord damage consists of only frontal and horizontal beam lateral plain radiographs obtained in the emergency center, followed by CT with appropriate image reformations and MRI of the injured area whenever clinically appropriate. Trauma patients with definite myelopathy but negative plain radiograph results are best served by performing MRI or, if MRI is unavailable, myelography and CT myelography as the next study.

Occasionally, the definitive evaluation of the spinal injury in major trauma patients must be superseded by

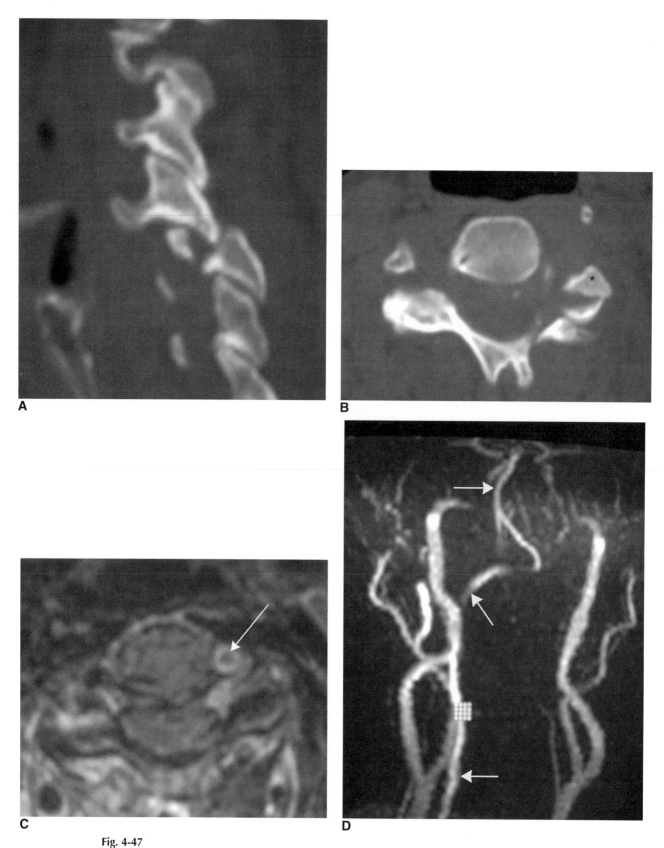

Fig. 4-47
Unilateral facet dislocation with vascular injury. **A**, Parasagittal multiplanar reformation image shows a fracture dislocation at C4-5 with a fracture through the C5 articular mass. **B**, An axial image through the level of dislocation shows three fragments on the left corresponding to the articular processes and a free fracture (*asterisk*). The left articular processes are jumped. **C**, MR image shows no signal void for the left vertebral artery (*arrow*). **D**, MR angiogram confirms occlusion of the left vertebral artery with a patent right vertebral artery (*arrows*).

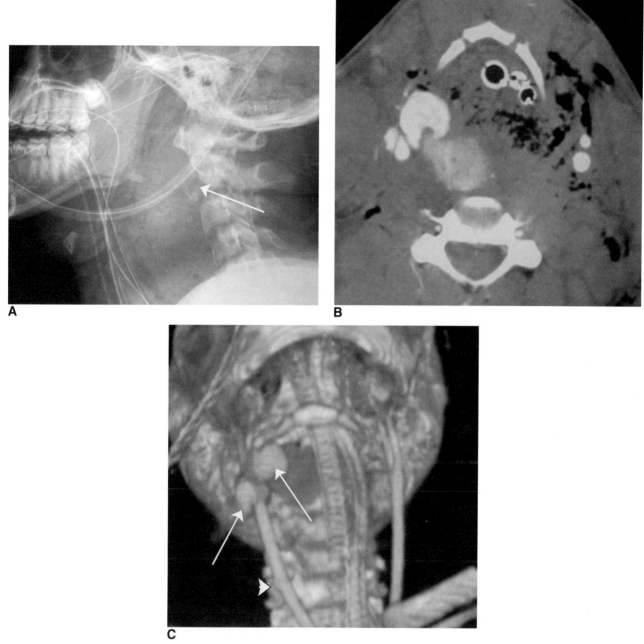

Fig. 4-48
CT angiography of penetrating carotid artery injury. **A**, Lateral cervical spine radiograph obtained after a gunshot wound to the neck shows marked prevertebral swelling. There is a fracture of the anteroinferior aspect in C2 *(arrow)*. **B**, Axial CT through the level of the right carotid bifurcation shows a large, bilobed pseudoaneurysm. **C**, Volume-rendered 3D view from anteroinferior aspect nicely illustrates bilobed pseudoaneurysm *(arrows)* in relation to the carotid artery bifurcation.

the evaluation and management of more urgent clinical problems, such as a low Glasgow Coma Scale score, a tension pneumothorax, a suspected aorta injury, or massive or progressive hemoperitoneum. In such instances, and whenever possible, AP and lateral radiographs of the injured region of the spine should be obtained concurrent with initial patient evaluation and stabilization procedures. If the spine cannot be declared negative for injury on the basis of this screening examination, it must be immobilized until the patient has been stabilized and the evaluation of the spinal injury can be concluded. If possible, MRI should be obtained as the next examination if plain radiographs do not reveal the cause of the neurologic deficit.

Alert Trauma Patient with Cervical Spine Pain. Radiographic examination of the spine clearly is not indicated in every patient who complains of minimal symptoms after minor trauma. The attending physician, however, must have a high index of suspicion for spinal injury, because failure to recognize and treat a clinically subtle dislocation, fracture, or fracture-dislocation can lead to devastating, irreparable cord injury. Therefore, a history of trauma that could produce spinal injury or the presence of objective physical signs consistent with spinal injury are of particular importance in determining which patients should undergo imaging evaluation.

The appropriate radiologic evaluation of the cervical spine is controversial, particularly with regard to the number of views that constitute an adequate radiologic assessment.[1-4,22,23,123-126] Whereas a single lateral radiograph will detect 74% to 86% of cervical spine injuries, sensitivity increases to nearly 100% when an AP and an OMO projection are added.[1] In the neurologically intact, alert trauma patient with a complaint of neck pain, physical findings of pain or point tenderness elicited on palpation of the cervical spine, a minimum of two views, typically a cross-table lateral and an AP view, are obtained. Additional views, including the OMO projection and supine oblique views, can be obtained also and may increase diagnostic yield slightly. If the results of AP and lateral views obtained with the patient in a rigid collar are negative from the occiput to the C7-T1 level, the collar can be removed to facilitate obtaining the OMO and oblique views. If all plain radiograph findings are normal, the possibility of a significant missed skeletal cervical spine injury is minimal. However, ligamentous injuries, including potentially neurologically unstable injuries such as reduced bifacet dislocations or reduced hyperflexion or hyperextension subluxations, still may not be demonstrated (Figs. 4-49 and 4-50). It is impor-

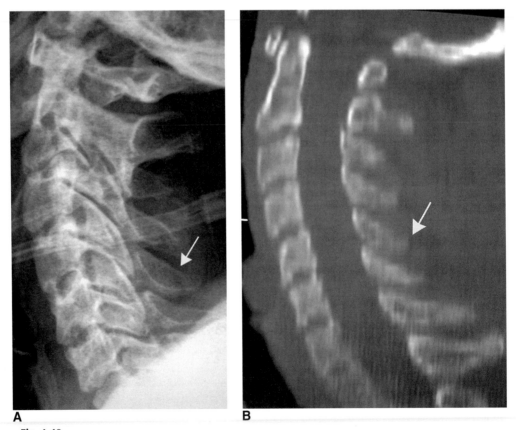

A **B**

Fig. 4-49
Delayed instability. **A,** Initial admission lateral radiograph shows anatomic alignment of spine through C6-7. There is a nondisplaced C5 spinous process fracture (*arrow*). **B,** Midsagittal multiplanar reformation shows same fracture (*arrow*) but normal alignment from the skull base to T1.

Continued

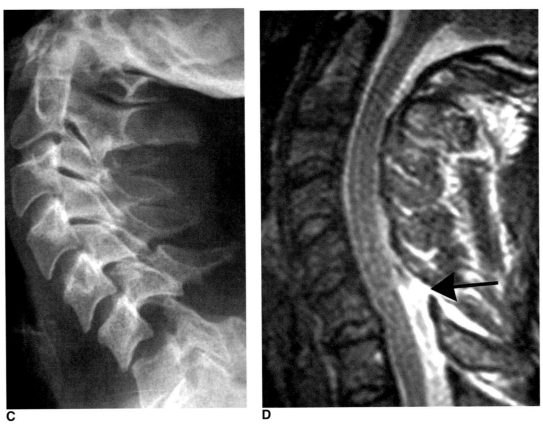

Fig. 4-49, cont'd
C, Delayed (1 week) follow-up with increasing neck pain shows obvious subluxation at C6-7. There is widening of the intraspinous and intralaminar distance, opening of the facet joints, and disruption of the posterior annulus longitudinal ligament complex, permitting angulation and displacement. **D,** The ligamentum flavum is clearly torn on the T2-weighted MR image (*arrow*).

tant to remember that on spinal radiographs obtained only with the patient supine, patient body habitus may obscure some spinal injuries.

A physician skilled in the interpretation of spinal radiographs should examine initial radiographs, obtained with spinal immobilization in place. At the University of Maryland Shock Trauma Center (UMSTC), clinically stable, alert, cooperative patients with cervical pain and normal initial cervical spine radiographs may undergo flexion-extension lateral radiography to assess ligamentous stability after the cervical collar is removed. On occasion, in the experience of that center, flexion and extension subluxations may be identified that are not evident on neutral cross-table lateral or AP cervical radiographs obtained in the supine position.[127] The use of routine flexion and extension lateral cervical radiographs is by no means universal and should not be considered standard practice.[33] This procedure should be *carefully supervised by a physician* and never should be performed

by a radiography technologist alone. The patient should flex and extend the neck to the limit of pain tolerance or onset of subjective neurologic symptoms. Obviously, any suggestion of an onset of neurologic impairment mandates return to the neutral position and reapplication of cervical immobilization. If adequate flexion and extension views are acquired with visualization of the spine through C7-T1, the vast majority of potentially unstable injuries are excluded. Flexion and extension lateral cervical views should not be performed in uncooperative patients or those with decreased mental acuity and should not be obtained with passive movement of the patient's cervical spine by a physician.

Alternatively, spiral CT can be used to screen patients with neck pain for subtle fractures that may be difficult or impossible to diagnose from radiographs. Increasingly, spiral CT is being used as a primary screening test in patients with cervical spine symptoms after blunt trauma. Patients with neck pain who will undergo CT scanning of

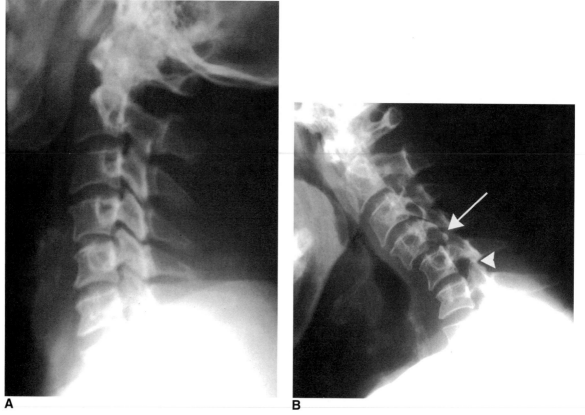

Fig. 4-50
Instability demonstrated in flexion. **A**, Limited lateral radiograph shows no abnormality of align-ment through C6. **B**, A flexion stress view demonstrates offset of the articular pillars (*arrow*) at C4 and above, as compared with C5 and below, indicating rotation consistent with a unilateral facet subluxation or dislocation. Also, there is loss of the facet coverage at C5 on C6 (*arrowhead*) as com-pared with normal levels indicating a hyperflexion sprain. (**A** from Mirvis SE, Harris JH Jr: Spinal imaging. In Browner BD, Jupiter JB, Levine AM, Trafton PG, eds: *Skeletal trauma*, ed 2, vol 1, Philadelphia, 1998, WB Saunders; **B** from Mirvis SE, Shanmuganathan K: *J Intensive Care Med* 10:15, 1995.)

other body regions may also undergo cervical spine CT to assess the region of neck pain or the entire cervical spine.[128] Although it is well established that CT is more sensitive than plain radiography in detecting cervical spine injury,* a positive cost-benefit ratio has not been determined for CT performed in trauma patients with neck pain whose radiographic findings are normal. Increasingly, spiral CT and multidetector CT are being used to perform screening studies of the entire cervical spine rather than depend on plain radiographic interpre-tation for alert patients with cervical spine symptoms. This development is based on the recognized improved accuracy of CT over radiography for traumatic osseous

pathology, the increased use of CT in general for assess-ing stable blunt trauma patients in multiple body regions, the increasing speed of image acquisition and processing, and its general cost and time effi-cacy.[43,50,128,130-133]

The accuracy of spiral CT to detect all potentially unstable ligament injuries is not known, although some of these injuries would be suggested by soft tissue swelling or subtle abnormalities of alignment. For this reason active flexion-extension views still are needed to ensure cervical spine ligament integrity.

Trauma Patient with an Unreliable Physical Examination. Trauma patients who lack evidence of myelopathy but in whom physical examination cannot be considered reliable constitute a major challenge with

---

*References 38, 41, 43, 45, 48, 50-52, 128, 129.

regard to potential spinal injury. All such patients should be regarded as having unstable spinal injuries until proven otherwise. The radiographic assessment of such patients should include at least lateral and AP radiographic views. Open-mouth views are often difficult to obtain and technically suboptimal in this population. In addition, supine oblique views of the cervicothoracic junction region can be performed, if needed. Often, CT is used to assess the cervicocranial junction if not well demonstrated by radiography, depending upon its availability and indication for CT of other body regions. If injuries are identified, spine immobilization is maintained and further imaging workup performed when clinically feasible. The potential role of spiral CT scanning for screening the entire cervical spine for patients with an unreliable clinical examination is undergoing study and appears as a likely future development.

If all radiographic evaluations of the spine are negative, the vast majority of injuries are excluded but, again, the potential for a neurologically unstable injury persists. D'Alise[134] performed limited cervical spine MRI within 48 hours of trauma in 121 patients who had no obvious injury by plain radiography. Thirty-one patients (25.6%) had significant injury to paravertebral ligamentous structures, the intervertebral disc, or bone. Eight of these patients required surgical fixation of the injury. If MRI is not available, an alternative approach is to perform erect AP and lateral cervical radiographs, with the patient in collar stabilization to allow limited physiologic stress on the cervical spine. If these film findings are normal, erect AP and lateral views are repeated out of the collar, with the cervical spine slightly extended and the head supported by a pillow. If the results of these views are normal, the cervical collar is removed permanently. Although the above approaches are considered prudent to avoid missing a cervical spine injury, they are by no means universally followed. At some sites, the cervical collar is removed based on negative AP and lateral supine radiography alone, suggesting the rarity with which neurologically unstable cervical spine injuries occur with normal-appearing cervical radiographs.[135]

Some authors have suggested the use of passive flexion and extension imaging under fluoroscopic guidance for patients in whom one cannot obtain a reliable physical examination.[131,136-138] Almost all patients studied in this manner have been normal, as would be expected from the extremely low pretest probability of an unstable injury. The limited data available do not provide sufficient evidence to support routine use of this technique. Complications of this procedure have been reported.[139] A number of cervical spine injuries will not be detected by this method, including herniated intervertebral discs and EDHs. These lesions may cause spinal cord compression that creates or worsens a neurologic deficit without evidence of overt subluxation on fluoroscopy. Cervical disc herniation is a more common cause of central cord syndrome than previously suspected.[140] Benzel et al.[141] found 27 acute cervical disc herniations among 174 trauma patients with negative cervical radiograph results who underwent cervical MRI. Rizzolo et al.[88a] observed acute cervical disc herniation in 42% of 55 patients with blunt cervical trauma who had cervical fractures or neurologic deficits. In addition, either congenital or acquired spinal stenosis can produce spinal cord lesions in association with blunt trauma when there is no radiographic evidence of injury.[97] Flexion and extension in this population could aggravate cord compression and ischemia. To date, only MRI has proven diagnostic accuracy for direct diagnosis of ligament injury from blunt spinal trauma.[134,141-144]

Alert Trauma Patient with Normal Cervical Spine Examination Findings. The need to perform imaging in alert, oriented trauma victims without evidence of cervical pain, tenderness to palpation of the cervical spine, or major distracting injuries has been highly controversial. Most patients admitted to emergency centers from the scene of a major blunt force trauma are placed in cervical immobilization and are presumed to have a cervical injury until proven otherwise. This scenario places a great deal of pressure on the admitting physician to exclude an injury with an extremely high degree of certainty. There are case reports describing so-called *painless cervical spine fractures*. A close review of many such articles typically reveals that the patient either had symptoms or was not truly alert.[1,22,145-148] Many large series indicate that alert trauma patients without major distracting injuries and without subjective complaints of neck pain or positive physical findings invariably have normal imaging evaluations.[1,149-151] A prospective series of alert trauma patients without symptoms who underwent cervical spine CT to clear the cervicothoracic junction revealed one nondisplaced C7 transverse process fracture in 146 patients at a cost of more than $58,000.[125] Diliberti and Lindsey[1] recommend omission of radiologic assessment of the cervical spine in any trauma patient with class 1 level of consciousness (i.e., able to follow complex commands, responds immediately) and without evidence of intoxication, neurologic deficit, cervical spine pain, or pain elicited on palpation. Gonzalez et al.[152] found that clinical assessment was more sensitive than radiography in detecting cervical spine injury, even in intoxicated patients. A prospective study involving 21 medical centers and over 34,000 patients (National X-ray Utilization Study [NEXUS]) found that the absence of five preset criteria, including no midline cervical spine tenderness, no neurologic deficit, normal alertness, no intoxication, and no distracting painful injury, had a negative predictive value of 99.8% (95% confidence interval, 99.6% to 100%) for excluding cervical spine injury, and use of these criteria would have avoided radiographic imaging in 12.6% (n = 4309) of all patients evaluated in the study.[150]

Concomitant Cervical Spine and Life-Threatening Injuries

As stated throughout this chapter, the imaging evaluation of the spine must be performed in the context of the trauma patient's overall management. Radiographic examination of patients with concomitant acute spinal injury and life- threatening injuries should consist of only AP and horizontal beam lateral projections obtained in the emergency center during the clinical evaluation. If a radiologic diagnosis can be made from this limited study (e.g., traumatic spondylolisthesis, bilateral facet dislocation, burst fracture), management of the injury consistent with the patient's clinical condition can be initiated. If results of the initial limited examination are equivocal or if the spinal injury is one that requires additional evaluation by CT or MRI, the spine must be immobilized appropriately until the life-threatening injury has been stabilized and the radiologic evaluation can continue.

SPECIFIC INJURY PATTERNS OF THE CERVICAL SPINE
Atlantooccipital Dissociation

Atlantooccipital dissociation (AOD) is an uncommon injury to encounter in the clinical setting but may be responsible for at least 6% to 8% of deaths related to motor vehicular trauma in adults and a higher percentage, 17.5%, in children.[153-155] Most fatal AOD is due to posterior cranial distraction, believed related to severe hyperextension and lateral bending.[156] AOD has been described in three forms, including anterior and superior displacement of the cranium relative to C1, the most common pattern, pure superior displacement (distraction) of the cranium and, rarely, posterior and superior displacement, the least common and mostly likely fatal (Figs. 4-51 to 4-53). Although these injuries have shown an increased likelihood of survivability in recent years given improved emergency medical services, injury recognition, and management, these patients are prone to a variety of neurologic injuries. Patients may have brainstem deficits, including asymmetric paralysis or paresis, respiratory depression or arrest, labile blood pressure, cardiac rhythm instability, lower cranial nerve deficits, and variable sensory disturbances.[156,157] Children are at relatively increased risk for this injury due to their relatively large head size, shallow C1-2 articulations, and ligament laxity.[155]

The diagnosis may be suspected clinically, but neurologic findings often are attributed to brain injury. The screening lateral cervical spine radiograph is the test most likely to reveal the injury in the primary imaging survey.

A wide variety of measurements have been used to attempt to define an abnormal atlantooccipital relationship. The Power ratio and Lee x-line require identification of the basion and opisthion that are often obscure on the lateral cervical radiograph.[14-16,153,158] The Kaufman method measures the width of the C1 occipital articulation which normally should be less than 5 mm, but this method is compromised by head rotation or tilt. More recently, Harris et al.[14,15] have proposed two measurements that appear to have both high sensitivity and specificity for the diagnosis of AOD and are based on readily identified landmarks. By this method, the basion-dental measurement (see Fig. 4-11) should not exceed 12 mm in the adult, and a line drawn along the margin of the posterior axis (posterior axial line) extended cephalad to the basion should not be further than 12 mm distant (see Figs. 4-11, 4-51, and 4-52). Three other anatomic relationships are noteworthy. A line drawn along the clivus should intercept the top, typically posterior, one half of the odontoid process; a curved line extending through the C1 spinolaminar line should intersect the opisthion; and there should be no visible space between the condyle and condylar fossa of C1 (see Fig. 4-10).[159] One or more of these relationships can be assessed quickly to indicate possible AOD (Fig. 4-54; see Figs. 4-51 to 4-53). In very subtle cases in which there is minimal displacement (subluxation) of the occipital condyles, prevertebral soft tissue swelling extending from the skull base inferiorly may be a suggestive sign. Thin collimation CT with multiplanar reformation (MPR) can demonstrate beautifully even subtle AOD, as well as any associated fractures (see Figs. 4-51, 4-52, and 4-54). MRI can show the extent of damage to ligaments between C1 and the occiput, as well as the transverse atlantal ligament, using axial images (see Figs. 4-21 and 4-53). MRI can further depict EDH, cord compression, and direct cord or brainstem injury, and widening of the atlantooccipital articulations (Fig. 4-55; see Figs. 4-51 to 4-53).

Importantly, the distraction forces responsible for AOD can also produce simultaneous atlantoaxial displacement or distraction, as well as potential distraction injury, at lower cervical levels. This information is vital for planning the appropriate levels for internal fixation, required management for AOD. Other fractures and ligament injuries, particularly involving the atlas and axis, should be sought in association with atlantooccipital distraction (see Figs. 4-54 and 4-55).

Occipital Condyle Fractures

Occipital condyle fractures (OCF) can result from a variety of forces applied to the craniocervical junction. The injury was first reported in 1817 by Sir Charles Bell based on autopsy findings, described radiographically in 1962, and by CT in 1983.[160] Since the introduction of CT imag-

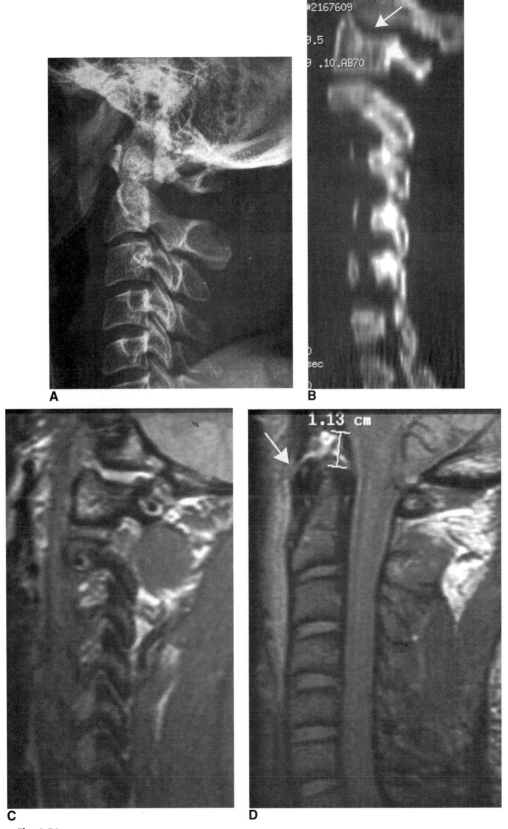

Fig. 4-51
Subtle atlantooccipital dissociation. **A**, Lateral cervical spine radiograph shows prevertebral soft tissue edema extending from the skull base to the midcervical level, but no definite injury. **B**, A parasagittal multiplanar reformation shows slight widening of one atlantooccipital joint (*white arrow*). **C**, Parasagittal T2-weighted MR image also shows widening of the joint space with increased joint fluid. **D**, A midsagittal proton-density MR image shows a top normal distance from the tip of the clivus to the top of the dens, prevertebral edema, and a possible tear in the anterior occipital membrane (*arrow*).

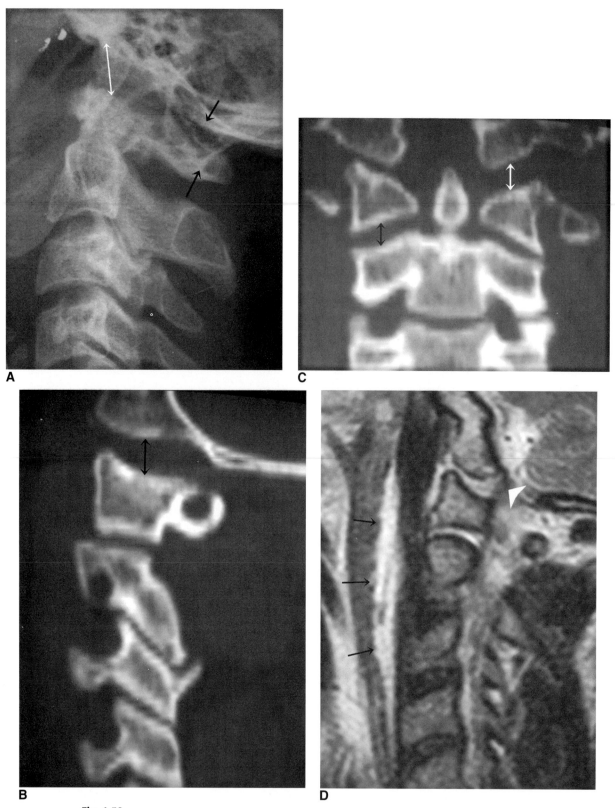

Fig. 4-52

Atlantooccipital dissociation. **A,** Lateral cervical radiograph in trauma patient illustrates increased distance between the tip of the clivus and the top of the dens (*two-headed white arrow*). There is offset between the C1 spinolaminar line and the opisthion (*black arrows*). Slight separation between the inferior occipital condyles and the top of the atlas is suggested. **B,** Parasagittal multiplanar reformation image demonstrates a widened atlantooccipital articular joint (*two-headed arrow*). **C,** A coronal multiplanar reformation shows a widened left atlantooccipital joint (*two-headed white arrow*) but also a widened right atlantoaxial joint, indicating at least two-level involvement (*two-headed black arrow*). **D,** Parasagittal T2-weighted MRI confirms a widened atlantooccipital joint (*arrowhead*), suggests a wide atlantoaxial joint below, and shows prevertebral edema (*arrows*).

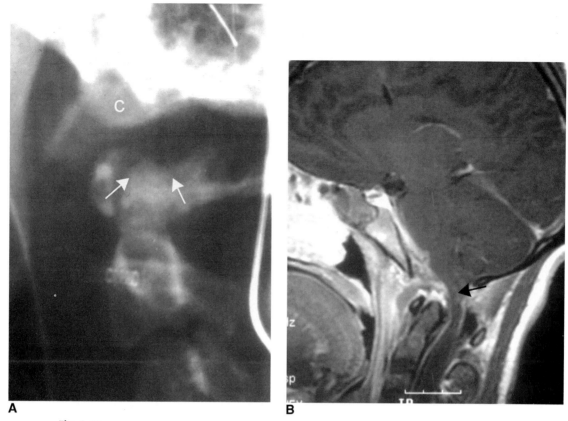

Fig. 4-53
Atlantooccipital dissociation. **A**, Lateral cervical spine radiograph shows marked anterior distraction of the occipital condyles (C) in relation to the C1 condylar fossae (arrows). **B**, Midsagittal MRI shows interruption of all ligaments between the skull base and the axis and atlas, with marked anterior occipital distraction and displacement. The spinal canal is compromised at C1 and the lower brainstem, and a medullary contusion is observed (arrow).

ing, numerous small series and case reports have appeared describing the mechanisms, clinical manifestations, and imaging features of OCF.[51,160-168]

CT has revealed that OCF is more common than was suspected before the CT era. Clinical reports indicate that OCF may occur in 16% to 19% of trauma victims sustaining high-energy injury to the craniocervical junction.[161,162] However, two postmortem radiologic studies demonstrated the injury in only 2 patients of 186 with head and neck injury sustained in traffic accidents[169] and 2 of 26 patients with cervical spine injury.[170] Thus, the precise incidence is unclear and based on the population studied and the study methods used.

The major importance of an OCF is the close proximity of the occipital condyles to the brainstem, lower cranial nerve exiting foramen, and vertebral arteries, any of which may be involved in OCF, particularly when associated with fracture fragment displacement or instability at the craniocervical junction.[160]

The classification mechanism most commonly used for OCF is the Anderson-Montesano system.[171] Using this system, the type I injury is a loading fracture of the occipital condyle (Jefferson-type), in which the condyle typically is fractured in a vertical sagittal plane(s) but there is no fracture displacement or associated craniocervical instability (Figs. 4-56 and 4-57). Craniocervical stability is based primarily on the integrity of the alar ligaments and the tectorial membrane. The type II injury is a skull-base fracture that propagates into one or both occipital condyles. The injury results from direct skull-base trauma and is usually stable at the craniocervical junction. Type III injuries result in an inferomedial avulsion fracture of

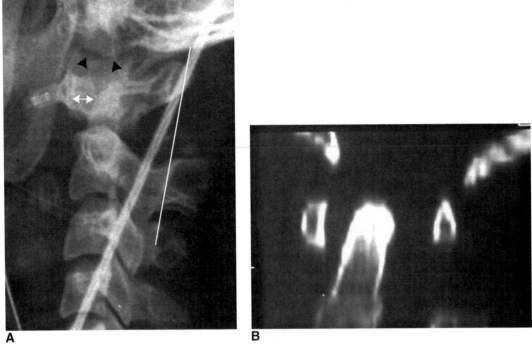

Fig. 4-54
Atlantooccipital dissociation with additional injury. **A**, The admission lateral view of this blunt trauma patient shows a widened anterior atlantodental space (*two-headed arrow*), anterior offset of the C1 spinolaminar line, and a widened atlantooccipital joint space (*arrowheads*). These findings indicate two contiguous levels of injury, not uncommon in atlantooccipital distracting injuries. **B**, A midsagittal CT multiplanar reformation confirms the occipital-atlas-axis relationship.

the condyle, with medial displacement of the fragment into the foramen magnum. There is usually associated strain or tearing of the contralateral alar ligament and possible avulsion of the inferior tip of the clivus (Fig. 4-58). The type III injury is believed secondary to combined rotation and lateral bending forces and is considered unstable.[160]

Tuli et al.[172] proposed another classification system. The type I injury is a stable, nondisplaced OCF, the type IIA injury is mechanically stable with displacement of the OCF, and type IIB has a displaced OCF associated with ligamentous instability. The author favors the latter system as being more general and directly related to the occipital condyles, craniocervical junction stability, and management planning.

In many cases, the clinical diagnosis of OCF is not established, particularly in unresponsive or unreliable patients. Potential clinical findings include persistent upper cervical pain despite an absence of a radiologic abnormality, spasmatic torticollis, limitation of skull mobility, dysphagia, and lower cranial nerve deficits. In severe cases, brainstem injury may occur, or there may be

injury to the vertebral arteries and resulting posterior fossa ischemia.[51,160,163] Cranial nerve deficits are often delayed, perhaps weeks to months in onset.[166,172] Involvement of cranial nerves 9 through 12 is referred to as *Collet-Sicard syndrome*.[160]

The radiologic diagnosis of OCF is all but impossible, due to overlapping of the bony structures of the face, upper cervical spine, and skull base.[160,167,172] Prevertebral soft tissue swelling at the craniocervical junction may be a secondary finding but is nonspecific. Other injuries that may be more apparent radiologically such as odontoid fractures, Jefferson fracture of the atlas, or atlantooccipital distraction injuries should also raise concern regarding the occipital condyles, because these injuries often are associated. Axial CT supplemented by MPR in the sagittal and coronal plane is extremely accurate for demonstrating this injury (see Fig. 4-27), as well as accompanying fractures. MRI is an excellent adjunctive study to assess the major ligaments and other soft tissues of the craniocervical junction, spinal cord, and adjacent vascular structures using both MRI and MRA.[173]

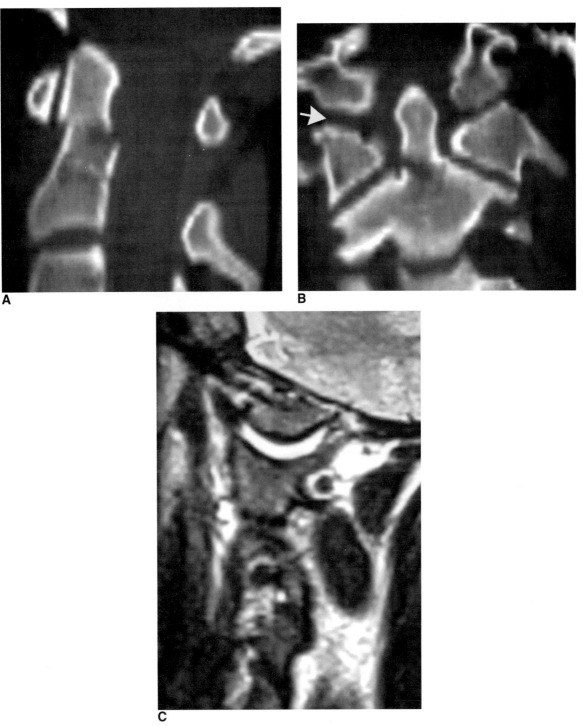

Fig. 4-55
Odontoid fracture with atlantooccipital distraction. **A**, Sagittal CT multiplanar reformation shows a type II odontoid fracture. **B**, The coronal CT multiplanar reformation also shows the fracture at the odontoid base but also indicates widening of the right atlantooccipital articulation (*arrow*). **C**, A T2-weighted parasagittal MR image confirms the distraction injury.

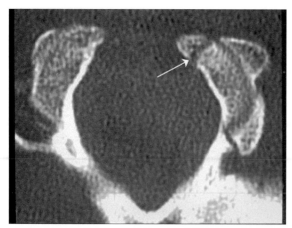

Fig. 4-56
Type I occipital condyle fracture. Axial CT shows a fracture (*arrow*), with minimal displacement from the medial left occipital condyle.

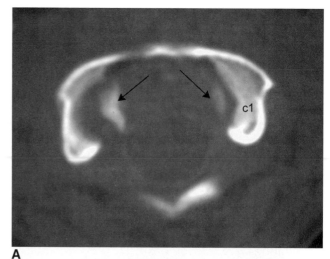

A

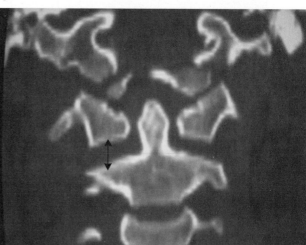

B

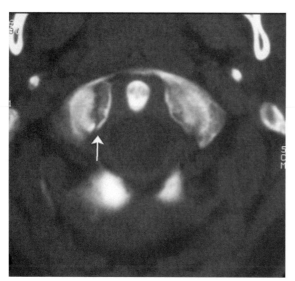

Fig. 4-57
Type I occipital condyle fracture. Axial CT of a different patient shows a similar minimally displaced fracture (*arrow*) of the right occipital condyle.

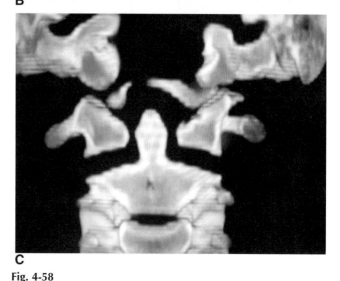

C

Because the clinical and radiographic diagnosis is so difficult, the injury should be excluded in any patient sustaining high-energy injury to the head and neck region.[160,164,165] For this reason, several authors recommend inclusion of C1 and perhaps C2 in standard brain imaging for trauma. Leone et al.[160] recommend 5-mm axial images to include the craniocervical junction and, if warranted, direct evaluation of the craniocervical junction alone, using 1- to 2-mm collimation and 1-mm table incrementation.[160]

In general, OCF without instability as indicated by CT and MRI studies is managed by rigid or semirigid external stabilization. OCF associated with instability requires either traction reduction with traction-halo stabilization

Fig. 4-58
Type III occipital condyle fracture. **A,** An axial CT image demonstrates medial dislocation of the occipital condyles (*arrows*) relative to the atlas. The condyles appear incomplete. **B,** This coronal CT multiplanar reformation shows avulsion of portions of both condyles which fuse posteriorly. Note the distraction between C1-2 (*arrow*), indicating the injury is "distributed" over at least two levels. **C,** A volume-rendered 3D image confirms the multiplanar reformation appearance.

or surgical internal fixation using occipital-atlantal-axial posterior fusion.[160]

The reader is referred to the excellent review of this injury written by Leone et al.[160] for further details of the epidemiology of OCF and anatomic details of the ligaments supporting the craniocervical region.

Axial Compression

Axial compression gives rise to crush or burst fractures in the lower cervical spine (see Fig. 4-31), Jefferson's fracture of the ring of C1 (Fig. 4-59; see Figs. 4-18 and 4-30), OCF (see Figs. 4-27, 4-56, and 4-57), and lateral loading fractures of the vertebral bodies (see Figs. 4-20 and 4-21) and articular pillars. The importance of burst fractures lies in the resulting displacement of the fracture fragments and their relationship to the spinal cord. Displacement of bone fragments into the spinal canal leads to impingement upon the cord (see Figs. 4-29 and 4-40), with a variable neurologic deficit. Although posteriorly displaced (retropulsed) fragments may be seen on high-quality lateral radiographs, CT is the method of choice for evaluating the exact location of fragments and degree of overall spinal canal compromise. MRI is used for its ability to define spinal ligament integrity, epidural mass effects, and spinal cord injury.

In the author's experience, axial compression or "bursting fractures" of the subaxial cervical spine are very uncommon. These injuries appear very similar to those in the lumbar spine, with loss of vertebral body height anteriorly and posteriorly, retropulsion of posterior cortical fragments, and fractures of the posterior elements (see Fig. 4-31). Most patients sustaining this fracture pattern show major neurologic deficits as a result of direct cord compression. Even if the spinal canal appears of normal dimension at the fracture site, the transient occlusion occurring at the time of loading produces far greater canal occlusion than that measured after injury.[174]

The classic Jefferson fracture, described in a 1920 article by Sir Geoffrey Jefferson, is a four-part injury with fractures occurring at the junctions of the anterior and posterior arches with the lateral masses, the weakest structural portion of the atlas.[27] By its nature, this is a decompressive injury, because the bony fragments are displaced radially away from the neural structures. As an isolated injury, the classic Jefferson pattern is both mechanically and neurologically stable. The diagnosis most often is made on the OMO radiograph, which shows bilateral offset of the lateral masses of the atlas relative to the lateral C2 vertebral body (see Figs. 4-18 and 4-59). On the lateral radiographic view, the diagnosis can be quite difficult. A fracture of the posterior arch that is displaced may be apparent but represents only a part of the total injury (Fig. 4-60). Depending upon stability of the atlantoaxial articulation, the C1 spinolaminar line

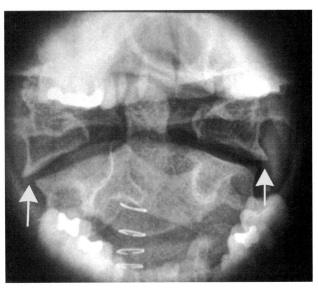

Fig. 4-59
Jefferson fracture. Open-mouth view shows lateral displacement of the lateral masses of the atlas relative to the lateral margins of the axis (*arrows*).

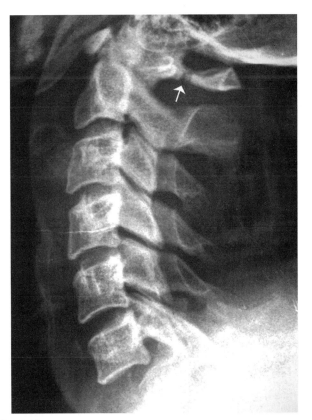

Fig. 4-60
Jefferson fracture. A lateral cervical radiograph shows a fracture of the C1 posterior arch (*arrow*) representing a part of a Jefferson fracture. There is marked prevertebral edema. Also, there is a bilateral facet dislocation at C6-7.

may also be displaced either anteriorly or posteriorly. The retropharyngeal soft tissue may be abnormal in both contour and thickness, suggesting the diagnosis.[175] Often the OMO view is difficult to obtain or of limited quality in the acute trauma setting. For this reason, the Jefferson fracture can be overlooked easily, particularly in the unresponsive patient. CT very accurately identifies the injury and establishes the exact sites of fracture, fracture displacement, and associated injuries. In most cases, a stable Jefferson injury can be managed successfully with external rigid collar stabilization, with a high likelihood of healing without long-term complications.[176,177]

Although the typical Jefferson fracture behaves in a stable fashion, variant injury patterns can be or are mechanically unstable, putting the patient at risk for neurologic injury. Lee and Woodring[27] described a group of patients with axial loading injuries, with less than four-part fractures and fractures through the ring in atypical locations. Two anterior ring fractures or disruption of the posterior longitudinal ligament, or both, could permit C1-2 subluxation (Fig. 4-61; see Fig. 4-21). If there is separation between the fracture fragments of the atlas by more than 6 to 7 mm, the injury is considered unstable, because this separation implies disruption of the transverse atlantal ligament.[100,178] The fragment separation can be ascertained from the OMO view by adding the amount of lateral displacement of each C1 lateral mass or by direct measurement on CT. In all Jefferson injuries, it is important to assess carefully the atlantodental space to be sure that it does not exceed 3 mm in the adult patient. A greater distance would imply transverse ligament tearing. CT can show direct injury to the transverse ligament by indicating avulsion of the C1 tubercle where the ligament inserts (Fig. 4-62). For unstable Jefferson-type injuries, reduction of the displaced fragments in traction and internal fixation with C1-2 articular screws typically is performed.[179] It is also important to recognize that the Jefferson fracture is associated not uncommonly with concurrent injuries of the upper cervical spine, particularly the high and low odontoid and hangman's fracture patterns. The association of these additional injuries effects both frequency and severity of neurologic injury and management. The Jefferson fracture rarely is associated with vertebral artery injury.[180]

Pitfalls in the diagnosis of the Jefferson fracture include clefts and aplasias in the atlas ring that simulate fractures on both radiographs and CT, but they typically are differentiated by smooth, well-defined corticate bone margins (Fig. 4-63). Gehweiler et al.[181] described two patients with posterior midline clefts (rachischisis) with 1 mm of bilateral atlantoaxial offset that could further suggest the diagnosis. In addition, in young children the atlas may normally overlap the axis laterally due to differential growth rates. A specific measured index described by Suss et al.[182] can be used to differentiate this

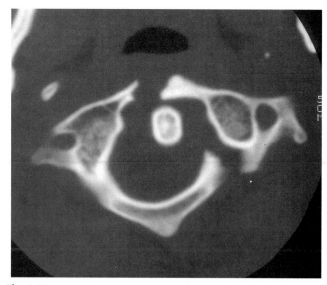

Fig. 4-61
Atypical Jefferson fracture. Axial CT shows a fracture of the midline anterior arch and left lateral atlas ring. This atypical two-part pattern often is associated with a transverse atlantal ligament tear and instability. (From Mirvis SE, Harris JH Jr: Spinal imaging. In Browner BD, Jupiter JB, Levine AM, Trafton PG, eds: *Skeletal trauma*, ed 2, vol 1, Philadelphia, 1998, WB Saunders.)

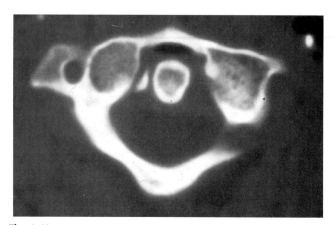

Fig. 4-62
Transverse atlantal ligament tear. Axial CT image through the atlas shows an avulsion fracture from the right lateral mass. The anterior atlantodental space is widened and there is gas in the joint space, indicating loss of transverse ligament integrity.

normal lateral spread from the Jefferson injury. Overall, the Jefferson fracture rarely is seen in children.[183]

Atlantoaxial Dissociation

Atlantoaxial subluxation and dislocation are uncommon injuries. The C1 ring can be displaced in several patterns, including bilateral anterior or posterior translation and rotation about the odontoid peg, producing either subluxation or dislocation of one or both C1 articular masses but in opposite directions[184] (Fig. 4-64). Rotation also can occur centered at one articular mass, leading to

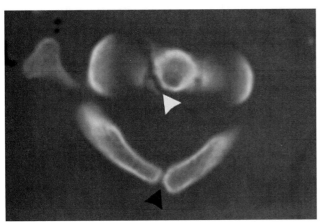

Fig. 4-63
Partial nonossifications of C1. Axial CT image shows smooth margins of partially nonossified posterior atlas ring (*black arrowhead*). There is a fracture at the base of the dens noted (*white arrowhead*). Midline clefts in the atlas ring often are mistaken for fractures by inexperienced observers.

unilateral anterior or posterior subluxation or dislocation of the contralateral side[184] (Fig. 4-65). Each of these patterns falls under the catch-all term of *atlantoaxial dissociation*. All of these injuries can be associated with concurrent fractures, transverse atlantal ligament injury, neurologic deficits, or vertebral artery injury that will, in part, determine the method of stabilization and need for internal fixation.

The radiographic diagnosis of atlantoaxial dissociation may be difficult, particularly in the rotational forms. Rotational injury may be suggested from the OMO view due to asymmetry of the C1 lateral masses, C1-2 joint height discrepancy, and asymmetry of the distance between the odontoid and atlas lateral masses. The LADS is usually symmetric on a normally positioned OMO view (see Fig. 4-17), but 2 to 5 mm of asymmetry can exist, mainly due to congenital variations of odontoid and lateral mass shape.[185,186] Any LADS asymmetry must be correlated with other findings that suggest injury. Head rotation alters the shape of the lateral masses of the atlas, the LADS, and the C1-2 joint width. As the head is turned to the right, the left C1 lateral mass appears to increase in width, the LADS decreases, and the joint space appears to widen, while the right lateral mass appears truncated, the right LADS increases, and the joint space appears to narrow (Fig. 4-66). On the lateral cervical radiograph, rotation causes loss of the normal hemispheric shape of the anterior C1 arch, indistinctness of the anterior atlantodental space, and C1 tilting into an oval configuration with loss of superimposition of the articular masses (Fig. 4-67). The mandible appears superimposed over the upper cervical spine, even in a true lateral projection. On the AP view, the chin is both rotated and tilted (see Fig. 4-67). These changes are similar to those seen with physiologic head rotation but become more exaggerated with rotatory subluxation or dislocation.

Atlantoaxial rotational injury must be distinguished from torticollis. Torticollis can be associated with minor

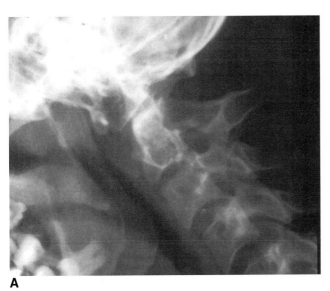

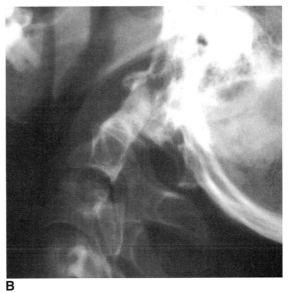

A   **B**

Fig. 4-64
Atlantoaxial dissociation. **A,** Patient with upper cervical pain shows marked anterior displacement of the atlas, with flexion suggesting injury to both the primary check ligament (transverse atlantal ligament) and accessory ligaments (alar and apical-dental) allowing this degree of anterior translation of the atlas. **B,** In extension, the displacement is reduced completely and would not be suspected in this position.

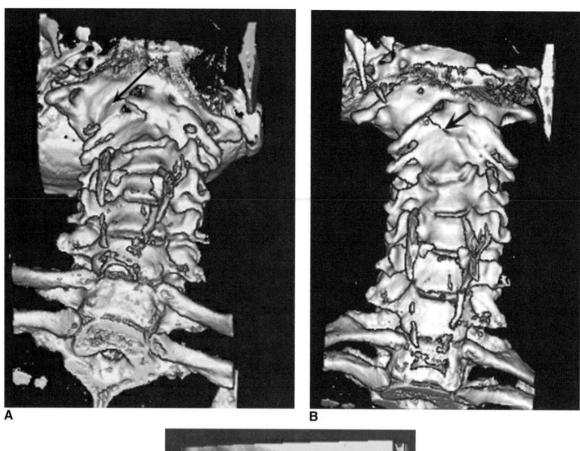

A

B

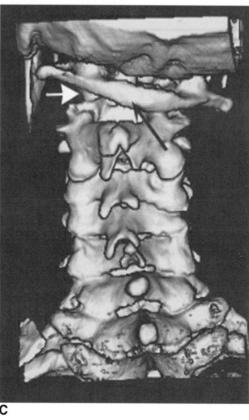

C

Fig. 4-65

Atlantoaxial rotatory subluxation. **A**, 3D surface-rendered view from anteroinferior perspective shows the undersurface of the anteriorly offset right lateral mass of C1 (*arrow*). The left lateral mass appears to move posteriorly. **B**, The rotational subluxation is shown from the anterior perspective. In addition, there is an oblique fracture in the C2 body (*arrow*). **C**, The posterior perspective nicely shows the rotation and exaggerated tilt of the atlas (*black arrow*) related to hyperrotation. The posteriorly displaced left C1 lateral mass is observed, also (*white arrow*).

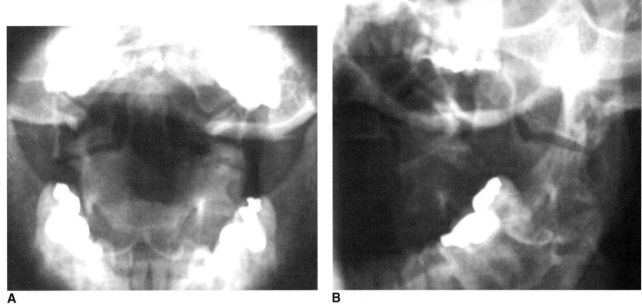

Fig. 4-66
Change in lateral mass appearance with normal rotation (open-mouth odontoid view). **A,** Normal open-mouth view shows symmetry in size and shape of the lateral masses of the atlas and symmetry of the atlantoaxial joint spaces and lateral atlantodental space. **B,** Upon rotation of the head to the right, the left lateral mass moves anteriorly and appears larger, closer to the odontoid, and the left articular space appears to narrow. The opposite changes occur on the right.

trauma, muscle spasm, upper respiratory tract infection or related inflammatory conditions, is termed *atlantoaxial rotatory displacement*, and occurs mainly in children to young adolescents.[187] The head rotation is physiologic and symmetric, with anterior movement of one lateral mass associated with equivalent posterior movement of the contralateral articular mass. Torticollis is usually self-limited, but displacement that fails to resolve even after abatement of symptoms is termed *atlantoaxial rotatory fixation*.[188]

A major traumatic force can cause nonphysiologic rotation of the C1 lateral masses in relation to the C2 articular pillars, with disruption of the articular capsules and, potentially, other adjacent major support ligaments.

The patient may be unable to rotate the head due to a "locked" dislocation, with a C1 lateral mass completely displaced anterior to the subjacent C2 articular mass (see Fig. 4-67) or simply from severe cervical pain. CT using thin 1- to 2-mm slice thickness with MPR is ideal for establishing the diagnosis of C1-2 dissociation. This study will show the relationship of the C1-2 joints and any associated fractures. On occasion, CT with 3D rendering may be useful for confirming or better illustrating the diagnosis (Fig. 4-68; see Fig. 4-65). In cases of suspected rotatory subluxation, "dynamic" axial CT imaging can be performed, with the patient scanned with the head in a neutral position and maximally rotated in each direction. This study may show evidence of injury by revealing asymmetric movement of the C1 lateral masses or shifting position of the odontoid process in relation to the lateral masses[186] (Fig. 4-69).

Widening of the anterior atlantodental space should be sought as a clue to concurrent transverse ligament injury.[184] In subluxation and dislocation, the amount of maximal rotation of C1 relative to C2 typically exceeds the normal maximal 45 degrees[189] and may approach 90 degrees in dislocation. MRI can assess the integrity of the C1-2 and alar ligaments,[190] as well as reveal evidence of cord injury, assess the size of the cervical spinal canal at the injured level, and detect sources of spinal canal impingement such as EDH. Findings from MRI may help determine the need for or type of surgical fixation required. Patients sustaining AOD injuries may have concurrent atlantoaxial dissociation, and this additional injury should be sought to plan appropriate surgical fixation (Fig. 4-70; see Figs. 4-55 and 4-58).

Another injury that may occur as a result of atlantoaxial dissociation involves the vertebral artery, which can undergo severe torsion or stretching along its course between C1 and C2. Although patients with vertebral artery injury often remain asymptomatic, particularly if the vessel is occluded, distal embolization with posterior

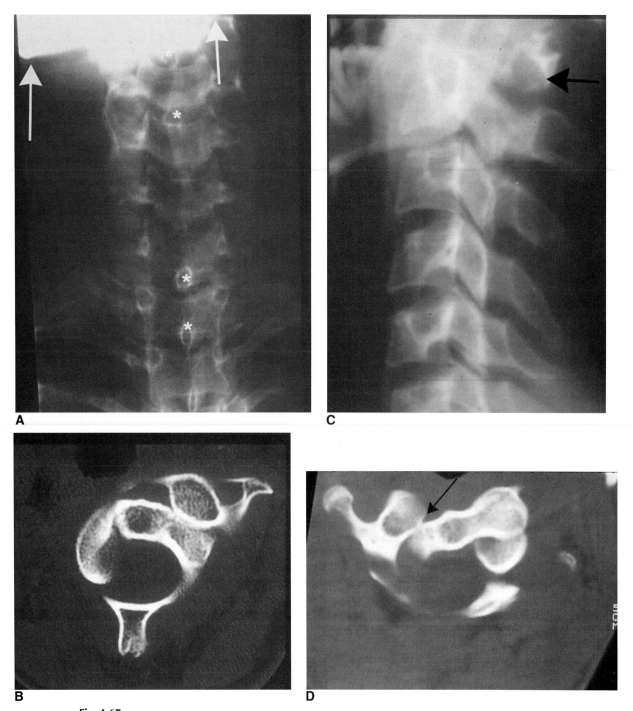

Fig. 4-67
Rotation dislocation of C1 on C2. **A,** Anteroposterior view of trauma patient shows tilting and rotation of the chin (*arrows*) and gradual deviation of the spinous processes to the right with rostral progression (*asterisks*). **B,** Axial CT shows left articular mass of the atlas locked anterior to the C2 lateral body. **C,** Lateral radiograph of a different patient with atlantoaxial rotational dislocation shows the mandible superimposed over the cervical spine. The atlas has an oval configuration due to tilt and rotation (*arrow*). **D,** Axial CT shows the right C1 lateral mass is locked in front of the C2 lateral body (*arrow*). The opposite joint is subluxed.

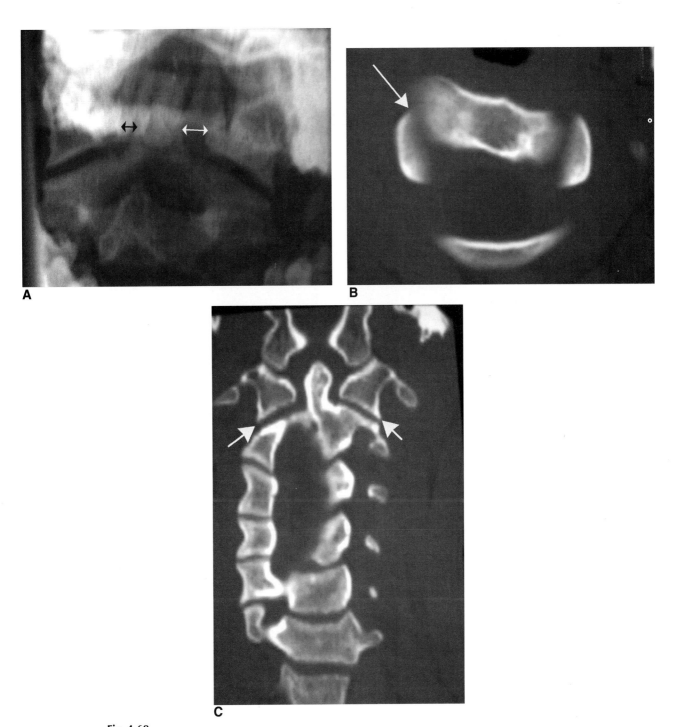

Fig. 4-68
Atlantoaxial rotatory subluxation. **A,** Open-mouth odontoid view of blunt trauma patient with neck pain shows asymmetry of the lateral atlantodental space indicating rotation (*two-headed arrows*). **B,** Axial CT image through the C1-2 level shows asymmetric offset of the right joint (*arrow*). **C,** Coronal multiplanar reformation shows acute alteration of rotation between C1 level and above and C2 level and below, indicating abrupt rotation. Note difference in the atlantoaxial joint spaces (*arrows*) from rotational malalignment.

Continued

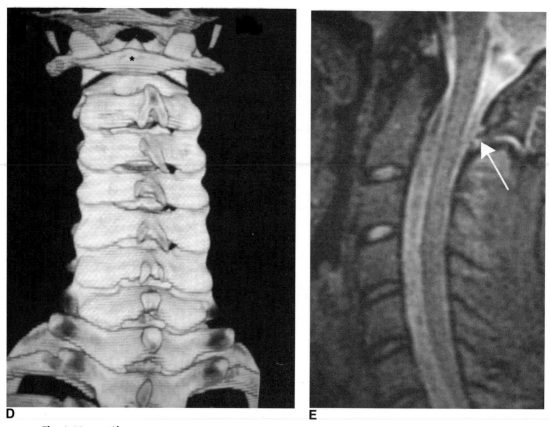

Fig. 4-68, cont'd
D, Posterior view of 3D volume rendering shows abrupt offset of posterior C1 tubercle (*asterisk*) and spinous processes below. **E**, T2-weighted sagittal MR image shows disruption of posterior ligaments (*arrow*) as a result of rotational stress at the atlantoaxial joint.

fossa infarction may occur if the vessel is injured but remains patent.[184] For this reason, screening of all patients with atlantoaxial dissociation for evidence of vertebral artery trauma is advised using MRA, if available, or direct angiography.

Odontoid Fractures

Fractures of the odontoid process arise as a result of diverse mechanisms. Fractures of the axis represent 15% to 20% of all cervical fractures and most of these (57%) involve the dens.[191-193] The classification of odontoid fractures most commonly used is by Anderson and D'Alonzo[194] and describes three types of fractures. The type I injury is an oblique fracture from the tip of the odontoid process and is an extremely uncommon injury (<1% of odontoid fractures), most likely related to a distracting force with avulsion of the odontoid fragment by a portion of the alar ligament.[195] This injury may indicate atlantooccipital dislocation and should be regarded as a sign of instability.[195] The type II injury (also referred to as a *high odontoid fracture*) is a horizontal fracture that crosses the tapered base of the dens and is the most common injury occurring in 60% of odontoid fractures[191]

(Figs. 4-71 to 4-73). The type III pattern (also referred to as *low odontoid fracture*) is typically an oblique fracture, which starts at the base of the odontoid process and extends into the body of C2 as single or multiple fractures, representing about 40% of odontoid fractures[191] (Figs. 4-74 to 4-76).

Another classification of odontoid fractures by Althoff et al. includes an "A" pattern equivalent to the classic type II, a "B" pattern that crosses the superior portion of the axis above the facet plane, a "C" pattern that equals the classic type III and extends into one superior facet, and a "D" pattern that extends into both superior facets.[191] Because the B through D patterns behave like the classic type III (low) odontoid fracture, the high and low designations are adequate. The author has noted that the Althoff "B" pattern is a very common form of low odontoid fracture and may be mistaken for a type II injury (Fig. 4-77).

It is important to recognize that odontoid fractures can be associated with a variety of other fractures as was seen in 117 (34%) of 340 patients with odontoid fractures reviewed by Greene et al.[191] Commonly associated injuries occur at the craniocervical junction and include anterior and posterior atlas ring fractures, Jefferson

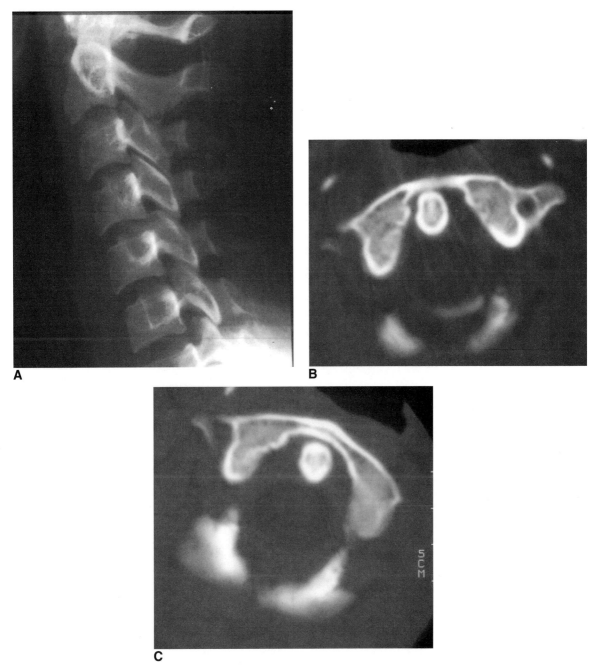

Fig. 4-69
Rotatory subluxation of C1-2. **A**, Neutral lateral view of trauma patient with upper cervical pain is normal. **B**, Rotation of the head to the right shows offset of the odontoid process toward the right. **C**, Rotation of the head to the left shows restoration of central position of the odontoid between the C1 lateral masses.

fracture, atlantoaxial dislocation, and atlantooccipital distraction injuries[196-200] (Fig. 4-78; see Fig. 4-39). These injuries must be specifically excluded whenever an odontoid fracture is diagnosed. Any injury in which the transverse atlantal ligament is potentially disrupted is critical to recognize, because this factor strongly influences management.[191]

Differentiation of the high from low odontoid fractures is of major significance, because it bears strongly on prognosis for healing and management. The high odontoid fracture tends to occur in older adults, usually from relatively minor trauma such as falls of limited height, and usually is displaced posteriorly on the lateral cervical radiograph.[191,201-203] Ryan and Taylor[202] described 35 patients over 60 years of age with odontoid fractures, of which 82% were classic type II injuries. A fall in the domestic setting was the cause of injury in 53% of cases, and the dens was displaced posteriorly in 88%.[202] There is a strong tendency for the type II fracture to heal without bony union, permitting delayed development of cervical myelopathy (Fig. 4-79).[197,202,204-206] A biomechanical study performed by Amling et al.[207] showed that the base of the odontoid was predisposed to fracture, because this portion contained 55% less trabecular bone than the axis body or odontoid process, had poorer trabecular connections, and had only one third the cortical thickness of the odontoid process. Cadaver specimens showed microcallus formation at the odontoid base, indicating microfractures from stress and relative bone insufficiency.[207] The pathophysiologic explanation for this high rate of nonunion of low odontoid fractures is not clear. Crockard et al.[206] indicate that the transverse ligament may be interposed between fracture margins. Microangiographic studies in dogs show that ischemic necrosis is not likely to be etiologic. What is clear is that advanced patient age, increased distance

between fracture fragments, degree of fracture angulation, and residual mobility at the fracture site all increase the chance for nonunion.[191,197,203] If fractures are displaced by more than 5 mm, a 75% nonunion rate results[197] and increases to 86% with more than 6 mm of displacement.[191]

The radiologic diagnosis of odontoid fractures usually is established using the lateral cervical and OMO radiograph. If there is significant fracture displacement, the diagnosis is straightforward; however, when minimally displaced these fractures can be extremely subtle and are often a source of missed diagnosis. A number of radiographic signs can be useful to detect the subtle injury. First, a careful inspection of the prevertebral soft tissues anterior to C1 and C2 may indicate bulging, straightening, or loss of the expected normal contour, suggesting hematoma or edema[10,208] (see Figs. 4-33, 4-71, and 4-75). Harris et al.[11] have described the *axis ring sign*. The axis ring is a composite shadow seen in the lateral view, composed of cortical bone of the axis that lies along the margins of the neurocentral synchondrosis (see Fig. 4-6). This cortical bone creates a somewhat elliptical or comet-

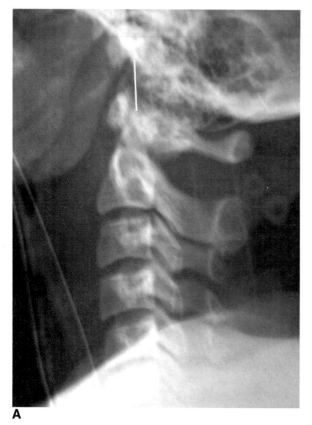

A

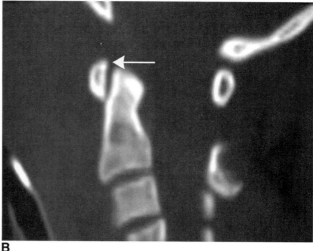

B

Fig. 4-70
Combined atlantooccipital and atlantoaxial distraction injury. **A,** Lateral radiograph of cervical spine shows increased separation between the basion and superior tip of the odontoid (*white line*) exceeding 12 mm. The anterior ring of the atlas also lies partially above the top of the odontoid process. **B,** Midsagittal CT multiplanar reformation shows the increased distance from the basion to the odontoid tip and the elevated position of the anterior atlas (*arrow*).

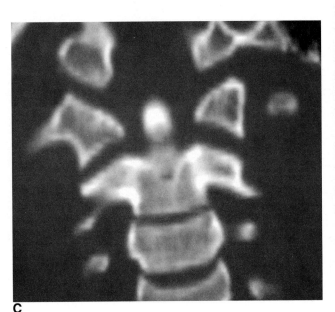

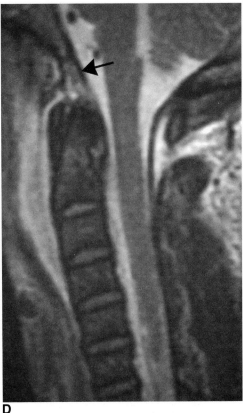

Fig. 4-70, cont'd
C, Coronal CT multiplanar reformation confirms widening of the atlantooccipital and atlantoaxial joint spaces. **D,** Midsagittal T2-weighted MRI shows upper cervical prevertebral edema and widened atlantooccipital distance. The bridging tectorial membrane appears stretched, but intact, at this point (*arrow*).

shaped density on the lateral view over the C2 body that is interrupted in its inferoposterior margin by the vertebral artery foramen (Fig. 4-80). Any other interruption of this composite shadow is indicative of a low odontoid or atypical hangman's fracture (see below) (see Figs. 4-8, 4-9, and 4-74 to 4-76), usually seen across the superior margin of the axis ring. Alternatively, areas of increased density may result if fractures of the axis overlap due to fracture displacement. If two parallel axis rings are seen, this indicates rotation of the axis from the lateral projection (Fig. 4-81). Another radiographic sign that may be seen with odontoid fracture is called the *tilted dens sign* (see Fig. 4-19). Normally a line bisecting the odontoid process vertically forms a right angle with a line drawn horizontally across the axis body at the level of its superior lateral margin. Thomeier et al.[209] showed that in uninjured patients this angle was always greater than or equal to 87 degrees, while in 8 of 12 patients with odontoid fractures the angle was less than or equal to 85 degrees. Seybold et al.[210] have described the posterior axial cortical margin sign. Normally, the odontoid process aligns with the posterior cortical margin of the axis body to within 3 mm. An anterior "step-off"

of the posterior cortex of the odontoid of 3 mm or more relative to the axis body posterior cortical margin suggests an odontoid fracture, usually type II (see Figs. 4-71 to 4-75 and 4-78). The step-off sign can be mimicked by C2 rotation and is not present with all odontoid fractures. Finally, careful review of the C1 spinolaminar line and its relationship to that of C2 often is useful to detect odontoid and hangman's injuries (see Figs. 4-8, 4-9, 4-71, 4-72, 4-74, and 4-75). In the author's experience, a line drawn along the C2 spinolaminar line should fall on or within 2 mm of the C1 spinolaminar line; a displacement greater than 2 mm suggests a possible anteriorly or posteriorly displaced odontoid fracture, with the C1 ring moving with the odontoid process. Hypoplasia or posterior aplasia of the C1 ring nullifies this sign. Concomitant fracture of the C1 body, as with traumatic spondylolisthesis, also abrogates the sign, because the C2 spinolaminar line is potentially out of anatomic position.

Often the OMO projection may be difficult to obtain in the acute trauma setting or is of poor quality. The necessity of having the OMO view to diagnose odontoid injury in the child has been questioned,[24,211,212] as long

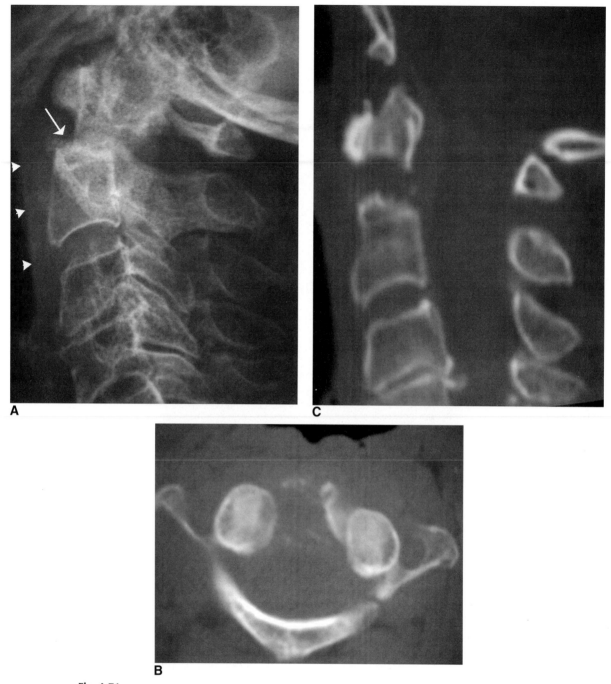

Fig. 4-71
High odontoid fracture. **A**, Lateral cervical radiograph shows interruption of the anterior cortical margin of the C2 (*arrow*) and posterior displacement of the dens relative to the C2 body. Note straightening of prevertebral soft tissue from edema or hemorrhage (*arrowheads*). **B**, Axial CT across the base of the dens shows absence of bone, indicating distraction at the fracture site. **C**, Distracted odontoid process is seen well on the midsagittal CT multiplanar reformation.

as the AP and lateral views are available. If the diagnosis is questioned in the adolescent or adult patient, thin-collimation CT with sagittal and coronal MPR is the next study of choice (see Figs. 4-73 and 4-77). Although flexion-extension views in the alert, oriented patient could be performed, there is some potential danger, because these are unstable injuries. If there is concern of either concurrent injury to the transverse ligament or other ligamentous injury to the craniocervical junction, then MRI is indicated as well. If, however, the diagnosis is clear on

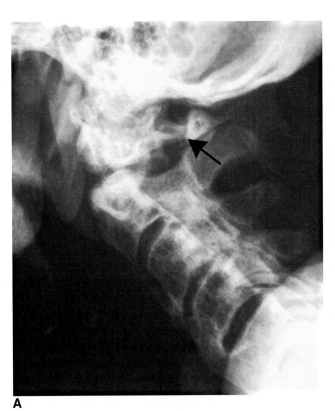

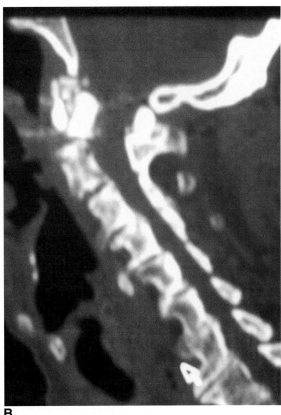

A

B

Fig. 4-72
High odontoid fracture. **A,** Lateral cervical radiograph shows posterior displacement of the odontoid process and posterior offset of the C1 spinolaminar line (*arrow*). **B,** Midline sagittal CT multiplanar reformation confirms fracture and posterior displacement of the dens.

radiography without suggestion of additional injury, then CT and MRI serve no purpose.

Other, less common injury patterns involving the odontoid process have been described. A vertical fracture can occur through the odontoid process, which some speculate occurs from extension and axial loading.[193,213] Another atypical odontoid fracture is produced by lateral bending force, creating an oblique fracture through the odontoid peg, associated with a fracture of a superior articular process on the side of lateral loading.[214-216] This pattern can produce angulation of the odontoid toward the side of injury, downward sloping of the involved articular mass, asymmetric atlantoaxial joints, and compression of the articular mass.[214-216] Hadley et al.[217] have described a comminuted fracture at the base of the dens, with free fragments, which requires surgical fixation. They have designated this as a type IIA pattern.

Several variants of anatomy can be mistaken for acute odontoid fractures. Incomplete ossification of the atlas can project lucent areas over the dens on the OMO view, simulating fractures.[218] Accessory ossicles may occur in

close relationship to the odontoid tip and could be mistaken for avulsion injuries if their smooth corticate contour is not appreciated.[219] The ununited dens fracture (Fig. 4-82; see Fig. 4-79) could be thought to represent an acute injury but usually shows marked sclerosis at the margins of the fracture and no evidence of prevertebral edema or abnormal marrow signal by MRI.[198] Holt et al.[220] have suggested that hypertrophy of the anterior C1 arch, related to chronic stress at a mobile articulation, is a useful sign that can accompany chronic conditions such as the os odontoideum (congenital nonfusion of the odontoid) from an acute injury.[220] It must be remembered that the os odontoideum or chronic posttraumatic nonunion can both be unstable and require internal fixation (Figs. 4-83 and 4-84).

The management of acute odontoid fractures depends on the injury type and any associated cervical injuries. Usually the type III pattern is managed with external alignment with halo or other rigid immobilization, with a high likelihood of success at over 90%.[191] The type II injury can be managed by external stabilization in a halo device if near-anatomic alignment at the fracture can be maintained. This approach is more likely to be successful in patients younger than 60 years old.[191,192,201,204,221-223] The type II injury can be managed by placement of an odontoid screw from an anterior approach that preserves

axial rotation. In older patients with the type II injury or patients with associated transverse ligament injury, posterior transarticular screw fixation usually is required. This fixation significantly limits axial rotation but is better tolerated than external halo stabilization in elderly

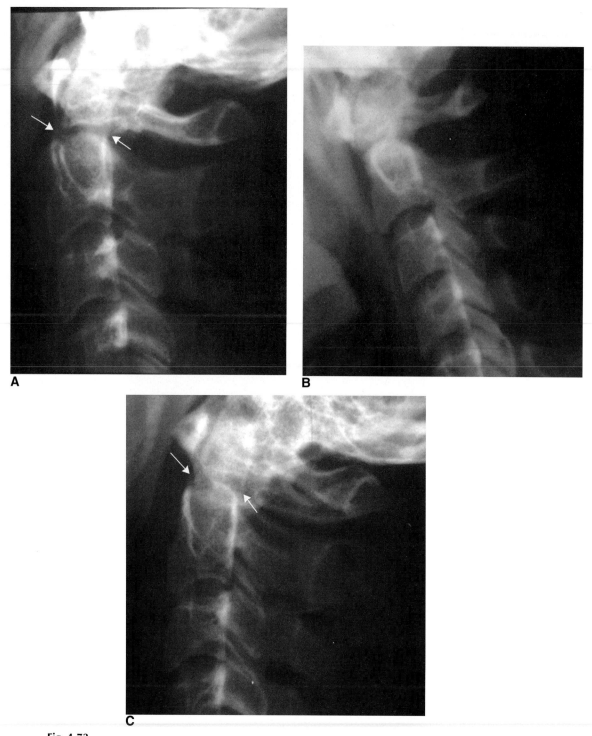

Fig. 4-73
High odontoid fracture—subtle. **A,** Lateral cervical radiograph of blunt trauma patient with neck pain shows subtle defects in the Harris ring (*arrows*). Flexion (**B**) and extension (**C**) views show movement of the dens and cortical defects (*arrows*).

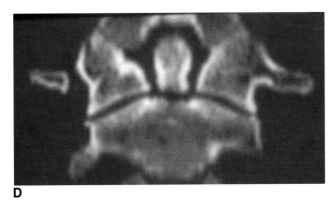

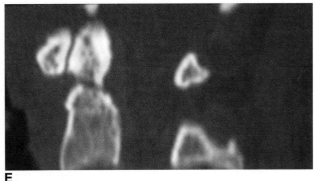

Fig. 4-73, cont'd
High-resolution (thin-section) CT multiplanar reformation in the coronal (**D**) and sagittal (**E**) planes clearly delineates fracture at the odontoid base. (From Mirvis SE, Harris JH Jr: Spinal imaging. In Browner BD, Jupiter JB, Levine AM, Trafton PG, eds: *Skeletal trauma*, ed 2, vol 1, Philadelphia, 1998, WB Saunders.)

individuals.[191,192,201,204,221-223] It is important to recognize the entire spectrum of craniocervical injuries which may be associated with the odontoid fracture to select the optimal form of management.

Traumatic Spondylolisthesis of C2 (Hangman's Fracture)

Traumatic spondylolisthesis of C2 is commonly known as the *hangman's fracture*, because it bears some radiographic resemblance to that injury produced as a product of the hangman's art. Of course, it is not the hangman whose neck is broken, but the unfortunate fellow with the rope around his neck. If performed correctly, the knot under the chin,[224] with fall, will sever the victim's cervical spine through the pars interarticularis of C2 and tear the upper spinal cord and lower medulla oblongata as a result of cervical distraction combined with hyperflexion and rotation. Although the common name for this injury is perhaps unfortunate, it is so ingrained in the medical lexicon that it seems inappropriate not to maintain it, hopefully with the kind understanding of any residual "hangmen" still hanging about.

In actuality, the hangman's fracture is a group of injuries with variable mechanisms that have different radiographic appearances. The most common form of this injury results from extension combined with axial loading. Excessive hyperextension of the upper cervical spine often results from deceleration injuries, with the head striking the windshield of a car, producing posterior rotation of the skull, set against anterior movement of the cervical spine. This motion causes the occiput to be driven downward onto the upper cervical spine. The fracture which often results from the inferior displacement of the occiput occurs bilaterally through the pars interarticularis of C2 and may continue obliquely

through the axis body[225] (Fig. 4-85 to 4-88; see Figs. 4-8, 4-39, and 4-46). There is variable forward displacement of the cervicocranium with respect to the spine below C2. Spinal cord damage is uncommon despite often significant fracture displacement, due to the wide spinal canal at this level.[225-230] Prevertebral soft tissue swelling or hematoma related to the hyperextension mechanism may be apparent at C1 to C3 or beyond but is often absent.[8,9] The fracture usually is diagnosed readily on lateral radiographs in more then 90% of cases unless nondisplaced, in which thin-section CT may identify the injury.[100] Fractures which extend through the pars interarticularis only are considered typical, while those extending to involve the posterior cortex of the axis and, perhaps, foramen transversarium are called *atypical*, even though they are actually quite common (Figs. 4-89 to 4-91; see Fig. 4-8). CT usually provides no useful additional information as to the nature of the hangman's fracture[225] but can be valuable to exclude or verify fracture line extension into the vertebral foramina, which can damage the vertebral arteries,[231] or to detect subtle concurrent adjacent injuries. At the University of Maryland Shock Trauma Center, screening MRA is performed to assess the vertebral arteries for patients with transvertebral foraminal involvement.

Levine and Edwards,[230] modifying the work of Effendi et al.,[232] have divided hangman's fractures into four types. Type I injury results from hyperextension with axial loading, as described above. Radiographically, the fracture is confined to the posterior elements (pars or lamina), with no displacement or angulation of the C2 body and with preservation of a normal C2-3 disc space (Fig. 4-92; see Fig. 4-85). These injuries are often subtle and easily missed radiographically but, fortunately, are stable. Type II injuries, the most commonly

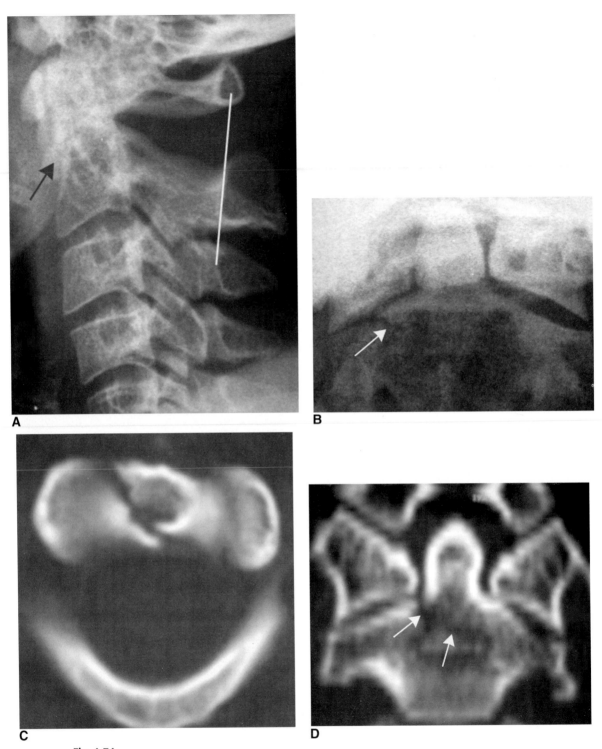

Fig. 4-74
Low odontoid fracture. **A,** Lateral cervical radiograph shows a subtle disruption in the anterior cortical line of C2 (*arrow*) and slight anterior tilt of the dens. The spinolaminar line of the atlas is anterior to its expected location (*white line*). **B,** Fracture extending into the C2 body is seen on the open-mouth radiograph (*arrow*). **C,** Fracture is seen well on the axial CT through the base of the dens. **D,** Extension of the fracture into the body is seen well on the coronal CT multiplanar reformation (*arrows*).

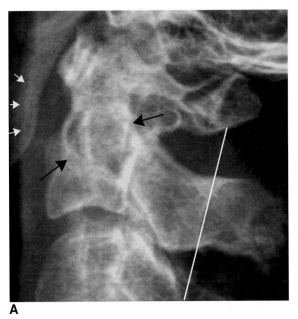

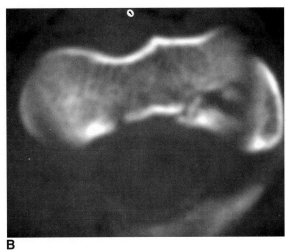

Fig. 4-75
Low odontoid fracture. **A,** Lateral cervical radiograph shows disruption of Harris ring (*black arrows*), with minimal anterior displacement of the dens. Note anterior displacement of the spinolaminar line of the atlas (*white line*) and minimal prevertebral edema anterior to C1-2 level. Also note soft tissue convex bulging anterior to C1-2 (*white arrows*). **B,** Axial CT image clearly shows fracture extending into the axis body.

seen,[227,229,231,233] are produced by combined hyperextension with axial loading and hyperflexion, resulting in disruption of the C2-3 disc, disc space widening, anterior angulation of C2 and, typically, a wide fracture separation (see Fig. 4-86). Type IIA injuries occur from flexion and distraction, leading to oblique fractures anterior to the articular facets with marked angulation of the axis body, disruption of the middle column ligaments, and hinging of the body from the anterior longitudinal ligament (see Fig. 4-87). Type III injuries result from hyperflexion and compression, producing anterior displacement of the axis facets in front of those of C3[226] (see Fig. 4-88). Mechanical instability and potential for neurologic injury increase with type IIA and type III hangman's fractures.[230] Type I injuries are considered stable and type II unstable, but both usually are managed successfully with external immobilization in collar or halo vest. Type IIA injuries require reduction by extension and gentle compression and halo-vest immobilization. Type III injuries are unstable and typically stabilized internally.[230] In fatal motor vehicle accidents, the appearance of high-grade hangman's-type fractures is exceeded in frequency only by atlantooccipital dislocations.[234]

As noted above, most hangman's fractures are diagnosed readily on the lateral cervical radiograph, but they can be overlooked easily if minimally displaced or nondisplaced. Clues to detection of these more subtle

fractures include use of the axis ring sign,[11] which will show posterior ring disruption from atypical fractures extending into the posterior C2 cortex (see Figs. 4-89 and 4-91). The axis body may appear widened in the AP dimension compared with that of C3 from an atypical fracture producing the "fat C2" sign[235] (see Fig. 4-89). Another clue useful when diagnosing a hangman's fracture is posterior displacement of the C2 spinolaminar line of more than 2 mm, compared with a line drawn between the spinolaminar line of C1 and C3 (Fig. 4-93; see Figs. 4-89 and 4-91). Of course, the suggestion or finding of prevertebral soft tissue contour abnormality or fullness in the upper cervical region also provides a clue indicating need for careful clinical or CT study of the region (see Figs. 4-85 and 4-91 to 4-93). Other fractures which occur commonly with the hangman's patterns include odontoid fractures (Fig. 4-94),[236] posterior C1 arch fractures,[225] and hyperextension tear drop fractures of C2 (Fig. 4-95). Other hyperextension injuries in the subaxial cervical spine should be sought also.

Injuries of the Subaxial Cervical Spine

Axial Compression or Burst Fracture. The subaxial cervical "burst" fracture (see above) is a relatively uncommon injury caused by axial compression of the cervical spine. Typically, in response to axial loading forces the cervical

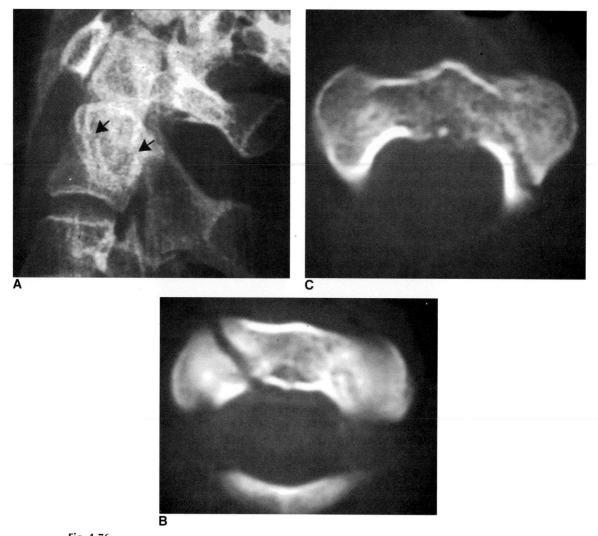

Fig. 4-76
Subtle low odontoid fracture. **A,** Magnified lateral view of cervicocranial region shows subtle defects of the Harris ring (*arrows*), indicating a low odontoid fracture. **B** and **C,** Axial CT views confirm fracture through axis body.

spine is driven into flexion or extension. In some cases the cervical spine maintains its axial alignment and absorbs the force along the vertical vertebral body axis. The rate of vertical load application may have some influence on the generation of pure axial load versus flexion or extension injuries combined with axial loading. A fast loading time favors production of an axial load pattern.[237]

Vertical force is absorbed initially by the intervertebral discs, which bulge outward in response. The annular fibers resist this expansion and refocus energy inward. The nucleus pulposus relieves pressure by rupturing into the inferior endplate of the superior vertebral body. The explosive deposition of energy within the center of the

body produces outward expansion of the vertebra, producing bone comminution and outward displacement.[238] Although usually one level is involved primarily, other cervical levels may sustain lesser degrees of injury. The primary determinant of neurologic outcome is the extent of posterior bone fragment displacement into the thecal sac and cord. One study on this subject concluded that all patients with less than 50% of residual AP canal diameter developed permanent tetraplegia, while those with greater than 50% canal compromise had incomplete tetraplegia and improvement in function.[239] However, studies performed using cadaver cervical spine models demonstrate that the maximal extent of canal compression is underestimated based on

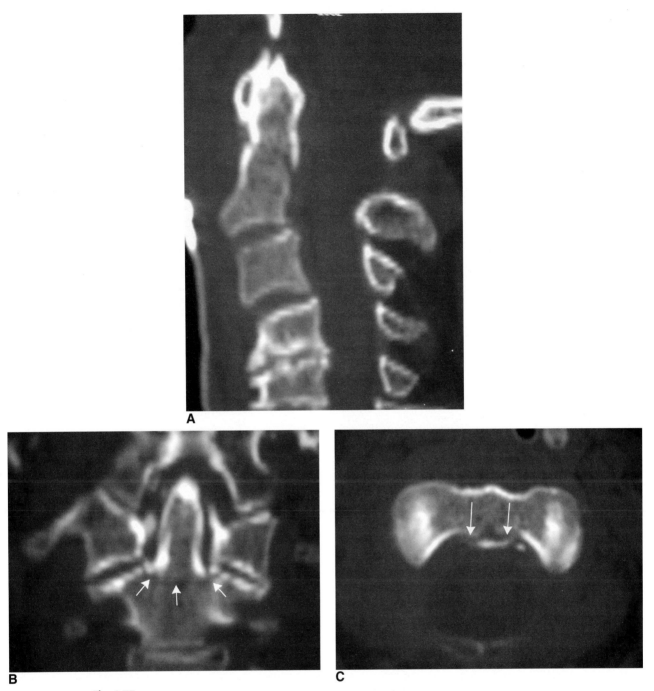

Fig. 4-77
Althoff type C odontoid fracture. Sagittal **(A)** and coronal **(B)** CT multiplanar reformation images show a fracture line in the C2 body below the typical plane of the high odontoid fracture, which involves the medial articular facets of the axis bilaterally consistent with the type C pattern described by Althoff. **C,** Axial CT image near the base of the odontoid shows fracture extension into the axis body (*arrows*).

posttrauma radiographs and that the neurologic outcome is related to canal compromise at the time of maximal spine loading during injury.[237,240] The amount of force applied to produce an axial compression load injury in the subaxial spine appears to be about one half of that

required for flexion and extension injuries based on cadaver models.[241]

Radiographically, the burst fracture demonstrates an overall loss of height compared with normal adjacent levels (Fig. 4-96; see Fig. 4-31). The AP view often shows a

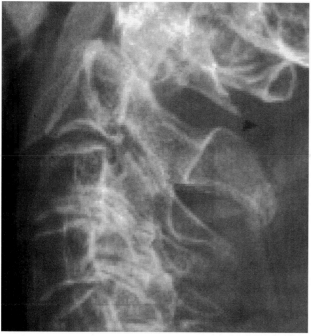

Fig. 4-78
Odontoid plus atlas fracture. Lateral cervical radiograph shows posteriorly displaced high odontoid fracture with associated displaced posterior C1 arch fracture (*arrowhead*).

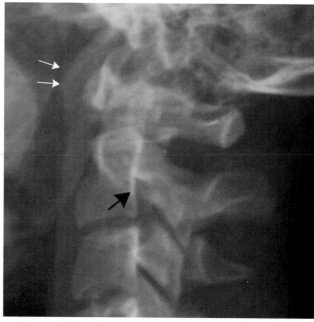

Fig. 4-80
Harris ring. The normal Harris ring has an interruption in the posteroinferior margin created by the foramen transversarium (*black arrow*). Note normal convex bulge of prevertebral soft tissue at the C1 arch (*white arrows*), with shallow concavity below.

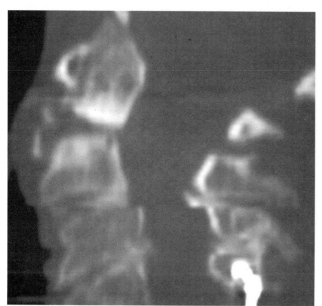

Fig. 4-79
Nonunion of remote type II odontoid fracture. Midsagittal CT multiplanar reformation shows a nonunion of a remote odontoid fracture. Note the sclerosis along the fracture margins, indicating attempted new bone formation and residual gap between fragments. Previous posterior internal fixation was performed caudally.

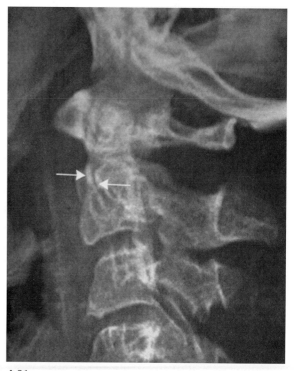

Fig. 4-81
Offset Harris ring. Rotation of the axis from the true lateral projection will create the appearance of two separate, but parallel, Harris rings (*arrows*) from each side of the axis.

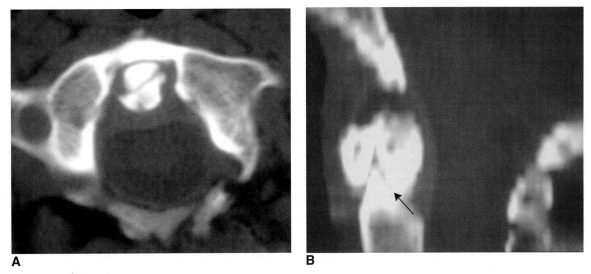

Fig. 4-82
Ununited high odontoid fracture. **A**, CT axial view shows smooth sclerotic margins of odontoid without evidence of bony bridging. **B**, Midsagittal CT multiplanar reformation shows same finding (*arrow*). Note marked sclerosis along fracture margins and close apposition of fragments.

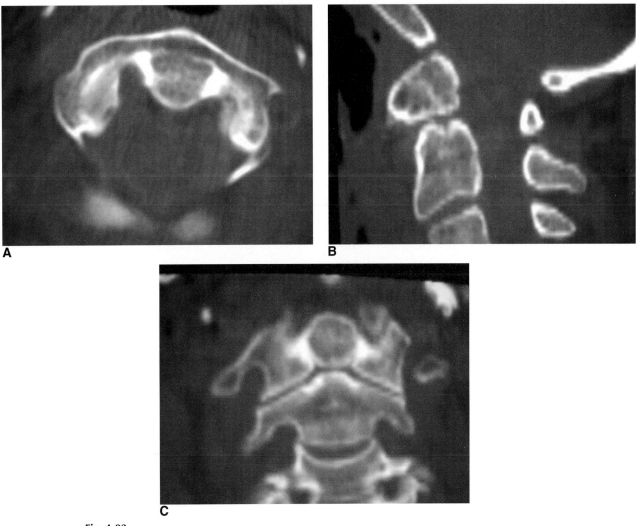

Fig. 4-83
Unstable os odontoideum. **A**, Axial CT image of trauma patient demonstrates hypertrophy of the dens that is fused to the anterior arch of the atlas. Sagittal (**B**) and coronal (**C**) CT multiplanar reformation images show smooth margins of odontoid and body of C2 without sclerosis. Again note fusion of dens to atlas.

Continued

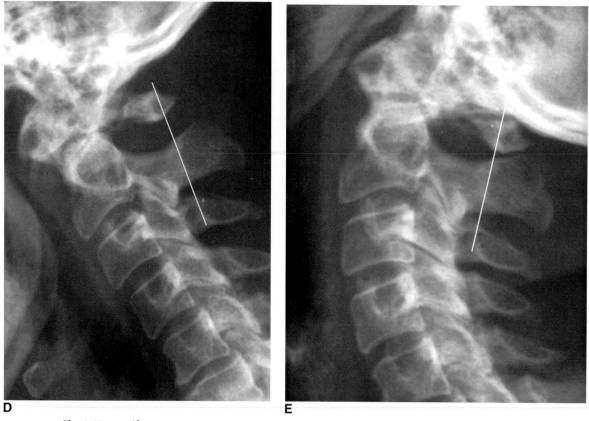

Fig. 4-83, cont'd
Flexion (**D**) and extension (**E**) lateral cervical views show about 2 to 3 mm of movement of the dens based on position changes of the C1 spinolaminar line (*white lines*).

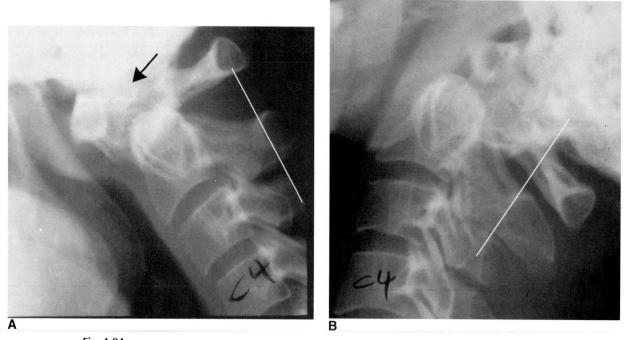

Fig. 4-84
Unstable os odontoideum. Flexion (**A**) and extension (**B**) lateral cervical views show smoothly corticate, nonsclerotic os odontoideum (*arrow*), showing significant movement between positions (*white lines*) and indicating instability of fibrous union. (From Mirvis SE, Harris JH Jr: Spinal imaging. In Browner BD, Jupiter JB, Levine AM, Trafton PG, eds: *Skeletal trauma*, ed 2, vol 1, Philadelphia, 1998, WB Saunders.)

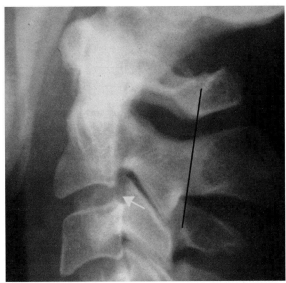

Fig. 4-85
Traumatic spondylolysis of the axis (hangman's). Type I hangman's fracture demonstrates offset of the C2 spinolaminar line (*black line*) and slight anterior displacement of the axis body without angulation (*arrow*). The fracture is not seen directly. There is prevertebral soft tissue swelling with a straight contour.

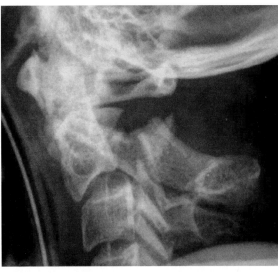

Fig. 4-87
Type IIA hangman's fracture. Lateral cervical radiograph demonstrates a hangman's fracture similar to the one shown in Fig. 4-39, but with greater angulation and displacement. This type might be more likely to be unstable (due to ligament damage) and to require internal fixation than types I and II and may involve a component of flexion in its mechanism.

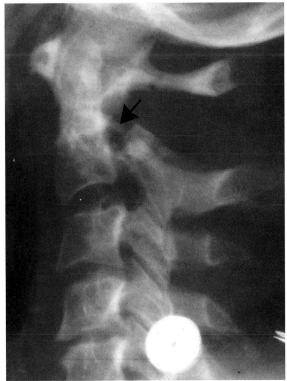

Fig. 4-86
Type II hangman's fracture. Lateral cervical radiograph shows clear fracture plane crossing the pars interarticularis (*arrow*), with disruption of the C2-3 disc and angulation and displacement of the axis. There is also a minimally displaced fracture of the posterior arch of the atlas.

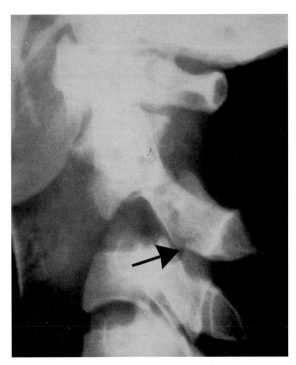

Fig. 4-88
Type III hangman's fracture-dislocation. Lateral cervical radiograph shows a high-grade (type III) hangman's pattern associated with complete dislocation of the articular facets (*arrow*). There is significant displacement and angulation, and the injury is unstable. This pattern most likely results from combined flexion and extension forces.

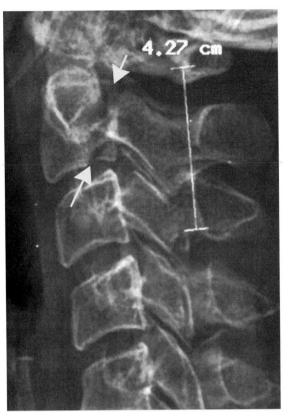

Fig. 4-89
Atypical hangman's fracture. Lateral cervical radiograph shows fracture line extending from pars through the posterior cortex of the axis body (*arrows*), which disrupts Harris's ring. The spinolaminar line of the axis is displaced posteriorly (*white line*).

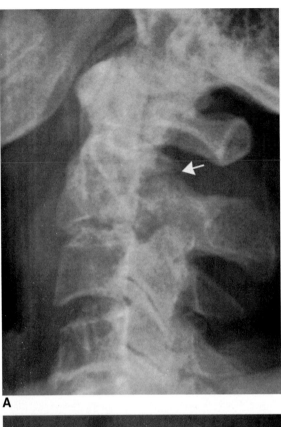

A

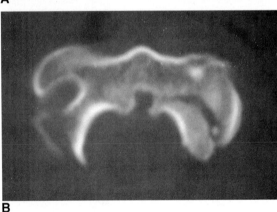

B

Fig. 4-90
Subtle atypical hangman's fracture. **A**, Lateral radiograph reveals a subtle fracture line through the top of the pars (*arrow*). Note the tilted axis of the C2 spinolaminar line compared with those of adjacent vertebra due to the fracture. **B**, Axial CT shows fracture lines extending into the posterior axis body, with right fracture progressing into the foramen transversarium.

midline or parasagittal vertical fracture line.[242] Also, on the AP view the body appears widened laterally, usually greater at the top than bottom. Importantly, on the lateral view, the posterior elements show no evidence of distraction injury such as widening of the interspinous or interlaminar distance or subluxation or dislocation of the facet joints. This lack of posterior distraction helps differentiate the axial compression, or burst, from the flexion tear drop pattern (see below), which it superficially may otherwise resemble. In an axial burst fracture, the spine appears in a neutral position or slightly kyphotic alignment but does not show a flexed orientation. A triangular inferoanterior bone fragment, which is similar in appearance to the tear drop fragment, may be present with a burst fracture. It is very important to distinguish between these two injury patterns. The flexion tear drop injury usually produces an immediate and complete neurologic deficit. The axial burst fracture may lead to a transient paraplegia or tetraplegia, which can show significant improvement with time. It is vital to maintain the stability of the spine so as not to aggravate the neurologic injury and diminish the extent of functional recovery.

CT will reveal fractures of one or both laminae, which result from compression of the posterior arches, that usually are not evident radiographically. CT also can demonstrate or exclude fractures which may result from axial loading to the articular pillars, particularly if there is a component of cervical lateral bending in the injury mechanism. Subtle fractures involving other

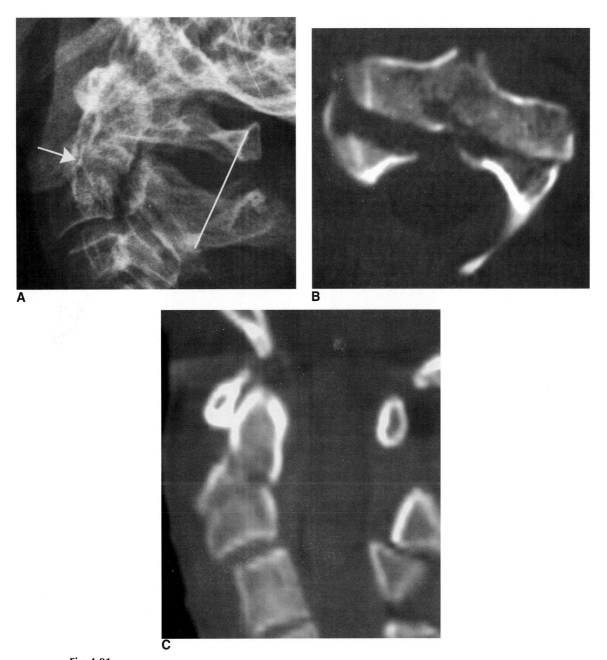

Fig. 4-91
Atypical hangman's fracture with odontoid fracture. **A,** Lateral cervical radiograph demonstrates an atypical hangman's fracture, with posterior displacement of the posterior aspect of the Harris ring (posterior axis cortex). A concurrent low odontoid fracture is posteriorly displaced (*arrow*). Again, note offset of C2 spinolaminar line (*white line*). **B,** Axial CT image shows fracture plane involving posterior cortex of the axis body. **C,** Midsagittal CT multiplanar reformation shows low odontoid fracture.

adjacent vertebrae may be revealed also. CT is not mandatory if a clear axial bursting pattern is evident radiographically.

Patients with neurologic deficits resulting from axial loading injuries should undergo MRI to assess for the presence of other lesions, such as EDH or herniation of disc material, which may impact the spinal cord and affect management. The major spinal ligaments should appear intact, although some stripping of the posterior and anterior longitudinal ligaments may occur as the anterior and posterior cortical fragments are displaced outward.

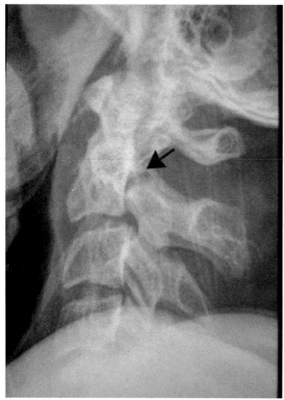

Fig. 4-92
Typical type I hangman's fracture. Lateral cervical radiograph demonstrates fractures through the pars interarticularis (*arrow*) without evidence of extension to the Harris ring. There is no angulation or displacement of the axis body. There is mild prevertebral soft tissue swelling.

Hyperextension Injuries

Overview. Extension force plays a role in a number of cervical spine injuries but is the predominant mechanism of injury responsible for the patterns considered in this section. Hyperextension injures represent 7% to 26% of all cervical spine injuries.[243] There is a continuum of injury severity, beginning with the hyperextension "sprain" that is stable, and progressing to the hyperextension-dislocation that is mechanically unstable and accompanied by major neurologic deficits. These injuries result from a direct AP force striking the head, face, or mandible. The result reflects the injurious force, and these fractures frequently are associated with mandibular, facial, or frontal bone injury. These injuries are usually evident on the admission lateral cervical spine radiograph; however, it must be remembered that stabilization of the head and neck with a cervical collar by emergency providers in the field may reduce gross displacements, giving rise to a virtually normal-appearing spine on the lateral radiograph. Even in such cases, however, there is usually some asymmetry of an intervertebral disc space, with widening anteriorly[244] (Fig. 4-97).

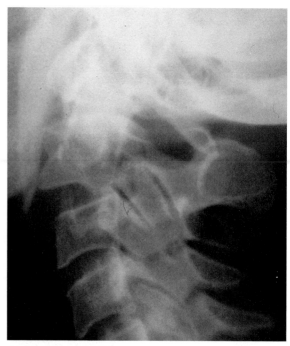

Fig. 4-93
Typical type III hangman's fracture. Lateral cervical radiograph shows a fracture line traversing the pars interarticularis. There is associated anterior displacement and moderate angulation of the C2 body, indicating disc disruption. The spinolaminar line of the axis is displaced posteriorly. There is an abnormal contour and fullness of the prevertebral soft tissues.

In general, hyperextension injuries tend to occur in the lower cervical levels, usually where there is degenerative disease of the facets and discs.[245,246] Individuals with preexisting cervical spine disease which creates spinal rigidity, such as ankylosing spondylitis, disseminated idiopathic skeletal hyperostosis (DISH), or severe degenerative disease, are at increased risk for hyperextension injuries from a given trauma.[243,247] In these patients, the fracture plane may cross either disc space or bone and usually is accompanied by gross dislocation of the spine. On some occasions and due, in part, to the underlying diseases, the injury may be radiographically subtle. For this reason, patients sustaining blunt trauma with these underlying conditions who have neck pain should undergo thin-section CT with sagittal reformation and, possibly, MRI to exclude fracture. Although most such patients have major neurologic deficits, others will remain intact and seek treatment subsequently when subluxation or dislocation occurs.

Hyperextension Sprain. The hyperextension sprain produces injury to the anterior longitudinal ligament, anterior annulus fibers, and disc. Radiographically, the injury is recognized by widening of the anterior disc space, possible acute vacuum disc, linear avulsion fractures from the vertebral endplate, and adjacent prevertebral

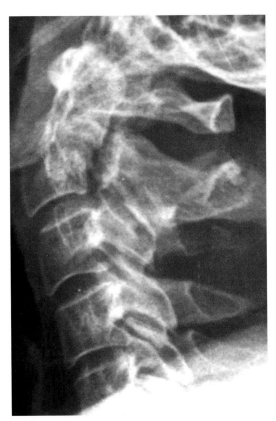

Fig. 4-94
Atypical hangman's fracture associated with low odontoid fracture.

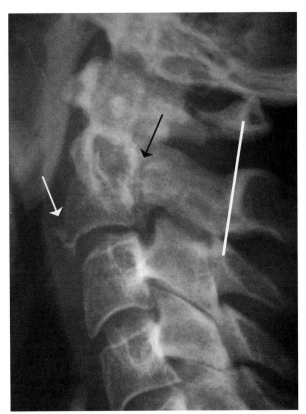

Fig. 4-95
Hangman's and commonly associated fractures. Lateral cervical spine view shows a typical type I hangman's fracture (*black arrow*), associated with a hyperextension tear drop fracture of the axis (*white arrow*) and a posterior C1 arch fracture. All injuries are secondary to hyperextension force. Again, note posterior offset of spinolaminar line of the axis (*white line*).

swelling[248] (Fig. 4-98). Although the extension sprain is not associated with neurologic deficits, it may occur with greater frequency in older adults due to a combination of posterior osteophytes and hypertrophied ligamentum flavum that compress the cord, usually leading to a central cord syndrome or anterior cord syndrome.[245,248] Also, cord injury is more likely in those with congenital spinal stenosis, with or without degenerative spondylosis. The diagnosis of hyperextension sprain assumes that the middle (posterior annulus and posterior longitudinal ligament) and posterior (joint capsules, intraspinous, and intralaminar ligaments) columns of the spine remain intact and, therefore, that the injury is stable. On radiography this is suggested by a normal relationship of the facet joints, lack of AP vertebral body displacement, and a normal posterior disc space height. In questionable cases, MRI is useful to verify ligament integrity.[19,77,249] MRI has increased sensitivity for detection of prevertebral edema or hematoma, longitudinal ligament and annulus injury, endplate avulsion fractures, posterior disc herniation which may impact the cervical cord, and other extension injuries at adjacent levels.[77,249,250]

Hyperextension-Posterior Dislocation. The hyperextension-posterior dislocation injury results from an impacting force of sufficient magnitude to disrupt the anterior and middle ligament supports of the cervical spine, including the facet joint capsules. The superior portion of the spine is driven backward and rostrally (Fig. 4-99). The pattern can occur as a pure ligamentous injury but usually is associated with avulsion fractures from the anterior aspects of the involved vertebrae (Fig. 4-100). If the injurious force acts in a circular vector, the posterior spinal elements (articular pillars, laminae, and spinous processes) may experience impacting forces, producing concurrent loading fractures in these areas (Fig. 4-101). Rarely, a laminar-pedicle separation will result from this impact. Also, fractures through the pedicles or posterior vertebral body, similar in appearance to the hangman's fracture of C2, can occur from this extension-posterior axial loading combination. If there is clear disruption of both anterior and middle ligament supports based upon the radiographic appearance, the injury is clearly unstable. In questionable cases, stability can be best determined by MRI assessment.[251]

Hyperextension-Anterior Dislocation. As noted above, a hyperextension force can rotate around the cervical

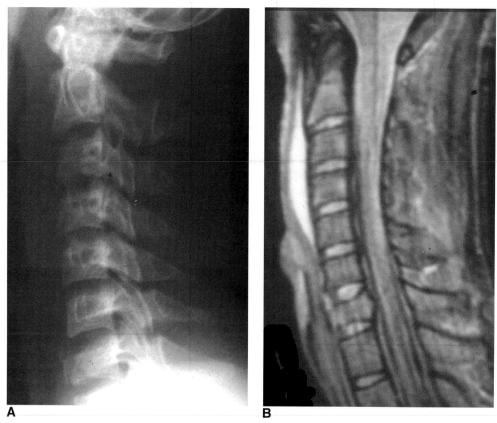

Fig. 4-96
Cervical spine burst fracture. **A**, Lateral cervical spine shows uniform loss of height of C7, with apparent preservation of the posterior elements. **B**, Proton-weighted midsagittal MR image demonstrates loss of height of body and buckling of posterior cortex, with prevertebral edema in upper cervical spine.

spine to produce force acting from the posterior direction. In such a case, the force can act on the injured anterior longitudinal ligament, annulus fibers, and posterior longitudinal ligament to displace the vertebral body "anteriorly" at the involved level. Usually, the vertebral body will appear intact and may be completely displaced anterior to the subjacent vertebral body (see Fig. 4-101). Although appearing to be a major dislocation, the decompressive nature of this injury may permit complete spinal cord integrity. There are usually associated compression fractures of posterior bony elements. This injury needs to be differentiated from hyperflexion dislocations, which might have a similar radiographic appearance related to anterior displacement of the injured vertebral body but are more likely to produce major neurologic deficits.

Extension Tear Drop Fracture. The extension tear drop fracture is an avulsion fracture at the site of the attachment of the anterior longitudinal ligament, usually involving the anteroinferior aspect of the vertebral body (Figs. 4-102 and 4-103; see Fig. 4-95). It is associated with

widening of the anterior intervertebral disc space and precervical soft tissue swelling and usually is differentiated easily from the tear drop fracture produced by hyperflexion.[49] Neurologic deficits rarely result from isolated hyperextension tear drop fractures, but they may be seen when this injury occurs in combination with other hyperextension fractures. There is a high incidence of concurrent cervical spine injuries.[252] The most frequent site of the hyperextension tear drop fracture is the C2 level, but a similar injury at C3 also occurs. The pattern appears to be mechanically stable in the vast majority of cases.[49,252] There is no indication for CT for this injury unless the diagnosis is uncertain or other extension injuries are suspected.

Atlas Anterior Ring Avulsion. Another rare extension mechanism injury is the avulsion fracture of the anterior atlas ring, which results from the pull of attached ligaments from below (Fig. 4-104). A horizontal fracture line extends through the midportion of the anterior atlas, with inferior displacement of the avulsed fragment and prevertebral edema at the injury site. Finally, rarely, the

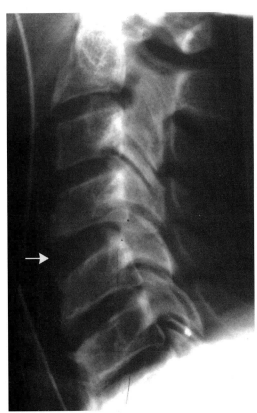

Fig. 4-97
Extension sprain. Lateral cervical radiograph shows anterior widening of the C4-5 disc space (*arrow*), with slight retrolisthesis of the C4 body. The integrity of the middle column support is unknown.

hyperextension cervical spine injury pattern can produce tears in the posterior cervical esophagus, usually related to impaction of large anterior osteophytes or irregular fracture margins into the adjacent esophagus or by entrapment of the esophagus within hyperextended disc spaces.[253,254]

Hyperflexion Injuries

Hyperflexion Subluxation or Sprain. Anterior subluxation is an injury important to understand, because its radiographic appearance is often subtle, yet a missed diagnosis can have significant negative consequences for the patient. The injury is primarily ligamentous, involving the posterior ligament complex (interspinous, interlaminar, capsular ligaments) and the posterior longitudinal ligament. The injury also extends into the posterior portion of the intervertebral disc. Although considered stable because most of the disc at the injury level and the anterior longitudinal ligament remain intact, delayed diagnosis and failure to treat results in persistent pain, potential kyphotic deformity (because

the ligaments heal inadequately to support physiologic stress), and the potential for neurologic injury. Green has described at least a 20% incidence of delayed cervical spine instability resulting from missed AS.[255]

The radiologic diagnosis requires careful inspection of spinal alignment. Several radiographic signs as seen on the lateral view have been described[255] (Figs. 4-105 to 4-107).

- "Fanning" of the spinous processes
- Lack of coverage of the facet surfaces compared with adjacent levels
- Widened facet joints with incongruous facet surfaces, lack of parallelism of facets
- Increased interlaminar and interspinous distance
- Anterior displacement or anterior rotation of one vertebra on its anteroinferior corner
- Focal spinal kyphosis
- Widening of the posterior portion of the intervertebral disc and narrowing of the anterior portion

If the displacement of the vertebral body anteriorly exceeds 3.5 mm or the body shows greater than 20 degrees of angulation, or more than 11 degrees of angulation compared with adjacent vertebral body pairs, the injury is considered unstable.[256]

When the lateral radiographs are taken of a patient with AS, these signs may be subtle or apparent (see Fig. 4-50). If there is suspicion of injury due to clinical signs and symptoms, flexion-extension lateral stress views can be useful (see Fig. 4-50). This study must be performed with an experienced physician in attendance and with an alert and cooperative patient. The radiographic signs should become far more obvious in flexion and resolve in extension. If the patient cannot achieve adequate degrees of flexion and extension during clinical assessment, usually due to spasm or pain, there is probably no utility to performing the radiographic study, because it would show only the application of limited stress on the cervical ligaments. In this case, alternatives include immobilization in a rigid cervical collar and return in 2 to 3 weeks for follow-up radiography with flexion-extension study at that time or, if available, MRI can be used to diagnose or exclude AS definitively using static imaging.

Harris[257] has pointed out that both positioning of the head and neck, as in a military posture or cervical collar and anatomic variants, can mimic AS. He emphasizes the relationship of the articular facets as key in differentiating such mimics from AS, which usually is managed with open fixation with articular mass Camille-Roy plate and screw.[258,259]

It is not uncommon for patients with AS to have mild anterior superior compression fractures of the vertebral body at the injury level, also. This is a minor component of the overall injury and should not distract from appreciation of the much more significant ligamentous injury posteriorly.

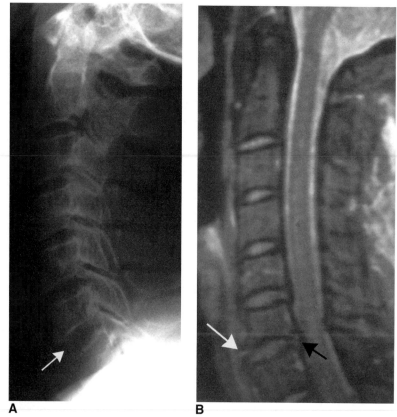

Fig. 4-98
Extension injury shown by MRI. **A**, Lateral cervical radiograph shows widening of the anterior disc space at C6-7 (*arrow*). Alignment otherwise appears anatomic. **B**, T2-weighted MR image shows tear in the anterior longitudinal ligament (*white arrow*) at this level and posterior disc herniation (*black arrow*), indicating acute annulus fibrosis injury.

It is unlikely that CT would be of significant value in either the initial diagnosis of AS or in further clarifying the injury. However, patients with posttrauma cervical pain without a radiologically apparent cause are likely to be the first studied by CT, due to its greater availability and in the search for a radiographically occult fracture. The facet relationships may be better revealed using thin-section MPR than by radiography. Also, a subtle compression fracture may more likely be detected, pointing to the possibility of AS.

MRI will show directly ligament disruptions and soft tissue edema and hemorrhage, fluid within the damaged facet joints and possibly within the intervertebral disc (Figs. 4-108 and 4-109; see Fig. 4-49). Other levels of more subtle injury may be revealed, information that is essential for planning the extent of internal fixation (see Fig. 4-109). Disc herniation and EDH can occur, also, with AS and would be diagnosed on MRI (see Figs. 4-42 and 4-43).

When the injury to the posterior ligament complex is only partial, an incomplete sprain, a stable injury results. This injury may show minimal degrees of AS due to liga-

ment stretching or partial tears, but these injuries should not be exaggerated by flexion and should reduce to normal alignment with extension. Again, a delayed flexion-extension study or MRI may be needed to attempt to separate partial from complete hyperflexion sprain.

Clay Shoveler's Fracture. The classic "clay shoveler's" fracture is a fatigue or stress injury involving the lower cervical and upper thoracic spinous processes from application of strong flexion force occurring with long-term lifting of heavy loads by shovel.[260] The injury is seen less commonly since the introduction of earth-moving machinery. Sudden severe hyperflexion force with resistance of the posterior paraspinal muscles can produce a similar injury from acute trauma (Fig. 4-110). It is important to distinguish spinous process fractures that arise from flexion from those sustained by impaction of adjacent spinous processes occurring with extension mechanisms and to recognize that such patterns often are unstable. It is also important to determine if spinous process fractures extend to cross the spinolaminar line,

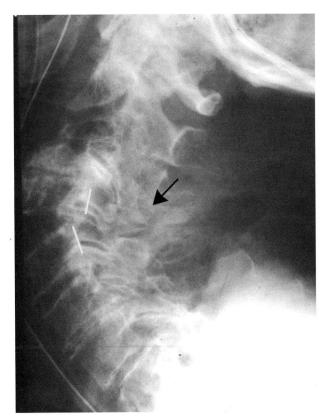

Fig. 4-99
Hyperextension-dislocation. Lateral cervical radiograph of patient after blunt trauma shows marked widening of the disc space at C4-5 and posterior displacement and angulation of the C4 (*white lines* mark posterior cortex). There is impaction, with fractures among the posterior elements (*arrow*).

indicating possible bilateral laminar breach. This feature implies concurrent injury to the posterior ligament complex, with disruption and potential for acute or delayed instability.[261]

Flexion Compression Fracture. A simple wedge fracture occurs as a result of compression of the anterior aspect of a vertebral body, between its flexed adjacent vertebrae. This results in loss of height, predominantly anteriorly, but is not associated with ligamentous disruption per se (Fig. 4-111). In practice, this commonly occurs in association with hyperflexion sprain and signs of posterior ligamentous injury, and instability should be sought if not already apparent from the neutral cervical radiographs. A variation of this fracture is a compression corner fracture of the superior anterior corner of the vertebral body, again resulting from hyperflexion force. Although seen among patients with hyperflexion sprain, this can also occur among patients with facet dislocation and may be associated with significant ligamentous injury.[248,256]

Hyperflexion Tear Drop Fracture. The hyperflexion tear drop fracture is among the most serious of all cervi-

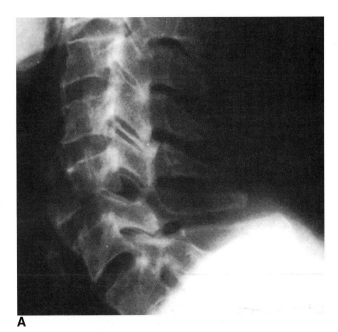

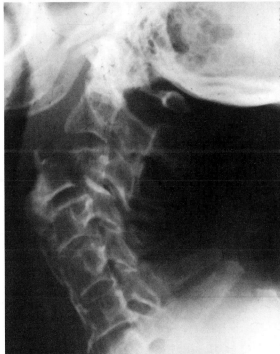

Fig. 4-100
Extension injury with avulsion fracture. **A**, Lateral cervical radiograph shows a hyperextension injury at C5-6, with an avulsion fracture arising from the C5 anteroinferior endplate. The fragment is longer in width than it is in height. Note the diastasis of the facet joints. **B**, Lateral cervical spine view of a different patient shows an extension fracture traversing the C3 body, with retrolisthesis of C3 and opening of the facet joints.

cal spine injuries. It is caused by high-energy axial loading of the flexed spine, resulting in a fracture-dislocation of one of the vertebrae, usually with retropulsion of the dorsal fragment of the dislocated vertebral body

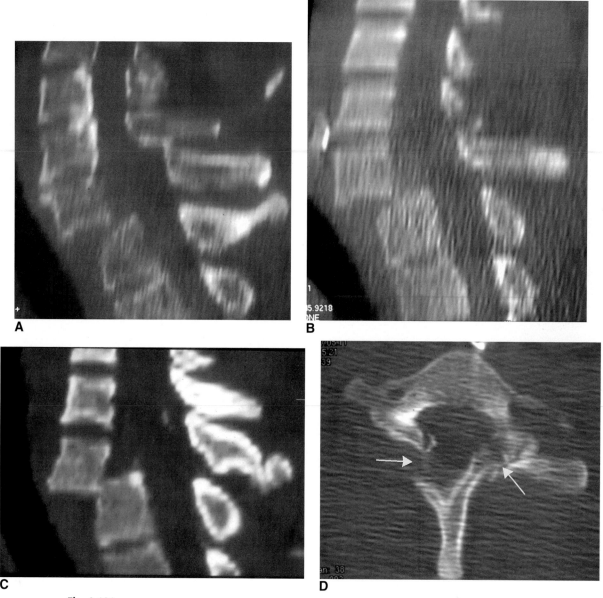

Fig. 4-101
Extension injury with anterior body displacement. **A** to **C**, Three different patients illustrating severe hyperextension force acting in a circular fashion, ultimately producing anterior vertebral body displacement. **D**, Axial CT image of patient B shows breaks in the lamina bilaterally, allowing ring separation and forward movement of the vertebral body. Patients may be neurologically intact following such an injury.

(Figs. 4-112 and 4-113; see Figs. 4-29 and 4-40).[262-264] It frequently is associated with an acute anterior cervical cord syndrome, with quadriplegia and loss of pain, touch, and temperature sensation. Cord compression most likely occurs as a result of the severe kyphotic angulation of the spine at the time of injury, coupled with simultaneous retropulsion of the dorsal vertebral body. Kim et al.[264] described 45 patients with hyperflexion tear drop fracture-dislocations and noted several classic features, including (1) posterior displacement of the upper cervical spine, (2) retropulsion of the posterior fragment from the involved vertebral body, (3) widening of the interlaminar and interfacet spaces, and (4) residual kyphotic deformity of the cervical spine. The fracture complex includes a sagittal fracture of the vertebral body in 87% of patients,[264] a displaced fracture(s) from the anteroinferior body, and simple or complex fractures of the laminae and facets. Of the 45 patients evaluated, 39

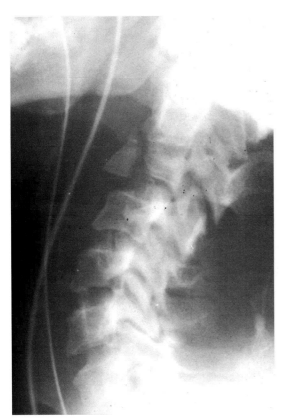

Fig. 4-102
Extension tear drop fracture. Large triangular bone fragment is avulsed from the axis body, representing the tear drop fragment. The C2-3 disc space appears intact.

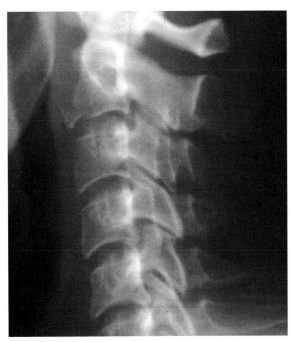

Fig. 4-103
Extension tear drop fracture in another patient shows apparent loss of integrity of C2-3 disc space.

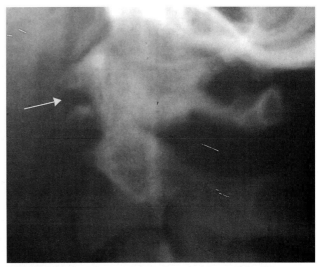

Fig. 4-104
Atlas extension fracture. Lateral cervical spine view focused at the C1-2 level shows an avulsion fracture of the anterior atlas arch (*arrow*).

(87%) had complete or incomplete neurologic deficits and 38 of these 39 (97%) had associated sagittal body and posterior element fractures, whereas 5 (83%) of 6 patients without these findings were neurologically intact. Despite the severe extent of injury produced by this fracture-dislocation complex, 8 (18%) patients in this series exhibited no precervical soft tissue edema, and only questionable edema was observed in an additional 10 (22%) patients.[264]

Hyperflexion tear drop fractures usually occur in the lower cervical spine, most commonly at C5.[264,265] The injury is usually apparent radiographically as the tear drop–shaped fragment of the anteroinferior portion of the vertebral body is displaced from the larger dorsal fragment. The tear drop fragment maintains alignment with the cervical spine below the injury level, although the posterior fragment and cervical spine above move as a unit. The distraction forces acting on the posterior elements produce one or more contiguous levels of widening of the interspinous and interlaminar spaces. Occasionally, the laminar fractures create a free bone segment that may displace inferiorly, causing a narrowing of the interlaminar space. Laminar and spinous process fractures may be indicated by interruption of the spinolaminar line or increased or decreased bone density in the laminar space as seen on the lateral radiograph. The posterior complex fractures may not be apparent on radiographs, particularly in the lateral radiographic view, but are seen easily with CT (Fig. 4-114; see Figs. 4-29, 4-40, and 4-112). Typically, there is also narrowing of the intervertebral disc space between the retropulsed posterior body and vertebral body below. Rarely, a flexion tear drop fracture appears quite subtle radiographically due to

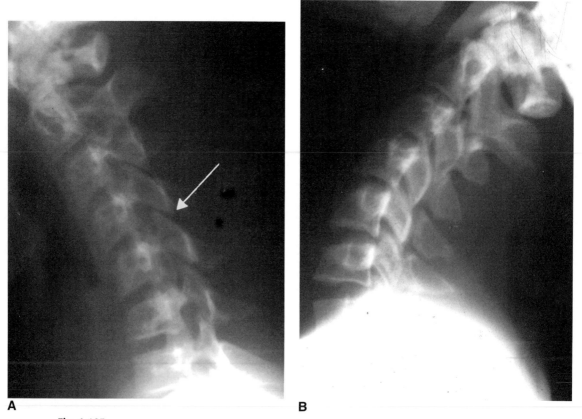

A　　　　　　　　　　　　　　　　　　　　　　　**B**

Fig. 4-105
Hyperflexion sprain. **A**, Lateral cervical radiograph in flexion shows a focal kyphosis at C4-5, with slight uncovering of the facets (*arrow*). **B**, The lateral view in extension shows complete reduction of the injury.

minimal or no retrolisthesis of the body. However, the patient may still exhibit a major neurologic deficit, because the degree of retropulsion and cord compression may have been far greater at the moment of impact but subsequently reduced afterward. In general, CT adds little to the diagnostic information provided by radiographs, except in subtle or atypical cases, but may show additional levels of injury unsuspected from the radiographic assessment. Because these injuries are highly unstable, they almost always require internal fixation. MRI is useful to observe the extent and type of cord injury and assess for disc herniation and other epidural mass effects, nerve root involvement, and extent of ligament injury. Findings that may permit improvement of neural function at even a single nerve root level ultimately can result in significant gains in motor function. Usually MRI shows a spindle-shaped cord contusion with central hemorrhage at the level of the retropulsed body fragment (see Figs. 4-29, 4-40, and 4-112 to 4-114). Functional recovery is quite uncommon when there is a complete motor deficit at diagnosis.

Bilateral Interfacet Dislocation. Given sufficient combined flexion and distraction forces, both inferior articular facets from one vertebral body can dislocate anterior to the superior facets of the subjacent vertebra. The bifacet dislocation causes disruption or stripping of all major support ligaments and facet capsules between the levels (Figs. 4-115 to 4-117). This injury most commonly occurs in the lower cervical spine, but can occur as high as C2 (see Fig. 4-88). The affected vertebral body is dislocated anteriorly by 50% or more of the AP diameter of the subjacent vertebral body. Severe and complete neurologic deficits are common, even if a simultaneous "decompressing" fracture has occurred through the posterior arch[241,266,267] of the dislocated vertebra. Despite the term *locked facets*, the bifacet dislocation is highly unstable, given injury to all major support ligaments, as well as the intervertebral disc[266,268] (see Figs. 4-116 and 4-117). Small, usually transverse fractures commonly arise from the articular facet tips due to impaction during injury.[47] These fractures are usually of no major clinical consequence but are not commonly visualized on plain

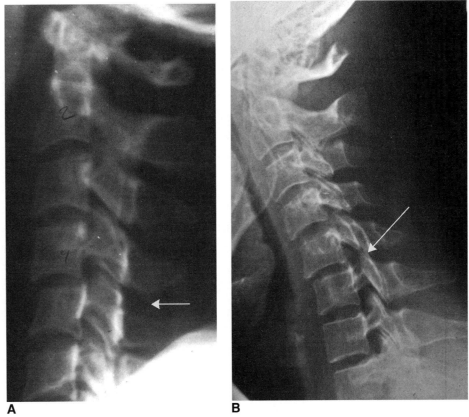

Fig. 4-106
Hyperflexion sprain. **A**, Lateral cervical radiograph shows slight anterolisthesis of C4, narrowing of the C4-5 disc space, and widening of the interspinous distance (*arrow*). **B**, Lateral cervical radiograph of another patient shows similar narrowing of the C5-6 disc space and near perching of the facet tips (*arrow*).

radiographs. Occasionally, a larger facet fracture may prevent closed reduction of the injury.[267]

Radiographic findings are usually obvious given the marked degree of anterior displacement of the cervical vertebral body. In rare cases, however, the injury can reduce spontaneously and the spine appear physiologically aligned on the initial "in- collar" lateral radiographs. Typically, there is little or no evidence of rotational injury such as a sudden change in the laminar space, because the amount of dislocation of the facets is symmetric. In some cases, one facet may dislocate while the other perches atop the subjacent facet tip, leading to subtle signs of rotation on the lateral or AP radiograph. Although fractures involving the displaced vertebra may be difficult to appreciate in standard lateral and AP radiographic views due to overlapping bone, CT reveals details of bony injury that may involve the posterior arch or articular facets. Other levels of injury adjacent to the major dislocation are also more apparent. MPR images clearly show the facet, articular pillar, and vertebral body relationships and are improved by use of thin and overlapping axial scans (see Figs. 4-115 and 4-117).

In general, MRI shows stripping of the anterior longitudinal and posterior longitudinal ligaments off the vertebral bodies (see Fig. 4-116), rather than frank disruption. Tearing of the posterior ligament complex is evident as increased signal on T2-weighted spin-echo and gradient-echo sequences crossing the low-signal ligaments (see Fig. 4-116). Herniated or extruded disc material is commonly present and, along with EDH, may contribute to anterior spinal cord compression. There is debate regarding the importance of diagnosing and removing herniated or extruded disc material prior to attempting injury reduction, because some believe that this contributes to neurologic deterioration,[266] while others do not share this view.[93,269] The spinal cord is compressed between the lamina of the displaced upper vertebra and superior posterior corner of the lower vertebra. In most cases, a cord contusion with hemorrhage is centered at this point. Screening MRA is important for patients sustaining bifacet dislocation given the extent of displacement of the vertebral arteries that occurs with this injury[270,271] (see Figs. 4-116 and 4-117). In the authors' experience, the vertebral arteries

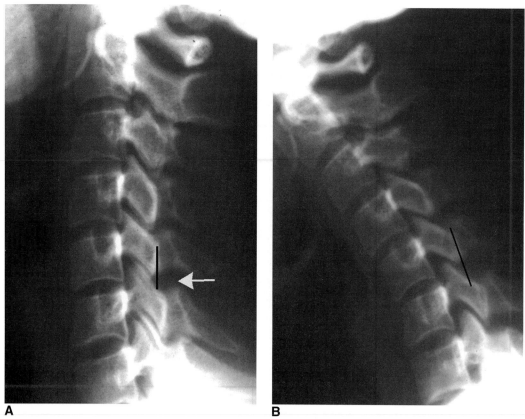

Fig. 4-107
Hyperflexion sprain.Neutral (**A**) and flexion (**B**) lateral cervical spine views of trauma patient demonstrate a widened C5-6 interlaminar and interspinous distance (*arrow*), a narrowed disc space, and partial uncovering of the facet articulations (*black line*). (From Mirvis SE, Harris JH Jr: Spinal imaging. In Browner BD, Jupiter JB, Levine AM, Trafton PG, eds: *Skeletal trauma*, ed 2, vol 1, Philadelphia, 1998, WB Saunders.)

typically are displaced abruptly at the injury level but remain intact (see Fig. 4-117).

Rotational Displacement Injuries of the Subaxial Cervical Spine

Unilateral Facet Fracture, Subluxation, Dislocation. Rotational forces producing flexion combined with distraction can cause injury to the facet joints that is *primarily* unilateral. The type of injury sustained depends on the magnitude, vector, and duration of the applied force. Rotational injuries of the cervical facets constitute about 5% to 17% of cervical spine injuries and often are missed or incorrectly characterized initially.[20,272-275] The facet surfaces can lose contact partially (subluxation) or completely (dislocation). Fractures of the articular facets and pillars may occur with either subluxation or dislocation. If the inferior articular process of a vertebral body is distracted above and translated anterior to the superior articular process of the subjacent vertebra, a "locked" facet joint results (Figs. 4-118 and 4-119; see Fig. 4-36,). In this

case, the dislocated articular process falls into the neural foramen between the vertebral bodies and is fixed in this position without application of external traction. The contralateral facet capsule and, potentially, several other major adjacent cervical support ligaments must be disrupted to permit such marked displacement to occur. Alternatively, the energy applied to the cervical spine may cause an inferior articular process to move cephalad and anteriorly, but not completely over the companion superior articular process (Figs. 4-120 and 4-121; see Figs. 4-32, 4-36, and 4-49). This subluxed facet joint could remain in an abnormal orientation or reduce spontaneously to physiologic alignment. The injury might, therefore, not be recognized either by radiography or CT. In many cases, the edges of the articular processes act like wedges,[20,273,276] producing vertical fractures through the facet surfaces into the articular pillars (see Figs. 4-32, 4-36, 4-49, 4-118, 4-120, and 4-121). One or both articulating facets can be fractured in this manner. In a study of 40 patients with rotational facet injuries, Shanmuganathan et al.[20] found that 11 patients (27%)

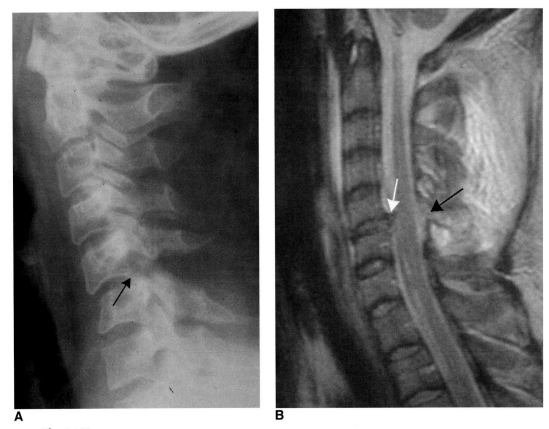

A **B**

Fig. 4-108
Hyperflexion subluxation. **A**, Lateral cervical radiograph reveals a flexion subluxation at C 5-6, with a widened interlaminar and interspinous distance, loss of facet coverage, and anterolisthesis of C5 (*arrow*). **B**, MRI at this level shows disruption of the ligamentum flavum (*black arrow*) and middle column ligament support, posterior longitudinal ligament and posterior annulus fibers (*white arrow*), indicating mechanical instability. There is prevertebral edema.

had pure unilateral facet dislocation with ligamentous injuries only, and 29 patients (73%) had facet subluxations with fractures. Fractures involved either the inferior articular process of the rotated vertebra (n = 13), the superior facet of the subjacent vertebra (n = 9), or both (n = 7). Based on this result, cervical facet fracture-subluxation occurs 3 times more frequently than classic unilateral facet dislocations.[20] In most patients with unilateral facet fracture-subluxation, the fracture has a vertical orientation through the articular pillar.[20,276] The pattern suggests that there is a contribution of lateral axial loading in the production of this injury. Other isolated fractures or extension of articular pillar fractures into the ipsilateral lamina and pedicle can occur, as well as fractures involving the contralateral facets. The most common associated fracture seen in the series of Shanmuganathan[20] was an avulsion fracture of the posteroinferior cortex of the rotating vertebral body which

occurred in 10 patients (25%), and 7 patients had an isolated articular pillar (see Fig. 4-121). Argenson et al.[273] reported that 25% of 47 patients with rotatory displacement injuries at one cervical level had another traumatic lesion of the cervical spine above or below that level.

Patients sustaining rotatory displacement injuries may be intact neurologically, may have radicular symptoms on the side of dislocation or subluxation, or may have major cord deficits.[273] In the Argenson series[273] of 47 patients with rotatory displacement injuries including unilateral facet fracture, unilateral facet dislocation, and fracture separation of the articular pillar, 30% had radicular symptoms. Patients with unilateral facet dislocation are more likely (P = .006) to have a spinal cord syndrome than patients with subluxation, with or without facet fracture.[20] In a study of 51 cases of unilateral facet dislocation by Shapiro et al.,[277] 73% had radiculopathy, 16% neck pain only, and 12% cord injury. Until recently, the

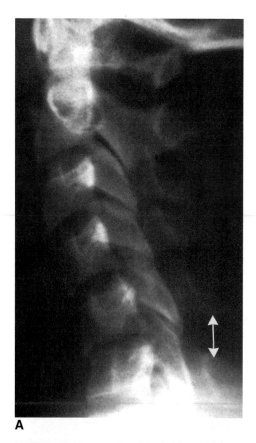

A

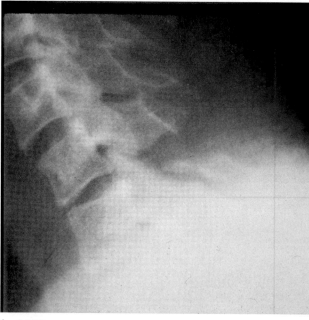

Fig. 4-110
Clay shoveler fracture. Lateral cervical radiograph focused on lower spine shows an inferiorly displaced avulsion from a portion of the C6 spinous process; a focal kyphosis is present at C6-7.

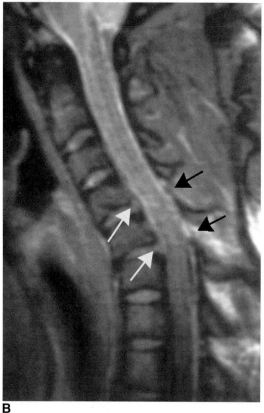

B

Fig. 4-109
Hyperflexion sprain. **A**, Lateral cervical radiograph shows widening of the interspinous distance at C5-6 (*two-headed arrow*), focal kyphosis, and a narrowed intervertebral disc. **B**, Proton-density MRI shows injury to the ligamentum flavum at C4-5 and C5-6 (*black arrows*), as well as the posterior longitudinal ligament and annulus fibers at the same levels (*white arrows*), creating instability.

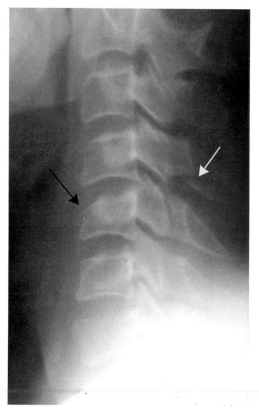

Fig. 4-111
Flexion compression fracture. Lateral cervical radiograph of trauma patient shows a flexion compression fracture of the anterior superior endplate of C5 (*black arrow*) and a fracture of the spinous process of C4 (*white arrow*). There is slight widening of the facet joint at C4-5.

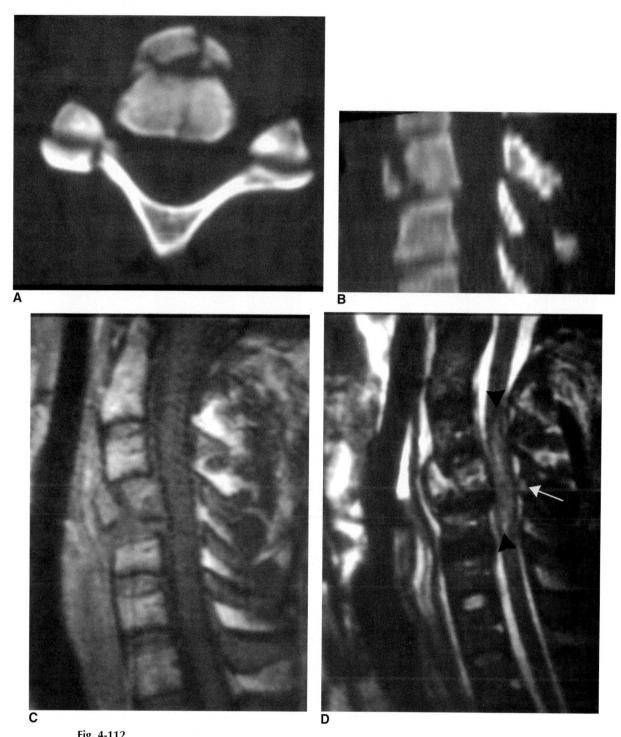

Fig. 4-112
Flexion tear drop fracture. Axial (**A**) and midsagittal (**B**) CT multiplanar reformations show typical hyperflexion tear drop fracture with anteriorly displaced fragments and retropulsion of the body. There is also a right lamina fracture and mild bilateral facet joint diastasis., T1-(**C**) and T2-(**D**) weighted midsagittal MR images show marked retropulsion of the C4 posterior body, a large cord contusion (*between arrowheads*), and ligamentum flavum disruption (*arrow*).

significant underlying soft tissue injuries often associated with rotational facet injures, as described below, were not appreciated.

The radiographic pattern seen with unilateral facet dislocation is well described.[275] On the lateral cervical radiograph, there is offset of the articular pillars at the level of injury due to the rotation. At one level they may appear superimposed, and at the adjacent level there is an abrupt offset (see Figs. 4-4, 4-32, and 4-119). This appearance has been referred to as the *bow-tie sign*. With

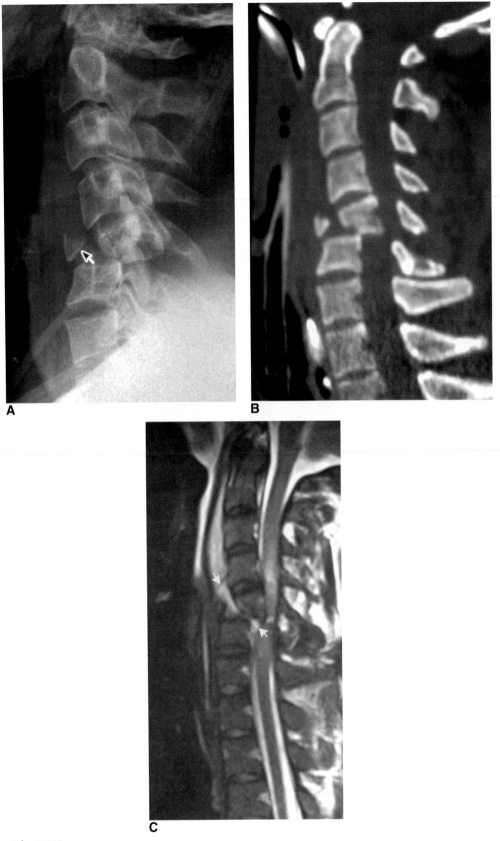

Fig. 4-113
Flexion tear drop fracture. **A,** Lateral cervical radiograph demonstrates a flexion tear drop fracture of C5, with marked retropulsion of the body and diastasis of the C5-6 facet articulations. **B,** CT multi-planar reformation in the midsagittal plane verifies the extent of retropulsion and canal occlusion. **C,** T2-weighted sagittal MR image shows stripping of the anterior and posterior longitudinal ligaments (*arrows*). An extensive cord contusion with hemorrhagic foci extends from C4 to C6.

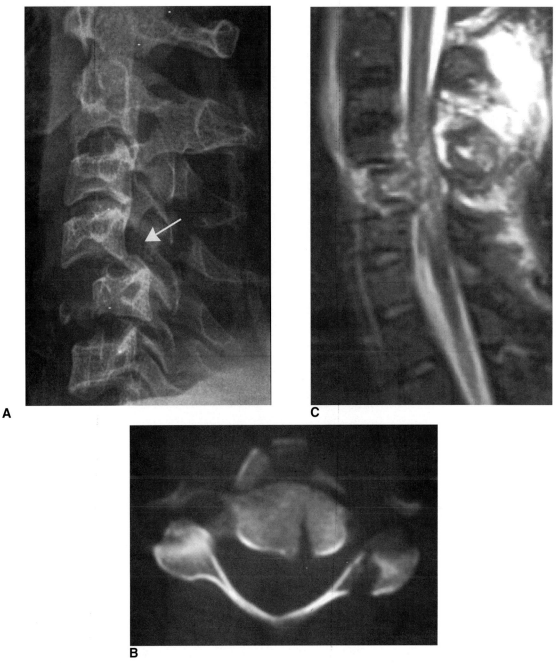

Fig. 4-114
Flexion tear drop and bilateral interfacet dislocation. **A,** Lateral cervical radiograph shows a tear drop fragment at C5, with marked retropulsion. There is a concurrent C4-5 bilateral facet dislocation (*arrow*) with fractures of the C3 and C4 spinous processes. **B,** Axial CT image through C5 shows classic pattern of radially oriented anterior fractures, midsagittal body fracture, and lamina fracture. **C,** Midsagittal T2-weighted MR image demonstrates extensive cord contusion with central hemorrhage at the C5 level.

complete dislocation there is usually anterior displacement of the rotated vertebra of 33% or less of the AP diameter of its body (see Figs. 4-32 and 4-119). Another useful sign of rotational injury is termed the *laminar space sign.*[278] The laminar space is that distance from the posterior margin of the articular pillars to the spinolaminar line (see Figs. 4-4 and 4-119). Normally this distance is nearly equivalent at adjacent levels or changes gradually due to head rotation. When there is an *abrupt* change in the laminar space, this indicates a

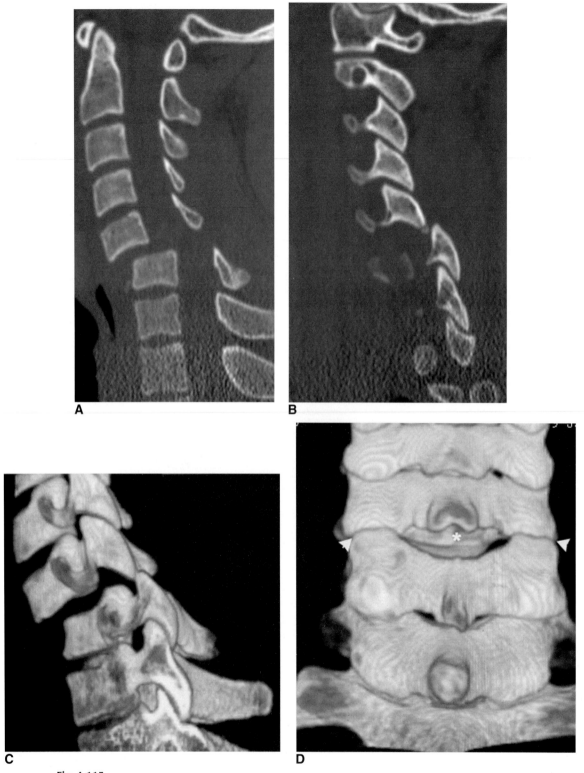

Fig. 4-115

Bilateral interfacet dislocation. **A**, Midsagittal CT multiplanar reformation shows about 50% displacement of C4 on C5, indicating a bilateral facet dislocation. There is marked interlaminar separation. **B**, A parasagittal CT multiplanar reformation shows the dislocation on one side, with a small articular process fracture of C5. **C**, A lateral perspective volume rendering nicely illustrates the dislocation of the facet joint. **D**, The posterior perspective shows the dislocated facets (*arrowheads*) and widened interspinous and interlaminar space (*asterisk*).

probable facet joint dislocation or subluxation.[278,279] On the AP radiograph, there is a sudden displacement in the orientation of the spinous processes. The spinous process of the involved level will shift toward the side of injury (see Figs. 4-36 and 4-120). Generally, associated articular process and facet fractures are not seen on plain radiographs; however, careful inspection of the laminar space on the lateral view at the involved level might show an extra density if a bone fragment from the articular pillar is displaced posteriorly. If the articular pillar is isolated by ipsilateral lamina and pedicle fractures, it may rotate so that the facet joint(s) above and below become visible on the AP radiograph (see below). Although prevertebral soft tissue swelling can accompany unilateral facet injuries, this is by no means reliably the case.[280]

In some ways, CT findings in these injuries can be more confusing than those of radiography. In classic unilateral facet dislocation, the injury is seen as a reversal of the nor- mal orientation of the articular process surfaces. Normally, the flat facet surface of the articular process articulates with its flat companion facet from the adjacent vertebra. The rounded, nonarticulating aspects of the artic- ular process face externally, away from the joint (see Figs. 4-49, 4-119, and 4-121). In a unilateral facet dislocation, the rounded nonfacet surfaces are in contact and the flat facet surfaces point externally outward. This appearance has been dubbed the *reverse hamburger bun sign* and seems very apropos. When fractures accompany either disloca- tion or subluxation of the facet joint, the picture gets more complex. In this case there may be three, four, or more bone fragments arising from the facets as seen in the axial CT plane. From this jumble, it can be hard to delineate the relationship of the articular processes and the origin of various bone fragments. Greater reliance on MPR parasagittal images can be quite useful to help understand the nature of the injury (see Figs. 4-32, 4- 118, and 4-121). CT will reveal additional fractures, which may not be seen

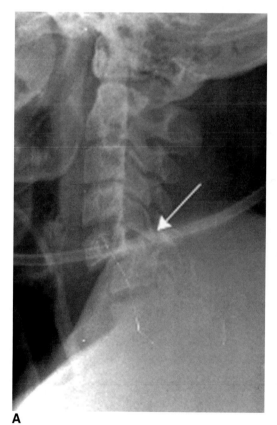

A

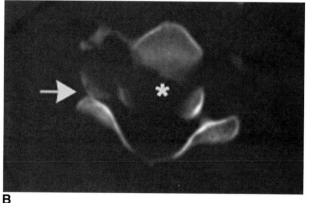

B

Fig. 4-116
Bilateral interfacet dislocation. **A,** Lateral cervical radiograph demonstrates C5-6 bilateral facet dis- location (*arrow*), with greater than 50% anterolisthesis. **B,** Axial CT image shows facet lock on the right (*arrow*) and exposed intervertebral disc (*asterisk*) due to anterolisthesis.

Continued

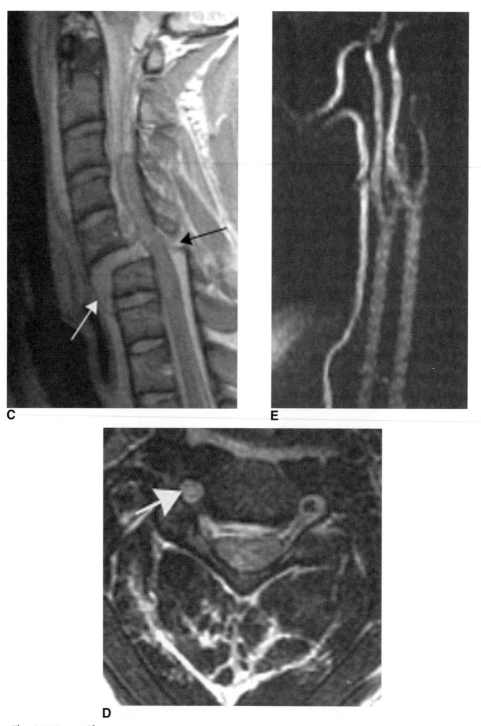

Fig. 4-116, cont'd
C, Midsagittal T2-weighted MR image shows stripping of the anterior longitudinal ligament (*white arrow*), disruption of the ligamentum flavum (*black arrow*), and tearing or stripping of the posterior longitudinal ligament. There is a diffuse increase in cord signal due to contusion. **D,** Axial fast T2-weighted spin echo shows occlusion of the right vertebral artery (*arrow*) marked by loss of flow void. **E,** Only one vertebral artery is seen on MR angiogram.

on the plain radiographs involving laminae, pedicles, and the vertebral body (see Fig. 4-121). As mentioned above, in about 10% of cases of rotatory displacement there is an avulsion fracture of the posterior cortex of the involved vertebra[20] (see Fig. 4-121). Most likely this injury results

from the rotational torque applied to the vertebral body, in which the posterior longitudinal ligament avulses a posterior cortical fragment. CT demonstrates diastasis of the contralateral facet joint which typically accompanies dislocation.

MRI may be warranted for patients with rotational facet displacement who manifest neurologic symptoms or progression of a neurologic deficit, and it is valuable to predict stability of the injury and, therefore, management planning.[281] In cases of dislocation, MRI typically shows evidence of injury to the disc and annular fibers, anterior longitudinal ligament, posterior longitudinal ligament, and ligamentum flavum at the level of rotation. The author believes that the powerful torque applied to the spinal column increases the vulnerability of these structures to tearing or avulsion. Because of the common association of rotational injuries with major cervical ligament tears, rotational facet injuries should be regarded as mechanically unstable. MRI will be valuable to assess any cord injury or epidural cord compression from herniated disc material or hematoma. In addition, MRI or MRA can evaluate flow in the vertebral arteries, which are prone to damage in patients sustaining this injury pattern[115,270,271,276] (see Fig. 4-48).

Isolated Articular Pillar. A combined fracture of the lamina and ipsilateral pedicle produces the laminar-pedicle separation fracture or isolated articular pillar (IAP) (Figs. 4-122 to 4-124; see Figs. 4-15 and 4-41). In this injury, disruption of the superior and inferior facet joints occurs, permitting the pillar to rotate freely. Some studies,[282-285] principally by Forsyth[282] and Allen et al.,[285] have suggested this injury is the result of combined rotation and compressive hyperextension. They support a mechanism in which a horizontal fracture usually is created at the base of the superior articular process of the involved vertebra due to extension and rotation. Although this combination of forces may produce the IAP, a review of cases conducted by Shanmuganathan et al.[286] demonstrates that hyperflexion and axial loading is the most common mechanism. In that study of 21 patients, IAP was observed at 24 levels. The patients had a clear hyperflexion mechanism with rotation (typically a unilateral rotatory facet displacement) in 17 (81%) and a

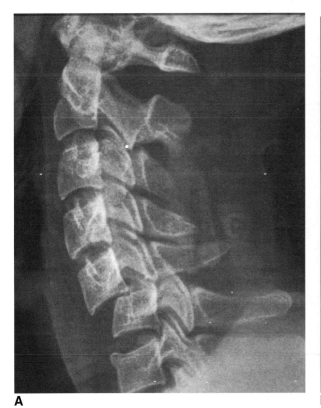
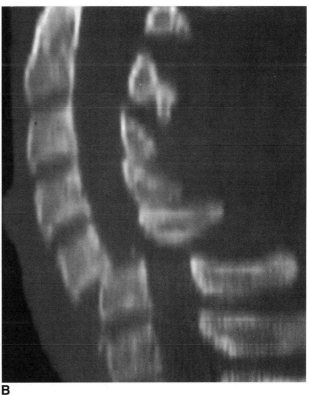

A **B**

Fig. 4-117
Bilateral interfacet dislocation. **A,** Lateral cervical spine radiograph of quadriplegic blunt trauma patient shows bilateral facet dislocation of C5-6, with greater than 50% anterolisthesis and interspinous flaring. **B,** Midsagittal CT multiplanar reformation confirms radiographic evaluation and demonstrates severe narrowing of the spinal canal.

Continued

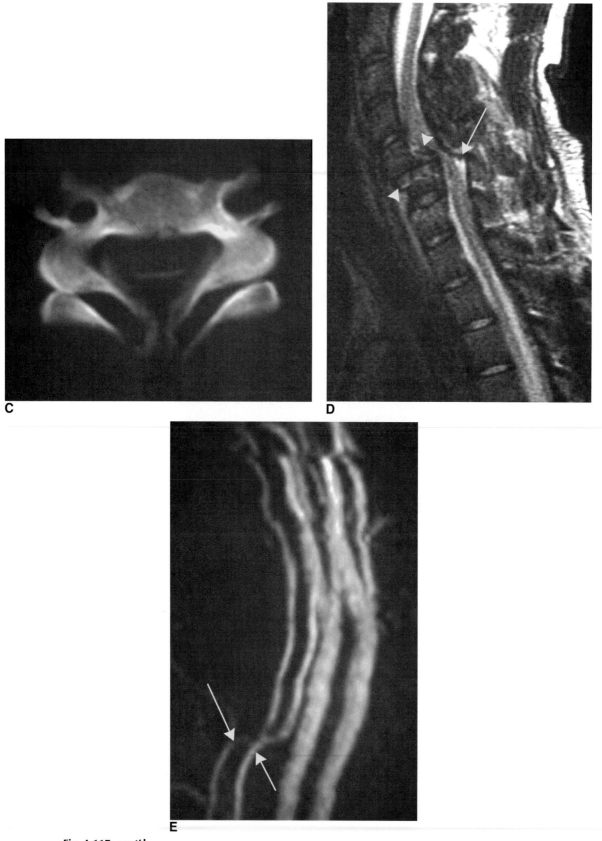

Fig. 4-117, cont'd
C, Axial CT image shows bilateral facet dislocations. **D,** Midsagittal T2-weighted MR image demonstrates marked narrowing of spinal canal at level of dislocation and disruption or stretching of ligamentum flavum (*arrow*). The anterior longitudinal and posterior longitudinal ligaments are avulsed
from the adjacent bodies (*arrowheads*). **E,** MR angiogram shows gentle bending of vertebral arteries (*arrows*) at level of the injury but no occlusion or overt injury.

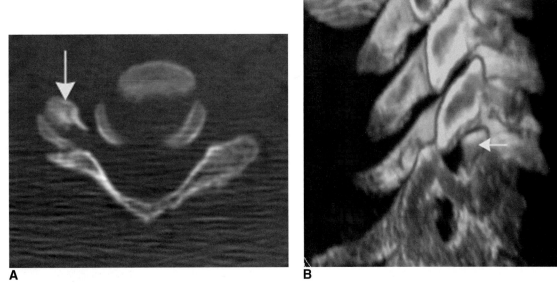

Fig. 4-118
Unilateral facet fracture-dislocation. **A**, Axial CT image shows a three-part right-sided facet fracture with subluxation. The most anterior fragment (*arrow*) is a free fragment from one articular process. **B**, Volume-rendered view from lateral perspective confirms facet dislocation, with a free fragment anteriorly (*arrow*).

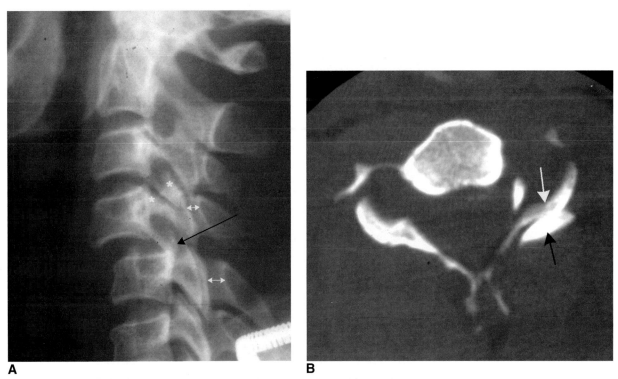

Fig. 4-119
Unilateral facet dislocation. **A**, A lateral cervical spine radiograph shows anterolisthesis of C4-5 with about 30% displacement. The articular pillars are offset from C4 and above (*asterisks*) but nearly superimposed below, indicating a rotational component. Also, the laminar space changes abruptly between C4 and C5 (*two-headed arrows*), also indicating sudden rotation. The locked facet joint is marked with a *black arrow*. A widened interspinous distance also marks the level of the unilateral facet dislocation. **B**, An axial view through one dislocated facet joint shows the "reverse hamburger buns" sign. The rounded, nonarticulating surfaces of the articular processes are opposed, while the flat articular surfaces face outward. Inferior left articular process of C4 (*white arrow*) and superior process of C5 (*black arrow*). The contralateral articular processes are not in contact at this axial level due to subluxation.

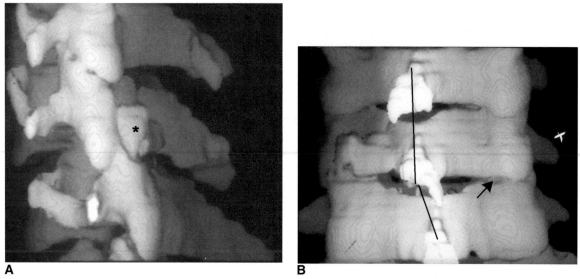

Fig. 4-120
Unilateral facet fracture-subluxation., Lateral (**A**) and posterior (**B**) volumetric image perspectives show a superior articular process "impaling" the adjacent right superior articular process and producing a fracture (*asterisk*) from the articular pillar to the lamina. Note the abrupt offset of the spinous processes at the injury level (*black lines*) and diastasis of the contralateral facet joint (*black arrow*). (From Shanmuganathan K, Mirvis SE, Levine AM: *AJR Am J Roentgenol* 163:1165, 1994.)

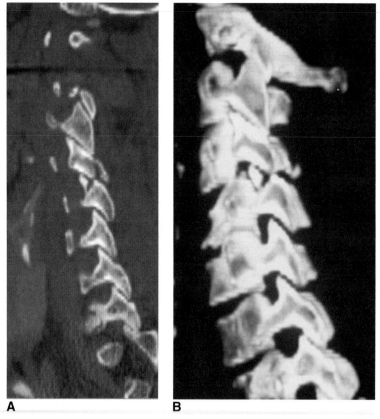

Fig. 4-121
Unilateral facet fracture-subluxation. **A,** Parasagittal CT multiplanar reformation image shows unilateral facet fracture subluxation at C4-5, with fractures of both articular pillars caused by impingement of the adjacent articular process. **B,** Volume-rendered lateral view shows a free bone fragment arising from the C5 articular pillar in the adjacent neural foramen.

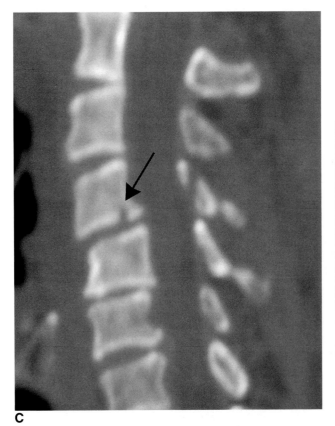

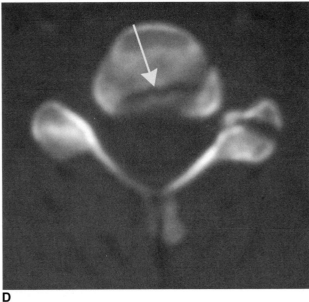

Fig. 4-121, cont'd
C, Midsagittal CT multiplanar reformation shows a posterior avulsion fracture from the C4 posterior cortex (*arrow*) that is not uncommon with rotational displacement. **D,** Axial CT through the lower C4 level shows the same avulsion fracture (*arrow*) and widening of the left C4-5 facet articulation.

bilateral facet dislocation in 3 (14%).[286] Only 1 patient (7%) had an extension-rotation pattern. Importantly, 19 of the 21 patients (90%) had fractures which extended across the ipsilateral foramen transversarium, 14 (67%) had contralateral osseous injury, and 13 (62%) had a neurologic deficit, including 10 with spinal cord syndromes and 3 with radiculopathy.[286] In most cases of IAP, the fracture of the articular pillar was oriented vertically, in keeping with a pattern of flexion, rotation, and axial loading. Bilateral IAP injury occurs (see Fig. 4-123) but was not seen in this study. Woodring et al.[287] observed that articular process fractures, in general, are isolated but often occur concurrently with unilateral facet or bilateral facet dislocation.[287]

The mechanism of injury proposed in the study by Shanmuganathan et al.[286] suggests that as hyperflexion occurs, the inferior articular process above the injury level moves anteriorly and impacts against the subja-

cent superior articular facet of the injured level. Simultaneously, the inferior articular process of the injured level moves anteriorly and impacts the superior articular process of the subjacent vertebra (Fig. 4-125). Both forces act to rotate the articular pillar by placing stress on the connecting lamina and pedicle. If there is sufficient flexion and axial loading force, the lamina and pedicle will fracture, permitting the pillar to rotate. Fractures, usually vertically oriented, can occur among any of the involved articular processes. Typically, other flexion-rotation displacement injuries will be concurrent with the IAP.

The articular facet joints normally are inclined about 35 degrees[283] from the horizontal plane. Thus, an AP view does not show the joint space unless the beam is angled such as for a pillar view. If the pillar is isolated, it can rotate into a position in which the joint space is more horizontally oriented so that the joint is visualized directly on the AP view (see Figs. 4-15 and 4-124). Detection of associated fractures into the lamina, pedicle, or transverse process is difficult radiographically due to usual minimal displacement and overlapping bone. Fractures associated with IAP are seen best by CT.[281] It is important to appreciate the transverse foraminal fracture to exclude vertebral artery injury. As is seen commonly with all types of rotatory facet displacement injuries, there is often disruption of the intervertebral disc, with possible herniation and ligament injury at the level of the

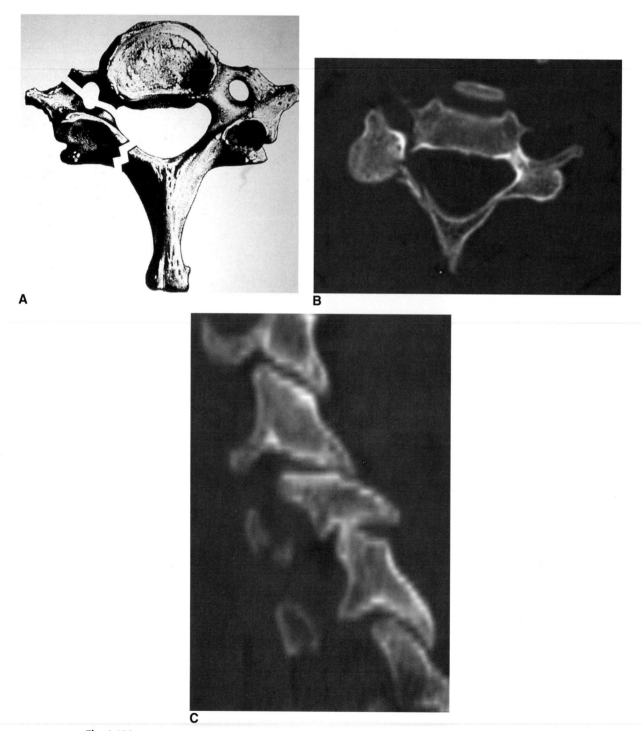

Fig. 4-122
Isolated articular pillar (IAP) or laminopedicular separation. **A,** Typical IAP showing laminar and ipsilateral pedicle fracture that crosses foramen transversarium. **B,** Axial CT shows example of IAP on the right. **C,** Parasagittal CT multiplanar reformation indicates rotation and malalignment of IAP, with horizontally oriented joint.

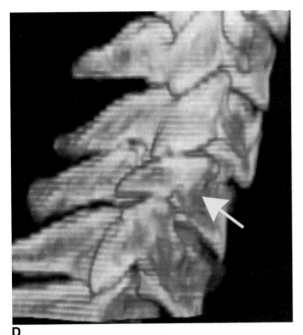

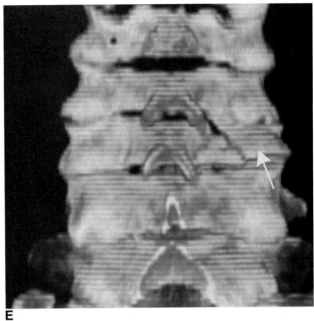

D   E

Fig. 4-122, cont'd
D, Volume-rendered image from a lateral perspective shows same finding (*arrow*). **E**, Posterior perspective of volume image shows right lamina fracture and articular pillar rotation (*arrow*). (From Shanmuganathan K, Mirvis SE, Dowe M, Levine AM: *AJR Am J Roentgenol* 166:897, 1996.)

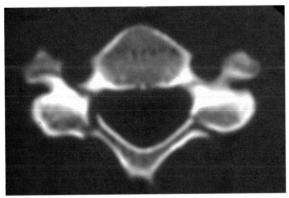

Fig. 4-123
Bilateral isolated articular pillars. Axial CT image shows laminar and bilateral pedicle fractures isolating both articular pillars. (From Shanmuganathan K, Mirvis SE, Levine AM: *AJR Am J Roentgenol* 163:1165, 1994.)

IAP. Both are best appreciated by MRI (see Fig. 4-124). The IAP injury creates instability laterally at three contiguous levels and requires a three-level lateral fixation for stabilization (Fig. 4-126).[286]

Imaging Spinal Trauma in Preexisting Pathologic Conditions

Patients with degenerative changes (spondylosis) of the cervical spine can experience vertebral anterolisthesis or retrolisthesis on lateral cervical radiographs which may

mimic the appearance of hyperflexion or hyperextension subluxation. It is not unusual for the apparent vertebral body displacement to exceed 5 mm or more. Lee et al.[288] have shown that patients with degenerative olisthesis usually will exhibit narrowed facet joints due to worn-down cartilage and thinning of the articular facets (see Fig. 4-26), while patients with traumatic olisthesis have normal or widened facet joints or facet fractures. Asymmetric loss of height from the anterior portion of the intervertebral disc at the level with facet joint degeneration favors anterolisthesis, while asymmetric substance loss of the posterior disc favors retrolisthesis.[289]

Trauma patients with various conditions that lead to fusion of the spine are at increased risk for spinal injury compared with patients with normal spine mobility. Patients with ankylosing spondylitis can sustain spinal injury from minimal amounts of blunt force impact. Because the spine has undergone bony ankylosis, it is very fragile and will fracture equally easily across the bone or disc spaces. Usually these injuries completely traverse all supporting ossified spinal ligaments, creating marked instability (Figs. 4-127 to 4-129). In the author's experience, these injuries typically are evident in extension or extension-dislocation patterns. It has been noted that spinal fractures among patients with underlying ankylosing spondylitis are not uncommonly occult radiographically. Fractures and dislocations most typically occur in the lower cervical spine, followed by the thoracic spine. This may occur due to spontaneous reduction of

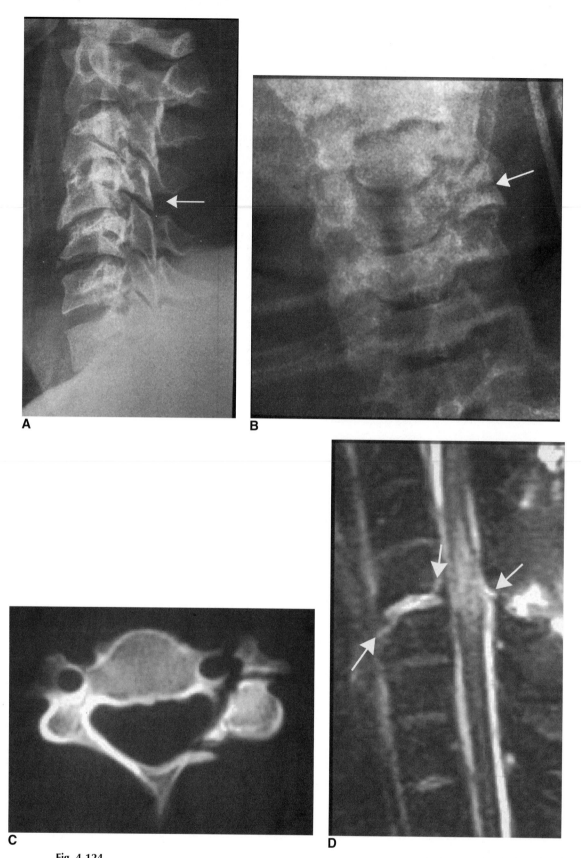

Fig. 4-124
Isolated articular pillar. **A**, Lateral cervical radiograph in blunt trauma patient with paralysis shows widened interlaminar and interspinous space at C4-5 (*arrow*), narrowing of the disc space, and loss of anterior height of C5. There is diffuse prevertebral soft tissue edema. **B**, The anteroposterior radiograph shows rotation of the left C4 articular pillar (*arrow*), with visualization of the facet joints. **C**, Axial CT shows left C4 lamina and pedicle fracture with transverse process extension typical of isolated articular pillar. **D**, Midsagittal inversion recovery MR image shows disruption of all major ligamentous supports (*arrows*) and a large cord contusion.

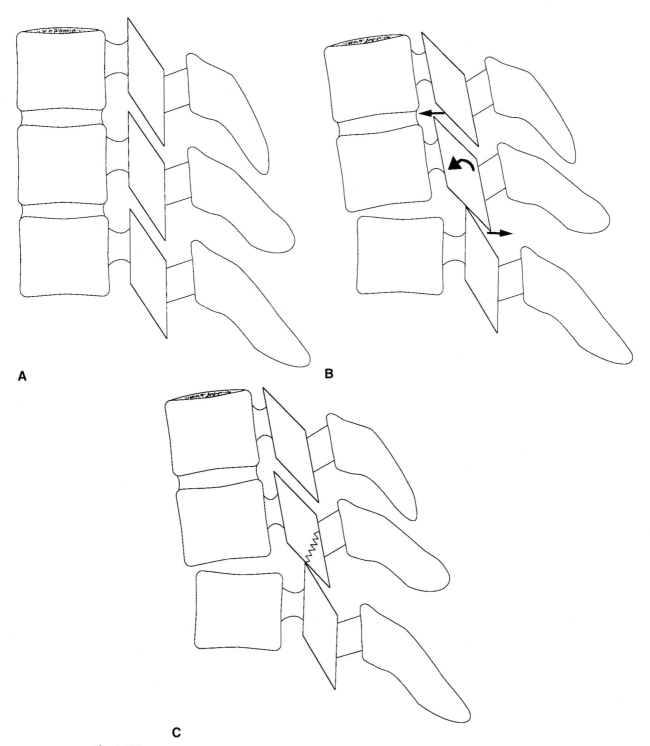

A

B

C

Fig. 4-125
Mechanism of isolated articular pillar fracture from flexion stress. **A**, Normal arrangement of artic-ular pillars from lateral view. **B**, A flexion force applies torque to the middle vertebral body by appli-cation of forward motion by the inferior articular process above against the superior articular process below. **C**, Depending on the relative forces (vectors) of forward movement and distraction, a fracture-dislocation or fracture-subluxation can result. Alternatively, the torque can result in both pedicle and laminar fractures, allowing rotation of the articular pillar. (From Shanmuganathan K, Mirvis SE, Dowe M, Levine AM: *AJR Am J Roentgenol* 166:897, 1996.)

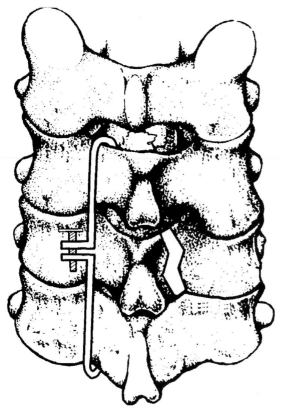

Fig. 4-126
Three-level fixation is required for proper management of the isolated articular pillar injury. (From Shanmuganathan K, Mirvis SE, Dowe M, Levine AM: *AJR Am J Roentgenol* 166:897, 1996.)

the fracture, generalized osteoporosis that often occurs in patients with advanced disease, and failure to appreciate second, noncontiguous injuries. Although patients with ankylosing spondylitis may have well-established neurologic deficits and obvious imaging abnormalities, about one third have a delayed onset of neurologic deficits as a result of failure to diagnose or properly immobilize the very unstable spine. In general, patients who suffer blunt trauma and have ankylosing spondylitis should be regarded as having unstable injuries until definitely proven otherwise. If radiographs appear normal, further evaluation by thin-section CT is recommended to detect subtle fractures. CT may also assist in differentiating acute fractures from pseudoarthrosis related to previous injury. If the patient has cervical pain, further assessment by MRI to detect subtle soft tissue edema or bone marrow edema is indicated, also, so as not to misdiagnose a highly unstable injury.

Other preexisting conditions which may cause an increased risk of spinal fracture with lower energy blunt trauma include DISH, also called *Forestier disease, ankylosing hyperostosis, spinal spondylosis,* and *osteoporosis.* DISH is similar to ankylosing spondylitis in the sense that the spine contains a segment of bony fusion. DISH may be differentiated from ankylosing spondylitis by the absence of squared vertebral body corners, the larger, coarser, and predominantly anterior syndesmophytes of DISH, and lack of sacroiliac and apophyseal changes that occur in ankylosing spondylitis. Fractures in DISH may occur through the midportion of a fused segment or at the top or bottom through a disc space or odontoid process. The long lever arm created by the fused segment focuses all the energy of the applied force onto a single disc space, increasing the risk of injury. Similarly, spines fused due to multiple contiguous levels of degenerative spondylosis also are at increased risk for injury because of inability to distribute straining forces across multiple spinal levels.

Patients with severe osteoporosis are at increased risk for fracture from minor injury or activities of daily living. In the spine, such injuries may appear as minor loss of height of a vertebral body. The age of this injury may not be apparent and it may be assumed in some cases to be a remote lesion. Compression fractures in patients with structural bone weakness can progress to significant compression with physiologic loading and acute or delayed onset of radicular deficits or complete neurologic deficits. The lack of density of demineralized bone associated with suboptimal film technique renders radiographic interpretation of the spine difficult and insensitive to detection of subtle fractures. If the patient has persistent spinal pain, examination by thin-section CT is recommended initially. This often will demonstrate subtle endplate fractures and paraspinal hematoma not detected by radiography. If clinical symptoms remain unexplained or CT is not definitive, MRI is suggested. MRI will show paraspinal edema, hematoma, and bone edema with high sensitivity, improving the level of confidence for injury detection or exclusion. Nuclear bone scintigraphy also can play a role in diagnosing fractures in this setting. However, acute fractures may not have abnormal bone turnover activity during the acute phase, particularly in the elderly. Also, foci of increased nuclide deposition in the spine may be due to chronic abnormalities such as seen with spondylosis or subacute injuries, as well as acute pathology, making this examination less useful. In general, very careful attention to imaging these subsets of patients combined with a low threshold to perform additional diagnostic studies in symptomatic patients is warranted.

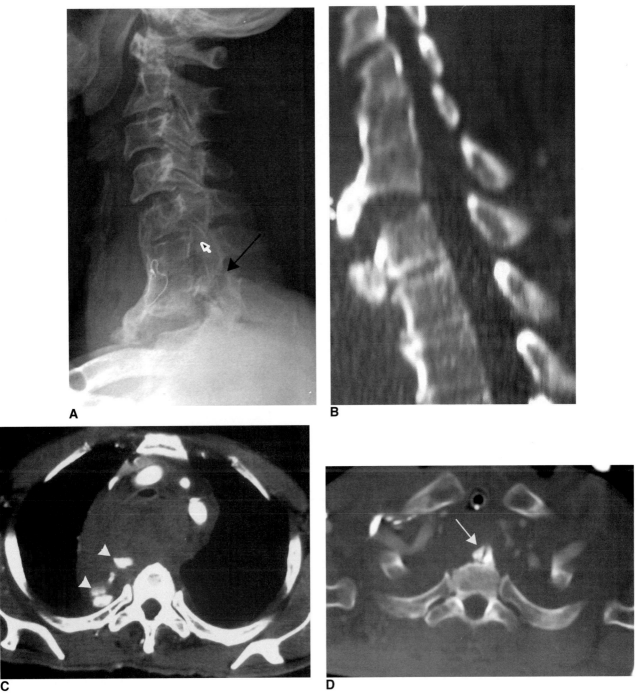

Fig. 4-127

Hyperextension of fused cervical spine. **A**, Lateral cervical radiograph of elderly blunt trauma patient shows fusion of the lower three vertebral bodies, a fractured prominent osteophyte at C7-T1, and an extension-distraction injury at C7-T1. There is a fracture plane obliquely crossing one or both laminae of C7 (*black arrow*). Note marked prevertebral swelling. Ignore small arrow in image. **B**, The parasagittal CT multiplanar reformation verifies fusion of lower cervical vertebrae, extension-distraction injury at C7-T1, and laminar fracture. **C**, Upper thoracic axial CT shows huge mediastinal hematoma, with sites of active bleeding (*arrowheads*). Angiography was negative for bleeding sites from major arteries in the region, but upper intercostal arteries were not studied. The bleeding ceased without direct intervention and the patient remained stable. **D**, The very sharp anterior osteophyte (*arrow*) was suspected of injuring adjacent artery at time of trauma.

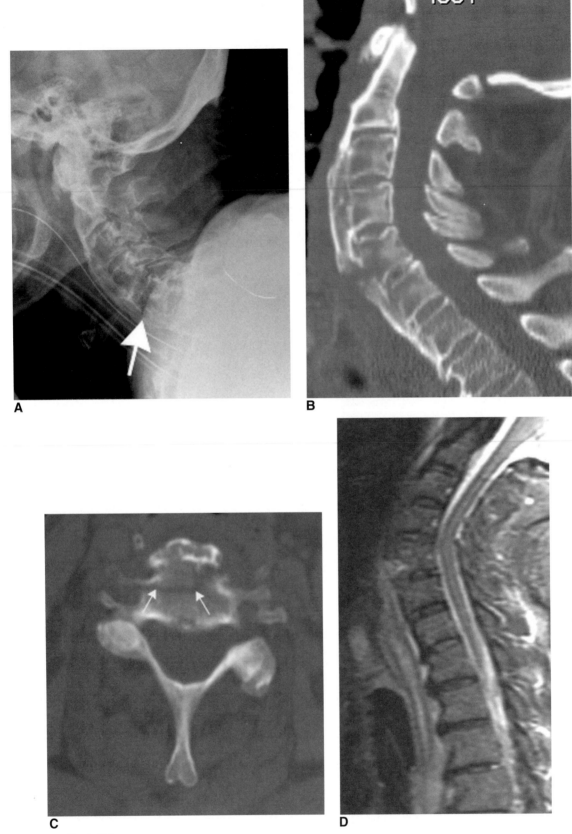

Fig. 4-128
Extension injury in cervical ankylosing spondylitis. **A**, Lateral cervical radiograph of blunt trauma patient shows bridging anterior osteophytes in a flowing pattern consistent with ankylosing spondylitis. There is a fracture through the C5 body (*arrow*). **B**, Midsagittal CT multiplanar reformation shows fracture plane across C5 through anterior osteophyte. **C**, Axial CT shows fracture line (*arrows*). **D**, Midsagittal T2-weighted MR image shows intact cord and spinal canal at injury level.

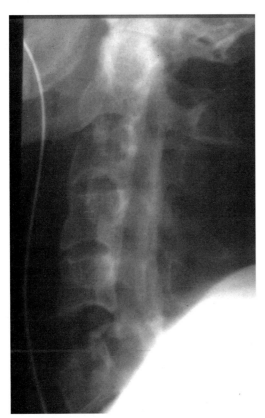

Fig. 4-129
Extension injury in a patient with cervical ankylosing spondylitis. Note bony fusion along anterior vertebral bodies and facet joints. Fracture occurs through the C5-6 disc.

REFERENCES

1. Diliberti T, Lindsey RW: Evaluation of the cervical spine in the emergency setting: who does not need an X-ray? *Orthopedics* 15:179, 1992.
2. MacDonald RL, Schwartz ML, Mirich D, et al: Diagnosis of cervical spine injury in motor vehicle crash victims: how many X-rays are enough? *J Trauma* 30:392, 1990.
3. Rizzolo SJ, Vaccaro AR, Cotler JM: Cervical spine trauma, *Spine* 19:2288, 1994.
4. Ross SE, Schwab CW, David ET, et al: Clearing the cervical spine: initial radiologic evaluation, *J Trauma* 27:1055, 1987.
5. Harris JH Jr: The normal cervical spine. In Harris JH Jr, Mirvis SE, eds: *The radiology of acute cervical spine trauma*, ed 3, Baltimore, 1996, Williams & Wilkins.
6. Seybold EA, Dunn EJ, Jenis LG, Sweeney CA: Variation in the posterior vertebral contour line at the level of C-2 on lateral cervical roentgenograms: a method for odontoid fracture detection, *Am J Orthop* 28:696, 1999.
7. Young WF, Rosenwasser RH, Getch C, Jallo J: Diagnosis and management of occipital condyle fractures, *Neurosurgery* 34:257, 1994.
8. Herr CH, Ball PA, Sargent SK, Quinton HB: Sensitivity of prevertebral soft tissue measurement of C3 for detection of cervical spine fractures and dislocations, *Am J Emerg Med* 16:346, 1998.
9. Templeton PA, Young JW, Mirvis SE, Buddemeyer EU: The value of retropharyngeal soft tissue measurements in trauma of the adult cervical spine. Cervical spine soft tissue measurements, *Skeletal Radiol* 16:98, 1987.
10. Harris JH Jr: Abnormal cervicocranial retropharyngeal soft tissue contour in the detection of subtle acute cervicocranial injuries, *Emerg Radiol* 7:11, 2000.
11. Harris JH, Burke JT, Ray RD, et al: Low (type III) odontoid fracture: a new radiographic sign, *Radiology* 153:353, 1984.
12. Benzel EC, Hart BL, Ball PA, et al: Fractures of the C-2 vertebral body, *J Neurosurg* 81:206, 1994.
13. Anderson LD, D'Alonzo RT: Fractures of the odontoid process of the axis, *J Bone Joint Surg Am* 56:1663, 1974.
14. Harris JH, Carson GC, Wagner LK: Radiologic diagnosis of traumatic occipitovertebral dissociation: 1. Normal occipitovertebral relationships on lateral radiographs of supine subjects, *AJR Am J Roentgenol* 162:881, 1994.
15. Harris JH, Carson GC, Wagner LK, Kerr N: Radiologic diagnosis of traumatic occipitovertebral dissociation: 2. Comparison of three methods of detecting occipitovertebral relationships on lateral radiographs of supine subjects, *AJR Am J Roentgenol* 162:887, 1994.
16. Powers B, Miller MD, Kramer RS, et al: Traumatic anterior atlanto-occipital dislocation, *Neurosurgery* 4:12, 1979.
17. Christenson PC: The radiologic study of the normal spine, *Radiol Clin North Am* 15:133, 1977.
18. Dickman CA, Mamourian A, Sonntag VK, Drayer BP: Magnetic resonance imaging of the transverse atlantal ligament for the evaluation of atlantoaxial instability, *J Neurosurg* 75:221, 1991.
19. Warner J, Shanmuganathan K, Mirvis SE, et al: Magnetic resonance imaging of ligamentous injury of the cervical spine, *Emerg Radiol* 3:9, 1996.
20. Shanmuganathan K, Mirvis SE, Levine AM: Rotational injury of cervical facets: CT analysis of fracture patterns with implications for management and neurologic outcome, *AJR Am J Roentgenol* 163:1165, 1994.
21. Forsyth HF: Extension injuries of the cervical spine, *J Bone Joint Surg Br* 46:1792, 1964.
22. Holliman CJ, Mayer JS, Cook RT Jr, Smith JS Jr: Is the anteroposterior cervical spine radiograph necessary in initial trauma screening? *Am J Emerg Med* 9:421, 1991.
23. West OC, Anbari MM, Pilgram TK, Wilson AJ: Acute cervical spine trauma: diagnostic performance of single-view versus three-view radiographic screening, *Radiology* 204:819, 1997.
24. Iannacone WM, DeLong WG Jr, Born CT, et al: Dynamic computerized tomography of the occiput-atlas-axis complex in trauma patients with odontoid lateral mass asymmetry, *J Trauma* 30:1501, 1990.
25. Thomeier WC, Brown DC, Mirvis SE: The laterally tilted dens: a sign of subtle odontoid fracture on plain radiography, *AJNR Am J Neuroradiol* 11:605, 1990.
26. Murray JB, Ziervogel M: The value of computed tomography in the diagnosis of atlanto-axial rotatory fixation, *Br J Radiol* 63:894, 1990.
27. Lee C, Woodring JH: Unstable Jefferson variant atlas fractures: an unrecognized cervical injury, *AJNR Am J Neuroradiol* 12:1105, 1991.
28. Ireland AJ, Britton I, Forrester AW: Do supine oblique views provide better imaging of the cervicothoracic junction than swimmer's views? *J Accid Emerg Med* 15:15, 1996.
29. Jenkins MG, Curran P, Rocke LG: Where do we go after the three standard cervical spine views in the conscious trauma patient? A survey, *Eur J Emerg Med* 6:215, 1999.
30. Bettinger BI, Eisenberg RL: Improved swimmer's lateral projection of the cervicothoracic region, *AJR Am J Roentgenol* 164:1303, 1995.
31. Weir DC: Roentgenographic signs of cervical injury, *Clin Orthop* 109:9, 1975.
32. Lee C, Woodring JH, Rogers LF, Kim KS: The radiographic distinction of degenerative slippage (spondylolisthesis and retrolisthesis) from traumatic slippage of the cervical spine, *Skeletal Radiol* 15:439, 1986.

33. Grossman MD, Reilly PM, Gillett T, Gillett D: National survey of the incidence of cervical spine injury and approach to cervical spine clearance in U.S. trauma centers, *J Trauma* 47:684, 1999.

34. Brady WJ, Moghtader J, Cutcher D, et al: ED use of flexion-extension cervical spine radiography in the evaluation of blunt trauma, *Am J Emerg Med* 17:504, 1999.

35. Knopp R, Parker J, Tashjian J, Ganz W: Defining radiographic criteria for flexion-extension studies of the cervical spine, *Ann Emerg Med* 38:31, 2001.

36. Wang JC, Hatch JD, Sandhu HS, Delamarter RB: Cervical flexion and extension radiographs in acutely injured patients, *Clin Orthop* 8:111, 1999.

37. Dwek JR, Chung CB: Radiography of cervical spine injury in children: are flexion-extension radiographs useful for acute trauma? *AJR Am J Roentgenol* 174:1617, 2000.

38. Acheson MB, Livingston RR, Richardson ML, Stimac GK: High-resolution CT scanning in the evaluation of cervical spine fractures: comparison with plain film examinations, *AJR Am J Roentgenol* 148:1179, 1987.

39. Angtuaco EJ, Binet EF: Radiology of thoracic and lumbar fractures, *Clin Orthop* 189:43, 1984.

40. Bauer RD, Errico TJ, Waugh TR, Cohen W: Evaluation and diagnosis of cervical spine injuries: a review of the literature, *Cent Nerv Syst Trauma* 4:71, 1987.

41. Dorwar RH, LaMasters DL: Applications of computed tomographic scanning of the cervical spine, *Orthop Clin North Am* 16:381, 1985.

42. Ebraheim NA, Rupp RE, Savolaine ER, Reinke D: Use of titanium implants in pedicular screw fixation, *J Spinal Disord* 7:478, 1994.

43. Handel SF, Lee YY: Computed tomography of spinal fractures, *Radiol Clin North Am* 19:69, 1981.

44. Harris JH Jr: Radiographic evaluation of spinal trauma, *Orthop Clin North Am* 17:75, 1986.

45. Lynch D, McManus F, Ennis JT: Computed tomography in spinal trauma, *Clin Radiol* 37:71, 1986.

46. McAfee PC, Yuan HA, Fredrickson BE, Lubicky JP: The value of computed tomography in thoracolumbar fractures. An analysis of one hundred consecutive cases and a new classification, *J Bone Joint Surg Am* 65:461, 1983.

47. Post MJ, Green BA: The use of computed tomography in spinal trauma, *Radiol Clin North Am* 21:327, 1983.

48. Post MJ, Green BA, Quencer RM, et al: The value of computed tomography in spinal trauma, *Spine* 7:417, 1982.

49. Erb R, Schucany WG, Shanmuganathan K, et al: Extension corner avulsion fractures of the cervical spine, *Emerg Radiol* 3:96, 1996.

50. Nunez D Jr: Value of complete cervical helical computed tomographic scanning in identifying cervical spine injury in the unevaluable blunt trauma patient with multiple injuries: a prospective study, *J Trauma* 48:988, 2000.

51. Clayman DA, Sykes CH, Vines FS: Occipital condyle fractures: clinical presentation and radiologic detection, *AJNR Am J Neuroradiol* 15:1309, 1994.

52. Brant-Zawadski MH, Minagi H: CT in the evaluation of spine trauma. In Federle MP, ed: *Computed tomography in the evaluation of trauma*, Baltimore, 1982, Williams & Wilkins.

53. Cooper PR, Cohen W: Evaluation of cervical spinal cord injuries with metrizamide myelography-CT scanning, *J Neurosurg* 61:281, 1984.

54. Kaufman HH, Harris JH Jr, Spencer JA, et al: Metrizamide-enhanced computed tomography and newer techniques of myelography. In Bailey RW, Sherk HH, Dunn EJ, et al, eds: *The cervical spine*, Philadelphia, 1983, Lippincott.

55. Leo JS, Bergeron RT, Kricheff II, Benjamin MV: Metrizamide myelography for cervical spinal cord injuries, *Radiology* 129:707, 1978.

56. Streiter ML, Chambers AA: Metrizamide examination of traumatic lumbar nerve root meningocele, *Spine* 9:77, 1984.

57. Morris RE, Hasso AN, Thompson JR, et al: Traumatic dural tears: CT diagnosis using metrizamide, *Radiology* 152:443, 1984.

58. Kassel EE, Cooper PW, Rubenstein JD: Radiology of spinal trauma—practical experience in a trauma unit, *J Can Assoc Radiol* 34:189, 1983.

59. Denis F, Burkus JK: Diagnosis and treatment of cauda equina entrapment in the vertical lamina fracture of lumbar burst fractures, *Spine* 16(suppl 8):433, 1991.

60. Herman GT, Liu HK: Display of three-dimensional information in computed tomography, *J Comput Assist Tomogr* 1:155, 1977.

61. Vannier MW, Marsh JL, Warren JO: Three- dimensional CT reconstruction images for craniofacial surgical planning and evaluation, *Radiology* 150:179, 1984.

62. Banna, M: *Clinical radiology of the spine and spinal canal*, Rockville, Md, 1985, Aspen Systems Corporation.

63. Hall AJ, Wagle VG, Raycroft J, et al: Magnetic resonance imaging in cervical spine trauma, *J Trauma* 34:21, 1993.

64. Kulkarni MV, McArdle CB, Kopanicky D, et al: Acute spinal cord injury: MR imaging at 1.5 T, *Radiology* 164:837, 1987.

65. Mirvis SE, Geisler FH, Jelinek JJ, et al: Acute cervical spine trauma: evaluation with 1.5-T MR imaging, *Radiology* 166:807, 1988.

66. Mirvis SE, Nessavier M: MRI of cervical spine trauma. In Harris JH Jr, Mirvis SE eds: *The radiology of acute cervical spine trauma*, ed 3, Baltimore, 1996, Williams & Wilkins.

67. Modic MT, Masaryk TJ, Ross JS: *Magnetic resonance imaging of the spine*, ed 3, Chicago, 1989, Year Book Medical.

68. Pomerantz SJ: *Craniospinal magnetic resonance imaging*, Philadelphia, 1989, WB Saunders.

69. Tarr RW, Drolshagen LF, Kerner TC, et al: MR imaging of recent spinal trauma, *J Comput Assist Tomogr* 11:412, 1987.

70. Killeen KL, Shanmuganathan K, Lefkowitz D, et al: Inversion recovery versus T2-weighted sagittal MR imaging in cervical cord injury, *Emerg Radiol* 8:15, 2001.

71. Katzberg RW, Benedetti PF, Drake CM, et al: Acute cervical spine injuries: prospective MR imaging assessment at a level 1 trauma center, *Radiology* 213:203, 1999.

72. McArdle CB, Nicholas DA, Richardson CJ, Amparo EG: Monitoring of the neonate undergoing MR imaging: technical considerations. Work in progress, *Radiology* 159:223, 1986.

73. McArdle CB, Wright JW, Prevost WJ, et al: MR imaging of the acutely injured patient with cervical traction, *Radiology* 159:273, 1986.

74. Mirvis SE, Borg U, Belzberg H: MR imaging of ventilator-dependent patients: preliminary experience, *AJR Am J Roentgenol* 149:845, 1987.

75. Shellock FG, Lipczak H, Kanall E: Monitoring patients during MR procedures, *Appl Radiol* 24:11, 1995.

76. Shellock FG, Morisoli S, Kanal E: MR procedures and biomedical implants, materials, and devices: 1993 update, *Radiology* 189:587, 1993.

77. Davis SJ, Teresi LM, Bradley WG Jr, et al: Cervical spine hyperextension injuries: MR findings, *Radiology* 180:245, 1991.

78. Bradley WG Jr: MR appearance of hemorrhage in the brain, *Radiology* 189:15, 1993.

79. Chakeres DW, Flickinger F, Bresnahan JC, et al: MR imaging of acute spinal cord trauma, *AJNR Am J Neuroradiol* 8:5, 1987.

80. Flanders AE, Schaefer DM, Doan HT, et al: Acute cervical spine trauma: correlation of MR imaging findings with degree of neurologic deficit, *Radiology* 177:25, 1990.

81. Mascalchi M, Dal Pozzo G, Dini C, et al: Acute spinal trauma: prognostic value of MRI appearances at 0.5 T, *Clin Radiol* 48:100, 1993.

82. Schaefer DM, Flanders AE, Osterholm JL, Northrup BE: Prognostic significance of magnetic resonance imaging in the acute phase of cervical spine injury, *J Neurosurg* 76:218, 1992.

83. Quencer RM, Bunge RP, Egnor M, et al: Acute traumatic central cord syndrome: MRI-pathological correlations, *Neuroradiology* 34:85, 1992.

84. Weirich SD, Cotler HB, Narayana PA, et al: Histopathologic correlation of magnetic resonance imaging signal patterns in a spinal cord injury model, *Spine* 15:630, 1990.

85. Brightman RP, Miller CA, Rea GL, et al: Magnetic resonance imaging of trauma to the thoracic and lumbar spine. The importance of the posterior longitudinal ligament, *Spine* 17:541, 1992.

86. Kerslake RW, Jaspan T, Worthington BS: Magnetic resonance imaging of spinal trauma, *Br J Radiol* 64:386, 1991.

87. Silberstein M, Tress BM, Hennessy O: Prevertebral swelling in cervical spine injury: identification of ligament injury with magnetic resonance imaging, *Clin Radiol* 46:318, 1992.

88. Warner J, Shanmuganathan K, Mirvis SE, et al: Magnetic resonance imaging of ligamentous injury of the cervical spine, *Emerg Radiol* 3:9, 1996.

88a. Rizzolo SJ, Piazza MR, Cotler JM, et al: Intervertebral disc injury complicating cervical spine trauma, *Spine* 16(6 Suppl):S187, 1991.

89. Doran SE, Papadopoulos SM, Ducker TB, Lillehei KO: Magnetic resonance imaging documentation of coexistent traumatic locked facets of the cervical spine and disc herniation, *J Neurosurg* 79:341, 1993.

90. Berrington NR, van Staden JF, Willers JG, van der Westhuizen J: Cervical intervertebral disc prolapse associated with traumatic facet dislocations, *Surg Neurol* 40:395, 1993.

91. Hall AJ, Wagle VG, Raycroft J, et al: Magnetic resonance imaging in cervical spine trauma, *J Trauma* 34:21, 1993.

92. Pratt ES, Green DA, Spengler DM: Herniated intervertebral discs associated with unstable spinal injuries, *Spine* 15:662, 1990.

93. Grant GA, Mirza SK, Chapman JR, et al: Risk of early closed reduction in cervical spine subluxation injuries, *J Neurosurg* 90(1 Suppl):13, 1999.

94. Garza-Mercado R: Traumatic extradural hematoma of the cervical spine, *Neurosurgery* 24:410, 1989.

95. Olshaker JS, Barish RA: Acute traumatic cervical epidural hematoma from a stab wound, *Ann Emerg Med* 20:662, 1991.

96. Regenbogen VS, Rogers LF, Atlas SW, Kim KS: Cervical spinal cord injuries in patients with cervical spondylosis, *AJR Am J Roentgenol* 146:277, 1986.

97. Koyanagi I, Iwasaki Y, Hida K, et al: Acute cervical cord injury without fracture or dislocation of the spinal column, *J Neurosurg* 93(suppl 1):15, 2000.

98. Taylor AR, Blackwood W: Paraplegia in hyperextension cervical injuries with normal radiographic appearance, *J Bone Joint Surg Br* 30:245, 1948.

99. Cheng CL, Wolf AL, Mirvis SE, Robinson WL: Bodysurfing accidents resulting in cervical spinal injuries, *Spine* 17:257, 1992.

100. Pathria MN, Petersilge CA: Spinal trauma, *Radiol Clin North Am* 29:847, 1991.

101. Quencer RM, Sheldon JJ, Post MJ, et al: MRI of the chronically injured cervical spinal cord, *AJR Am J Roentgenol* 147:125, 1986.

102. Takahashi M, Yamashita Y, Sakamoto Y, Kojima R: Chronic cervical cord compression: clinical significance of increased signal intensity on MR images, *Radiology* 173:219, 1989.

103. Castillo M, Harris JH Jr: MRI of the spine: recent applications, *Mediguide Orthop* 10, 1991.

104. Mirvis SE, Geisler F, Joslyn JN, Zrebeet H: Use of titanium wire in cervical spine fixation as a means to reduce MR artifacts, *AJNR Am J Neuroradiol* 9:1229, 1988.

105. Ebraheim NA, Rupp RE, Savolaine ER, Reinke D: Use of titanium implants in pedicular screw fixation, *J Spinal Disord* 7:478, 1994.

106. Deen HG Jr, McGirr SJ: Vertebral artery injury associated with cervical spine fracture. Report of two cases, *Spine* 17:230, 1992.

107. Demetriades D, Charalambides K, Chahwan S, et al: Nonskeletal cervical spine injuries: epidemiology and diagnostic pitfalls, *J Trauma* 48:724, 2000.

108. Gambee MJ: Vertebral artery thrombosis after spinal injury: case report, *Paraplegia* 24:350, 1986.

109. Giacobetti FB, Vaccaro AR, Bos-Giacobetti MA, et al: Vertebral artery occlusion associated with cervical spine trauma. A prospective analysis, *Spine* 22:188, 1997.

110. Jabre A: Subintimal dissection of the vertebral artery in subluxation of the cervical spine, *Neurosurgery* 29:912, 1991.

111. Parent AD, Harkey HL, Touchstone DA, et al: Lateral cervical spine dislocation and vertebral artery injury, *Neurosurgery* 31:501, 1992.

112. Vaccaro AR, Klein GR, Flanders AE, et al: Long term evaluation of vertebral artery injuries following cervical spine trauma using magnetic resonance imaging, *Spine* 23:789, 1998.

113. Reid JD, Weigelt JA: Forty-three cases of vertebral artery trauma, *J Trauma* 28:1007, 1988.

114. Schwarz N, Buchinger W, Gaudernak T, et al: Injuries to the cervical spine causing vertebral artery trauma: case reports, *J Trauma* 31:127, 1991.

115. Veras LM, Pedraza-Gutiérrez S, Castellanos J, et al: Vertebral artery occlusion after acute cervical spine trauma, *Spine* 25:1171, 2000.

116. Weller SJ, Rossitch E Jr, Malek AM: Detection of vertebral artery injury after cervical spine trauma using magnetic resonance angiography, *J Trauma* 46:660, 1999.

117. Biffl WL, Moore EE, Elliott JP, et al: The devastating potential of blunt vertebral arterial injuries, *Ann Surg* 231:672, 2000.

118. Price RF, Sellar R, Leung C, O'Sullivan MJ: Traumatic vertebral arterial dissection and vertebrobasilar arterial thrombosis successfully treated with endovascular thrombolysis and stenting, *AJNR Am J Neuroradiol* 19:1677, 1998.

119. Matin P: The appearance of bone scans following fractures, including immediate and long-term studies, *J Nucl Med* 20:1227, 1979.

120. Spitz J, Lauer I, Tittel K, Wiegand H: Scintillometric evaluation of remodeling after bone fractures in man, *J Nucl Med* 34:1403, 1993.

121. Barton D, Allen M, Finlay D, Belton I: Evaluation of whiplash injuries by technetium 99m isotope scanning, *Arch Emerg Med* 10:197, 1993.

122. Hildingsson C, Hietala SO, Toolanen G: Scintigraphic findings in acute whiplash injury of the cervical spine, *Injury* 20:265, 1989.

123. Wales LR, Knopp RK, Morishima MS: Recommendations for evaluation of the acutely injured cervical spine: a clinical radiologic algorithm, *Ann Emerg Med* 9:422, 1980.

124. Streitwieser DR, Knopp R, Wales LR, et al: Accuracy of standard radiographic views in detecting cervical spine fractures, *Ann Emerg Med* 12:538, 1983.

125. Mirvis SE, Diaconis JN, Chirico PA, et al: Protocol-driven radiologic evaluation of suspected cervical spine injury: efficacy study, *Radiology* 170:831, 1989.

126. Shaffer MA, Doris PE: Limitation of the cross table lateral view in detecting cervical spine injuries: a retrospective analysis, *Ann Emerg Med* 10:508, 1981.

127. Lewis LM, Docherty M, Ruoff BE, et al: Flexion-extension views in the evaluation of cervical spine injuries, *Ann Emerg Med* 20:117, 1991.

128. Nunez DB, Zuluaga A, Fuentes-Bernardo DA, et al: Cervical spine trauma: how much more do we learn by routinely using helical CT? *Radiographics* 16:1307, 1996.

129. Hanson JA, Blackmore CC, Mann FA, Wilson AJ: Cervical spine injury: a clinical decision rule to identify high-risk patients for helical CT screening, *AJR Am J Roentgenol* 174:713, 2000.

130. Berne JD, Velmahos GC, El-Tawil Q, et al: Value of complete cervical helical computed tomographic scanning in identifying cervical spine injury in the unevaluable blunt trauma patient with multiple injuries: a prospective study, *J Trauma* 47:896, 1999.

131. Blackmore CC, Ramsey SD, Mann FA, Deyo RA: Cervical spine screening with CT in trauma patients: a cost-effectiveness analysis, *Radiology* 212:117, 1999.

132. Daffner RH: Cervical radiography for trauma patients: a time-effective technique? *AJR Am J Roentgenol* 175:1309, 2000.

133. Leidner B, Adiels M, Aspelin P, et al: Standardized CT examination of the multitraumatized patient, *Eur Radiol* 8:1630, 1998.

134. D'Alise MD, Benzel EC, Hart BL: Magnetic resonance imaging evaluation of the cervical spine in the comatose or obtunded trauma patient, *J Neurosurg* 91(suppl 1):54, 1999.

135. Gupta KJ, Clancy M: Discontinuation of cervical spine immobilisation in unconscious patients with trauma in intensive care units—telephone survey of practice in south and west region, *BMJ* 314:1652, 1997.

136. Davis JW, Parks SN, Detlefs CL, et al: Clearing the cervical spine in obtunded patients: the use of dynamic fluoroscopy, *J Trauma* 39:435, 1995.

137. Scarrow AM, Levy EI, Resnick DK, et al: Cervical spine evaluation in obtunded or comatose pediatric trauma patients: a pilot study, *Pediatr Neurosurg* 30:169, 1999.

138. Sees DW, Rodriguez Cruz LR, Flaherty SF, Ciceri DP: The use of bedside fluoroscopy to evaluate the cervical spine in obtunded trauma patients, *J Trauma* 45:768, 1998.

139. Davis JW, Kaups KL, Cunningham MA, et al: Routine evaluation of the cervical spine in head-injured patients with dynamic fluoroscopy: a reappraisal, *J Trauma* 50:1044, 2001.

140. Dai L, Jia L: Central cord injury complicating acute cervical disc herniation in trauma, *Spine* 25:331, 2000.

141. Benzel EC, Hart BL, Ball PA, et al: Magnetic resonance imaging for the evaluation of patients with occult cervical spine injury, *J Neurosurg* 85:824, 1996.

142. Katzberg RW, Benedetti PF, Drake CM, et al: Acute cervical spine injuries: prospective MR imaging assessment at a level 1 trauma center, *Radiology* 213:203, 1999.

143. Klein GR, Vaccaro AR, Albert TJ, et al: Efficacy of magnetic resonance imaging in the evaluation of posterior cervical spine fractures, *Spine* 24:771, 1999.

144. Paleologos TS, Fratzoglou MM, Papadopoulos SS, et al: Posttraumatic spinal cord lesions without skeletal or discal and ligamentous abnormalities: the role of MR imaging, *J Spinal Disord* 11:346, 1998.

145. Fischer RP: Cervical radiographic evaluation of alert patients following blunt trauma, *Ann Emerg Med* 13:905, 1984.

146. Mace SE: Unstable occult cervical-spine fracture, *Ann Emerg Med* 20:1373, 1991.

147. McNamara RM, Heine E, Esposito B: Cervical spine injury and radiography in alert, high-risk patients, *J Emerg Med* 8:177, 1990.

148. Roth BJ, Martin RR, Foley K, et al: Roentgenographic evaluation of the cervical spine. A selective approach, *Arch Surg* 129:643, 1994.

149. Graber MA, Kathol M: Cervical spine radiographs in the trauma patient, *Am Fam Physician* 59:331, 1999.

150. Hoffman JR, Mower WR, Wolfson AB, et al: Validity of a set of clinical criteria to rule out injury to the cervical spine in patients with blunt trauma. National Emergency X-Radiography Utilization Study Group, *N Engl J Med* 343:94, 2000.

151. Zabel DD, Tinkoff G, Wittenborn W, et al: Adequacy and efficacy of lateral cervical spine radiography in alert, high-risk blunt trauma patient, *J Trauma* 43:952, 1997.

152. Gonzalez RP, Fried PO, Bukhalo M, et al: Role of clinical examination in screening for blunt cervical spine injury, *J Am Coll Surg* 189:152, 1999.

153. Ferrera PC, Bartfield JM: Traumatic atlanto-occipital dislocation: a potentially survivable injury, *Am J Emerg Med* 14:291, 1996.

154. DiBenedetto T, Lee CK: Traumatic atlanto-occipital instability: a case report with follow-up and a new diagnostic technique, *Spine* 15:595, 1990.

155. Shamoun JM, Riddick L, Powell RW: Atlanto-occipital subluxation/dislocation: a "survivable" injury in children, *Am Surgeon* 65:317, 1999.

156. Bools JC, Rose BS: Traumatic atlantooccipital dislocation: two cases with survival, *AJNR Am J Neuroradiol* 7:901, 1986.

157. Ahuja A, Glasauer FE, Alker GJ Jr, Klein DM: Radiology in survivors of traumatic atlanto-occipital dislocation, *Surg Neurol* 41:112, 1994.

158. Lee C, Woodring JH, Goldstein SJ, et al: Evaluation of traumatic atlantooccipital dislocations, *AJNR Am J Neuroradiol* 8:19, 1987.

159. Deliganis AV, Baxter AB, Hanson JA, et al: Radiologic spectrum of craniocervical distraction injuries, *Radiographics* S237, 2000.

160. Leone A, Cerase A, Colosimo C, et al: Occipital condylar fractures: a review, *Radiology* 216:635, 2000.

161. Bloom AI, Neeman Z, Floman Y, et al: Occipital condyle fracture and ligament injury: imaging by CT, *Pediatr Radiol* 26:786, 1996.

162. Bloom AI, Neeman Z, Slasky BS, et al: Fracture of the occipital condyles and associated craniocervical ligament injury: incidence, CT imaging and implications, *Clin Radiol* 52:198, 1997.

163. Stroobants J, Fidlers L, Storms JL, et al: High cervical pain and impairment of skull mobility as the only symptoms of an occipital condyle fracture. Case report, *J Neurosurg* 81:137, 1994.

164. Kelly A, Parrish R: Fracture of the occipital condyle: the forgotten part of the neck, *J Accid Emerg Med* 17:220, 2000.

165. Noble ER, Smoker WR: The forgotten condyle: the appearance, morphology, and classification of occipital condyle fractures, *AJNR Am J Neuroradiol* 17:507, 1996.

166. Urculo E, Arrazola M, Arrazola M Jr, et al: Delayed glossopharyngeal and vagus nerve paralysis following occipital condyle fracture. Case report, *J Neurosurg* 84:522, 1996.

167. Young WF, Rosenwasser RH, Getch C, Jallo J: Diagnosis and management of occipital condyle fractures, *Neurosurgery* 34:257, 1994.

168. Ide C, Nisolle JF, Misson N, et al: Unusual occipitoatlantal fracture dissociation with no neurological impairment. Case report, *J Neurosurg* 88:773, 1998.

169. Alker GJ Jr, Oh YS, Leslie EV: High cervical spine and craniocervical junction injuries in fatal traffic accidents: a radiological study, *Orthop Clin North Am* 9:1003, 1978.

170. Bucholz RW, Burkhead WZ: The pathological anatomy of fatal atlanto-occipital dislocations, *J Bone Joint Surg Am* 61:248, 1979.

171. Anderson PA, Montesano PX: Morphology and treatment of occipital condyle fractures, *Spine* 13:731, 1988.

172. Tuli S, Tator CH, Fehlings MG, Mackay M: Occipital condyle fractures, *Neurosurgery* 41:368, 1997.

173. Schweitzer ME, Hodler J, Cervilla V, Resnick D: Craniovertebral junction: normal anatomy with MR correlation, *AJR Am J Roentgenol* 158:1087, 1992.

174. Carter JW, Mirza SK, Tencer AF, Ching RP: Canal geometry changes associated with axial compressive cervical spine fracture, *Spine* 25:46, 2000.

175. Scher AT: The value of retropharyngeal swelling in the diagnosis of fractures of the Atlas, *S Afr Med J* 58:451, 1980.

176. Han SY, Witten DM, Mussleman JP: Jefferson fracture of the atlas. Report of six cases, *J Neurosurg* 44:368, 1976.

177. Kesterson L, Benzel E, Orrison W, Coleman J: Evaluation and treatment of atlas burst fractures (Jefferson fractures), *J Neurosurg* 75:213, 1991.

178. Fielding JW, Cochran G, Lawsing JF III, Hohl M: Tears of the transverse ligament of the atlas. A clinical and biomechanical study, *J Bone Joint Surg Am* 56:1683, 1974.

179. Scharen S, Jeanneret B: [Atlas fractures], *Orthopade* 28:385, 1999.

180. Song WS, Chiang YH, Chen CY, et al: A simple method for diagnosing traumatic occlusion of the vertebral artery at the craniovertebral junction, *Spine* 19:837, 1994.

181. Gehweiler JA, Daffner RH, Roberts L: Malformations of the atlas vertebra simulating the Jefferson fracture, *AJR Am J Roentgenol* 140:1083, 1983.

182. Suss RA, Zimmerman RD, Leeds NE: Pseudospread of the atlas: false sign of Jefferson fracture in young children, *AJR Am J Roentgenol* 140:1079, 1983.

183. Marlin AE, Williams GR, Lee JF: Jefferson fractures in children. Case report, *J Neurosurg* 58:277, 1983.

184. Moore KR, Frank EH: Traumatic atlantoaxial rotatory subluxation and dislocation, *Spine* 20:1928, 1995.

185. Iannacone WM, DeLong WG Jr, Born CT, et al: Dynamic computerized tomography of the occiput-atlas-axis complex in trauma patients with odontoid lateral mass asymmetry, *J Trauma* 30:1501, 1990.

186. Mirvis SE: How much lateral atlantodental interval asymmetry and atlantoaxial lateral mass asymmetry is acceptable on an open-mouth odontoid radiograph, and when is additional investigation necessary? *AJR Am J Roentgenol* 170:1106, 1998.

187. Maheshwaran S, Sgouros S, Jeyapalan K, et al: Imaging of childhood torticollis due to atlanto-axial rotatory fixation, *Childs Nerv Syst* 11:667, 1995.

188. Fielding JW, Hawkins RJ: Atlanto-axial rotatory fixation. (Fixed rotatory subluxation of the atlanto-axial joint), *J Bone Joint Surg Am* 59:37, 1977.

189. Kathol MH: Cervical spine trauma. What is new? *Radiol Clin North Am* 35:507, 1997.

190. Niibayashi H: Atlantoaxial rotatory dislocation: a case report, *Spine* 23:1494, 1998.

191. Greene KA, Dickman CA, Marciano FF, et al: Acute axis fractures: analysis of management and outcome in 340 consecutive cases, *Spine* 22:1843, 1997.

192. Hadley MN, Dickman CA, Browner CM, Sonntag VK: Acute axis fractures: a review of 229 cases, *J Neurosurg* 71:642, 1989.

193. Kokkino AJ, Lazio BE, Perin NI: Vertical fracture of the odontoid process: case report, *Neurosurgery* 38:200, 1996.

194. Anderson LD, D'Alonzo RT: Fractures of the odontoid process of the axis, *J Bone Joint Surg Am* 56:1663, 1974.

195. Scott EW, Haid RW Jr, Peace D: Type I fractures of the odontoid process: implications for atlanto-occipital instability. Case report, *J Neurosurg* 72:488, 1990.

196. Guiot B, Fessler RG: Complex atlantoaxial fractures, *J Neurosurg* 91(suppl 2):139, 1999.

197. Hanssen AD, Cabanela ME: Fractures of the dens in adult patients, *J Trauma* 27:928, 1987.

198. Blacksin MF, Lee HJ: Frequency and significance of fractures of the upper cervical spine detected by CT in patients with severe neck trauma, *AJR Am J Roentgenol* 165:1201, 1995.

199. Graziano G, Colon G, Hensinger R: Complete atlanto-axial dislocation associated with type II odontoid fracture: a report of two cases, *J Spinal Disord* 7:518, 1994.

200. Przybylski GJ, Welch WC: Longitudinal atlantoaxial dislocation with type III odontoid fracture. Case report and review of the literature, *J Neurosurg* 84:666, 1996.

201. Pepin JW, Bourne RB, Hawkins RJ: Odontoid fractures, with special reference to the elderly patient, *Clin Orthop* 193:178, 1985.

202. Ryan MD, Taylor TK: Odontoid fractures in the elderly, *J Spinal Disord* 6:397, 1993.

203. Muller EJ, Wick M, Russe O, Muhr G: Management of odontoid fractures in the elderly, *Eur Spine J* 8:360, 1999.

204. Clark CR, White AA III: Fractures of the dens: a multicenter study, *J Bone Joint Surg Am* 67:1340, 1985.

205. Lennarson PJ, Mostafavi H, Traynelis VC, Walters BC: Management of type II dens fractures: a case-control study, *Spine* 25:1234, 2000.

206. Crockard HA, Heilman AE, Stevens JM: Progressive myelopathy secondary to odontoid fractures: clinical, radiological, and surgical features, *J Neurosurg* 78:579, 1993.

207. Amling M, Hahn M, Wening VJ, et al: The microarchitecture of the axis as the predisposing factor for fracture of the base of the odontoid process: a histomorphometric analysis of twenty-two autopsy specimens, *J Bone Joint Surg Am* 76:1840, 1994.

208. Andrew WK, Wilkinson AE: Prevertebral soft-tissue swelling as a sign of undisplaced fracture of the odontoid process, *S Afr Med J* 53:672, 1978.

209. Thomeier WC, Brown DC, Mirvis SE: The laterally tilted dens: a sign of subtle odontoid fracture on plain radiography, *AJNR Am J Neuroradiol* 11:605, 1990.

210. Seybold EA, Dunn EJ, Jenis LG, Sweeney CA: Variation in the posterior vertebral contour line at the level of C-2 on lateral cervical roentgenograms: a method for odontoid fracture detection, *Am J Orthop* 28:696, 1999.

211. Swischuk LE, John SD, Hendrick EP: Is the open-mouth odontoid view necessary in children under 5 years? *Pediatr Radiol* 30:186, 2000.

212. Buhs C, Cullen M, Klein M, Farmer D: The pediatric trauma C-spine: is the "odontoid" view necessary? *J Pediatr Surg* 35:994, 2000.

213. Castillo M, Mukherji SK: Vertical fractures of the dens, *AJNR Am J Neuroradiol* 17:1627, 1996.

214. Hahnle UR, Wisniewski TF, Craig JB: Shear fracture through the body of the axis vertebra, *Spine* 24:2278, 1999.

215. Craig JB, Hodgson BF: Superior facet fractures of the axis vertebra, *Spine* 16:875, 1991.

216. Abel MS, Teague JH: Unilateral lateral mass compression fractures of the axis, *Skeletal Radiol* 4:92, 1979.

217. Hadley MN, Browner CM, Liu SS, Sonntag VK: New subtype of acute odontoid fractures (type IIA), *Neurosurgery* 22:67, 1988.

218. Glasser SA, Glasser ES: Rare congenital anomalies simulating upper cervical spine fractures, *J Emerg Med* 9:331, 1991.

219. Schwarz N, Putz R, Buchinger W: [Isolated ossicle of the dens axis. Case reports and differential diagnosis], *Unfallchirurg* 99:223, 1996.

220. Holt RG, Helms CA, Munk PL, Gillespy T III: Hypertrophy of C-1 anterior arch: useful sign to distinguish os odontoideum from acute dens fracture, *Radiology* 173:207, 1989.

221. Morandi X, Hanna A, Hamlat A, Brassier G: Anterior screw fixation of odontoid fractures, *Surg Neurol* 51:236, 1999.

222. Andersson S, Rodrigues M, Olerud C: Odontoid fractures: high complication rate associated with anterior screw fixation in the elderly, *Eur Spine J* 9:56, 2000.

223. Muller EJ, Wick M, Russe O, Muhr G: Management of odontoid fractures in the elderly, *Eur Spine J* 8:360, 1999.

224. Fielding JW, Francis WR Jr, Hawkins RJ, et al: Traumatic spondylolisthesis of the axis, *Clin Orthop* 239:47, 1989.

225. Mirvis SE, Young JW, Lim C, Greenberg J: Hangman's fracture: radiologic assessment in 27 cases, *Radiology* 163:713, 1987.

226. Roda JM, Castro A, Blazquez MG: Hangman's fracture with complete dislocation of C-2 on C-3. Case report, *J Neurosurg* 60:633, 1984.

227. Muller EJ, Wick M, Muhr G: Traumatic spondylolisthesis of the axis: treatment rationale based on the stability of the different fracture types, *Eur Spine J* 9:123, 2000.

228. Francis WR, Fielding JW, Hawkins RJ, et al: Traumatic spondylolisthesis of the axis, *J Bone Joint Surg Br* 63:313, 1981.

229. Hadley MN, Dickman CA, Browner CM, Sonntag VK: Acute axis fractures: a review of 229 cases, *J Neurosurg* 71:642, 1989.

230. Levine AM, Edwards CC: The management of traumatic spondylolisthesis of the axis, *J Bone Joint Surg Am* 67:217, 1985.

231. Veras LM, Pedraza-Gutiérrez S, Castellanos J, et al: Vertebral artery occlusion after acute cervical spine trauma, *Spine* 25:1171, 2000.

232. Effendi B, Roy D, Cornish B, et al: Fractures of the ring of the axis: a classification based on the analysis of 131 cases, *J Bone Joint Surg Br* 63:319, 1981.

233. Burke DC: Hyperextension injuries of the spine, *J Bone Joint Surg Br* 53:3, 1971.

234. Bucholz RW, Burkhead WZ: The pathological anatomy of fatal atlanto-occipital dislocations, *J Bone Joint Surg Am* 61:248, 1979.

235. Smoker WR, Dolan KD: The "fat" C2: a sign of fracture, *AJR Am J Roentgenol* 148:609, 1987.

236. Gleizes V, Jacquot FP, Signoret F, Feron JM: Combined injuries in the upper cervical spine: clinical and epidemiological data over a 14-year period, *Eur Spine J* 9:386, 2000.

237. Carter JW, Mirza SK, Tencer AF, Ching RP: Canal geometry changes associated with axial compressive cervical spine fracture, *Spine* 25:46, 2000.

238. Roaf R: A study of the mechanics of spinal injuries, *J Bone Joint Surg* 42B:810, 1960.

239. Sapkas G, Korres D, Babis GC, et al: Correlation of spinal canal post-traumatic encroachment and neurological deficit in burst fractures of the lower cervical spine (C3-7), *Eur Spine J* 4:39, 1995.

240. Chang DG, Tencer AF, Ching RP, et al: Geometric changes in the cervical spinal canal during impact, *Spine* 19:973, 1994.

241. Maiman DJ, Sances A Jr, Myklebust JB, et al: Compression injuries of the cervical spine: a biomechanical analysis, *Neurosurgery* 13:254, 1983.

242. Harris JH Jr: Mechanistic classification of cervical spine fractures. In Harris JH Jr, Mirvis SE, eds: *The radiology of acute cervical spine trauma*, ed 3, Baltimore, 1996, Williams & Wilkins.

243. Kiwerski J: Extension injuries of the cervical spine, *Chir Narzadow Ruchu Ortop Pol* 41:233, 1976.

244. Cintron E, Gilula LA, Murphy WA, Gehweiler JA: The widened disk space: a sign of cervical hyperextension injury, *Radiology* 141:639, 1981.

245. Scher AT: Hyperextension trauma in the elderly: an easily overlooked spinal injury, *J Trauma* 23:1066, 1983.

246. Shea M, Wittenberg RH, Edwards WT, et al: In vitro hyperextension injuries in the human cadaveric cervical spine, *J Orthop Res* 10:911, 1992.

247. Murray GC, Persellin RH: Cervical fracture complicating ankylosing spondylitis: a report of eight cases and review of the literature, *Am J Med* 70:1033, 1981.

248. Edeiken-Monroe B, Wagner LK, Harris JH Jr: Hyperextension dislocation of the cervical spine, *AJR Am J Roentgenol* 146:803, 1986.

249. Schweighofer F, Ranner G, Schleifer P, et al: [Hyperextension injury of the lower cervical spine and diagnosis of dorsal unstable motion segments], *Langenbecks Arch Chir* 380:162, 1995.

250. Le Hir PX, Sautet A, Le Gars L, et al: Hyperextension vertebral body fractures in diffuse idiopathic skeletal hyperostosis: a cause of intravertebral fluidlike collections on MR imaging, *AJR Am J Roentgenol* 173:1679, 1999.

251. Harris JH Jr, Yeakley JW: Hyperextension-dislocation of the cervical spine. Ligament injuries demonstrated by magnetic resonance imaging, *J Bone Joint Surg Br* 74:567, 1992.

252. Korres DS, Zoubos AB, Kavadias K, et al: The "tear drop" (or avulsed) fracture of the anterior inferior angle of the axis, *Eur Spine J* 3:151, 1994.

253. Reddin A, Mirvis SE, Diaconis JN: Rupture of the cervical esophagus and trachea associated with cervical spine fracture, *J Trauma* 27:564, 1987.

254. Stringer WL, Kelly DL Jr, Johnston FR, Holliday RH: Hyperextension injury of the cervical spine with esophageal perforation: case report, *J Neurosurg* 53:541, 1980.

255. Green JD, Harle TS, Harris JH: Anterior subluxation of the cervical spine: hyperflexion sprain, *AJNR Am J Neuroradiol* 2:243, 1981.

256. White AA, Punjabi IMM: *Clinical biomechanics of the spine 2*, Philadelphia, 1991, JB Lippincott.

257. Harris JH Jr: Hyperflexion injuries. In Harris JH Jr, Mirvis SE, eds: *The radiology of acute cervical spine trauma*, ed 3, Baltimore, 1996, Williams & Wilkins.

258. Barquet A, Dubra A: Occult severe hyperflexion sprain of the lower cervical spine, *Can Assoc Radiol J* 44:446, 1993.

259. Laporte C, Laville C, Lazennec JY, et al: Severe hyperflexion sprains of the lower cervical spine in adults, *Clin Orthop* 363:126, 1999.

260. Dellestable F, Gaucher A: Clay-shoveler's fracture. Stress fracture of the lower cervical and upper thoracic spinous processes, *Rev Rhum Engl Ed* 65:575, 1998.

261. Matar LD, Helms CA, Richardson WJ: "Spinolaminar breach": an important sign in cervical spinous process fractures, *Skeletal Radiol* 29:75, 2000.

262. Scher AT: "Tear-drop" fractures of the cervical spine-radiological features, *S Afr Med J* 61:355, 1982.

263. Schneider R, Kahn E: Chronic neurologic sequelae of acute trauma to the spine and spinal cord. Part 1: the significance of the acute flexion or "tear-drop" fracture-dislocation of the cervical spine, *J Bone Joint Surg Am* 38:985, 1956.

264. Kim KS, Chen HH, Russell EJ, Rogers LF: Flexion teardrop fracture of the cervical spine: radiographic characteristics, *AJR Am J Roentgenol* 152:319, 1989.

265. Fuentes JM, Bloncourt J, Vlahovitch B, Castan P: [Tear drop fractures. Contribution to the study of the mechanism of osteo-discoligamentous lesions], *Neurochirurgie* 29:129, 1983.

266. Doran SE, Papadopoulos SM, Ducker TB, Lillehei KO: Magnetic resonance imaging documentation of coexistent traumatic locked facets of the cervical spine and disc herniation, *J Neurosurg* 79:341, 1993.

267. Sonntag VK: Management of bilateral locked facets of the cervical spine, *Neurosurgery* 8:150, 1981.

268. Wolf A, Levi L, Mirvis SE: Operative management of bilateral facet dislocation, *J Neurosurg* 75:883, 1991.

269. Vaccaro AR, Falatyn SP, Flanders AE, et al: Magnetic resonance evaluation of the intervertebral disc, spinal ligaments, and spinal cord before and after closed traction reduction of cervical spine dislocations, *Spine* 24:1210, 1999.

270. Louw JA, Mafoyane NA, Small B, Neser CP: Occlusion of the vertebral artery in cervical spine dislocations, *J Bone Joint Surg Br* 72:679, 1990.

271. Willis BK, Greiner F, Orrison WW, Benzel EC: The incidence of vertebral artery injury after midcervical spine fracture or subluxation, *Neurosurgery* 34:435, 1994.

272. Hadley MN, Fitzpatrick BC, Sonntag VK, Browner CM: Facet fracture dislocation injuries of the cervical spine, *Neurosurgery* 30:661, 1992.

273. Argenson C, Lovet J, Sanouiller J, Lde Peretti F: Traumatic rotatory displacement of the lower cervical spine, *Spine* 13:767, 1988.

274. Scher AT: Unilateral locked facet in cervical spine injuries, *AJR Am J Roentgenol* 129:45, 1977.

275. Key A: Cervical spine dislocations with unilateral facet interlocking, *Paraplegia* 13:208, 1975.

276. Sim E: Vertical facet splitting: a special variant of rotary dislocations of the cervical spine, *J Neurosurg* 82:239, 1995.

277. Shapiro S, Snyder W, Kaufman K, Abel T: Outcome of 51 cases of unilateral locked cervical facets: interspinous braided cable for lateral mass plate fusion compared with interspinous wire and facet wiring with iliac crest, *J Neurosurg* 91:19, 1999.

278. Young JW, Resnik CS, DeCandido P, Mirvis SE: The laminar space in the diagnosis of rotational flexion injuries of the cervical spine, *AJR Am J Roentgenol* 152:103, 1989.

279. Lintner DM, Knight RQ, Cullen JP: The neurologic sequelae of cervical spine facet injuries. The role of canal diameter, *Spine* 18:725, 1993.

280. Herr CH, Ball PA, Sargent SK, Quinton HB: Sensitivity of prevertebral soft tissue measurement of C3 for detection of cervical spine fractures and dislocations, *Am J Emerg Med* 16:346, 1998.

281. Halliday AL, Henderson BR, Hart BL, Benzel EC: The management of unilateral lateral mass/facet fractures of the subaxial cervical

spine: the use of magnetic resonance imaging to predict instability, *Spine* 22:2614, 1997.

282. Forsyth H: Extension injuries of the cervical spine, *J Bone Joint Surg Am* 46:1792, 1964.

283. Scher AT: Articular pillar fractures of the cervical spine: diagnosis on the anteroposterior radiograph, *S Afr Med J* 60:968, 1981.

284. Harris JH Jr: Hyperextension injuries. In Harris JH Jr, Mirvis SE, eds: *The radiology of acute cervical spine trauma*, ed 3, Baltimore, 1996, Williams & Wilkins.

285. Allen BL, Ferguson RL, Lehmann TR, O'Brien RP: A mechanistic classification of closed, indirect fractures and dislocations of the lower cervical spine, *Spine* 7:1, 1982.

286. Shanmuganathan K, Mirvis SE, Dowe M, Levine AM: Traumatic isolation of the cervical articular pillar: imaging observations in 21 patients, *AJR Am J Roentgenol* 166:897, 1996.

287. Woodring JH, Goldstein SJ: Fractures of the articular processes of the cervical spine, *AJR Am J Roentgenol* 139:341, 1982.

288. Lee C, Woodring JH, Rogers LF, Kim KS: The radiographic distinction of degenerative slippage (spondylolisthesis and retrolisthesis) from traumatic slippage of the cervical spine, *Skeletal Radiol* 15:439, 1986.

289. Pellengahr C, Pfahler M, Kuhr M, Hohmann D: Influence of facet joint angles and asymmetric disk collapse on degenerative olisthesis of the cervical spine, *Orthopedics* 23:697, 2000.11

Stuart E. Mirvis

The emergency imaging evaluation of the thorax has consisted primarily of a supine chest radiograph obtained in the primary radiographic survey of blunt trauma patients. This study is relatively easy to obtain at the bedside, is inexpensive, and provides substantial information concerning potentially life-threatening conditions. The chest radiograph has high sensitivity in detecting medium to large pneumothoraces, tension pneumothorax, medium to large pleural fluid collections, pneumomediastinum, injury to the lung parenchyma and diaphragm, distortions of the mediastinal contour that indicate possible mediastinal bleeding, and most displaced fractures of the thoracic skeleton. The quality of the supine radiograph is often compromised by a variety of factors including patient motion, exposure factors limited by the use of portable x-ray generators, tubes, lines, backboards, and other objects lying under or over the patient, limited or no patient cooperation with inspiration or breath holding, and lack of a grid to intercept scatter radiation. During the past decade the deficiencies of chest radiography have been heightened by the increasingly common use of thoracic CT for acute trauma. Thoracic CT has shown improved accuracy over radiography in the diagnosis of small and radiographically occult pneumothorax, small pleural fluid collections, hemopericardium and pneumopericardium, details of lung parenchymal injury, subtle fractures, and both mediastinal hemorrhage and direct vascular injury, among other injuries.[1-22] Many of these CT findings greatly influence clinical management decisions. The overall cost-benefit

and clinical efficacy of CT in the acute evaluation of blunt thoracic trauma as compared with radiography alone is not known, although studies do indicate a cost-benefit for CT in the assessment of mediastinal hemorrhage.[23,24] With the increasing reliance on CT to assess the mediastinum, when mediastinal hemorrhage cannot be reliably excluded by radiography, use of admission thoracic CT in blunt trauma cases is anticipated to continue to increase. It is well within the realm of probability that admission chest radiographs will be replaced by frontal CT digital scout images combined with complete chest CT using multidetector CT scanners as these scanners become ubiquitous in trauma and emergency departments.

This chapter reviews the appearance of common and uncommon thoracic injuries diagnosed by radiography and CT primarily as a result of blunt force trauma. Some general comments address penetrating thoracic injury, but this topic is discussed more fully in Chapter 11. The impact of particular CT findings on management decisions is emphasized, and algorithms concerning imaging for particular diagnostic problems are suggested.

CHEST WALL INJURY

Isolated fractures of the ribs, clavicle, or scapula seldom represent significant injuries in and of themselves, but they do reflect the magnitude and location of the force imparted, especially in older patients with noncompliant chest walls. The more compliant chest walls of children and younger adults may allow transmission of significant energy into the thorax without producing fractures, so severe chest trauma can be present in the absence of rib or other thoracic skeletal injury.[25] Fractures of the first three ribs in particular indicate significant energy transfer. Brachial plexus or vascular injury accompanies fractures involving the thoracic outlet, upper ribs, upper sternum, and clavicles in 3.0% to 15.0% of patients.[26-30] Subclavian vascular injury should be suspected with fractures of the first three ribs, clavicle, and scapula. However, subclavian vascular injuries usually are accompanied by significant fracture displacement, apical extrapleural hematoma, brachial plexus neuropathy, radiographic evidence of mediastinal hemorrhage, posterior displacement of the first rib fracture, or fracture of the anterior subclavian groove.[29] Performing angiography in the absence of these signs or hard clinical findings, such as an upper extremity pulse deficit or expanding hematoma, yields very few significant vascular injuries and probably is not warranted on an emergency basis.[29-31] Gupta et al.[29] showed that first rib fractures associated with concomitant head, chest, abdominal, or long bone injury had a 24% incidence of subclavian vascular injury. Fractures of the lower ribs should increase suspicion of splenic, hepatic, or renal injury, confirmation of which should then be sought by appropriate diagnostic investigations, usually CT.

Single rib fractures are of limited clinical significance, and precise localization and quantification of these injuries are of dubious clinical use. Double fractures in three or more adjacent ribs or adjacent combined rib and sternal or costochondral fractures can produce a focal area of chest wall instability (Fig. 5-1). Paradoxic movement of this "flail" segment during the respiratory cycle can impair respiratory mechanics, promote atelectasis, and impair pulmonary drainage. Although usually recognized by physical inspec-

tion, a flail segment involving the upper ribs may be hidden by the chest wall musculature.[32] Fractured ribs accompanied by lacerations of intercostal arteries can cause major intrapleural hemorrhage, often requiring angiographic identification and embolization. The irregular etches of fractured and displaced ribs can lacerate the pleural lung and abdominal organs directly. In rare cases an anterior rib fragment can directly puncture the heart[33] (Fig. 5-2).

Rib fractures are often accompanied by extrapleural hematomas (EPH) that present as focal lobulated areas of increased density on a chest radiograph. Due to their extrapleural nature, such hematomas indent the parietal pleura focally and maintain a convex margin toward the lung (Fig. 5-3). Development of EPH over the apices may accompany fractures of the upper ribs or hemorrhage from the subclavian vessels from blunt trauma or iatrogenic causes. EPH will not change configuration with changes in patient position, as will free pleural space fluid collections. Rashid et al.[34] found EPH in 34 (7.1%) of 477 blunt trauma patients, and more than half of these had associated hemothorax. The localization of a hematoma to the pleural or extrapleural space is usually straightforward on CT because of the shape of the collection, but occasionally it may be uncertain. Incorrect localization may lead to extrapleural chest tube placement. EPH produces medial displacement of a fat layer that is just external to the parietal pleura deep to the endothoracic fascia and inner intercostal muscles. This medially displaced fat layer aids in localization of hematoma to the extrapleural region.[35]

Fractures of the sternum are infrequent, occurring in 1.5% to 4% of blunt chest trauma cases.[36] The diagnosis may be made by clinical inspection or chest wall palpation but typically is established by imaging. Although a properly exposed lateral chest radiograph will detect sternal

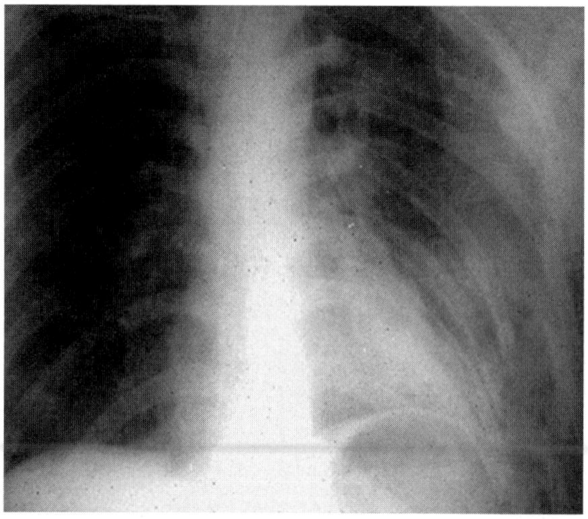

Fig. 5-1
Flail chest. Supine chest radiograph shows multiple comminuted left rib fractures in continuity. Most likely this segment of chest wall would move paradoxically with respiration.

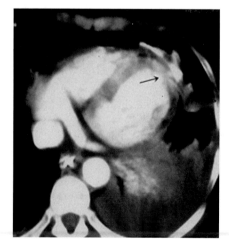

Fig. 5-2
Cardiac perforation by rib fracture. CT image shows contrast leak from the left apex (*arrow*) and left thoracic hemothorax. The cause of the perforation was found at emergency surgery to be the edge of a fractured rib. (From Shanmuganathan K, Mirvis SE: *Radiol Clin North Am* 37:548, 1999.)

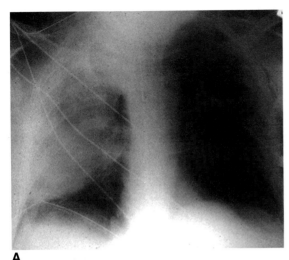

A

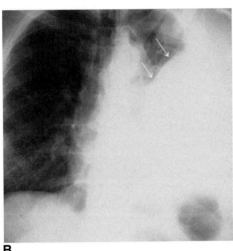

B

Fig. 5-3
Radiographs of extrapleural hematomas. **A**, Density over the right chest with convex margin toward lung is typical of extrapleural source of bleeding. Collection has a sharp margin and obtuse angle with the chest wall. **B**, A similarly shaped density in another patient shows convex curvature (*arrows*) toward lung. This hematoma resulted from a bleeding intercostal artery. Mass effect on mediastinum and heart suggests arterial bleeding as the source, as does the ability to dissect parietal pleura away from the inner chest wall.

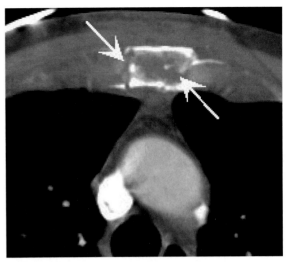

Fig. 5-4
CT of coronal sternal fractures. CT image shows slightly oblique coronally oriented fracture plane (*arrows*) through the sternal body. Substernal blood is minimal.

fractures with reasonably high sensitivity, this view is seldom obtained in a routine acute trauma assessment.[37] The frontal view misses essentially all sternal fractures unless these are associated with significant transverse displacement.[22] CT should permit detection of most sternal fractures unless they are nondisplaced and occur in the axial plane. Sternal fractures often have a coronal orientation or have a component in that axis, allowing easy CT recognition (Fig. 5-4). A limited series by Huggett and Roszler[37] suggested that the detection of a retrosternal hematoma by CT is specific for the diagnosis of sternal fracture (Fig. 5-5), but this is insensitive and was seen in only 44% of nine cases.

Although sternal fractures have been associated with major injuries to the heart and great vessels, this appears

to be quite uncommon, especially with isolated, nondisplaced, and nondepressed patterns.[38,39] Cardiac injury arising as a direct result of sternal fracture has been reported in 1.5% to 6% of patients.[36] However, a review of 70 patients with sternal fractures, of which 50% were isolated, showed no significant association with cardiac injury.[38] Laceration of the innominate artery caused by a displaced fracture of the sternum has been reported but appears to be quite rare.[40] Crestanello et al.[36] noted that fractures of the manubrium require higher force and are likely to be associated with more severe thoracic injuries than sternal body fractures. They described sternal fractures occurring as a result of direct impact, but also arising indirectly from flexion and axial loading forces associated with thoracic spine wedge compression fractures. They also noted a threefold increase in the incidence of this injury pattern with use of the shoulder–lap belt restraint system.

Most sternoclavicular dislocations are anterior and have no major clinical significance. However, posterior dislocations of the clavicle relative to the manubrium can damage the great vessels, superior mediastinal nerves, trachea, and esophagus. Although sternoclavicular dislocations are demonstrable using angled chest radiographs (tube angled 35 degrees cranially), they are most easily diagnosed using axial CT (Fig. 5-6). Posterior dislocation can result from a posterior and laterally directed force into the shoulder, moving the lateral clavicle forward and pivoting the medial clavicle posteriorly. Thoracic angiography and esophagography are warranted to exclude injury.

Isolated fractures of the scapula are frequently overlooked in interpretation of both chest radiographs and thoracic CT.[4] These injuries are important because they indicate the likelihood of significant chest wall impact

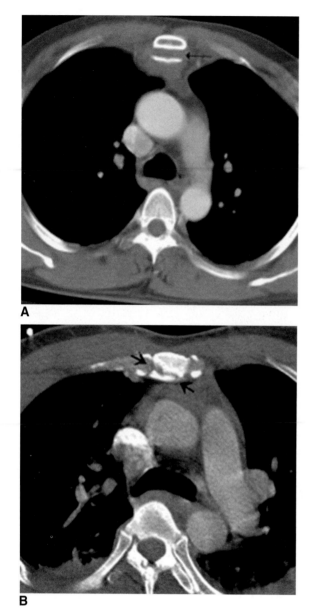

Fig. 5-5
CT of sternal fractures. **A**, CT image of coronal fracture (*arrow*) with more retrosternal hematoma. **B**, Another patient with oblique coronal fracture (*arrows*) as seen on CT with anterior mediastinal hematoma.

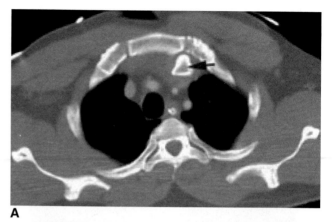

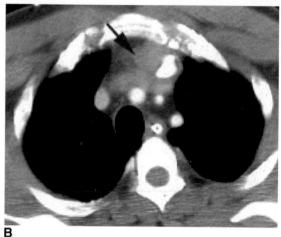

Fig. 5-6
CT of sternoclavicular dislocation. **A** and **B**, The left clavicular head is dislocated posteriorly (*arrow*). There is compression of the left brachiocephalic vein and rightward displacement of the trachea. Injury to the trachea, esophagus, and major vessels in the region needs to be considered. A small adjacent hematoma is present (*arrow* in **B**).

and may be a cause of pain and limitation of shoulder girdle motion (Fig. 5-7). Scapulothoracic dissociation (STD) is a rare and serious injury characterized by a lateral displacement of the entire forequarter with intact overlying skin, complete acromioclavicular separation, and usually multiple ipsilateral upper extremity fractures[42] (Fig. 5-8). Avulsion injuries to the brachial plexus and subclavian nerves always accompany the injury. Vascular injuries are also common and should be sought even if the distal pulse is normal, which may be maintained by collateral flow. Usually there is a large hematoma over the involved shoulder, and the injury is

clinically apparent. The diagnosis may be suggested on chest radiography or CT initially, both of which typically demonstrate lateral displacement and often an abnormal orientation of the involved scapula[43] (Fig. 5-9). In a review of five cases of STD, Sheafor and Mirvis[43] found that the mean lateral displacement of the injured scapula was 3.76 cm (standard deviation, 2.2 cm). The lateral scapular displacement ratio a/n (where n = distance from medial margin of normal scapula to the midline and a = distance from medial border of the abnormal scapula to the midline) was 1.54 (standard deviation, 0.36).

Fractures of the thoracic spine may be easily overlooked when interpreting the frontal chest radiograph in acute blunt trauma patients. The admission chest radiograph is often suboptimally exposed in the acute trauma setting and is frequently compromised by patient motion, overlying support lines and tubes, and scatter radiation. More overt findings can easily distract

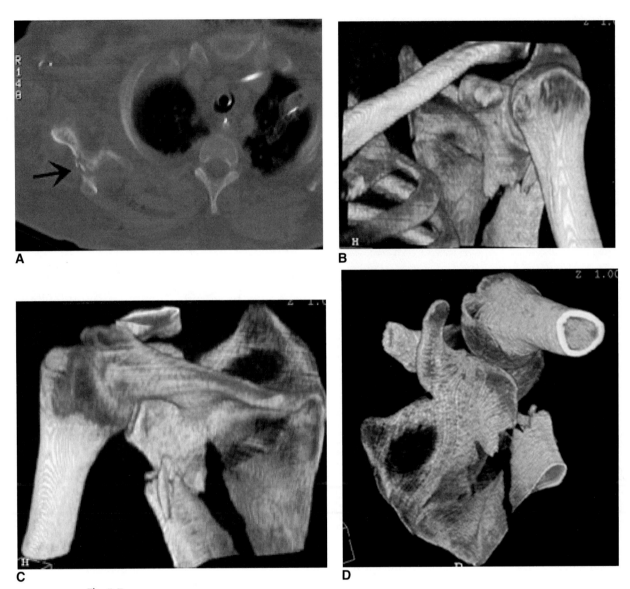

Fig. 5-7
CT of scapula fracture. Arrow marks fracture at base of scapular spine. Information about the degree of comminution and involvement of the glenoid fossa is important because surgical intervention may be required. These fractures are frequently overlooked.

a reader from a careful review of the radiograph for evidence of paraspinal hematoma and abnormalities of spinal alignment. A substantial percentage of thoracic injuries will be fracture-dislocations that will present with profound neurologic deficits, but many others will be amenable to reduction and stabilization before the onset or exacerbation of neurologic dysfunction. Similarly, review of thoracic CT images for bone detail, in addition to the traditional lung and soft tissue window surveys, can often detect unsuspected thoracic spine injuries. Diffuse mediastinal hemorrhage associated with lower cervical, thoracic, or upper lumbar spine fractures should not be assumed to arise strictly from the skeletal injury, and concurrent major vas-

cular injury must also be considered. However, if a paraspinal hematoma surrounds a spine fracture more or less symmetrically, displaces the aorta, and the great vessels appear normal on high-quality intravenous contrast-enhanced thoracic CT, aortography is not required.[12,23]

ECTOPIC AIR AND FLUID
Pneumomediastinum

Complete disruption of air-containing structures within the thorax including the tracheobronchial tree to the distal alveoli and the esophagus can permit air to enter the mediastinum. Rupture can occur as a result of

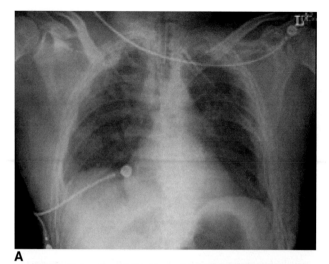

A

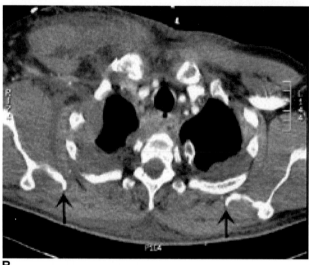

B

Fig. 5-8
Thoracoscapular dissociation. **A,** Supine chest radiograph shows displaced fracture of the proximal clavicle and marked increased soft tissue density over the lateral right chest and shoulder. **B,** CT of same patient shows lateral displacement of the medial border of the right scapula as compared with the left (*arrows*).

increased intraluminal pressure, as may be seen with sudden chest compression, stretching, shearing, or direct puncture of air-containing structures. Air may also enter the mediastinum from extrathoracic sources (e.g., the larynx, cervical trachea, and from penetrating wounds of the chest wall from a knife or missile) and rarely retroperitoneal sources (e.g., a posterior perforated duodenal ulcer). The most common origin of pneumomediastinum in trauma is a result of the Macklin effect[44] in which air enters the pulmonary interstitium from ruptured alveoli and subsequently dissects centrally along the connective tissues around the airways into the hila and mediastinum.[45]

Pneumomediastinum is appreciated radiographically as lucent streaks of air outlining the inner aspect of the

parietal pleura that is pushed laterally away from the mediastinum. Normally the pleura forms a border with the air-filled lung, but the introduction of air into the mediastinum leads to air density on both sides of the parietal pleura, thus creating a line of soft tissue density dividing the air-filled lung laterally and the air-containing mediastinum medially (Fig. 5-10). The parietal pleural is most commonly seen along the left superior mediastinum and is often visualized paralleling the left cardiac border and fading below the left hemidiaphragm. It is important to observe that the parietal pleural line created by pneumomediastinum does not sweep around the heart, as would be seen with pneumopericardium. The parietal pleural line to the right of the superior mediastinum can be seen, but less consistently, often lost against the density of the spine. Air within the mediastinum outlines numerous structures including the aorta and its proximal branches, the brachiocephalic veins, the proximal abdominal aorta, the thymus, and the costal and sternal attachments of the diaphragm.[46] Specific radiologic signs attributed to pneumomediastinum include the "continuous diaphragm sign" (Fig. 5-11), the "V" sign of Naclerio, and the "ring-around-the-artery" sign.[46] The descending aorta is sharply outlined by air and can usually be followed into the upper abdomen because of adjacent air density. The space separating the aortic arch from the main pulmonary artery segment, the aortico-pulmonary window, is also sharply defined due to the contrast created by adjacent air density. On the lateral chest radiograph, pneumomediastinum can best be appreciated as retrosternal lucency and as streaks of air density in the middle mediastinum paralleling the trachea and esophagus. Pneumomediastinum can mimic and coexist with pneumopericardium. The distinction is important because of the potential for pneumopericardium to progress to cardiac tamponade.[47]

Due to its extended contrast range, CT is more sensitive than radiography to the presence of small quantities of air in the mediastinum.[46] Pneumomediastinum typically appears as retrosternal lucency with intervening streaks of mediastinal fat and is adjacent to the aorta and esophagus. The laterally displaced parietal pleura is usually seen on the left side (Fig. 5-12).

It is common for mediastinal air to extend into the cervical and supraclavicular soft tissues and chest wall. This progression is exacerbated if the patient is receiving positive pressure ventilatory support. Air within the mediastinum occasionally tracks into the retroperitoneum through transdiaphragmatic fascial communication or rupture directly into the peritoneal cavity. Air from a mediastinal leak can also dissect into the anterior abdominal wall deep to the rectus sheath or within the mesentery (Fig. 5-13). It is important to attempt to distinguish air in extraperitoneal spaces from pneumoperi-

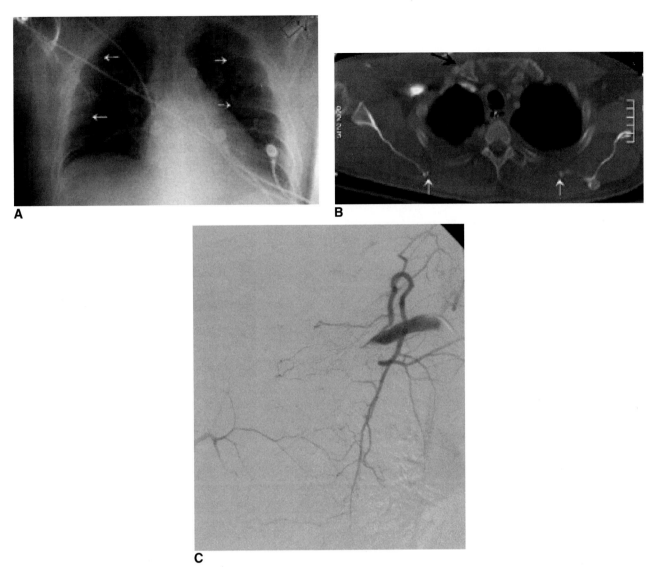

Fig. 5-9
Thoracoscapular dissociation. **A,** Supine chest radiograph demonstrates slight lateral displacement of the right scapula in blunt trauma patient (*arrows*). **B,** CT image shows lateral displacement of the right scapula and a difference in orientation compared with left (*white arrows*). A proximal right clavicle fracture is noted (*black arrow*). **C,** A selective right subclavian arteriogram performed for diminished right upper extremity pulses showed complete proximal axillary artery occlusion. The patient had a bypass graft but had major damage to the innervation of the right arm.

toneum, since the latter raises concern regarding primary or delayed full-thickness bowel injury.

Pneumothorax

Pneumothorax occurs commonly after blunt and penetrating chest trauma. Air can collect in the pleural space either from a leak in the proximal or distal airway or from penetrating trauma, with air entering from outside the chest. In addition to traumatic events, pneumothorax is often a complication of early resuscitation efforts related to central line placement and positive pressure ventilator support. Although a relatively small pneumothorax is unlikely to contribute to significant respiratory impairment, its potential to enlarge and to develop tension is a major risk. Thus the detection of even a small pneumothorax is important. Small pneumothoraces are not initially recognized either by clinical findings or by the admission chest radiograph in 30% to 55% of trauma patients[2,18,48,49] and may be diagnosed only after thoracic CT. Up to one third of trauma patients with simple pneumothorax will progress to tension pneumothorax if untreated.[48,50,51] The clinical significance of an occult pneumothorax in a trauma patient has been questioned

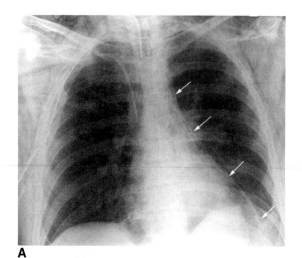

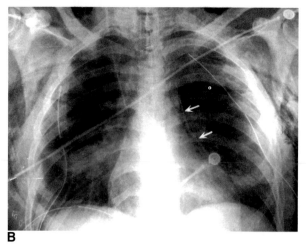

Fig. 5-10
A, Radiograph of pneumomediastinum. Left parietal pleural line is marked by arrows. Soft tissue air is seen bilaterally in the chest wall and neck. **B,** Another patient with clear left parietal pleural line (*arrows*) and bilateral soft tissue air.

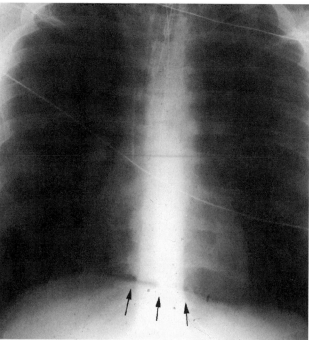

Fig. 5-11
Continuous diaphragm sign. A straight line of air is seen beneath the pericardium and above the central tendon of the diaphragm within the mediastinum (*arrows*). In some cases this is the only sign of mediastinal air. (From Shanmuganathan K, Mirvis SE: *Radiol Clin North Am* 37:536, 1999.)

by others.[11,52] Compared with radiography, chest CT is much more sensitive in detecting pneumothorax.* For this reason, CT scans obtained through the abdomen should routinely include the lung bases with review of these images in lung windows.[49,51]

Air in the pleural space can have a variety of radiographic appearances depending on the size of the pneumothorax, patient position, presence of pleural effusion, atelectasis, and previous pleural disease and adhesions. Most commonly, in the anteroposterior erect chest radiograph, pleural space air distributes to the superior and superolateral portion of the thoracic cavity outlining the thin visceral pleural line. No lung markings are seen peripheral to the visceral pleural line (Fig. 5-14). The visceral pleural line can be simulated by skin folds, tape on the skin, bedclothes, overlying tubes and

lines, subcutaneous air, and subpleural lung cysts, among others. The difference between the aerated lung and air-filled pleural space is accentuated by expiratory views that increase lung density while not affecting the pleural air density, maximizing contrast between lung and pneumothorax. Trauma patients are most commonly studied in the supine position. In this orientation, air collects in the anteroinferior aspect of the pleural space. In this location air creates hypodensity over the lower chest and upper abdomen. Air can fill the lateral costophrenic sulcus, creating the so-called deep costophrenic sulcus sign (Fig. 5-15) first described by Gordon.[55-58] Also, in a supine patient air outlines the anterior costophrenic recess, resulting in an abrupt curvilinear change in density projected over the right or left upper quadrant, which is normally convex inferiorly.[56,58] Air in this location can outline the inferior visceral pleura, confirming its subpulmonic position (Fig. 5-16). Since pleural air can outline the anteroinferior insertion of the diaphragm as well as the dome, both edges of the diaphragm may be projected on the frontal radiograph, producing a "double diaphragm" appearance (Fig. 5-17). Air in the left inferior pleural space produces a sharply defined cardiac apex or pericardial fat pad. The presence of pleural adhesions or lobar collapse may cause a pneumothorax to collect in an atypical

---

*References 2, 11, 18, 50, 51, 53, 54.

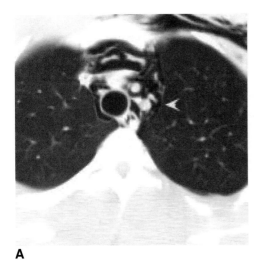

A

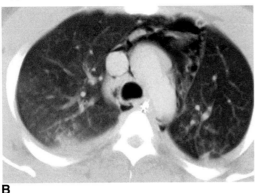

B

Fig. 5-12
CT of pneumomediastinum. **A** and **B,** Two images from the same patient show air within the mediastinum outlining the trachea, esophagus, great vessels, and anterior mediastinum. An arrowhead marks the distended left parietal pleura.

distribution such as around the collapsed lobe or subpulmonically. If there is a question regarding the presence of a pneumothorax, additional studies such as an expiratory view or altered positioning such as a decubitus view or lateral view may be helpful. CT is likely to be definitive. Potentially, air in a supine patient can collect in the ventral pleural space, even producing tension pneumothorax, and still not be apparent from frontal radiographs.[59] Other locations where pneumothorax can collect are behind the pulmonary ligament[60] and minor fissure.[61]

Tension pneumothorax is a medical emergency that can develop when air enters the pleural space but does not egress during expiration. High intrathoracic pressure produces displacement of the mediastinum and heart, flattening of the ipsilateral hemidiaphragm, spreading of the ipsilateral ribs, and compression of the ipsilateral lung (Figs. 5-18 and 5-19). Tension pneumothorax can persist despite chest tube placement if the tube is malpositioned or occluded or if there is a major airway injury allowing air to leak into the pleural space as quickly as it can be evacuated by chest tube.[62] Pleural adhesions may prevent the chest tube from communicating with the pneumothorax. High intrapleural pressure impairs venous blood return, potentially leading to cardiac arrest.

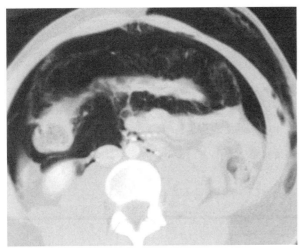

Fig. 5-13
Dissection of air from the chest. This patient was intubated and then received positive pressure ventilation. Air has dissected through soft tissue planes into the anterior abdominal subcutaneous tissue and into the retroperitoneal and peritoneal spaces and along the mesentery. An abdominal compartment syndrome potentially could arise in this situation.

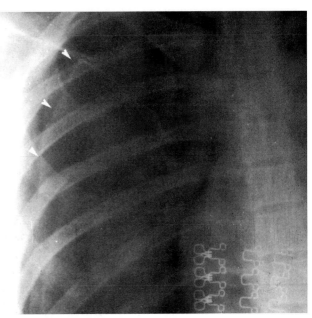

Fig. 5-14
Radiograph of pneumothorax. In the erect patient air will rise to the upper chest and outline the visceral pleura of the partially collapsed lung. No lung markings should be seen beyond the visceral pleura (*arrowheads*). The appearance can be confused with skin folds, external lines, tubes, tape, and other objects on or around the patient.

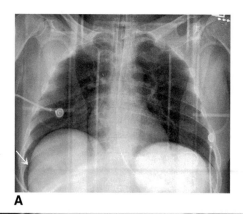

A

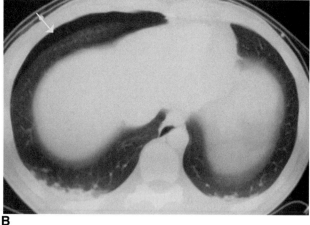

B

Fig. 5-15
Pneumothorax. **A**, Supine chest radiograph demonstrates air outlining deep recess created by costophrenic sulcus laterally (*arrow*), as well as hyperlucency over the right upper abdomen. **B**, CT image shows tendency of pneumothorax to collect in the anteroinferior pleural space in the supine patient (*arrow*).

Pleural Effusion and Hemothorax

Pleural fluid appearing after acute thoracic trauma usually is caused by hemorrhage and is present in about 50% of major thoracic trauma victims.[63] Hemothorax can

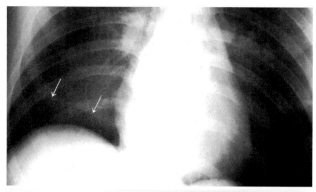

Fig. 5-16
Subpulmonic pneumothorax. Chest radiograph demonstrates hyperlucent lung bases bilaterally due to bilateral pneumothorax. On the right the air collection is beneath the lung and demarcates the visceral pleura of the undersurface (*arrows*).

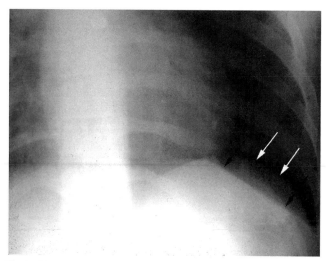

Fig. 5-17
Double diaphragm sign. View of the left base in a supine patient shows an air-diaphragm interface between pneumothorax and anterior diaphragm (*black arrows*) and between the lung and dome of the diaphragm (*white arrows*).

result from injury to the visceral pleura with lung contusion or laceration or from injury to the chest wall with tearing of the parietal pleura. A small amount of hemorrhage typically occurs, with a traumatic pneumothorax presenting as an air-fluid level on erect chest radiographs. Bleeding of venous origin is of low pressure, likely to be self-limited, and is unlikely to exert mass effect sufficient to displace the heart or mediastinum. Bleeding of arterial origin such as from an intercostal, internal mammary, or subclavian artery branch is under higher pressure and can cause mass effect on the heart and mediastinum.

In an erect patient, chest radiographs typically show a meniscus sign and obliteration of the costophrenic

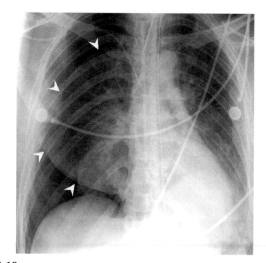

Fig. 5-18
Tension pneumothorax. Chest radiograph in a supine patient shows collapse of the right lung (*arrowheads*) and displacement of the heart and mediastinum to the left, indicating tension.

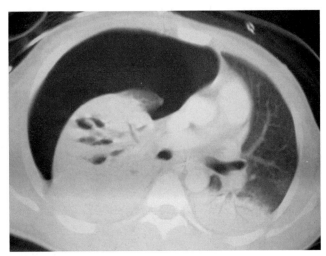

Fig. 5-19
CT of tension pneumothorax. The right lung is markedly collapsed with surrounding pneumothorax. The mediastinum is shifted to the left, indicating tension. Note lacerations (linear lucent areas) in the right lung.

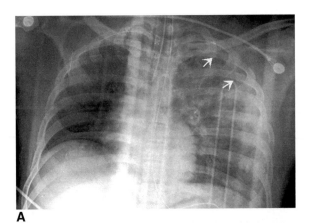

A

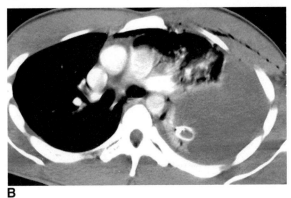

B

Fig. 5-20
Large hemothorax—supine patient. **A**, Chest radiograph shows increased density over the entire left hemithorax with the highest density laterally (*arrows*). **B**, CT of the same patient shows a large pleural fluid collection with posterior left lower lobe collapse and a chest tube in the hemothorax. The mediastinum is shifted to the right, indicating high pressure in the left chest (i.e., arterial bleed).

and cardiophrenic angles as fluid fills these spaces. A uniform band of increased density occurs wherever the lung is displaced away from the chest wall by fluid as a result of the presence of pleural fluid only without intervening lung. Bronchovascular markings should be clearly discerned through pleural fluid that is anterior or posterior to the lung if there is no primary lung disease. In a supine patient, pleural effusion may produce a uniform increase in density over the entire hemithorax that might be attributed to technique factors. If the amount of pleural fluid is relatively equal bilaterally, it may not be possible to discern and may be attributed to uniform underexposure. Blood in the pleural space may clot and therefore not follow the gravity-dependent movement expected of free fluid, but in an acute trauma setting, this is somewhat uncommon in the author's experience. Blood may also collect beneath the lung (subpulmonic), especially in an upright-positioned patient, producing a pseudodiaphragm that mimics the normal diaphragm but that appears elevated and flattened along its medial aspect. The peak of this pseudodiaphragm occurs lateral to the peak of the normal diaphragm in the midclavicular line[64] (Fig. 5-21). This classic subpulmonic fluid configuration is more likely to be recognized on an expiratory radiograph.[64] Fluid may collect within the pleural fissures, in the medial pleural space, and behind the pulmonary ligaments and may be marginated by pleural adhesions, creating atypical distribution patterns.

Other origins of pleural fluid should also be considered besides hemorrhage in an acute trauma setting. Uncommon fluid sources include a bilo-pleural fistula,[65] occurring with right hemidiaphragm and liver laceration,[62] chylothorax from thoracic duct injury,[66] urothorax,[67] preexisting serous pleural effusion, and enteric fluid as may occur from a torn hemidiaphragm and concurrent gastric or small bowel perforation. The distinction of fluid of various sources is aided by use of CT density. Hemothorax measures 30 HU to about 70 HU depending on the extent of clot retraction and hematocrit. Chyle and bile may appear less than 0 HU due to fat content. Active bleeding into the pleural space from an arterial source will have a high density, probably greater than 90 HU, if the patient receives intravenous contrast enhancement[68] (Fig. 5-22).

The sensitivity of chest radiography to pleural fluid improves as the quantity of fluid increases. Still, relatively large quantities of pleural fluid may not be appreciated by frontal radiography when filling the posterior costophrenic and subpulmonic spaces.[69] CT has greater sensitivity for detection of small pleural fluid collections in any location and often can determine the type of fluid based on CT attenuation. Bedside sonography is also very sensitive in detecting minimal quantities of pleural fluid and is ideal for use in acute settings,

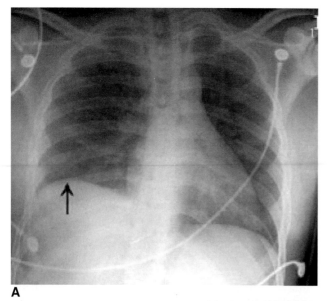

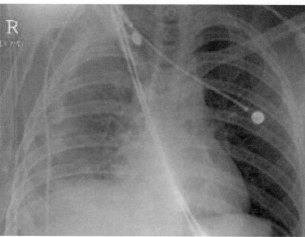

Fig. 5-21
Subpulmonic pleural effusion. **A**, Erect chest radiograph shows a gradually rising right hemidiaphragm moving medial to lateral with a peak lateral to the typical midclavicular location (*arrow*). This is a pseudodiaphragm created by pleural effusion beneath the lung. **B**, The supine film of the same patient shows the large amount of pleural fluid filling the dependent pleural space.

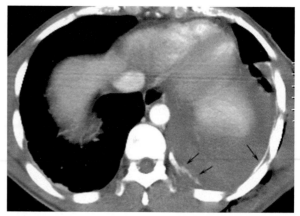

Fig. 5-22
Hemorrhage into the pleural space. CT through the lower chest of a stabbing victim demonstrates high-density arterial contrast extravasation (*arrows*) and hemothorax. Most likely the bleeding is from an adjacent injured intercostal artery.

TRAUMA TO THE LUNG
Pulmonary Contusion

Pulmonary contusion represents the most common primary lung injury caused by nonpenetrating trauma, occurring in 30% to 70% of blunt chest trauma victims.[20,27,72] The injury is produced by direct transmission of energy through the chest wall to the underlying lung.[73] Lung contusion is usually present on the initial admission chest radiograph, but its appearance may be delayed up to 6 hours.[74] The lesion appears as a fluffy, air space–occupying process that is typically nonsegmental, "geographic," and frequently peripheral in its distribution (Figs. 5-23 and 5-24). Contusions tend to occur adjacent to solid structures such as the ribs, sternum, and vertebral bodies. Contusion patterns often reflect the site and configuration of blunt impact

especially in an unstable patient who may not undergo CT study.[70,71]

Hemorrhage of extrapleural origin (epipleural) is typically associated with rib fractures. Bleeding of arterial origin strips the parietal pleura away from the inner chest wall and creates a convex bulge toward the lung (see Fig. 5-3). The hematoma is contained and therefore is not gravity-dependent in position and does not change location with patient movement. A thin layer of subpleural fat may be seen along the outer margin of an extrapleural hematoma.[35]

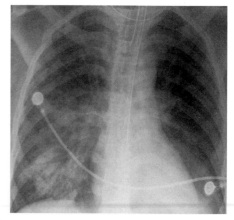

Fig. 5-23
Radiograph of pulmonary contusion. Radiograph shows consolidation at the right mid and lower lung with few air-bronchograms. There is left lower lobe atelectasis.

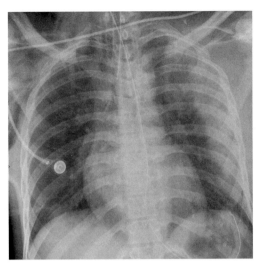

Fig. 5-24
Radiograph of pulmonary contusion. There is an area of uniform increased density in the periphery of the left lung after blunt chest trauma. No air-bronchograms are seen. The contusion corresponds to the shape of the impacting object and tends to be nonlobar and nonsegmental in its pattern. No rib fractures are seen.

on the thoracic cage. The lesions may be unilateral or bilateral, focal, multifocal, or diffuse. The opacification of lung is caused by hemorrhage and edema in the alveoli as a result of disruption of small blood vessels and damage to the alveolar-capillary membrane, permitting increased fluid leakage into the alveolar space.[27,32] Air bronchograms may be seen within lung contusions but are frequently absent due to filling of the adjacent bronchi with blood or secretions. Although adjacent rib fractures may accompany lung contusion, they are often not present.[74]

Clearing of contusions is usually detected radiographically within 48 to 72 hours but may not appear for 5 to 7 days with more extensive injuries. Complete resolution usually requires 10 to 14 days.[74] Failure of the density of the contusion to resolve during this time suggests either the wrong initial diagnosis or superimposition of another pathologic process such as pneumonia, aspiration, atelectasis, or adult respiratory distress syndrome (ARDS).[75] The impaired ability of the contused lung to clear secretions, diminished regional lung compliance, and the presence of intraalveolar blood and edema fluid provide a focus for the development of infection and sepsis.[32] Although local, discrete contusions do not appear to have a significant impact on morbidity and mortality, they can contribute to respiratory insufficiency of a variable degree. Diffuse pulmonary contusions can lead to severe ARDS, possibly because of extensive damage to alveolar-capillary membranes.[27,75] CT is much more sensitive than chest radiography at demonstrating and quantifying pulmonary contusion, as discussed later (Figs. 5-25 and 5-26).

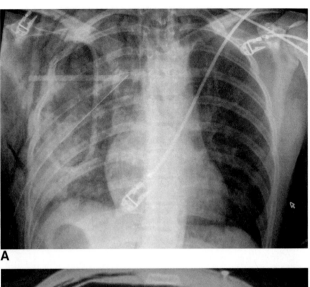

A

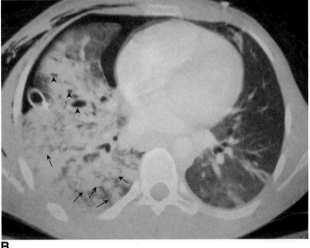

B

Fig. 5-25
CT of pulmonary contusions. **A,** Diffuse increased density in the right lung after blunt trauma on chest radiograph. A second right rib fracture is noted. **B,** CT scan confirms the marked extent of the injury and shows numerous small uniform density hematomas (*arrows*) and multiple small lung lacerations (*arrowheads*). There is a residual pneumothorax.

Lacerations, Pneumoceles (Pseudocysts), and Hematomas

Pulmonary lacerations have been considered unusual sequelae of blunt chest trauma, but studies using CT have suggested that they are in fact quite common, although frequently overlooked.[20] Pulmonary laceration is a disruption of the alveolar spaces with subsequent formation of a cavity filled with blood or air resulting from blunt or penetrating injury.[22] A variety of mechanisms have been proposed to explain the creation of pulmonary laceration. A concussion wave from blunt trauma may produce a shearing injury due to differential inertia between different lung segments. Sudden closure of the glottis or compression of a

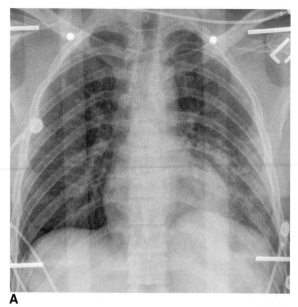

A

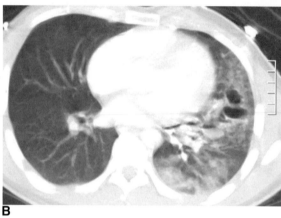

B

Fig. 5-26
CT of pulmonary contusion. **A**, Chest radiograph after blunt trauma shows only faint increased density in the left lower lobe. **B**, CT demonstrates a large area of lung contusion containing at least two lacerations on this single slice. These are seldom demonstrated on radiography, especially soon after injury.

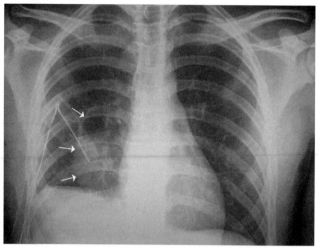

Fig. 5-27
Radiograph of traumatic lung laceration. The study shows a lesion (*arrows*) in the right lung composed of a lucent portion superiorly and a solid portion below. The solid component could be hematoma or consolidated lung tissue. Note the thin pseudomembrane of the cavitated portion (*top arrow*). This lesion was created by ballistic cavitation.

bronchus may produce high intraluminal airway pressures that rupture distal alveoli. Rib fractures can penetrate directly into the lung. Impact against the lower ribs or adjacent vertebral bodies can compress paraspinal segments of the lung. Finally, pleural adhesions may avulse peripheral portions of the lung.[20,74] Pulmonary lacerations generally occur in patients under 30 years of age, when the elasticity of the ribs and lung are optimal.[74]

Pulmonary lacerations may communicate with the visceral pleura, leading to pneumothorax. When intraparenchymal in location, lacerations of the lung are often masked by surrounding contusion and may not become radiographically visible until the contusion begins to resolve.[74] Lacerations of the lung, although initially linear in configuration, tend to assume an ovoid or elliptical shape due to the elastic recoil of the lung. Pathologically,

lacerations are lined by a pseudomembrane composed of alveolar remnants and may be monolocular or multilocular, generally varying from 2 to 14 cm in diameter.

Radiographically, lacerations appear as ovoid radiolucencies (cysts) surrounded by a thin 2- to 3-mm rim of increased density representing the pseudomembrane (Fig. 5-27). When hemorrhage occurs into the cavity, an air-fluid level may appear if the cavitation communicates with an airway. When a clot forms, a thin crescent of air may persist over the clot, producing a so-called air-meniscus sign. The laceration may completely fill with clotted blood (a pulmonary hematoma) and present as a uniform mass on a chest radiograph (Fig. 5-28). Lung lac-

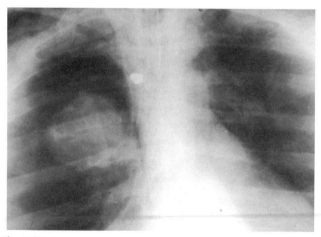

Fig. 5-28
Radiograph of pulmonary hematoma. This solid, rounded area of density in the right upper lobe resulted from passage of the adjacent bullet. Typically, such a lesion gradually shrinks over weeks to months and mimics a "coin" lesion (soft tissue).

erations usually resolve over 3 to 5 weeks but may persist for months as a slowly shrinking "coin lesion" on a chest radiograph. It is important to note such a development before discharge of the patient to prevent misidentification of the resolving contusion as a potential malignancy. Lung lacerations may persist for months in the presence of continued pulmonary pathology such as ARDS and positive-pressure ventilation, but generally these lesions resolve, since the cavity is not lined by a true epithelium.[76]

Kato et al.[76] followed traumatic pulmonary pseudocysts in 12 patients who had sustained blunt chest injury. They established that CT was superior to supine chest radiography in identifying and following the evolution of these lesions and in establishing the presence of complications such as infection or hemorrhage. All pseudocysts resolved in 1 to 4 months (mean, 1.8 months). Lesions began to show resolution usually within 2 weeks. They did not recommend surgical resection of pulmonary pseudocysts unless a superimposed infection developed that was resistant to standard nonsurgical therapy.

Pulmonary lacerations are generally benign injuries but occasionally can cause complications. A laceration may communicate with an adjacent bronchus and the visceral pleura, producing a bronchopleural fistula and a persistent air leak. On rare occasions, infection within a pulmonary laceration can progress to an abscess[76,77] (Fig. 5-29). Carroll et al.[77] described this complication in four patients and noted difficulty in curing lesions using typical postural drainage and antibiotic therapy. Large lung lacerations can expand under positive airway pressure and produce compression of adjacent normal lung by their mass effect. Traumatic lung lacerations can be diagnostically confused

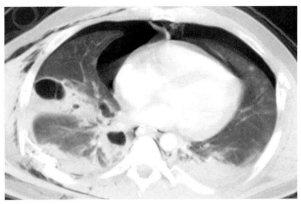

Fig. 5-30
CT of pulmonary laceration. Several focal lucent areas in the right lower lobe are lung lacerations with surrounding consolidation-hematoma. There are bilateral pneumothoraces and displaced posterior and left lateral rib fractures. Contusion or atelectasis is present at the left posterior lung base.

with congenital lung cysts or pulmonary sequestrations, lung abscesses, postpneumonic pneumatocele, and cavitations caused by fungus or tuberculous infection.

Parenchymal Lung Injury: Computed Tomography

Many studies have suggested that CT offers greater sensitivity in identifying a variety of pulmonary injuries and in demonstrating the extent of disease than does radiography.* Wagner et al.[20] demonstrated that CT detects pulmonary lacerations with far greater accuracy than radiography. In their series of 85 consecutive chest trauma victims, CT detected 99 lung lacerations compared with 5 detected by radiography. They suggested that lung lacerations are so frequently present in nonpenetrating chest trauma that they probably constitute the major underlying lesion accompanying lung contusion (Fig. 5-30). Trupka et al.[18] compared CT and plain chest radiographic findings in 103 patients with chest trauma (average injury severity score of 30). In 67 (65%) of the patients CT detected a major injury that was missed by the corresponding chest radiograph including lung contusion in 33 patients and pneumothorax in 27 patients. In 42 patients (41%) the additional thoracic CT findings resulted in a change of therapy. The patient group with CT diagnosis of chest injury was compared with a historical control group without CT diagnosis. The rate of respiratory failure (36% vs. 56%) was not statistically different between the two groups, but the rates of adult respiratory distress syndrome (8% vs. 20%; p < 0.05) and mortality (10% vs. 21%; p < 0.05) were significantly reduced in the group having thoracic CT. In a report regarding the classification and quantification of pathologic conditions, Kunisch-Hoppe et al.[80] concluded that CT assessment of

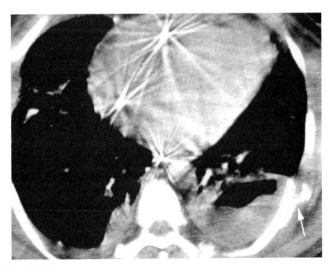

Fig. 5-29
CT of infected lung laceration. Cavitary lesion in the left posterior lower lobe resulted from an initial laceration probably created by fractured rib fragment (*arrow*) resulting from a 30-ft fall. The laceration became secondarily infected and proved resistant to antibiotics and drainage. In some cases these lesions may require surgical resection.

---

*References 8, 15, 18, 20, 53, 68, 78, 79, 81.

the lungs of patients on respiratory support correlated better with the duration and pressure of respiratory support and prognosis than did a radiographic assessment.

A segment of the peripheral lung rarely can herniate outside the confines of the thoracic cavity either as a result of blunt or penetrating trauma.[82-84] Herniation can occur at sites of penetrating wounds or chest tubes or as a result of multiple rib fractures that create a partial chest wall defect. The anterior thorax is a favored site of herniation because of a general lack of muscular support[82] (Figs. 5-31 and 5-32). Radiographically, the herniated lung appears as a well-circumscribed loculation of subcu-

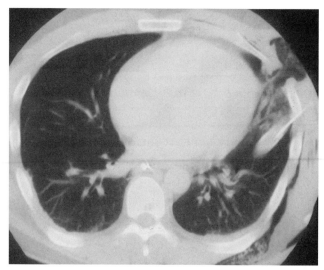

Fig. 5-32
Lung herniation. CT shows transthoracic wall lung herniation of a contused segment of the lingula.

taneous air and may be better appreciated on projections tangential to the hernia. On frontal views the hernia may project over the lung and be indistinguishable from the lung or a loculated pneumothorax. CT provides a straightforward diagnosis, clearly showing the herniated lung projecting through the chest wall.[82] Surgical reduction of intercostal lung hernias with narrow necks is recommended because of the potential for incarceration or strangulation, especially in mechanically ventilated patients, or because of a threat of tension pneumothorax.[83] The entrapped segment of lung can interfere with respiratory dynamics by tethering the affected lung in place. Supraclavicular hernias, secondary to sternoclavicular dislocation, usually reduce spontaneously as a result of a larger thoracic wall defect and the absence of associated perforating bone fragments. These are therefore usually observed.

RUPTURE OF THE HEMIDIAPHRAGM
Blunt Trauma

Overview. Rupture of the hemidiaphragm occurs in approximately 3.0% to 8.0% of patients undergoing celiotomy after blunt abdominal trauma[85-90] and in 0.8% to 5.8% of patients with a major thoracic injury from blunt force.[88-90] Motor vehicle accidents are responsible for up to 90% of all diaphragmatic injuries from blunt trauma.[88] Several mechanisms have been proposed as causes of diaphragm tearing, including sudden increase in intraabdominal pressure transmitted throughout the abdomen at impact, avulsion of the diaphragm from its attachments, penetration by rib fracture fragments, and shearing of the stretched diaphragm dome. Kearney et al.[88] demonstrated that patients sustaining left

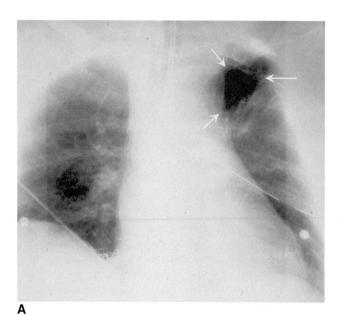

A

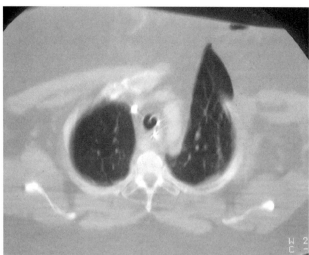

B

Fig. 5-31
Lung herniation. **A,** Supine chest radiograph shows irregular area of lucency projecting over the left upper lobe but projecting beyond the chest wall (*arrows*). **B,** CT image shows a portion of the left upper lobe herniating through the anterior chest wall. This lung was entrapped and causing respiratory distress and was surgically reduced.

lateral impact are at three times higher risk of diaphragmatic rupture than those receiving a frontal impact, supporting a role for chest wall deformation and shearing forces in producing this injury. Right hemidiaphragmatic injuries occurred in 50% of patients after right lateral impact, whereas 91% of left hemidiaphragmatic ruptures occurred after left lateral impact. Left hemidiaphragmatic rupture predominates in blunt injury, representing 75% of 44 diaphragmatic injuries diagnosed at thoracotomy by Morgan et al.[85] and 72.3% of 83 patients studied by Kearney et al.[88] Rodriguez-Morales et al.[89] reported a 70% incidence of left hemidiaphragmatic rupture among a series of 60 patients with ruptured diaphragms from blunt trauma. Herniation of abdominal viscera into the thorax occurs in 95.0% of cases through the left hemidiaphragm.[91]

Several factors account for the increased incidence of left hemidiaphragmatic rupture from blunt trauma. The left hemidiaphragm is relatively unprotected by abdominal viscera, such as the liver on the right side, and therefore it represents an area of relative weakness among the structures containing the abdominal viscera. The right diaphragm is stronger than the left and consistently requires a greater force to rupture.[92,93] The left hemidiaphragm is weaker because of a line of embryonic fusion between the costal and lumbar parts, predisposing this site to injury.[94] Finally, right hemidiaphragmatic injuries are underdiagnosed in nonsurgical series.[88] A positive pressure gradient of 7 to 20 cm of water exists between the peritoneal and pleural spaces. This gradient facilitates herniation of abdominal viscera through tears of the left diaphragm. Herniation markedly increases the potential for imaging diagnosis of the injury. On the right, the bulk of the liver blocks herniation of abdominal viscera unless the entire liver or a substantial portion herniates through a large gap in the right hemidiaphragm. The lack of herniated viscera markedly decreases the chances of direct imaging diagnosis. Tears of the left hemidiaphragm tend to be 10 cm or more in length and are usually located along the posterolateral aspect between the spleen and abdominal aorta, extending medially in a radial orientation toward the central tendon. Cardiac subluxation through a simultaneous tear in the diaphragm and pericardium has been described.[86] Also, visceral herniation into the pericardial space can occur through the same combination of injuries[95] (Fig. 5-33). Bilateral injuries and injuries into the central tendon of the diaphragm are uncommon and have been reported in 2% to 6% of patients with diaphragmatic injury.[90]

The central location of the diaphragm and its close proximity to other structures accounts for the frequent association of diaphragmatic rupture with other injuries that are present in 52% to 100% of cases.[85,89,96-98] Common concurrent injuries include pelvic fractures

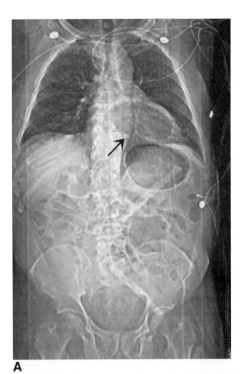

A

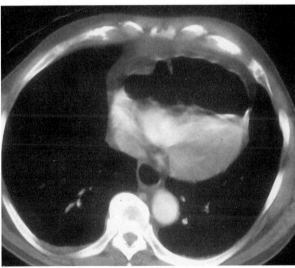

B

Fig. 5-33
Intrapericardial gastric herniation. **A,** CT scout digital radiograph shows peculiar lucent shadow overlying the heart with collar sign (*arrow*) leading to some diaphragmatic round gas shadows. **B,** CT through the heart shows air-filled stomach within pericardium anterior to the heart that is compressed by the air-filled stomach. (From Glaser DL, Shanmuganathan K, Mirvis SE: *Radiographics* 18:799, 1998.)

(40% to 55%), splenic injury (60%), and renal injury. Liver trauma occurs in 93% of patients with right and 24% of patients with left hemidiaphragmatic rupture. Intrathoracic injuries commonly associated with diaphragmatic rupture include multiple rib fractures, pneumothorax and hemothorax, and lung contusion.[97,99] Displaced left lower rib fractures should particularly increase concern for possible left hemidiaphragmatic tears. Aortic injuries have a weak association with diaphragmatic tears, occurring in about 5% of cases.[92,100]

Clinical Diagnosis. Unfortunately the clinical diagnosis of rupture of the diaphragm is difficult and is missed in 7% to 66% of patients.[88] Morgan et al.[85] established the diagnosis preoperatively in only 43% of 44 patients with this injury. Physical findings were nonspecific, consisting primarily of chest and abdominal wall contusions (only 16% of patients) and respiratory distress (52% of 60 patients) reported by Rodriguez-Morales et al.[85,89] As noted earlier, the force rupturing the hemidiaphragm often produces significant associated injuries. In the series of Morgan et al.[85] 59% of patients had major intraabdominal visceral injury and 45.5% had major intrathoracic injury. Voeller et al.[98] reported associated abdominal injuries in 82% of 33 patients with hemidiaphragmatic rupture. These injuries draw attention away from and delay recognition of diaphragmatic rupture. If there are no indications for celiotomy, the diagnosis can be further delayed, since direct inspection of the diaphragm is not performed.[101] Diagnostic peritoneal lavage (DPL) is falsely negative in up to 34% of patients with diaphragm disruption, perhaps as a result of negative intrapleural pressure drawing blood into the pleural space rather than the peritoneal cavity.[98,102,103]

Imaging Diagnosis of Hemidiaphragmatic Rupture

Chest Radiograph. Many radiologic methods have been advocated for the diagnosis of traumatic hemidiaphragmatic rupture, but the chest radiograph serves as the initial imaging study for evaluating the integrity of the hemidiaphragm after trauma.[104] The preoperative radiographic diagnosis of traumatic diaphragmatic rupture (TDR) caused by blunt trauma is often difficult, especially if no herniation of abdominal contents has occurred through the tear in the hemidiaphragm.[109] Initial chest radiographs may be completely normal or nonspecifically abnormal in 25% to 50% of patients.[103] Admission radiographs are diagnostic for TDR in 27% to 62% of patients with left-sided diaphragmatic injury and in 33% of right-sided injuries[89,103,106,107] and are suggestive of the diagnosis in another 18% of cases.[103,108]

Plain radiographic findings suggestive of the diagnosis of TDR include elevation of the apparent hemidiaphragm, obliteration or distortion of the diaphragm contour, contralateral displacement of the heart and mediastinum, and an ipsilateral pleural effusion[103] (Figs. 5-34 to 5-37). The demonstration of gas-containing

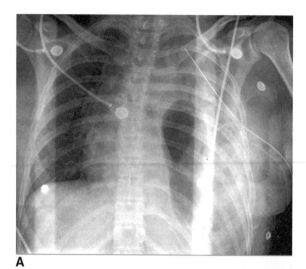

A

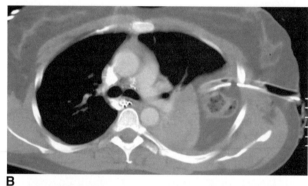

B

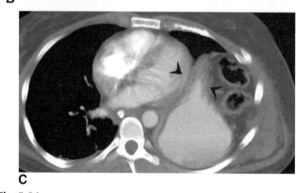

C

Fig. 5-34
Left hemidiaphragmatic rupture with gastric herniation. **A,** Chest radiograph after blunt trauma demonstrated a gastric bubble in the left lower chest with cardiac and mediastinal displacement. The left hemithorax is opacified, and a left thoracostomy tube is in place. **B,** CT through the mid chest shows atelectatic left lower lobe, splenic flexure, intraabdominal fat, and chest tube at the same level. **C,** CT through the lower chest shows sections of colon and surrounding fat. The stomach narrows as it crosses the rent in the diaphragm (*arrowheads*), producing the collar sign.

viscera within the thorax, particularly with a focal constriction ("the collar sign") across the air-containing structure, is pathognomonic of the diagnosis (Fig. 5-37). Clear demonstration of the stomach or nasogastric tube in the lower thorax in the setting of acute blunt trauma should be regarded as diagnostic of the injury

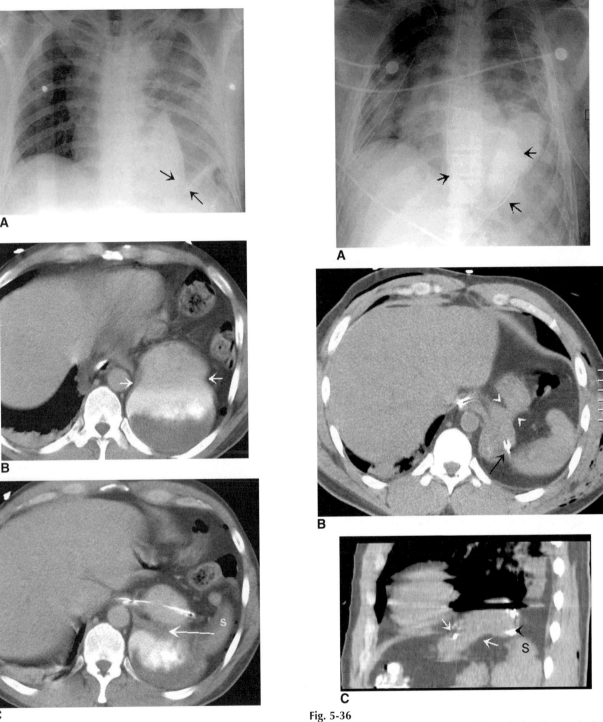

Fig. 5-35
Left hemidiaphragmatic rupture with gastric herniation. **A**, Supine chest radiograph shows gastric shadow projecting over left lower chest. Note narrowing of stomach as it crosses diaphragm tear (*arrows*). **B**, CT across lower chest shows focal minimal narrowing of stomach (*arrows*). **C**, A more caudal image shows the stomach divided across the torn diaphragm (*arrow*), with a nasogastric tube in the lower portion and contrast in the upper (fundic) portion, which is herniated. A portion of the spleen *(s)* and abdominal fat extend into the left thorax.

Fig. 5-36
Left hemidiaphragmatic rupture with gastric herniation. **A**, Supine chest radiograph demonstrated an elevated apparent left hemidiaphragm. The nasogastric tube tip (*black arrows*) projects over the lower left chest. **B**, CT across the upper abdomen shows the nasogastric tube tip in the fundus (*black arrow*), but the stomach shows a focal constriction (*white arrowheads*). **C**, A sagittal MPR shows the nasogastric tube in the stomach (*black arrowhead*) with a focal constriction of the gastric body (*white arrows*) as it ascends through the torn diaphragm. A portion of the superior pole of the spleen *(S)* also projects above the level of the hemidiaphragm.

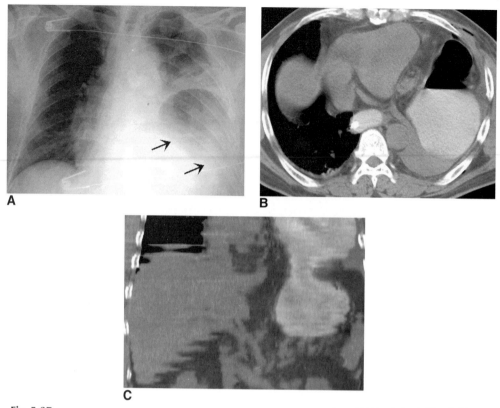

Fig. 5-37
Left hemidiaphragmatic rupture with gastric herniation. **A,** Chest radiograph shows elevation of the gastric bubble into the left lower chest and focal narrowing in the body region (*arrows*). There are fractures of left ribs and the left clavicle. The heart is displaced to the right. **B,** Chest CT indicates elevation of the stomach and surrounding fat with cardiac shift to the right. There is left posterior lower lobe atelectasis and minimally displaced rib fractures. **C,** Coronal MPR shows clearly that the stomach is herniated into the left chest with a focal collar sign at the level of the hemidiaphragm.

until proved otherwise (see later discussion). Herniation of the gastric fundus into the chest cavity may be misdiagnosed as a loculated pneumothorax and treated with placement of a thoracostomy tube (Fig. 5-36). Rupture of the diaphragm can be mimicked or masked on chest radiography by superimposed lung pathology. Confusing pathology includes atelectasis of the lower lobe (Fig. 5-38) elevating the stomach and hemidiaphragm, pleural effusion, pulmonary contusion with multiple traumatic lung cysts, aspiration, total or partial diaphragm eventration (Figs. 5-39 to 5-41), acute gastric distension, phrenic nerve palsy, loculated hemopneumothorax, subpulmonic fluid collections, and chronic esophageal or paraesophageal hernias.[13] In some cases serial chest radiographs demonstrate herniation of abdominal contents as a result of the persistent negative intrapleural pressure gradually pulling abdominal contents into the thoracic cavity. Also, some acute pulmonary and pleural abnormalities will have resolved or diminished on follow-up studies and may improve recognition of superimposed diaphragm injury. Positive pressure ventilatory support may delay herniation of abdominal viscera and postpone recognition of the

injury (Fig. 5-42). Postextubation radiographs should be performed in blunt trauma patients to exclude delayed herniation after intrapleural pressure reverts from positive to negative.

Gastrointestinal Contrast Studies. The introduction of an esophagogastric tube may be very helpful in diagnosing intrathoracic gastric herniation. A nasogastric tube serves to outline the location of the gastric fundus in relation to the hemidiaphragm. The addition of barium contrast through hand injection into the stomach through the esophagogastric tube will outline the stomach in relation to the lower thorax and occasionally can reveal constriction of the stomach at the level of the torn hemidiaphragm. Of course, barium should be suctioned from the stomach after the diagnostic study to prevent aspiration. If air-fluid levels are detected in the lower thorax by radiography and are not attributed to the stomach or proximal small bowel after an upper gastrointestinal contrast study, a barium enema should be given to exclude herniation of the colon. A drawback to the use of barium contrast is that its high density creates artifacts during subsequent CT studies. For this reason, diluted

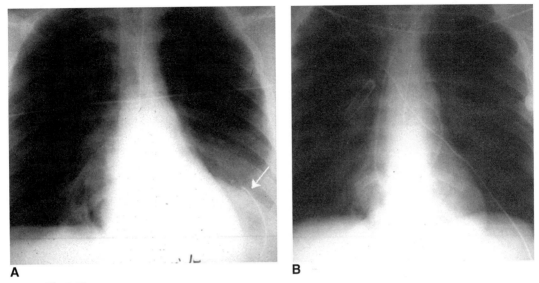

Fig. 5-38
Atelectasis mimics herniation across left hemidiaphragm. **A**, Increased density is seen in the left lower lobe on a chest radiograph of a blunt trauma patient with elevation of the apparent left hemidiaphragm and stomach as demarcated by nasogastric tube (*arrow*). This appearance could suggest left hemidiaphragmatic rupture with herniation, but note cardiac shift toward the left, which is more typical of atelectasis. **B**, After physical therapy the left base has cleared, indicating atelectasis as the cause of the original finding.

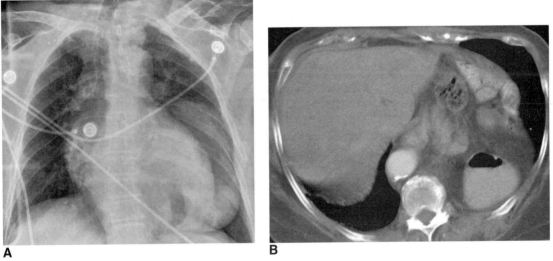

Fig. 5-39
Eventration mimics hemidiaphragmatic rupture. **A**, Chest radiograph on admission of a trauma patient shows masslike left lower chest density. Lateral rib fractures are present, but the diaphragm contour appears intact and there is no effusion or mass effect on the mediastinum. **B**, CT shows elevation of left upper abdominal contents, but these appear confined within abdomen. This appearance is due to eventration (congenital weakness) of a portion of the diaphragm without disruption.

water-soluble contrast is the preferred gastrointestinal contrast agent; otherwise CT should be obtained before barium contrast studies.

Cross-sectional Imaging. Use of sonography to diagnose acute diaphragmatic rupture may be limited by the presence of gas in the splenic flexure and stomach, creating an acoustic barrier to the more frequently injured left hemidiaphragm. In several instances in the current author's experience, subcutaneous emphysema accompanying chest trauma has limited the use of sonography in imaging either hemidiaphragm. Ideally, if the entire hemidiaphragm contour can be imaged sonographically, then a defect or herniation can be detected.[109,110] Of

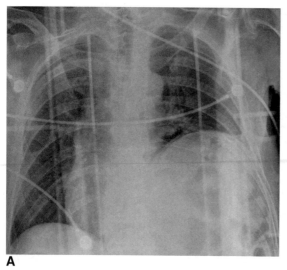 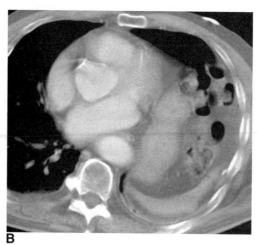

A **B**

Fig. 5-40
Possible palsy of the left hemidiaphragm. **A,** Admission chest radiograph of a trauma patient shows elevation of apparent left hemidiaphragm without effusion but with significant mass effect on the heart. Diaphragmatic rupture was considered. **B,** CT showed elevation of upper abdominal contents but contained within abdomen. Appearance was attributed to an abnormality of an intact hemidiaphragm due to palsy, contusion, or congenital weakness.

course, this method is highly dependent on the skill and expertise of the examiner and requires some degree of patient cooperation. In general, sonography has not been used extensively for diagnosis of acute injury of the left hemidiaphragm, but its successful use on the right, with the liver acting as an acoustic window, has been reported.[111,112]

Both CT and MRI have been used successfully to diagnose or exclude TDR[21,22,113] Cross-sectional imaging is most successful at assessing injury of the left hemidiaphragm, since herniation of abdominal contents is more common on this side. Both CT and MRI have been used successfully to demonstrate right hemidiaphragmatic rupture with herniation of bowel or liver and for the rare intrapericardial herniation as well (see Fig. 5-33). In cases in which the diagnosis of TDR is suspected based on plain radiographs, spiral CT is performed after administration of diluted oral contrast material. A special "diaphragm protocol" is used with spiral scanning from the lung bases to the upper abdomen with a 5 mm effective slice thickness and 3 to 5 mm/sec table increments. Axial images are reformatted from 2 to 3 mm reconstructed images into the sagittal and coronal planes.

Whenever possible, patient breath-hold through the scan is encouraged to minimize diaphragm motion. Axial and reformatted 2D sagittal and coronal plane images can show direct localized disruption of the diaphragm with herniation of abdominal contents. Using multidetector helical CT (MX 8000, Philips CT Systems, Cleveland, Ohio) images are acquired at 2.5 mm as part of the routine chest-abdomen-pelvis protocol and used directly to reformat into the coronal and sagittal planes. Conventional (nonspiral) CT with an 8 to 10 mm slice profile is often compromised by motion artifact and inadequate 2D reformations, limiting its diagnostic value for reliably diagnosing TDR. However, interpretation of even high-quality

Fig. 5-41
Lacerations and contusion mimicking diaphragmatic rupture with herniation. Chest radiograph of a trauma patient reveals irregular lucent areas in the left lower chest. The appearance could be confused with gastric herniation, but note that the diaphragm contour is intact, there is no obvious effusion or mass effect, and the nasogastric tip is below the hemidiaphragm. CT (not shown) revealed this finding as multiple adjacent lacerations and a contusion of the left lower lobe.

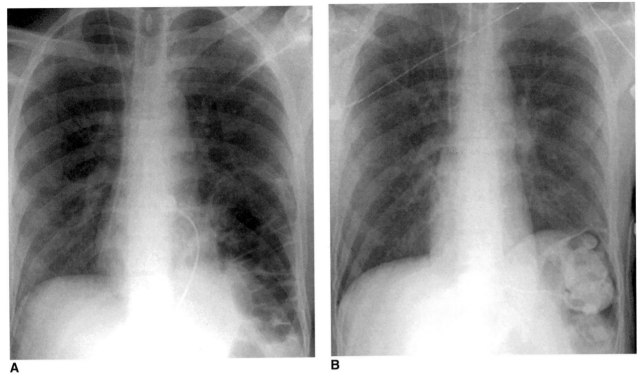

Fig. 5-42
Delayed bowel herniation through a torn left hemidiaphragm. **A,** Initial chest radiograph of a blunt trauma patient shows elevation of the left hemidiaphragm with the colon clearly herniated into the left lower chest. **B,** After institution of ventilatory support, the colon is significantly depressed with only a small portion projecting above the left hemidiaphragm contour.

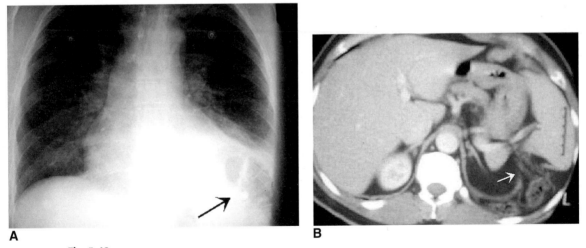

Fig. 5-43
Left hemidiaphragmatic rupture with colon herniation. **A,** Chest radiograph of a blunt trauma patient on admission indicates potential herniation of colon (*arrow*). **B,** CT of upper abdomen clearly shows torn left hemidiaphragm (*arrow*) with herniation of colon and surrounding fat into the left chest.

Continued

spiral axial and 2D CT can also be confounded by concurrent pulmonary or pleural-based pathology. CT signs of diaphragm injury include herniation of abdominal contents across a disrupted diaphragm, usually accompanied by the collar sign (Figs. 5-34 to 5-37 and 5-43 to 5-45), a focal discontinuity of the diaphragm (Figs. 5-43 to 5-45), or thickening of the hemidiaphragm due to hemorrhage[21,114,115] (see Fig. 5-43). Hemorrhage into fat adjacent to the diaphragm on the abdominal side also often accompanies diaphragmatic rupture.

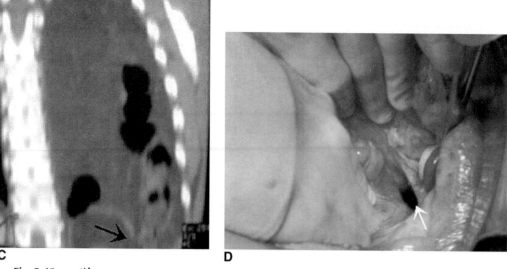

Fig. 5-43, cont'd
C, Coronal MPR demonstrates tear in left hemidiaphragm directly (*arrow*) and herniation of colon into the left chest. **D,** Intraoperative appearance of diaphragm rent (*arrow*) after bowel reduced.

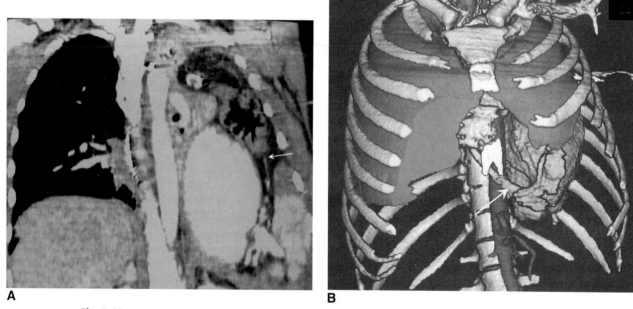

Fig. 5-44
MPR of left diaphragm injury. **A,** MPR coronal view obtained from multislice CT data set clearly shows gastric and left colon herniation. Note torn edge of left hemidiaphragm (*arrow*). **B,** 3D volumetric rendering of the chest shows herniated stomach. Note nasogastric tube (*arrow*) entering fundus that is inferior to remainder of the stomach, indicating gastric rotation about the coronal plane.

Conventional single-slice CT is 14% to 61% sensitive and 76% to 99% specific for diagnosing diaphragmatic rupture.[21,98,103,108,116] A focal defect in the diaphragm is the most sensitive sign described on conventional CT and is seen in 71% to 73% of patients with TDR.[21,108] Care must be taken not to mistake an interruption in the diaphragm, which is a normal variant (Fig. 5-46) seen particularly in elderly women,[21,117] or an acquired Bochdalek hernia[118] as an acute injury. Usually hemorrhage is seen at the site of an acute diaphragm injury.

Conventional CT is limited in the diagnosis of TDR because of relative thick, 8 to 10 mm slice thickness and

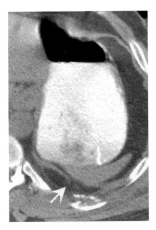

Fig. 5-45
Direct CT finding of diaphragm tear. CT of blunt trauma patient demonstrates focal tear in the posterior left hemidiaphragm (*arrow*).

patient motion. These thick sections make it difficult to distinguish a diaphragmatic injury from adjacent lung or pleural space pathology. Also, the multiplanar reformations are compromised by poor spatial resolution. Spiral CT improves detection of diaphragmatic injury mainly by improving the quality of multiplanar reformations (MPR) based on thinner or overlapping axial sections with decreased patient motion. Significant improvement of MPR images results in improved accuracy for confident diagnosis of TDR by permitting evaluation of the entire contour of the diaphragm and its relationship to the abdominal viscera.[15,95] It is anticipated that multidetector spiral scanning will further improve CT accuracy.

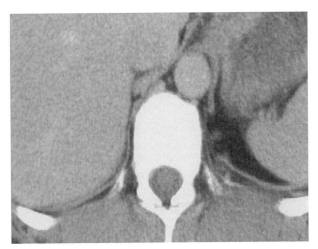

Fig. 5-46
Defects in diaphragm due to normal variant. CT of nontrauma patient shows congenital defects in the medial left hemidiaphragm and crus region. Note lack of hemorrhage in adjacent fat of thickening of diaphragm that would be expected with an acute tear.

A retrospective study was conducted at the Maryland Shock Trauma Center to evaluate spiral CT in 41 patients with suspicion of TDR based on radiographs. The study group included 32 patients with possible left-sided injury, 10 with possible right-sided injury, and one with suspected bilateral injury. Spiral CT was 78% sensitive for left-sided injury and 50% sensitive for right-sided injury with 100% specificity on both sides.[10] The collar sign was the single most common diagnostic finding, with 63% sensitivity and 100% specificity for TDR. MPR images were particularly helpful in establishing the diagnosis on the right side (see Fig. 5-52). A similar study performed by Murray et al.[108] analyzed preoperative abdominal CT scans in 11 patients with diaphragmatic rupture (eight left and three right) and 21 patients with intact diaphragms after major acute blunt abdominal trauma. CT studies were reviewed independently by three observers without knowledge of surgical findings. Diaphragmatic discontinuity was seen in eight of the 11 cases of diaphragmatic rupture, visceral herniation was seen in six, and the "collar sign" was seen in four. Hemoperitoneum of hemothorax completely obscured visualization of the ruptured diaphragm in three cases. Individual diagnostic sensitivity among the three reviewers to detect diaphragmatic rupture was 54% to 73% and specificity was 86% to 90%. Average sensitivity for the three observers was 61% (95% confidence interval, 41% to 81%), and average specificity was 87% (95% confidence interval, 76% to 99%).

Whenever the interpretation of radiographic and CT studies is equivocal for diaphragm injury, MRI provides a useful alternative procedure.[119,120] Among 16 patients studied by MRI for potential diaphragm injury at the UMSTC, seven had the diagnosis confirmed with surgical verification, nine patients had no evidence of diaphragm injury, and none had clinical sequelae of a missed injury.[113] T1-weighted coronal and sagittal images through the hemidiaphragm in question are quickly obtained and typically are adequate for diagnosis (Figs. 5-47 to 5-51). Fast gradient-echo and inversion recovery MR pulse sequences have also been used, but in the author's experience these do not improve on the information obtained from the T1 spin-echo images. On MRI the diaphragm appears as a continuous dark curvilinear line. Atelectatic lung or pleural fluid usually marginates the superior aspect of the hemidiaphragm when injured. The undersurface is contrasted against the liver on the right and the retroperitoneal fat, omentum, and viscera on the left. When ruptured the hemidiaphragm shows discontinuity in the dark curvilinear line and extension of abdominal contents above the disruption. Typically, a collar sign is seen at the point where the abdominal structure crosses the diaphragm tear. MRI is very useful to confirm an intact diaphragm in trauma patients in cases of eventration or dysfunction (Fig. 5-50).

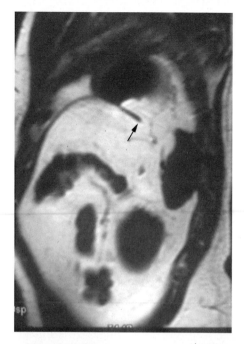

Fig. 5-47
MRI of diaphragmatic rupture. Sagittal T1-weighted study demonstrates a clear disruption of the left hemidiaphragm (*arrow*). Intraperitoneal fat and stomach have herniated into the left chest. Fat on either side clearly outlines the dark signal of the diaphragm. (From Shanmuganathan K, Mirvis SE, White CS, Pomerantz SM: *AJR* 167:402,1996.)

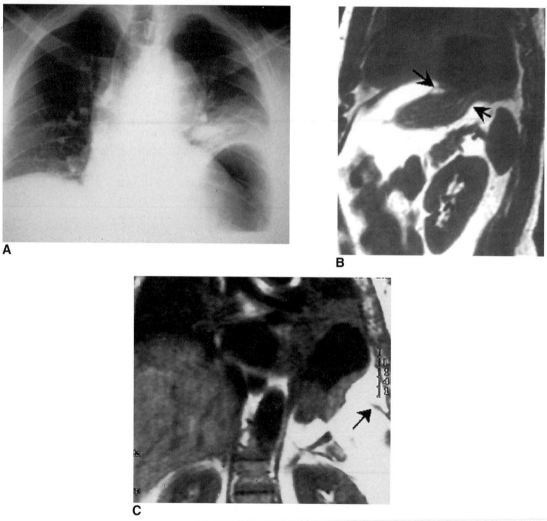

Fig. 5-48
MRI diaphragmatic rupture. **A,** Chest radiograph taken at admission shows apparent elevation of the left hemidiaphragm, distended stomach projecting over the left hemithorax, and shift of the mediastinum to the right. Sagittal **(B)** and coronal **(C)** MR images show herniation of omentum, the fundus of the stomach, and the superior aspect of the spleen herniating through a posterior diaphragm tear. The stomach shows the collar sign (*arrows*) on the sagittal view and the torn edge of the diaphragm (*arrow*) on the coronal view. (From Shanmuganathan K, Mirvis SE, White CS, Pomerantz SM: *AJR* 167:402, 1996.)

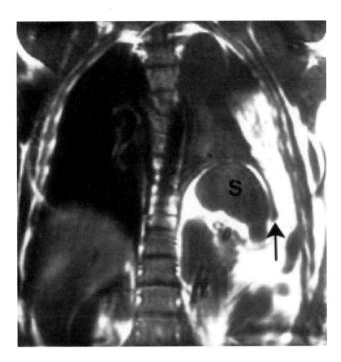

Fig. 5-49

MRI of diaphragmatic rupture. Coronal T1-weighted MRI of a trauma patient shows free edge of the left hemidiaphragm (*arrow*) that was avulsed from the left chest wall. Omental fat has herniated into the left hemithorax, producing left lung atelectasis and mediastinal shift to the right. The spleen *S* appears in an ectopic position just beneath the mid-diaphragm, indicating avulsion from its peritoneal attachments. (From Gelman R, Mirvis SE, Gens D: *AJR* 156:56, 1991.)

Nuclear Scintigraphy. Isotopic techniques are available for imaging the lung, liver, and spleen to detecting transdiaphragm herniation. Injection of technetium 99m (Tc 99m)–sulfur colloid demonstrates the location of the liver and spleen and may detect either constriction of the parenchyma at the site of herniation or displacement of either organ into the thorax. Injection of Tc 99m–macroaggregated albumin permits simultaneous localization of the lung bases, liver, and spleen (liver-spleen-lung scan). Currently, nuclear scintigraphy is

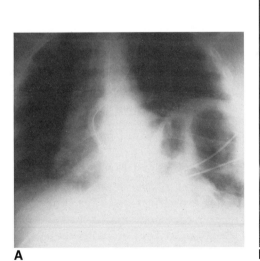

A

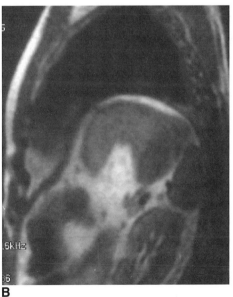

B

Fig. 5-50

MRI of elevated left hemidiaphragm. **A**, Admission chest radiograph in a blunt trauma victim shows smooth but quite elevated apparent left hemidiaphragm with bowel loops projecting beneath the apparent diaphragm. **B**, Sagittal T1-weighted MRI clearly shows the low-intensity signal of the elevated left diaphragm with abdominal contents beneath. The appearance suggests eventration or hemidiaphragm paralysis.

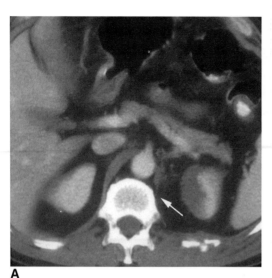

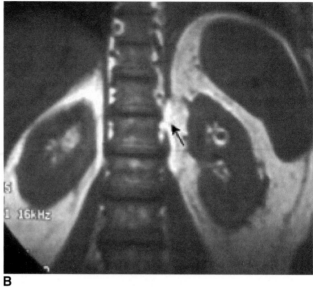

A **B**

Fig. 5-51
Tear in crus of left hemidiaphragm on MRI. **A**, CT image of a patient who had sustained blunt trauma shows loss of substance of crus of the left hemidiaphragm (*arrow*) and left renal upper pole infarct. **B**, T1-weighted coronal MRI confirms tear in the left crus with some fat herniation (*arrow*). The injury was managed clinically and was not surgically verified. (From Shanmuganathan K, Mirvis SE, White CS, Pomerantz SM: *AJR* 167:401, 1996.)

infrequently used for diagnosing acute hemidiaphragmatic rupture.

The typical diagnostic approach as practiced at the UMSTC for possible diaphragm injury in blunt torso trauma is shown in Fig. 5-52.

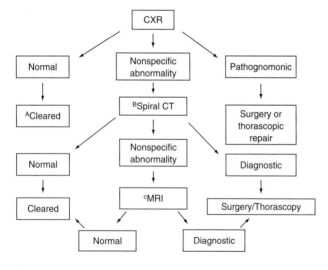

ASome injuries with initial normal radiographs will manifest radiographically in a delayed fashion; a normal spiral CT or MRI may not completely exclude injury.
BSlice thickness of 5 mm or less with overlap and suspended breathing. Requires review of sagittal and coronal multiplanar reformations.
CUse T1-weighted coronal and sagittal of side(s) of suspected injury.

Fig. 5-52
Diagnostic algorithm for diaphragm injury at UMSTC.

Penetrating Trauma (see Chapter 11)

Injury to the diaphragm occurs in up to 10% of patients with penetrating chest trauma.[100] Diagnostic imaging has played a less significant role in diagnosing injury to the diaphragm from penetrating trauma than from blunt force injury. Usually the diagnosis is made surgically during exploration of the abdomen or chest for common associated injuries or by thoracoscopy. The diagnosis must be suspected whenever there is penetrating trauma to the torso between the nipple and costal margins, a wounding trajectory that might traverse the diaphragm, or a hemothorax or pneumothorax on chest radiography after penetrating injury. Since up to 84% of tears of the diaphragm resulting from penetrating trauma are less than 2 cm long,[121] acute transdiaphragmatic herniation is rare, making acute preoperative imaging diagnosis uncommon.[100,116,121] Herniation can certainly occur acutely or subacutely after a penetrating trauma (Fig. 5–53), especially with a large defect or more likely with a delayed presentation after a small diaphragmatic tear is undiagnosed in the acute setting. Diaphragm injury appears to be common after left-sided penetrating thoracoabdominal trauma, is frequently associated with other injuries, may be clinically occult, and is often accompanied by a normal chest radiograph.[121]

Although most trauma surgeons elect surgical exploration of patients with penetrating thoracoabdominal trauma, including stable patients, to view the location

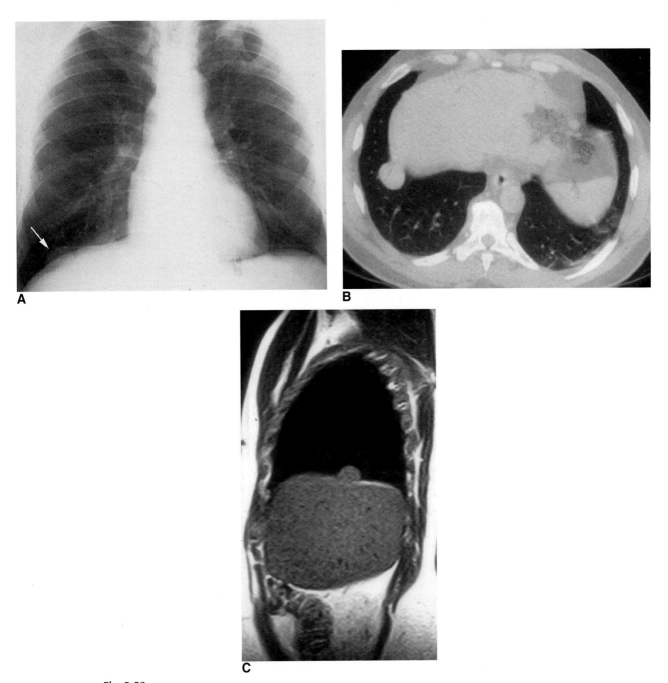

Fig. 5-53
Delayed herniation after remote stab wound. **A,** Routine chest radiograph in nontrauma patient shows pulmonary nodule at the right lung base *(arrow)* suspicious for neoplasm. **B,** Chest CT image shows rounded nodule at the right lung base adjacent to the diaphragm. Prior to a lung biopsy a scar was noted over the left lower lateral chest. The patient described a stab wound to the region 7 years before without medical intervention. **C,** Sagittal T1-weighted MRI verifies that the mass is herniated liver presumably related to the remote stab wound. (From Pomerantz SM, Shanmuganathan K, Siegel EL, et al: *Emerg Radiol* 3:205, 1996.)

and extent of injury directly, selective use of CT for penetrating trauma to the right upper quadrant has been attempted in stable patients.[122] CT can directly show involvement of the lung, pleural space, solid abdominal viscera, and the diaphragm either directly or indirectly by demonstrating injury on both sides. The presence or absence of intraperitoneal air and blood can assist in determining the need for celiotomy. Renz et al.[122]

studied 13 consecutive patients with a gunshot wound between the right nipple, costal margin, right posterior axillary line, and anterior midline by CT. No patient had or developed more than local wound tenderness clinically. All patients had a right hemothorax treated with a chest tube. CT scanning was performed within 8 hours of admission in 12 of the 13 patients, and demonstrated the following injuries: pulmonary contusion (12), hepatic laceration (seven), spinal cord transection (two), and a renal laceration (one). CT was used to follow the hepatic and renal injuries to resolution. The patients were all managed successfully without surgery. Selective CT examination for penetrating trauma to the right upper quadrant and lower chest is used at the UMSTC to help determine the requirement for surgical exploration. A detailed discussion of penetrating torso trauma including the diaphragm is found in Chapter 11.

MEDIASTINAL INJURY
Esophageal Injury in Trauma

Esophageal rupture from blunt trauma is very rare, occurring in less than 1% of patients.[22,73,123] A review by Beal et al.[124] from 1900 to 1988 found only 96 cases reported, mostly occurring in violent vehicular trauma. Blunt and penetrating injury together, excluding iatrogenic causes, accounted for only 10% of esophageal perforations occurring in 127 patients over a 47-year period reviewed by Bladergroen et al.[125] Blunt force injury to the esophagus occurs most commonly in the cervical and upper tho-

racic portions, as well as just above the gastroesophageal junction.[22,126] The author has observed one case in which the midthoracic esophagus was torn and occluded within a thoracic spine fracture-subluxation[127] (Fig. 5-54). In most cases, blunt esophageal rupture is accompanied by other significant intrathoracic injury.[123] A variety of mechanisms account for acute esophageal injury after blunt thoracic trauma, including crushing between the spine and trachea, tearing due to hyperextension-traction force (particularly at the level of the diaphragmatic hiatus), and direct penetration by cervical spine fracture fragments (Fig. 5-55). Radiographic signs are often not immediately present or relate to associated injuries such as to the adjacent airway. Radiographic findings seen with complete esophageal wall disruption include persistent pneumomediastinum and cervical emphysema (60%),[123] left pleural effusion, and an abnormal mediastinal contour caused by leakage of fluid or associated mediastinum hemorrhage. The role of CT scan for primary diagnosis of esophageal perforation in blunt trauma has not been described in any series because of the rarity of the injury. Hypothetically, spiral CT should be more sensitive for detection of small air bubbles or fluid collections adjacent to the torn esophagus, as well as minimal contrast leaks (Figs. 5-56 and 5-57). Development of complete esophageal perforation can be postponed as a result of delayed breakdown of an ischemic segment of the esophagus or an occluding periesophageal hematoma.[73] The diagnosis of esophageal injury from blunt trauma is also potentially delayed

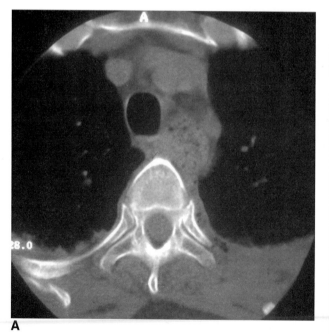
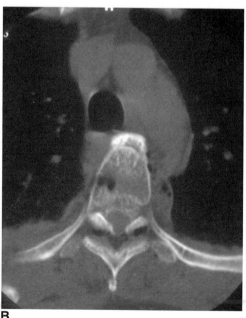

A   **B**

Fig. 5-54
Esophageal entrapment after blunt trauma. **A**, CT of an elderly blunt trauma patient with T3-T4 subluxation shows dilated fluid-filled mass in mediastinum interpreted as an occluded esophagus. **B**, A more caudal CT image shows air in T3-T4 disc space and facet joints and in paraspinal soft tissue. Widening of the facet joints and no definite esophagus.

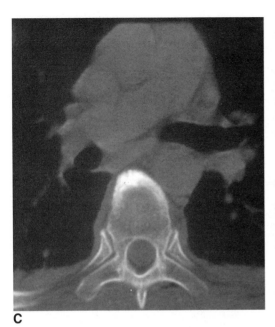

C

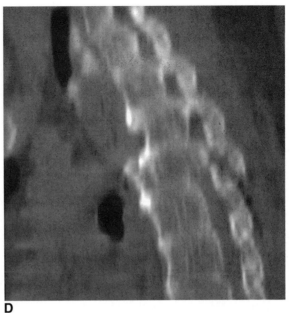

D

Fig. 5-54, cont'd
C, More caudal CT shows no evidence of the esophageal lumen. **D**, CT was performed after the patient swallowed minimal oral contrast with difficulty. Sagittal reformation shows distended esophagus containing minimal oral contrast entrapped in the thoracic spine injury at the T3-T4 disc level. (From Maroney M, Mirvis SE, Shanmuganathan K: *AJR* 167:714, 1996.)

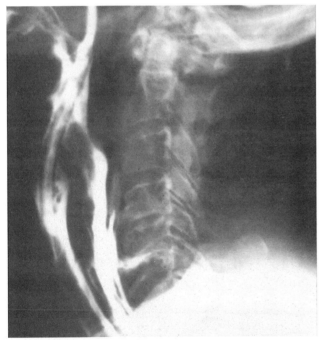

Fig. 5-55
Cervical esophageal perforation. Lateral cervical radiograph obtained during Gastrografin swallow demonstrated extravasation of contrast for a posterior esophageal tear into ruptured C5-C6 and prevertebral soft tissue. An anterior osteophyte at this level combined with cervical hyperextension (note anterior widening of C5-C6 disc space) was believed to be etiologic. (From Reddin A, Mirvis SE, Diaconis JN: *J Trauma* 27:565, 1987.)

because of a lack of a specific symptom complex, symptoms attributed to other causes, and an incomplete diagnostic evaluation.[124] Delay in diagnosis leads to an increased risk of mediastinitis, sepsis, and death.

Iatrogenic causes of esophageal injury that may occur in the acute trauma setting include nasogastric tube placement, esophageal intubation, and manipulation of esophagoscopy tubes. Any potential penetrating trauma to the mediastinum can produce injury to the esophagus, vascular structures, and the airway and must be excluded by appropriate direct inspection or diagnostic imaging. Spiral CT scan of the mediastinum has been used recently to define the track of a missile through the chest and its precise relationship to the mediastinal structures. Any wound in which the missile's course is in close proximity to the mediastinum would mandate a diagnostic workup. However, if the course is definitely not near the mediastinum, the workup could be safely skipped. In a study of 24 patients with missile injury to the thorax, the mediastinal diagnostic workup was changed in 12 (50%) on the basis of CT study findings.[128] In general, this method is not applicable to knife wounds of the thorax, since knife tracks usually are more difficult to define with certainty than ballistic objects.

Once suspected, esophageal rupture can be confirmed radiologically. Contrast esophagogram, initially performed with water-soluble contrast media and then, if negative, barium sulfate, is about 90% sensitive in establishing the diagnosis,[125] with greater diagnostic accuracy reported in the thoracic than in the cervical esophagus[123] (Fig. 5-57).

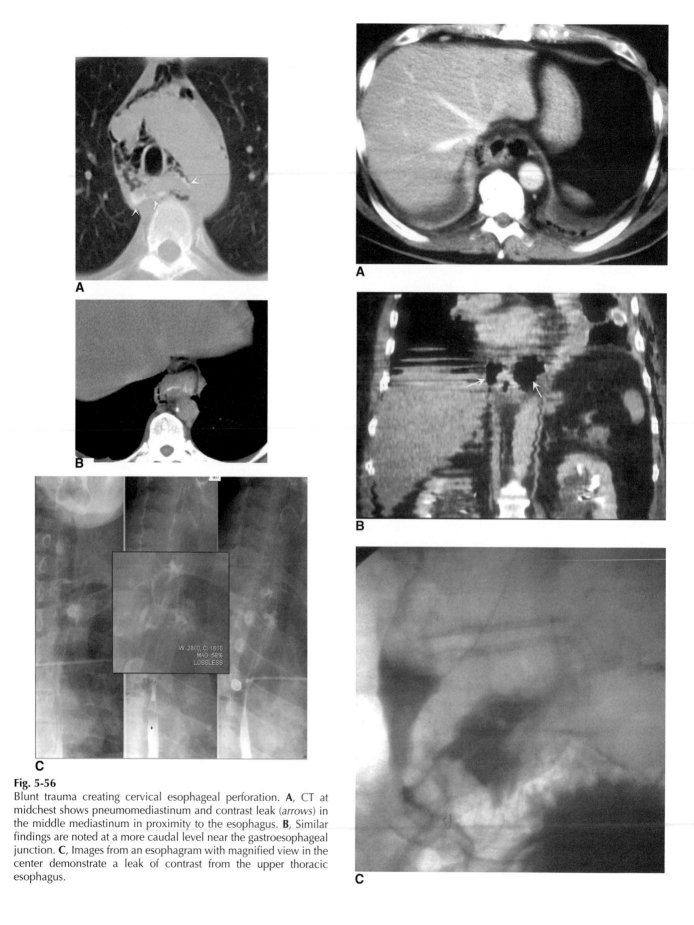

Fig. 5-56
Blunt trauma creating cervical esophageal perforation. **A**, CT at midchest shows pneumomediastinum and contrast leak (*arrows*) in the middle mediastinum in proximity to the esophagus. **B**, Similar findings are noted at a more caudal level near the gastroesophageal junction. **C**, Images from an esophagram with magnified view in the center demonstrate a leak of contrast from the upper thoracic esophagus.

Fig. 5-57
Esophageal tear from blunt trauma. **A,** CT shows small collections of air in the lower mediastinum near the esophagus; the patient had foul-smelling left chest tube drainage. **B,** Coronal MPR confirms mediastinal gas pockets (*arrows*). **C,** Esophagram confirms leak near the gastroesophageal junction.

Esophagoscopy has similar diagnostic sensitivity. Both studies together probably offer better diagnostic accuracy than either one alone. Flowers et al.[129] reported on the use of flexible fiberoptic esophagogastroduodenoscopy (EGD) for detection of esophageal injury from blunt and penetrating trauma in 31 patients (24 penetrating). They found 100% sensitivity, 96% specificity, and 97% accuracy and recommended the method highly.

Tracheobronchial Rupture

Tracheobronchial rupture (TBR) is an uncommon injury after blunt trauma, occurring in 0.4% to 1.5% of blunt trauma victims in clinical series[130-133] and in 2.8% to 5.4% in autopsy series of trauma victims.[134] Prehospital mortality is up to 78% with an early mortality of 20% to 30% for initial survivors.[135-137] Early mortality is higher for patients with complete thoracic tracheal transection than cervical tracheal trauma, and it is lowest for those with small tears or perforations.[137-139] Thoracic tracheal injuries are more common than cervical injuries, and right mainstem bronchus injuries are somewhat more common than left mainstem injury.[140]

About 60% to 80% of TBR occurs within 2.5 cm of the carina[73] with a predominance of right-sided injuries.[32,141] Injuries to the trachea from blunt injury usually involve the membranous portion.[3] A number of mechanisms have been proposed to explain TBR from blunt force. A sudden AP compression of the thorax causes lateral displacement of the lungs and mainstem bronchi, tearing the mainstem bronchi near the carina. Compression of the air-containing tracheobronchial tree against a reflexively closed glottis can generate a rapid rise in intraluminal pressure, bursting the airway. The trachea can be directly crushed between the depressed sternum and thoracic spine. The cervical trachea can directly impact the rigid steering wheel or dashboard. Rapid deceleration can produce shearing forces at the relatively fixed cricoid cartilage and carina. Finally, exaggerated hyperextension of the cervical spine applies longitudinal traction on the trachea.[73,130,133,142-144] Animal studies performed by Lloyd et al.[144] show that an 11 kg distracting force is required to tear the trachea when acting along its long axis, but only a 3 kg force will tear the carina transversely

at the mainstem bronchi, suggesting that a transverse force most likely accounts for clinical injury. The trachea can also be injured by a "clothes-line" type impact with ropes, tree limbs, wires, or cables, typically by individuals riding recreational vehicles or running, producing an impacting force between the cartilage rings or at the laryngotracheal junction.[145]

The clinical diagnosis of TBR is not established acutely in up to 68% of patients.[134] The diagnosis may be obscured by other major or more overt injuries that may not have any external manifestations. A number of clinical signs may be present including respiratory distress (57% to 85%), cough, hemoptysis (26% to 54%), cyanosis, and subcutaneous air (37% to 100%). However, these signs are neither highly sensitive nor specific for the diagnosis. Other signs include sternal tenderness, Hamman's sign (xiphisternal crunching sound synchronous with cardiac motion), and hoarseness or aphonia related to recurrent laryngeal nerve injury.[135,137,146-150] Clinical signs and symptoms are more likely to be present with tracheal than bronchial injury. Cervical tracheal injury is likely to be accompanied by external abrasions, lacerations, and contusions to direct clinical attention. Larger tears in the airway would be expected to produce earlier and more profound symptoms. Pathologically, TBR is most commonly a transverse tear between the tracheal rings (75%) or a longitudinal tear (18%) in the membranous segment with 8% combined tears. Complete separation of the trachea may occur, but airway continuity can still be maintained by peritracheobronchial tissue. This situation is tenuous and can quickly deteriorate to severe airway compromise and a surgical emergency.

Acutely, the radiographic findings of TBR are often subtle and nonspecific. Radiographic signs of TBR commonly include pneumomediastinum that is often severe, persistent, and progressive (Fig. 5-58). Air, particularly delivered by positive pressure ventilation, can dissect widely from the mediastinum into the neck and subcutaneous tissues. Unilateral or bilateral pneumothorax is common and may not be relieved by thoracostomy tube evacuation (Fig. 5-59), indicating a persistent source of air leak into the pleural space.[137] In most cases (79%) pneumothoraces will respond, so reexpansion of the lung does not exclude TBR.[151] Air can dissect into the peribronchial adventitia, forming a "sleeve of air" that permits visualization of both inner and outer surfaces of the airway by chest radiography.[152,153] Signs of a major airway leak may also be noted on the initial or subsequent lateral cervical spine radiograph as air ascends through the deep cervical fascial planes. Air may also dissect into the retroperitoneum, peritoneal cavity, spinal canal, and pericardium.[154,155] Atelectasis may develop acutely or in delayed fashion in the lung distal to an interrupted

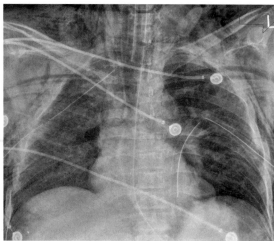

Fig. 5-58
Chest radiograph of a blunt trauma patient with tracheobronchial rupture. Supine chest radiograph shows pneumomediastinum and diffuse soft tissue air. There are bilateral rib fractures and bilateral chest tubes. The appearance is not specific for major airway injury but should increase suspicion. A right mainstem bronchus injury was found at surgery.

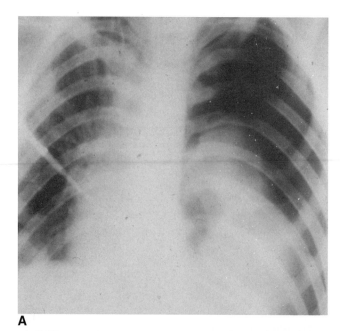

A

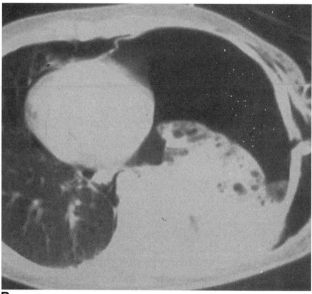

B

Fig. 5-59
Chest radiograph of "fallen" lung. **A**, Supine chest radiograph shows a left tension pneumothorax with cardiac and mediastinal displacement. The left lung is collapsed and has fallen into a gravity-dependent position in the lower left chest. **B**, CT image shows collapse of the left lung into the posterior thoracic cavity. There is a marked left tension pneumothorax despite a chest tube because of a large airway leak from the left mainstem bronchus.

bronchus as a result of partial or complete obstruction of the bronchus and is likely to persist.[73,156] In about 10.0% of patients with TBR, no radiographic signs are evident acutely, indicating that a partially or completely transected airway is maintained by an intact peritracheal or peribronchial adventitia. An endotracheal tube balloon or blood/fibrin clot may also seal the airway injury.[73,74,157,158] Such patients may present with delayed or persistent atelectasis after occlusion of the airway by fibrous stricture. If transection of the bronchus is complete in the acute setting, the lung may collapse away from the mediastinum and settle into the posterolateral or inferior thorax, depending on patient position—the so-called fallen lung sign (Fig. 5-59). The disrupted end of a torn mainstem bronchus may appear to terminate or taper abruptly (the "bayonet" sign) and is best demonstrated using thin section CT with coronal reformation. An overdistended endotracheal (ETT) balloon (Fig. 5-60) or an abnormally positioned endotracheal tube in relation to the airway also indicates tracheal disruption. The ETT balloon appears overinflated because of diminished resistance by the injured tracheal walls, requiring more volume to seal the airway. The balloon may assume an atypical rounded or elliptical shape (see Fig. 5-60). If the trachea around the balloon is disrupted, the balloon diameter exceeds 2.8 cm. The normal diameter measured 2 cm above the aortic arch is 13 to 25 mm in men and 10 to 21 mm in women.[3,159] Focal portions of the balloon may

herniate beyond the tracheal walls through small tears (Fig. 5-61). Transection of the cervical trachea or cricotracheal junction permits elevation of the hyoid bone above the superior endplate of the C3 vertebral body due to the unopposed pull of the suprahyoid musculature. This finding, typically noted on the lateral cervical

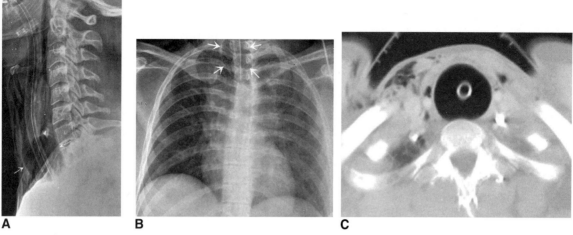

Fig. 5-60
Overdistended endotracheal tube balloon as sign of tracheal injury. **A,** Lateral cervical radiograph of blunt trauma patient shows a markedly overdistended endotracheal tube balloon just below the larynx (*arrows*). The lower cervical trachea was ruptured at surgery. **B,** A chest radiograph of the same patient also shows a markedly distended balloon in the upper thoracic trachea (*arrows*). **C,** CT confirms the finding, showing the balloon uniformly distended around endotracheal tube. This appearance suggests a large trachea defect that permits uniform distension of the balloon. (From Chen JD, Shanmuganathan K, Mirvis SE, et al: *AJR* 176:1273, 2001.)

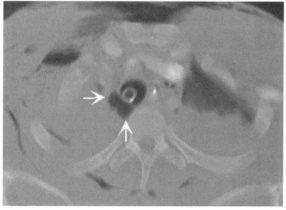

Fig. 5-61
Focal endotracheal tube balloon herniation. CT through the superior mediastinum shows a focal herniation of the endotracheal tube, indicating focal disruption of the posterolateral tracheal wall (*arrows*). (From Chen JD, Shanmuganathan K, Mirvis SE, et al: *AJR* 176:1273, 2001.)

radiograph, is strongly suggestive, if not pathognomonic, of tracheal transection.[160,161]

In a review of nine patients with tracheal or bronchial tears caused by blunt chest trauma, Unger et al.[162] suggested that the "fallen lung" sign or an ectopic or overdistended ETT balloon was the most specific radiographic finding of TBR; however both are uncommon. Distal

bronchial tears are more likely to be associated with pneumothorax and proximal tears with pneumomediastinum.[163] Spencer et al.[147] also suggested that thoracic tracheal injury is most likely to produce massive mediastinal air and deep cervical emphysema, and bronchial injury is more likely than tracheal injury to produce a pneumothorax. In a study by Chen et al.,[3] patients with tracheal disruption were significantly less likely (p=0.01) to have a pneumothorax than a control population of patients with pneumomediastinum but an intact trachea. They proposed that the injury to the trachea spared the mediastinal pleura and limited the air leak to the mediastinum. The resolution of pneumomediastinum and subcutaneous emphysema after its initial appearance does not exclude airway injury.[161]

TBR is typically suspected on the admission or early chest radiograph by the findings already described. Spiral CT will also demonstrate findings associated with TBR but may provide a precise diagnosis. Diagnostic CT signs include visualization of direct discontinuity of the airway fracture and deformity of a tracheal ring(s), continuity between intraluminal and extraluminal air (Figs. 5-62 and 5-63), and overdistension (see Fig. 5-60), partial herniation (see Fig. 5-61), or ectopic positioning of the ETT balloon. Among 14 patients with proven tracheal injury studied by Chen et al.[3] by spiral CT, tracheal injury was directly visualized in 71% (10/14). Five of seven intubated patients had overdistension of the ETT balloon (range, 2.8 to 4.2 cm; mean, 3.4 cm; control population range, 1.7 to 2.7 cm).

The balloon shape was abnormal (ovoid or elliptical) in three, and a portion of the balloon was herniated beyond the tracheal wall in two. Among intubated patients the presence of paratracheal mediastinal air was significantly more likely to occur (p less than or equal to 0.05) in patients with tracheal rupture than in a control population of patients with pneumomediastinum but no tracheal injury. In a study reported by Kunisch-Hoppe et al.,[153] routine CT was diagnostic of TBR in only one of ten patients. Thus further studies using spiral and multidetector spiral CT with volumetric and virtual "fly-through" imaging are needed to better define the potential accuracy of state-of-the-art CT for this diagnosis (Fig. 5-64).

Once suspected either clinically or by imaging studies, the diagnosis of TBR is best confirmed using laryngoscopy or fiberoptic bronchoscopy.[152,163] Early diagnosis of TBR improves the opportunity for successful primary surgical reanastomosis and offers the best chance for a successful long-term outcome with fewest complications.[73] The presence of upper rib fractures is not associated with tracheal injury with a positive predictive value of only 2%.[28] Combined injuries of the esophagus or major thoracic arteries and the trachea are most likely to occur after penetrating mediastinal trauma.[137] A wide variety of injuries occur in association with TBR from blunt trauma, with extrathoracic system injury seen in 75% of patients.[25,145] Tracheal injury can result from trachea intubation, although this is a rare complication.[164,165] Predisposed patients include those with tracheomalacia, as may occur in the elderly, or those with tracheal stenosis.[165-167] The membranous trachea appears most susceptible to this injury mechanism because this portion resists the tip of the tube as it is

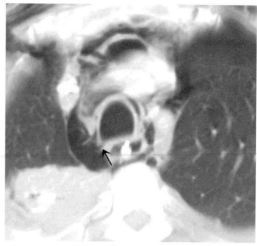

Fig. 5-63
CT of tracheal injury. Image through the upper chest shows direct connection between trachea posterolaterally and mediastinal air (*arrow*). Right anterior displaced rib fracture noted. (From Chen JD, Shanmuganathan K, Mirvis SE, et al: *AJR* 176:1273, 2001.)

positioned.[165] The injury may also result when intubation is performed by an inexperienced care provider or is attempted while working under extremely stressful or poor conditions. Other factors that may contribute include use of the wrong tube size or inappropriate use of the stylet. There are reports of tracheal injury resulting from overdistension of the ETT balloon.[168,169] Overdistension of the ETT balloon may occur in patients with underlying tracheomalacia in which the resistance of the trachea to expansion is diminished. However, cadaver studies performed by Chen et al.[3] indicate that extremely high cuff pressures using 70 to 80 ml of inflation are needed to rupture the trachea. There is high resistance to inflation of the intubated cadaver trachea after 50 ml of air is injected into a standard cuff. In most cases it is the ETT balloon that expands to fill a low-resistance disrupted airway rather than an overdistended balloon that actually ruptures the airway.

Traumatic Aortic Injury and Mediastinal Hemorrhage

Traumatic aortic injury (TAI) accounts for 16% of the fatalities resulting from motor vehicle accidents. The mortality from TAI before treatment can be provided at a medical facility has been reported at 85% to 90% but can be expected to improve with increasing use of regional trauma centers and rapid helicopter transportation.[170] The danger of rapid exsanguination remains a constant risk among patients who initially survive aortic injury. The study of Parmley et al.[171] emphasized the need for prompt diagnosis of TAI and surgical management. Of 35 patients who

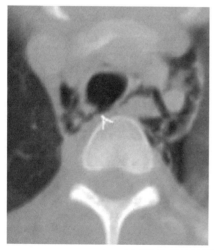

Fig. 5-62
Direct CT sign of tracheal injury. A direct connection of air is present between the posterior trachea and the surrounding mediastinal soft tissues (*arrowhead*). The injury was surgically verified. (From Chen JD, Shanmuganathan K, Mirvis SE, et al: *AJR* 176:1273, 2001.)

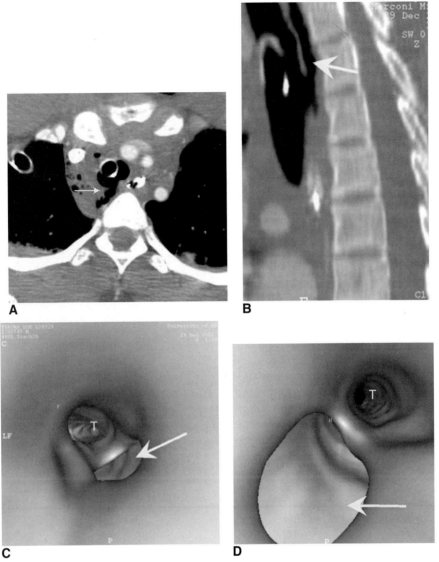

Fig. 5-64
CT and "Voyager 3D" of tracheal injury. **A**, Axial CT image in a blunt trauma patient shows air extending from posterior trachea into adjacent soft tissue *(arrow)*. **B**, Sagittal reformation shows collection of mediastinal air posterior to trachea *(arrow)*. **C**, Voyager fly-through (MX 8000, Phillips Medical Systems) shows large collection of air *(arrow)* directly adjacent to trachea *(T)* at site of tear. **D**, Another Voyager image shows posterior tracheal wall defect *(arrow)*.

survived to reach a medical facility but whose aortic injuries were not diagnosed, 30% died within 6 hours, rising to 40% by 24 hours after admission. Unfortunately, this often-cited study is based on a small population of autopsied patients. The study was conducted before the era of modern thoracic angiography and does not consider the possible influence of undiagnosed aortic ruptures with prolonged survival on the overall natural history of this injury. Although the need for early diagnosis of aortic injury is undeniable, the true natural history of this injury, if untreated, is not well known. A study at the UMSTC

reviewed mortality from undiagnosed TAI measured from the time of the injury, including both directly admitted and transferred patients. During the second 30 minutes after injury, mortality peaked at 30% of remaining survivors per hour but decreased to 1.7% of remaining untreated survivors per hour from 1 to 17 hours after injury (personal communication, Dr. Stephen Turney, Professor of Surgery, University of Maryland Shock Trauma Center, 1995). This mortality pattern indicates a very unstable patient subgroup, perhaps with near-complete rupture or tamponade of bleeding only by the mediastinal pleura and a more stable population with bleeding confined to the aortic wall, in whom diagnostic testing is practicable if performed expeditiously. A study performed by Duhaylongsod et al.[172] also indicated a bimodal risk of death from TAI. In that study, 66% of 42 deaths occurred within 4 hours after injury from free aortic rupture, and 14 (33%) late deaths (4 to14 days) were attributed to unrelated causes.

The mechanism of TAI is debated, and a number of hypotheses have been advanced. A sudden influx of blood from the compressed heart could increase intraluminal aortic pressure and cause a tear in the relatively weak isthmic region. The aorta may be compressed between the "anterior bony complex" (manubrium, first rib, and clavicle) and the spine, resulting in a transverse tear, the so-called osseous pinch mechanism.[173] A combination of rapid deceleration and compression producing rotational and shearing forces and transverse laceration at the vulnerable isthmic region of the aorta is the most commonly proposed theory in the literature.[174] The rate of chest wall deformation at impact rather than the absolute amount of chest wall compression related to a given impact is correlated more strongly with TAI. Lateral and frontal impacts appear equally common among patients sustaining TAI in motor vehicular trauma.[126] The incidence of TAI in pedestrian fatalities at 12.7% is similar to its incidence in fatal motor vehicle accidents.[175]

After the proximal descending aorta, the next most common site of aortic injury based on autopsy studies is the ascending aorta (Figs. 5-65 to 5-67), accounting for 2% of fatalities from road traffic accidents.[176] This injury is rarely encountered clinically because of the high mortality, most likely from concurrent injuries.[176] Patients with ascending aortic injury usually manifest mediastinal

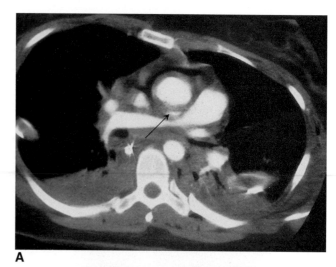

A

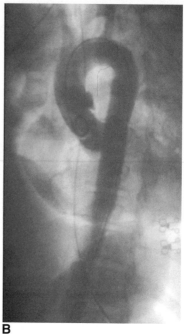

B

Fig. 5-66
CT of ascending aortic injury. **A**, CT image through the ascending aorta in a patient who had fallen 70 feet shows a small pseudoaneurysm arising from the proximal ascending aorta (*arrow*). **B**, Aortogram confirms the injury.

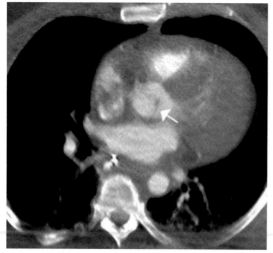

Fig. 5-65
CT of ascending aortic injury. Image through the proximal ascending aorta shows an intimal flap (*arrow*).

hemorrhage by radiography and CT but may rarely have a normal mediastinal appearance.[177] Clinical signs of cardiac tamponade or aortic regurgitation suggest this injury.[177] In the UMSTC experience the aortic arch is the third most common site (Figs. 5-68 and 5-69), followed by the distal descending aorta above the diaphragmatic hiatus (Fig. 5-70).

Patients sustaining TAI do not have clinical signs and symptoms sufficiently sensitive or specific to dictate the need for thoracic angiography or other imaging evaluation.

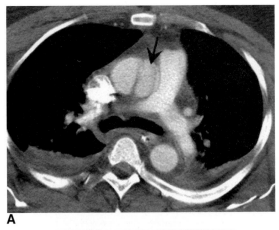

A

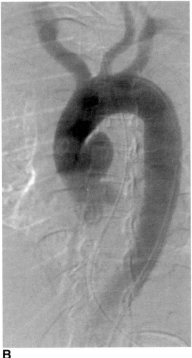

B

Fig. 5-67
CT of ascending aortic injury. **A,** CT through the ascending aorta reveals a large pseudoaneurysm near the root *(arrow).* There is mass effect on the aortic lumen and proximal pulmonary artery. **B,** Angiogram demonstrating the pseudoaneurysm.

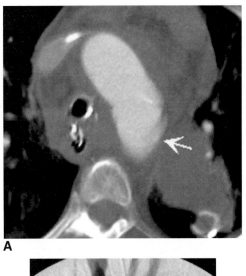

A

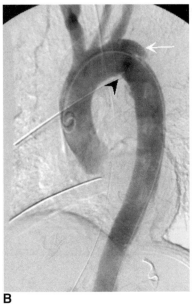

B

Fig. 5-68
CT of injury to aortic arch. **A,** A pseudoaneurysm arises from the aortic arch just distal to the subclavian origin *(arrow).* These injuries can be difficult to detect on axial CT with thick sections (8 to 10 mm) because of their orientation to the plane of section. There is abundant, diffuse mediastinal hemorrhage and mass effect on the trachea and esophagus. **B,** Aortogram confirms mushroom-shaped pseudoaneurysm *(arrow)* arising from the top of the arch. Note small intimal flap along the inferior margin of the arch *(arrowhead).*

Overall, suggestive clinical findings are present in less than half of patients with TAI, and up to one third of patients have no evidence of external thoracic trauma.[143,178,179]

Radiographic Signs of Mediastinal Hemorrhage. Over the past three decades, a wide variety of radiographic signs have been promoted for their value as indicators of mediastinal hemorrhage and potential great vessel injury. A retrospective analysis of chest radiographs and thoracic aortograms of more than 200 patients, including 42 with

arteriographically diagnosed and surgically confirmed great vessel ruptures, was conducted at the UMSTC to determine the value of these signs (Table 5-1). Mediastinal hemorrhage is a direct indicator of mediastinal trauma but an indirect indicator of TAI. Bleeding in the mediastinum is believed to originate from tears in small veins and arteries, perhaps including the vaso vasorum of the aorta. The majority of patients with

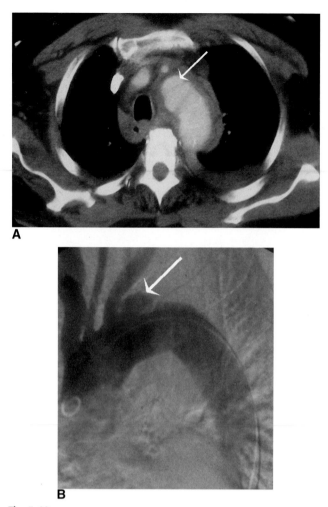

Fig. 5-69
CT of injury to the aortic arch. **A,** Pseudoaneurysm arises from the top of the aortic arch (*arrow*) at the level of the origins of the great vessels and could be mistaken for a major branch vessel. Note periaortic mediastinal hematoma and displacement of the trachea and esophagus to the right. **B,** Aortogram confirms the pseudoaneurysm (*arrow*) just distal to the left subclavian origin from ectatic aorta.

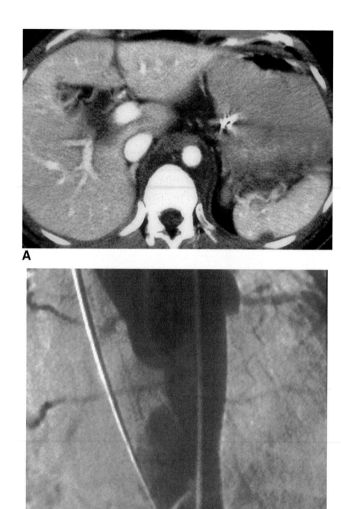

Fig. 5-70
Distal thoracic aortic injury. **A,** CT through the lower chest shows periaortic retrocrural hemorrhage. A small splenic laceration and perihilar liver lacerations also are present. The study was an abdominal CT. **B,** Aortogram shows pseudoaneurysm of the descending thoracic aorta accounting for the adjacent hematoma.

radiographic evidence of mediastinal hemorrhage will not have major thoracic arterial injury.[6,12,23,178]

Radiographic assessment of the mediastinal contour should be based, whenever possible, on the "true erect view of the thorax." Ayella et al.[180] argued that an AP projection with the patient erect and leaning 10 degrees to 15 degrees beyond the vertical most closely simulated the routine posteroanterior chest radiograph. The true erect view provides a more accurate display of the anatomy of the superior mediastinum than either supine or semierect projections. Schwab et al.[181] assessed the effect of patient position on the plain radiographic diagnosis of TAI. In their study, 21 of 55 patients (38%) had apparent "widened mediastinums" on supine chest radiographs

obtained after blunt chest trauma but were considered to have normal radiographs in the erect position. All these patients had normal aortograms; however, 4 of 12 patients with widened mediastinal contours on both views had TAI. These authors recommended the use of the erect view to avoid unnecessary aortography.[181] The oversensitivity of the supine view for mediastinal hemorrhage was illustrated in a retrospective study performed at the UMSTC. In this study the supine chest radiograph was falsely positive for mediastinal hemorrhage in 80%

Table 5-1
Sensitivity, Specificity, and Predictive Values of the Signs of Traumatic Aortic Rupture*

| | INCIDENCE | | | | PREDICTIVE VALUES | |
Sign	Positive Diagnosis	Negative Diagnosis	Sensitivity (%)	Specificity (%)	Positive (%)	Negative (%)
Aortic knob outline	113	323	72	47	26	87
Widened mediastinum[†]	82	249	53	59	25	83
Tracheal shift[‡]	31	48	20	92	39	82
Left mainstem bronchus[§]	5	5	3	99	50	80
Left hemothorax	7	16	5	97	30	80
Nasogastric tube displaced to right	14	23	9	96	38	80
Left apical cap						
Fracture	3	31	2	95	9	79
No fracture	14	27	9	96	34	80
Rib fracture first through fourth	24	98	15	84	20	79
Widened left paraspinal stripe[‖]						
Fracture	4	24	3	96	14	79
No fracture	18	21	12	97	46	81
Widened right paraspinal stripe[¶]						
Fracture	3	4	2	99	43	80
No fracture	3	7	2	99	30	80
Lung contusion	18	88	12	86	17	79
Loss of descending aorta	98	283	63	53	26	85
Loss of aortico-pulmonary window	65	101	42	83	39	85
Opacified medial left lung field	18	32	12	95	36	81
Pneumothorax or pneumomediastinum	18	69	12	89	21	80
Displaced superior vena cava to right[¶]	11	23	7	96	32	80
Negative	2	84	—	—	—	98

From Mirvis SE, Bidwell JK, Buddemeyer EU, et al: *Radiology* 163:487, 1987.
*Total of all examiners. Based on 156 total positive and 606 total negative studies.
[†]Subjective impression, or >8 cm at the aortic knob, or >0.25 mediastinal width/chest width.
[‡]Left tracheal wall to the right of the T4 spinous process.
[§]Subjective impression, or shifted >40 degrees below horizontal.
[‖]Greater than 5 mm or greater than one half the width of descending aorta, or greater than one half the distance from the spine to the left margin of the descending aorta.
[¶]Subjective impression.

of patients with normal aortograms, whereas the true erect view in the same patients suggested mediastinal hemorrhage in only 52%.[165,182]

Selected Radiographic Signs of Mediastinal Hemorrhage

Mediastinal Widening. In 1975, Marsh and Sturm[184] concluded that a mediastinal width greater than 8 cm at the level of the aortic arch on a 100-cm AP chest radiograph constituted a highly sensitive sign of aortic injury. However, in a later publication, Sturm et al.[185] demonstrated significant overlap in the measured mediastinal width of traumatized patients with and without TAI, thus diminishing the value of this sign. In 1981, Seltzer et al.[186] introduced the concept of the mediastinal width/chest width (M/C) ratio, suggesting that a ratio ranging from 0.25 to 0.28 on an AP supine chest radiograph was 95.0% sensitive and 75.0% specific for aortic injury. Subsequent studies by Marnocha et al.[187] challenged this concept; they found an M/C ratio greater than 0.38 to be only 40.0% sensitive and 60.0% specific for great vessel injury. In the UMSTC experience, an M/C ratio greater than 0.25 was 53.0% sensitive and 59.0% specific as an indicator of aortic injury.[182] The measurement of the mediastinal width does not take into account variations produced by body habitus (mediastinal fat), respiratory phase, X-ray target to film distance effects, and patient positioning, among other factors. A number of normal variants and trauma-related pathologies such as mediastinal lipomatosis, congenital vascular anomalies, acquired aortic disease, atelectasis, medial lung contusion, and medial pleural effusion could create a falsely positive M/C ratio.

Although the observation of a "widened mediastinum" was somewhat sensitive for detection of mediastinal hematoma and potential aortic injury, patients with TAI can certainly manifest a narrow mediastinal width by chest radiography (Fig. 5-71). In these cases it is the abnormal contour of the mediastinum rather than a single measurement that is crucial in recognizing the potential for TAI.

Progressive widening of the superior mediastinum on serial radiographs due to a gradually expanding hematoma has been suggested as another sign of TAI. Applebaum et al.[188] recommended serial chest radiographs during the first 48 hours after admission to detect delayed mediastinal bleeding. Ayella et al.[180] challenged this concept because in their extensive clinical experience no patient with an aortic rupture exhibited a gradually expanding hematoma. They argued that lysis of a mediastinal hematoma initially containing an aortic rupture or rupture of the adventitia would result in a sudden, massive hemorrhage that would not permit time for serial radiographs. They suggested that the gradually widening mediastinum was caused by nonaor-

tic sources of bleeding or by technical difficulties in attempting to produce equivalent chest radiographs. The UMSTC experience over the past 15 years has validated this impression.

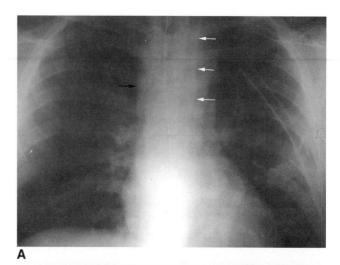

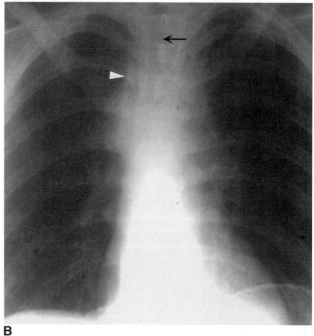

Fig. 5-71

Mediastinal hemorrhage with near-normal mediastinal width. **A,** Chest radiograph in a supine trauma patient shows a right paratracheal stripe (*black arrow*), a widened left paraspinal stripe (*white arrows*) ascending above the aortic arch, and an ill-defined aortic arch. These findings are all indicative of mediastinal hemorrhage in the trauma setting. The mediastinal width was less than 8 cm, or 25% of the thoracic width at the level of the arch. A torn aorta was repaired. **B,** An admission radiograph from a different patient also demonstrates a right paratracheal stripe (*white arrowhead*) and rightward tracheal deviation (*black arrow*). The mediastinal width is mildly widened. (From White CS, Mirvis SE, Templeton PA: *Emerg Radiol* 1:72,1994.)

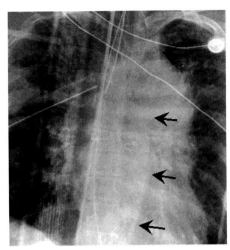

Fig. 5-72
Abnormal mediastinal contours with aortic injury. Supine radiograph shows very abnormal mediastinal contour with loss of aortic outline and very wide left paraspinal stripe representing posterior mediastinal blood (*arrows*). Left paraspinal stripe continues to form an apical extrapleural cap.

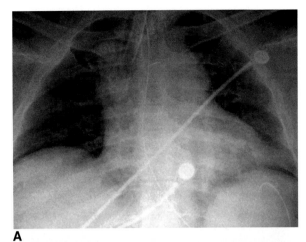

A

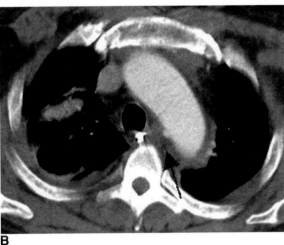

B

Fig. 5-73
Abnormal mediastinal contours with aortic injury. **A,** Supine chest radiograph shows a generally poorly defined mediastinal contour. The aortic outline is difficult to perceive. The trachea appears displaced to the right, but this could be caused by patient rotation. Suffice it to say, the mediastinal contour cannot be "cleared." **B,** CT shows a small pseudoaneurysm arising from the posterior arch (*arrow*) with minimal surrounding mediastinal hemorrhage. Note right anterior costochondral chest wall fracture.

Mediastinal hemorrhage can arise from lower cervical, thoracic, and upper lumbar vertebral fractures. Dennis and Rogers[189] observed that superior mediastinal widening caused by thoracic spinal fractures could mimic widening seen with TAI. They concluded that mediastinal widening in the presence of thoracic fractures made the diagnosis of aortic injury unlikely in the absence of clinical signs and symptoms to support the diagnosis. Although the concurrence of both injuries appears relatively uncommon, the presence of a spinal fracture alone cannot, in any manner, exclude TAI in the presence of mediastinal hemorrhage. Further imaging evaluation in all patients with unequivocal radiographic evidence of mediastinal contour abnormality after blunt thoracic trauma is therefore recommended.

Abnormal Aortic Arch and Descending Aorta Contour. Several authors have stressed the importance of abnormalities of the contour or obscurity of the aortic outline as an indicator of mediastinal hemorrhage and possible TAI[178,190,191] (Figs. 5-72 to 5-75). Marsh and Sturm[184] reported this sign in all of their patients with aortic rupture but also in 45% of patients with normal aortas. Marnocha et al.[187] reported this sign to be a sensitive (88%) but nonspecific (42.0%) indicator of TAI. They observed that the outline of the aorta could appear blurred if the radiograph is underexposed or if there is excessive patient motion. Adjacent lung infiltrates due to aspiration or pulmonary contusion can obscure the aortic outline, as can venous hemorrhage into the mediastinum. Overall, previous series have found a sensitivity

of 53% to 100% and specificity of 20% to 53% for this sign as an indicator of TAI. The UMSTC study found 72% sensitivity and 40% specificity for this sign.[192]

Shift of the Trachea and Nasogastric Tube. By virtue of anatomic proximity, a contained hematoma or pseudoaneurysm of the proximal descending aorta might be expected to affect the position of adjacent structures such as the trachea or esophagus. Gerlock et al.[193] reported that, if both the trachea and esophagus were shifted to the right on an AP chest radiograph (using the thoracic spinous process at T4 as a midline landmark), then the patient had a 96% probability of TAI (see Figs. 5-74 and 5-75). In a series of 45 patients, no patient without a

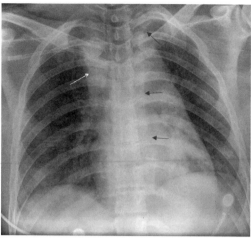

Fig. 5-74
Abnormal mediastinal contours with aortic injury. Supine chest radiograph demonstrates mediastinal hemorrhage causing a right paratracheal stripe (*white arrow*) and a wide left paraspinal stripe that extends above the aortic arch level (*black arrows*). The trachea is slightly displaced to the right.

shifted nasogastric tube had a ruptured aorta. Wales et al.[194] demonstrated rightward deviation of the nasogastric tube in only five of eight patients with TAI. A study by Dart and Braitman[195] found normal tracheal position in many patients with TAI.

Pitfalls in determining the presence of tracheal and/or esophageal displacement include positioning of the chest for radiography, failure to place a nasogastric tube, and the potential of a balancing hematoma in the right mediastinum. In a previous series, deviation of the trachea

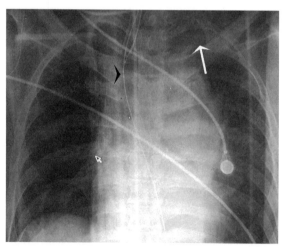

Fig. 5-75
Abnormal mediastinal contour and aortic injury. Supine chest radiograph of trauma patient struck by car. Image shows large amount of soft tissue density obscuring the aortic arch. A widened left paraspinal stripe extends to an apical pleural cap (*arrow*). The nasogastric tube is markedly bowed to the right (*arrowhead*). The patient sustained a fatal traumatic aortic injury.

demonstrated a poor sensitivity (12% to 53%) but better specificity (80% to 89%) for diagnosing TAI, whereas deviation of a nasogastric tube to the right has a higher sensitivity (40% to 71%) and specificity (90% to 94%). In the UMSTC experience, tracheal shift to the right of the spinous process of the T4 vertebra was 20% sensitive and 92% specific, whereas rightward displacement of the nasogastric tube was 9% sensitive and 96% specific for TAI.[182]

The Apical Pleural Cap Sign. In 1975, Simeone et al.[196] stressed the value of an extrapleural left apical cap as a sign of an aortic isthmus region aortic injury (see Figs. 5-71, 5-72, and 5-75). Blood from a mediastinal hematoma could extend along the left subclavian artery into the potential space between the left parietal pleura and the extrapleural soft tissue, producing an apical soft tissue density. In the original study by Simeone et al. this sign was present in 25 of 27 patients with TAI.[196] However, in their subsequent evaluation in 1981, Simeone et al.[197] noted that the apical cap was usually accompanied by other signs of TAI such as a widened mediastinum or a poorly defined aortic arch. They believed that aortography was not indicated if an apical cap was the only positive radiographic sign. Other series indicate a sensitivity of 20% to 63% and a specificity of 75% to 76% for this sign.

The false-positive rate of the apical pleural cap sign is increased by the similar radiographic appearance produced by hematoma arising from adjacent rib or clavicle fractures or by an ectatic subclavian artery. In the UMSTC experience, Mirvis et al.[182] observed this sign in only 9% of the patients with TAI; however, half of the patients with an apical pleural cap without associated fractures had aortic injury diagnosed. In agreement with Simeone et al.,[196,197] no patient was observed in whom an apical pleural cap was the only sign of TAI.

Widened Paraspinal Lines. Bleeding within the posterior mediastinum can distend the paraspinal stripes. Barcia and Livoni[178] reported a displaced left paraspinal line, defined as greater than half of the distance from the spine to the left margin of the descending aorta, in 83.0% of patients with aortic injury (see Figs. 5-72 and 5-74 to 5-76). This sign was also 83% specific without concomitant spine or sternal fractures. Other series have determined a somewhat lower sensitivity of 40% to 62%. Barcia and Livoni[178] found widening of the right paraspinal stripe to be less sensitive (seen in only 4 of 14 patients with TAI) but 94% specific without spine or sternal fractures. Peters and Gamsu[198] found this sign in 8 of 14 patients with TAI and in none without this injury.

The sensitivity of the paraspinal stripe sign is likely to be compromised by the failure to visualize even widened

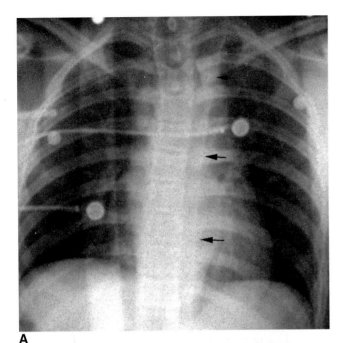

A

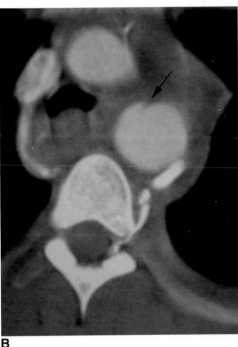

B

Fig. 5-76
Abnormal left paraspinal stripe. **A**, Chest radiograph in supine position shows a wide left paraspinal stripe (typically less than 5-7 mm) that extends to apex (*arrows*). The aortic arch and descending aorta are ill defined. **B**, CT image through the proximal descending aorta shows intimal flap (*arrow*) and medially projecting pseudoaneurysm. There is surrounding mediastinal hematoma and the carina is deviated to the right.

paraspinal lines on underexposed chest radiographs, and specificity is decreased by paraspinal hematomas arising from concomitant spinal fractures. Mirvis et al.[182] reported widening of the right and left paraspinal stripes

without associated thoracic fracture in only 2% to 12%, respectively, of patients with TAI. The extension of a left paraspinal stripe above the level of the aortic arch is more likely to occur in the presence of aortic injury (see Figs. 5-72, 5-75, and 5-76).

Depression of the Left Mainstem Bronchus. Hematoma or pseudoaneurysm arising from the aortic isthmus may depress the left mainstem bronchus and narrow the carinal angle. Barcia and Livoni[178] measured the carinal angle in 113 patients with blunt chest trauma. In 17 patients with aortic injury, the carinal angle varied from 56 to 92 degrees (mean, 75 degrees) and in patients without vascular injury, the range was 49 to 108 degrees (mean, 71 degrees). They believed this measurement had no predictive value. Other series using various criteria to measure left mainstem bronchus depression have shown a low sensitivity (4% to 41%) but high specificity (80% to 100%) for this sign. Decreased sensitivity may be related in part to difficulty in accurately visualizing the mainstem bronchi on underexposed portable chest radiographs. This sign was present in only 3% of patients with TAI seen at the UMSTC, but 50% of patients with this sign had TAI diagnosed angiographically.[182]

Injury to Ribs, Lungs, and Pleura. Other signs (pulmonary contusion, rib fractures, pneumothorax, and hemothorax) present on chest radiographs after blunt chest trauma have been assessed for potential association with TAI. In general, these signs have not shown sufficient sensitivity or specificity to be of diagnostic value in dictating the need for thoracic CT or angiography. Specifically, Poole[31] in a collective review of 1390 patients did not demonstrate a high probability of aortic or great vessel injury associated with first- or second-rib fractures. He pointed out that TAI is more likely to occur with no rib fractures or with other than first- or second-rib fractures and suggested that other radiographic evidence of mediastinal hemorrhage was almost always present on the chest radiograph of patients with TAI. Kram et al.[199] also indicated that upper rib fractures at any level did not increase the likelihood of TAI.

Combining Radiographic Signs: Diagnostic Value. Analysis of the study performed at the UMSTC, as well as that of previous studies, demonstrates that no single plain chest radiographic sign is either completely sensitive or specific in diagnosing TAI (see Table 5-1). Thus some authors have suggested that any patient with a history of blunt decelerating chest trauma should have thoracic angiography despite the appearance of the chest radiograph.[200,201] This approach would result in an excessive number of normal aortograms that might delay diagnoses and treatment of other life-threatening craniocerebral or abdominal injuries. The use of thoracic CT for diagnosing TAI, as discussed later, offers an alternative imaging procedure to thoracic aortography. Mirvis et al.[182] noted that the simultaneous absence of certain combinations of radiographic signs has a high negative predictive value for TAI (see Table 5-1). For instance, a normal aortic arch, normal descending aorta, and clear aorticopulmonary window had a 91.0% negative predictive value on both supine and erect radiographs of the chest. A normal aortic arch and normal descending aorta had an 87% negative predictive value on the erect view and a 91% negative predictive value on the supine study. A normal chest radiograph had a 98.0% negative predictive value. It must be recalled, however, that these statistics are derived from a population of patients whose radiographs were already "suspicious" enough to warrant aortography. Patients with a normal mediastinal contour by radiologists' interpretation did not undergo thoracic CT or angiography. A large number of aortograms have been safely eliminated without any known adverse outcome based on the analysis of the chest radiograph.

Computed Tomography for Potential Traumatic Aortic Injury. During the past decade CT has become increasingly well established as a secondary screening study, following chest radiography, to demonstrate both the presence or absence of mediastinal hemorrhage and direct findings of aortic injury.[4,6,12,23,202-206] In 1983 Heiberg et al.[207] described a small series of 10 patients, four of whom demonstrated direct CT evidence of aortic injury; normal aortas were identified in the other six. However, other studies subsequently cited both a lack of sensitivity and specificity for CT in diagnosing TAI, citing problems with motion and volume averaging in identifying intimal injuries, interobserver differences, and missed branch vessel injuries.[208-210] It is clear from the literature that the introduction of spiral CT, increased familiarity

with CT findings of aortic injury, and use of multiplanar and 3D imaging has markedly improved the accuracy of CT for diagnosis of TAI. Table 5-2 lists results of several recently published studies using spiral CT in the assessment of possible TAI.

Thoracic CT is optimally performed after bolus injection of at least 90 ml of 60% intravenous contrast. Helical scanning begins typically after a 25 second delay but may be controlled using bolus-tracking technology. Slice thickness of 5 to 7 mm through the chest is obtained, and images are reformatted at every 2 to 3 mm. Using multidetector CT, thinner slices (2 to 3 mm) reformatted with overlap are more readily obtained, providing improved z-axis resolution. Two-dimensional reformations should be performed through the long axis of the aorta, as well as in standard coronal or sagittal planes. Three-dimensional imaging using maximal intensity projection (MIP) or volume rendering is required if an aortic injury is evident. These presentations enhance appreciation of the pathologic anatomy and the relationship of the injury site to adjacent important vascular structures and landmarks. The major thoracic arteries should be reviewed from the base of the neck to the diaphragm. The study should assess the presence and location of mediastinal hemorrhage, the presence, location, and extent of aortic injury, and the relationship of an injury to adjacent vessels such as the left subclavian artery. It is important to search all major vascular structures because multiple injuries can occur involving both the aorta and its major branches. At the UMSTC, nonenhanced thoracic CT is not obtained as an initial screening study.

In most cases of TAI, the injury is readily apparent on axial CT images as a pseudoaneurysm that typically projects anteriorly or anteromedially from the aortic lumen at the level of the left pulmonary artery (Figs. 5-77 to 5-87).

There is typically a collar of surrounding mediastinal blood that is believed to arise from small veins, arteries,

Table 5-2
Studies of Helical CT Diagnosis of Traumatic Aortic Injury

Author	CT	TAI	Sensitivity(%)	Specificity(%)	PPV(%)	NPV(%)	Accuracy(%)
Dyer et al.[238]	1561	30	NA	NA	100	100	100
Mirvis et al.[12]	1104	24	100	99.7*	89	100	99.7
Raptopoulos et al.[202]	326	8	100	86†	19	100	87
Fabian et al.[205]	494	71	100	83	50	100	86
Biquet et al.[204]	28	12	92	100	NA	NA	NA
Wicky et al.[203]	487	14	90	99	NA	NA	NA
Wicky et al.[203] (meta-analysis)	NA	NA	97	99.8	NA	NA	NA
Gavant et al.[6]	1518	21	100	81.7	47.4‡	100	84

*Only patients with an equivocal or suboptimal chest radiograph underwent CT.
†No adverse sequelae were seen at clinical follow-up in patients with a negative scan, which was deemed to be true-negative.
‡No adverse sequelae were seen at clinical follow-up in patients with a negative scan, which was deemed to be true-negative. Data are listed only for patients with abnormal CT findings who underwent angiography.

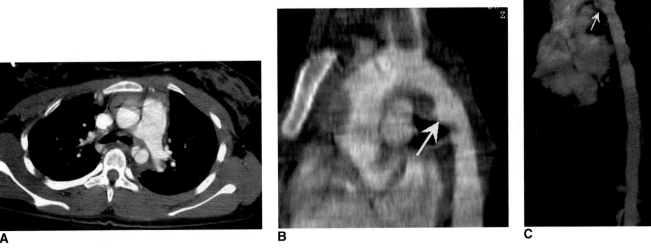

Fig. 5-77
CT of aortic injury. **A,** Axial CT shows abnormal contour of proximal descending aorta at the level of the left pulmonary artery with surrounding mediastinal hemorrhage. **B,** 2D reformation through pseudoaneurysm (*arrow*). **C,** 3D volume rendering showing irregular pseudoaneurysm (*arrow*) adjacent to left pulmonary artery.

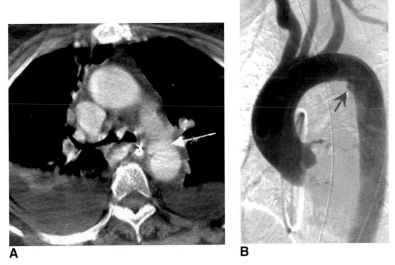

Fig. 5-78
CT of aortic injury. **A,** CT image through the proximal descending aorta shows a pseudoaneurysm (*arrow*) arising from the anteromedial aspect at the level of the left pulmonary artery. Note there is minimal perivascular hemorrhage. **B,** A portion of the injury is barely visualized on the LAO projection aortogram (*arrow*).

or the vaso vasorum of the aorta. Periaortic blood distorts the normal contour of the aortic arch and proximal descending aorta on frontal chest radiographs. In many cases a large quantity of mediastinal blood displaces the trachea and esophagus anteriorly and to the right. In some cases compression of both the pulmonary arteries and mainstem bronchi is clearly seen, suggesting a high-pressure (arterial) component to some of the mediastinal bleeding (see Fig. 5-79). Another sign of aortic injury

is distortion in the shape of the lumen that may appear gradually over several slices or abruptly over only a few. The contour of the aorta is altered both by tearing of the wall and compression from the adjacent pseudoaneurysm or hematoma (see Figs. 5-86 and 5-87). Linear intimal flaps and clot may also be observed at the injury site (see Figs. 5-82, 5-86, and 5-87). If there is significant compression of the aortic lumen, the aorta below the compression point becomes atypically narrow in caliber,

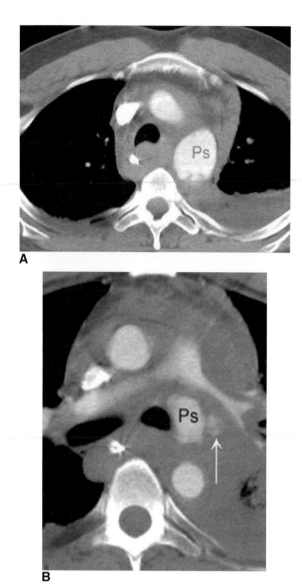

A

B

Fig. 5-79
CT of aortic injury. **A**, CT study of the patient in Fig. 5-80 shows a huge pseudoaneurysm (*Ps*) with marked mediastinal hemorrhage. The aortic lumen is not seen clearly at this level. **B**, A more caudal image shows the aortic lumen and the bottom of the pseudoaneurysm (*Ps*). A small amount of contrast is seen leaking into the mediastinum (*arrow*) and represents bleeding from the pseudoaneurysm.

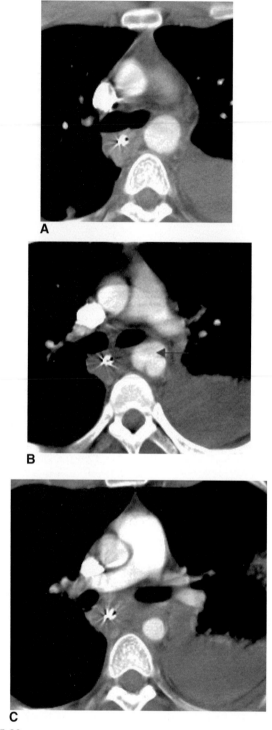

A

B

C

Fig. 5-80
CT of aortic injury. **A**, CT shows slightly irregular-shaped proximal descending aorta with surrounding mediastinal hemorrhage and carinal shift to the right. **B**, Slightly more caudal image shows pseudoaneurysm (*arrow*) that compresses the aortic lumen. **C**, Another more caudal image shows a smaller aortic diameter than above, indicating a probable coarctation effect from the more proximal pseudoaneurysm.

corresponding with a diminished distal pulse (femoral)—so-called pseudocoarctation (see Figs. 5-83, 5-86, and 5-87). Posttraumatic pseudocoarctation occurs in 5% to 10% of patients with TAI. The diagnosis can be suspected if the abdominal aorta appears atypically small on abdominal CT images (see Figs. 5-86 and 5-87). In some cases the aortic injury appears as a simple intimal flap that may be difficult or impossible to verify angiographically.

Published data on the use of CT for aortic branch injuries are relatively limited. These are far less common

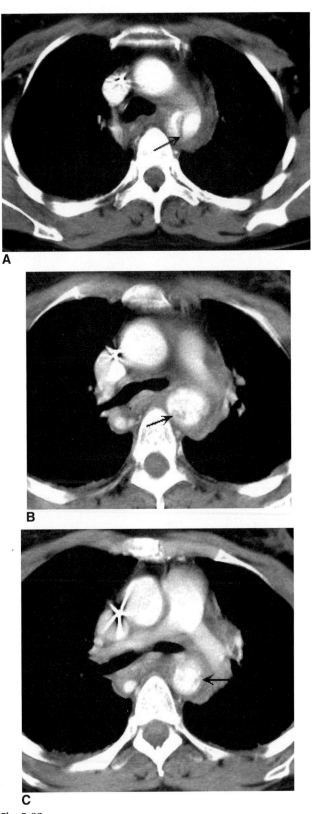

A

B

C

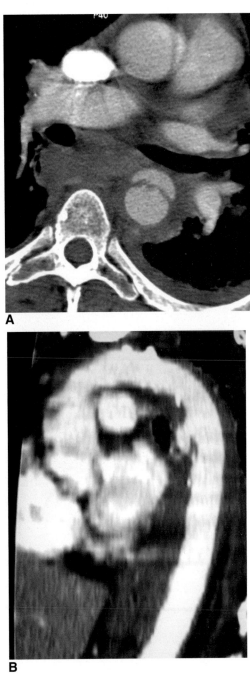

A

B

Fig. 5-81
CT of aortic injury. **A**, CT at level of pulmonary artery bifurcation shows anterior pseudoaneurysm arising from aorta with adjacent hematoma displacing carina anteriorly. **B**, MPR performed through the long axis of the thoracic aorta shows pseudoaneurysm projecting from inferior anterior proximal descending aorta.

Fig. 5-82
CT of aortic injury. **A**, CT shows intimal flap separating aortic lumen from medial pseudoaneurysm (*arrow*). Note surrounding hemorrhage and carinal shift to the right. **B**, A more caudal image shows irregular contour to the aortic lumen with a probable clot (*arrow*) at injury site. **C**, A still more caudal image shows a smaller aortic lumen with intimal flaps (*arrow*), indicating an element of coarctation.

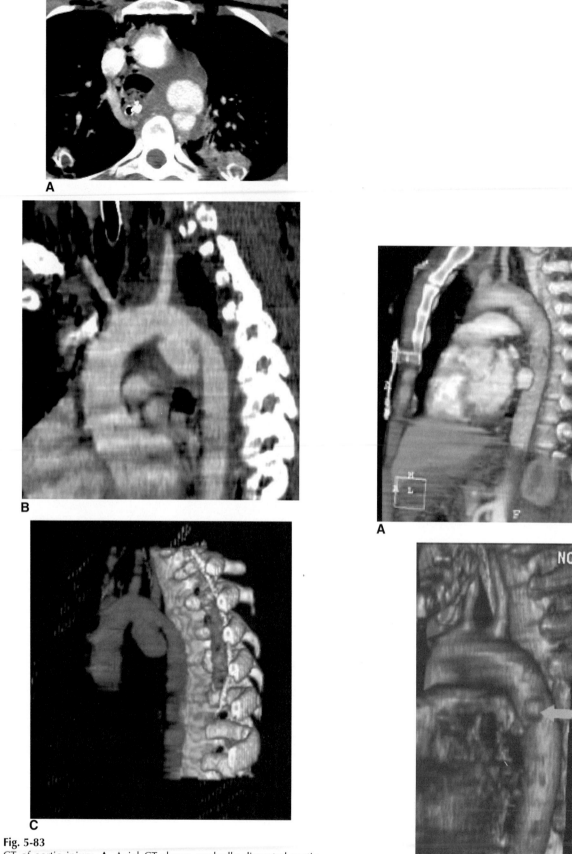

Fig. 5-83
CT of aortic injury. **A,** Axial CT shows markedly disrupted aortic lumen surrounding mediastinal hemorrhage and tracheal and esophageal displacement to the right. **B,** Curved MPR shows a large pseudoaneurysm projecting from the inferior aspect of the arch. **C,** Volumetric 3D of the pseudoaneurysm. MPR and volumetric 3D show size of pseudoaneurysm and relationship to major branches.

Fig. 5-84
Volume CT of aortic injury. Volume render 3D-CT demonstrates a small pseudoaneurysm at the level of the left pulmonary artery, several centimeters distal to left subclavian origin.

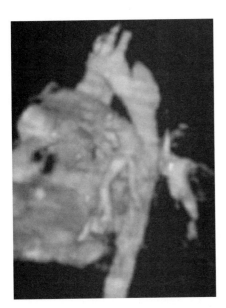

Fig. 5-85
Volume rendering of traumatic aortic injury.

than aortic injuries, making large series difficult to perform. The brachiocephalic artery is the most commonly injured major aortic branch[211,214] (Fig. 5-88). Aortic branch vessel injury should be suspected in the presence of a primary aortic injury and in patients with superior mediastinal thoracic inlet hemorrhage. The injured vessel may appear abnormally small due to spasm or may demonstrate direct luminal irregularity. Careful review of axial images through the lower neck may show absence of a normal vessel, suggesting more proximal traumatic interruption (Fig. 5-89). A number of other pathologic processes and variants of anatomy can make the CT diagnosis of TAI challenging. Aortic injuries that occur in atypical locations such as the ascending aorta, branch vessels, or aortic arch may be particularly confusing on axial CT. Injuries that arise from the superior aspect of the arch are in close proximity to aortic branch origins and can be difficult to distinguish (see Figs. 5-68 and 5-69). Anatomic variants such as the ductus diverticulum (Fig. 5-90) or a diverticular origin of the bronchial artery[213] (Fig. 5-91) can also be mistaken for aortic injury, particularly if seen adjacent to mediastinal blood. These entities and other anatomic variants can also be confusing and be a source of diagnostic error by arteriographic evaluation.[214-218]

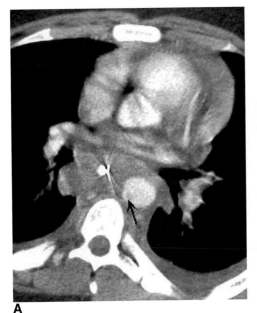

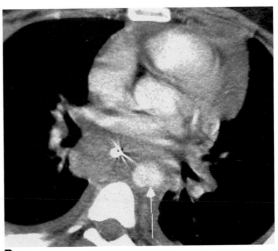

A   B

Fig. 5-86
CT of aortic injury with pseudocoarctation. **A,** CT through the proximal descending aorta shows an irregular contour with probable clot (*arrow*) and surrounding hematoma. Nasogastric tube is displaced to the right. **B,** A more caudal adjacent image shows irregular-shaped lumen (*arrow*) suggesting a focal pseudoaneurysm that is not well demarcated from aortic lumen.

Continued

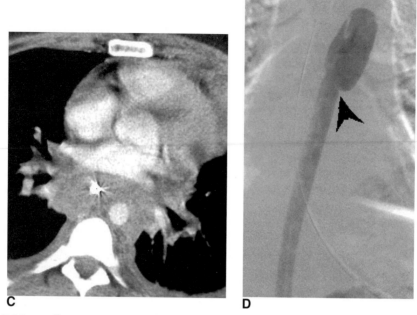

Fig. 5-86, cont'd
C, A still more caudal adjacent image shows a well-rounded but smaller aortic lumen suggesting some coarctation above. **D**, Limited aortogram shows a large pseudoaneurysm paralleling the proximal descending aorta with a tapered aorta below the injury level (*arrowhead*).

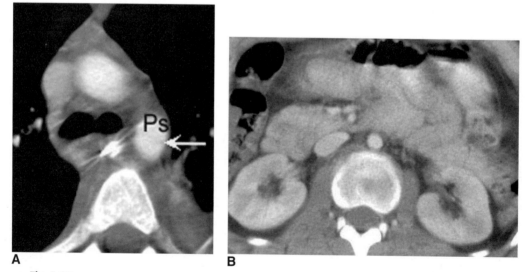

Fig. 5-87
CT of aortic injury with pseudocoarctation. **A**, CT shows intimal flap (*arrow*) crossing between aortic lumen and pseudoaneurysm (*Ps*). There is surrounding mediastinal blood and nasogastric tube and carina shift to the right. **B**, CT of the upper abdomen reveals a small-caliber aorta for an adult, indicating aortic coarctation effect from pseudoaneurysm.

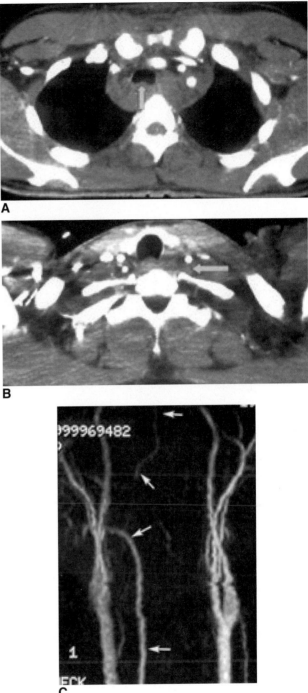

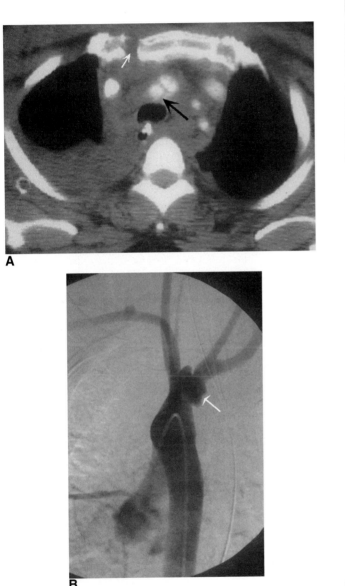

Fig. 5-88
Traumatic injury of the brachiocephalic artery. **A**, CT through the superior mediastinum shows a pseudoaneurysm arising from the proximal right innominate artery (*black arrow*). There is marked diffuse mediastinal hemorrhage. A costochondral anterior chest wall fracture is present on the right (*white arrow*). **B**, Arteriogram confirms pseudoaneurysm (*arrow*).

Fig. 5-89
Traumatic occlusion of the left vertebral artery. **A**, CT shows a large superior mediastinal hematoma with displacement of the trachea to the right (*arrow*). **B**, CT image of a chest trauma patient demonstrates no evidence of a left vertebral artery (*arrow*). **C**, MRI confirms occlusion of the left vertebral artery with a patent right vertebral artery (*arrows*). The patient remained without symptoms related to this injury.

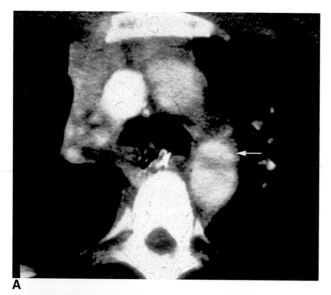

A

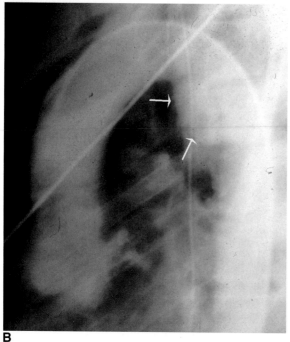

B

Fig. 5-90
Ductus diverticulum. **A**, CT image shows a smooth contoured "bump" (*arrow*) arising from the anterior aspect of the proximal descending aorta without adjacent hemorrhage. Hemorrhage is present in the anterior right mediastinum. **B**, Aortogram demonstrates a typical ductus bump (*arrows*) with smooth contour and obtuse margins with aortic lumen.

Transesophageal Echocardiography for Potential Aortic Injury. Transesophageal echocardiography (TEE) has been promoted in the past several years as an alternative to CT and angiography for the diagnosis of TAI.[219-225] Direct sonographic signs of aortic injury include thickened vessel walls, dissection, intimal flap, wall hematoma, aneurysm, and aortic obstruction (Fig. 5-92).

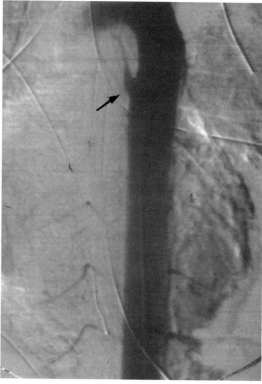

Fig. 5-91
Diverticular origin of bronchial artery. A normal variant of anatomy (*arrow*) that can be mistaken for an injury if the vessel is not followed beyond its origin to confirm branching.

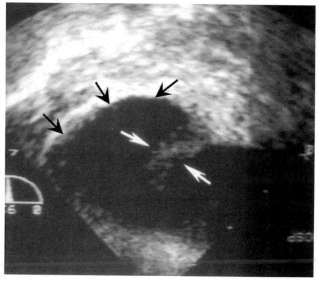

Fig. 5-92
Transesophageal sonogram of traumatic aortic injury. Sonogram demonstrates intimal flap (*white arrows*). The pseudoaneurysm (*black arrows*) causes some compression of the lumen.

Indirect signs include impaired aortic flow as shown by color Doppler, an increased aorta probe distance, and increased aortic diameter.[219] Advantages of TEE over catheter angiography include portability, short procedure time, relative safety, and lower cost. Some limitations of TEE include the inability to view the distal ascending aorta and arch, operator expertise and availability, the potential for complications related to the technique such as aspiration, esophageal injury, or arrhythmia, need for patient cooperation, and inferior delineation of the exact point of damage.[219]

Some studies have shown very accurate results using TEE for assessing the aorta of the blunt trauma victim. Vignon et al.[225] compared TEE with aortography in 32 patients with historical and radiographic suspicion of aortic injury. There were 13 positive and 18 negative results based on angiogram, with a single intimal injury missed by TEE. TEE was 91% sensitive and 100% specific and was recommended as a first-line study. Ahrar et al.[220] described a series of 72 patients with major thoracic arterial injuries that included the distal ascending aorta in one and aortic branch vessels in 17 (exclusively in 14). They emphasized that these injuries, representing 20% of all arterial injuries, may be suboptimally seen or missed entirely by TEE. Saletta et al.[224] studied results of TEE performed by "experienced" cardiologists on 114 trauma patients. The result was indeterminate in 17 patients and falsely negative for TAI in three. TEE was 63% sensitive and 84% specific in their study. Finally, Nagy et al.,[222] in a comprehensive literature review of aortic injury, suggested that TEE be used to follow small intimal injuries or for patients too unstable to leave the admission area for CT or angiography. The accuracy of TEE performed by well-trained individuals is still debated, given the "relative blind spot" of the distal ascending aorta and branches. TEE does not appear to be gaining widespread popularity as a screening study but may have a role in special situations as suggested by Nagy et al.[222] TEE has not been commonly used at the UMSTC to diagnose TAI.

Intravascular Sonography. Intravascular ultrasonography (IVUS) may also have potential application for the diagnosis or further assessment of aortic injury.[226,227] IVUS can identify intimal flaps, intramural hemorrhage, pseudoaneurysms, and perivascular hemorrhage. The high-frequency, high-resolution catheters can distinguish the three walls of the normal aorta (hyperechoic intima, hypoechoic media, and hyperechoic outer layer). After angiographic evaluation, Uflacker et al.[227] used a 6F, 12.5 mHz sonographic catheter to evaluate the aorta in 20 consecutive patients with suspected aortic injury. Five patients had a surgically confirmed TAI. IVUS was positive in seven, with one false positive due to a ductus diverticulum and one unconfirmed intramural hematoma. Digital subtraction angiography was falsely positive in one (the ductus diverticulum) and falsely negative in one. The authors emphasized the learning curve associated with using IVUS in this application. The potential value of IVUS performed after thoracic angiography as an adjunct study to supply information for potential intravascular stent placement was considered but not defined by the study.[227-229]

Thoracic Angiography. Thoracic angiography for trauma is discussed in detail in Chapter 12. Thoracic angiography has been the primary study used to diagnose traumatic aortic injury for more than three decades. The technique has high sensitivity and specificity and relatively low associated morbidity. Improved technology using digital subtraction and rotational angiography have contributed to improved overall accuracy.[230] The major drawbacks to aortography include high cost, invasiveness, availability in a timely fashion, and removal of the patient from direct clinical care for a potentially extended time. In addition, many vascular abnormalities, both congenital and acquired, can lead to interpretive errors,[214-218,231-233] including ductus diverticulum (see Fig. 5-90) and variants, atherosclerotic disease, atypical injury location (see Figs. 5-65 to 5-70), diverticular origin of the bronchial-intercostal trunk (see Fig. 5-91), and subtle injuries, among others. The use of thoracic angiography as a screening study results in a large number of normal studies for each vascular injury detected.[4-6,23,205,222,234-238] There is some debate regarding the cost efficacy of screening for TAI using angiography versus CT,[4,23,24,202,239] with most studies indicating a cost savings with CT screening in selecting patients for angiography. There is less information on cost efficacy of CT versus screening angiography, since that relates to years of quality adjusted by years of life gained.[24,239]

Magnetic Resonance Imaging. To date, MRI has been used to demonstrate congenital anomalies of the aorta and chronic pseudoaneurysm resulting from aortic rupture. MRI also can be used to assess the aorta after surgical repair of thoracic aortic ruptures or as a method to follow injuries that are being managed nonoperatively.[240] Currently, MRI is limited in its application to acutely injured patients because of difficulties with hemodynamic monitoring and support in the magnetic field around the MRI device, as well as the potential for sudden hemodynamic deterioration. Further developments in MRI-compatible physiologic support and monitoring devices and the increasing availability of fast-imaging and motion-suppression techniques will undoubtedly facilitate direct MRI imaging of the great vessels in appropriately selected patients. At this time MRI should serve as an adjunct study in hemodynamically stable trauma patients in whom the diagnosis of TAI is uncertain despite CT and angiography studies or in patients for whom intravenous contrast is strictly contraindicated. Perhaps MRI can be used to follow aortic injuries that are treated nonoperatively when repeat CT scans are considered less suitable (e.g., severe renal insufficiency).

Mediastinal Hemorrhage Without Aortic Injury.

As described earlier, mediastinal hemorrhage is essentially always seen in association with TAI but may be relatively limited in quantity. By comparing results of chest radiography with thoracic aortography, it has been found that mediastinal hemorrhage commonly occurs without major arterial injury[23,182,183,202,241] (Figs. 5-93 to 5-95). Other sources of mediastinal bleeding should be considered. In most cases mediastinal bleeding in trauma patients arises from low-pressure veins and small arteries and often is associated with thoracic skeletal fractures.[36,189] Injuries to major venous structures can occur, including the azygous vein and vena cavae (Fig. 5-96), especially near their insertion into the right atrium as they are invested by pericardium.[242,243] Injuries can occur to nonaortic branch vessels such as the internal mammary arteries (Fig. 5-97)

that can cause high-pressure mediastinal hemorrhage to the extent of producing cardiac tamponade and constriction of the airway.[244] Of course, blunt trauma to nonaortic mediastinal structures such as the airway and esophagus typically leads to mediastinal hemorrhage. In general, chest radiography cannot distinguish mediastinal hemorrhage from other sources of bleeding, since they all have a similar appearance, with blood tracking into essentially the same regions of the mediastinum. CT permits more precise localization of the source of bleeding in some cases. Mediastinal blood that is substernal alone most likely is caused by a sternal fracture and does not require further investigation if the major vessels appear normal on a high-quality CT study. In this case the anterior mediastinal hemorrhage is typically separated from the aorta by a fat plane.

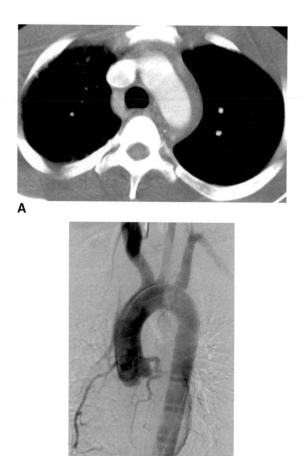

Fig. 5-93
A, Mediastinal blood without major arterial injury. CT through the aortic arch shows periaortic hemorrhage but no definite aortic lesion. B, Aortogram confirms normal aorta and proximal branch vessels.

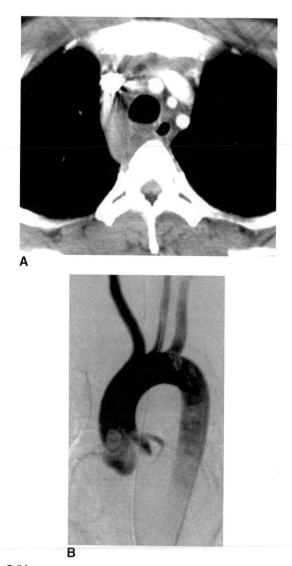

Fig. 5-94
Normal aorta with periaortic hemorrhage. A, CT through the superior mediastinum shows hemorrhage around the trachea and major aortic branches. B, Aortogram is normal.

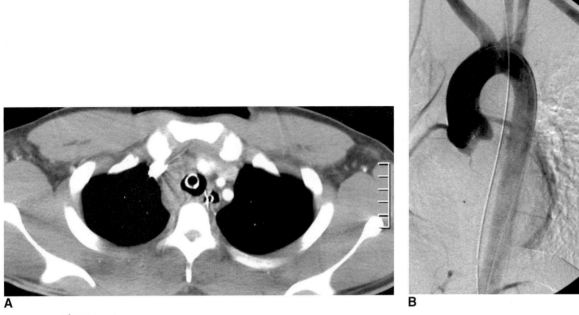

Fig. 5-95
Normal aorta with superior mediastinal hemorrhage. **A**, CT through the superior mediastinum reveals hemorrhage in the paratracheal region primarily. **B**, Aortogram is normal.

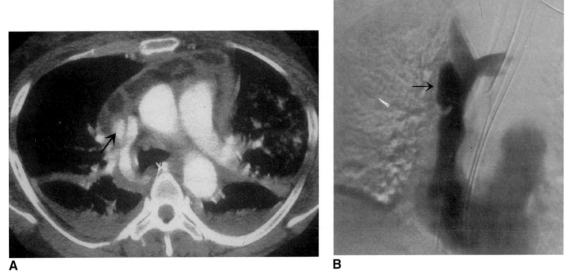

Fig. 5-96
Injury to the superior vena cava (SVC) from blunt trauma. **A**, CT through the roots of the aorta and pulmonary artery shows a linear lucent line in the SVC with a pseudoaneurysm projecting laterally from the lumen (*arrow*). There is diffuse mediastinal hemorrhage. **B**, SVCgram confirms pseudo-aneurysm (*arrow*) arising from lateral SVC.

Continued

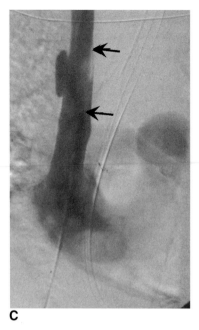

Fig. 5-96, cont'd
C, Repeat SVCgram after stent placement (*arrows*) compresses pseudoaneurysm. The injury was not a further clinical concern.

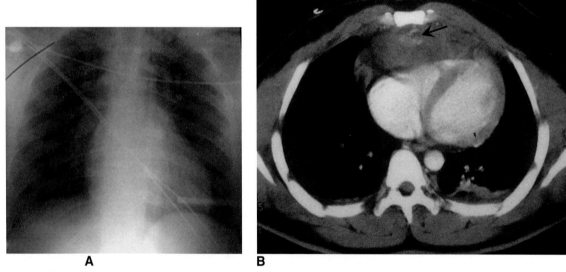

Fig. 5-97
Internal mammary arterial bleeding. **A**, Admission chest radiograph is unremarkable. **B**, CT shows a large anterior mediastinal hematoma compressing the heart. There is arterial extravasation in the center of the hematoma (*arrow*). At surgery, the source was a torn internal mammary artery. (From Killeen KL, Poletti PA, Shanmuganathan K, Mirvis SE: *Emerg Radiol* 6:343, 1999.)

Similarly, if a posterior hematoma is more or less centered on a vertebral body fracture and is displacing the aorta and the major vessels appear normal, then the spine is the source of bleeding and further assessment of the aorta is not required. In cases in which mediastinal bleeding is seen in the middle or superior mediastinum adjacent to major vessels, the possibility of major arterial injury still must be considered. If the major arteries appear normal on a high-quality, intravenous contrast-enhanced CT, the possibility of an arterial injury would appear to be remote. However, to some degree this determination depends on the quality of the CT scanner and the experience of the

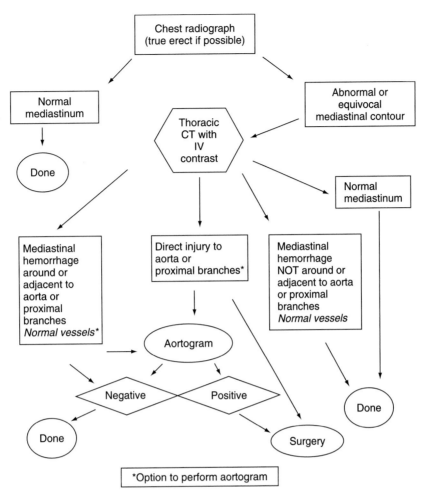

Fig. 5-98
Algorithm for diagnosing potential aortic injury.

interpreter. With the development of multislice CT scanning, the chance of missing a significant direct arterial injury would appear even more remote. Some centers with extensive experience dealing with potential aortic injury may have a high enough "comfort" level with single or multislice CT to avoid aortography despite the presence of periarterial blood if the major mediastinal vessels appear normal, whereas others would prefer to perform aortography in this circumstance. Thus the standard of care is somewhat site dependent and in evolution.

Recommended Approach To Exclude TAI. An algorithm recommended for imaging management of blunt trauma victims with a mechanism of injury compatible with producing aortic injury is shown in Fig. 5-98. As noted above, differences in local experience, facilities, and staffing may require adjustment of this approach to one that is optimized to the site.

TRAUMA TO THE HEART AND PERICARDIUM
Pneumopericardium

Pneumopericardium is a relatively uncommon consequence of blunt thoracic trauma.[47] Pneumopericardium may develop as a consequence of prolonged positive airway pressure, in which case air under pressure presumably enters the pericardium around the pulmonary perivascular connective tissue or ostia of the pulmonary veins.[245] Direct communication from a ruptured trachea or tension pneumothorax with the adjacent pericardium may result from either blunt or penetrating trauma.[47,245]

The identification of pneumopericardium by chest radiography was described by Wenkebach in 1910 and elaborated upon by Cimmino.[246] Chest radiographs obtained in either posteroanterior or lateral projections show the heart partially or completely surrounded by air with the pericardium sharply outlined by air density (Figs. 5-99 to 5-101). Pneumopericardium usually can be distinguished from pneumomediastinum, since air in the pericardial sac should not rise above the anatomic limits of the pericardial reflection on the proximal great vessels. On radiographs obtained with the patient in the decubitus position, air in the pericardial sac will shift in location immediately, whereas air confined to the mediastinum will not move during a short interval. On occasion, it may not be possible to distinguish between pneumopericardium and pneumomediastinum with certainty. The pericardium appears as a thicker line than the parietal pleura and curves around the heart rather than disappearing below the diaphragm, as is typical of the parietal pleura in cases of pneumomediastinum.

Pneumopericardium, although generally innocuous, can lead to sufficient intrapericardial pressure to produce cardiac tamponade, so-called tension pneumopericardium.[47,245,247] Tension pneumopericardium can present acutely, within several hours after admission, or as a consequence of severe pulmonary disease and respiratory support. Presumably, under conditions of elevated airway pressure, air can be forced into the pericardium through connective tissue around the pulmonary veins but may not egress, a one-way valve mechanism. Mirvis et al.[47] described five patients who developed tension pneumopericardium after closed chest trauma. Each patient

exhibited a global decrease in the area of the cardiac silhouette on serial chest radiography with at least a 2 cm decrease in the transverse cardiac diameter, corrected for target-film distance, at the time of physiologic cardiac tamponade as compared with a baseline measurement (Figs. 5-99 to 5-101). Higgins et al.[248] showed that symptoms of severe hemodynamic compromise from tension pneumopericardium are accompanied by a perceptible decrease in the size of the cardiac silhouette in neonates with respiratory distress syndrome receiving positive pressure ventilatory support.

Clinical signs of cardiac tamponade, such as pulsus paradoxus, tachycardia, low-voltage electrocardiogram, increasing central venous pressure with decreasing cardiac output, muffled heart sounds, and worsening pulmonary function, may indicate developing cardiac tamponade. However, concurrent conditions, such as cardiac contusion, shock lung, intravascular volume depletion, tension pneumothorax, and sepsis, may confuse the clinical picture. Furthermore, measures to maintain normal blood pressure (e.g., vasopressors and volume support) can potentially mask early hemodynamic indicators of cardiac tamponade. In the presence of pneumopericardium, the development of a radiographic "small heart" sign (see Figs. 5-99 and 5-101) should raise the suspicion of cardiac tamponade.

CT scans can demonstrate pneumopericardium and also suggest the presence of a tension component with cardiac tamponade.[47,245,247] Air surrounds the heart

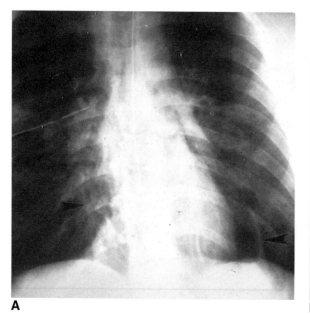

A

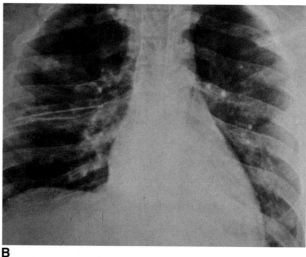

B

Fig. 5-99

Pneumopericardium with tamponade. **A,** Radiograph of a blunt trauma patient shows air around the heart displacing the pericardium outward (*arrowheads*). The cardiac shadow is atypically uniformly small, indicating tamponade. Pericardial air will not ascend above the root of the great vessels at the pericardial reflection. **B,** After a pericardial window with the release of air, the cardiac silhouette returns to normal. (From Mirvis SE, Indeck I, Schorr RM, Diaconis JN: *Radiology* 158:667, 1986.)

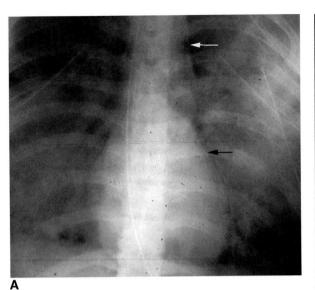
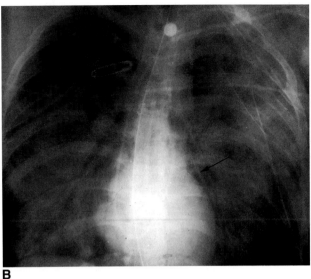

Fig. 5-100
Pneumopericardium with tamponade. **A**, Chest radiograph acquired early after admission of a young man with severe chest trauma shows bilateral pulmonary contusions and bilateral chest tubes. The parietal pleura is seen on the left (*white arrow*), and the pericardium is outlined by air (*black arrow*), indicating pneumopericardium. Note the proximity of the parietal pleura and pericardium. The cardiac size is normal. **B**, Follow-up radiograph obtained with clinical signs of cardiac tamponade shows uniform decrease in cardiac size, indicating increased intrapericardial pressure. Pericardium is again noted (*arrow*). Tamponade was relieved by intrapericardial drain insertion. (From Mirvis SE, Indeck I, Schorr RM, Diaconis JN: *Radiology* 158:665, 1986.)

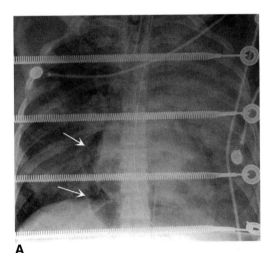
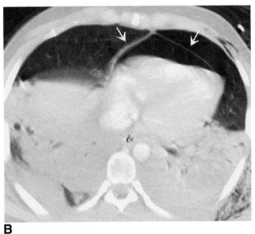

Fig. 5-101
Chest radiograph of traumatic pneumopericardium. **A**, Radiograph obtained on a Stryker frame shows diffuse lung consolidation that is compatible with contusion and ARDS. A halo of air is seen surrounding the heart, indicating pericardial air (*arrows*). The combination of severe, diffuse lung injury and high-pressure ventilation predisposes to pneumopericardium. **B**, The finding is verified by CT study through the heart, showing pericardium outlined by air on either side and some flattening of the anterior right heart, indicating some direct cardiac compression. There is a left pneumothorax apparent and severe bilateral lower lobe consolidation.

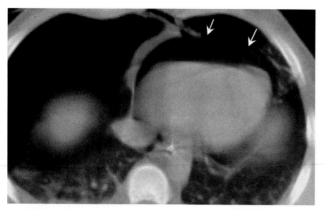

Fig. 5-102
CT of cardiac tamponade. CT demonstrates intrapericardial air distending the pericardium (*arrows*) and compressing the anterior heart. There is a right tension pneumothorax and pneumomediastinum.

and displaces the pericardium away (Fig. 5-102). Mediastinal emphysema may be present concurrently with pneumopericardium, but in most cases it should be clearly distinguishable. The pericardium is thicker than the parietal pleura and surrounds the heart. If intrapericardial pressure is elevated, the anterior heart (right ventricle) may appear "flattened"[245] (Fig. 5-103). Other CT signs of pericardial tamponade include distension of the inferior and superior vena cava, periportal lymphatic distension within the liver, distension of the renal veins, pericholecystic fluid, and other signs of increased central venous pressure within the abdomen[7] (Fig. 5-103).

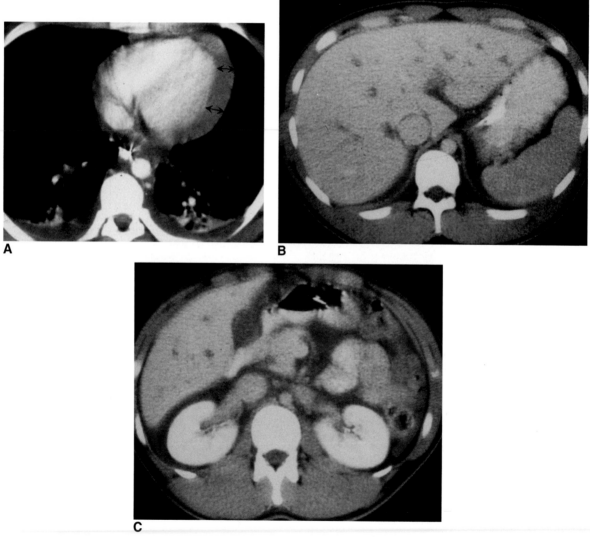

Fig. 5-103
Secondary CT signs of cardiac tamponade. **A**, Admission CT shows pericardial hemorrhage (*double-headed arrows*) in a blunt trauma patient. **B**, CT through the upper abdomen shows distended inferior vena cava (IVC), periportal lymphatic distension (black circles around portal vein branches), and a small aorta. These effects are caused by high venous return pressure in the IVC and decreased returning blood volume to the heart. **C**, Image obtained more caudal than **B** shows distension of renal veins and retroperitoneal and mesenteric edema, also reflecting elevated venous pressures. (From Goldstein L, Mirvis SE, Kostrubiak IS, Turney SZ: *AJR* 152:740,1989.)

Hemopericardium

Hemopericardium may develop acutely as a direct consequence of blunt trauma to the anterior chest and from severe crush injuries, but more typically it results from penetrating injury to the heart or severe blunt chest trauma and cardiac rupture.[249] A rapid accumulation of blood in the pericardial space often causes cardiac tamponade and severe hemodynamic compromise without significantly altering the radiologic appearance of the cardiac silhouette; however, it may manifest as a nonspecific enlargement of the cardiopericardial contour.[250,251] Bedside sonographic evaluation of the heart rapidly and noninvasively permits detection of even small quantities of pericardial fluid and is the study of choice to assess for hemopericardium on admission.[251-253] Simultaneously, cardiac function, chamber size, and valvular integrity can be assessed by appropriately skilled personnel.[254] CT is also highly sensitive for diagnosing intrapericardial fluid and may incidentally detect pericardial hemorrhage, as indicated by high CT attenuation fluid between the epicardial and pericardial fat during evaluation of the thorax for trauma[7,255,256] (Figs. 5-104 and 5-105). Cardiac tamponade from hemorrhage is reflected on CT, as with tension pneumopericardium, by distension of the inferior vena cava and hepatic and renal veins and by development of periportal lymphatic distension within the liver (see Fig. 5-103 and 5-104). Harries et al.[256] described reflux of contrast material into the azygous vein from the heart as an indication of cardiac tamponade. The author noted contrast reflux into the hepatic and renal veins due to the same mechanism associated with concurrently diminished arterial pressure (Fig. 5-106).

Rarely, extracardiac mediastinal hematoma resulting from blunt chest trauma can cause compression of the right ventricle and extrapericardial tamponade.[244,257,258] CT has identified mediastinal hemorrhage from the internal mammary artery as a cause of cardiac compression and physiologic tamponade[258] (see Fig. 5-98). Herniation of abdominal content into the pericardium through the central tendon of the diaphragm could also conceivably lead to tamponade[95] (see Fig. 5-33).

Pericardial Rupture

Pericardial rupture is a rare consequence of serious thoracic trauma and was diagnosed in only 22 (0.11%) of 20,000 admissions to UMSTC over a 10-year period.[259] Rupture may involve the diaphragmatic pericardium or the pleuropericardium. In the series of Fulda et al.[259] the majority (64%) of tears involved the left pleuropericardium. Typically, the diagnosis is established intraoperatively during resuscitation or surgery for associated injuries or at autopsy, but pericardial rupture can be indicated by chest radiograph with herniation of air-containing

abdominal viscera into the pericardium accompanying diaphragmatic rupture. Pneumopericardium may appear in the presence of pneumothorax as air enters through the pericardial disruption. Finally, cardiac luxation into the pleural cavity (predominantly left sided) may occur after large pericardial tears and present as gross cardiac displacement by radiography or CT[260,261] (Fig. 5-107). These patients have hypotension without evidence of persistent blood loss. Combined pericardial and diaphragmatic tears can lead to cardiac subluxation into the peritoneal cavity.[86] In the series of Fulda et al.[259] the mortality rate was 63% for patients with traumatic pericardial rupture, but was 100% for the 5 of 22 patients with associated cardiac injury.

Cardiac Contusion or Dysfunction

Cardiac contusion may result from blunt chest trauma in 8% to 76% of patients,[262] but functional cardiac abnormalities occur in less than 20% of patients with blunt chest trauma.[263] Significant myocardial injury presents radiographically as a spectrum of findings related to injury to the heart and to the chest. The cardiac findings may be similar to those occurring from acute myocardial infarction, such as congestive heart failure, ventricular aneurysm, or massive cardiac enlargement. The presence of anterior rib and sternal fractures should raise suspicion of a possible myocardial injury, although no clear relationship exists between the extent of chest wall injury and the degree of underlying cardiac damage. Myocardial injury can range from mild cardiac contusion to severe transmural contusion. Pathologically, blunt myocardial trauma produces a wide spectrum of injury, ranging from small, subepicardial, or subendocardial petechiae or ecchymoses to full-thickness contusion.[264] The right ventricle is most frequently injured, since it makes up almost three times more exposed anterior surface of the heart than does the left ventricle.

Clinically, mild myocardial dysfunction can produce low cardiac output and acute cardiac arrhythmias, whereas more severe injury can lead to congestive failure or cardiac rupture. Cardiac dysfunction after blunt chest trauma is one of the most frequently missed or delayed diagnoses made after severe injury and is frequently masked by more obvious injury.[264]

Although nuclear isotopic imaging with technetium 99m pyrophosphate (infarct avid agent) may detect severe myocardial injury, it may not detect smaller areas of damage. Holness and Waxman[262] demonstrated the reliability of thallium 201 scanning and single photon emission CT (SPECT) in diagnosing cardiac contusion. In 125 patients with blunt chest trauma undergoing SPECT evaluation, 75 (60%) had positive scans, demonstrating a focus of diminished perfusion. Of these 75, 11 had serious

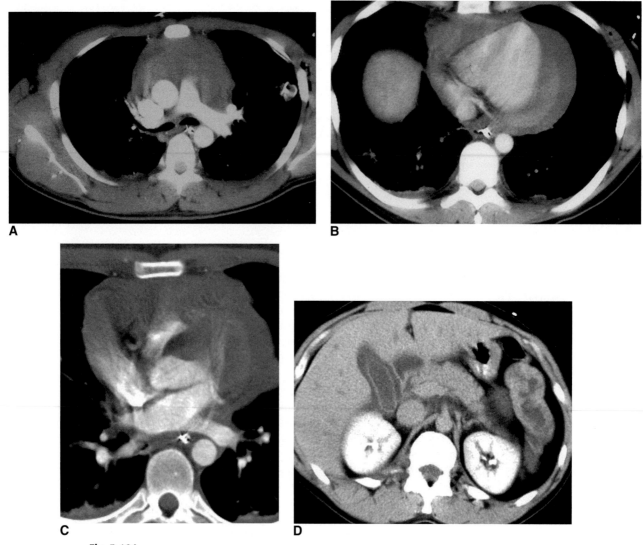

A

B

C

D

Fig. 5-104
CT of pericardial hemorrhage. **A,** CT through the base of the heart shows a large amount of hematoma anterior to the aorta and pulmonary trunks. The shape of the hematoma suggests that it is confined by a distended pericardium. **B** and **C,** Lower images show extensive blood and clot in the pericardial space compressing the heart. The patient had a biatrial rupture from blunt trauma found at surgery and survived. **D,** Secondary signs of cardiac tamponade in this patient include pericholecystic fluid, periportal lymphedema, a distended inferior vena cava, a small caliber aorta, and bowel wall thickening. (From Killeen KL, Poletti PA, Shanmuganathan K, Mirvis SE: *Emerg Radiol* 6:342, 1999.)

cardiac arrhythmias. Three patients with negative SPECT studies also had arrhythmias, but two of these patients had previous cardiac disease and were taking antiarrhythmic medications.

Two-dimensional transthoracic and transesophageal echocardiography are useful for evaluating cardiac valve function, cardiac wall function, cardiac chamber size, papillary muscle function, and the anatomy of the aortic valve and root.[265-267] In general the use of serial cardiac isoenzymes, including cardiac troponin, has

not been particularly sensitive for detection of cardiac contusion.[268,269]

Direct injury to the coronary arteries after blunt trauma to the chest can occur and lead to pseudoaneurysm formation, intimal injury, and occlusion. In the presence of ECG changes of myocardial infarction, cardiogenic shock, or recurrent arrhythmias after blunt thoracic trauma, early catheterization to evaluate the coronary artery anatomy is indicated.[270] Cardiac sonography, intravascular coronary sonogra-

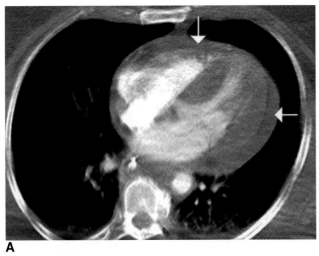

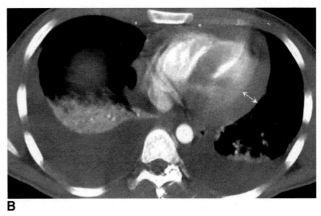

A   B

Fig. 5-105
CT of pericardial hemorrhage. **A**, CT image shows blood surrounding both ventricles *(arrows)* without obvious cardiac chamber compression. **B**, CT of another patient reveals a larger hemopericardium after trauma *(double-headed arrow)* with suggestion of left ventricular compression.

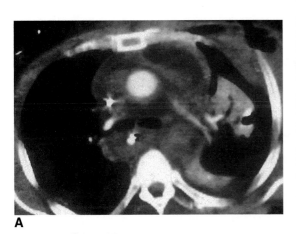

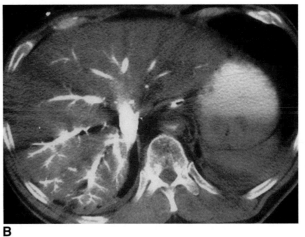

A   B

Fig. 5-106
CT of aortic transection. **A**, CT through the ascending aorta reveals mediastinal hemorrhage. There is no evidence of a descending aorta. **B**, CT through the liver shows marked venous reflux in the hepatic veins with injection into the inferior vena cava. This is due to lack of arterial inflow pressure and reversal of the normal pressure gradient with power injection. A small amount of contrast is seen in the abdominal aorta. The patient did not survive.

phy, and MRI have also been used to evaluate posttraumatic coronary artery injury.[271,272]

CONCLUSION

Technical advances in CT imaging, especially spiral and multislice spiral CT, have contributed significantly to the practical application of chest CT in the setting of blunt chest trauma. The increased sensitivity of CT over chest radiography has been shown to be substantial for many common diagnoses. Findings from CT in many cases change treatment decisions that were based solely on information acquired from radiography. CT has had a major influence on decreasing the need for angiography for investigation of potential aortic injury.

It is likely that CT will become as indispensable and routine for evaluation of the chest in blunt trauma as it is currently for the abdomen and pelvis.

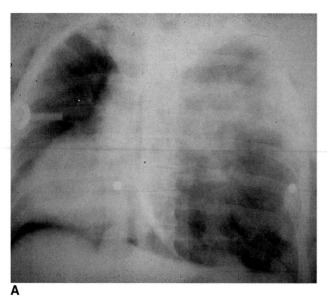

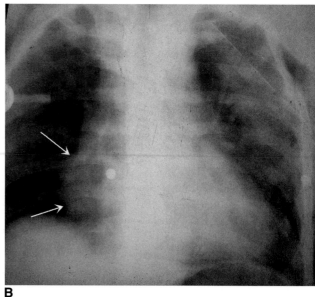

A   B

Fig. 5-107
Chest radiograph of cardiac herniation. **A,** Image shows right-sided cardiac apex in a man who had
fallen from a height of 30 feet onto his left side. There are minimally displaced left-sided lower rib
fractures. There is no evidence of pneumothorax. The patient was in extremis. **B,** During placement
of a left chest tube for a presumed pneumothorax, the patient improved, but no air was vented from
the tube. Repeat chest radiograph shows heart in typical location, but there is an abnormal contour
to the right cardiac border (*arrows*) suggesting a herniated portion. At surgery a 6 cm tear in the
right pericardium was found that had permitted the heart to be completely herniated into the right
chest. The heart returned to the pericardial sac during maneuvering of the patient for the chest tube.
(From Mirvis SE: Imaging of thoracic trauma. In Turney SZ, Rodriguez A, Cowley RA, eds:
Management of cardiothoracic trauma, Baltimore, 1990, Williams & Wilkins.)

Further research in elucidating the accuracy of
CT for diagnosing diaphragm injuries and nonaortic arterial vascular injuries within the chest is needed.

REFERENCES

1. Blostein PA, Hodgman CG: Computed tomography of the chest in
   blunt thoracic trauma: results of a prospective study, *J Trauma* 43:13,
   1997.
2. Bridges KG, Welch G, Silver M, et al: CT detection of occult pneumothorax in multiple trauma patients, *J Emerg Med* 11:179, 1993.
3. Chen JD, Shanmuganathan S, Mirvis SE et al: Using CT to diagnose
   tracheal rupture, *AJR* 176:1273, 2000.
4. Dyer ES, Moore EE, Mestek MF, et al: Can chest CT be used to exclude
   aortic injury? *Radiology* 213:195, 1999.
5. Demetriades D, Gomez H, Velmahos GC, et al: Routine helical computed tomographic evaluation of the mediastinum in high-risk
   blunt trauma patients, *Arch Surg* 133:1084, 1998.
6. Gavant ML, Menke PG, Fabian T, et al: Blunt traumatic aortic
   rupture: detection with helical CT of the chest, *Radiology* 197:125,
   1995.
7. Goldstein L, Mirvis SE, Kostrubiak IS, et al: CT diagnosis of acute
   pericardial tamponade after blunt chest trauma, *AJR* 152:739,
   1989.
8. Kang EY, Muller NL: CT in blunt chest trauma: pulmonary, tracheobronchial, and diaphragmatic injuries, *Semin Ultrasound CT MR*
   17:144, 1996.
9. Kerns SR, Gay SB: CT of blunt chest trauma, *AJR* 154:55, 1990.
10. Killeen KL, Mirvis SE, Shanmuganathan K: Helical CT of diaphrag-
    matic rupture caused by blunt trauma, *AJR* 173:1611, 1999.
11. Marts B, Durham R, Shapiro M: Computed tomography in the diag-
    nosis of blunt thoracic injury, *Am J Surg* 168:688, 1994.
12. Mirvis SE, Shanmuganathan K, Beull J: Use of spiral computed
    tomography for the assessment of blunt trauma patients with
    potential aortic injury, *J Trauma* 45:922, 1994.
13. Mirvis S, Shanmuganathan K: Trauma radiology. II. Diagnostic
    imaging of thoracic trauma: review and update, *J Intensive Care Med*
    9:179, 1994.
14. Poole GV, Morgan DB, Cranston PE: Computed tomography
    in the management of blunt thoracic trauma, *J Trauma* 35:296,
    1993.
15. Shanmuganathan K, Mirvis SE: Imaging diagnosis of nonaortic tho-
    racic injury, *Radiol Clin North Am* 37:533, 1999.
16. Sliker CW, Mirvis SE, Shanmuganathan K: Blunt cardiac rupture:
    value of contrast-enhanced spiral CT, *Clin Radiol* 10:805, 2000.
17. Tello R, Munden RF, Hooton S, et al: Value of spiral CT in hemo-
    dynamically stable patients following blunt chest trauma, *Comput
    Med Imaging Graph* 22:447, 1998.
18. Trupka A, Waydhas C, Hallfeldt KK, et al: Value of thoracic com-
    puted tomography in the first assessment of severely injured
    patients with blunt chest trauma: results of a prospective study, *J
    Trauma* 43:405, 1997.
19. Van Hise ML, Primack SL, Israel RS, et al: CT in blunt chest trauma:
    indications and limitations, *Radiographics* 18:1071, 1998.
20. Wagner RB, Crawford WO Jr, Schimpf PP: Classification of
    parenchymal injuries of the lung, *Radiology* 167:77, 1988.

21. Worthy SA, Kang EY, Hartman TE, et al: Diaphragmatic rupture: CT findings in 11 patients, *Radiology* 194:885, 1995.

22. Zinck SE, Primack SL: Radiographic and CT findings in blunt chest trauma, *J Thorac Imaging* 15:87, 2000.

23. Mirvis SE, Shanmuganathan K, Miller BH: Traumatic aortic injury: diagnosis with contrast-enhanced thoracic CT—five-year experience at a major trauma center, *Radiology* 200:413, 1996.

24. Hunink MG, Bos JJ: Triage of patients to angiography for detection of aortic rupture after blunt chest trauma: cost-effectiveness analysis of using CT, *AJR* 165:27, 1995.

25. Shorr RM, Crittenden M, Indeck M, et al: Blunt thoracic trauma: analysis of 515 patients, *Ann Surg* 206:200, 1987.

26. Bowers VD, Watkins GM: Blunt trauma to the thoracic outlet and angiography, *Am Surg* 49:655, 1983.

27. Greene R: Lung alterations in thoracic trauma, *J Thorac Imaging* 2:1, 1987.

28. Woodring JH, Fried AM, Hatfield DR: Fractures of first and second ribs: predictive value for arterial and bronchial injury, *AJR* 138:211, 1982.

29. Gupta A, Jamshidi M, Rubin JR: Traumatic first rib fracture: is angiography necessary? A review of 730 cases, *Cardiovasc Surg* 5:48, 1997.

30. Fermanis GG, Deane SA, Fitzgerald PM: The significance of first and second rib fractures, *Aust N Z J Surg* 55:383, 1985.

31. Poole GV: Fracture of the upper ribs and injury to the great vessels, *Surg Gynecol Obstet* 169:275, 1989.

32. Henry D: Thoracic trauma: triage of the chest radiograph. Paper presented at the Eighty-seventh American Roentgen Ray Society, 1987.

33. Patetsios P, Priovolos S, Slesinger TL: Lacerations of the left ventricle from rib fractures after blunt trauma, *J Trauma* 49:771, 2000.

34. Rashid MA, Wikstrom T, Ortenwall P: Nomenclature, classification, and significance of traumatic extrapleural hematoma, *J Trauma* 49:286, 2000.

35. Aquino SL, Chiles C, Oaks T: Displaced extrapleural fat as revealed by CT scanning: evidence of extrapleural hematoma [see comments], *AJR* 169:687, 1997.

36. Crestanello JA, Samuels LE, Kaufman MS: Sternal fracture with mediastinal hematoma: delayed cardiopulmonary sequelae, *J Trauma* 47:161, 1999.

37. Huggett JM, Roszler MH: CT findings of sternal fracture, *Injury* 29:623, 1998.

38. Gouldman JW, Miller RS: Sternal fracture: a benign entity? *Am Surg* 63:17, 1997.

39. Harley DP, Mena I: Cardiac and vascular sequelae of sternal fractures, *J Trauma* 26:553, 1986.

40. Ben-Menachem Y: Avulsion of the innominate artery associated with fracture of the sternum, *AJR* 150:621, 1988.

41. Collins J: Chest wall trauma, *J Thorac Imaging* 15:112, 2000.

42. Oreck SL, Burgess A, Levine AM: Traumatic lateral displacement of the scapula: a radiographic sign of neurovascular disruption, *J Bone Joint Surg [Am]* 66:758, 1984.

43. Sheafor DH, Mirvis SE: Scapulothoracic dissociation: report of five cases and review of the literature, *Emergency Radiology* 2:279, 1995.

44. Macklin MI: Malignant interstitial emphysema of the lungs and mediastinum as important occult complications in many respiratory diseases and other conditions: interpretation of clinical literature in light of laboratory experiment, *Medicine* 23:281, 1944.

45. Mirvis SE, Rodriguez A: Diagnostic imaging of thoracic trauma. In Mirvis SE, Young JWR, eds: *Imaging in trauma and critical care*, Baltimore, 1992, Williams & Wilkins.

46. Bejvan SM, Godwin JD: Pneumomediastinum: old signs and new signs, *AJR* 166:1041, 1996.

47. Mirvis SE, Indek M, Schorr RM: Posttraumatic tension pneumopericardium: the "small heart" sign, *Radiology* 158:663, 1986.

48. Tocino IM, Miller MH, Fairfax WR: Distribution of pneumothorax in the supine and semirecumbent critically ill adult, *AJR* 144:901, 1985.

49. Neff MA, Monk JS Jr, Peters K, et al: Detection of occult pneumothoraces on abdominal computed tomographic scans in trauma patients, *J Trauma* 49:281, 2000.

50. Rhea JT, Novelline RA, Lawrason J, et al: The frequency and significance of thoracic injuries detected on abdominal CT scans of multiple trauma patients, *J Trauma* 29:502, 1989.

51. Wall SD, Federle MP, Jeffrey RB, et al: CT diagnosis of unsuspected pneumothorax after blunt abdominal trauma, *AJR* 141:919, 1983.

52. Brasel KJ, Stafford RE, Weigelt JA, et al: Treatment of occult pneumothoraces from blunt trauma, *J Trauma* 46:987, 1999.

53. Tocino IM, Miller MH, Frederick PR, et al: CT detection of occult pneumothorax in head trauma, *AJR* 143:987, 1984.

54. Khodadadyan C, Hoffmann R, Neumann K, et al: Unrecognized pneumothorax as a cause of intraspinal air, *Spine* 20:838, 1995.

55. Ziter FM Jr, Westcott JL: Supine subpulmonary pneumothorax, *AJR* 137:699, 1981.

56. Rhea JT, vanSonnenberg E, McLoud TC: Basilar pneumothorax in the supine adult, *Radiology* 133:593, 1979.

57. Gordon R: The deep sulcus sign, *Radiology* 136:25, 1980.

58. Chiles C, Ravin CE: Radiographic recognition of pneumothorax in the intensive care unit, *Crit Care Med* 14:677, 1986.

59. Vermeulen EG, Teng HT, Boxma H: Ventral tension pneumothorax, *J Trauma* 43:975,1997.

60. Friedman PJ: Adult pulmonary ligament pneumatocele: a loculated pneumothorax, *Radiology* 155:575, 1985.

61. Spizarny DL, Goodman LR: Air in the minor fissure: a sign of right-sided pneumothorax, *Radiology* 160:329, 1986.

62. Campbell-Smith TA, Bendall SP, Davis J: Tension pneumothorax in the presence of bilateral intercostal chest drains, *Injury* 29:556, 1998.

63. Stark P: Chest cage injuries. In Stark P, ed: *Radiology of thoracic trauma*, Boston, 1993, Andover Medical Publishers.

64. Bryk D: Intrapulmonary effusion. Effect of expiration on the pseudodiaphragmatic contour, *Radiology* 120:33, 1976.

65. Franklin DC, Mathai J: Biliary pleural fistula: a complication of hepatic trauma, *J Trauma* 20:256, 1980.

66. Benhaim P, Streat C, Knudson M: Posttraumatic chylous ascites in a child: recognition and management of an unusual condition, *J Trauma* 39:1175, 1995.

67. Hase T, Kodama M, Domasu S: A case of urothorax that manifested as posttraumatic pleural effusion after a motorcycle crash, *J Trauma* 46:967, 1999.

68. Cerva DS Jr, Mirvis SE, Shanmuganathan K: Detection of bleeding in patients with major pelvic fractures: value of contrast-enhanced CT, *AJR* 166:131, 1996.

69. Mirvis SE, Tobin KD, Kostrubiak I: Thoracic CT in detecting occult disease in critically ill patients, *AJR* 148:685, 1987.

70. Sisley AC, Rozycki GS, Ballard RB, et al: Rapid detection of traumatic effusion using surgeon-performed ultrasonography, *J Trauma* 44:291, 1998.

71. Ma OJ, Mateer JR: Trauma ultrasound examination versus chest radiography in the detection of hemothorax, *Ann Emerg Med* 29:312, 1997.

72. Mirvis SE, Templeton PA: Imaging in acute thoracic trauma, *Semin Roentgenol* 27:184, 1992.

73. Maltby JD: The post-trauma chest film, *Crit Rev Diagn Imaging* 14:1,1980.

74. Goodman LR, Putman CE: The SICU chest radiograph after massive blunt trauma, *Radiol Clin North Am* 19:111, 1981.

75. Allen GS, Cox CS Jr: Pulmonary contusion in children: diagnosis and management, *South Med J* 19:1099, 1998.

76. Kato R, Horinouchi H, Maenaka Y: Traumatic pulmonary pseudocyst: report of twelve cases [see comments], *J Thorac Cardiovasc Surg* 97:309, 1989.

77. Carroll K, Cheeseman SH, Fink MP, et al: Secondary infection of post-traumatic pulmonary cavitary lesions in adolescents and young adults: role of computed tomography and operative debridement and drainage [see comments], *J Trauma* 29:109, 1989.

78. Roddy LH, Unger KM, Miller WC: Thoracic computed tomography in the critically ill patient, *Crit Care Med* 9:515, 1981.

79. Karaaslan T, Meuli R, Androux R et al: Traumatic chest lesions in patients with severe head trauma: a comparative study with computed tomography and conventional chest roentgenograms, *J Trauma* 39:1081, 1995.

80. Kunisch-Hoppe M, Bachmann G, Hoppe M, et al: [CT quantification of pleuropulmonary lesions in severe thoracic trauma], *Rofo Fortschr Geb Rontgenstr Neuen Bildgeb Verfahr* 167:453, 1997.

81. Toombs BD, Sandler CM, Lester RG: Computed tomography of chest trauma, *Radiology* 140:733, 1981.

82. Allen GS, Fischer RP: Traumatic lung herniation, *Ann Thorac Surg* 63:1455, 1997.

83. Francois B, Desachy A, Cornu E, et al: Traumatic pulmonary hernia: surgical versus conservative management, *J Trauma* 44:217, 1998.

84. Sadler MA, Shapiro RS, Wagreich J: CT diagnosis of acquired intercostal lung herniation, *Clin Imaging* 21:104, 1997.

85. Morgan AS, Flancbaum L, Esposito T, et al: Blunt injury to the diaphragm: an analysis of 44 patients, *J Trauma* 26:565, 1986.

86. Bogers AJ, Zweers DJ, Vroom EM, et al: Cardiac subluxation in traumatic rupture of diaphragm and pericardium, *Thorac Cardiovasc Surg* 34:132, 1986.

87. Simpson J, Lobo DN, Shah AB, et al: Traumatic diaphragmatic rupture: associated injuries and outcome, *Ann R Coll Surg Engl* 82:97, 2000.

88. Kearney PA, Rouhana SW, Burney RE: Blunt rupture of the diaphragm: mechanism, diagnosis, and treatment, *Ann Emerg Med* 18:1326, 1989.

89. Rodriguez-Morales G, Rodriguez A, Shatney CH: Acute rupture of the diaphragm in blunt trauma: analysis of 60 patients, *J Trauma* 26: 438, 1986.

90. Shanmuganathan K, Killeen KS, Mirvis SE , et al: Imaging of diaphragmatic injuries, *J Thorac Imaging* 15:104, 2000.

91. Putman CE, Goodman LR: Thoracic trauma. In Teplick HM, ed: *Surgical radiology*, Philadelphia, 1981, WB Saunders.

92. Estrera AS, Landay MJ, McClelland RN: Blunt traumatic rupture of the right hemidiaphragm: experience in 12 patients, *Ann Thorac Surg* 39:525, 1985.

93. Beal SL, McKennan M: Blunt diaphragm rupture: a morbid injury, *Arch Surg* 123:828, 1988.

94. Lucido JL: Rupture of the diaphragm due to blunt trauma, *Arch Surg* 86:989, 1963.

95. Glasser DL, Shanmuganathan K, Mirvis SE: General case of the day: acute intrapericardial diaphragmatic hernia, *Radiographics* 18:799, 1998.

96. Boulanger BR, Milzman DP, Rosati C, et al: A comparison of right and left blunt traumatic diaphragmatic rupture, *J Trauma* 35:255, 1993.

97. Ilgenfritz FM, Stewart DE: Blunt trauma of the diaphragm: a 15-county, private hospital experience, *Am Surg* 58:334,1992.

98. Voeller GR, Reisser JR, Fabian TC: Blunt diaphragm injuries: a five-year experience, *Am Surg* 56:28,1990.

99. Ball T, McCrory R, Smith JO, et al: Traumatic diaphragmatic hernia: errors in diagnosis, *AJR* 138:633, 1982.

100. Meyers BF, McCabe CJ: Traumatic diaphragmatic hernia: errors in diagnosis, *Ann Surg* 218:783, 1993.

101. Guth AA, Pachter HL, Kim U: Pitfalls in the diagnosis of blunt diaphragmatic injury, *Am J Surg* 170:5, 1995.

102. Freeman T, Fischer RP: The inadequacy of peritoneal lavage in diagnosing acute diaphragmatic rupture, *J Trauma* 16:538, 1976.

103. Gelman R, Mirvis SE, Gens D: Diaphragmatic rupture due to blunt trauma: sensitivity of plain chest radiographs [see comments], *AJR* 156:51, 1991.

104. Toombs BD, Sandler CM, Lester RG: Computed tomography of chest trauma, *Radiology* 140:733, 1981.

105. Wiencek RG Jr, Wilson RF, Steiger Z: Acute injuries of the diaphragm: an analysis of 165 cases, *J Thorac Cardiovasc Surg* 92:989, 1986.

106. Shackleton KL, Stewart ET, Taylor AJ: Traumatic diaphragmatic injuries: spectrum of radiographic findings, *Radiographics* 18:49, 1998.

107. Pagliarello G, Carter J: Traumatic injury to the diaphragm: timely diagnosis and treatment, *J Trauma* 33:194, 1992.

108. Murray JG, Caoili E, Gruden JF, et al: Acute rupture of the diaphragm due to blunt trauma: diagnostic sensitivity and specificity of CT, *AJR* 166:1035, 1996.

109. Rao KG, Woodlief RM: Grey scale ultrasonic demonstration of ruptured right hemidiaphragm, *Br J Radiol* 53:812, 1980.

110. Ammann AM, Brewer WH, Maull KI, et al: Traumatic rupture of the diaphragm: real-time sonographic diagnosis, *AJR* 140:915, 1983.

111. Somer JM, Gleeson FV, Flower CD: Rupture of the right hemidiaphragm following blunt trauma: the use of ultrasound in diagnosis, *Clin Radiol* 42:97, 1990.

112. Nilsson PE, Aspelin P, Ekberg O, et al: Radiologic diagnosis in traumatic rupture of the right diaphragm: report of a case, *Acta Radiol* 29:653, 1988.

113. Shanmuganathan K, Mirvis SE, White CS, et al: MR imaging evaluation of hemidiaphragms in acute blunt trauma: experience with 16 patients, *AJR* 167:397, 1996.

114. Shanmuganathan K, Killeen K, Mirvis SE, et al: Imaging of diaphragmatic injuries, *J Thorac Imaging* 15:104, 2000.

115. Leung JC, Nanace ML, Schwab CW, et al: Thickening of the diaphragm: a new computed tomography sign of diaphragm injury, *J Thorac Imaging* 14:126, 1999.

116. Chen JC, Wilson SE: Diaphragmatic injuries: recognition and management in sixty-two patients, *Am Surg* 57:810, 1991.

117. Caskey CI, Zerhouni EA, Fishman EK: Aging of the diaphragm: a CT study, *Radiology* 171:385, 1989.

118. Gale ME: Bochdalek hernia: prevalence and CT characteristics, *Radiology* 156:499, 1985.

119. Mirvis SE, Keramati B, Buckman R: MR imaging of traumatic diaphragmatic rupture, *J Comput Assist Tomogr* 12:147, 1988.

120. Boulanger BR, Mirvis SE, Rodriguez A: Magnetic resonance imaging in traumatic diaphragmatic rupture: case reports, *J Trauma* 32:89, 1992.

121. Murray JA, Demetriades D, Cornwell EE III, et al: Penetrating left thoracoabdominal trauma: the incidence and clinical presentation of diaphragm injuries, *J Trauma* 43:624, 1997.

122. Renz BM, Feliciano DV: Gunshot wounds to the right thoracoabdomen: a prospective study of nonoperative management, *J Trauma* 37:737, 1994.

123. Van Moore A, Ravin CE, Putman CE: Radiologic evaluation of acute chest trauma, *Crit Rev Diagn Imaging* 19:89, 1983.

124. Beal SL, Pottmeyer EW, Spisso JM: Esophageal perforation following external blunt trauma, *J Trauma* 28:1425, 1988.

125. Bladergroen MR, Lowe JE, Postlethwait RW: Diagnosis and recommended management of esophageal perforation and rupture, *Ann Thorac Surg* 42:235, 1986.

126. Ketai L, Brandt MM, Schermer C: Nonaortic mediastinal injuries from blunt chest trauma, *J Thorac Imaging* 15:120, 2000.

127. Maroney MJ, Mirvis SE, Shanmuganathan K: Esophageal occlusion caused by thoracic spine fracture or dislocation: CT diagnosis, *AJR* 167:714, 1996.

128. Hanpeter DE, Demetriades D, Asensio JA, et al: Helical computed tomographic scan in the evaluation of mediastinal gunshot wounds, *J Trauma* 49:689, 2000.

129. Flowers JL, Graham SM, Ugarte MA, et al: Flexible endoscopy for the diagnosis of esophageal trauma, *J Trauma* 40:261, 1996.

130. Bertelsen S, Howitz P: Injuries of the trachea and bronchi, *Thorax* 27:188, 1972.

131. Conn JH, Hardy JD, Fain WR, et al: Thoracic trauma: analysis of 1022 cases, *J Trauma* 3:22, 1963.

132. Lee RB: Traumatic injury of the cervicothoracic trachea and major bronchi, *Chest Surg Clin N Am* 7:285, 1997.

133. Kiser AC, O'Brien SM, Detterbeck FC: Blunt tracheobronchial injuries: treatment and outcomes, *Ann Thorac Surg* 71:2059, 2001.

134. Chu CP, Chen PP: Tracheobronchial injury secondary to blunt chest trauma: diagnosis and management, *Anaesth Intensive Care* 30:145, 2002.

135. Halttunen PE, Kostiainen SA, Meurala HG: Bronchial rupture caused by blunt chest trauma, *Scand J Thorac Cardiovasc Surg* 18:141, 1984.

136. Ecker RR, Libertini RV, Rea WJ, et al: Injuries of the trachea and bronchi, *Ann Thorac Surg* 11:289, 1971.

137. Anderson JN: Major airway injury in closed chest trauma, *Chest* 72:63, 1977.

138. Kelly JP, Webb WR, Moulder PV, et al: Management of airway trauma. I. Tracheobronchial injuries, *Ann Thorac Surg* 40:551, 1985.

139. Kirsh MM, Orringer MB, Behrendt DM, et al: Management of tracheobronchial disruption secondary to nonpenetrating trauma, *Ann Thorac Surg* 22:93, 1976.

140. Urschel HC Jr, Razzuk MA: Management of acute traumatic injuries of tracheobronchial tree, *Surg Gynecol Obstet* 136:113, 1973.

141. Symbas PN, Justicz AG, Ricketts RR: Rupture of the airways from blunt trauma: treatment of complex injuries, *Ann Thorac Surg* 54:177, 1992.

142. Tanaka H, Endoh Y, Kobayashi K: Urgent thoracotomy for injuries to the tracheobronchial tree due to blunt trauma: a seven cases report and a literature review of 32 cases in Japan, *Nippon Kyobu Geka Gakkai Zasshi* 45:851, 1997.

143. Kirsh MM, Behrendt DM, Orringer MB: The treatment of acute traumatic rupture of the aorta: a 10-year experience, *Ann Surg* 184:308, 1976.

144. Lloyd HD Jr, Klassen KP, Roettig LC: Rupture of the main bronchi in closed chest injury, *Arch Surg* 77:597, 1958.

145. Mason AC, Mirvis SE, Templeton PA: Imaging of acute tracheobronchial injury: review of the literature, *Emergency Radiology* 1:250, 1994.

146. Offiah CJ, Endres D: Isolated laryngotracheal separation following blunt trauma to the neck, *J Laryngol Otol* 111:1079, 1997.

147. Spencer, JA, Rogers CE, Westaby S: Clinico-radiological correlates in rupture of the major airways [published erratum appears in *Clin Radiol* 44:214, 1991; see comments], *Clin Radiol* 43:371, 1991.

148. Baumgartner F, Sheppard B, de Virgilio C, et al: Tracheal and main bronchial disruptions after blunt chest trauma: presentation and management, *Ann Thorac Surg* 50:569, 1990.

149. Grover FL, Ellestad C, Arom KV, et al: Diagnosis and management of major tracheobronchial injuries, *Ann Thorac Surg* 28:384, 1979.

150. Jones WS, Mavroudis C, Richardson JD: Management of tracheobronchial disruption resulting from blunt trauma, *Surgery* 95:319, 1984.

151. Mathisen DJ, Grillo H: Laryngotracheal trauma, *Surgery* 95:319, 1984.

152. Burke JF: Early diagnosis of traumatic rupture on the bronchus, *JAMA* 181:682, 1962.

153. Kunisch-Hoppe M, Hoppe M, Rauber K, et al: Tracheal rupture caused by blunt chest trauma: radiological and clinical features, *Eur Radiol* 10:480, 2000.

154. Major CP, Floresguerra CA, Messerschmidt WH, et al: Traumatic disruption of the cervical trachea, *J Tenn Med Assoc* 85:517, 1992.

155. Chitre VV, Prinsley PR, Hashmi SM: Pneumopericardium: an unusual manifestation of blunt tracheal trauma, *J Laryngol Otol* 111:387, 1997.

156. Romano L, Rossi G, Pinto A, et al: [A case of tracheal rupture caused by blunt trauma associated with pneumoretroperitoneum and intraspinal gas], *Radiol Med (Torino)* 92:642, 1996.

157. Ramzy AI, Rodriguez A, Turney SZ: Management of major tracheobronchial ruptures in patients with multiple system trauma, *J Trauma* 28:1353, 1988.

158. Pratt LW, Smith RJ, Guite LA Jr, et al: Blunt chest trauma with tracheobronchial rupture, *Ann Otol Rhinol Laryngol* 93:357, 1984.

159. Wiot JF: Tracheobronchial trauma, *Semin Roentgenol* 18:15, 1983.

160. Tobias ME, Sack AD, Carter G, et al: Cricotracheal separation in blunt neck injury—the sign of hyoid bone elevation: a case report, *S Afr J Surg* 27:189, 1989.

161. Polansky A, Resnick D, Sofferman RA, et al: Hyoid bone elevation: a sign of tracheal transection, *Radiology* 150:117, 1984.

162. Unger JM, Schuchmann GG, Grossman JE, et al: Tears of the trachea and main bronchi caused by blunt trauma: radiologic findings [see comments], *AJR* 153:1175, 1989.

163. Hosny A, Bhendwal S, Hosni A: Transection of cervical trachea following blunt trauma, *J Laryngol Otol* 109:250, 1995.

164. Harris R, Joseph A: Acute tracheal rupture related to endotracheal intubation: case report, *J Emerg Med* 18:35, 2000.

165. Marty-Ane CH, Picard E, Jonquet O, et al: Membranous tracheal rupture after endotracheal intubation, *Ann Thorac Surg* 60:1367, 1995.

166. Thompson DS, Read RC: Rupture of the trachea following endotracheal intubation, *JAMA* 204:995, 1968.

167. Massard G, Rouge C, Dabbagh A, et al: Tracheobronchial lacerations after intubation and tracheostomy, *Ann Thorac Surg* 61:1483, 1996.

168. Striebel HW, Pinkwart LU, Karavias T: [Tracheal rupture caused by overinflation of endotracheal tube cuff], *Anesthetist* 44:186, 1995.

169. Tornvall SS, Jackson KH, Oyanedel E: Tracheal rupture, complication of cuffed endotracheal tube, *Chest* 59:237, 1971.

170. Stark P: Traumatic rupture of the thoracic aorta: a review, *Crit Rev Diagn Imaging* 21:221, 1984.

171. Parmley LF, Marion WC, Jahnke EJ: Nonpenetrating traumatic injury of the aorta, *Circulation* 17:1086, 1958.

172. Duhaylongsod FG, Glower DD, Wolfe WG: Acute traumatic aortic aneurysm: the Duke experience from 1970 to 1990, *J Vasc Surg* 15:331, 1992.

173. Cohen AM, Crass JR, Thomas HA, et al: CT evidence for the "osseous pinch" mechanism of traumatic aortic injury, *AJR* 159:271, 1992.

174. Shkrum MJ, McClafferty KJ, Green RN, et al: Mechanisms of aortic injury in fatalities occurring in motor vehicle collisions, *J Forensic Sci* 44:44, 1999.

175. Brundage SI, Harruff R, Jurkovich GJ, et al: The epidemiology of thoracic aortic injuries in pedestrians, *J Trauma* 45:1010, 1998.

176. Pretre R, LaHarpe R, Cheratakis A, et al: Blunt injury to the ascending aorta: three patterns of presentation, *Surgery* 119:603, 1996.

177. Symbas PJ, Horsley WS, Symbas PN: Rupture of the ascending aorta caused by blunt trauma, *Ann Thorac Surg* 66:113, 1998.

178. Barcia TC, Livoni JP: Indications for angiography in blunt thoracic trauma, *Radiology* 147:15, 1983.

179. Symbas PN, Tyras DH, Ware RE, et al: Traumatic rupture of the aorta, *Ann Surg* 178:6, 1973.

180. Ayella RJ, Hankins JR, Turney SZ, et al: Ruptured thoracic aorta due to blunt trauma, *J Trauma* 17:199, 1977.

181. Schwab CW, Lawson RB, Lind JF, et al: Aortic injury: comparison of supine and upright portable chest films to evaluate the widened mediastinum, *Ann Emerg Med* 13:896, 1984.

182. Mirvis SE, Bidwell JK, Buddemeyer EU, et al: Value of chest radiography in excluding traumatic aortic rupture, *Radiology* 163:487, 1987.

183. Richardson P, Mirvis SE, Scorpio R, et al: Value of CT in determining the need for angiography when findings of mediastinal hemorrhage on chest radiographs are equivocal, *AJR* 156:273, 1991.

184. Marsh DG, Sturm JT: Traumatic aortic rupture: roentgenographic indications for angiography, *Ann Thorac Surg* 21:337, 1976.

185. Sturm JT, Marsh GD, Bodily KC: Ruptured thoracic aorta: evolving radiological concepts, *Surgery* 85:363, 1979.

186. Seltzer SE, D'Orsi C, Kirshner R, et al: Traumatic aortic rupture: plain radiographic findings, *AJR* 137:1011, 1981.

187. Marnocha KE, Maglinte DD, Woods J, et al: Mediastinal-width/chest-width ratio in blunt chest trauma: a reappraisal, *AJR* 142:275. 1984.

188. Appelbaum A, Karp RB, Kirklin JW: Surgical treatment for closed thoracic aortic injuries, *J Thorac Cardiovasc Surg* 71:458, 1976.

189. Dennis LN, Rogers LF: Superior mediastinal widening from spine fractures mimicking aortic rupture on chest radiographs, *AJR* 152:27, 1989.

190. Creasy JD, Chiles C, Routh WD, et al: Overview of traumatic injury of the thoracic aorta, *Radiographics* 17:27, 1997.

191. Savastano S, Feltrin GP, Miotto D, et al: Value of plain chest film in predicting traumatic aortic rupture, *Ann Radiol* 32:196, 1989.

192. Mirvis SE, Bidwell JK, Buddemeyer EU, et al: Imaging diagnosis of traumatic aortic rupture: a review and experience at a major trauma center, *Invest Radiol* 22:187, 1987.

193. Gerlock AJ, Muhletaler CA, Coulam CM, et al: Traumatic aortic aneurysm: validity of esophageal tube displacement sign, *AJR* 135:713, 1980.

194. Wales LR, Morishima MS, Reay D, et al: Nasogastric tube displacement in acute traumatic rupture *of* the thoracic aorta: a postmortem study, *AJR* 138:821, 1982.

195. Dart CH Jr, Braitman HE: Traumatic rupture of thoracic aorta: diagnosis and management, *Arch Surg* 111:697, 1976.

196. Simeone JF, Minagi H, Putman CE: Traumatic disruption of the thoracic aorta: significance of the left apical extrapleural cap, *Radiology* 117:265, 1975.

197. Simeone JF, Deren MM, Cagle F: The value of the left apical cap in the diagnosis of aortic rupture: a prospective and retrospective study, *Radiology* 139:35, 1981.

198. Peters DR, Gamsu G: Displacement of the right paraspinous interface: a radiographic sign of acute traumatic rupture of the thoracic aorta, *Radiology* 134:599, 1980.

199. Kram HB, Wohlmuth DA, Appell PL: Clinical and radiographic indications for aortography in blunt chest trauma, *J Vasc Surg* 6:168, 1987.

200. Smith RS, Chang FC: Traumatic rupture of the aorta: still a lethal injury, *Am J Surg* 152:660, 1986.

201. Woodring JH, King JG: The potential effects of radiographic criteria to exclude aortography in patients with blunt chest trauma: results of a study of 32 patients with proved aortic or brachiocephalic arterial injury, *J Thorac Cardiovasc Surg* 97:456, 1989.

202. Raptopoulos V, Shieman RG, Phillips DA: Traumatic aortic tear: screening with chest CT, *Radiology* 182:667, 1992.

203. Wicky S, Capasso P, Meuli R: Spiral CT aortography: an efficient technique for the diagnosis of traumatic aortic injury, *Eur Radiol* 8:828, 1998.

204. Biquet JF, Dondelinger RF, Roland D: Computed tomography of thoracic aortic trauma, *Eur Radiol* 6:25, 1996.

205. Fabian TC, Davis KA, Gavant ML: Prospective study of blunt aortic injury: helical CT is diagnostic and antihypertensive therapy reduces rupture, *Ann Surg* 227:666, 1998.

206. Pate JW, Gavant ML, Weiman DS: Traumatic rupture of the aortic isthmus: program of selective management. *World J Surg* 23:59, 1999.

207. Heiberg E, Wolverson MK, Sundaram M, et al: CT in aortic trauma, *AJR* 140:1119, 1983.

208. Miller FB, Richardson JD, Thomas HA, et al: Role of CT in diagnosis of major arterial injury after blunt thoracic trauma, *Surgery* 106:596, 1989.

209. Durham RM, Zuckerman D, Wolverson M, et al: Computed tomography as a screening exam in patients with suspected blunt aortic injury, *Ann Surg* 220:699, 1994.

210. Fabian TC, Richardson JD, Croce MA, et al: Prospective study of blunt aortic injury: multicenter trial of the American Association for the Surgery of Trauma, *J Trauma* 42:374, 1997.

211. Rosenberg JM, Bredenberg CE, Marvasti MA, et al: Blunt injuries to the aortic arch vessels, *Ann Thorac Surg* 48:508, 1989.

212. Petre R, Chilcott M, Murith N: Blunt injury to the supra-aortic arteries, *Br J Surg* 84:603, 1997.

213. Oxorn D, Saibil E, Boulanger B: The ductus diverticulum: false-positive angiographic diagnosis of traumatic aortic disruption, *J Cardiothorac Vasc Anesth* 11:86, 1997.

214. Morse SS, Glickman MG, Greenwood LH, et al: Traumatic aortic rupture: false-positive aortographic diagnosis due to atypical ductus diverticulum, *AJR* 150:793, 1988.

215. Fisher RG, Sanchez-Torres M, Wingham CJ, et al: "Lumps" and "bumps" that mimic acute aortic and brachiocephalic vessel injury, *Radiographics* 17:825, 1997.

216. Fisher RG, Sanchez-Torres M, Thomas JW: Subtle or atypical injuries of the thoracic and brachiocephalic vessels in blunt thoracic trauma, *Radiographics* 17:835, 1997.

217. Mirvis SE, Pais SO, Shanmuganathan K: Atypical results of thoracic aortography performed to exclude aortic rupture, *Emerg Radiol* 0:42, 1988.

218. Orron DE, Porter DH, Kim D, et al: False-positive aortography following blunt chest trauma: case report, *Cardiovasc Intervent Radiol* 11:132, 1988.

219. Goarin JP, Catoire P, Jacquens Y, et al: Use of transesophageal echocardiography for diagnosis of traumatic aortic injury, *Chest* 112:71, 1997.

220. Ahrar K, Smith DC, Bansal RC, et al: Angiography in blunt thoracic aortic injury, *J Trauma* 42:665, 1997.

221. Cohn SM, Pollak JS, McCarthy S, et al: Detection of aortic tear in the acute trauma patient using MRI, *Magn Reson Imaging* 12:963, 1994.

222. Nagy K, Fabian T, Rodman G, et al: Guidelines for the diagnosis and management of blunt aortic injury: an EAST Practice Management Guidelines Work Group, *J Trauma* 48:1128, 2000.

223. Sparks MB, Burchard KW, Marrin CA, et al: Transesophageal echocardiography: preliminary results in patients with traumatic aortic rupture, *Arch Surg* 126:711, 1991.

224. Saletta S, Lederman E, Fine S, et al: Transesophageal echocardiography for the initial evaluation of the widened mediastinum in trauma patients, *J Trauma* 39:137, 1995.

225. Vignon P, Gueret P, Vedrinne JM, et al: Role of transesophageal echocardiography in the diagnosis and management of traumatic aortic disruption, *Circulation* 92:2959, 1995.

226. Read RA, Moore EE, Moore FA, et al: Intravascular ultrasonography for the diagnosis of traumatic aortic disruption: a case report, *Surgery* 114:624, 1993.

227. Uflacker R, Horn J, Phillips G, et al: Intravascular sonography in the assessment of traumatic injury of the thoracic aorta, *AJR* 173:665, 1999.

228. Semba CP, Kato N, Kee ST, et al: Acute rupture of the descending thoracic aorta: repair with use of endovascular stent-grafts, *J Vasc Intervent Radiol* 8:337, 1997.

229. Kramer S, Gorich J, Rilinger N, et al: [Therapy of acute traumatic vascular injuries using covered stents], *Rofo Fortschr Geb Rontgenstr Neuen Bildgeb Verfahr* 167:486, 1997.

230. Mirvis SE, Pais SO, Gens DR: Thoracic aortic rupture: advantages of intraarterial digital subtraction angiography, *AJR* 146:987, 1986.

231. Ferrera PC, Ghaemmaghami PA: Ductus diverticulum interpreted as traumatic aortic injury, *Am J Emerg Med* 15:371, 1997.

232. Cordoba Lopez A, Lopez-Sanchez L, Lopez Rodriguez A: [False positive aortography in the diagnosis of aortic rupture], *Rev Clin Esp* 197:856, 1997.

233. Broux C, Lavagne P, Ferretti G, et al: [Aortic diverticulum: differential diagnosis of traumatic lesions of the thoracic aorta], *Ann Fr Anesth Reanim* 18:1065, 1999.

234. Patel NH, Stephens KE Jr, Mirvis SE, et al: Imaging of acute thoracic aortic injury due to blunt trauma: a review, *Radiology* 209:335, 1998.

235. Mayberry JC: Imaging in thoracic trauma: the trauma surgeon's perspective, *J Thorac Imaging* 15:76, 2000.

236. Mirvis SE, Kostrubiak I, Whitley NO, et al: Role of CT in excluding major arterial injury after blunt thoracic trauma, *AJR* 149:601, 1987.

237. Fishman JE: Imaging of blunt aortic and great vessel trauma, *J Thorac Imaging* 15:97, 2000.

238. Dyer DS, Moore EE, Ilke DN, et al: Thoracic aortic injury: how predictive is mechanism and is chest computed tomography a reliable screening tool? A prospective study of 1561 patients, *J Trauma* 48:673, 2000.

239. Brasel KJ, Weigelt JA: Blunt thoracic aortic trauma: a cost-utility approach for injury detection, *Arch Surg* 131:619, 1996.

240. Fattori R, Celletti F, Bertaccini P, et al: Delayed surgery of traumatic aortic rupture: role of magnetic resonance imaging, *Circulation* 94:2865, 1996.

241. Harris JH Jr, Horowitz DR, Zelitt DL: Unenhanced dynamic mediastinal computed tomography in the selection of patients requiring thoracic aortography for the detection of acute traumatic aortic injury, *Emergency Radiology* 2:67, 1995.

242. Chaumoitre K, Zapp M, Portier F, et al: Rupture of the right atrium-superior vena cava junction from blunt thoracic trauma: helical CT diagnosis, *AJR* 169:1753, 1997 [letter].

243. Walsh A, Snyder HS: Azygos vein laceration following a vertical deceleration injury, *J Emerg Med* 10:35, 1992.

244. Irgau I, Fulda GJ, Hailstone D, et al: Internal mammary artery injury, anterior mediastinal hematoma, and cardiac compromise after blunt chest trauma, *J Trauma* 39:1018, 1995.

245. Hernandez-Luyando L, Gonzalez de las Heras E, Calvo J, et al: Posttraumatic tension pneumopericardium, *Am J Emerg Med* 15:686, 1997.

246. Cimmino CV: Some radio-diagnostic notes on pneumomediastinum, pneumothorax, and pneumoperitoneum, *Va Med* 94:205, 1967.

247. Baksaas ST, Fosse E, Pillgram-Larsen J: [Traumatic pneumopericardium with cardiac tamponade], *Tidsskr Nor Laegeforen* 112:2085, 1992.

248. Higgins CB, Broderick TW, Edwards DK, et al: The hemodynamic significance of massive pneumopericardium in preterm infants with respiratory distress syndrome: clinical and experimental observations, *Radiology* 133:363, 1979.

249. Brathwaite CE, Rodriguez A, Turney SZ, et al: Blunt traumatic cardiac rupture. A 5-year experience, *Ann Surg* 212:701, 1990.

250. Grumbach K, Mechlin MB, Mintz MC: Computed tomography and ultrasound of the traumatized and acutely ill patient, *Emerg Med Clin North Am* 3:607, 1985.

251. Whye D, Barish R, Almquist T, et al: Echocardiographic diagnosis of acute pericardial effusion in penetrating chest trauma, *Am J Emerg Med* 6:21, 1988.

252. Mazurek B, Jehle D, Martin M: Emergency department echocardiography in the diagnosis and therapy of cardiac tamponade, *J Emerg Med* 9:27, 1991.

253. Carrillo EH, Guinn BJ, Ali AT: Transthoracic ultrasonography is an alternative to subxyphoid ultrasonography for the diagnosis of hemopericardium in penetrating precordial trauma, *Am J Surg* 179:34, 2000.

254. Chong HH, Plotnick GD: Pericardial effusion and tamponade: evaluation, imaging modalities, and management, *Compr Ther* 21:378, 1995.

255. Frantz KM, Fishman EK: Hemopericardium leading to cardiac tamponade in the traumatized pediatric patient: discovery by CT, *Clin Imaging* 16:180, 1992.

256. Harries SR, Fox BM, Roobottom CA: Azygos reflux: a CT sign of cardiac tamponade [see comments], *Clin Radiol* 53:702, 1998.

257. Coleman GM, Fischer R, Fuentes F: Blunt chest trauma: extrapericardial cardiac tamponade by a mediastinal hematoma, *Chest* 95:922, 1989.

258. Braatz T, Mirvis SE, Killeen KL, et al: CT diagnosis of internal mammary artery injury caused by blunt trauma, *Clin Radiol* 56:120 2001.

259. Fulda G, Rodriguez A, Turney SZ: Blunt traumatic pericardial rupture: a ten-year experience 1979 to 1989, *J Cardiovasc Surg (Torino)* 31:525,1990.

260. Deslandes V, Jacob JP, Chapillon M, et al: [Early diagnosis of traumatic extra-pericardial luxation of the heart. Value of tomodensitometry. Apropos of a case (see comments)]. *Ann Fr Anesth Reanim* 13:734, 1994.

261. Carrillo EH, Heniford BT, Dykes JR, et al: Cardiac herniation producing tamponade: the critical role of early diagnosis, *J Trauma* 43:180, 1992.

262. Holness R, Waxman K: Diagnosis of traumatic cardiac contusion utilizing single photon-emission computed tomography, *Crit Care Med* 18:1, 1990.

263. Hossack KF, Moreno CA, Vanway CW, et al: Frequency of cardiac contusion in nonpenetrating chest injury, *Am J Cardiol* 61:391, 1988.

264. Rosenbaum RC, Johnston GS: Posttraumatic cardiac dysfunction: assessment with radionuclide ventriculography, *Radiology* 160:91, 1986.

265. Hilton T, Mezei L, Pearson AC: Delayed rupture of tricuspid papillary muscle following blunt chest trauma, *Am Heart J* 119:1410, 1990.

266. Helling TS, Duke P, Beggs CW, et al: A prospective evaluation of 68 patients suffering blunt chest trauma for evidence of cardiac injury, *J Trauma* 29:961, 1989.

267. Weiss RL, Brier JA, O'Connor W, et al: The usefulness of transesophageal echocardiography in diagnosing cardiac contusions, *Chest* 109:73, 1996.

268. Bertinchant JP, Polge A, Mohty D, et al: Evaluation of incidence, clinical significance, and prognostic value of circulating cardiac troponin I and T elevation in hemodynamically stable patients with suspected myocardial contusion after blunt chest trauma, *J Trauma* 48:924, 2000.

269. Ferjani M, Droc G, Dreux S, et al: Circulating cardiac troponin T in myocardial contusion, *Chest* 111:427, 1997.

270. Grieco JG, Montoya A, Sullivan HJ, et al: Ventricular aneurysm due to blunt chest injury, *Ann Thorac Surg* 47:322, 1989.

271. Blessing E, Wolpers HG, Hausmann D, et al: Posttraumatic myocardial infarction with severe coronary intimal dissection documented by intravascular ultrasound, *J Am Soc Echocardiogr* 9:906, 1996.

272. Dougherty JE, Gabram SG, Glickstein MF, et al: Traumatic intramyocardial dissection secondary to significant blunt chest trauma: a case report, *J Trauma* 34:300,1993.

6 Imaging of Abdominal Trauma

K. Shanmuganathan and Karen L. Killeen

Motor vehicle crashes are the leading cause of death for Americans between the ages of 1 and 34.[1] In 1999 the rate for all age groups of deaths involving mechanically or electrically powered highway-transport vehicles in motion was 15.1 per 100,000 people. The death rates are especially high among 15- to 24-year-olds (27 per 100,000) and people 80 years and older (28 per 100,000).[1,2] Motorcycle riders, who lack the protection of enclosed vehicles, are 16 times more likely to be killed per mile traveled than someone in a car.[3] In 1999, 41,661 people died from injuries in 37,043 crashes involving 56,668 motor vehicles,[1,2] and there were 2.2 million nonfatal injuries from motor vehicle crashes. The total cost of these nonfatal crashes exceeded $150 billion.[1,2] Although the number of registered vehicles in the United States has increased to more than 218 million (about four vehicles for every five people), the death rates for all age groups have generally decreased since World War II.[1,2] The National Highway Traffic Safety Administration estimates that at least one driver or nonoccupant had a blood alcohol level concentration of 0.10 percent or more in all traffic deaths that occurred in 1999. The death rate from falls was 6.3 per 100,000 and a total of 17,100 falls from height occurred in 1999.[2]

From 1998 through 2000, 13,703 blunt trauma patients were admitted to the University of Maryland Medical Shock Trauma Center (UMSTC), and 14% (1976) of the patients required inpatient care for their injuries. The average Injury Severity Score (ISS) was 16.4 for persons requiring inpatient care. The mechanism of blunt abdominal injury was motor vehicle collision in 63% (1243) of the 1976 patients, falls 12% (215), pedestrian struck 9% (183), motorcycle collision 6% (120), assaults 5% (97), and other mechanisms 5% (93). Exploratory laparotomies were performed in 11% (214) of all blunt abdominal trauma patients admitted. The majority of laparotomies (65% or 139) were performed within 24 hours of admission to the trauma center.

Diagnosis and treatment of patients admitted to a trauma center with potential blunt abdominal injury have been a difficult and challenging task for the trauma surgeon and emergency radiologist. Unlike penetrating injury, the associates multisystem injuries often seen with blunt trauma may divert attention from the abdomen to more obvious injuries, making diagnosis and triage more difficult and complex. Until the early 1960s physical examination and abdominal radiographs were the mainstay of diagnosing abdominal injuries and determining the need for laparotomy in blunt trauma patients.[4-7] Based on clinical examination alone, the decision to perform a celiotomy in these patients resulted in an accuracy ranging from 17% to 87%,[4,5,8,9] compared with findings at surgery. Peritoneal signs or shock may be absent in one-third of patients with intraabdominal injuries after blunt trauma. A significant number of these patients are intoxicated or have suffered injuries to the brain or spinal cord, rendering the physical examination less reliable.[10] Mackersie et al.[11] reported a significant correlation between major abdominal visceral injuries and hypotension on hospital arrival, presence of major chest trauma, and a base deficit of ≥ 3 mEqL in a large series of blunt trauma patients. The constant introduction and further development of new technology and diagnostic studies—such as diagnostic peritoneal lavage (DPL), sonography, single- or multislice spiral computed tomography (CT), angiography, and laparoscopy—in most level I trauma centers in the United States, coupled with the emerging popularity and success rate of nonoperative management of solid organ injury, have modified the traditional approach of depending on physical examination alone to triage hemodynamically stable blunt trauma patients.[12-23]

The optimal method of triage of a blunt trauma patient is determined by hemodynamic stability, physical examination results, local familiarity, and clinical expertise with the multiple diagnostic modalities, including DPL, sonography, CT, and laparoscopy. At our level I trauma center hemodynamically unstable patients are initially evaluated by sonography or DPL for the presence of free intraperitoneal blood. A grossly positive DPL as a result of aspiration of 10 ml of blood or evidence of a large amount of free intraperitoneal blood on sonography are indications for celiotomy. CT is the imaging modality of choice in hemodynamically stable patients with abdominal pain, tenderness, or a positive ultrasound examination for free intraperitoneal fluid.

DIAGNOSTIC METHODS
Diagnostic Peritoneal Lavage

In the past, to increase diagnostic accuracy in hemodynamically stable patients, four-quadrant paracentesis of the peritoneal cavity was used as an adjunct to physical examination. This technique, however, was associated with a 36% false-negative rate.[24,25] In 1965 Root et al.[26] described DPL as a highly sensitive diagnostic test to detect blood within the peritoneal cavity. Trauma centers currently use an open, semi-open, or closed technique to perform this test after decompression of the bladder and stomach.[27-33] The entry site is below the umbilicus unless a space of Retzius or preperitoneal hematoma is clinically suspected or encountered during dissection, especially in patients with pelvic fractures.[29,34] If the peritoneal tap is negative or equivocal for aspiration of gross blood, a liter of crystalloid solution is introduced into the peritoneum and the lavage effluent is sent for analysis. All three techniques are used at our trauma center. The closed method uses a Seldinger technique with an infraumbilical puncture with a 21 G needle to enter the peritoneal cavity.[31] A catheter is introduced into the peritoneal cavity over a guide wire after tract dilation. The semi-open technique is performed using an initial incision down to the fascia, and then the Seldinger technique is used.[29] The open technique is performed through a longitudinal incision made down to the peritoneum. A dialysis catheter is introduced into the peritoneal cavity through an incision made under direct inspection of the peritoneal lining. Studies suggest the closed technique is faster, less invasive, and equal in sensitivity and specificity to the open technique.[27,28,35,36] Proponents of the open technique claim insertion of the catheter under direct vision provides a sense of security and ability to visualize an extraperitoneal hematoma tracking along the abdominal wall,[28,35] avoiding insertion of the catheter through a hematoma. Complication rates vary from 0.8% to 1% in large series, and complications include perforation of bowel or bladder, mesenteric injuries, infusion of crystalloids into the abdominal wall (Fig. 6-1) or retroperitoneum, laceration of the ovary, and vascular injuries.[29,37] Relative contraindications for DPL include pregnancy, coagulopathy, and history of multiple abdominal surgeries or peritonitis.

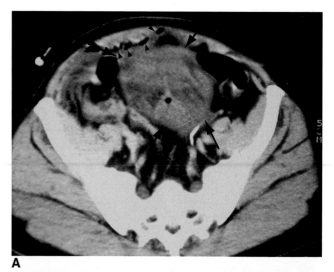

A

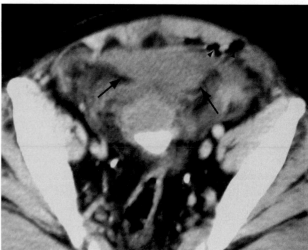

B

Fig. 6-1
Infusion of diagnostic peritoneal lavage (DPL) fluid into anterior abdominal wall. **A** and **B**, CT images show extraperitoneal air (*arrowheads*) and fluid (*arrows*) in preperitoneal space after attempted DPL. No DPL fluid is seen in peritoneal cavity.

Box 6-1 lists criteria for a positive DPL for blunt trauma patients used at the UMSTC. Table 6-1 summarizes the results of DPL from different trauma centers. Most of these studies base their sensitivity, specificity, and accuracy on diagnosing an intraperitoneal injury. Although sensitive to the presence of free intraperitoneal hemorrhage, DPL is not specific regarding the quantity of blood, its site(s) of origin, or the extent of injury. Thus, even relatively minor injuries that could potentially be treated nonsurgically may produce a positive DPL result. Celiotomy on the basis of a positive DPL (>100,000 red blood cells/mm^3) or aspiration of 10 ml of blood from the peritoneal cavity will result in a nontherapeutic celiotomy rate of 3% to 6%.* Nontherapeutic laparotomies

---

*References 4, 6, 8, 26, 38, 39.

Table 6-1
DPL Evaluation in Blunt Abdominal Trauma

Study	No. of Subjects	DPL Technique	Sensitivity (%)	Specificity (%)
Nagy et al.[29]	969	Closed	95	100
Menedez et al.[34]	286	Open	94	99
Velmahos et al.[28]	55	Closed	100	97
Velmahos et al.[28]	75	Open	92	100
Henneman et al.[30]	608	*	87	97
Hawkins et al.[47]	414	Open	96	98
Fabian et al.[5]	91	Open	90	100

*Cannot determine

Box 6-1
Criteria for Positive DPL

1. Aspiration of gross blood
2. Red blood cell count >100,000
3. White blood cell count >500
4. Presence of bile
5. Presence of feces
6. Presence of food material

performed for positive DPL results have been associated with 12% morbidity and 3.5% mortality.[26] This policy may have been appropriate before the era of nonoperative management of solid organ injuries, when the belief was that every injured spleen or liver required hemostasis and repair.[40] The availability of ultrasound, CT, and transcatheter angiographic embolization techniques has relegated the role of DPL to diagnosis of peritoneal hemorrhage in unstable blunt trauma patients or in patients requiring immediate surgical intervention for severe head injuries.[29]

False-positive DPL results can occur from faulty technique, passage of the catheter through an abdominal wall hematoma, leakage of retroperitoneal or pelvic hemorrhage into the abdominal cavity, and incisional bleeding.[5,37,41-43] Pelvic fractures can cause false-positive DPL results in 12% to 28% of patients.[41,42] By using an open technique in patients with pelvic fracture, the possibility of passing the catheter through an anterior abdominal wall hematoma can be avoided by a DPL performed from a supraumbilical position. Using this technique Menedez et al.[34] reported a false-positive rate of 0.7% and sensitivity of 94% for DPL. False-negative DPL results can occur when parenchymal hematomas or lacerations are contained within the capsule of an organ such as the liver or spleen.[44,45] DPL can also be falsely negative in patients with diaphragmatic rupture, especially if the bleeding occurs into the thoracic cavity as

might be expected from a negative intrapleural pressure gradient.[46,47] Freeman and Fischer[46] reported false-negative DPL results in 29.4% (10/34) of patients with diaphragm rupture. In a retrospective review of 50 patients with surgically documented diaphragmatic rupture, 21% (8/38) of patients undergoing DPL had false-negative results.[48] Retroperitoneal injuries such as injuries to the duodenum, pancreas, and kidneys are usually not detected by DPL, unless associated with concomitant intraperitoneal injury.[49-51] A false-negative DPL may also result from extraperitoneal insertion of the lavage catheter (Fig. 6-1) or recovery of an inadequate volume (<600 ml) of peritoneal lavage effluent, leading to low cell counts.[52-54] Overall, DPL has proved falsely negative in 1% to 1.3% of patients with significant abdominal injuries.[47,52]

Bowel injuries may also be missed if DPL is performed within a few hours of injury, as these injuries may bleed minimally, and leukocytosis ($\geq$500 white blood cells/mm^3) requires about 4 to 6 hours to develop within the peritoneal fluid.[5,9,32,46,47] Since the initial report by Perry et al.[55] suggesting that the presence of $\geq$500 white cells/mm^3 in the peritoneal lavage effluent should be a criterion for laparotomy, other studies have also confirmed this criterion.[5,9,56,57] However, a critical review of this criterion by Jacobs et al.[58] described 29 blunt trauma patients with a lavage white blood cell (WBC) count of $\geq$500 /mm,^{3} of whom only four patients had laparotomy. Only one of the four patients actually had a bowel injury. Reviewing the indications for laparotomy and the peritoneal lavage cell counts of 27 patients with intestinal injury in this study, nine patients underwent laparotomy on the basis of clinical examination, the lavage was positive for gross blood in 17 patients, and only one patient had an elevated WBC count. This study concluded that an elevated WBC count in the peritoneal effluent is a nonspecific finding for intestinal injury after blunt abdominal trauma.

A recent study performed by Fang et al.[59] demonstrated that using the DPL "cell count ratio" was 100%

sensitive and 97% specific in diagnosing hollow organ perforation. In this study DPL was performed between 1.5 to 5 hours after injury and the cell count ratio was determined by dividing the ratio of the WBC and red blood cell (RBC) count in the lavage effluent by that of a peripheral blood sample. A cell count ratio of one or greater was considered to predict intestinal perforation.

The value of determining peritoneal lavage enzymes including amylase and alkaline phosphate levels in the lavage fluid is controversial.[9,59-61] Attempts were made to measure lavage enzyme levels to improve on the sensitivity and limitations of DPL cell counts alone for the early diagnosis of hollow visceral injury. Some clinicians advocate routine lavage amylase level determinations,[62] whereas others believe that elevation of the amylase level in an otherwise clear lavage effluent has no predictive value for injury, is not cost-effective, and is not alone an indication for laparotomy.[38] Studies report that a lavage amylase level of 20 IU/L or higher had a sensitivity of 87% and a specificity of 75% in predicting significant abdominal injuries.[60] In a prospective study of 672 patients undergoing DPL, all 12 patients with small bowel injury and three of the four patients with large bowel injury had a lavage alkaline phosphatase level >10 IU/L.[61] This study recommended selective use of the alkaline phosphatase level in the lavage effluent for patients with equivocal DPL results to help to improve diagnostic accuracy for bowel injury.

Sonography

The advantages of using sonography for evaluation of patients with potential abdominal trauma are that it is noninvasive, can be performed at the bedside rapidly during resuscitation, does not involve ionizing radiation, and is an inexpensive method to detect free intraperitoneal fluid when performed by a well-trained sonographer.[63-81] Serial sonographic examinations may also be performed at regular intervals if clinically warranted. Sonography has been recognized as a valuable primary imaging modality in Europe and Asia for more than 20 years but did not gain popularity in the United States for evaluation of trauma patients until the 1990s.[63-81] Historically, most trauma centers in the United States have used DPL and/or CT to diagnose abdominal injuries in acute blunt trauma patients. Now U.S. surgeons and emergency physicians have developed an interest in sonography and have incorporated it as an initial diagnostic screening study in the workup of blunt trauma patients, or as an ancillary study to either CT or DPL.

Most studies on sonography for blunt trauma have used the finding of free intraperitoneal fluid as the sole criterion of abdominal organ injury after blunt torso trauma. The premise for using bedside sonography as an imaging modality to evaluate blunt trauma patients is based on the assumption that clinically significant abdominal injuries are associated with free intraperitoneal fluid or hemoperitoneum. Using this indirect method of predicting organ injury the reported sensitivity and negative predictive value for sonography in detecting free intraperitoneal fluid varies from 78% to 99% and 93% to 99%, respectively.[70-72,75,77,78,82-86] Most trauma centers in the United States are using sonography for screening blunt trauma patients for free fluid and not to evaluate the source of the fluid. The ultrasound findings are categorized as positive, negative, or indeterminate. Very few studies have confirmed the true sensitivity, specificity, and accuracy of sonography to detect free intraperitoneal fluid by comparing the result with a "reference standard" study (laparotomy, DPL, or CT) for the entire study population to verify results.[76,87] Many studies have used clinical improvement or a negative clinical examination to confirm a true negative study for free intraperitoneal fluid. The few studies that have compared sonographic results with CT or DPL report lower sensitivity (63% to 69%) for detecting free intraperitoneal fluid by sonography.[63,88] Table 6-2 summarizes the results of sonography from various trauma centers.

Our experience at the UMSTC with CT for evaluating blunt trauma patients suggests that a high number of significant abdominal organ injuries occur *without* associated hemoperitoneum. Multiple studies performed at the

Table 6-2 Results of FAST from Various Trauma Centers				
Authors	**Method of Confirmation***	**No. of Patients**	**Sensitivity (%)**	**Specificity(%)**
McKenney et al.[78]	CT	899	86	99
Rozycki et al.[114]	Clinical	371	81	99
Yoshii et al.[109]	Clinical	1239	95	95
Bode et al.[86]	Clinical	1671	88	100
Gruessner et al.[83]	DPL	71	84	89
Boulanger et al.[82]	CT or DPL	400	81	97

*Method of confirmation of free intraperitoneal fluid.
Clinical, Clinical examination; *FAST,* focused abdominal sonography for trauma.

UMSTC have shown that from 26% to 34% of patients with visceral injury after blunt trauma demonstrate no free intraperitoneal fluid on admission CT.[89-91] A large retrospective study performed by Shanmuganathan et al.[91] demonstrated 34% (157/467) of visceral injuries including 27% (57/210) of the splenic (Fig. 6-2), 34% (71/206) of the liver (Fig. 6-3), 48% (30/63) of the renal, 11% (4/35) of the mesenteric, and 17% (1/6) of bowel injuries (Fig. 6-4) had no hemoperitoneum on admission CT. Significant injuries needing surgical or angiographic intervention (see Figs. 6-2 and 6-4) were diagnosed in 17% (26/157) of patients without hemoperitoneum or free fluid. Combined abdominal injuries including intraperitoneal visceral or intraperitoneal and extraperitoneal injuries were diagnosed in 18% (29/157) of patients without free fluid. Transcatheter angiographic embolization or laparotomy was needed in 41% (12/29) of patients with combined injuries. The major injury site should be identified in patients with combined injuries to plan prompt appropriate treatment (Figs. 6-5 to 6-7) that may include transcatheter embolization or laparotomy.

A prospective study performed by Ballard et al.[92] to reduce the number of false-negative focused abdominal sonography for trauma (FAST) studies confirmed our finding that sonography does not readily differentiate between concurrent retroperitoneal and intraperitoneal injuries or hemorrhage. FAST was falsely negative in 19% (13/70) of patients with pelvic fractures, including pelvic ring fracture (n=9), acetabular fracture (n=1), and isolated pelvic fracture (n=1). Nonoperative management of

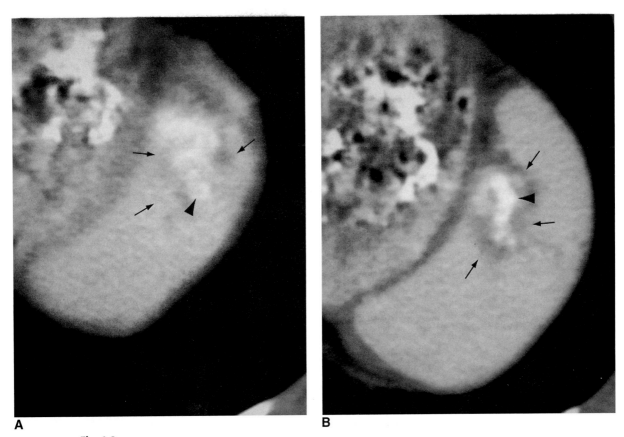

A   **B**

Fig. 6-2
Splenic vascular injury without intraperitoneal fluid in blunt trauma patient who was discharged from hospital after negative sonography and minimal abdominal pain. Patient was readmitted to hospital for persistent left upper quadrant abdominal pain. A multislice helical CT was obtained on readmission. **A** and **B**, CT images obtained in portal venous phase show a well-circumscribed vascular lesion (*arrowhead*) similar in density to contrast seen within splenic artery (not shown) and a grade III splenic laceration (*arrows*). No free fluid is seen around spleen or within the peritoneal cavity.

Continued

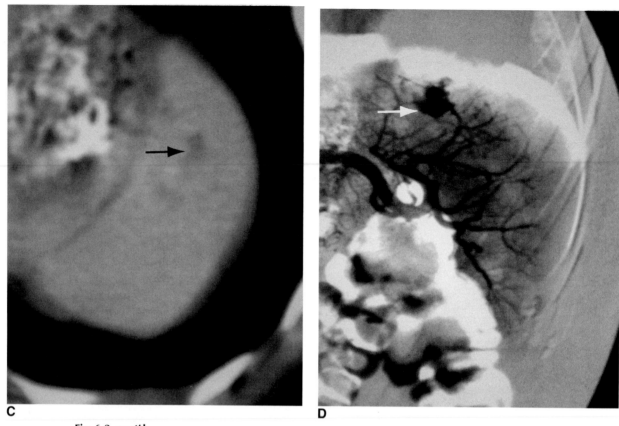

C   D

Fig. 6-2, cont'd
C, Delayed image obtained in the renal excretory phase of a similar anatomic region of the spleen shows complete washout of contrast. Splenic laceration (*arrow*) is seen less well from filling with contrast from periphery. These findings are diagnostic of a splenic pseudoaneurysm. **D,** Selective splenic arteriogram shows a splenic pseudoaneurysm (*arrow*). This vascular lesion was successfully embolized.

solid organ injury was successful in 69% (9/13) of patients, and 31% (4/13) needed surgery. This study concluded that CT is the imaging modality of choice to diagnose all intraperitoneal and retroperitoneal injuries in patients with pelvic ring fractures.

Recent prospective and retrospective studies performed in children and adults at other trauma centers demonstrated a sensitivity for FAST ranging from 47% to 82% and a negative predictive value of 50% to 79% when CT was used to confirm the presence of organ injury and free intraperitoneal fluid.[92-97] These studies concluded that significant numbers of injuries occur without hemoperitoneum, and the absence of free fluid alone is not reliable to exclude blunt intraabdominal injury in stable patients. Brown et al.[97] reported 26% (44/172) of patients with intraperitoneal injuries after blunt trauma had no free fluid. However, the screening ultrasound was positive in 43% (19/44) of these patients as a result of parenchymal abnormalities or small amounts of retroperitoneal fluid. Sonography did not show any abnormalities in the remaining 25 patients. This study recommended routine organ parenchymal evaluation to improve on the high false-negative rate of screening ultra-

sonography. At our institution the high yield of associate injuries seen with patients who have chest injuries (lower rib fractures, pulmonary contusion, pneumothorax, hemothorax), pelvic fractures, hematuria, and thoracolumbar spine fractures has led to a more aggressive diagnostic workup of the abdomen.[89-91]

Studies have attempted to define the role of screening sonography to predict the need for laparotomy by estimating the volume of free intraperitoneal fluid in blunt trauma patients.[73,79,98-100] These studies have taken into account the different locations of free fluid and measured fluid levels in a supine abdomen by devising a scoring system. Huang et al.[73] assessed four areas and gave one point for each location that contained fluid less than 2 mm in depth and an additional point for more than 2 mm fluid depth in Morison's pouch, in the pelvis, and for the presence of "floating bowel." Ninety-six percent (24/25) of patients with ultrasound scores >3 underwent therapeutic laparotomy. To determine the ultrasound hemoperitoneum score, McKenney et al.[79] added the maximum depth of fluid to the number of different locations of free intraperitoneal fluid. One point was given for each location of free fluid (maximum of four areas).

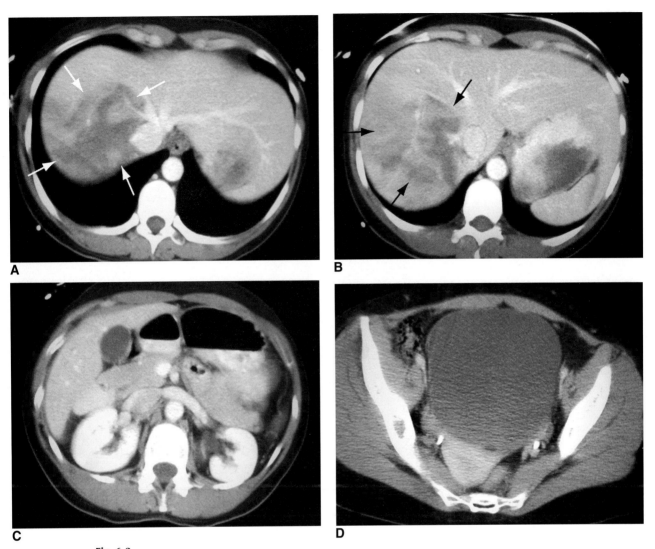

Fig. 6-3
Grade IV liver injury without free intraperitoneal fluid in a patient admitted after motor vehicle collision. **A** and **B**, CT images show grade IV liver lacerations and hematoma (*arrows*) involving "bare area" and posterior segment of right lobe of liver. No free blood is seen around liver or spleen. **C** and **D**, CT images in paracolic region and pelvis show no free intraperitoneal fluid.

In this prospective study the systolic blood pressure, base deficit, and ultrasound scores were all available to the surgical team to make the operative decision. Among the eight patients with systolic blood pressure ≥90 mm Hg and low ultrasound score <3, five therapeutic operations were done. Among patients presenting with systolic blood pressure ≤90 mm Hg and ultrasound scores ≥3 overall sensitivity was 83% and specificity was 85% in predicting need for laparotomy. The sensitivity in predicting need for laparotomy in normotensive patients with ultrasound score ≥3 was 89% (32/36) in this study.

In the setting of trauma, the presence of free intraperitoneal fluid usually indicates hemoperitoneum. A small amount of free fluid is most commonly seen in the hepatorenal fossa or Morison's pouch, the most dependent area in a supine patient.[101] Other common sites for free fluid include the pelvis, perisplenic space, subphrenic space, or paracolic gutters. Free blood is seen as a hypoechoic region within the peritoneal cavity (Fig. 6-8). Fluid may be differentiated from fluid-filled bowel loops by observing for peristalsis. A large amount of blood in the peritoneal space may have echogenic areas representing clotted blood or debris.[76,100] Clotted blood may be isoechoic with parenchyma and may be missed on sonography. Controversy exists concerning the minimum amount of fluid that can be detected by FAST. Branney et al.[102] performed a study to determine the minimum amount of free intraperitoneal fluid that could be detected in Morison's pouch by infusing known volumes of lavage fluid while scanning the hepatorenal fossa.

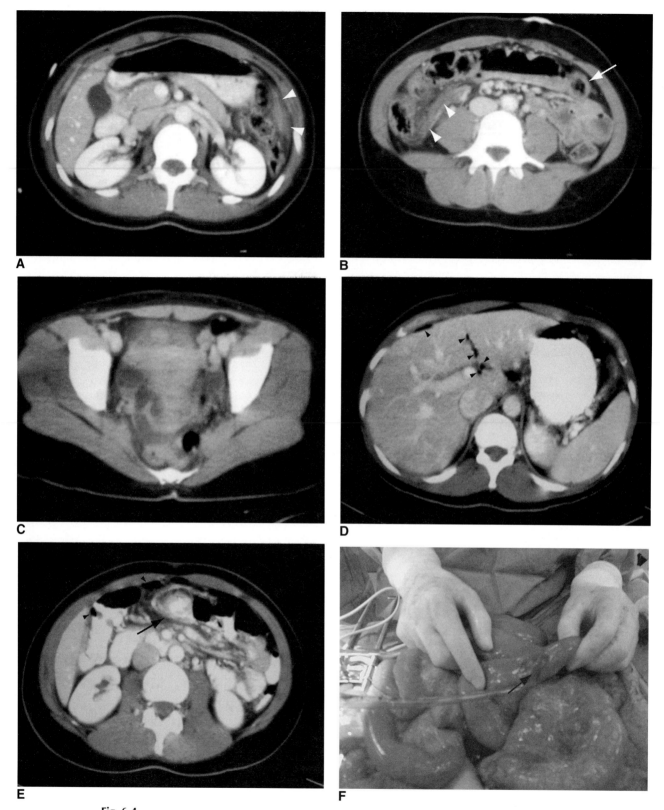

Fig. 6-4
Bowel injury without free intraperitoneal fluid. Admission CT images of upper abdomen (**A**), mid abdomen (**B**), and pelvis (**C**) show infiltration of mesentery (*arrowheads*) and a loop of thick-walled bowel (*arrow*). No free intraperitoneal fluid is seen in peritoneum. **D** and **E**, Images from CT obtained on following day show free intraperitoneal air (*arrowheads*) and bowel wall thickening (*arrow*). **F**, At surgery perforation and contusion (*arrow*) of small bowel was seen.

Only 10% of study participants could detect less than 400 ml. The overall ability to detect fluid in the Morison's pouch increased to 97% when a liter of fluid was infused into the peritoneal cavity. However, studies performed by Paajanen et al.[103] demonstrated that from 10 ml to 50 ml of fluid could be detected adjacent to an injured organ.

Appearances of parenchymal injuries on ultrasound vary greatly and include disorganization of the normal parenchymal architecture, cystic (see Fig. 6-8), mixed (Fig. 6-9), or hyperechoic areas[76,100,104,105] (Fig. 6-10). Among the intraabdominal organs ultrasound has the highest sensitivity for detection of splenic injuries.[76,88,104] The most common parenchymal abnormality seen after blunt splenic trauma is a diffuse heterogeneous parenchyma.[104] With time, splenic injuries are more easily visualized on sonography.[106] A study performed by McGahan et al.[88] to assess the use of sonography in blunt trauma reported that

69% (9/13) of splenic, 14% (1/7) of liver, 25% (1/4) of renal, and no bowel injuries were diagnosed. The study concluded that current sonographic technique is not sensitive enough to diagnose organ injury.

Wong et al.[107] performed a prospective study at the UMSTC to evaluate the ability of sonography to grade blunt liver injuries in 36 patients. The sonography and CT grades of liver injury were compared. A single radiologist performed the ultrasound examination within 24 hours of CT after review of the CT scan. Sonography injury grades were similar to CT in 31% (11) of the 36 patients, undergraded by sonography in 53% (19), and overgraded by sonography in 6% (2). Sonography missed the injury in 11% (4). A prospective study to evaluate the sensitivity and the parenchymal abnormalities seen by sonography in patients with blunt hepatic trauma performed by Richards et al.[108] reported that sonographic

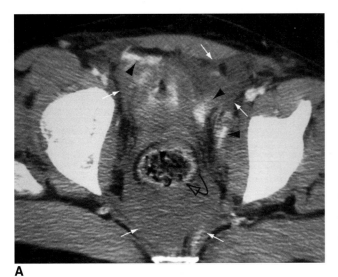

A

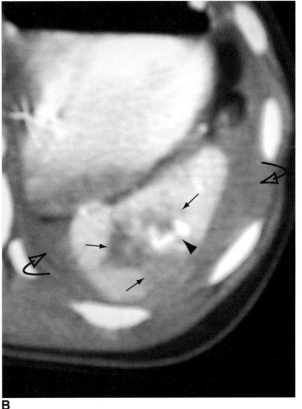

B

Fig. 6-5
Active bleeding in spleen and pelvis in a 22-year-old woman admitted after motor vehicle collision. **A,** Multislice helical CT image shows a moderate size pelvic hematoma (*arrows*) with multiple sites of active bleeding (*arrowheads*). The rectum (*curved arrow*) is displaced anteriorly by presacral hematoma. **B** and **C,** CT images taken of upper abdomen during portal venous phase show a grade IV splenic laceration (*arrow*) with vascular lesion within parenchyma (*black arrowheads*) and peritoneum (*white arrowheads*). Perisplenic clot (*curved arrows*) is also seen. **D** and **E,** CT images of same region in upper abdomen in renal excretory phase show significant increase in amount of active bleeding (*arrowheads*) into peritoneum. Demonstration of profuse ongoing hemorrhage from spleen during CT was helpful in planning splenectomy before pelvic arteriography.

Continued

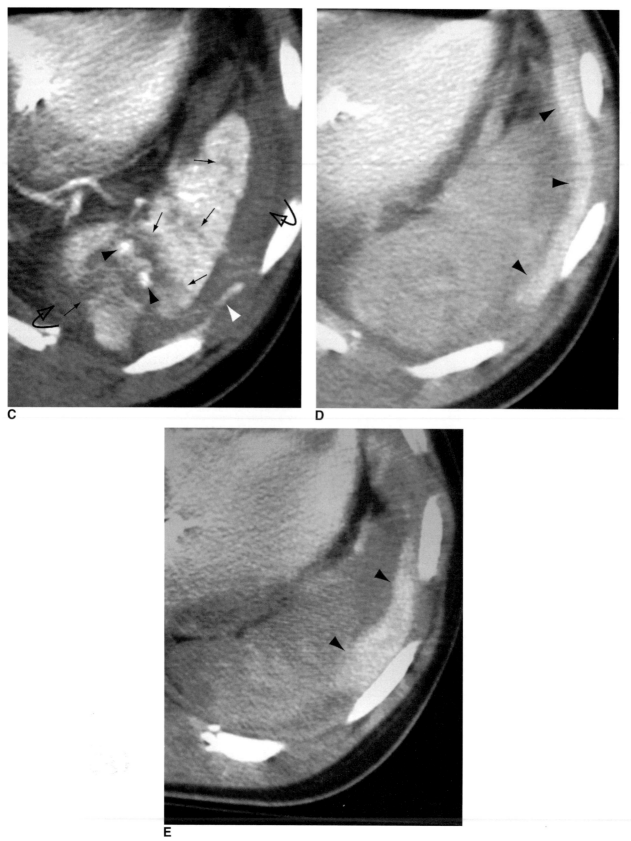

Fig. 6-5, cont'd
For legend see p. 377.

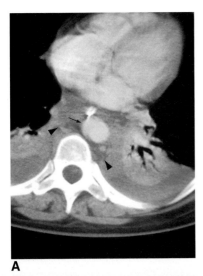

A

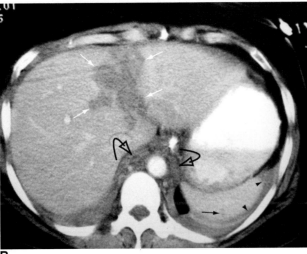

B

Fig. 6-6
Combined injury to aorta, liver, and spleen in a 48-year-old blunt trauma patient. **A,** Helical CT image through lower chest shows an abnormal contour (*arrow*) of the lower thoracic aorta adjacent to diaphragmatic hiatus. Periaortic blood (*arrowheads*) is also seen. **B,** CT image in upper abdomen shows a grade III liver laceration (*white arrows*) and a grade I splenic laceration (*black arrow*). A minimal amount of free fluid (*arrowheads*) is seen adjacent to spleen. Periaortic blood (*curved arrows*) tracks from aortic injury along abdominal aorta. CT shows a small amount of intraperitoneal hemorrhage but no active bleeding from solid organ injury; it was helpful in decision to select conservative management of abdominal injuries. The aortic injury was repaired immediately after CT.

abnormalities in the liver parenchyma were seen in 57% (40/70) of patients with isolated hepatic injury. However, all grades IV and V injuries were detected by sonography. The most common hepatic parenchymal abnormality seen by sonography was discrete or diffuse hyperechoic area(s) within the parenchyma. Low sensitivity was attributed to the large volume of liver parenchyma that

has to be scanned with the rapid FAST technique and the subtle parenchymal architectural and echo pattern changes that are difficult to detect by this technique. These two studies demonstrate the limited utility of sonography as the sole imaging modality to evaluate blunt trauma patients for liver injury.

Further limitations of sonography for blunt trauma include its rapid performance under suboptimal conditions, strong operator-dependence with reliance on training and experience, and the need for a thorough understanding of the equipment. FAST does not evaluate the retroperitoneum nor generally identify the intraperitoneal source(s) of hemorrhage.[109] Screening sonography performed by Yoshii et al.[109] evaluated six regions for free fluid in the abdomen and individual organs, including the liver, spleen, kidney, pancreas, and bowel, for injury. Sonography showed high sensitivity and specificity for solid organ injury. The overall sensitivity of sonography in detecting gastrointestinal injuries was 35%, with an even lower sensitivity (18%) for small bowel injuries. Small bowel perforation in 22% (11/49) of patients was not detected by FAST. Fifty-two percent (10/19) of false-negative sonographic examinations included bowel injury without free fluid detected by sonography. In an era of increasing nonoperative management of solid organ injuries it is *imperative* to diagnose patients with bowel and mesenteric injuries to optimize the success rate of nonsurgical solid organ injury management.[110-112]

Other potential limitations of sonography include its inability to distinguish hemorrhage in the retroperitoneum and intraperitoneal compartment that may result in incorrect patient triage to surgery or angiography.[89-91] Cystic lesions on the surface of solid organs or pelvic adnexa may mimic free fluid. Fat between the kidney and liver may mimic free intraperitoneal fluid in Morison's pouch. The optimal time to perform a repeat sonogram has not been determined. If repeat examinations need to be performed at regular intervals, requiring hospital admission for further observation and repeat FAST examination, this approach would significantly escalate the cost of sonographic screening of stable blunt trauma patients.

Considerable controversy exists in the United States as to what constitutes "adequate training" to be credentialed for FAST performed by nonradiologists.[113-117] In Asia and Europe ultrasound training is part of the surgery residency, is required for board certification, and includes theory, practical instructions, and 400 examinations performed under direct supervision.[117] An international consensus conference held by a panel of experts in trauma ultrasound recommended that the minimum training requirement to learn FAST is 4 hours each of theory and practical instruction with a minimum of 200 supervised patient examinations.[117]

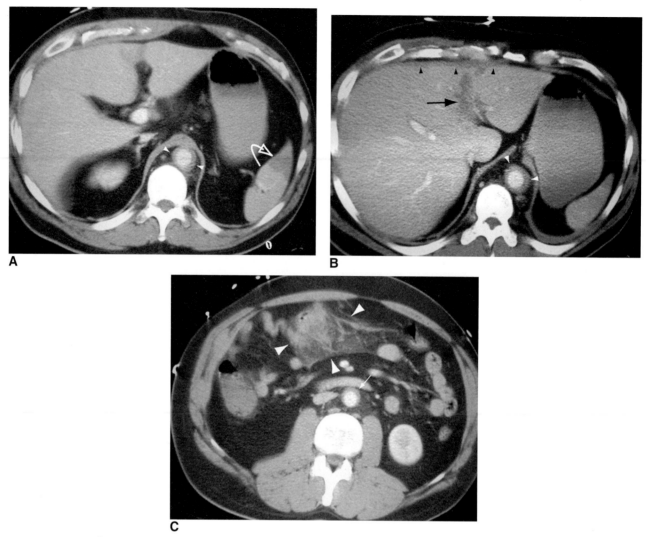

Fig. 6-7
Combined solid organ and mesenteric injury in a blunt trauma patient with traumatic aortic injury. **A** and **B**, Multislice helical CT image shows a well-demarcated, low-attenuation area (*curved arrow*) in the anterior spleen, compatible with an infarct. Liver laceration (*arrow*) and a small subcapsular liver hematoma (*black arrowheads*) are also seen. Aortic wall thickening (*white arrowheads*) is seen from blood tracking along aorta secondary to traumatic aortic injury (not shown). No free intraperitoneal fluid is seen. **C**, CT image shows a mesenteric contusion (*arrowheads*) without bowel wall thickening. Aortic wall thickening (*arrow*) without free fluid is also seen. Conservative management of abdominal injuries was successful.

At the UMSTC the FAST study is performed in the admitting area during initial evaluation by a trauma surgeon using a 3.5 or 5.0 MHz probe to detect free intraperitoneal fluid. Overhead lights are eliminated during the examination. The hepatorenal fossa (Morison's pouch) and right subphrenic space, left upper quadrant with attention to left subphrenic space and splenorenal recess, and pelvis with attention to rectovesicle pouch in males and pouch of Douglas in females are visualized to detect free fluid. If free intraperitoneal fluid is identified in any of these regions, FAST is considered positive, and negative if no free fluid is found. The study is considered

indeterminate if the sonographer cannot definitely judge the results as negative or positive. Indeterminate studies may result from inadequate examination as a result of morbid obesity, soft tissue emphysema, bowel gas obscuring an acoustic window, poorly distended bladder making it difficult to evaluate the pelvis, or extensive soft tissue injury making it difficult to obtain an optimal view.

In our opinion FAST should replace DPL to rapidly triage blunt trauma patients with unstable vital signs and examine the peritoneal cavity as a site of major hemorrhage to expedite exploratory laparotomy. CT should

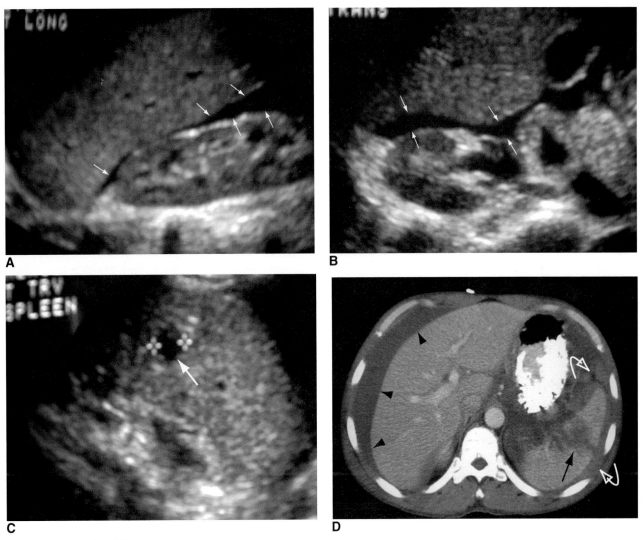

Fig. 6-8
Free intraperitoneal blood on sonography. Longitudinal (**A**) and transverse (**B**) ultrasound images in Morison's pouch show hypoechoic blood (*arrows*) between liver and kidney. **C**, Longitudinal ultrasound image of spleen shows a hypoechoic splenic laceration (*arrow*). **D**, CT image shows a grade IV splenic laceration (*arrow*), a moderate amount of perihepatic free blood (*arrowheads*), and perisplenic clot (*curved arrows*). Transcatheter splenic embolization was performed to control hemorrhage.

evaluate hemodynamically stable patients with multisystem blunt trauma who are admitted to a trauma center with CT in close proximity to the admitting area.

Computed Tomography (CT)

CT has become the imaging modality of choice, replacing abdominal radiography, nuclear medicine, and intravenous pyelography since the early 1980s and DPL in the 1990s in evaluating hemodynamically stable patients after blunt trauma.* All level I trauma centers in the United

States have a CT scanner available to scan trauma patients immediately on arrival. CT is comparable in accuracy to DPL for diagnosing intraperitoneal visceral injury, but is noninvasive, able to survey both the intraperitoneal and retroperitoneal viscera for injury. CT can help to prioritize optimal management by diagnosing the major or most life-threatening site of hemorrhage or injury. Level I trauma centers admit up to 89% of their admissions with low injury severity scores (<4).[131] These patients with minor injury may account for 52% of the direct medical expenditures for trauma care because of the current standard practice of hospitalization of trauma patients with minor injury for observation[131,132] A negative CT after blunt trauma can reliably exclude a significant injury that

*References 4, 5, 16, 39, 40, 43, 118-130.

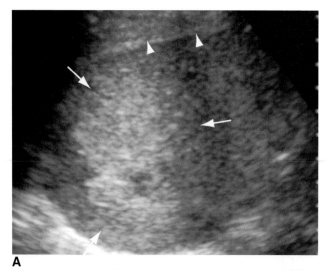

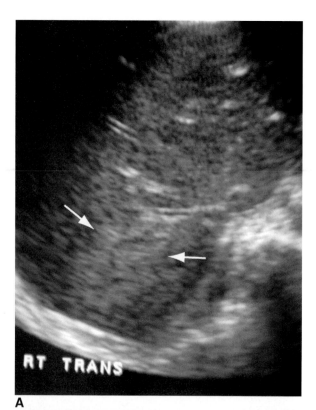

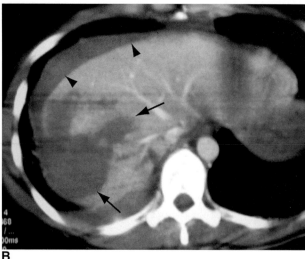

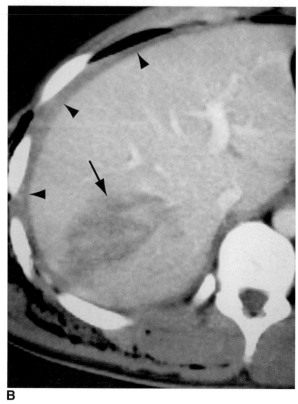

Fig. 6-9

Mixed echogenic liver injury on sonography. **A**, Transverse ultrasound image through right lobe of liver shows a predominantly hyperechoic right lobe liver laceration (*arrows*) with a small central hypoechoic area. Hyperechoic clotted blood (*white arrowheads*) is also seen anterior to liver. **B**, CT image obtained before sonography confirms a grade IV liver laceration (*arrows*) and mixed density blood (*arrowheads*) along the convexity of right lobe.

may require surgery and enable discharge of the patient from the hospital without further observation.[122] Use of CT to triage these patients with minor injuries would help reduce the cost of hospitalization and labor-intensive observation. A prospective multiinstitutional study performed by Livingston et al.[122] determined the negative predictive value of CT to identify blunt trauma patients who may be safely discharged without observation or hospitalization. CT was obtained in 2299 patients, was negative in 1809 patients and positive for organ injury in 389 patients. Nine celiotomies, including six therapeutic, two nontherapeutic, and one negative celiotomy, were performed in patients with negative CT. Based on the prelim-

Fig. 6-10

Hyperechoic liver laceration. **A**, Transverse ultrasound image through right lobe of liver shows a hyperechoic laceration (*arrows*). **B**, CT image shows a grade III posterior right lobe liver laceration (*arrow*) and small amount of perihepatic blood (*arrowheads*).

inary readings of CT scans, CT had a 99.63% negative predictive value defined by the need for surgery. The high negative predictive value of CT indicated hospital admission or observation is not necessary for blunt trauma patients with negative abdominal CT.

The advances that have occurred in CT technology since the early 1980s—with progression from fast conventional CT to single-slice helical CT and to currently available multislice spiral CT—have reduced scanning and image reconstruction time. The ability to scan with thinner collimation has improved image resolution and decreased partial volume and motion artifacts. These factors have helped significantly in providing rapid access to optimum quality images required for triaging blunt trauma patients in a busy trauma center. The accuracy of CT diagnosis of abdominal injury is determined by the experience of the radiologist interpreting the study combined with optimal technical quality and use of oral and intravenous contrast opacification. At the UMSTC we use a multislice spiral CT adjacent to the patient admitting area with facilities for intensive care monitoring and resuscitation equipment provided in the CT suite.

CT scans are obtained from the lower chest to the symphysis pubis after administration of intravenous contrast material unless there is a known history of major allergic reaction to contrast material or renal insufficiency. The value of routine administration of oral contrast material to opacify bowel for CT evaluation of blunt abdominal trauma remains controversial in trauma centers in the United States.[133-138] Proponents for administration of oral material believe bowel opacification is necessary for optimal interpretation of the CT, increasing conspicuity of free intraperitoneal fluid, intramesenteric fluid, and bowel and mesenteric injuries (Fig. 6-11). Oral contrast material may be administered safely without aspiration of the contrast material and does not delay the patient workup.[133,137,138] Federle et al.[137,138] performed a retrospective study of 510 consecutive blunt trauma patients evaluated with abdominal CT with both oral and intravenous contrast material for potential risk of aspiration pneumonitis. Patients were administered a 2.5% solution of diatrizoate meglumine and sodium orally if awake or by means of a nasogastric tube after intubation if obtunded or uncooperative. None of the 510 patients developed an aspiration pneumonitis as a result of the oral contrast material. Nastanski et al.[133] reported similar results in a study of 1173 abdominal CT examinations performed immediately after administration of oral contrast material. Aspiration pneumonia developed in only one patient after administration of oral contrast material.

Opponents of routine use of oral contrast material in the blunt trauma setting believe that administration of oral contrast may delay obtaining the CT study, may increase the risk of oral contrast aspiration in obtunded

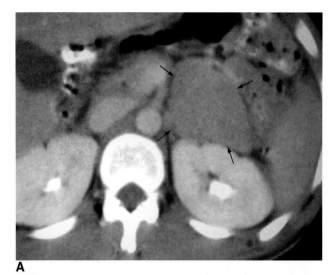

A

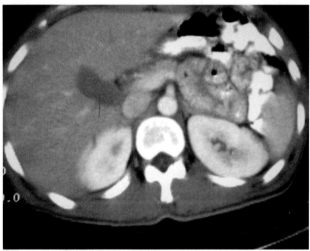

B

Fig. 6-11
Value of administration of oral contrast material in a patient admitted after blunt trauma. **A,** CT image shows a high-density area (*arrows*) in the left abdomen that may represent a moderate size mesenteric or peripancreatic hematoma. **B,** Follow-up CT obtained 4 hours after initial CT shows high-density lesion represents unopacified bowel loops (these bowel loops are filled with oral contrast material), not a hematoma.

patients, and does not improve or accelerate the CT diagnosis of bowel injury.[134,136] At our institution, oral contrast material is routinely administered before abdominal CT.

The CT parameters used at our institution for conventional, helical, and multislice spiral CT and for administration of intravenous contrast material are shown in Table 6-3. A total volume of 600 ml of 2% sodium diatrizoate (Hypaque sodium, Nycomed Inc., Princeton, NJ) oral contrast material is administered orally or per nasogastric tube 30 minutes and immediately before the scan. Patients who require urgent CT on arrival to the

Table 6-3
CT Parameters for Conventional, Helical, and Multislice Spiral CT

	Volume of IV Contrast (ml)	Delay (sec)	Injection Rate (ml/sec)	Collimation Speed	Table (mm)	Pitch
Conventional CT	150	20	1.5	10	—	—
Single-slice spiral CT	150	60	3	8	8	1
Multislice spiral CT	150	70	3	2.5 × (4)	10	1

admitting area may be scanned immediately after administration of one dose of oral contrast material. This usually permits opacification of the stomach and proximal small bowel. Delayed images are obtained routinely about 2 to 3 minutes after injection of intravenous contrast material to evaluate the renal collecting system for injuries. Rectal contrast is not routinely used to study blunt trauma patients.

CT Findings

Active Bleeding, Hemoperitoneum, and Free Fluid. CT is extremely sensitive in detecting even small quantities of intraperitoneal fluid or hemoperitoneum.[126] Small amounts of blood or free fluid are usually seen in the most gravity-dependent portions of the peritoneal cavity. In the supine position the most dependent region of the peritoneal cavity is the hepatorenal fossa (Morison's pouch) (Fig. 6-12). Other areas where free fluid or blood is often seen include the pelvis adjacent to the bladder (Fig. 6-13), paracolic gutters (Fig. 6-14), and perihepatic and perisplenic spaces. Careful inspection of these areas is necessary to identify small quantities of fluid or blood that may be the only CT sign of peritoneal violation and a subtle or occult intraperitoneal visceral injury.

By using density measurements of intraperitoneal fluid, CT can help distinguish between free fluid, blood, hematoma, bile, and active bleeding (see Figs. 6-12 to 6-14).* Hematomas or clotted blood are often seen adjacent to the site of injury. Orwig and Federle[140] demonstrated that the highest density blood among several areas of intraperitoneal blood is adjacent to the injured organ, a concept they referred to as the "sentinel clot" sign (Figs. 6-15 to 6-17). The sentinel clot sign was the only finding indicating the source of hemorrhage in 14% of 120 blunt trauma patients. On contrast-enhanced CT, free intraperitoneal fluid usually measures between 0 and 15 HU, free blood between 20 and 40 HU, clotted blood or hematoma between 40 and 70 HU, and active bleeding measures within 10 HU of the density of vascular contrast material seen within an adjacent major artery.[129,139] The significant difference in the attenuation value of extravasated contrast material (range, 85 to

350 HU; mean, 132 HU) and hematoma (range, 40 to 70 HU; mean, 51 HU) is helpful in differentiating active bleeding from clotted blood.[130] This attenuation difference between clotted blood and active bleeding may often be appreciated on inspection, with no need for measuring attenuation values using a region of interest (ROI) (Figs. 6-17 and 6-18).

The extended scanning range permitted by multislice spiral CT during various phases of contrast enhancement (arterial, portal venous, and excretory) helps demonstrate active hemorrhage during the scan as compared to single-slice spiral CT. On multislice CT, active hemorrhage may be seen as an increase in the amount of intravenous

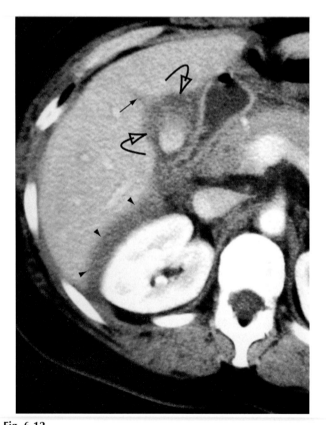

Fig. 6-12
Fluid in hepatorenal fossa. CT image shows small amount of fluid in Morison's pouch (*arrowheads*) and pericholecystic (*curved arrows*) region. A liver laceration (*arrow*) is seen extending into gallbladder fossa.

*References 123, 126, 130, 133, 139, 140.

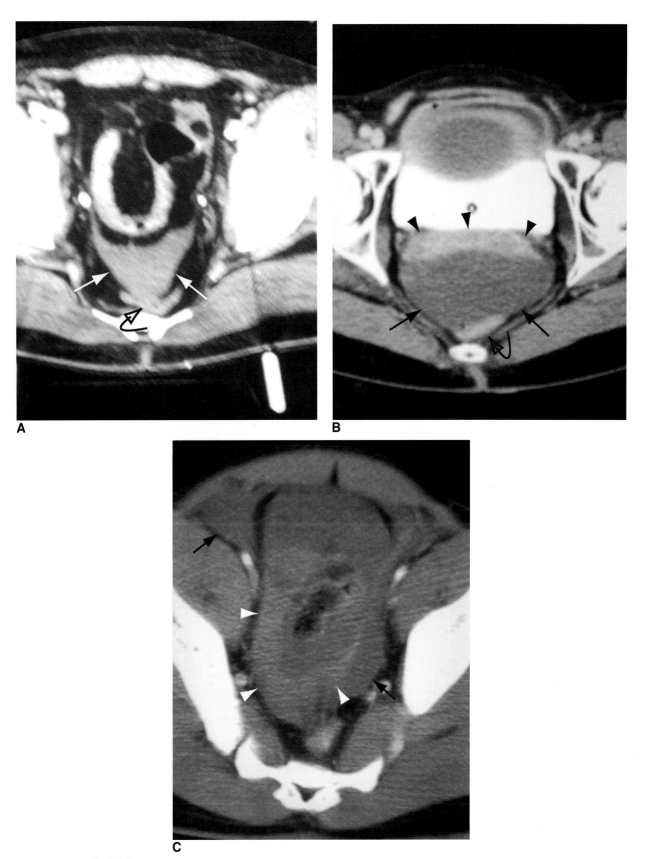

Fig. 6-13
Free blood in pelvis in three patients admitted after blunt trauma. **A**, Small amount of blood (*arrows*) is seen anterior to rectum (*curved arrow*). Unlike a extraperitoneal hematoma that displaces rectum anteriorly (compare to Fig. 6-5, *A* and *B*), free intraperitoneal blood is usually seen anterior to rectum. **B**, CT image shows blood (*arrows*) between seminal vesicles (*arrowheads*) and rectum (*curved arrow*). **C**, CT image shows hematocrit effect; higher density clot (*arrowheads*) is seen in more dependent region of pelvis within lower density nonclotted blood (*arrows*).

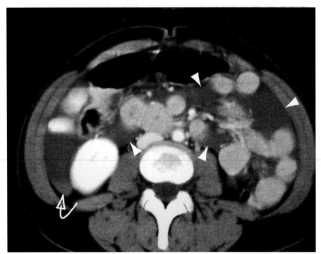

Fig. 6-14
Paracolic blood with hematocrit effect. CT image shows right paracolic blood with a hematocrit effect (*curved arrow*) from contrast and red cells seen in most dependent region. Mesenteric blood (*arrowheads*) is also seen.

contrast material extravasated on images obtained in the identical anatomic region during the early arterial and delayed renal excretion phases of contrast administration (Figs. 6-19, 6-20; see Fig. 6-5). On contrast-enhanced CT scans, blood and fluid are hypodense compared to the parenchyma of solid organs (see Figs. 6-17 to 6-20). Blood appears hyperdense compared to parenchyma on unenhanced CT (Figs. 6-21 and 6-22). Blood or hematoma may appear isodense to suboptimally enhancing parenchyma, making it difficult to diagnose on CT. To avoid this pitfall and optimize diagnosis of small quantities of intraperitoneal fluid and blood, it is important to scan during peak parenchymal enhancement after administration of an adequate volume and concentration of intravenous contrast material. Administration of gastrointestinal contrast material helps to opacify bowel and to distinguish small quantities of intermesenteric blood, fluid, or hematoma (Fig. 6-23).

Density measurements should be obtained in all fluid collections identified by CT to help characterize its origin. Care should be taken to avoid volume averaging in measuring the density of the fluid. When DPL is performed before CT the lavage fluid can decrease the attenuation value of hemoperitoneum by dilution. This knowledge is required for accurate interpretation of hemoperitoneum. At our institution, whenever DPL is performed before CT, any fluid that measures more than 10 HU is considered to have admixed with blood, oral, or rectal contrast material.[141]

The CT attenuation value of bile is usually below zero because of its high cholesterol content (Fig. 6-24). Intraperitoneal or combined intraperitoneal and extraperitoneal bladder injuries could result in urine leaking into the peritoneal cavity (Fig. 6-25). Unopacified

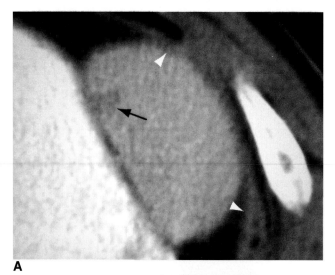

A

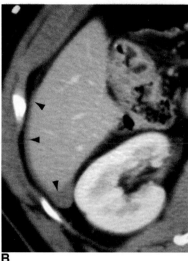

B

Fig. 6-15
Splenic injury with "sentinel clot" sign. **A** and **B**, Multislice helical CT images show a subtle splenic contusion (*arrow*) with minimal amount of high-density perisplenic clot (*white arrowheads*) and less dense perihepatic blood (*black arrowheads*).

urine is usually similar in density to fluid and measures between 0 and 15 HU. However, on delayed images obtained during the excretory phase the density of urine may increase in value as a result of admixing of extravasated urinary contrast material and unopacified urine in the peritoneal cavity, or may be similar in attenuation values to urinary contrast material seen within the bladder.[139]

Isolated Free Intraperitoneal Fluid. Free intraperitoneal fluid identified as the sole CT finding (Fig. 6-26) in blunt abdominal trauma may indicate a significant occult injury. This has been investigated in the trauma literature.[142-148] Studies suggest important factors that should be taken into consideration in planning management of patients with isolated free intraperitoneal fluid on CT

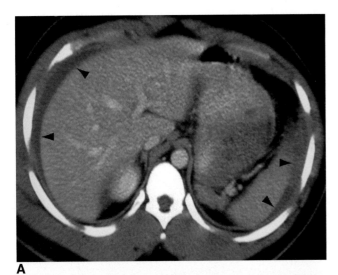

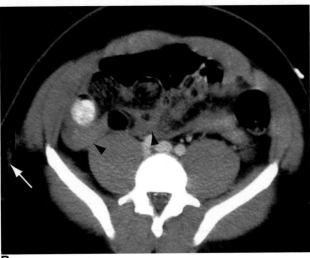

Fig. 6-16
"Sentinel clot" sign in a 24-year-old man involved in a motor vehicle accident. **A**, Multislice helical CT image in upper abdomen shows free intraperitoneal blood (*arrowheads*) around spleen and liver. No solid organ injury was seen. **B**, CT image in lower abdomen shows right paracolic gutter and intermesenteric blood (*arrowheads*). Highest density blood is seen within mesentery (confirmed by attenuation values not shown). Right abdominal wall muscle and subcutaneous fat (*arrow*) contusion is also seen. At surgery a mesenteric injury was repaired. No solid organ injury was seen.

include the quantity and location of the free intraperitoneal fluid, the sex of the patient, the result of physical examination, and the presence of leukocytosis (Fig. 6-27). There is no clear consensus among the various trauma centers how these patients should be managed to identify occult injury.[143,145,147,148] Some studies consider that isolated intraperitoneal fluid represents an occult bowel or mesenteric injury and provides a strong indication for laparotomy.[143-147] Other etiologies for free fluid include previous intraperitoneal fluid not associated with trauma (ascites), occult surface lacerations to solid

organs, intraperitoneal bladder injury (see Fig. 6-25), and decompression or diapedesis of red blood cells from the retroperitoneal space to the peritoneal cavity. Female patients of reproductive age may have a small amount of "physiologic" free fluid in the cul-de-sac related to menstruation (Fig. 6-28).[145,147,148] In a retrospective review by Cunningham et al.[145] of CT scans of 126 patients with injury, isolated free intraperitoneal fluid was found in 25% (31/126) of patients. Those 31 patients underwent laparotomy, and 94% (29/31) were therapeutic. Bowel (n=21) and mesenteric (n=7) injuries were commonly identified. Other injuries seen were intraperitoneal bladder rupture (n=5) and undetected solid organ injury (n=2). Studies performed by Brasel et al.[144] and Levine et al.[147] indicate that an isolated finding of minimal intraperitoneal fluid (one to three images) in the pelvis is generally treated conservatively. Only up to 2% (1/37) of patients with small amount of free fluid required a laparotomy. These two studies concluded patients with moderate to large amounts of isolated free fluid, small amounts of fluid in multiple locations, or intermesenteric fluid require aggressive follow up with DPL or laparotomy.

At our institution, routine follow-up CT is not routinely obtained in asymptomatic female patients with a small amount of isolated free fluid in the pelvis (see Fig. 6-28). Male patients without pelvic fractures who have isolated free intraperitoneal fluid (irrespective of magnitude) (see Fig. 6-13), female patients with moderate or large amounts of pelvic fluid, and free fluid in multiple locations or between the mesenteric leaves (see Fig. 6-26), require further careful observation with serial physical examinations, follow-up CT in 4 to 6 hours, DPL, or laparoscopy to determine the etiology of the fluid. In our opinion it is important for the trauma surgeon and trauma radiologist to discuss the radiologic and clinical findings in these patients on an individual patient basis to plan management better. After consultation at our trauma center, serial physical examination, follow-up CT in 4 to 6 hours (see Figs. 6-26 to 6-28), DPL, or laparoscopy is performed based on the individual circumstances of the patient.

Splenic Injury. The spleen is the most commonly injured solid abdominal organ after blunt trauma. Over a 3-year period 522 patients were admitted to the UMSTC with splenic injury. Associate injuries to the liver occurred in 25% (129) of the patients, to the kidney in 9% (46), and to the pancreas in 3% (16). Only recently has the vital role played by the spleen in the immune defense system been fully appreciated, and this understanding has led to a more conservative approach in the management of splenic injury both in adults and children.[12-15,22,23,149-155] Over the past two decades, CT use of power injection of intravenous contrast material has been shown to be highly accurate (98%) in diagnosing

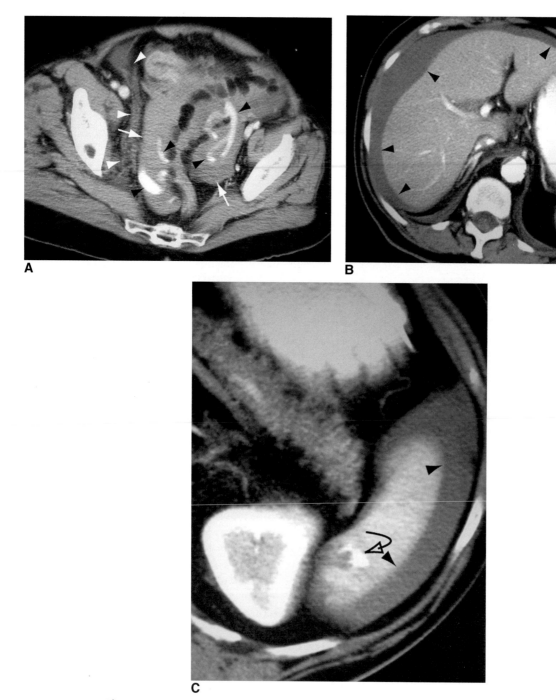

Fig. 6-17
Active bleeding mesenteric injury and pseudoaneurysm of spleen in an adult patient involved in a motor vehicle collision. **A**, Multislice helical CT image in mid pelvis shows multiple areas of active bleeding (*black arrowheads*) similar in density to contrast material seen in iliac vessels. Less dense clotted blood (*arrows*) is seen adjacent to areas of active bleeding. A right pelvic wall hematoma (*white arrowheads*) without active bleeding is seen because of right-sided pelvic fractures (not shown). **B** and **C**, CT images in upper abdomen show hemoperitoneum (*arrowheads*) around liver and spleen lower in density than clotted blood seen within mesentery (**A**). A grade III splenic injury (*arrows*) and an area of high density (*curved arrow*) is seen in splenic parenchyma.

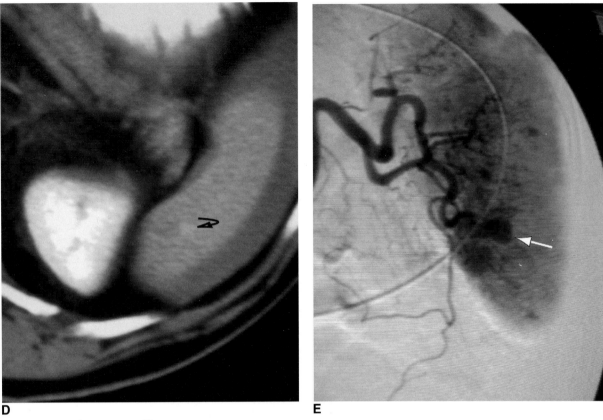

D   **E**

Fig. 6-17, cont'd
D, Excretory phase CT images show washout of high-density area seen within splenic parenchyma, confirming the diagnosis of a splenic vascular lesion. **E,** Selective splenic arteriogram shows a pseudoaneurysm (*arrow*). Patient initially underwent celiotomy, and mesenteric bleeding was stopped. The splenic injury was not bleeding at surgery. Splenic arteriography and transcatheter embolization were performed to salvage splenic function.

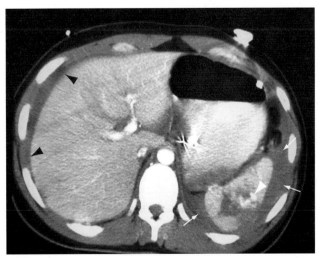

Fig. 6-18
Active bleeding from splenic injury. CT image shows active bleeding (*white arrowhead*) similar in density to vascular contrast material seen within abdominal aorta. Perisplenic clotted blood (*arrows*) and less dense hemoperitoneum (*black arrowheads*) around liver are also seen. Splenectomy was performed for bleeding.

acute spleen injuries. This has had a significant impact in helping to implement a new conservative approach to management of blunt splenic trauma.[16,156-165]

Splenic Anatomy and Function. The spleen is located in the left upper quadrant of the abdomen covered completely by peritoneum. The splenic capsule is 1 to 2 mm thick. The capsule is formed by the external serosal coat derived from the peritoneum and fibroelastic internal coat. The spleen is closely related to the diaphragm on its superior and posterolateral aspect, the left kidney and adrenal gland posteromedially, the stomach medially and anterolaterally, the splenic flexure of the colon on its inferior aspect, and the pancreatic tail medial to its hilum. The spleen receives approximately 5% of cardiac output. Its primary blood supply is from the splenic artery. The splenic artery divides into multiple branches before entering the splenic parenchyma. These branch vessels enter the splenic parenchyma perpendicular to the long axis of the spleen. This arrangement allows segmental resection used to perform splenorrhaphy. A rich

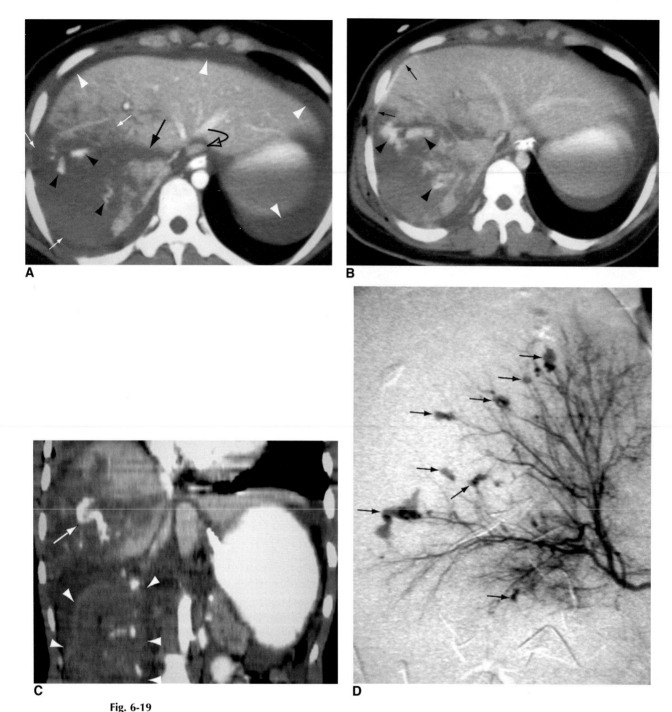

Fig. 6-19

Ongoing hemorrhage from liver seen on multislice helical CT in a 19-year-old woman admitted after blunt trauma. **A**, CT image obtained in portal venous phase shows multiple sites of active bleeding (*black arrowheads*) within a large hepatic hematoma (*white arrows*). The liver laceration (*black arrow*) extends into the region of right hepatic vein and intrahepatic inferior vena cava (*curved arrow*). A large amount of hemoperitoneum (*white arrowheads*) is seen in upper abdomen. **B**, Delayed CT image obtained in same region during renal excretory phase shows increased intra-parenchymal hemorrhage (*arrowheads*). Some of the extravasated intravenous contrast material (*arrows*) is now seen anterior to liver. **C**, Multiplanar reformatted image in coronal plane shows active bleeding (*arrow*) in posterior lobe of liver. Major right renal injury with large retroperitoneal hematoma (*arrowheads*) is seen. **D**, Selective arteriogram of right hepatic artery obtained after laparotomy performed for "damage control" shows multiple sites of hemorrhage (*arrows*). Transcatheter embolization was attempted to control hemorrhage.

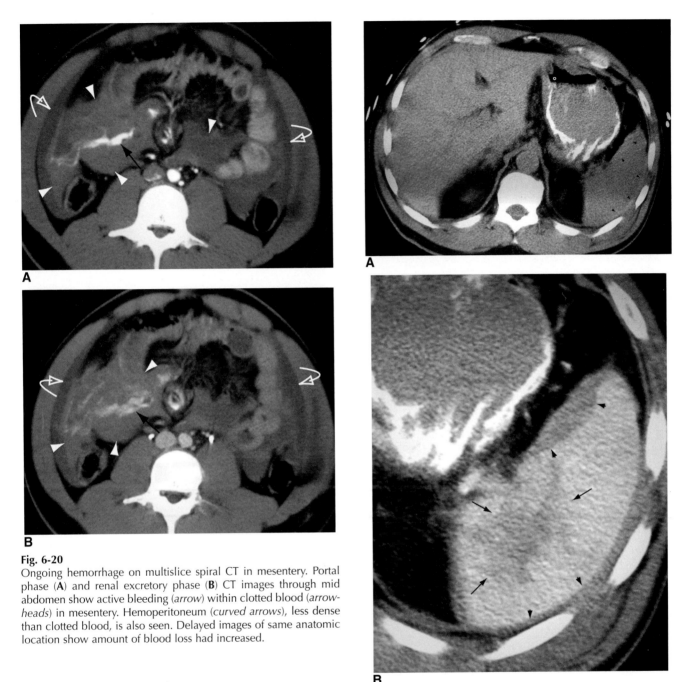

Fig. 6-20
Ongoing hemorrhage on multislice spiral CT in mesentery. Portal phase (**A**) and renal excretory phase (**B**) CT images through mid abdomen show active bleeding (*arrow*) within clotted blood (*arrowheads*) in mesentery. Hemoperitoneum (*curved arrows*), less dense than clotted blood, is also seen. Delayed images of same anatomic location show amount of blood loss had increased.

Fig. 6-21
Appearance of splenic blood on unenhanced and enhanced CT. **A**, Unenhanced CT image shows a small subcapsular hematoma (*arrowheads*) that is hyperdense compared to splenic parenchyma. **B**, Contrast-enhanced CT (CECT) image shows subcapsular hematoma (*arrowheads*) as hypodense compared to enhancing normal splenic parenchyma. Splenic contusion and laceration (*arrows*) are only seen after administration of intravenous contrast material.

collateral circulation of the splenic artery from the left gastric, the gastroepiploic, and pancreatic branches helps to keep the spleen viable after occlusion of the proximal main splenic artery.

The spleen plays a major role in clearing intravascular antigens as the plasma traverses the white pulp coming into contact with lymphocytes and neutrophils.[150] The unique circulation of the spleen with a perfusion of 200 ml of blood per minute, its 25% of the total reticuloendothelial cell mass, and production of IgM and tuftsin are all factors that greatly facilitate removal of poorly opsonic bacteria.[166,167] In asplenic patients, though the liver assumes the reticuloendothelial function of the spleen, it usually cannot provide the environment necessary to clear intravascular antigens, the source for overwhelming postsplenectomy infection (OPSI).

The rationale for splenic preservation by nonoperative management is based on the observation that the spleen

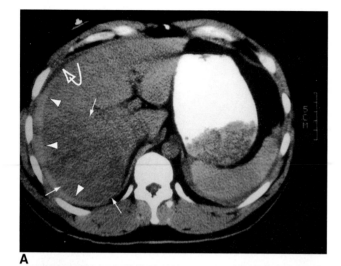

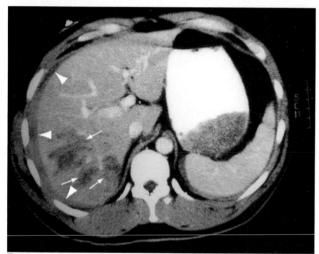

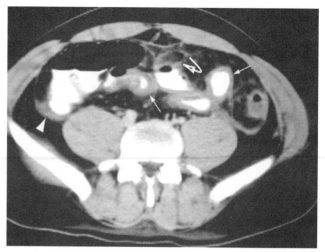

Fig. 6-23
Value of oral contrast material in detecting small quantities of intraperitoneal fluid. CT image shows multiple loops of thick wall small bowel (*arrows*) and mesenteric contusion (*curved arrow*). Small amount of free intraperitoneal fluid (*arrowhead*) is seen posterior to small bowel in right mid abdomen.

Fig. 6-22
Appearance of hepatic blood on unenhanced and enhanced CT. **A,** Unenhanced CT image shows a small subcapsular hematoma (*arrowheads*) that is hyperdense compared to hepatic parenchyma with minimal amount of free intraperitoneal fluid (*curved arrow*). Poorly defined area (*arrows*) in posterior aspect of right lobe of liver may represent contusion, fatty infiltration, or neoplasm. **B,** CECT image shows subcapsular hematoma (*arrowheads*) hypodense compared to enhancing normal hepatic parenchyma. Liver lacerations (*arrows*) are clearly seen after administration of intravenous contrast material. (From Shanmuganathan K, Mirvis SE: *Crit Rev Diagn Imaging* 36:73. 1995.)

plays an important role in removing immunocompetent bacteria from the blood and provides a source of IgM and opsonins that enhance clearance of vascular antigens and bacteria.

Splenic Injury CT Grading Systems. Many systems have been proposed to grade splenic injury after trauma. The splenic injury grades may be based on the extent of injury seen at laparotomy, CT, or autopsy.[128,164,168-172] Lack of consistency of various splenic injury grading systems

have made it difficult to compare outcome and treatment protocols and to standardize reporting of splenic injuries among patients in the same trauma center over a period of time or to compare this information across different centers. To rectify this problem the American Association for the Surgery of Trauma (AAST) formed a committee to develop an injury severity score.[169,173,174] This injury scale (Table 6-4) is based on an anatomic depiction of splenic disruption including the length and number of lacerations, the surface area involved, and the extent of subcapsular or intraparenchymal hematoma(s) seen at laparotomy, among other factors. This surgical classification system is used by most trauma centers in the United States.

Based on the AAST splenic injury scale, investigators have developed various CT classifications of splenic injury to predict outcome of nonoperative management.[128,164,168,172,175] Although contrast-enhanced CT is highly accurate in diagnosing splenic injury, CT grading systems have been generally unreliable in predicting outcome after blunt splenic injury in adults[127,164,175] (Figs. 6-29 to 6-31). In a study performed at our trauma center by Mirvis et al.[128] a CT-based classification system of splenic injury similar to the surgical system in design was applied to 39 patients with isolated splenic injury. Nonoperative management was initially attempted in 61% (24/39) of patients including 10 grade I injuries, five grade II injuries, four grade III injuries, and five grade IV injuries. Nonsurgical management was successful in all five patients with grade IV splenic injury. Among the 13% (5/39) of patients in whom nonoperative management failed as a result of splenic hemorrhage, four patients had a grade I injury classified initially by CT.

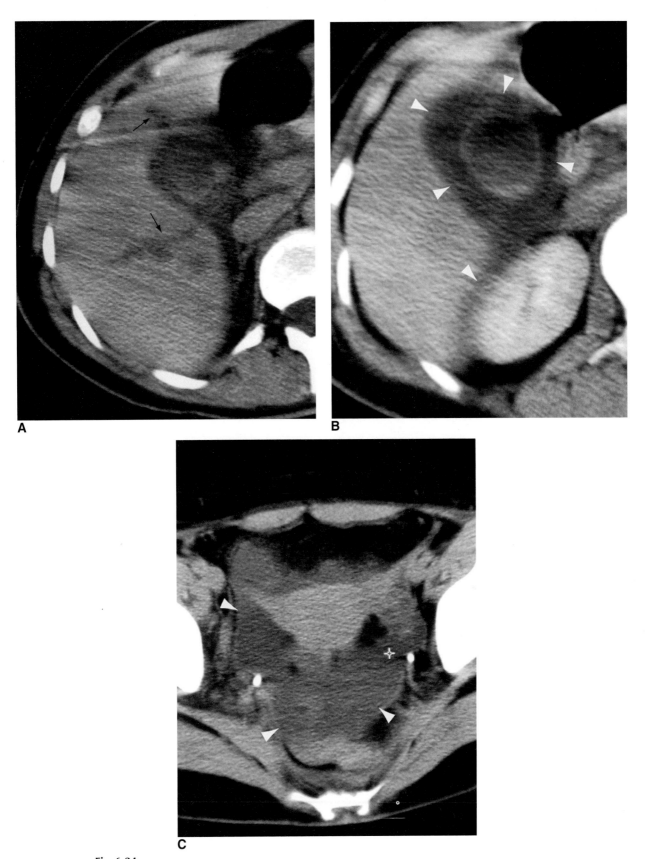

Fig. 6-24
Free intraperitoneal bile from gallbladder injury. **A** to **C**, Conventional CT images show liver lacerations (*arrows*) extending into gallbladder fossa. Low-attenuation free intraperitoneal fluid (*arrowheads*) is seen around gallbladder fossa and in pelvis. Attenuation values of this fluid were below zero, suggesting intraperitoneal bile. At surgery cholecystectomy was performed for gallbladder perforation. (From Shanmuganathan K, Mirvis SE: CT evaluation of the liver with acute blunt trauma, *Crit Rev Diagn Imaging* 36:73, 1995.)

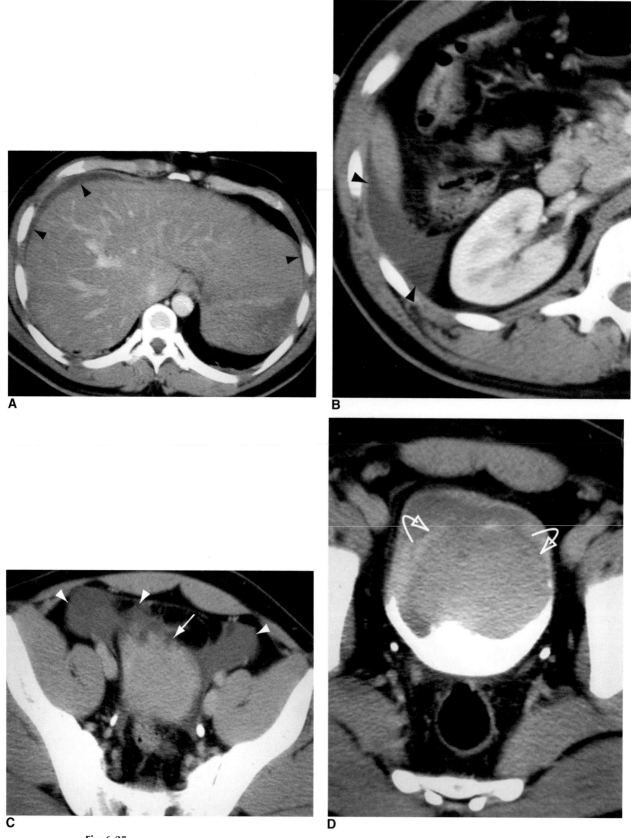

Fig. 6-25
Urine in peritoneal cavity from intraperitoneal bladder rupture in a 33-year-old man admitted after blunt trauma. **A** and **B**, Multislice helical CT images show low-density free intraperitoneal fluid (*arrowheads*) around liver and in right paracolic gutter. **C** and **D**, CT images through pelvis show deformity in dome of the bladder (*arrow*) with blood clot (*curved arrows*) within lumen. Free intraperitoneal fluid (*arrowheads*) more dense than fluid in upper abdomen is seen adjacent to bladder, indicating admixture of opacified and unopacified urine. An intraperitoneal bladder rupture was repaired at surgery.

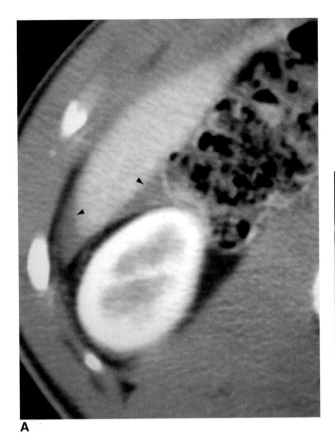

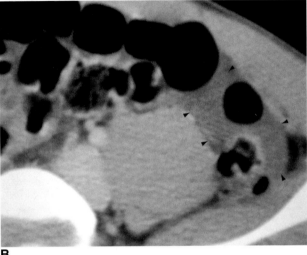

Fig. 6-26
Isolated free intraperitoneal fluid with indeterminate etiology. **A,** CT image shows minimal amount of fluid (*arrowhead*) adjacent to inferior aspect of liver. **B,** CT image shows free intraperitoneal fluid (*arrowheads*) in left iliac fossa between bowel loops. Patient was managed with observation and serial clinical examination. Follow-up CT showed no interval change in amount of free intraperitoneal fluid or other CT findings of bowel injury. Patient was discharged from hospital after second CT examination.

Using a CT-based grading system to predict outcome in 36 patients with splenic injury, Becker et al.[164] reported similar results with failed conservative management in 20% (5/25) of low-grade splenic injuries (grade I or II).

None of the current surgical or CT-based splenic injury grading systems has taken into consideration the importance of some CT findings now typically seen on contrast-enhanced studies, including active splenic bleeding, pseudoaneurysms, or posttraumatic arteriovenous fistulas in grading spleen injury. Recent radiologic and surgical literature suggests that these three CT findings have a high association with failed nonoperative management.* At the UMSTC we use a new CT-based grading system proposed by Mirvis et al. (Table 6-5) that takes these major vascular CT findings into account, in addition to

the extent of anatomic disruption of the spleen, including depth and number of lacerations, subcapsular, or intraparenchymal hematomas, and extent of tissue devitalization seen on CT. Prospective studies are needed to validate the accuracy of this new classification system in predicting outcome of nonsurgical management of blunt splenic injuries.

Nonoperative Management of Blunt Splenic Injury. Pediatric trauma surgeons have managed blunt splenic injury with observation alone since the late 1960s.[180-182] The ability to accurately diagnose splenic injuries using CT, recognition of lifelong susceptibility to infectious complications after splenectomy, the high postoperative complications rates, and the longer hospital stays reported in patients undergoing splenic surgery have been a major impetus to increase splenic salvage.[183-186] Other factors that should be taken into consideration in

---

*References 16, 130, 139, 155, 156, 176-179.

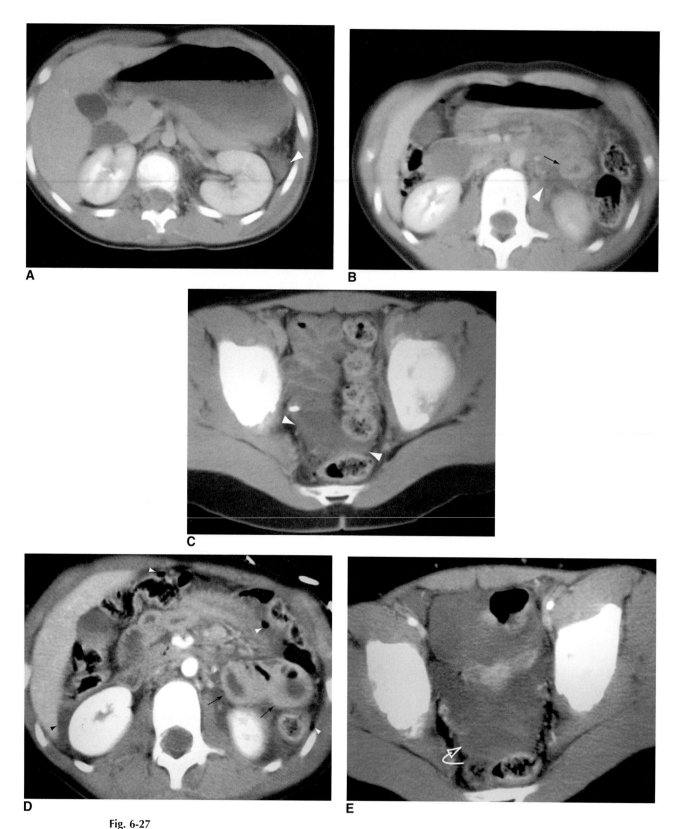

Fig. 6-27
Isolated free intraperitoneal fluid as a result of bowel injury in a 19-year-old woman admitted after blunt trauma. **A** and **B**, Admission CT images show bowel wall thickening (*arrow*) and free intraperitoneal fluid (*arrowheads*) in upper left abdomen and pelvis. No solid organ injury was seen. **C** to **E**, Follow-up CT images show free intraperitoneal air (*white arrowheads*), increase in extent of bowel wall thickening (*arrows*), and pelvic free intraperitoneal fluid (*curved arrow*). New free fluid (*black arrowhead*) is seen in right upper abdomen. At surgery small bowel perforation was repaired.

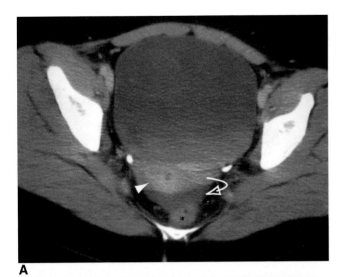

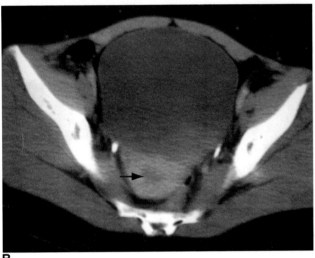

Fig. 6-28
Physiologic fluid in 22-year-old woman admitted after blunt trauma. **A** and **B**, CT images show minimal amount of free intraperitoneal fluid (*curved arrow*) between rectum (*asterisk*) and uterus (*arrowhead*). Some menstrual fluid (*arrow*) is seen within uterine cavity. Patient did not have abdominal pain and was discharged without any further follow-up studies.

making this decision include evidence of ongoing splenic hemorrhage, blood transfusion requirement, possible missed injuries that require surgery, and potential complications associated with nontherapeutic laparotomy.

During much of the last decade splenorrhaphy was the method of choice in adults for splenic salvage.[183,187,188] More recently, attempted nonoperative management is being firmly established as the primary method of splenic salvage in adult patients when other medical considerations permit.* A retrospective multicenter study was performed in 1997 by Peitzman

et al.[197] for the Eastern Association for the Surgery of Trauma (EAST) involving 1,488 adults (age >15 years) with blunt splenic injuries to determine factors that predicted successful outcome by observation alone. Planned observation of splenic injuries was attempted in 63% (913/1448) of blunt splenic injuries. Failed nonoperative management occurred in 11% (97/913) of patients selected for observation. Factors associated with successful outcome in this study included a low splenic injury grade, a small amount of hemoperitoneum, a blood pressure >100 mm Hg, and a near normal hematocrit. Laparotomy was performed in 25% of grade I, 30% of grade II, 51% of grade III, 83% of grade IV, and 99% of grade V splenic injuries. The majority of failures (61%) occurred within 24 hours of admission as a result of hemorrhage. A high failure rate was observed in the patients with grade IV and grade V splenic injuries. Compared with the observation rate of only 13% reported in studies performed in the 1980s, 63% of patients with blunt splenic injuries were observed during this study, demonstrating a major change in approach among trauma surgeons to primarily nonoperative management of blunt splenic injuries.[13,188]

Criteria used to select patients for nonoperative management of splenic injuries described in the literature include hemodynamic stability on admission, grade of splenic injury, amount of hemoperitoneum seen on CT, age <55 years, ability to elicit reliable physical signs on serial physical examination, limited blood transfusion requirements, and exclusion of other injuries that may require laparotomy.* Controversy has been described in the literature regarding the association of failure rates of nonoperative management with grade of splenic injury, patient age, and Glasgow Coma Scale (GCS).[191-194,197-206] Studies performed by Gaunt et al.[200] and Myers et al.[193] evaluating nonoperative management of splenic injuries in all age groups recommended loosening of the traditional criteria, including age >55 as a significant factor predicting failure. In the study of Gaunt et al.,[200] 4% of 100 patients who failed nonoperative management were all <55 years old. A 94% (17/18) success rate for observation of splenic injuries in patients >55 in the study of Myers et al.[193] was similar to that in other age groups. However, other studies dispute these results and have reported high failure rates (30% to 100%) among patients age >55.[192,194,203] A multivariate analysis performed by Bee et al.[192] to identify independent predictors of failure of nonoperative management of splenic injury showed a failure rate of 22% (11/55) in patients >55, even though their splenic injuries were less severe than patients <50, who had only a 6% failure rate of nonoperative management. The failure rate was significantly higher in patients >55 (p=0.0006).

---

*References 13, 22, 23, 157, 162, 189-195

*References 13, 19, 155, 156, 160, 178, 179, 188-193

Table 6-4
AAST Spleen Injury Scale (1994 Revision)

Grade*	Type	Description of Injury
I	Hematoma	Subcapsular, <10% surface area
	Laceration	Capsular tear, <1 cm parenchymal depth
II	Hematoma	Subcapsular, 10% to 50% surface area; Intraparenchymal, <5 cm in diameter
	Laceration	1 to 3 cm parenchymal depth that does not involve a trabecular vessel
III	Hematoma	Subcapsular, >50% surface area or expanding, ruptured subcapsular or parenchymal hematoma
	Laceration	>3 cm parenchymal depth or involving trabecular vessels
IV	Laceration	Laceration involving segmental or hilar vessels producing major devascularization (>25% of spleen)
V	Laceration	Completely shattered spleen
	Vascular	Hilar vascular injury that devascularizes spleen

From Moore EE, Cogbill TH, Jurkovich GH, et al: *J Trauma* 38:323, 1995.
*Advance one grade for multiple injuries, up to grade III.

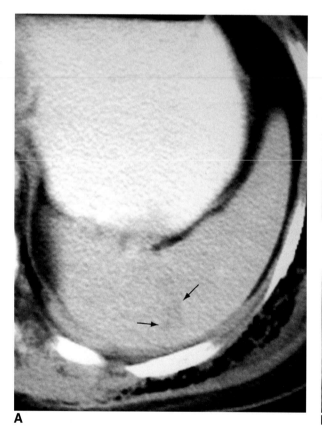 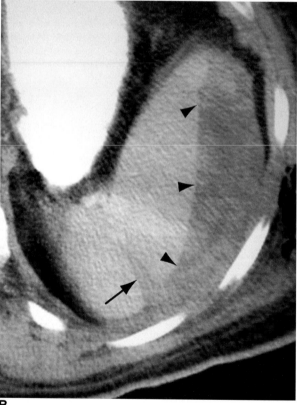

Fig. 6-29
Inability to predict outcome of blunt splenic injury using CT-based splenic injury grading system. **A**, Admission CT image shows a subtle contusion and laceration (*arrows*) in mid spleen (grade II). No free fluid is seen. **B**, Follow-up CT image 3 days postadmission shows progression of splenic injury. A new mixed-density perisplenic hematoma (*arrowheads*) and a laceration (*arrow*) are seen.

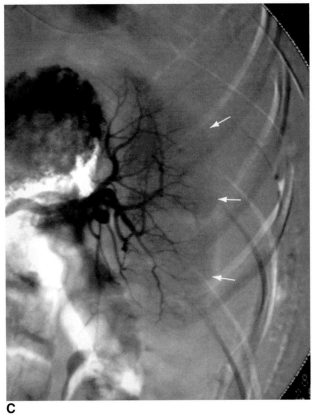

C

Fig. 6-29, cont'd
C, Selective splenic arteriogram shows displacement of spleen (*arrows*) from left lower ribs as a result of a perisplenic hematoma. No angiographic lesion was seen warranting transcatheter embolization. Splenectomy was performed for hemorrhage within 12 hours of angiogram.

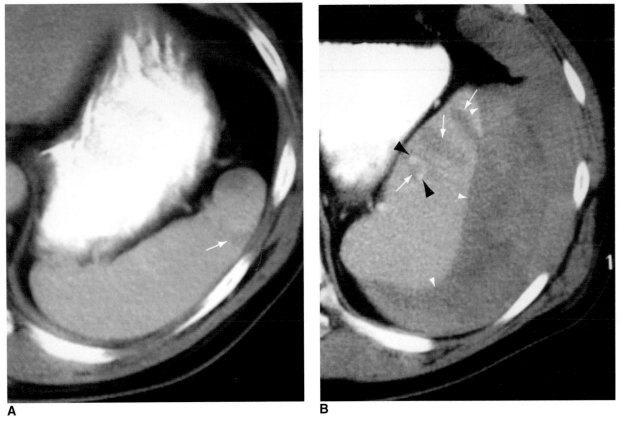

A   **B**

Fig. 6-30
Inability to predict outcome of blunt splenic injury using CT-based splenic injury grading system. **A,** Admission helical CT image shows a subtle grade I anterior splenic contusion (*arrow*) without free intraperitoneal fluid. **B,** Follow-up CT image taken because of fall in hematocrit level 5 days postadmission shows splenic rupture with active bleeding (*black arrowheads*), multiple new lacerations (*arrows*), and mixed-density perisplenic blood (*white arrowheads*).

Continued

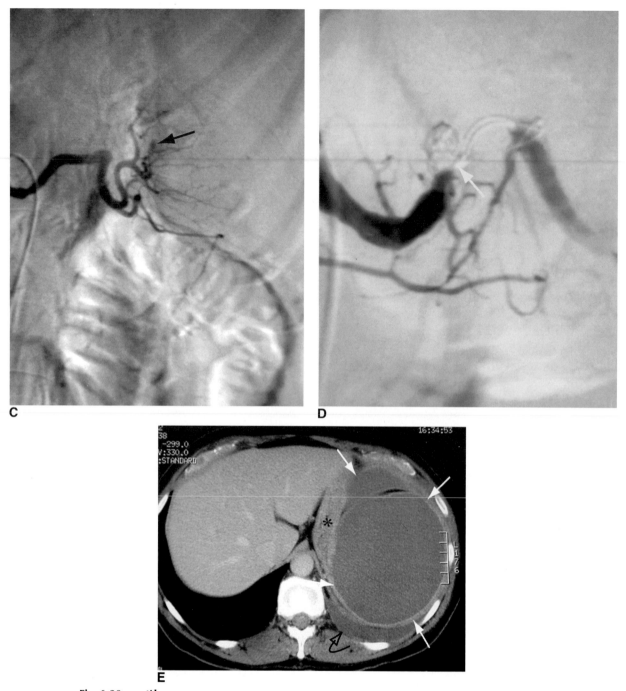

Fig. 6-30, cont'd
C, Splenic arteriogram shows a pseudoaneurysm (*arrow*). **D**, Transcatheter embolization (*arrow*) of main splenic artery was performed to arrest hemorrhage. **E**, CT image taken 2 weeks after splenic embolization because of abdominal distension and anorexia shows a large splenic hematoma (*arrows*) compressing stomach (*asterisk*). A small left sympathetic pleural effusion (*curved arrow*) is also seen. Splenectomy was performed to relieve symptoms.

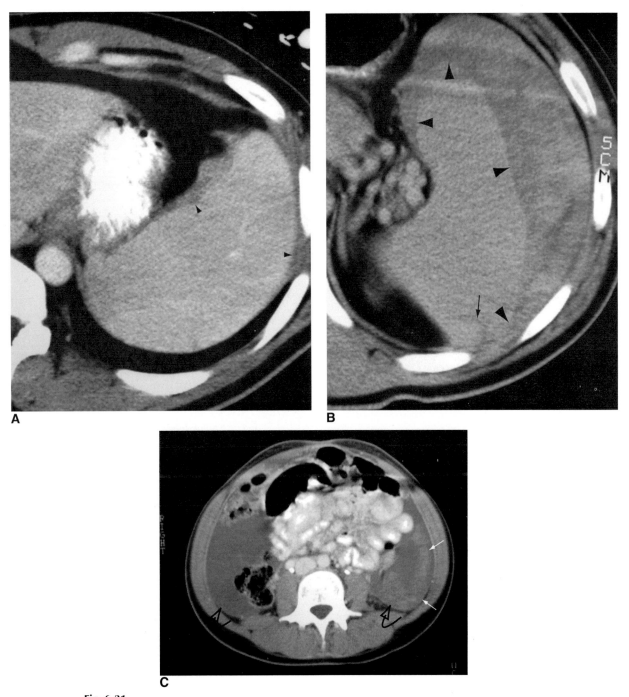

Fig. 6-31
Subcapsular hematoma of spleen in patient admitted after motor vehicle collision. **A**, Admission helical CT image shows minimal amount of perisplenic fluid (*arrowheads*), but no splenic injury is seen. **B** and **C**, Follow-up CT images taken because of transient hypotension show a large mixed-density subcapsular splenic hematoma (*arrowheads*) compressing normal splenic parenchyma. A small posterior laceration (*black arrow*) is also seen. Large amount of hemoperitoneum (*curved arrows*) with clotted blood (*white arrow*) in left paracolic gutter is seen.

The ability to reliably examine patients serially for signs of peritonitis has been considered an important factor in attempting nonoperative management. Concerns regarding the low sensitivity of CT for detection of gastrointestinal injuries, which can result in missed or delayed injuries in neurologically impaired patients, have precluded some trauma centers from considering such patients for conservative management[204] of splenic injury. Transient variation in blood pressure among patients with severe brain injury may also be a concern

Table 6-5
CT-Based Splenic Injury Scale

Grade	Criteria
I	Subcapsular hematoma <1 cm thick
	Laceration <1 cm parenchymal depth
	Parenchymal hematoma <1 cm in diameter
II	Subcapsular hematoma 1-3 cm thick
	Laceration 1-3 cm parenchymal depth
	Parenchymal hematoma 1-3 cm in diameter
III	Splenic capsular disruption
	Subcapsular hematoma >3 cm thick
	Laceration >3 cm parenchymal depth
	Parenchymal hematoma >3 cm in diameter
IV A	Active intraparenchymal and subcapsular splenic bleeding
	Splenic vascular injury (pseudoaneurysm or A-V fistula)
	Shattered spleen (fragmentation into three or more sections)
IV B	Active intraperitoneal splenic bleeding

Grade IV A requires surgery or splenic arteriography and embolization; Grade IV B requires immediate surgery or splenic arteriography and embolization.

for some trauma surgeons. However, recent studies suggest that patients with GCS <13 can be safely managed nonoperatively without high failure rates.[192,199,204]

Patients with high-grade splenic injuries (grades III to V) selected for nonoperative management are significantly more likely to fail than patients with low-grade injuries (grades I to II). However, more recent studies have demonstrated these high-grade splenic injuries can be managed nonoperatively with success rates of 87% to 96%.[156,191]

Sclafani et al.[16,176] and Hagiwara et al.[177] have shown that splenic arteriography can be used to diagnose and embolize traumatic splenic vascular lesions. They reported a 93% to 97% success rate for patients with all grades of blunt splenic injury diagnosed by CT followed by splenic arteriography to embolize splenic vascular injuries. Davis et al.[155] in a retrospective study demonstrated that aggressive pursuit of splenic pseudoaneurysms detected on contrast-enhanced CT with splenic angiography and embolization resulted in an improvement in the success rate of nonoperative management of blunt splenic injuries from 87% to 94%. Embolization of splenic aneurysms was successful in 78% (22/28) of patients during this study. Another prospective study was performed by Shanmuganathan et al.[156] to determine the accuracy of contrast-enhanced helical CT criteria to select patients with all grades of blunt splenic injury for splenic angiography and possible embolization. Nonoperative management was ultimately successful in 94% (73/78) of patients initially selected for conservative treatment.

At our institution, patients with all grades of splenic injury who are hemodynamically stable without CT evidence of surgical bowel or mesenteric injuries, irrespective of their GCS, are selected for initial nonoperative management. In an effort to improve the outcome of nonoperative management, splenic angiography is performed routinely in all patients with high grades of splenic injury (grades III to V) and in any grade of injury with CT evidence of active splenic bleeding, splenic pseudoaneurysm(s), or traumatic arteriovenous fistulas. Failed nonoperative management is defined as patients requiring laparotomy for missed nonsplenic injury or splenectomy or splenorrhaphy for persistent splenic hemorrhage despite embolization.

Computed Tomography Appearances of Splenic Injury. Many previous studies have shown that contrast-enhanced CT can accurately diagnose the four principal types of splenic injury—hematoma(s), laceration(s), active hemorrhage, and vascular injuries, including pseudoaneurysm and posttraumatic arteriovenous fistula.*

Hematomas and laceration. Single or multiple hematomas may be seen after blunt trauma. Splenic hematomas may be intraparenchymal or subcapsular (Figs. 6-31 to 6-33). On unenhanced CT subcapsular

---

*References 1, 3, 18, 19, 156, 178, 179.

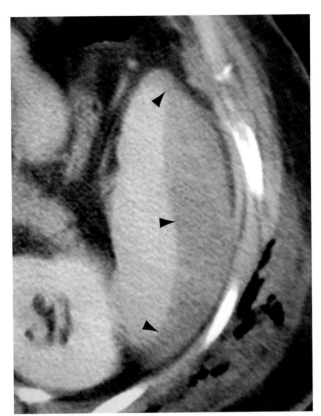

Fig. 6-32
Subcapsular hematoma of spleen of patient admitted after motor vehicle collision. CT shows 3-day-old subacute subcapsular hematoma (*arrowheads*) compressing normal splenic parenchyma.

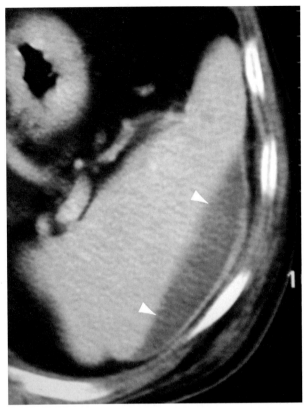

Fig. 6-33
Subcapsular hematoma of spleen of patient admitted after motor vehicle collision. CT shows a chronic low-attenuation subcapsular hematoma (*arrowheads*) with mass effect on normal splenic parenchyma. Compression of normal splenic parenchyma helps to differentiate subcapsular hematoma from free intraperitoneal blood adjacent to spleen.

hematoma is hyperdense relative to normal splenic parenchyma (see Fig. 6-21). Using contrast-enhanced CT, subcapsular hematomas are typically seen as a low-attenuation collection of blood between the splenic capsule and the enhancing splenic parenchyma (see Figs. 6-32 and 6-33). Unless there is recurrent hemorrhage the attenuation value of the subcapsular hematoma usually decreases with the age of the lesion (see Fig. 6-33). Subcapsular hematomas often compress the underlying splenic parenchyma, and this CT finding helps to differentiate subcapsular hematomas from small amounts of blood or fluid in the perisplenic space. Uncomplicated subcapsular hematomas typically resolve within 4 to 6 weeks. On contrast-enhanced CT, acute hematomas appear as irregular high- or low-attenuation areas within the parenchyma (Figs. 6-34 and 6-35). Acute splenic lacerations have sharp or jagged margins and appear as linear or branching low-attenuation areas on contrast-enhanced CT (Figs. 6-36 and 6-37). With time the margins of splenic lacerations and hematomas become less evident, and the lesions decrease in size until the area becomes isodense with normal splenic parenchyma. A peripheral "scar" or irregular margin may form along the contour of the spleen at the site of injury. In our expe-

rience the development of a posttraumatic cyst appears to be extremely uncommon in the normal healing process. Increase in number or extension of the lesion on follow-up CT should raise the possibility of injury progression warranting close clinical follow-up, further follow-up CT, or arteriography. Complete healing in CT appearance may take weeks to months depending usually on the initial size of the injury.

Active hemorrhage. On contrast-enhanced CT active hemorrhage in the spleen is seen as an irregular or linear area of contrast extravasation (Fig. 6-38; see Figs. 6-5 and 6-18,). Active splenic hemorrhage may be seen within the splenic parenchyma (Figs. 6-39 and 6-40), subcapsular space (Figs. 6-41 and 6-42), or intraperitoneally (Figs. 6-43 and 6-44; see Figs. 6-5 and 6-38). The significant difference between the attenuation value of extravasated contrast material (range, 85 to 350 HU; mean, 132 HU) and hematoma (range, 40 to 70 HU; mean, 51 HU) is helpful in differentiating active bleeding from clotted blood.[130] Ongoing hemorrhage on multislice spiral CT

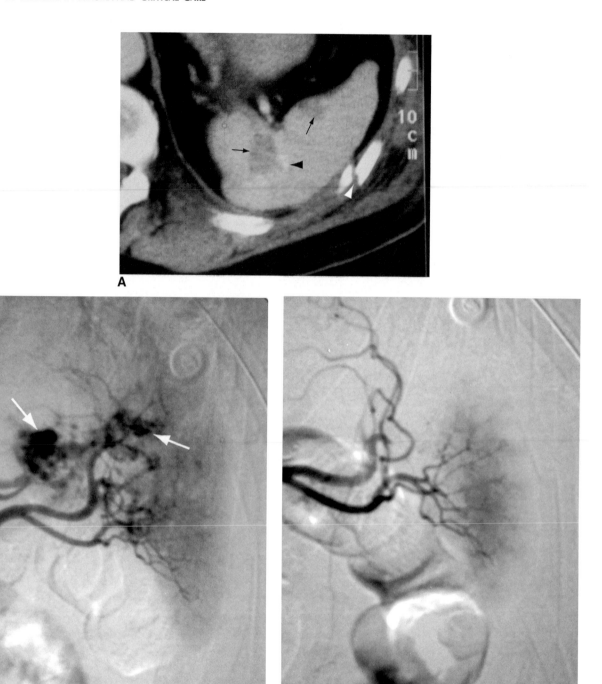

Fig. 6-34
Splenic hematoma in a patient admitted after blunt injury. Helical CT image shows two irregular areas of low-attenuation (*arrows*) hematoma. High-density area (*black arrowhead*) seen in peripheral region of hematoma represents a splenic vascular injury. Minimally displaced left lower rib fracture (*white arrowhead*) is also seen. Preembolization (**B**) and postembolization (**C**) splenic arteriograms show multiple pseudoaneurysms (*arrows*). These pseudoaneurysms were treated with distal transcatheter embolization.

may be seen as an increase in the amount of intravenous contrast material extravasated on images obtained in the identical anatomic region during the arterial and delayed renal excretion phases of contrast administration. The multislice spiral CT finding in our experience has

been helpful to differentiate active bleeding from posttraumatic splenic pseudoaneurysms or arteriovenous fistulas. Usually, posttraumatic vascular injuries are similar in attenuation value to active hemorrhage in the arterial phase but "wash out" in the excretory phase, becoming

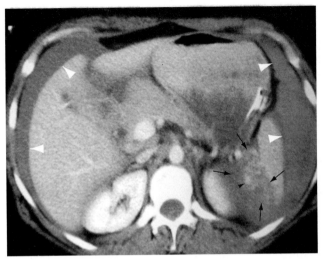

Fig. 6-35
Splenic hematoma with active bleeding in spleen. Helical CT image shows a high-attenuation irregular hematoma (*arrows*) with an area of active bleeding (*black arrowhead*). Large amount of hemoperitoneum (*white arrowheads*) is seen around spleen and liver in upper abdomen.

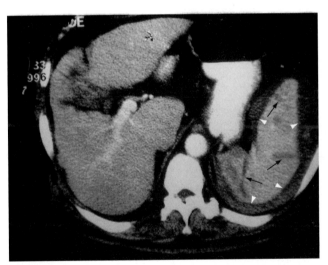

Fig. 6-36
Splenic laceration on CT. Multiple splenic lacerations in a patient admitted after blunt trauma. Helical CT image shows a grade III splenic injury with multiple lacerations (*arrows*) and a small amount of free intraperitoneal blood (*arrowheads*).

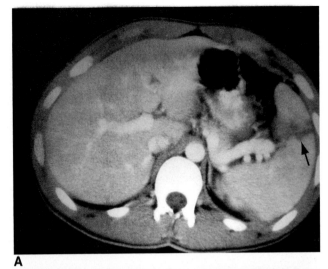

A

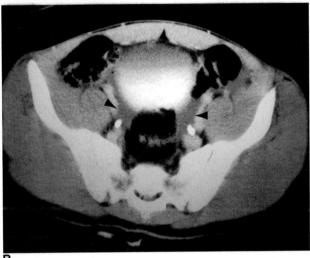

B

Fig. 6-37
Splenic laceration on CT. **A** and **B**, Conventional CT images show a grade III splenic laceration (*arrow*). Although there is no perisplenic blood, a minimal amount of free intraperitoneal blood (*arrowheads*) is seen in pelvis.

minimally hyperdense or isodense compared with normal splenic parenchyma (see Figs. 6-2 and 6-18).

Retrospective studies performed by Federle et al.[178] and Shanmuganathan et al.[130] have reported that demonstration of arterial contrast material extravasation or vascular abnormalities in the spleen seen on contrast-enhanced conventional and single-slice spiral CT have a statistically significant association with splenic hemorrhage at surgery. Among 28 patients diagnosed with active splenic hemorrhage on CT by Federle et al.,[178] 93% (26/28) underwent splenic surgery to control hemorrhage. All five patients with active splenic bleeding diagnosed on conventional CT by Shanmuganathan et al.[130] underwent splenectomy. However, in these two studies splenic angiography was not performed to confirm or treat splenic lesions seen on CT.

A prospective study was performed by Shanmuganathan et al.[156] at the UMSTC to determine accuracy of contrast-enhanced spiral CT criteria to select patients with all grades of blunt splenic injury for splenic angiography and possible endovascular treatment. Technically successful contrast-enhanced multislice spiral CT scans followed by splenic angiography were obtained in 40%

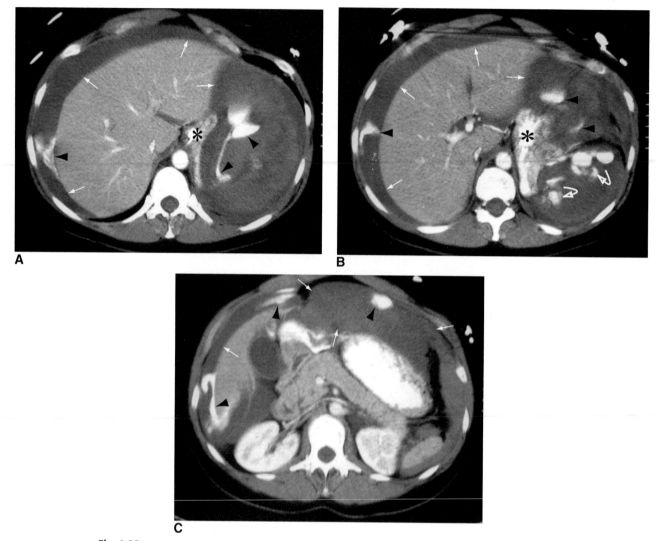

Fig. 6-38
Active intraperitoneal and intraparenchymal contrast material extravasation in a pedestrian struck by motor vehicle. **A** to **C**, Helical CT images show active bleeding into peritoneal cavity (*black arrowheads*) and splenic parenchyma from a grade V splenic injury. Large amount of hemoperitoneum (*arrows*) is seen with compression of stomach (*asterisk*) by perisplenic blood. Splenic parenchyma is not enhancing as a result of lack of perfusion due to profuse hemorrhage. Splenectomy was performed to stop hemorrhage.

(78/195) of patients admitted with blunt splenic injury who were hemodynamically stable and required no immediate surgery. Seven patients had vascular contrast extravasation on admission CT, and six had evidence of bleeding by angiography and were successfully embolized. One patient did not demonstrate splenic hemorrhage or vascular injury by angiography. However, this patient ultimately required a delayed splenectomy for persistent hemorrhage within 12 hours of the splenic angiography, indicating that a splenic arterial injury identified on admission CT may not have been detected by angiography or was not apparent at the time of angiography. In this study splenic vascular contrast extravasation was highly predictive of the need for transcatheter splenic embolization in patients with blunt splenic injury. This significant correlation of CT findings of active splenic hemorrhage and need for angiographic or surgical intervention to treat hemorrhage has led to an aggressive diagnostic and therapeutic pursuit at our institution of splenic vascular injury with multislice contrast-enhanced spiral CT and splenic angiography. Patients with *CT evidence of splenic vascular contrast extravasation without vascular injury on splenic arteriography* undergo prophylactic proximal main splenic artery embolization to prevent delayed splenic

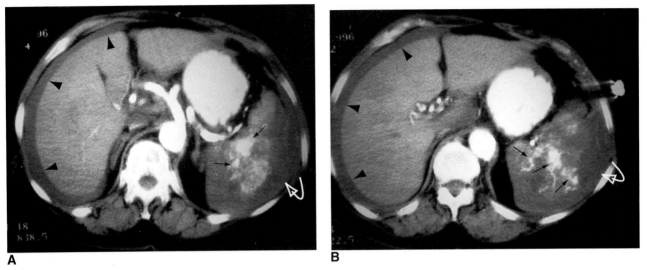

Fig. 6-39
Intraparenchymal active splenic bleeding in a patient admitted after blunt trauma. **A** and **B**, Helical CT images show intraparenchymal active bleeding (*arrows*) similar in density to intravenous contrast material seen within splenic artery. Perisplenic clot (*curved arrow*) and perihepatic hemoperitoneum (*arrowheads*) are also seen. Splenectomy was performed after CT.

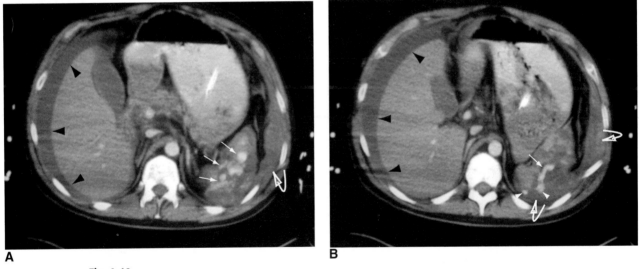

Fig. 6-40
Intraparenchymal and intraperitoneal active splenic bleeding in a 39-year-old woman admitted after motor vehicle collision. **A** and **B**, Helical CT images show both intraparenchymal (*arrows*) and intraperitoneal active bleeding (*white arrowheads*) from spleen. Intraperitoneal active bleeding is seen within perisplenic clot (*curved arrows*). Hemoperitoneum (*black arrowheads*) is seen adjacent to liver.

bleeding (see Fig. 6-44). This approach potentially increases the number of patients with blunt splenic injuries managed successfully without surgery.

Splenic vascular injuries. Posttraumatic pseudoaneurysms usually result from an injury to the arterial wall. The defect in the arterial wall, though small in size, allows blood to escape into the arterial wall or surrounding tissue. The adventitia and the perivascular tissues form the wall of the pseudoaneurysm. The rate of enlargement of the pseudoaneurysm depends not only on the integrity of the adventitial layer of the artery but also on the strength of the surrounding tissues resisting the expansion of the pseudoaneurysm.[207] Splenic arterial pseudoaneurysm may be seen on admission or follow-up CT. The natural progression of splenic pseudoaneurysm is not clearly known. Posttraumatic arteriovenous fistula may develop in the immediate

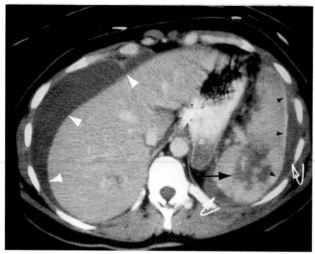

Fig. 6-41
Subcapsular active bleeding in a patient with grade III splenic injury. Helical CT image shows splenic laceration and contusion (*arrow*) with active intravenous contrast material extravasation in subcapsular space (*black arrowheads*). Free intraperitoneal blood (*white arrowheads*) and perisplenic clotted blood (*curved arrows*) is also seen.

posttraumatic period as a result of injury to the wall of both the artery and adjacent vein.[207] Although some splenic pseudoaneurysms heal by spontaneous thrombosis without intervention, recent studies have shown that up to 67% of these lesions may ultimately rupture and therefore represent a strong predictor for failed nonsurgical management.[155,207]

The appearance of posttraumatic splenic pseudoaneurysms (see Fig. 6-45) and arteriovenous fistulas (Figs. 6-46 and 6-47) are similar on contrast-enhanced CT and could only be differentiated using splenic angiography.[156] Both these lesions appear as well-circumscribed focal areas of increased CT density, higher in attenuation than the normal enhanced splenic parenchyma on contrast-enhanced CT.[156,178,179,208] On contrast-enhanced multislice CT (CE-MSCT), posttraumatic splenic vascular lesions (Fig. 6-48; see Fig. 6-2) are seen in the arterial phase as well-circumscribed foci of hyperdensity that measure within 10 HU of the density of an adjacent major artery.[130,139] On images obtained in the delayed

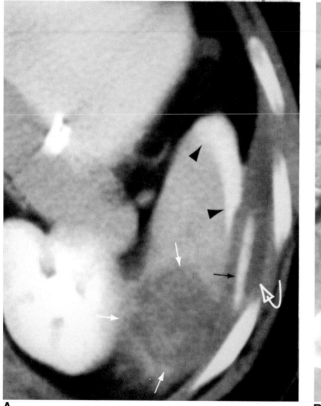

A

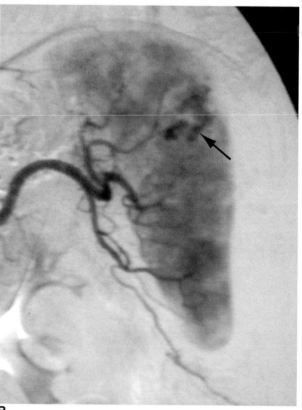

B

Fig. 6-42
Subcapsular and intraperitoneal active bleeding. **A,** Helical CT shows subcapsular (*arrowheads*) and intraperitoneal (*black arrow*) active bleeding seen within perisplenic hematoma (*curved arrow*). A posterior splenic hematoma (*white arrows*) is also seen. **B,** Selective splenic arteriogram shows active bleeding (*arrow*). (From Shanmuganathan K, Mirvis SE, Boyd-Kranis R, et al: *Radiology* 217:75, 2000.)

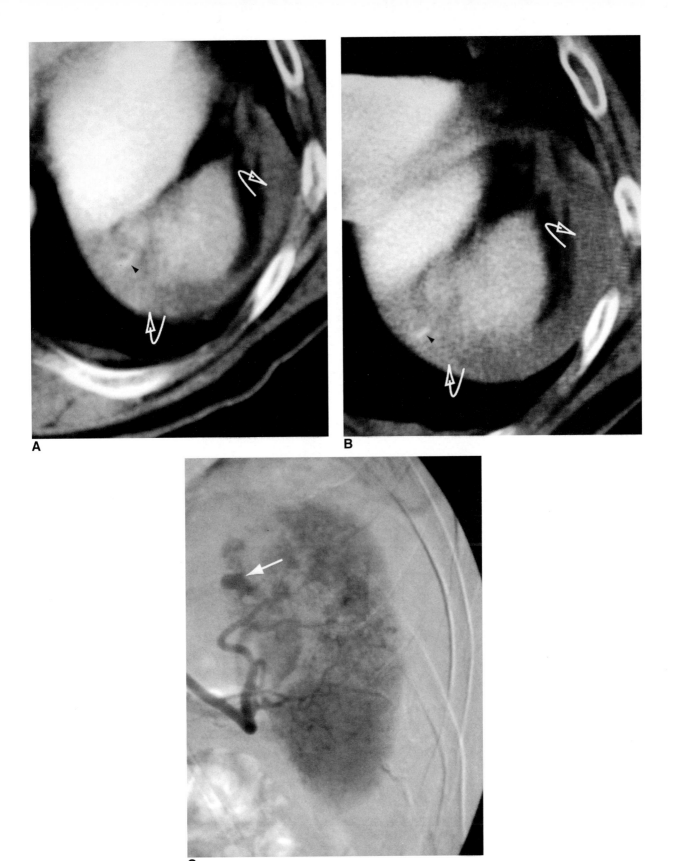

Fig. 6-43
Subtle amount of intraperitoneal vascular contrast extravasation. **A** and **B**, Helical CT images show small amount of vascular contrast material (*arrowheads*) within a perisplenic hematoma (*curved arrows*). **C**, Selective splenic arteriogram shows a bleeding pseudoaneurysm (*arrow*) in upper pole of spleen corresponding to CT findings of active bleeding. Transcatheter embolization was performed to manage hemorrhage.

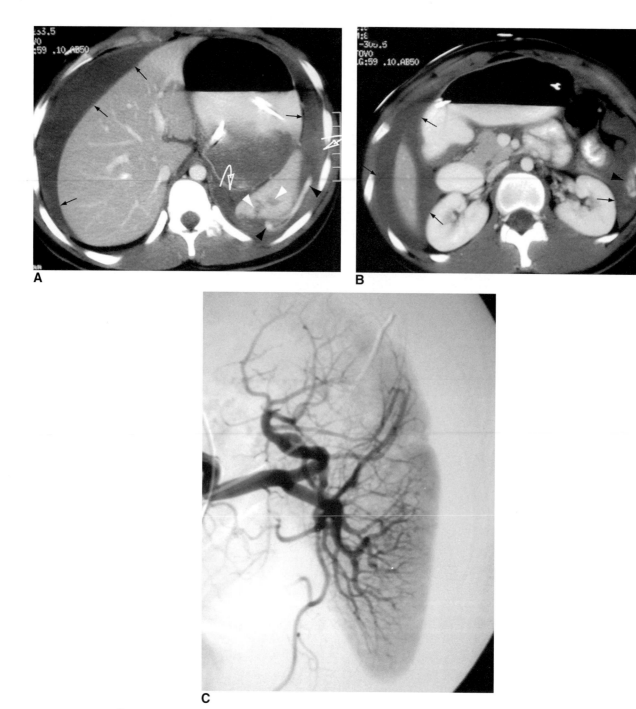

Fig. 6-44
CT evidence of active splenic hemorrhage confirmed at surgery. **A** and **B**, CT images show active bleeding (*black arrowheads*) from grade III splenic lacerations (*white arrowheads*). Large amount of hemoperitoneum is seen around liver and within paracolic gutters (*arrows*) with high-density hematoma (*curved arrows*) adjacent to the spleen. **C**, Selective splenic angiogram does not demonstrate hemorrhage or a posttraumatic vascular injury. At celiotomy for hemodynamic instability after angiography, splenectomy was performed to stop hemorrhage.

renal excretory phase these lesions become minimally hyperdense or isodense to the normal splenic parenchyma (see Figs. 6-47 and 6-48).

Gavant et al.[179] reported demonstration of arterial contrast material extravasation or vascular abnormalities in the spleen seen on contrast-enhanced conventional and single-slice spiral CT associated with an 82% (9/11) failure rate of nonoperatively managed blunt splenic injuries. In this retrospective study, among the 11 patients for whom nonoperative management failed, nine (82%)

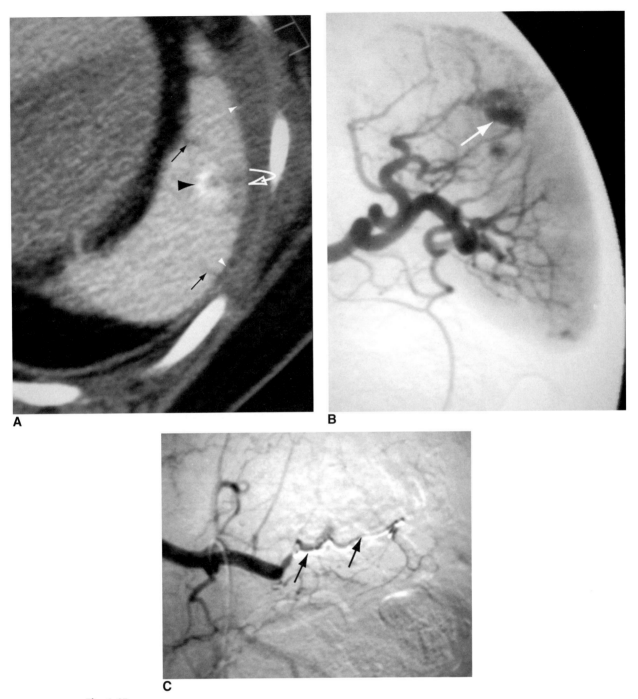

Fig. 6-45
Splenic pseudoaneurysm in a 40-year-old blunt trauma patient. **A,** Helical CT image shows multiple lacerations (*arrows*), area of contusion (*curved arrow*), and a splenic vascular injury (*black arrowhead*). Perisplenic blood (*white arrowheads*) is also seen. **B,** Selective splenic arteriogram shows a pseudoaneurysm (*arrow*). **C,** Completion splenic arteriogram shows total main splenic artery occlusion after embolization with coils (*arrows*).

had vascular injuries, including pseudoaneurysms in eight patients and active hemorrhage in one.

In a prospective study performed to correlate CT findings that might predict the need for arteriography in patients with blunt splenic injury at our institution, vascular lesions in the spleen, including pseudoaneurysm and arteriovenous fistulas, were seen on contrast-enhanced spiral CT in 24% (19/78) of patients who had both CT and splenic arteriography irrespective of injury grade.[156] Nine of the lesions were confirmed by splenic

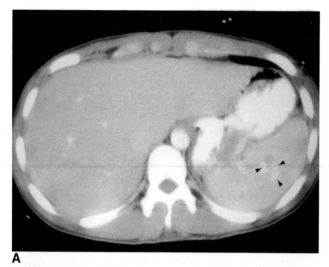

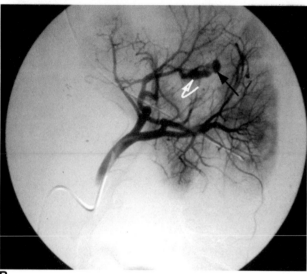

Fig. 6-46

Posttraumatic splenic arteriovenous fistula of patient admitted after blunt abdominal trauma. **A,** Helical CT image shows three high-attenuation areas (*arrowheads*) in a grade I splenic injury. No free intraperitoneal fluid was seen. **B,** Selective splenic arteriogram shows an arteriovenous fistula (*arrow*). Early filling of a splenic vein branch (*curved arrow*) also is seen. (From Shanmuganathan K, Mirvis SE, Boyd-Kranis R, et al: *Radiology* 217:75, 2000.)

angiography and embolized. In the other 10 patients the angiogram demonstrated irregular splenic parenchymal staining, but no focal vascular injury, and did not meet angiographic criteria for transcatheter embolization. Delayed splenectomy was performed for hemorrhage in one of the 10 patients with a splenic pseudoaneurysm diagnosed on admission CT who had a negative splenic angiogram for vascular injury. In two patients CT failed to detect vascular lesions that were diagnosed and embolized by angiography. The finding of a splenic vas-

cular lesion by contrast-enhanced spiral CT was 83.3% (10/12) sensitive and 56.2% (9/16) specific for predicting the need for splenic angiography and subsequent endovascular therapy or splenic surgery.

In a retrospective study performed by Omert et al.[209] 11% (30/274) of patients with splenic injury had splenic vascular lesions ("contrast blush"), and 25% (7/30) of these patients did not require surgical or angiographic intervention. The likelihood of surgical or angiographic intervention in patients with splenic vascular lesion was 9.2 times higher than in patients without this lesion. However, interestingly, in this study a univariate analysis (Fischer's exact *t* test) showed no significant difference in the rate of surgical intervention with or without splenic vascular injuries among patients with blunt splenic injury.

Posttraumatic splenic infarction. Injury to the intima of splenic artery branches from sudden deceleration at the time of impact can lead to thrombosis and infarction of the splenic parenchyma from lack of perfusion distal to the intimal injury. Similar injuries have been observed on CT of the kidneys after blunt trauma.[210] On contrast-enhanced CT, posttraumatic splenic infarcts are seen as well-demarcated segmental wedge-shaped low-attenuation areas with the base of the wedge toward the periphery of the splenic parenchyma (Fig. 6-49; see Fig. 6-7). These infarcts may be the only CT finding of blunt splenic trauma and occur without any adjacent free fluid. Splenic infarcts may also be seen in association with splenic lacerations and segmental infarcts in the kidney. Although the exact natural history of this injury is not known, the majority of these lesions that we have observed have healed without need for surgical or angiographic intervention. Delayed complications of posttraumatic splenic infarction include splenic abscess formation (Fig. 6-50) and delayed rupture of spleen.

Pitfalls in diagnosing splenic injury. Radiologists should be aware of and pay careful attention during interpretation of trauma CT to the multiple potential diagnostic pitfalls that may mimic splenic injuries. Splenic clefts or lobulations can mimic splenic laceration on CT. Clefts typically have smooth or rounded margins (Fig. 6-51) without adjacent free intraperitoneal fluid. Splenic lacerations have an irregular margin, usually with free intraperitoneal fluid adjacent to the spleen or other peritoneal recess. Patient motion and breathing during scanning may cause volume averaging and create a low-density artifact mimicking a subcapsular hematoma or small amount of perisplenic fluid (Figs. 6-52 and 6-53). Streak artifacts arising from cutaneous lines, tubes, monitors, and abrupt density changes, such as the gastric air-contrast level, may also simulate splenic lacerations. "Beam hardening" artifact arising from adjacent ribs pro-

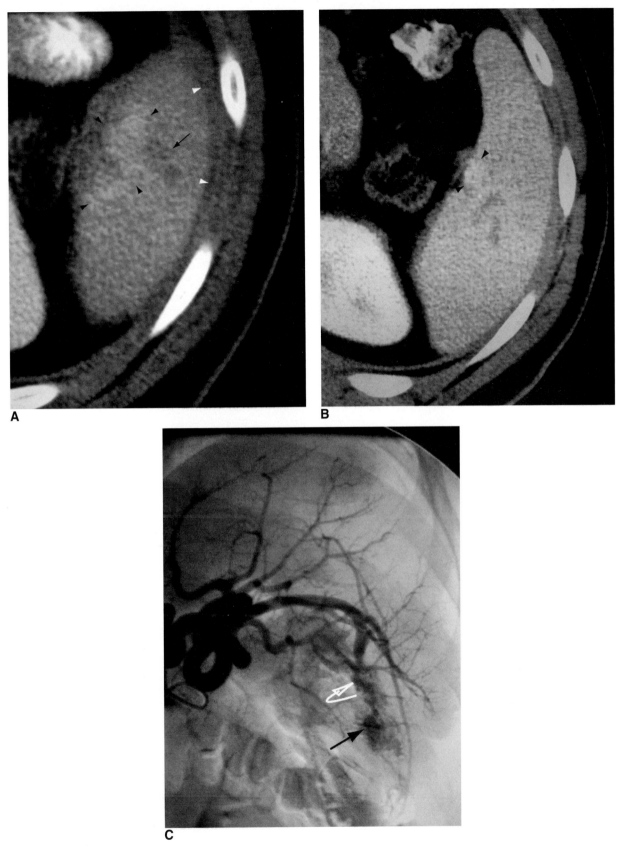

Fig. 6-47
Posttraumatic splenic arteriovenous fistula of patient admitted after blunt abdominal trauma. **A,** Multislice helical CT image obtained in portal venous phase shows a hyperdense lesion (*black arrowheads*) within a grade II splenic injury (*arrow*). Free blood (*white arrowheads*) is seen adjacent to spleen. **B,** Renal excretory phase image shows a minimally hyperdense area (*arrowheads*) compared to normal splenic parenchyma after partial washout of this hyperdense splenic vascular lesion. **C,** Selective splenic arteriogram shows an arteriovenous fistula (*arrow*) with early filling of draining vein (*curved arrow*).

ducing low-attenuation areas within the splenic parenchyma may mimic splenic lacerations or contusions. Scanning the spleen in the early arterial phase of intravenous contrast enhancement may produce a heterogeneous splenic parenchymal pattern that can also look like lacerations or contusions (Fig. 6-54).

Hematomas, lacerations, and posttraumatic splenic vascular lesions may become isodense with normal splenic parenchyma and easily missed by CT if delayed scanning is performed after the peak of parenchymal enhancement or if the volume or concentration of intravenous contrast material is inadequate, particularly in obese patients.[156] CT findings mimicking splenic vascular lesions include splenic hemangiomas, islands of viable enhancing splenic parenchyma surrounded by low-attenuation splenic laceration-contusions, and intact intrasplenic vessels traversing the center or periphery of parenchymal lacerations simulating a focal pseudoaneurysm. Understanding these

potential diagnostic pitfalls, use of an optimal volume and concentration of intravenous contrast material, scanning at the peak of visceral contrast enhancement, and use of objective contrast bolus timing techniques can reduce false-negative CT results and improve selection of patients for splenic angiography. In our opinion these artifacts are less likely to result with MSCT imaging systems using subsecond scanning that are obtained with efficient contrast bolus tracking.

Follow-up CT of the spleen. The role of follow-up CT for patients with splenic injury undergoing nonoperative management is controversial.[196,211-214] Usually patients who develop hemodynamic instability during nonoperative management or require multiple blood transfusions may either undergo follow-up CT, angiography, or proceed directly to laparotomy. Some studies indicate that routine follow-up CT is not necessary or useful in predict-

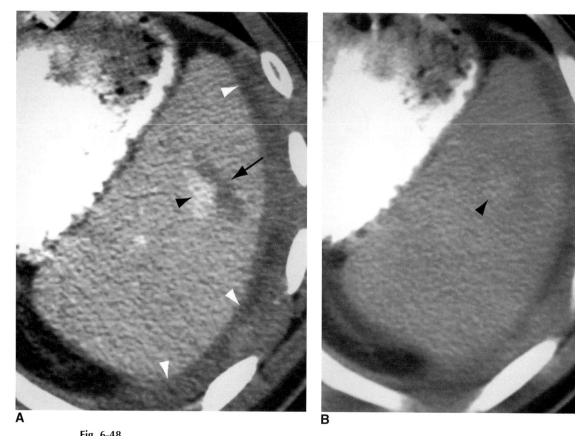

A   **B**

Fig. 6-48
Washout of splenic vascular lesion seen on renal excretory phase of multislice helical CT in a 17-year-old man admitted after motor vehicle collision. **A**, CT image obtained in portal venous phase shows a grade II splenic laceration (*arrow*) with a splenic vascular lesion (*black arrowhead*). Perisplenic blood (*white arrowheads*) is also seen. **B**, Delayed image obtained in renal excretory phase shows washout of splenic vascular lesion (*arrowhead*) that is isodense compared to normal splenic parenchyma. No splenic laceration is seen.

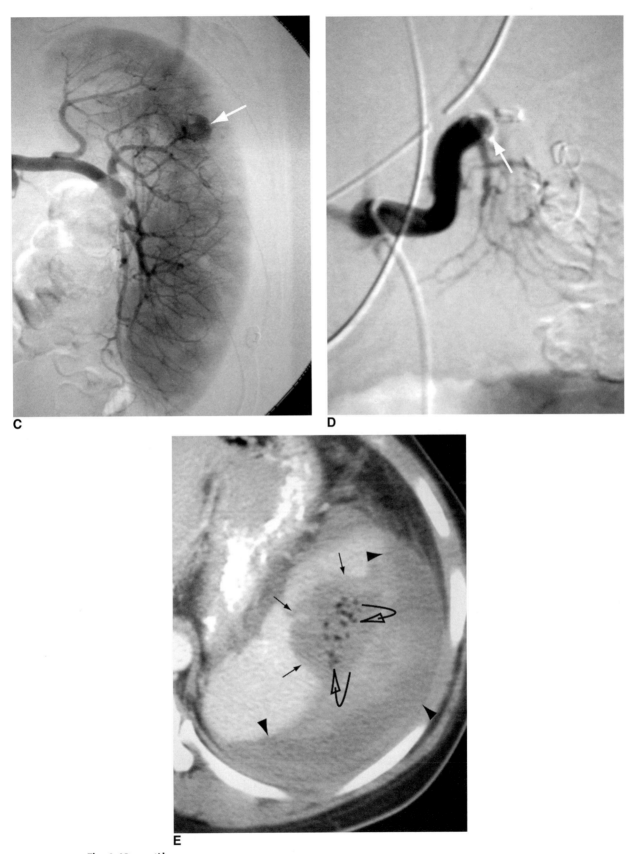

Fig. 6-48, cont'd
C, Selective splenic angiogram shows a pseudoaneurysm (*arrow*). **D,** This lesion was treated by transcatheter embolization (*arrow*) of the main splenic artery. **E,** Postembolization CT images show air (*curved arrows*) within splenic infarct (*arrows*) and a mixed-density subcapsular hematoma (*arrowheads*).

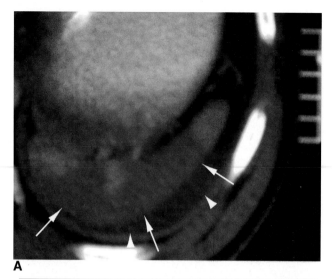

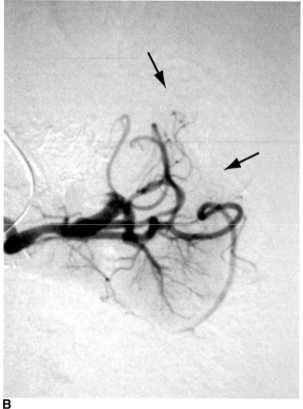

Fig. 6-49
Splenic infarction confirmed by splenic arteriography. **A**, CT image shows a well-demarcated area lacking parenchymal enhancement (*arrows*) as a result of infarction. Free intraperitoneal fluid (*arrowheads*) is also seen. **B**, Selective splenic arteriogram shows lack of arterial perfusion to mid and upper spleen (*arrows*) consistent with CT findings of splenic infarction.

ing delayed complications, such as ongoing hemorrhage, progression of extent of splenic parenchymal injury, abscess formation, or missed hollow viscus or solid organ injury that requires surgical intervention.[211,212,214] Contrary to this view other studies performed by Federle

et al.[213] and Davis et al.[155] report progression of splenic injury by early follow-up CT in 8% to 74% of blunt splenic injury patients. In a study performed by Davis et al.[155] of 31 splenic pseudoaneurysms identified by CT, 26% (8/31) were diagnosed on admission CT and 74% (23/31) were first detected on follow-up CT. The ability to identify these patients will prevent potential "delayed splenic rupture" by referring these patients for splenic arteriography and transcatheter embolization. Also, demonstration of normal healing (Fig. 6-55) of the splenic injuries on follow-up CT could be used as a criterion for resumption of normal physical activity.[213]

At the UMSTC we perform follow-up CT on patients with splenic injury within 48 to 72 hours postadmission to assess for CT signs of splenic injury progression, including development of new splenic vascular lesions (Fig. 6-56; see Fig. 6-29), increases in the number or extent of laceration(s) (Fig. 6-57; see Fig. 6-30), or the size of the hematoma(s). Our experience has shown no clinical evidence of injury progression in most cases with CT findings of injury progression on follow-up CT.

CT is useful to evaluate ongoing or recurrent active bleeding in the spleen after surgical or angiographic intervention (Fig. 6-58). Extravasated contrast from *a prior angiographic study can mimic active hemorrhage* on contrast-enhanced CT. Therefore, it is important to perform both precontrast and postcontrast CT scans of the spleen for a patient who has recently had splenic angiography to distinguish previously extravasated angiographic contrast from ongoing splenic bleeding.

Postembolization spleen. Splenic arteriography and transcatheter arterial embolization to stop splenic hemorrhage and treat posttraumatic vascular injuries are becoming more popular techniques to improve the success of nonoperatively managed blunt splenic injury.[16,155,156,177,178,215-217] At the UMSTC proximal main splenic artery embolization and distal branch vessel embolization are both performed to preserve splenic function and viability during the healing process.[156,218] Indications for follow-up CT after embolization include persistent hypotension, abdominal pain, and elevated white blood cell count or fever.

A retrospective review by Killeen et al.[218] of postembolization CT results in 53 patients with blunt splenic injury found that splenic infarcts occurred in 63% of patients after their proximal main splenic artery embolization (Fig. 6-59) and in all 22 patients who had distal splenic branch vessel embolization (Fig. 6-60). After proximal main splenic artery embolization in 15 patients, 80% (12) had infarcts involving less than 50% of the splenic parenchyma. These infarcts were typically multiple, small, and peripheral in location. The 22 patients who had distal splenic branch embolization had single infarcts peripheral to the embolized branch, and

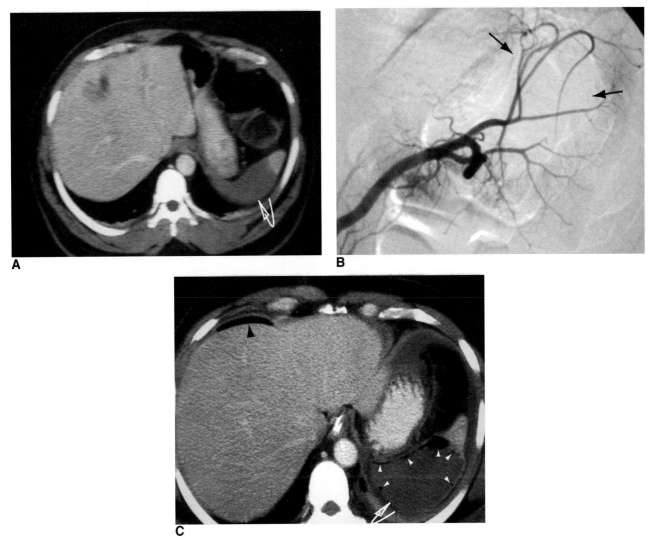

Fig. 6-50
Splenic necrosis after infarction of spleen in a 31-year-old man admitted following motor vehicle collision. **A**, Admission helical CT shows a wedge-shaped well-demarcated perfusion defect in splenic parenchyma (*curved arrow*) without perisplenic fluid. **B**, Selective splenic angiogram performed after CT shows a lack of perfusion to upper and mid aspect of spleen corresponding to CT findings. **C**, Follow-up CT obtained because of abdominal pain and fever 10 days after admission shows free intraperitoneal air (*black arrowhead*) and intrasplenic air (*white arrowheads*) within infarcted area (*curved arrow*) from splenic necrosis. Splenectomy was performed.

infarcts after distal embolization involved less than 50% of splenic parenchyma in 81% (20) of those patients. Gas was seen within the splenic parenchyma in 13% (7) of all 53 patients. The splenic gas was within the infarct (see Fig. 6-48) in four patients, within a subcapsular collection with an air-fluid level (Fig. 6-61) in two patients, and diffusely throughout the splenic parenchyma (Fig. 6-62) in one patient. Gelfoam material was used for embolization in six of the seven patients with splenic gas. Both patients with subcapsular collections of gas with air-fluid levels were febrile, had elevated white cell counts, and were percutaneously drained (Fig. 6-63) for apparent splenic abscess; one was sterile, and the other infected.

Liver Injury. Significant liver injury occurs in 3% to 12% of patients who are admitted to a major trauma center.[219] The liver is the second most commonly injured solid organ after blunt trauma. Over a 3-year period, 428 patients were admitted to UMSTC with liver injury. Associate injuries to the spleen occurred in 30% (127) of the patients, to the kidney in 9% (40), and to the

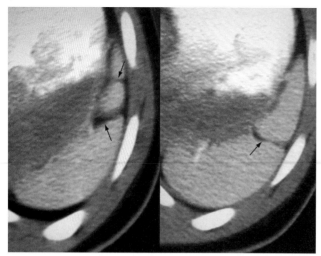

Fig. 6-51
Splenic cleft mimicking splenic laceration. Two contiguous axial CT images show splenic clefts (*arrows*) with rounded margins and no free intraperitoneal fluid adjacent to spleen.

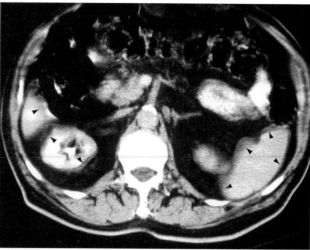

Fig. 6-53
Motion artifact mimicking free intraperitoneal fluid on conventional CT. CT image shows a low-attenuation area (*arrowheads*) surrounding spleen mimicking free fluid from motion artifact. Same artifact (*arrowheads*) is seen around liver and right kidney. Abdominal wall muscles are blurred from motion.

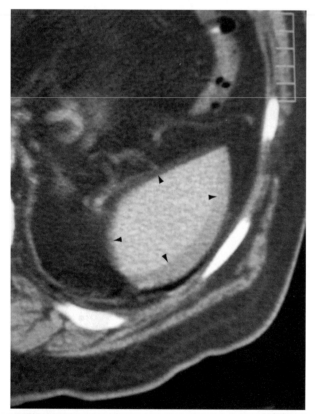

Fig. 6-52
Partial volume artifact mimicking free intraperitoneal fluid on multislice helical CT. CT image shows a low-attenuation area (*arrowheads*) surrounding spleen mimicking free fluid from partial volume artifact.

pancreas in 3% (14). Mortality rates may exceed 50% in patients with complex liver injuries who have hemodynamic instability from active bleeding.[220-227]

From 70% to 90% of hepatic injuries are minor and either do not require surgery or have stopped bleeding at the time of celiotomy.[19,129,221,223] CT has had a major influence, particularly since the 1990s, on the prevailing surgical philosophy that surgical intervention is the only acceptable way to successfully manage hepatic injuries.* The common availability of CT, the capacity to accurately diagnose the presence and extent of liver injury and concurrent abdominal organ injury, the ability to demonstrate active bleeding and vascular injuries, and the capacity to quantify hemoperitoneum have all been factors permitting gradual adoption of nonoperative treatment of stable patients with blunt liver injury.

Anatomy. The liver is a wedge-shaped organ occupying a large volume of the upper abdomen. It is enclosed anteriorly and laterally by the lower rib cage. The Glisson capsule is a thin though fibrous capsule that invests the entire surface of the liver deep to the peritoneum. The liver is covered by peritoneum except for the "bare area," a small rhomboid area on the posterior aspect between the triangular and coronary ligaments directly in contact with the retroperitoneum. The English literature divides the liver into right and left lobes by a vertical plane

---

*References 17, 19, 22, 23, 129, 130, 228-233

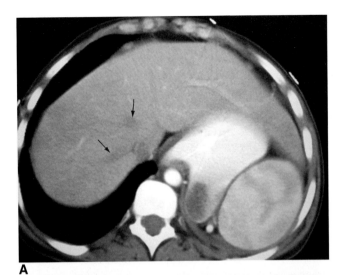

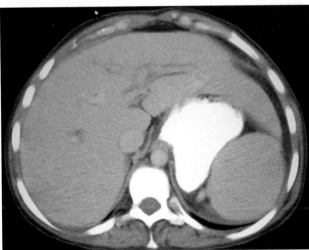

Fig. 6-54
Heterogeneous parenchymal enhancement pattern mimicking splenic injury in a patient with low cardiac output from congenital heart block. **A**, Helical CT image through upper abdomen obtained 60 seconds after initiation of intravenous contrast injection shows late arterial phase image with heterogeneous enhancement of splenic parenchyma. Note main hepatic veins (*arrows*) are void of intravenous contrast material. **B**, CT image in portal venous phase shows homogeneous enhancement of normal splenic parenchyma.

traversing the gallbladder and inferior vena cava at a 75-degree angle (Cantlie's line). This plane contains the middle hepatic vein. The caudate lobe is considered as a separate lobe because of the direct venous drainage into the inferior vena cava. Couinaud[234] divided the liver into eight discrete functional segments based on the hepatic venous drainage and portal branches.

Since the hepatic veins lie in rigid canals and contract poorly, the liver is incapable of achieving spontaneous hemostasis after injury.[235] The retrohepatic inferior vena cava is about 8 to 10 cm long and receives blood from

multiple hepatic veins. Exposure and vascular control can be challenging even to the most experienced trauma surgeon under the best of circumstances. The portal vein supplies 75% of the hepatic blood flow. There may be considerable variation in the origin and course of the hepatic arteries. The most common finding is the proper hepatic artery arising from the common hepatic artery after it gives off the gastroduodenal, right gastric, and supraduodenal arteries.

Nonoperative Management of Hepatic Injury. The published data suggest that a steady rise in the number of adults sustaining blunt hepatic injury that can be successfully managed without surgical treatment, and this rate has increased from about 20% in the 1980s to 80% in the 1990s.[19,236-247] This nonoperative approach requires hemodynamic stability and includes patients with all grades of liver injury, but without associate injuries requiring celiotomy.* In a retrospective study performed by Meredith et al.,[245] 92 hemodynamically stable patients with blunt liver injury had admission CTs and 78% (72/92) of them were successfully managed without surgery or complications. The nonoperatively managed patients included 11 grade I, 28 grade II, 16 grade III, 10 grade IV, and 5 grade V liver injuries. The CT grades were not predictive of the need for surgery. A prospective study performed by Croce et al.[19] studied 112 patients to determine the safety of conservative management of blunt hepatic injury. In the study 30% (35) of the patients had minor liver injuries (grades I and II) and 70% (77) had major liver injuries (grades III to V). Comparing the outcomes of patients with hepatic injuries managed without surgery with a control group of surgically managed liver injuries (n= 84) revealed no difference in length of hospital stay between the two groups. Transfusion requirements and intraabdominal complications were significantly lower in the patient group treated without surgery.†

The most common cause for failed nonoperative management of hepatic injury is ongoing bleeding.[19,239,245,249-251] To improve outcome of nonoperative management for patients with high-grade blunt hepatic injuries, Hagiwara et al.[248] used hepatic arteriography and embolization as alternatives to surgery. All 28 patients with high-grade injury in this study (Mirvis et al.[129] classification grades III to V) had hepatic arteriography. Arterial embolization was performed to manage hemorrhage in 54% (15/28) of the patients. Repeat hepatic arteriography was performed in six patients, and two of these needed repeat embolization. Although there was a significantly higher requirement for fluid resuscitation, nonsurgical

---

*References 19, 236, 237, 239, 246, 247.
†References 19, 241, 242, 245, 247, 248.

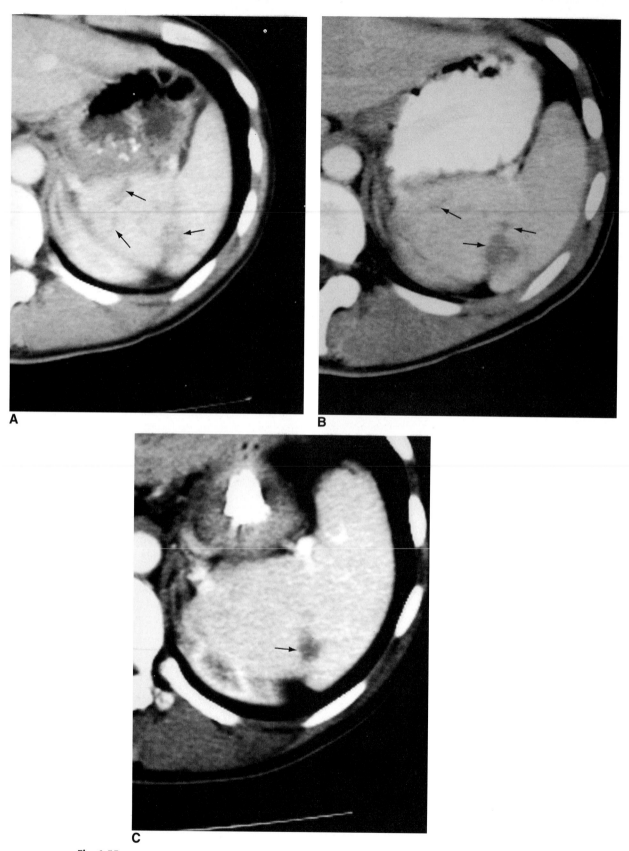

Fig. 6-55
Normal healing of splenic injury. **A**, Admission CT image shows acute splenic laceration (*arrows*) with jagged margins. **B**, Follow-up CT image about 10 days postinjury shows lacerations (*arrows*) have smoother margins and have become rounded. **C**, Follow-up CT image 3 months postinjury shows a single rounded area (*arrow*). Other lacerations have healed completely.

management ultimately did not fail for any of the patients with high-grade liver injury.

At the UMSTC, patients with all grades of liver injury who are hemodynamically stable without CT evidence of surgical bowel or mesenteric injuries, irrespective of their GCS, are initially nonoperatively managed. To optimize outcome, hepatic arteriography is performed for all patients with a high anatomic CT injury grade (grades III to V), with injuries extending into the hepatic veins, with all grades of hepatic injury with CT evidence of active bleeding, with pseudoaneurysms, or with traumatic arteriovenous fistulas, and for patients who require multiple blood transfusions attributable to the liver injury.[233]

Sites and Mechanisms of Hepatic Injury. Of all patients with blunt traumatic injury to the abdomen, some 15% to 20% involve the liver.[251] Isolated injuries of the liver occur in less than 50% of patients with blunt liver injury. Because the right lobe constitutes 80% of hepatic volume, it is the most frequently injured region. In one series reported by McClellan and Shiers,[251] of the 48 patients with injury to the superior aspect of right lobe, 33% had concurrent right-sided rib fractures and 23% also had pneumothoraces. Injuries to the left lobe of the liver are associated with duodenal and pancreatic injuries.

Its large size, the friability of the liver parenchyma, a thin capsule, and a fixed position anterior to the spine make it susceptible to injury.[252] A variety of biomechanical mechanisms have been proposed to explain hepatic injuries. Injuries occur to the posterior right lobe of the liver from simple compression against the fixed ribs, spine, or posterior abdominal wall. Pressure applied to the right thoracic cavity may propagate through the

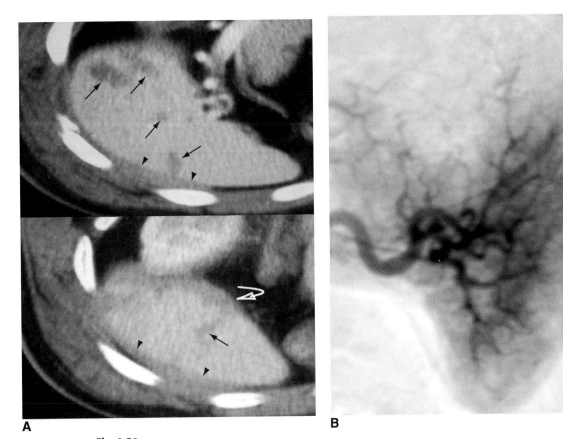

A **B**

Fig. 6-56
Value of follow-up CT in a 56-year-old man admitted after blunt trauma. **A,** Admission multislice CT images show a grade III splenic injury with multiple lacerations (*arrows*), subcapsular hematoma (*curved arrow*), and perisplenic fluid (*arrowheads*). **B,** Selective arteriogram after CT shows no active bleeding or vascular lesions.

Continued

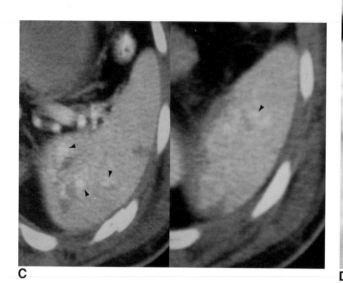

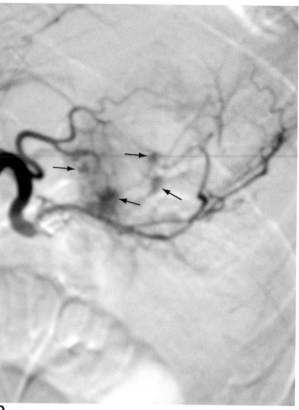

C

D

Fig. 6-56, cont'd
C, Routine follow-up CT images 3 days after admission show multiple vascular lesions (*arrowheads*) within some splenic lacerations. **D,** Selective splenic arteriogram performed after second CT study shows multiple pseudoaneurysms (*arrows*). These lesions were treated by transcatheter embolization.

diaphragm, creating a contusion of the dome of the right lobe. The liver's attachment by the coronary ligaments to the undersurface of the diaphragm and posterior abdominal wall can act as sites of shear injury created by motion of the liver relative to the rest of the body during rapid deceleration. Hepatic injuries can also result from transmission of excessively high venous pressure occurring at the time of impact to remote body sites.[252,253]

Hepatic Injury Grading System. To standardize reporting of liver injuries over time and to compare outcomes and treatment protocols in the same trauma center or between different centers the AAST formed a committee to develop an injury severity score.[169,173,174] This injury scale (Table 6-6) is based on the anatomic disruption of the liver, including the lengths and number of lacerations, and the surface area involved by the subcapsular or intraparenchymal hematoma seen at laparotomy. This classification system is scaled 1 to 6 indicating the least to

the most severe injury and is used by most trauma surgeons in the United States.

Based on the AAST liver injury scale, investigators have developed various CT classifications of liver injury to predict successful outcome of nonoperative management.[129,228,254] Based on the AAST liver injury scale, Mirvis et al.[129] developed an injury scale applicable to CT (Table 6-7) that was found to be valuable in predicting outcome and treatment in 37 patients with isolated blunt hepatic injury, 84% (31) of whom were managed nonoperatively, including three patients with grade IV injuries. For none of these patients selected initially for observation did nonoperative management fail. Surgical exploration was performed based on grossly positive DPL results in 16% (6/37) of the patients, but only one required surgical intervention to pack a stellate liver injury. This study demonstrated that hemodynamically stable patients with major liver injury, including grade IV based on this CT classification system, could usually be

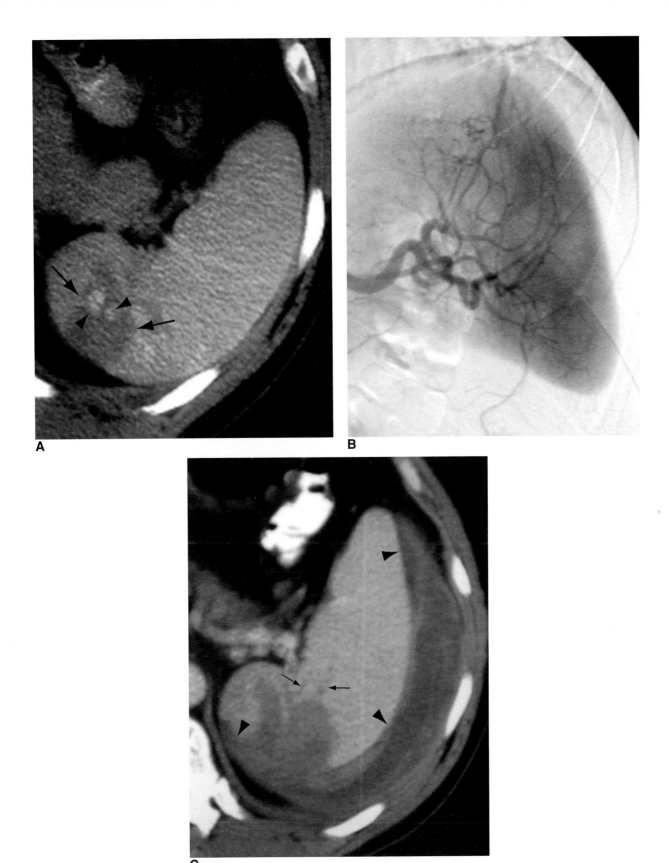

Fig. 6-57
Progression of splenic injury seen on follow-up CT in patient admitted after blunt force injury. **A,** Admission helical CT shows a grade III splenic injury (*arrows*) with a vascular lesion (*arrowhead*). **B,** Selective splenic arteriogram shows no vascular injury. **C,** Follow-up CT shows delayed splenic rupture, a new large subcapsular hematoma (*arrowheads*), and lacerations (*arrows*).

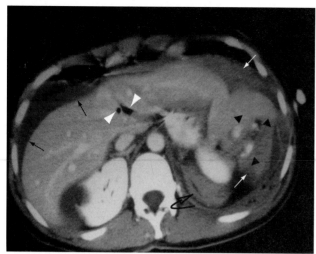

Fig. 6-58
Recurrent active bleeding in spleen after surgery. Conventional CT image because of hypotension after splenorrhaphy for blunt splenic injury shows three areas of active bleeding (*black arrowheads*) within splenic parenchyma. Perisplenic hematoma (*white arrows*) and hemoperitoneum (*black arrows*) around liver are seen. Free intraperitoneal air (*white arrowheads*) from recent surgery and a left adrenal hematoma (*curved arrow*) are also seen. Splenectomy was performed to arrest hemorrhage. (From Shanmuganathan K, Mirvis SE, Sover ER: *AJR Am J Roentgenol* 161:65, 1993.)

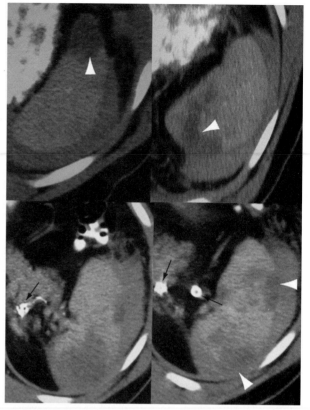

Fig. 6-59
Splenic infarction after proximal main splenic artery embolization. Four multislice helical CT images after proximal splenic embolization with coils (*arrows*) show multiple small peripheral infarcts (*arrowheads*).

managed without surgery. Poletti et al.[233] and Hagiwara et al.[248] have used the Mirvis classification to predict the need for hepatic arteriography in blunt hepatic injury. Both these studies demonstrated that high-grade (grades III to V) hepatic injuries were at a higher risk of ongoing or delayed bleeding and may benefit from early hepatic arteriography to improve the success rate of nonoperative management.

Contrary to these reports, a study performed by Becker et al.[254] to correlate CT-based grading system with treatment outcomes in 38 patients with liver injuries, demonstrated that though CT was helpful in reflecting the extent of parenchymal injury, it was unable to predict complications or need for surgery. Conservative management was complicated by hepatic rupture in 3% (1/38) of the patients, and arteriovenous fistula or biloma in 5% (2). Exploratory laparotomy was performed in 26% (10). However, only 1 of those 10 patients explored had active bleeding in this study.

Computed Tomography Appearance of Liver Injury. The four principal types of parenchymal liver injury shown by CT include hematoma(s), laceration(s), vascular injuries, and active hemorrhage.[2,4,35] Numerous previous studies have shown that CT can accurately diagnose these four types of injuries and guide management of blunt trauma patients with liver injuries.* A study by Poletti et al.[233] at

*References 17, 126, 129, 141, 233, 253-258.

the UMSTC reported that high-grade liver lacerations involving major hepatic veins or with active bleeding had an increased likelihood of major vascular injury and should undergo hepatic arteriography even without overt clinical signs of hemorrhage. Prior knowledge of lacerations extending into the region of the intrahepatic inferior vena cava (IVC) or the three major hepatic veins indicates an increased likelihood of IVC or hepatic vein disruption (see below). Prior knowledge of the potential for these major hepatic venous injuries allows the surgical team to prepare for possible hepatic venous isolation strategies should surgery become necessary.[225]

Hematoma. Hepatic hematomas may be intraparenchymal and/or subcapsular (Figs. 6-64 to 6-67; see Figs. 6-7, 6-19, and 6-22). Single or multiple hematomas may be seen after blunt trauma. Most subcapsular hematomas are seen along the anterolateral aspect of the right lobe of the liver. Subcapsular hematomas cause direct compression of underlying liver parenchyma, and this CT sign is helpful in differentiating subcapsular hematoma from small amounts of free intraperitoneal blood or fluid seen adjacent to the liver (perihepatic

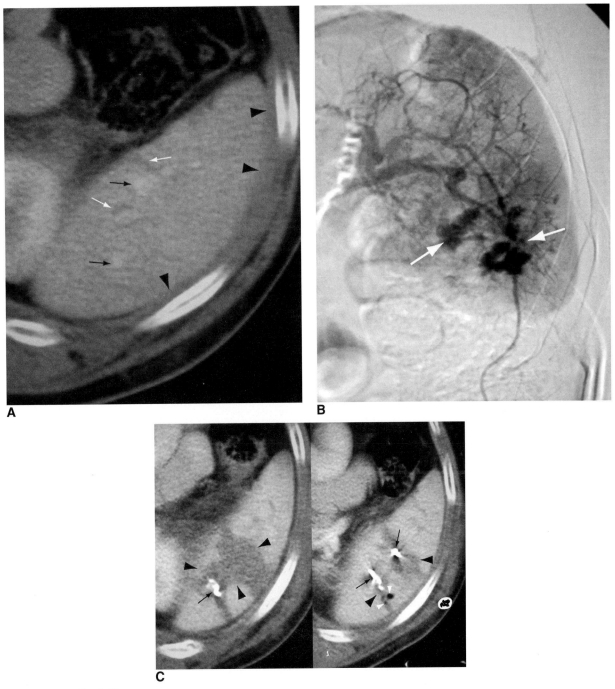

Fig. 6-60
Splenic infarction after distal splenic embolization. **A,** Admission multislice helical CT image shows a grade II splenic injury with lacerations (*white arrow*) and vascular lesions (*black arrows*). Minimal amount of perisplenic hematoma (*arrowheads*) is seen lateral to spleen. **B,** Selective splenic arteriogram shows multiple pseudoaneurysms (*arrows*). Distal embolization was performed to treat these two lesions. **C,** Postembolization CT images show infarcts (*black arrowheads*) in relation to embolization coils (*arrows*). Intraparenchymal air (*white arrowheads*) was introduced during the embolization procedure.

spaces) (see Fig. 6-65). On unenhanced CT scans the liver parenchyma appears hypodense relative to subcapsular hematomas (see Fig. 6-22). On contrast-enhanced CT, a subcapsular hematoma is typically seen as a low-attenuation, lens-shaped collection of blood between

Glisson's capsule and the enhancing liver parenchyma (see Fig. 6-22). The hemorrhage may appear as alternating bands of differing density most likely resulting from alternating areas of liquid blood and clot formation. Unless recurrent hemorrhage occurs, usually the

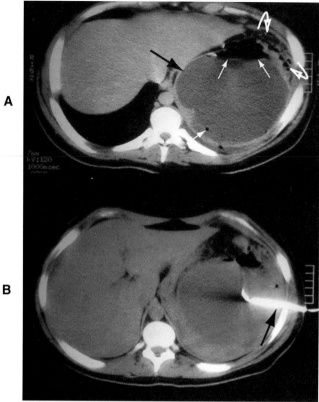

Fig. 6-61
Subcapsular air-fluid levels after splenic embolization. Patient was febrile and had an elevated white blood cell count. **A,** Helical CT image shows a large intrasplenic fluid collection (*black arrow*) with gas bubbles (*white arrows*). Free intraperitoneal air (*curved arrows*) is also seen. **B,** CT images after CT-guided drainage shows a catheter (*arrow*) within this collection.

attenuation value of a subcapsular hematoma decreases with the age of the injury. Follow-up CT typically shows resolution of uncomplicated subcapsular hematomas within 6 to 8 weeks.[259,260]

Contusion. Parenchymal contusions of the liver appear as irregular areas of low attenuation on contrast-enhanced CT with possible intermixed high-density blood (Figs. 6-67 to 6-69). On CT, acute hematomas appear as irregular high-attenuation regions of clotted blood surrounded by lower-density nonclotted blood or bile. Signs of healing may be evident as early as 3 or 4 days after trauma. With early healing the contusion may initially expand in size slightly and develop smoother, more regular margins, which should not be taken as a sign of injury worsening. With further resolution, the lesion demonstrates a gradual decrease in hematoma attenuation and size until blending with the background parenchyma. Even large, irregular injuries typically heal completely without residual abnormalities of hepatic contour or density. Infection within the injured area or

admixture of hematoma and bile in the contusion will delay the healing process.[260]

Laceration. On contrast-enhanced, CT liver lacerations appear as irregular linear or branching low-attenuation areas (see Figs. 6-3, 6-6, 6-7, 6-9, 6-10, 6-19, 6-65, and 6-70). Multiple parallel lacerations resulting from a compressive force are termed "bear claw" lacerations (see Fig. 6-70). Hepatic lacerations with a branching pattern could mimic the appearance of unopacified portal or hepatic veins or dilated bile ducts and may require careful evaluation of serial images to differentiate among these various structures. The location of laceration(s) and the relationship to the porta hepatis and biliary radicles may be important, because these deep lacerations may be more commonly associated with biliary system injury[260] (Figs. 6-69 and 6-70). Poletti et al.[233] found that 12% (6/49) of patients with blunt hepatic injury selected for nonoperative management developed a biloma, but found no significant association between biloma and extension of lacerations into the region of the porta hepatis. Lacerations can be classified into superficial (limited to 3 cm depth from the surface) and deep (>3 cm from the surface). The surgical grading system could underestimate the true extent of injury to the liver, because deep, central parenchymal lesions seen on CT may go unrecognized during laparotomy, particularly if the liver surface appears intact.

Liver lacerations that are limited to the posterior segment of the right lobe of the liver with extension to the "bare area" usually develop hematoma in the retroperitoneal compartment.[261] CT findings usually associated with isolated "bare area" hepatic lacerations include right-sided retroperitoneal hematomas (Figs. 6-71 and 6-72), right adrenal or periadrenal hematoma, right perirenal and subcapsular hematoma, and fluid around the intrahepatic inferior vena cava. False-negative DPL or sonography may be associated with this injury, as only a few of these patients will have free intraperitoneal blood.

Acute liver lacerations have sharp or jagged margins (Fig. 6-72). As the lesion heals, it enlarges, its margins become smoother, and it assumes a rounded to oval configuration (Figs. 6-73 and 6-74) on follow-up CT. Unlike subcapsular hematomas, intraparenchymal liver injuries can persist for several months and occasionally longer.[259,260] Savolaine et al.[260] have demonstrated that stasis of bile products at the margin of liver injuries prolongs blood clot resorption and also has an adverse effect on healing. These lesions may gradually decrease in size or remain as well-defined hepatic cysts.

Vascular injuries. Injuries to the major hepatic veins (Fig. 6-75) or retrohepatic vena cava are fortunately rarely seen after blunt abdominal trauma. Retrohepatic vena caval injuries are typically associated with very high

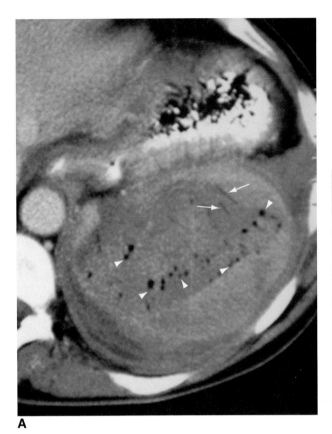

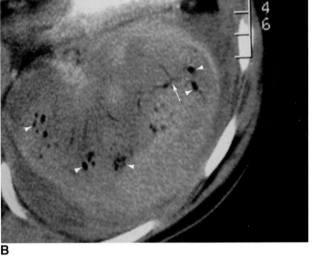

Fig. 6-62
Diffuse air within splenic parenchyma after transcatheter embolization in a 37-year-old man. **A** and **B**, Helical CT images after transcatheter embolization of spleen with Gelfoam material show air (*arrowheads*) seen diffusely throughout splenic parenchyma. Some of the air is linear and has a branching pattern (*arrows*).

mortality of 90% to 100%.[225,262-266] In most series this mortality has been attributed to excessive blood loss and the inevitable coagulopathy resulting from a long delay in recognizing that a juxtahepatic venous injury is present, ongoing bleeding, and the difficulty in obtaining surgical exposure to repair these injuries.[262-266] Retrohepatic vena caval injuries are suspected on CT when liver lacerations extend to the major hepatic veins or IVC, with profuse hemorrhage behind the right lobe of the liver, into the lesser sac, or near the diaphragm (Fig. 6-76; see Fig. 6-19). Prior suspicion of such vascular injuries can assist the surgeon in planning the best approach to control hemorrhage and to repair the vascular injury, typically through vascular isolation techniques requiring a combined thoracoabdominal approach. A combined therapeutic approach for high-grade liver lacerations with injury to the retrohepatic IVC often involves both the trauma surgeon and interventional radiologist. Initially the trauma surgeon attempts to control the massive hemorrhage by temporary peri-

hepatic packing. The angiographer can map the site and extent of venous injury and potentially control this by stent placement.[225]

Partial hepatic devascularization can result from an injury to the vessels in the perihilar region by a deep laceration or partial avulsion of the dual blood supply of the liver. On contrast-enhanced CT devascularized segments would appear as wedge-shaped regions extending to the periphery that fail to enhance with the normally perfused liver (Figs. 6-77 and 6-78).

Pseudoaneurysms of the hepatic artery and its branches (Fig. 6-79) may result from lacerations extending across the course of these vessels, as well as from shearing forces. Arteriovenous (see Fig. 6-79) or arterioportal fistulas (Fig. 6-80) may mimic the contrast-enhanced CT appearance of hepatic pseudoaneurysm. A retrospective study performed at the UMSTC on patients sustaining blunt hepatic injury, who had both contrast-enhanced single-slice spiral CT and hepatic arteriography, showed that single-slice contrast-enhanced helical CT

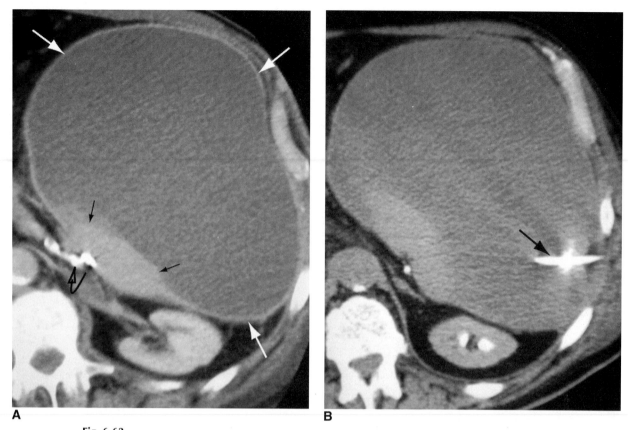

A   **B**

Fig. 6-63
Percutaneous CT-guided drainage of postembolization pneumococcal splenic abscess in 75-year-old man. Patient presented with overwhelming sepsis 30 days after main splenic artery embolization. **A**, Multislice helical CT image shows a large subcapsular collection (*white arrow*) compressing splenic parenchyma (*black arrow*). Embolization coils (*curved arrow*) are seen in main splenic artery. **B**, A percutaneous drainage catheter (*arrow*) was placed under CT guidance into this collection and drained about 3000 ml of altered blood. The fluid and blood cultures both grew Pneumococcus.

Table 6-6
AAST Liver Injury Scale

Grade*	Type	Description†
1	Hematoma	Subscapsular, nonexpanding, <10% surface area
	Laceration	Capsular tear, nonbleeding: <10 cm parenchymal depth
2	Hematoma	Subcapsular, non-expanding, 10%-50% surface area; intraparenchymal, non-expanding <2 cm diameter
	Laceration	Capsular tear, active bleeding; 1-3 cm in parenchymal depth, <10 cm in length
3	Hematoma	Subcapsular, >50% surface area or expanding: ruptured subcapsular hematoma with active bleeding; intraparenchymal hematoma >2 cm or expanding
	Laceration	>3-cm parenchymal depth
4	Hematoma	Ruptured intraparenchymal hematoma with active bleeding
	Laceration	
5	Hematoma	Parenchymal disruption involving >50% of hepatic lobe
	Vascular	Juxta venous injuries (i.e., retrohepatic vena cava/major renal veins)
6	Vascular	Hepatic avulsion

From Moore EE, Cogbill TH, Jurkovitch J, Shackford SR: *J Trauma* 38:333, 1995.
*Advance one grade for multiple injuries to the same organ.
†Based on most accurate assessment at autopsy, laparotomy, or radiologic study.

Table 6-7
CT-Based Injury Severity Grades for Blunt Hepatic Trauma

CT Grade	Criteria
I	Capsular avulsion, superficial laceration(s) <1 cm deep, subcapsular hematoma <1 cm maximal thickness
II	Laceration(s) 1-3 cm deep, central/subcapsular hematoma(s) 1-3 cm diameter
III	Laceration >3 cm deep, central/subcapsular hematoma(s) >3 cm in diameter
IV	Massive central/subcapsular hematoma >10 cm, lobar tissue destruction (maceration) or devascularization
V	Bilobar tissue destruction (maceration) or devascularization

Modified from Mirvis SE, Whitley NO, Vainwright JR, et al: *Radiology* 171:27, 1989.

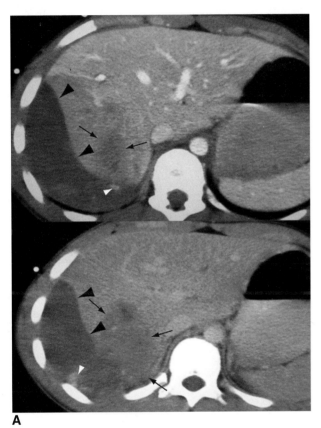

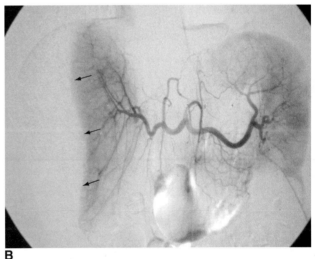

A
B

Fig. 6-64
Hepatic hematomas and active bleeding in a 26-year-old man involved in a motor vehicle collision. **A,** Multislice CT images show a moderate subcapsular hematoma (*black arrowheads*) compressing liver parenchyma. A mixed-density intraparenchymal hematoma (*arrows*) is also seen. Active bleeding (*white arrowheads*) is seen within subcapsular hematoma. **B,** Celiac axis arteriogram shows mass effect (*arrows*) on right lobe of liver from subcapsular hematoma. No active bleeding is seen. Surgical evacuation of subcapsular hematoma was performed.

had a sensitivity of 65% and a specificity of 85% for detecting hepatic arterial injury for all CT injury grades if arteriography was the gold standard. Sensitivity was 100% and specificity 94% if applied only to CT grades II and III. Thus, CT can provide a clear indication in many cases of whether to perform hepatic angiography.[233]

Active hemorrhage. CT can often distinguish a pseudoaneurysm from intraparenchymal extravasation

(Figs. 6-81 and 6-82; see Fig. 6-19) by comparing the appearance of the lesion during peak arterial enhancement and delayed "washout" imaging (renal collecting system phase). Pseudoaneurysms will show a more or less complete washout of contrast, whereas parenchymal contrast staining from local tissue extravasation will persist and may be seen to increase in quantity on the delayed scan. Studies performed at our institution to determine the value of contrast-enhanced conventional CT in

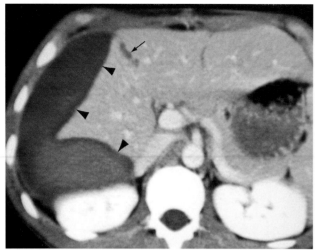

Fig. 6-65
Mixed-density subcapsular hematoma. Conventional CT image shows a large mixed-density 10-day-old subcapsular hematoma (*arrowheads*) with significant mass effect on normal liver parenchyma. A liver laceration (*arrow*) is also seen.

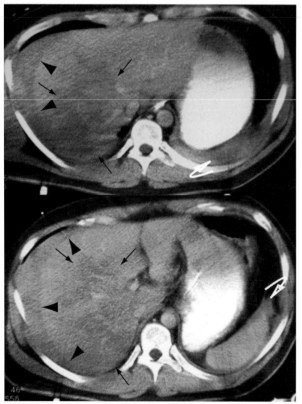

Fig. 6-66
Isodense subcapsular hematoma. Helical CT images show a moderate size isodense subcapsular hematoma (*arrowheads*) along anterolateral aspect of right lobe of liver. A right lobe low-attenuation hepatic contusion (*arrows*) is also seen in right lobe. Free intraperitoneal fluid (*curved arrow*) is seen in left upper abdomen.

detecting active hemorrhage found that CT showed the exact location of bleeding, helping to direct appropriate management.[130] Two of three patients who had evidence of active hepatic bleeding by conventional CT were found to be hemorrhaging at the time of angiographic embolization or ligation of the hepatic artery to control hemorrhage.[130] The third patient required multiple transfusions to maintain a near normal hematocrit. Studies performed by Fang et al.[267,268] using single-slice helical CT demonstrated that the presence of hepatic and intraperitoneal bleeding or parenchymal contrast extravasation with hemoperitoneum on CT had a significant correlation with rapid hemodynamic deterioration and need for surgical intervention. However, in the same study, patients who had only parenchymal contrast extravasation without hemoperitoneum (intact Glisson's capsule) remained hemodynamically stable and two out of three of these patients had no bleeding on hepatic arteriography.

Multiple studies and case reports have shown that hepatic arteriography is technically safe to perform, usually controls hepatic hemorrhage, and improves the success rate of nonoperative management of liver injury.[248-250,269-273] Schwartz et al.[269] reported their 11-year experience of embolization for controlling hemorrhage from hepatic injuries. They found this technique to be safe and effective in 21 of the 24 study patients. Angiographic embolization can be performed independently or as an adjunct to surgery. Follow-up CT is useful to assess the liver after surgical or angiographic intervention. Extravasated contrast from a prior angiographic study can mimic active hemorrhage on CT performed in this setting; therefore, it is important to perform both pre- and postcontrast CTs to distinguish previously extravasated angiographic contrast from current hepatic bleeding (Fig. 6-83). Liver lesions that could possibly mimic active bleeding on CT, other than retained extravasated arteriographic contrast, mainly include contrast enhancement seen in hepatic hemangiomas or other vascular tumors (Figs. 6-84 and 6-85). Other signs of hepatic trauma essentially always accompany bleeding of traumatic origin, but hemorrhage from vascularized hepatic tumors induced by trauma should also be considered.

Periportal low density. Periportal low density refers to regions of low attenuation that parallel the portal vein and its branches on CT (Figs. 6-86 and 6-87). This CT finding has been noted in several nontraumatic clinical conditions, such as acute transplant rejection, malignant neoplasm of the liver, liver transplantation, cardiac failure, and cardiac tamponade, and is usually attributed to dilation of the intrahepatic lymphatics from obstruction to the normal hepatic lymphatic drainage. Periportal low density seen alone in blunt trauma victims was attributed to hemorrhage tracking along the periportal connective

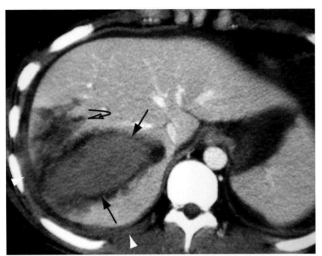

Fig. 6-67
Hepatic hematoma and lacerations in a 21-year-old man admitted after blunt trauma. Helical CT image shows a large hematoma (*arrows*) in right lobe of liver. Multiple lacerations (*curved arrow*) are seen adjacent to hematoma. A small amount of perihepatic clotted blood (*arrowheads*) is also seen.

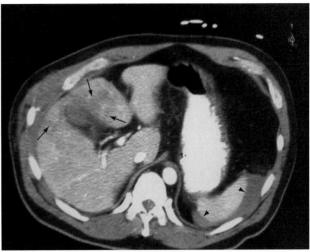

Fig. 6-69
Hepatic contusions in patient admitted after blunt force trauma. Multislice CT image shows contusions in both right and left lobes of liver adjacent to gallbladder fossa. Free intraperitoneal blood (*arrowheads*) is seen next to spleen.

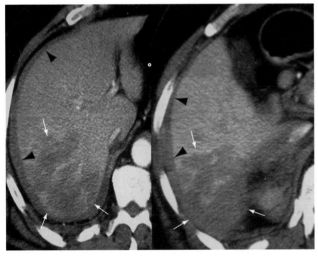

Fig. 6-68
Hepatic contusions in 71-year-old patient admitted after blunt force trauma. Multislice helical CT images show hepatic contusion as a poorly defined area of low attenuation (*arrows*) within right lobe of liver. Small amount of blood (*arrowheads*) is seen around liver.

tissues and was believed to represent an important, if subtle, CT sign of liver injury.[274,275] Macrander et al.[274] reported that periportal low density was seen on CT in 62% of patients and was indicative of liver injury. A study performed to determine the significance of periportal tracking in the liver on CT by Yokota et al.[275] reported that periportal tracking had a significant association with extrahepatic injuries beneath the liver and delayed complications, such as bile leak, hemobilia, and infected hematomas. However, studies performed by

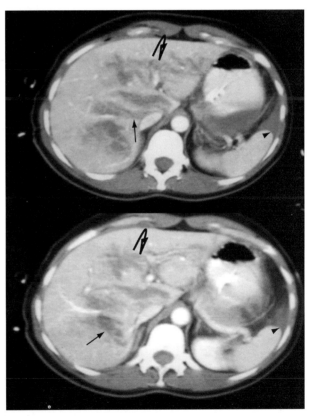

Fig. 6-70
"Bear claw" liver laceration. Helical CT images in a 39-year-old woman admitted after motor vehicle collision show multiple parallel lacerations in right and left lobes of liver. Lacerations extended into region of porta hepatis (*curved arrows*), inferior vena cava, and right hepatic vein (*arrows*). Minimal amount of free intraperitoneal blood (*arrowheads*) is seen next to spleen.

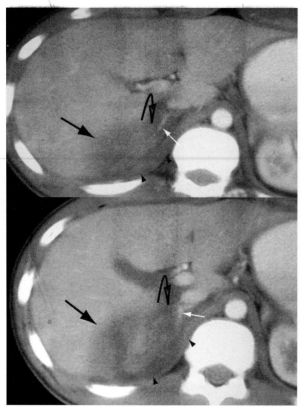

Fig. 6-71
"Bare area" liver injuries. Helical CT images show a contusion (*black arrows*) of "bare area" with retroperitoneal blood in posterior pararenal space (*arrowheads*), perinephric space (*curved arrows*), and surrounding right adrenal gland (*white arrow*). No free intraperitoneal blood was seen on other CT images.

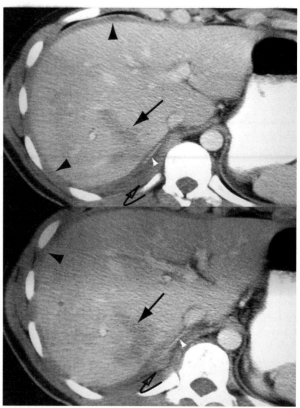

Fig. 6-72
"Bare area" liver injuries. Multislice helical CT images show lacerations (*arrows*) in bare area with retroperitoneal blood (*curved arrows*) around right adrenal gland (*white arrowheads*) and minimal amount of free intraperitoneal blood (*black arrowheads*).

Shanmuganathan et al.[276] in adult blunt hepatic injury patients and Patrick et al.[277] in children with blunt abdominal trauma suggest that periportal low density without parenchymal liver injury occurs as a result of an elevated central venous pressure (CVP). This elevation results from vigorous intravenous fluid administration before obtaining CT or from other trauma-related causes of elevated CVP, such as tension pneumothorax (Fig. 6-88) or pericardial tamponade (Fig. 6-89), that result in distention of the periportal lymphatic vessels.[276,277] At our institution, periportal low density seen on CT without evidence of parenchymal liver injury is not considered to represent hepatic injury and does not warrant hospital admission for observation or follow-up CT. Focal periportal low density seen in close proximity to a liver laceration may represent some focal hemorrhage dissecting into adjacent portal tracts.

CT grade, hepatic angiography, and outcome of blunt hepatic trauma. A retrospective study performed by Poletti et al.[233] at the UMSTC reviewed the contrast-enhanced

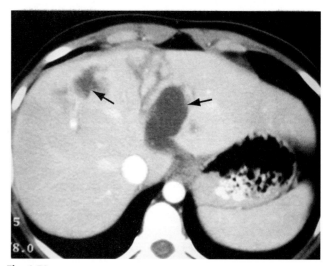

Fig. 6-73
Healing liver laceration. Conventional CT image 7 days after blunt force trauma shows healing lacerations with rounded margins in right and left lobes of liver.

single-slice helical CT and hepatic arteriographic findings for 72 patients with blunt hepatic trauma. Results of the CT and angiographic studies were compared as to management approach, surgical results, morbidity, and

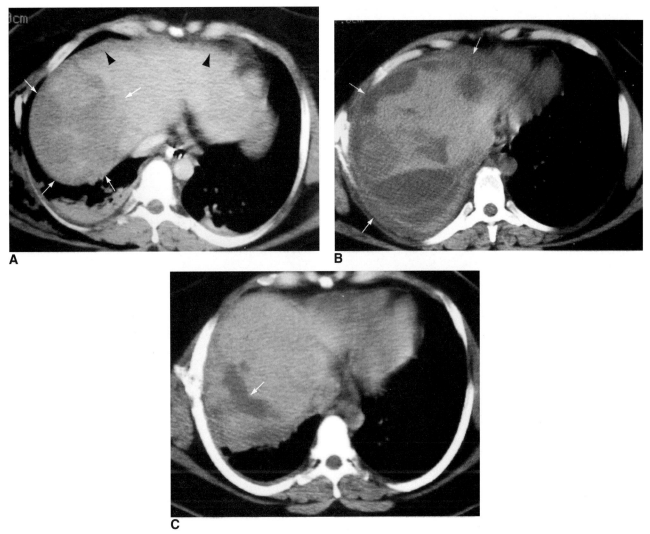

Fig. 6-74
Healing liver injury in 31-year-old woman admitted after motor vehicle collision. **A**, Admission conventional CT image shows a large area of contusion (*arrows*) in dome of liver with intraperitoneal blood (*arrowheads*) anterior to liver. **B**, Follow-up CT 4 weeks after admission shows multiple rounded low-attenuation areas (*arrows*) in area of healing, representing seroma-biloma. **C**, Follow-up CT 8 weeks after admission shows a residual small, well-defined area of low attenuation (*arrow*) in dome of right lobe.

mortality. The 72 admission CT studies were graded for extent of hepatic injury, using the classification of Mirvis et al. (Table 6-7). Because all patients selected for this study also had hepatic angiography, the overall CT injury grade was selectively *biased toward higher injury grades.* There were 8 grade II, 34 grade III, 29 grade IV, and 1 grade V liver injuries.

Active bleeding or pseudoaneurysm was diagnosed on CT in 22 patients. As noted above, using hepatic angiography (the reference standard), CT was 69% sensitive and 86% specific for diagnosing all hepatic arterial injury. When limited only to grade II and III injuries CT sensitivity was 100% and specificity was 94% with a positive

predictive value of 67% and negative predictive value of 100%. Involvement of one or more major hepatic veins in the injury was associated with an increased likelihood of a falsely negative CT interpretation for vascular injury, with an increased chance for recurrent postoperative hepatic hemorrhage, an increase in delayed hepatic-based complications, and an increased failure of nonoperative treatment (see Fig. 6-82). Speculatively, the false-negative CT result for arterial injury might indicate a venous origin to delayed hepatic bleeding not seen on the CT. Based on these findings hepatic arteriography was indicated for all patients with direct CT evidence of vascular injury (active bleed or pseudoaneurysm) and for patients with

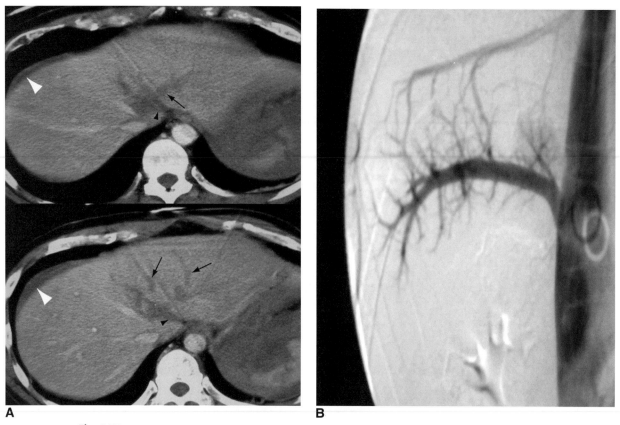

A **B**

Fig. 6-75
Hepatic vein thrombosis in a 36-year-old man admitted after motor vehicle collision. **A**, Helical CT images show a deep laceration (*arrowheads*) extending into region of left hepatic vein. Left hepatic vein and its branches (*arrows*) are not opacified as a result of thrombosis. Middle and right hepatic veins are normal. **B**, Hepatic venogram shows normal right hepatic vein. Left hepatic vein could not be cannulated or opacified by reflux of intravenous contrast material when inferior vena cavogram was performed.

CT grades IV and V, especially if associated with an injury involving a major hepatic vein. Clear management recommendations for patients with CT grades I, II, and III injuries associated with hepatic vein involvement and CT grade IV without hepatic venous involvement could not be ascertained based on the limited patient population. Interestingly, no correlation was found between liver injuries extending into the porta hepatis region, inferior vena cava, or gallbladder fossa and hepatic-related complications or ultimate outcome.

At the UMSTC patients with CT evidence of active hepatic hemorrhage or high-grade liver injury (grades III to V using the Mirvis classification) who do not promptly respond to intravenous fluid resuscitation are referred for urgent surgery or angiographic study, depending on the total injury complex.

Gallbladder Injury. Gallbladder injury after blunt abdominal trauma is uncommon with a reported incidence in the surgical literature of 2% to 8%.[278-289] In a review of 31 patients who sustained blunt gallbladder trauma, Soderstrom et al.[278] reported only one (3.2%) of the 31 patients had an isolated injury to the gallbladder. Possible predisposing factors contributing to gallbladder rupture include alcohol ingestion, causing an increased tone of the sphincter of Oddi and a normal but distended gallbladder.[284] Paradoxically, chronic cholecystitis leading to fibrosis of the gallbladder wall makes it somewhat less prone to rupture during blunt abdominal impact.[282]

Mechanisms proposed to cause gallbladder injury in blunt trauma include a direct blow resulting in rupture of a normal gallbladder, or an avulsion injury of the gallbladder from the gallbladder fossa due to shear stress resulting from deceleration forces. Sudden compression of a distended gallbladder at impact may also produce the injury. Gallbladder injuries are classified as contusion, laceration or perforation, and avulsion.[289] Contusions of the gallbladder are the most common injury after blunt trauma. Avulsion injuries are second most common with the gallbladder being partially or

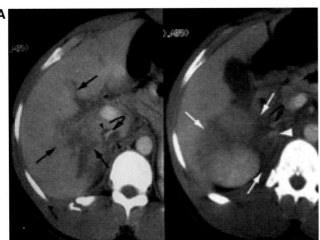

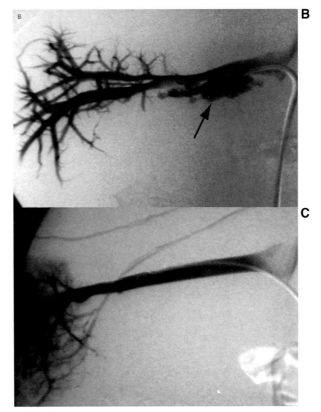

Fig. 6-76
Retrohepatic vena caval injury in a 26-year-old man admitted after a crush injury. **A,** Helical CT images show liver in right lobe lacerations (*black arrows*) with extension into area around IVC (*curved arrow*) and porta hepatis. Active bleeding (*white arrowhead*) is seen in retroperitoneum posterior to inferior vena cava. Intraperitoneal and retroperitoneal blood (*white arrows*) are seen inferior and posterior to liver. Blood (*black arrowheads*) is seen around intrahepatic vena cava as well. **B,** Hepatic venogram shows extravasation of contrast material (*arrow*) from a hepatic vein injury corresponding to area of active bleeding seen on CT. **C,** Hepatic venogram after stenting of injured hepatic vein shows no extravasation of contrast material.

completely torn from the gallbladder fossa. Concurrent intraabdominal injuries are very common, seen in 92% to 100% of patients; these injuries involve the liver (83%), duodenum (57%), and pancreas (17%).[283,286] Fortunately, however, associated injury to the intrahepatic or common bile duct is uncommon.[286,288] The diagnosis of traumatic gallbladder injury is typically made incidentally at laparotomy performed for associated injuries or is delayed until the onset of complications such as bile peritonitis.[283,288,289]

The diagnosis of gallbladder injury was rarely made preoperatively before the general availability of CT and sonographic imaging. Except for occasional case reports, only two series describe the CT findings of gallbladder injury secondary to blunt trauma.[281,287] The CT findings associated with gallbladder injury include an ill-defined or irregular wall contour, pericholecystic or subserosal fluid, nondistended or collapsed lumen (Fig. 6-90), wall thickening (Fig. 6-91), mass effect on the adjacent duo-

denum, and high-density intraluminal blood (Fig. 6-92). No combination of CT signs has been reported to be specific for the type of gallbladder injury. Other CT findings that may indicate gallbladder injury are a free mucosal flap projecting into the lumen, contrast enhancement of the gallbladder wall or mucosa (see Fig. 6-91), free intraperitoneal fluid isodense with bile (see Fig. 6-24), and apparent displacement of the gallbladder toward the midline.[290]

Bile Duct Injury. Injuries to the intrahepatic and extrahepatic bile ducts are uncommon injuries after blunt trauma.[291-300] Such injuries may be underestimated and may occur in up to 9% of patients with severe liver injury who are candidates for nonoperative management.[295] Transection of the extrahepatic bile duct (Fig. 6-93) most commonly occurs distally at a fixed point at the entrance of the common bile duct into the head of the pancreas.[292,297] Experimental studies by Fletcher et al.[300]

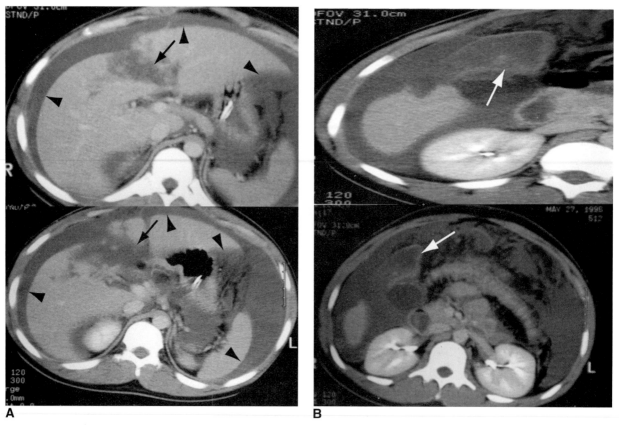

Fig. 6-77
Hepatic devascularization after blunt abdominal injuries. **A,** Admission helical CT images in a 17-year-old patient show a deep liver laceration (*arrows*) extending into region of porta hepatis. A large amount of free intraperitoneal blood (*arrowheads*) is seen in upper abdomen. Patient was managed nonoperatively. **B,** Follow-up CT images 5 days after admission show an area liver parenchyma (*arrows*) that does not enhance as the normal liver parenchyma as a result of infarction.

suggest that a simultaneous shearing force applied to the common bile duct, rapid emptying of gallbladder, and a short cystic duct are three factors essential to cause this injury. The more elastic and tortuous hepatic artery and the straight portal vein with no valves, though subjected to the same shearing force, more often escape injury.[292]

No clear correlation has been demonstrated between the hepatic parenchymal injury pattern seen on CT and intrahepatic bile duct injury[233,295] (Fig. 6-94). Intrahepatic bile duct injuries generally occur adjacent to the hilum.[297] Injuries to the first and second order intrahepatic bile ducts can result in serious complications.[299] Two distinct types of presentation of bile duct injuries have been described.[291,295,298] In the first type, other visceral injuries are diagnosed by CT, DPL, or sonography with no relevant findings to suggest a bile duct injury. Careful inspection of the hepatoduodenal ligament or lesser sac for bile staining at surgery may help diagnose a ductal injury. The second type is an isolated injury to the extrahepatic bile duct with no clinical symptoms.

Diagnosis and treatment are delayed until the chronic phase (see Fig. 6-93), when there is abdominal distention, jaundice, anorexia, and abdominal discomfort from biliary ascites. Endoscopic retrograde cholangiopancreatography (ERCP) has been useful in diagnosing and treating biliary duct injuries that persistently leak.[293,295] CT and ERCP were performed in 28 patients with blunt hepatic injury selected for nonoperative management by Sugimoto et al.,[249] and intrahepatic bile duct injuries were diagnosed in 21% (6/28) of them. CT scans only confirmed the location of liver injury. Five patients developed bilomas that were detected on follow-up CT.

Complications of Hepatic and Biliary Duct Injury. In general, complications of hepatic trauma are more common after surgical intervention, in patients with a high injury severity score (ISS), or among patients with severe hepatic injuries selected for nonoperative management.*

---

*References 19, 219, 233, 236, 239, 243, 245, 299, 301.

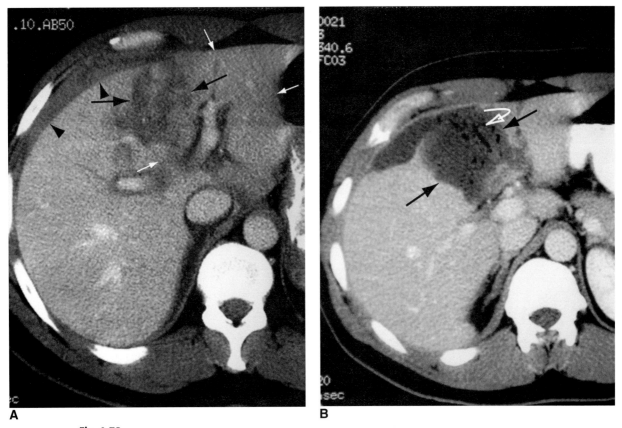

Fig. 6-78
Hepatic devascularization after blunt abdominal injuries. **A,** Admission helical CT image shows an area of low attenuation (*white arrows*) and deep lacerations (*black arrows*) involving left lobe of liver. Perihepatic intraperitoneal hematoma (*arrowheads*) is also seen. **B,** Follow-up CT image after angiography and embolization of a hepatic arterial injury shows liver necrosis (*arrows*) and intra-parenchymal air (*curved arrow*). Etiology of liver necrosis could be attributed to embolization or deep liver lacerations injuring dual hepatic blood supply.

About 11% to 24% of patients with hepatic injuries after blunt trauma develop nonfatal complications. Complications seen after blunt hepatic trauma include infection, delayed hemorrhage, biloma, biliary fistula, biliary ascites, and hemobilia. An increasing reliance has been placed on imaging techniques and endoscopic retrograde cholangiopancreatography to diagnose and treat late complications of major liver injuries.[293,295,299,302] CT can diagnose complications arising from liver trauma, monitor progression or resolution, and guide percutaneous drainage as an alternative to surgical management for a variety of complications of blunt hepatic trauma.[219,273,299] Carrillo et al.[273] performed a study of 135 patients with blunt hepatic trauma, of whom complications occurred in 24% (32/135). Of the patients with complications 6% (2/32) had grade III injury, 56% (18) grade IV injury, and 38% (12) grade V injury. Early and delayed hemorrhage requiring arteriography and

embolization developed in 37% (12). Perihepatic collections were seen in 31% (10), including five infected and five noninfected that were drained percutaneously by CT. Endoscopic sphincterotomy and endobiliary stenting were performed in 25% (8). In all, nonoperative interventional procedures were adequate to treat 85% (27) of the complications that developed in this population.

Infection. Blunt hepatic trauma is the third leading cause of hepatic abscess formation.[255] Olsen[303] observed that factors predisposing to liver abscess include capsular laceration, inadequate debridement of necrotic liver tissue, poor external drainage of deep hepatic hematomas, and drain tract contamination of hepatic wounds. Organisms seed the hematoma directly from the biliary system or via a hematogenous route. A higher incidence of liver abscess has been reported for patients managed operatively than nonoperatively.[19,236] Clinical

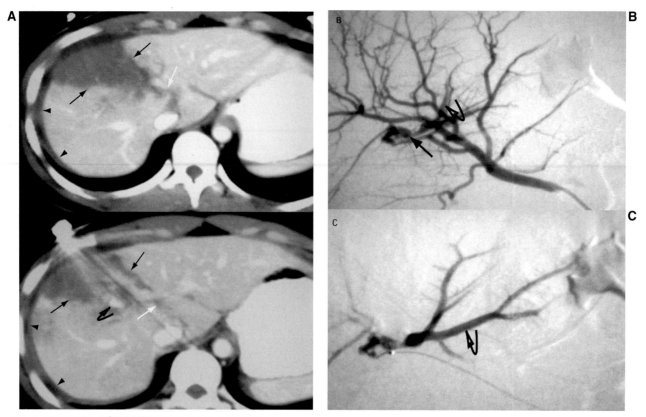

Fig. 6-79
Hepatic pseudoaneurysm and arteriovenous fistula in a 24-year-old woman admitted after motor vehicle collision. **A,** Helical CT images show a wedge-shaped area of nonperfusion in right lobe of liver (*black arrows*). An area of extravasated contrast material (*curved arrow*) is seen within this region. Adjacent liver lacerations (*white arrow*) and free intraperitoneal blood (*arrowheads*) are also seen. **B,** Selective right hepatic arteriogram shows a pseudoaneurysm (*arrow*) and early filling of a hepatic venous branch (*curved arrow*). **C,** Delayed images from hepatic arteriogram confirm an arteriohepatic venous fistula (*curved arrow*). Transcatheter embolization was performed to treat these two lesions.

presentation of hepatic abscess includes abdominal pain and tenderness, fever, and leukocytosis.

Hepatic abscess or subcapsular empyema is recognized on CT as a focal collection of fluid of near-fluid attenuation. Occasionally hepatic abscess may contain gas bubbles within it (Fig. 6-95) or be surrounded by a low-attenuation halo of edematous hepatic parenchyma. Depending on the age or prior treatment with antibiotics an enhancing wall may also be observed. Intrahepatic air has been described within an avulsed portion of liver resulting from ischemia that may mimic infection.[304] No CT findings described are specific for hepatic abscess, and the final diagnosis must depend on the clinical presentation of the patient and confirmed by percutaneous needle aspiration, drainage, or surgery.

Delayed hemorrhage. Delayed hemorrhage from liver injury requiring surgical or angiographic intervention (Fig. 6-96) is an uncommon complication in patients who are initially hemodynamically stable on admission and conservatively managed.[13,27,66] Delayed hepatic bleeding occurs in about 3% of patients initially managed nonoperatively within 2 to 4 days of admission.[16,19,59,233,299] Patcher et al.[246] described a multicenter study of 404 patients who sustained blunt hepatic trauma and were treated nonoperatively. Among this group 21 complications developed, including 14 patients with persistent bleeding, 3 with perihepatic abscesses, 2 with bilomas, and 2 with intestinal injuries. Six of the 14 patients with hepatic hemorrhage were managed with transfusions alone, four required angiographic embolization, and one patient was further observed without transfusion. Risk factors that increase the likelihood of delayed hemorrhage include severe initial hepatic injury, concurrent injury to other organs, and coagulopathy.

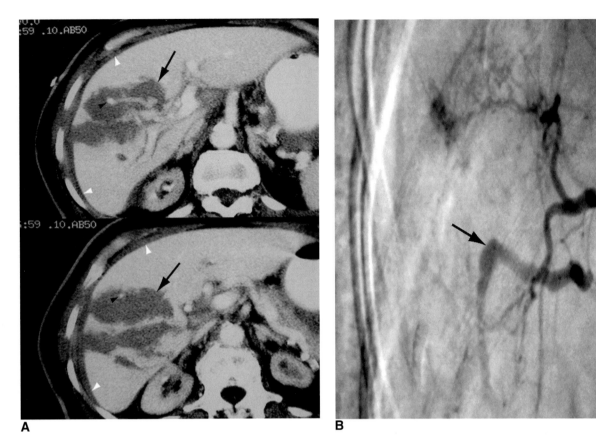

A **B**

Fig. 6-80
Arterioportal fistula of liver in a 66-year-old woman admitted after blunt injury. **A,** Helical CT images show a grade IV liver injury (*arrow*) with a well-defined area of high-density contrast material (*black arrowheads*) seen within the area of injury on multiple images, suggestive of a hepatic vascular injury. Small amount of free intraperitoneal blood (*white arrowheads*) is also seen. **B,** Delayed image obtained in the late phase of a selective right hepatic arteriogram shows arterioportal fistula (*arrow*). Transcatheter embolization was performed to treat this lesion.

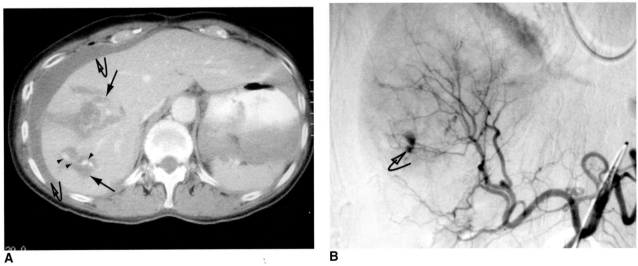

A **B**

Fig. 6-81
Active hemorrhage in liver of a 70-year-old woman involved in a motor vehicle collision. **A,** Admission helical CT image shows multiple lacerations (*arrows*) with active bleeding (*arrowheads*). A moderate amount of hemoperitoneum (*curved arrows*) is seen lateral to right lobe of liver. **B,** Hepatic arteriography confirms active bleeding (*curved arrow*) seen on CT. Transcatheter embolization was performed to manage hemorrhage.

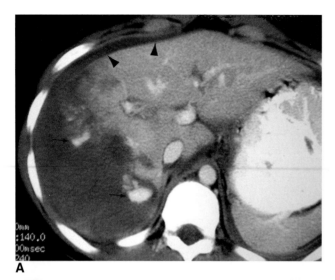

A

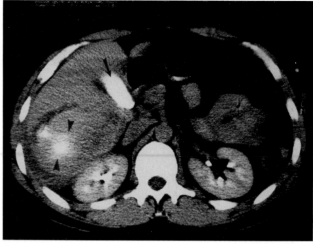

Fig. 6-83
Extravasation of intravenous contrast material from angiography. CT image postembolization of active bleeding liver for fall in hematocrit shows high-density intraparenchymal contrast (*arrowheads*) extravasation from prior hepatic arteriograms within resolving hepatic hematoma. Vicarious contrast excretion is seen within gallbladder (*arrow*).

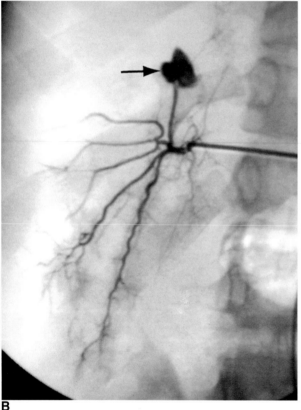

B

Fig. 6-82
Active bleeding in a 17-year-old girl admitted after a motor vehicle collision. **A**, Helical CT image shows two sites of active bleeding (*arrows*) in large right lobe hematoma. Hemoperitoneum (*arrowheads*) is present anterior to liver. **B**, Selective right hepatic arteriogram confirms active bleeding (*arrow*). After embolization of hepatic artery the patient required laparotomy to control hepatic bleeding. (From Poletti PA, Mirvis SE, Shanmuganathan K, et al: *Radiology* 216:418, 2000.)

Traumatic Budd-Chiari syndrome. A large quantity of hemorrhage into liver lacerations, and subcapsular or intraparenchymal hematomas can cause compression of the hepatic veins and inferior vena cava (Fig. 6-97). A posttraumatic Budd-Chiari syndrome, or one similar to it, can result from the proximity of an expanding hepatic hematoma to the hepatic veins and intrahepatic IVC leading to obstruction.[258] CT findings of posttraumatic Budd-Chiari syndrome include a large intrahepatic or subcapsular hepatic hematoma, nonvisualization or narrowing of one or more hepatic veins, compression or nonvisualization of the intrahepatic IVC, and accumulation of low-attenuation (6 to 15 HU) ascites. A slowly expanding hematoma confined by the hepatic capsule may lead to the gradual development of traumatic Budd-Chiari without presenting as an acute major blood loss.

Biloma and Bile Peritonitis. Transection of the intrahepatic biliary radicles is more likely to occur after high-grade liver injury. Interestingly, no correlation was found in a recent study between blunt liver injuries extending into the porta hepatis region, IVC, or gallbladder fossa and hepatic-related complications, including biloma.[233,295] Injuries to the extrahepatic or first or second order intrahepatic bile ducts are likely to result in serious complications such as biloma (Figs. 6-98 and 6-99), biliary fistula, bile peritonitis, and bile ascites.[295,299] A 2% to 8% incidence of biloma or biliary fistula has been reported after hepatic trauma.[293,305-307] Most bilomas are asymptomatic and serendipitously diagnosed, but if symptomatic, present with abdominal distention, pain and tenderness, fever, jaundice, or anorexia. As a result of the slow rate of bile leak, in most patients the

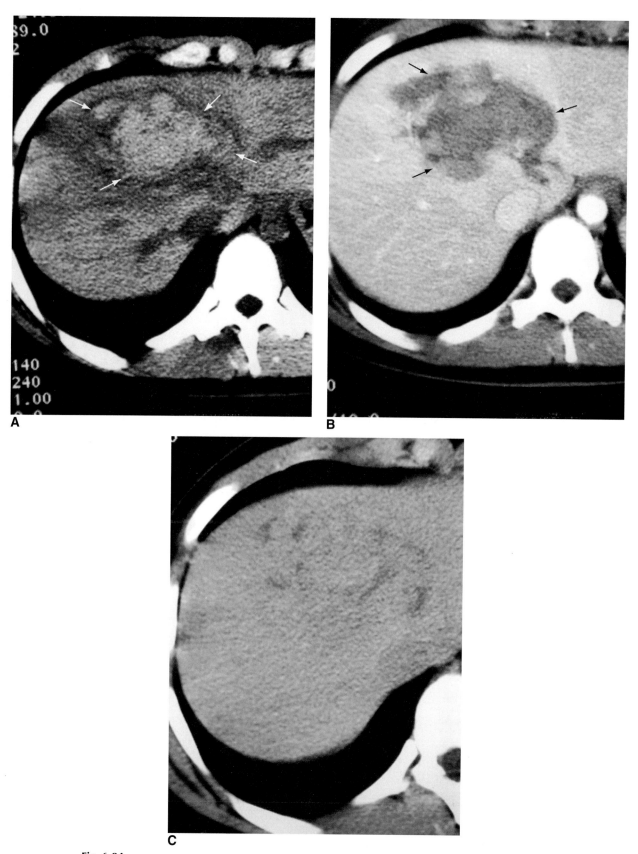

Fig. 6-84
Hemangioma of liver mimicking liver injury. **A,** Noncontrast helical CT image compared with normal liver parenchyma shows a large hyperdense area (*arrows*) in anterolateral aspect of liver. **B,** Postcontrast image shows a low-attenuation region (*arrows*) mimicking a hematoma or laceration of liver. **C,** Delayed images 5 minutes after injection of intravenous contrast material show filling in of this lesion with contrast. Lesion is isodense with normal liver parenchyma. Tc 99ᵐ red cell labeled isotope study of liver (not shown) confirmed this lesion was a liver hemangioma.

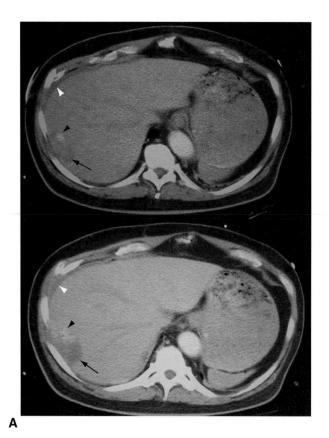
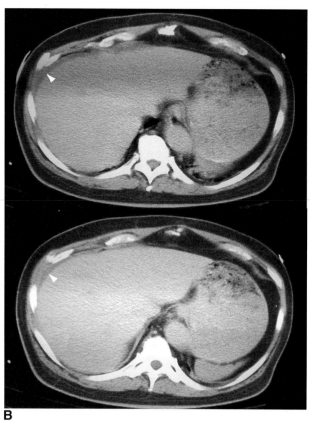

Fig. 6-85

Hemangioma of liver mimicking active bleeding. **A,** Postcontrast multislice CT images show a low-attenuation area (*arrows*) in lateral right lobe of liver with peripheral nodular enhancement (*black arrowheads*). Minimal amount of perihepatic fluid (*white arrowhead*) is seen. **B,** Delayed images in the renal excretory phase show a lesion isodense to normal liver parenchyma. CT findings are compatible with a hemangioma.

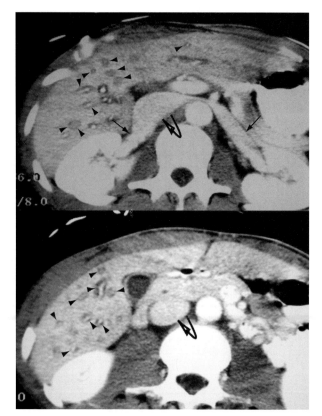

Fig. 6-86

Diffuse periportal edema from vigorous fluid resuscitation in a blunt trauma patient. Helical CT images show a large IVC (*curved arrow*), distended renal veins (*arrows*), and low-attenuation areas (*arrowheads*) paralleling the portal vein and its branches, which are related to vigorous fluid resuscitation before obtaining CT. No liver lacerations were seen on other CT images.

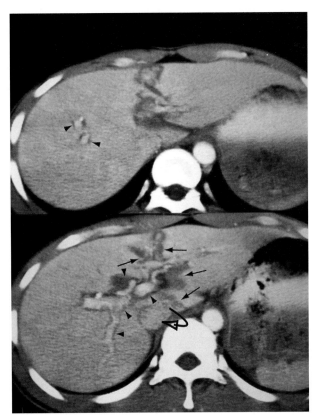

Fig. 6-87
Acute liver lacerations with periportal low density in a patient admitted after blunt trauma. Admission helical CT images show a jagged branching liver laceration (*arrows*) involving the left lobe of the liver. Laceration extends into porta hepatis and caudate lobe. The IVC (*curved arrow*) is distended from vigorous fluid resuscitation. Diffuse periportal edema (*arrowheads*) is seen from distention of intrahepatic lymphatics.

diagnosis of intrahepatic biloma is delayed until weeks to months after the initial trauma.[293,295,298,299,308]

CT findings of posttraumatic intrahepatic biloma or biliary cyst include a low-attenuation collection in or around the liver. A persistent and echo free well-defined collection seen in the clinical setting of hepatic trauma on sonography strongly suggests the diagnosis of biloma.[309] Bilomas may contain a small amount of debris or have a few septations. CT and sonographic signs of biloma are, however, nonspecific, as these findings may also be seen with resolving hematomas and abscess. Percutaneous CT or sonographically guided aspiration or accumulation of activity during hepatobiliary scintigraphy within the suspected collection is needed to confirm the diagnosis of biloma in symptomatic patients.[306]

Surgical repair of persistent biliary fistula after blunt liver injuries often is technically very difficult. Attempts have been made to treat these injuries less invasively with endoscopy with sphincterotomy and endobiliary stenting of the right or left hepatic duct to permit prompt closure of

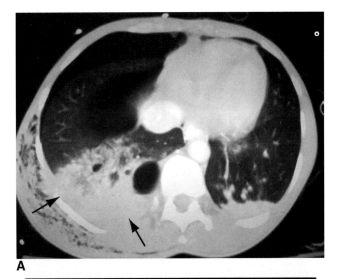

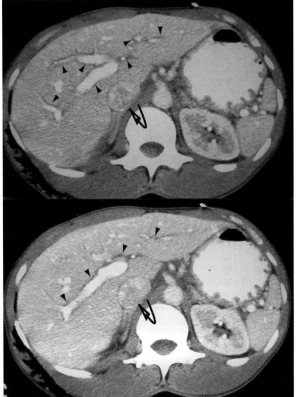

Fig. 6-88
Periportal lymphedema resulting from tension pneumothorax in a patient admitted after chest and abdominal trauma. **A,** Multislice helical CT image in lower chest shows right lung lacerations and contusions (*arrows*). A large inferior pneumothorax is seen with shift of mediastinum to left side. **B,** Images in upper abdomen show a distended IVC (*curved arrows*) with its transverse diameter twice the transverse diameter of abdominal aorta. Periportal low density is seen diffusely throughout the liver paralleling portal vein and its branches (*arrowheads*) as a result of high central venous pressure.

the biliary leak.[273,293,299,308] Sugiyama et al.[293] treated five patients with biliary endoscopic stenting for biliary fistula, none of whom required balloon dilation of the

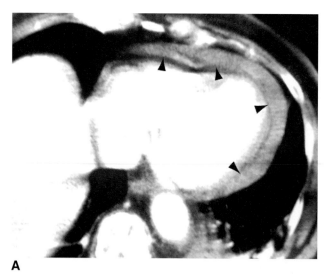

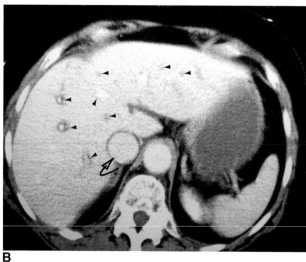

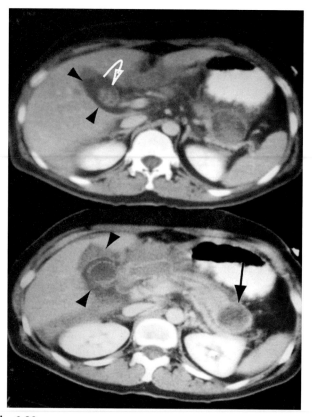

Fig. 6-90
Avulsion of gallbladder in a patient admitted after a motor vehicle collision. CT images show low-attenuation pericholecystic fluid (*arrowheads*), deformity of gallbladder (*curved arrow*), and pancreatic fluid collection (*arrows*). At surgery partial avulsion of gallbladder from gallbladder fossa resulted in cholecystectomy. (From Erb RE, Mirvis SE, Shanmuganathan K: *J Comput Assist Tomogr* 18:778, 1994.)

Fig. 6-89
Periportal lymphedema related to pericardial tamponade **A**, Helical CT image shows a high-density pericardial effusion (*arrowheads*). **B**, CT image shows diffuse periportal edema in liver as low-attenuation areas (*arrowheads*) paralleling portal vein and its branches from high central venous pressure as a result of pericardial tamponade. IVC (*curved arrow*) is also distended.

injured bile duct before stent and none of whom had late complications.

Although bile promotes bacterial infection, sterile bile itself causes minimal irritation of the peritoneum. Bile peritonitis is an uncommon complication seen after blunt hepatic trauma. The most likely source of intraperitoneal bile leak is injury to the intrahepatic bile ducts. Rupture of the extrahepatic bile ducts and gallbladder are other sources for intraperitoneal bile leak, but are uncommon injuries. The clinical signs and symptoms of biliary peritonitis include abdominal pain, nausea, and emesis. These signs may evolve gradually, making diagnosis difficult and leading to increased morbidity or mortality.

Findings on contrast-enhanced CT (CECT) suggest that indications for a diagnosis of biliary peritonitis are persistence or increasing amounts of low-attenuation free fluid in the peritoneal cavity and thickening of the peritoneal membrane that shows evidence of contrast enhancement. Bile peritonitis can be confirmed by diagnostic aspiration of bile from the peritoneum under sonographic or CT guidance. Laparoscopic irrigation of the peritoneal cavity, drainage of intraperitoneal collections, and perihepatic drain placement have been used to treat biliary peritonitis.[273]

Hemobilia. Communication between the hepatic arterial and biliary system results in hemobilia, an unusual complication of liver injury. At times the bleeding may arise directly from the gallbladder. The classical clinical triad of hemobilia is colicky abdominal pain, jaundice, and upper or lower gastrointestinal bleeding. Endoscopic visualization of bleeding from the ampulla of Vater or hepatic angiography can confirm the diagnosis. Although the standard treatment of hemobilia has been surgical ligation of the bleeding artery or hepatic resection, such treatment is associated with a high operative morbidity and mortality.[273,307] Selective embolization has been

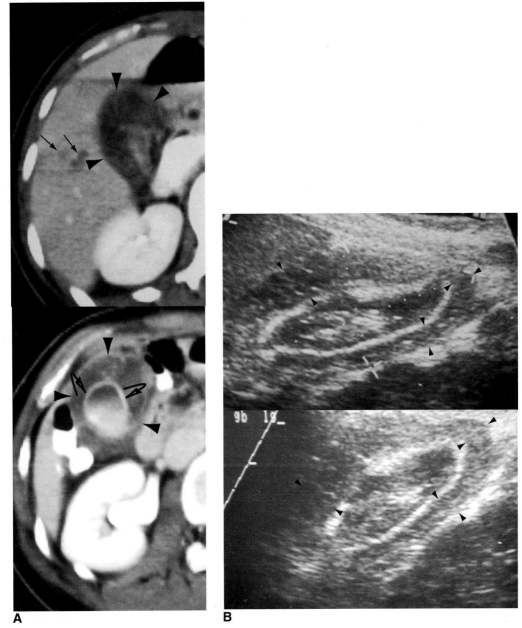

Fig. 6-91
Gallbladder wall contusion in a patient admitted after motor vehicle collision. **A,** CT images show diffuse thickening of gallbladder wall (*arrowheads*) with enhancement of mucosa (*curved arrows*). Liver lacerations (*arrows*) are seen adjacent to gallbladder fossa. **B,** Longitudinal ultrasound images of gallbladder after CT confirm diffuse gallbladder wall thickening (*arrowheads*). Patient was managed successfully without surgical intervention.

found to be an effective and safe treatment for patients with hemobilia.[310] On CT, hemobilia may cause mixed or uniform high-attenuation blood within the gallbladder lumen. However, high-density material within the lumen of the gallbladder on CT is seen with gallstones, gallbladder wall hematomas, vicarious excretion of intravenous contrast, biliary sludge, and milk of calcium bile. These entities need to be considered in the differential diagnosis of hemobilia.

Follow-up CT in Hepatic Trauma. CT is accurate in detecting an increase in the amount of intraperitoneal blood or expansion of an intrahepatic hematoma (see Figs. 6-96 and 6-97). Persistence or increase in the volume of hemoperitoneum may indicate ongoing bleeding or an intraperitoneal bile leak (see Figs. 6-93, 6-94, 6-98, and 6-99). The pediatric literature supports a single late follow-up CT at 3 to 6 months to document complete healing of the liver injury.[311,312] However, in the surgical

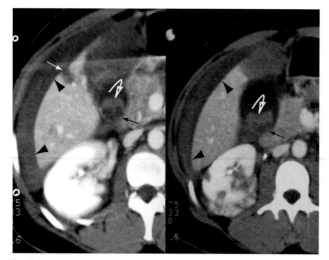

Fig. 6-92
High-density blood within gallbladder lumen in a 33-year-old woman admitted after blunt trauma. Conventional CT images show high-attenuation intraluminal hematoma (*curved arrows*) within gallbladder. Filling defects (*black arrows*) are seen within hematoma due to gallstones. Perihepatic blood (*arrowheads*) and a liver laceration (*white arrow*) adjacent to gallbladder fossa are also seen. Surgery was performed for hemorrhage from grade IV liver injury (not shown). A gallbladder wall contusion was seen at surgery and cholecystectomy was performed.

literature, a routine second CT for nonoperative management of adult blunt hepatic injury appears of limited value. None of the CT scans reported in two studies showed either progression of injury or new CT findings that influenced or changed treatment.[301,313] At the UMSTC a follow-up CT is obtained in blunt liver trauma patients who exhibit an unexplained fall in hematocrit, have persistent abdominal pain, abdominal distention, or jaundice.

Pancreatic Injury. Injuries to the pancreas occur infrequently after trauma. In the United States, though, most pancreatic injuries are associated with penetrating trauma; a third result from nonpenetrating trauma.[314-326] Pancreatic injuries occur in 0.2% to 12% of blunt trauma victims. Isolated injury to the pancreas is rare, but is seen more commonly after blunt trauma.[314] Associated injuries occur frequently and have been reported in 50% to 98% of patients with pancreatic injury[317,320,322] (Figs. 6-100 to 6-102). Motor vehicle collision is the most common mode of injury, and up to 60% of adult pancreatic injuries are caused by impact against the steering wheel.[314] The use of seat belts may also contribute to an increase in the incidence of this injury.[315,327] Other causes of pancreatic

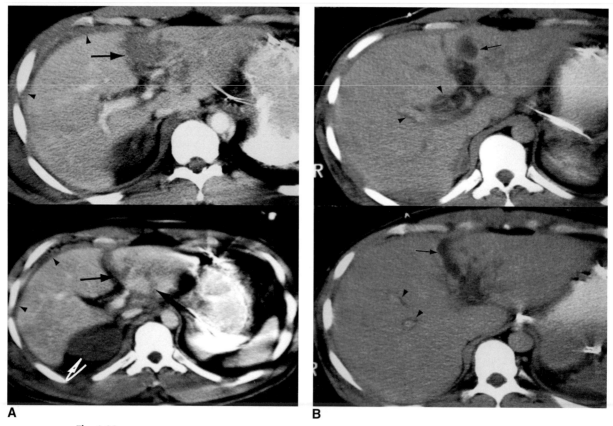

A **B**

Fig. 6-93
Delayed diagnosis of common bile duct injury in a 22-year-old man admitted after blunt force trauma.
A, Admission CT images show deep left lobe liver lacerations (*arrows*) extending into porta hepatis.
Perihepatic blood (*arrowheads*) and an infarcted right kidney (*curved arrow*) are seen.

Continued

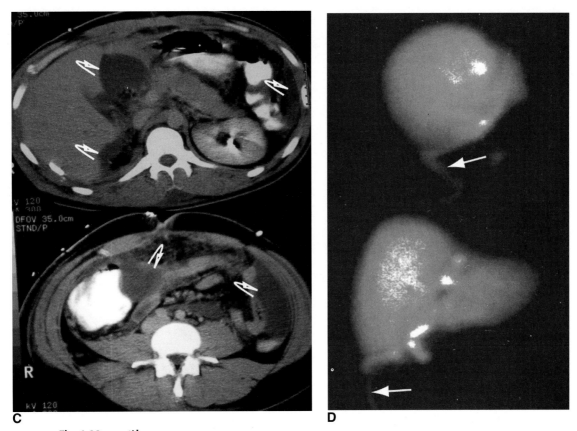

Fig. 6-93, cont'd

B and **C**, Follow-up CT images obtained because of jaundice and abdominal pain 10 days postadmission show intrahepatic bile duct dilation (*arrowheads*) and multiple collections of low-attenuation fluid (*curved arrows*) in peritoneal cavity. Healing liver lacerations (*arrows*) are also seen. These findings are highly suspicious for an injury to biliary tract. **D**, HIDA study shows free intraperitoneal extravasation of isotope (*arrows*) confirming diagnosis of biliary tract injury. At surgery a common bile duct injury was repaired.

injury from blunt trauma include a direct blow to the abdomen or falling across a rigid object with impact to the upper abdomen. At the UMSTC, 32 patients were admitted with blunt pancreatic injury over a 3-year period. Associated injuries occurred to the spleen in 53% (17/32) of patients, to the liver in 47% (15), and to the bowel in 47% (15), including small bowel (n=5), duodenum (n=3), stomach (n=2), and colon (n=5).

A mortality rate as high as 20% has been reported after pancreatic trauma.* Because the pancreas is closely related to a rich anastomosis of major vessels, concurrent vascular injuries are common, and hemorrhage contributes to the high injury mortality (see Figs. 6-100 and 6-102). Mortality may also vary with the location of the injury.[314,326,328] Injuries to the pancreatic head are twice as lethal to the body as injuries to the tail (28% versus 16%). Other factors that contribute to high mortality rate include hemorrhagic shock on admission, delay in treat-

ment, and the number of associate visceral injuries, especially involving the duodenum and colon.[314,325,326]

Mechanism and Classification. Depending on the site of impact of the blunt force in relation to the rigid spine three patterns of pancreatic injury, with other associate injuries to the adjacent viscera, have been observed.[317,322,329] An impacting force acting to the right of the spine results in a crush injury to the head of the pancreas. Crushing or rupture of the duodenum is common with this injury pattern (see Fig. 6-101). Other associate injuries to the liver, common bile duct, transverse mesocolon, gastroduodenal, and right and middle colic arteries, often accompany the pancreatic injury (see Fig. 6-103). Impact to the midline directly compresses the neck of the pancreas over the lumbar spine. This often results in a pancreatic transection to the left of the superior mesenteric vessels. Injuries commonly associated with the midline impact include injuries to stomach, transverse colon, liver (Fig. 6-103), major vessels (see Figs. 6-100 and 6-102), and gallbladder. If the impact acts

---

*References 314, 318, 319, 322, 324, 326.

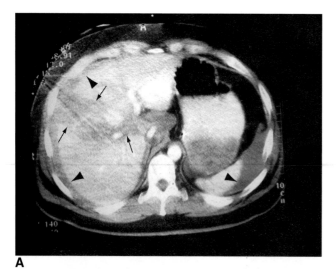

A

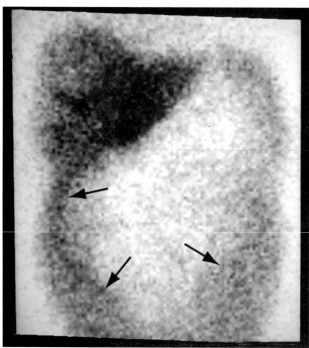

B

Fig. 6-94
Intrahepatic bile duct injury in a patient admitted after blunt trauma.
A, Admission helical CT image shows a grade IV liver laceration
(*arrows*) involving right lobe of liver with perihepatic and
perisplenic blood (*arrowheads*). **B**, HIDA scan performed because
of jaundice and abdominal pain shows extravasation of isotope into
peritoneal cavity. Retrograde cholangiography demonstrated an
injury to proximal right hepatic duct. Endobiliary stent was placed
across the injury.

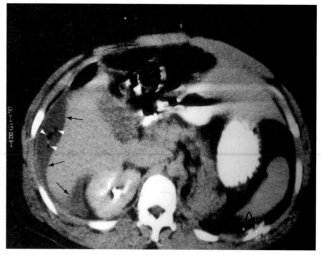

Fig. 6-95
Hepatic abscess with gas bubbles in a patient with elevated white
cell count and fever. Conventional CT image shows subcapsular
fluid collection (*arrows*) with gas bubbles (*arrowheads*). A rib fracture and bullet fragments (*curved arrow*) are seen on contralateral
side. Percutaneous CT-guided drainage of this collection confirmed
infection. (From Shanmuganathan K, Mirvis SE: *Radiol Clin North
Am* 36:399, 1998.)

Lucas[330]: (1) contusion or laceration of pancreas and
intact duct, (2) deep laceration or transection with duct
injury, (3) severe laceration or crush injury to head of the
pancreas, and (4) severe pancreaticoduodenal injuries.

Diagnosis. Clinical diagnosis of pancreatic injury may
be a challenge, especially in an isolated injury.[331,332]
Signs of peritonitis are subtle initially, evolve slowly, and
are less likely to be present on initial presentation, as the
pancreas is a retroperitoneal organ. Symptoms could
even be absent for up to 5 days after complete isolated
transection of the pancreas.[314] The most common findings in the immediate postinjury period after isolated
injury to the pancreas are minimal abdominal pain and
tenderness. These physical findings may decrease in
severity initially, but worsen again within 6 hours.[330]

Pancreatic enzyme levels. Serum and urinary amylase
levels have proven neither sensitive nor specific in diagnosing pancreatic injury.[330,333,334] Serum amylase levels
generally remain normal for 2 to 48 hours after injury
and may be normal in 30% to 35% of patients with pancreatic transection.[318,320,335] However, a rising serum
amylase level on serial serum amylase measurements in a
patient with abdominal tenderness and pain is a better
indicator of pancreatic injury.[330,336] Other causes for a
raised serum amylase level in a blunt trauma patient
include trauma to salivary glands, acute alcohol intake,
bowel infarction, and injury to duodenum, stomach, or
small bowel. Ryan et al.[337] performed a prospective study
in 100 patients admitted consecutively to an intensive

to the left of the spine, laceration or contusion to the
pancreatic tail may occur. This pattern of distal pancreatic
injury is often associated with injuries to spleen, left kidney, stomach, and colon. The type of treatment, morbidity, and mortality depend on the location and severity of
the pancreatic injury and concurrent injuries. Pancreatic
injuries are classified into four levels of severity by

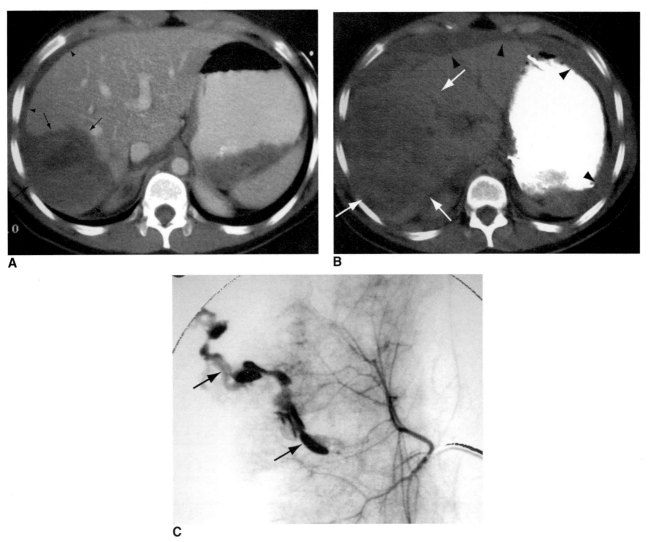

Fig. 6-96
Delayed hemorrhage in a 20-year-old woman admitted after a motor vehicle collision. **A,** Admission CT image shows a right lobe posterior hematoma (*arrows*) and hemoperitoneum (*arrowheads*). **B,** Follow-up CT obtained without intravenous contrast material because of abdominal distention and transient hypotension shows increase in the amount of hemoperitoneum (*arrowheads*) and size of parenchymal hematoma (*arrows*). Liver margins are less well defined. CT findings are consistent with delayed hemorrhage from rupture of a hepatic hematoma. **C,** Selective right hepatic arteriogram after CT shows active bleeding (*arrows*) from a distal branch of right hepatic artery. Transcatheter embolization was performed to control hemorrhage.

care unit to evaluate the natural history and the significance of elevated serum amylase and lipase levels in posttraumatic pancreatitis. At least one elevated pancreatic enzyme level occurred during the first 3 days after ICU admission in 38% (38/100) of patients. Persistent elevation of pancreatic enzyme levels (amylase and lipase levels) were seen in 17% (17) of patients. None of the 17 patients with persistent pancreatic enzyme levels had CT evidence of pancreatitis. Clinical symptoms of pancreatitis and persistent elevation of pancreatic enzymes were present in 29% (5/17) of these patients. In this study sporadic elevation of pancreatic enzyme levels after blunt trauma was not uncommon. The majority of patients

with persistent elevation of pancreatic enzyme levels also remained asymptomatic.

Bouwman et al.[334] performed a study to evaluate the role of serum amylase and its isoenzymes after blunt trauma for diagnosing pancreatic trauma. They reported that 33% (20/61) of patients had hyperamylasemia, but only two (3%) actually had pancreatic injury. The measurement of isoenzyme levels was not helpful to improve the diagnostic sensitivity or specificity for diagnosing pancreatic injury in this study. However, a retrospective study performed by Takishima et al.[338] evaluated serum amylase levels in 73 patients with blunt pancreatic injury. Hyperamylasemia was noted on admission in 84%

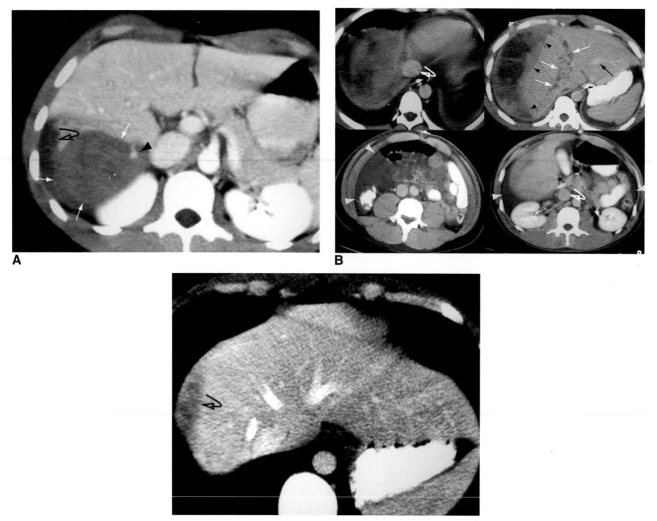

Fig. 6-97
Posttraumatic Budd-Chiari syndrome in a patient admitted after a blow to the right lower ribs in a boxing match. **A,** Admission CT image shows a hematoma (*arrow*) and active bleeding (*arrowhead*) in posterior right lobe of liver. A small subcapsular hematoma (*curved arrow*) is also seen. At laparotomy a hepatic hematoma was visualized through an intact Glisson's capsule. No free intraperitoneal blood was present. **B,** Follow-up CT image shows subcapsular hematoma (*black arrowheads*) has expanded and now compresses normal liver parenchyma, intrahepatic IVC, and right and middle hepatic veins. Only the left hepatic vein (*arrow*) is visualized. New lacerations (*white arrows*) are also seen in liver parenchyma. Infra- and suprahepatic vena cava (*curved arrows*) are distended, and there are low-attenuation ascites. Patient was managed without any further surgical intervention. **C,** Follow-up scan after discharge from hospital shows a residual small subcapsular hematoma (*curved arrow*) with no significant mass effect on normal liver parenchyma. All three hepatic veins are visualized. (From Markert DJ, Shanmuganathan K, Mirvis SE, et al: *Clin Radiol* 52:384 1997.)

(61/73) of the patients. The 12 patients with normal serum amylase level were all admitted 3 hours or less after the time of trauma. There was a significant correlation (p <0.001) between the time that had elapsed between the traumatic event and admission and serum amylase level. The study said determination of serum amylase levels more than 3 hours after blunt trauma may avoid false-negative results in detecting pancreatic injuries.

Diagnostic peritoneal lavage. DPL may not be helpful in diagnosing pancreatic injuries.[318,320,332,339] False-neg-

ative results are common even in patients with major isolated trauma to the pancreas. The high incidence of associate injuries to intraperitoneal organs results in a positive DPL and allows detection of the pancreatic injury at celiotomy. Lavage fluid amylase levels are nonspecific and are more often elevated as a result of bowel injury.[335,340]

Computed tomography. The majority of patients with blunt pancreatic injuries have associate injuries, and if these patients are hemodynamically stable, they will

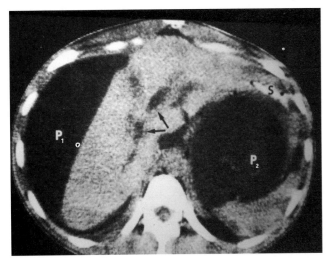

Fig. 6-98
Biloma complicating hepatic injury. Follow-up conventional CT image shows an intrahepatic (*P 1*) and a lesser sac biloma (*P 2*) with multiple lacerations (*arrows*) in liver. Mass effect is seen on stomach (*S*) and normal liver parenchyma because of bilomas.

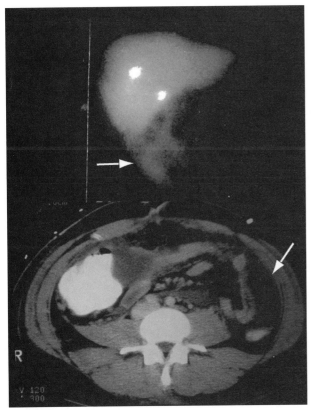

Fig. 6-99
Biloma complicating hepatic injury **A**, HIDA nuclear scintigraphy study obtained for abdominal distention and jaundice shows extravasation of isotope (*arrow*) into peritoneal cavity. **B**, Helical CT image shows a low-attenuation left paracolic biloma (*arrow*).

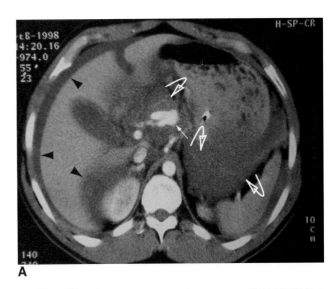

A

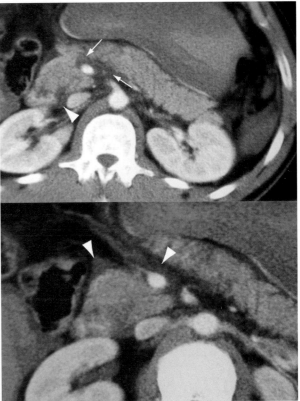

B

Fig. 6-100
Pancreatic injury with active bleeding from left gastric artery in a 36-year-old man admitted after blunt trauma. **A**, Helical CT image shows active bleeding (*arrows*) and free blood (*curved arrows*) in lesser sac. Moderate amount of free intraperitoneal blood (*arrowheads*) is also seen. **B**, CT images show fluid around superior mesenteric vein (*arrow*) and infiltration of peripancreatic fat (*arrowheads*) adjacent to the pancreatic head. Pancreatic contusion and active bleeding from left gastric artery were confirmed at surgery.

require CT. Therefore, CT has emerged as the imaging modality of choice to diagnose pancreatic injuries.[335,341-349] The CT findings of pancreatic injury may be subtle or normal in the immediate postinjury period (Figs. 6-104 and 6-105); controversy still exists concerning the accuracy

of CT for diagnosing pancreatic injuries.[335,342,346,348] Accurate determination of the integrity of the pancreatic duct is of major importance in planning manage-

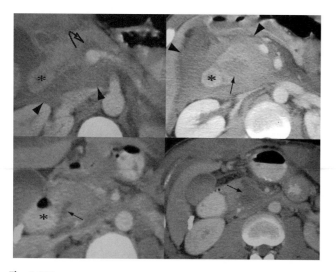

Fig. 6-101
Pancreaticoduodenal injury of patient admitted after motor vehicle collision. Multislice spiral CT images show a large retroperitoneal hematoma around pancreatic head (*arrowheads*) and thick-walled second part of duodenum (*asterisk*). Lacerations are seen in pancreatic head (*arrows*) with fluid seen around superior mesenteric vein (*curved arrow*). At laparotomy a pancreaticoduodenal injury was seen and repaired. (Images of duodenal injury shown in Fig. 6-116.)

ment.[321,342,348,350-354] Jeffrey et al.[335] reported that conventional CT diagnosed 85% (11/13) of surgically proven pancreatic injuries among 300 patients who underwent preoperative CT after blunt abdominal trauma. This series included two false-positive and two false-negative interpretations. CT was performed within 12 hours of injury in both patients with false-negative studies. Cook et al.[340] retrospectively evaluated the usefulness of CT in 83 blunt trauma victims and reported false-positive diagnosis of pancreatic injury in 9% (7/77) of patients, representing the most common cause of diagnostic error in interpretation of CT studies of blunt trauma patients.

On contrast-enhanced CT, findings of pancreatic trauma may be subtle, particularly in the immediate postinjury period and in adults with minimal retroperitoneal fat (see Figs. 6-104 and 6-105). Pancreatic contusion may appear as low-attenuation or heterogeneous focal or diffuse enlargement of the pancreas (see Fig. 6-103). Pancreatic lacerations are seen as linear irregular low-attenuation areas within the normal parenchyma. Unless the two edges of a fracture or transected pancreas are separated by low-attenuation fluid (Fig. 6-106) or

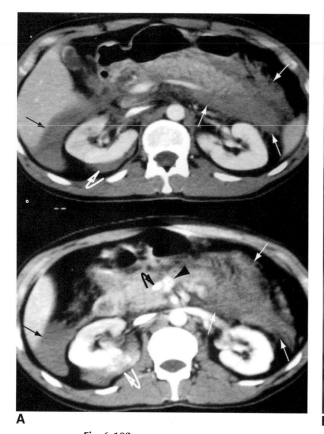

A

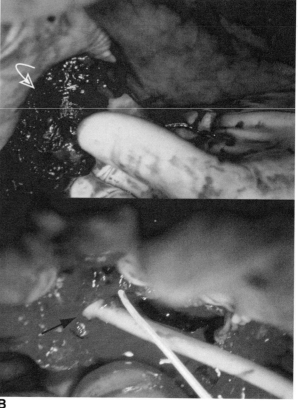

B

Fig. 6-102
Pancreatic injury with active bleeding in a patient involved in a motor vehicle collision. **A,** Conventional CT images show active bleeding (*arrowhead*) adjacent to superior mesenteric vein (*black curved arrow*). Peripancreatic hematoma (*white arrows*) is seen around body and tail of pancreas. Free intraperitoneal blood in right paracolic gutter (*black arrows*) and actively bleeding right perinephric hematoma (*white curved arrows*) are also seen. **B,** Intraoperative photographs show active bleeding arising from superior mesenteric vein (*arrow*). Distal pancreas was necrotic (*curved arrow*). A Foley catheter was inserted into superior mesenteric vein, and its balloon was inflated to control hemorrhage before repair of vascular injury.

Continued

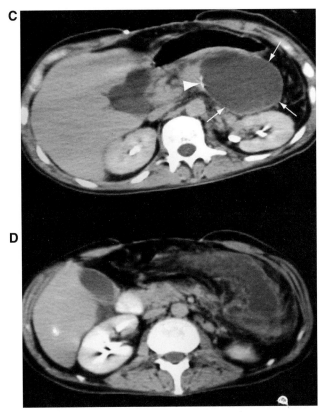

Fig. 6-102, cont'd
C, Follow-up CT obtained for abdominal pain and elevation of pancreatic enzymes shows a pseudocyst (*arrows*) adjacent to surgical clip (*arrowhead*) at site of distal pancreatectomy. **D,** CT obtained because of increase in abdominal pain shows rupture of pseudocyst and infiltration of peritoneal fat consistent with chemical peritonitis. (From Shanmuganathan K, Mirvis SE: Evaluation of liver and pancreas after blunt trauma. In Gazelle SG, Saini S, Mueller PR, eds: *Hepatobiliary and pancreatic radiology imaging and intervention*, New York, 1998, Thieme.)

hematoma (Fig. 6-107), the diagnosis of pancreatic transection may be difficult to recognize on CT. The location of the pancreatic laceration or fracture, whether to the left or right of the superior mesenteric artery, and the depth of the laceration(s) may help predict pancreatic duct disruption.[348] Wong et al.[348] performed a retrospective study to determine the ability of single-slice helical CT to predict pancreatic ductal disruption in 22 patients with pancreatic injury later confirmed at surgery. CT was 100% (10/10) accurate in predicting an intact duct and 89% (8/9) accurate in predicting ductal disruption. None of the 10 patients with lacerations that extended less than half (50%) of the anteroposterior diameter of the pancreas had an injury to the pancreatic duct. In this study ductal disruption was found in all five patients with lacerations of more than 50% of the anteroposterior diameter of the pancreas in the body or tail region and in four of the five patients with lacerations in the head region.

Hemorrhage from the abundant peripancreatic vascular anastomosis (see Figs. 6-100 and 6-102) may be identified on CT. Other nonspecific CT findings that alert the radiologist to possible pancreatic trauma include thickening of the anterior pararenal fascia, infiltration of the peripancreatic fat with fluid or hemorrhage (see Figs. 6-103 to 6-105), blood or fluid tracking along the mesenteric vessels (see Figs. 6-100 to 6-102), fluid in the lesser sac (see Fig. 6-100), or fluid between the pancreas and splenic vein (see Fig. 6-105). Among the nonspecific CT findings of pancreatic injury, thickening of the anterior pararenal fascia was the most commonly observed finding in the series reported by Jeffrey et al.[335] This finding was seen in 73% (8/11) of patients with pancreatic injury. Retrospectively evaluating the CT findings in 10 patients with blunt pancreatic injury, Lane et al.[344] noted fluid between the splenic vein and pancreas in 90% (9/10) of the patients. Often this finding was seen adjacent to the site of pancreatic injury and was helpful in directing the attention of the radiologist to more subtle CT signs at the site of the pancreatic injury.

Common CT findings that lead to pitfalls in diagnosing pancreatic injury include unopacified bowel (see Fig. 6-11) or fluid in the lesser sac mimicking focal pancreatic enlargement (contusion) and streak artifacts or focal

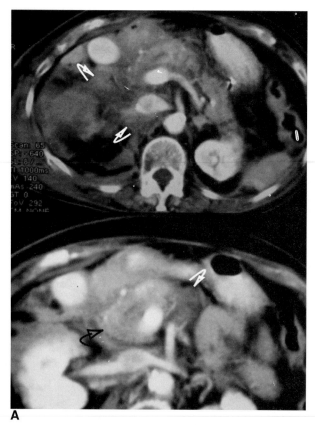

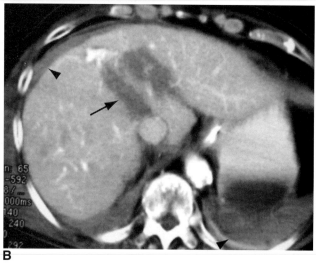

Fig. 6-103
Midline force vector causing liver and pancreatic injury in a 93-year-old woman admitted after motor vehicle collision. **A** and **B**, Admission helical CT images show a grade III liver laceration (*arrow*) and free intraperitoneal blood (*arrowheads*) in upper abdomen. Pancreatic head (*black curved arrow*) is enlarged with peripancreatic fluid and fat infiltration (*curved white arrows*) as a result of pancreatic contusion.

areas of fatty replacement of pancreatic parenchyma simulating pancreatic lacerations. Other CT findings that could mimic pancreatic injury include blood or fluid tracking around the pancreas arising from injuries to the adjacent duodenum, spleen, or left kidney, pelvic hematomas tracking superiorly in the retroperitoneum, and retroperitoneal edema from vigorous intravascular volume resuscitation[355] (Fig. 6-108).

Magnetic resonance cholangiopancreatography (MRCP). MRCP is a valuable new imaging modality recognized to play an increasingly important role in evaluating patients with pancreaticobiliary disease.[356-361] Although ERCP is considered to be the reference study to evaluate the integrity of the pancreatic duct, it is an invasive technique associated with complications including aspiration and pancreatitis in 3% to 5% of patients.[356,362] The results are operator-dependent, and failure to cannulate the ampullary duct or inadequate pancreatography may occur in 10% to 20% of patients.[363]

Only a limited experience concerning sensitivity and specificity of MRCP in diagnosing pancreatic ductal disruption has been reported.[356,358,359] Multislice, thick-slab coronal and axial images without fat suppression are used initially to localize the pancreatic duct. Once the duct has been localized, thin-slab (5 mm) images with fat suppression are obtained in a coronal-oblique plane parallel to the long axis of the pancreas with or without suspended respiration. Soto et al.[359] performed MRCP in seven patients with pancreatic injuries. MR showed duct disruption related to fractures in the neck (n=2), body (n=3), and tail (n=2) of the pancreas. MRCP findings indicating injury to the pancreatic duct included focal disruption of the duct, focal or diffuse dilation of the duct diameter greater than 2 mm, and apparent communication between the duct and intrapancreatic or peripancreatic fluid collections. Unlike retrograde pancreatography, MRCP was able to provide additional useful information concerning distal pancreatic duct architecture and injury even if it was not in continuity with the proximal duct.

Endoscopic retrograde cholangiopancreatography. Although injuries to the pancreatic duct may be diagnosed intraoperatively by cannulating the pancreatic duct directly, preoperative diagnosis may only be reliably

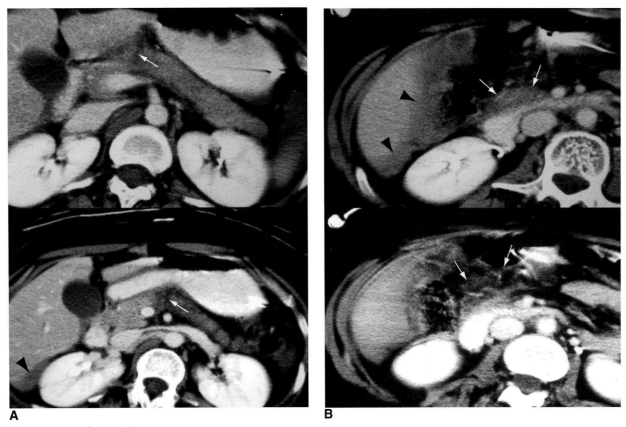

Fig. 6-104
Subtle CT findings in a patient with transection of pancreatic neck. **A,** Conventional CT images show a low-attenuation area (*arrow*) on two contiguous images in neck of pancreas. No peripancreatic fluid is seen adjacent to low-attenuation area in neck. Small amount of free blood (*arrowheads*) is seen adjacent to liver. **B,** CT images inferior to pancreas show fluid and fat infiltration in anterior pararenal space. Laparotomy was performed for abdominal tenderness and free intraperitoneal fluid in abdomen and pelvis (not shown) without a source seen on CT. Pancreatic neck was transected at surgery.

made by ERCP.[350-353,364-368] Recent reports suggest that pancreatic duct disruption is amenable to definitive treatment in selected patients by stent placement.[352,353,365,368] Untreated injuries of the pancreatic duct may result in pancreatitis, fistulas, ascites, pseudocyst, or abscess formation, thus, knowledge of the presence and location of duct injuries is vital.[314,350] Barkin et al.[351] described four patients with pancreatic duct rupture among 14 studied by emergency ERCP. All four injuries were confirmed at celiotomy. Three of the four duct disruptions were not evident on preoperative CT. In this limited study, emergent ERCP was 100% sensitive and specific in diagnosing pancreatic duct ruptures.

Pancreatic ductal injuries may be overlooked on ERCP from dilution of extravasated contrast material within a large retroperitoneal hematoma or if there is minimal contrast extravasation.[367] Takishima et al.[367] performed a retrospective study to determine the value of follow-up CT performed immediately after endoscopic retrograde pancreatography (ERP) to detect small quantities of extravasated contrast. CT was performed in six patients

after ERP and detected extravasated contrast material extending outside the pancreas in four and confined to the pancreatic parenchyma in one. All four patients with extrapancreatic contrast material extravasation had pancreatic duct injury confirmed at surgery. The patient with extravasation of ERP contrast material confined to the pancreas was managed conservatively. CT and ERP both missed a pancreatic duct injury in the other patient.

Complications. Complication rates in patients sustaining pancreatic injuries range from 28% to 77%.[318,325,336,369-371] Delayed complications can occur months to years after initial injury, usually resulting from strictures or disruption of the main pancreatic duct.[371] A higher incidence of complications has been attributed to inadequate drainage of pancreatic injuries, combined injuries to the pancreatic head and duodenum, and major pancreatic duct disruption.[314,318,336,369] Optimal drainage of the pancreatic injury site has helped significantly to reduce all complications resulting from pancreatic trauma from 26% to 2%.[316]

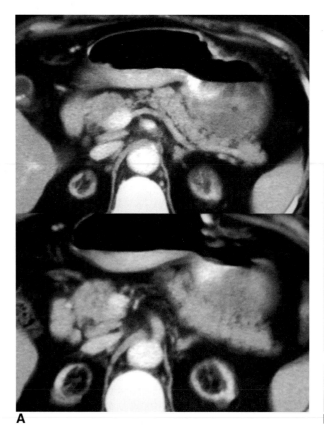

A

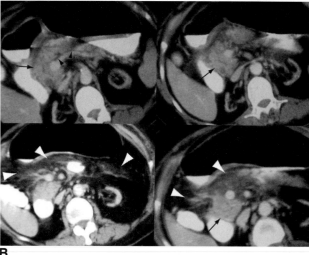

B

Fig. 6-105
Normal CT during immediate postinjury period for 54-year-old woman with pancreatic injury. **A**, Admission helical CT shows a normal pancreas with no peripancreatic fluid or fat stranding. **B**, Follow-up CT images 3 days after injury for abdominal pain and persistent elevation of pancreatic enzymes shows enlarged pancreatic head (*arrows*), peripancreatic fat infiltration (*white arrowheads*), and fluid (*black arrowheads*) between pancreas and splenic vein due to pancreatitis.

The most common complication to occur immediately after pancreatic trauma is a pancreatic fistula[318,325,326,372] (see Fig. 6-106). Fistulas are more likely in blunt trauma victims and usually develop in the first 3 weeks. Multivariate analysis indicates factors associated with fistula formation are the presence of duct injury and performance of a distal pancreatectomy.[325] Most pancreatic fistulas heal spontaneously or with treatment using somatostatin analogue.[325,372] Usually fistulas do not require imaging studies for diagnosis or management.

Other complications include pancreatitis (see Figs. 6-105 and 6-106), pseudocyst (see Fig. 6-102), and abscess formation. Serial CT scans can evaluate onset and monitor progression or resolution of these complications. Pseudocyst formation is the most common late complication after blunt trauma and has been reported in 3% to 10% of all pancreatic injuries.[314,316] Up to one-third of blunt trauma victims with pancreatic injury develop pseudocyst(s). Pancreatic pseudocysts are usually associated with pancreatic duct strictures or untreated disruption.[371] Lewis et al.[372] reported their experience in 15 patients with traumatic pancreatic

pseudocyst. All 15 patients had injuries to the pancreatic duct that were either missed at surgery (n=8) or among patients treated nonoperatively (n=7). The location of the pancreatic duct injury influenced the treatment approach. Posttraumatic pseudocyst resulting from proximal duct injuries required celiotomy. Distal duct injuries were managed by percutaneous drainage, and spontaneous resolution occurred with peripheral duct injuries.

Pseudocysts are round or oval collections of pancreatic fluid as imaged by CT (see Fig. 6-102) or sonography. The wall or capsule of the pseudocyst may vary in thickness and shows contrast enhancement. Complications of pseudocysts include pain, bile duct obstruction, infection, hemorrhage, and rupture (see Fig. 6-102).

Intraabdominal sepsis develops in 8% to 34% of patients after pancreatic injury.[314,317,318,328,336] Factors associated with pancreatic abscess formation are concurrent colonic injuries, duct injury, and distal pancreatic resection.[325] Typical CT findings of a pancreatic abscess are a thick-walled, focal fluid collection that may contain air bubbles (Fig. 6-109). Because CT findings are nonspecific for pancreatic abscess, clinical suspicion of pancre-

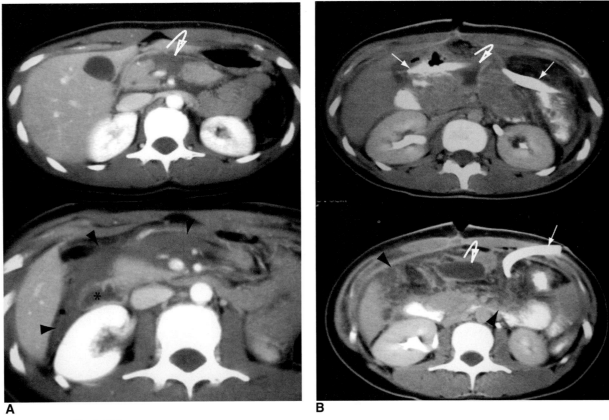

Fig. 6-106
Pancreatic transection in 17-year-old woman admitted after motor vehicle collision. **A**, Contiguous helical CT images show low-attenuation fluid (*curved arrow*) clearly separating pancreatic head and body. Peripancreatic and periduodenal (*asterisks*) hematoma (*arrowheads*) in anterior pararenal space is seen. Laparotomy confirmed transection of pancreatic neck. **B**, Follow-up CT for persistent high fluid output from pancreatic drain shows intrapancreatic and peripancreatic fluid collections (*curved arrows*). A pancreatic drain (*arrows*) is seen adjacent to fluid collection with infiltration of adjacent mesenteric fat (*arrowheads*) due to posttraumatic pancreatitis.

atic abscess warrants percutaneous needle aspiration or surgery to confirm the diagnosis. Pancreatitis is a common complication of pancreatic trauma and varies in its severity. Posttraumatic hemorrhagic pancreatitis is associated with high mortality.[317] The CT findings and treatment of pancreatitis developing after pancreatic injury are similar to those of any patient with pancreatitis.

Bowel and Mesenteric Injuries. Bowel and mesenteric injuries are found in approximately 5% of patients suffering from blunt abdominal trauma.[373] Unrecognized bowel injuries are associated with significant morbidity, including fatal peritonitis from perforation, sepsis, and life-threatening hemorrhage. Mesenteric injuries may produce significant blood loss or may result in bowel ischemia and necrosis with resultant delayed rupture or ischemic strictures. A recent study noted that a delay in diagnosis of only 8 hours was associated with increased morbidity and mortality.[185] This is especially concerning as nonoperative management for solid organ injury becomes more widely adopted and reliance on imaging

and physical examination increases. Unfortunately, findings on physical examination can initially be benign, with delayed onset of peritoneal signs, and the classic symptoms of rigidity, tenderness, and decreased or absent bowel sounds may be present in only one third of patients.[8,374,375]

In the past, diagnosis of bowel injury has been made by physical examination. However, drawbacks include requirement of repeat examination by the same observer to obtain the most consistent result, the need for admission to allow observation, and an unreliable examination in patients with neurologic impairment or significant distracting injuries. DPL has long been used as an adjunct to physical examination. However, this is an invasive procedure with a real, albeit small, risk of complications. Additionally, it offers no specific information regarding the site or severity of injury, and it is often not reliable in the detection of isolated retroperitoneal injuries.

CT is well established as a highly accurate imaging modality for detecting solid organ injury after blunt trauma. However, until recently, the role of CT in the

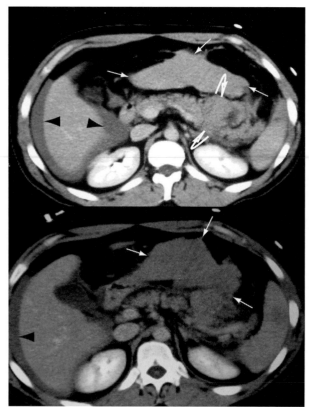

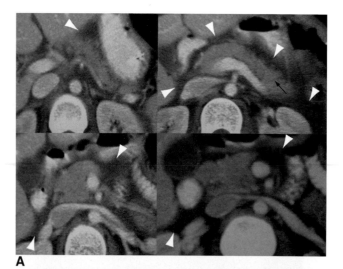

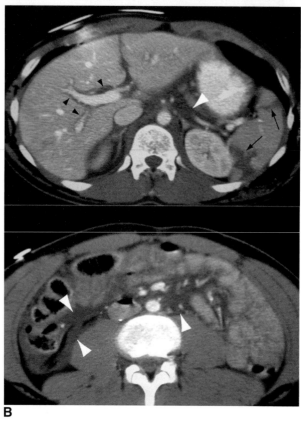

Fig. 6-107

Pancreatic transection separated by hematoma. Helical CT images show a hematoma (*curved arrows*) separating tail and distal body of pancreas. Hematoma of transverse mesocolon (*arrows*) and hemoperitoneum (*arrowheads*) are also seen. Distal pancreatectomy was performed. (From Shanmuganathan K, Mirvis SE: Evaluation of liver and pancreas after blunt trauma. In Gazelle SG, Saini S, Mueller PR, eds: *Hepatobiliary and pancreatic radiology imaging and intervention*, New York, 1998, Thieme.)

Fig. 6-108

Retroperitoneal fluid from volume overload mimicking pancreatic injury. **A,** Multislice helical CT images show retroperitoneal fluid (*arrowheads*) around pancreas with a linear area of fatty replacement (*arrow*) mimicking a pancreatic laceration. **B,** CT images also show other evidence of fluid overload including periportal lymphatic distention and edema (*black arrowheads*) and diffuse small bowel edema. Retroperitoneal edema (*white arrowheads*) and a grade III splenic injury (*arrows*) are also seen. Serial pancreatic enzyme levels remained normal.

diagnosis and evaluation of hollow viscus injury has remained controversial. Earlier studies that reviewed the use of conventional CT have reported both high diagnostic accuracy[373,376,377] and poor ability to detect such injuries.[39,378,379] More recent reviews using helical CT and larger patient populations have reported sensitivities ranging from 84% to 94% with accuracy from 84% to 99%.[380-382]

The CT scan appearance of bowel and mesenteric injuries has been well described.[376,378,383] Findings of a full-thickness bowel injury include extraluminal gas (Figs. 6-110 to 6-113), extraluminal oral contrast material (Figs. 6-110 and 6-114) or intestinal content (Fig. 6-115), discontinuity of bowel wall (Figs. 6-116 and 6-117), intramural air (Fig. 6-118), and a moderate to large amount of free peritoneal fluid (Fig. 6-119; see Fig. 6-27). Additionally, focal bowel wall thickening (>4 mm with mild distension) can suggest bowel contusion without transmural injury (Figs. 6-120 and 6-121). Evidence to suggest mesenteric injury includes active bleeding or

active extravasation of intravenous contrast into the mesentery (Figs. 6-122 and 6-123; see Figs. 6-17 and 6-20), bowel wall thickening associated with mesenteric

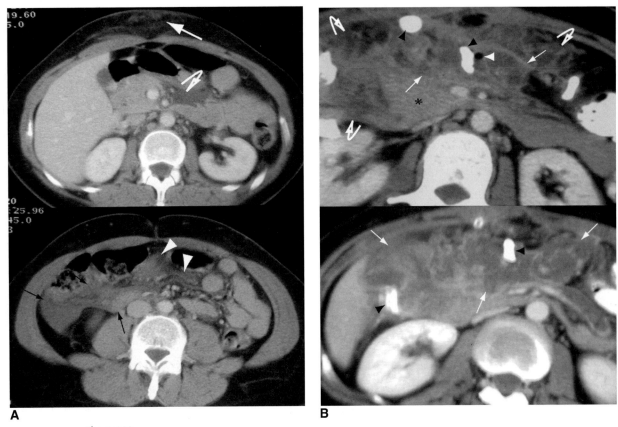

Fig. 6-109
Pancreatic abscess after laparotomy for blunt pancreatic and mesenteric injury. **A,** Admission CT images show peripancreatic fluid (*curved arrow*) medial to pancreatic head and a mesenteric contusion (*arrowheads*). Mesenteric contusion extends into root of mesentery and right retroperitoneum (*black arrows*). An anterior abdominal wall contusion (*white arrow*) from a seat belt injury is also seen. Laparotomy was performed for mesenteric injury, and at surgery a mesenteric injury was repaired. A pancreatic contusion was also seen at surgery, and a drain was placed adjacent to pancreas. **B,** Follow-up CT because of purulent drainage from pancreatic bed shows fluid collections (*arrows*) medial and inferior to pancreatic head (*asterisk*) with a gas bubble (*white arrowhead*) and surgical drain (*black arrowheads*). Infiltration of peritoneal fat (*curved arrow*) is also seen.

hematoma (Figs. 6-124 and 6-125), or focal mesenteric hematoma (Figs. 6-125 and 6-126) or infiltration (Figs. 6-127 and 6-128; see Figs. 6-7 and 6-109).

Recent reviews have attempted to demonstrate the ability of CT to differentiate between a full-thickness bowel injury, which would require surgical intervention, and a nonsurgical bowel injury, such as a serosal tear or bowel wall contusion. The ability to predict a full-thickness bowel injury was similar to the overall ability to detect bowel injury, with an accuracy ranging from 75% to 86%. Importantly, negative predictive values ranged from 89% to 96%, indicating that CT is capable of excluding such injuries with a reasonable level of certainty.

CT was found to be less reliable in determining the need for surgical intervention for mesenteric injuries, with an accuracy ranging from 54% to 75%. Active bleed-

ing and bowel wall thickening associated with mesenteric hematoma were found to be the most specific signs for surgical mesenteric injury. The significance of isolated mesenteric contusion or hematoma has not been clarified with certainty, as a number of the patients in recent studies did not undergo exploratory laparotomy. Many underwent follow-up CT scan examination with resolution of the mesenteric infiltrate or hematoma.

The significance of isolated intraperitoneal free fluid remains controversial. Recent reports suggest that the finding of a moderate or large amount of free fluid without evidence of solid organ injury is a strong indicator of full-thickness bowel or mesenteric injury and occasionally may be the only finding identified.[381,384,385] However, others note that only a small percentage (8%) have free fluid secondary to bowel injury[122] and that

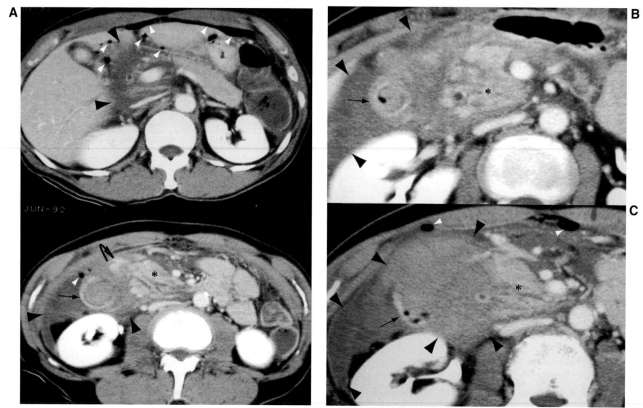

Fig. 6-110
Extraluminal air with bowel injury. Free intraperitoneal air in a 58-year-old woman kicked by a horse in upper abdomen. **A,** Conventional CT images show moderate amount of free intraperitoneal air (*white arrows*) and periduodenal and peripancreatic hematoma (*black arrowheads*). Second part of duodenum (*arrow*) is separated from pancreatic head (*asterisks*) as a result of a pancreaticoduodenal injury. Free oral contrast material (*curved arrow*) is seen with periduodenal hematoma. **B** and **C,** CT images show extent of periduodenal and peripancreatic hematoma (*black arrowheads*) and intraperitoneal air (*white arrowheads*). Hematoma separates pancreatic head (*asterisk*) and second part of duodenum (*arrows*). Duodenal wall is not seen between 10 and 5 o'clock positions medially.

exploratory laparotomy is not mandatory in this setting. Rather, patients can be observed clinically, with late DPL being used to diagnose intestinal injury in patients with worsening examinations by examining leukocyte influx into the peritoneal cavity.[386,387]

Radiologists should be familiar with abnormalities observed in the bowel in patients with hypoperfusion complex and fluid over-resuscitation.[355,388,389] These two entities can mask or mimic the diagnosis of bowel injury.[388,390] The CT findings of shock bowel or diffuse small bowel ischemia in hypotensive adult blunt trauma patients were described by Mirvis et al.[388] and include diffuse thickening of the small bowel wall (range, 7 mm to 15 mm), fluid-filled dilated small bowel loops, increased contrast enhancement of the small bowel wall from slow perfusion and interstitial leak of intravenous

contrast material, and a flattened inferior vena cava (Figs. 6-129 and 6-130). The large bowel usually appears normal. In the absence of focal bowel injury at celiotomy the small bowel appears normal on inspection. A small bowel can withstand prolonged ischemia without injury; follow-up CT obtained after adequate treatment of the cause of hypoperfusion shows complete resolution of small bowel changes.[391]

The bowel wall changes seen after vigorous fluid over-resuscitation may result in diffuse edema of the bowel wall, particularly the small bowel (Figs. 6-131 and 6-132).[355] Other CT findings of intravenous volume expansion—such as periportal low density, distension of the IVC, retroperitoneal fluid density, and occasionally ascites—usually accompany the bowel wall thickening (see Figs. 6-131 and 6-132). These CT findings result

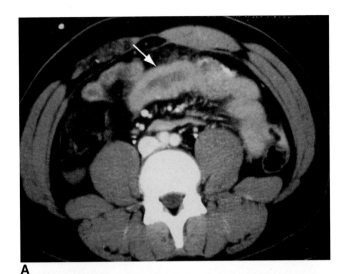

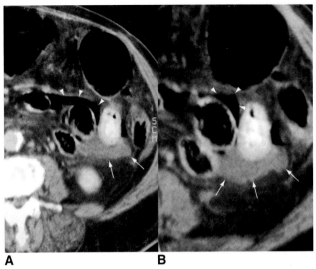

Fig. 6-112
Free intraperitoneal air and fluid in a 78-year-old man admitted after blunt force trauma. **A** and **B**, Conventional CT images show minimal amount of high-density free intraperitoneal fluid between bowel loops (*arrows*) and free intraperitoneal air (*arrowheads*). At celiotomy a proximal jejunal injury was repaired.

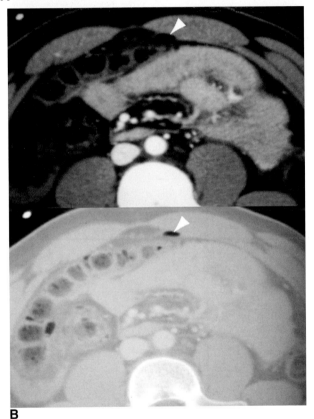

Fig. 6-111
Free intraperitoneal air seen better on lung window levels in 24-year-old man admitted after motor vehicle collision. Patient complained of abdominal pain. **A**, Helical CT image shows small bowel wall thickening (*arrow*) in mid abdomen. **B**, CT images on lung and soft tissue window levels show minimal amount of free intraperitoneal air (*arrowhead*) in anterior abdomen. A jejunal injury was repaired at celiotomy.

from lymphedema related to elevated central venous pressure produced by vigorous intravenous fluid administration.[355]

It is important to distinguish small bowel injury from these two entities. Small bowel injury usually appears as a focal rather than diffuse abnormality on CT, involving the entire small bowel, as seen in these two entities. Scrutinize the scans carefully for CT findings of pneumoperitoneum, mesenteric hematoma, oral contrast extravasation, and bowel wall or mesenteric air. Any one of these findings should indicate concurrent full-thickness bowel injury[355,388] (see Fig. 6-130). Follow-up CT should be routinely obtained in all patients suspected to have small bowel injury with CT findings of shock bowel or volume overexpansion (see Fig. 6-131).

Follow-up CT in Bowel and Mesenteric Injuries. No clear consensus appears among the radiologic or surgical literature on how to ideally manage patients with nonspecific CT findings of bowel or mesenteric injury.[142-148,392-395] These CT findings include bowel wall thickening (Figs. 6-133, 6-134; see Fig. 6-4) mesenteric hematoma, focal mesenteric infiltration (see Figs. 6-4 and 6-133), and a small amount of free intraperitoneal fluid (Fig. 6-135). At the UMSTC for all patients with nonspecific CT findings of bowel or mesenteric injury who cannot be observed with serial physical examinations to diagnose onset of peritonitis, a routine follow-up CT is obtained in 4 to 6 hours. The follow-up CT is carefully scrutinized for new onset of free intraperitoneal fluid, extravasation of oral contrast material or bowel wall thickening, increase in the amount of free intraperitoneal fluid, mesenteric infiltration, and bowel wall thickening when compared with the admission CT. For other patients with nonspecific CT findings of bowel or mesenteric injury, it is important

Text continued on p. 468.

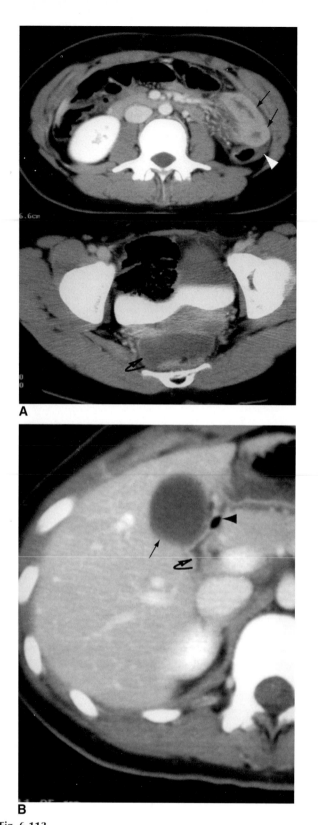

Fig. 6-113
Small amount of free air in a patient admitted after blunt trauma. **A,** Helical CT images show small bowel wall thickening (*arrows*) with adjacent mesenteric stranding (*arrowhead*). A small amount of low-attenuation free intraperitoneal fluid (*curved arrow*) is seen in pelvis. **B,** CT image shows a bubble of free air (*arrowhead*) between gallbladder (*arrow*) and duodenum (*curved arrow*). Small bowel perforation was confirmed at surgery.

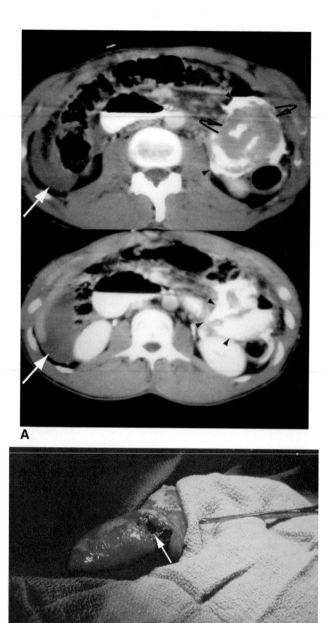

Fig. 6-114
Oral contrast material extravasation into peritoneum in a patient admitted after blunt abdominal trauma. **A,** Conventional CT images show free intraperitoneal oral contrast material extravasation (*arrowheads*). Some of the extravasated contrast material is seen adjacent to thick-walled small bowel (*curved arrows*). Free intraperitoneal fluid (*arrows*) is seen in right paracolic gutter. **B,** Intraoperative photograph shows a perforation (*arrow*) and adjacent contusion of proximal jejunum.

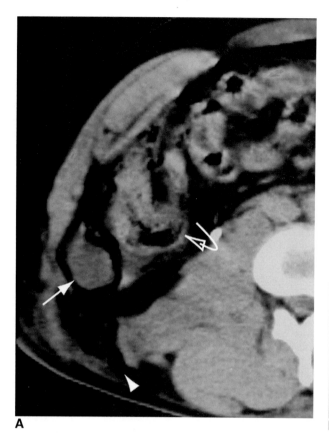

A

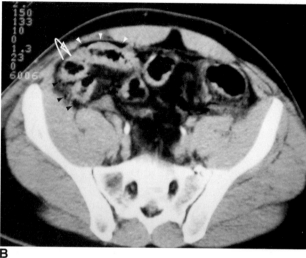

B

Fig. 6-115
Extraluminal fecal material in a 26-year-old man admitted after blunt injury. **A,** Conventional CT image shows fecal material (*arrow*) lateral to cecum (*curved arrow*) in retroperitoneum. A traumatic right lumbar hernia (*arrowhead*) is also seen. **B,** CT image in upper pelvis shows free intraperitoneal (*white arrowhead*) and retroperitoneal air (*black arrowheads*) with some thickening of terminal ileum (*curved arrow*). At surgery a cecal perforation was repaired.

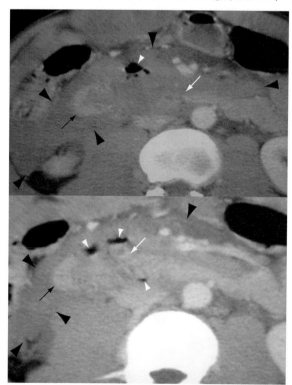

Fig. 6-116
Discontinuity of duodenal wall in a patient with pancreaticoduodenal injuries (see Fig. 6-101). Multislice helical CT images show a large retroperitoneal hematoma (*black arrowheads*) around pancreas and duodenum. Discontinuity of duodenal wall is seen between the proximal (*black arrow*) and third part (*white arrow*) of duodenum. Free retroperitoneal air (*white arrowheads*) is also seen. This injury was repaired at surgery.

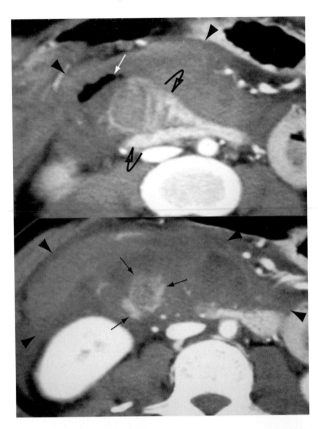

Fig. 6-117
Discontinuity of bowel wall with oral contrast extravasation in a 48-year-old woman admitted after motor vehicle collision. Helical CT images show disruption of walls of proximal third portion of duodenum (*curved arrows*). A large periduodenal hematoma (*arrowheads*) with oral contrast material extravasation (*black arrows*) within hematoma is observed. Free retroperitoneal air (*white arrow*) is also seen. Concurrent flexion-distraction injury of lumbar spine is not seen well on these images.

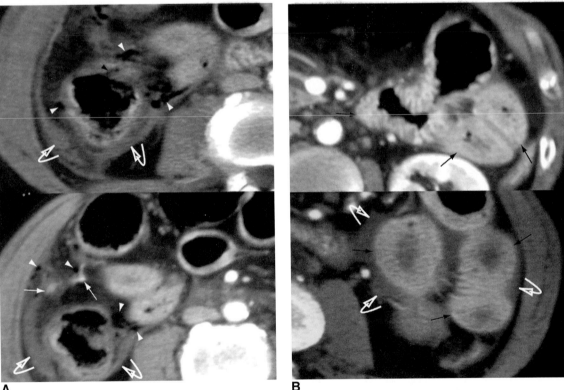

A **B**

Fig. 6-118
Subtle oral contrast extravasation and intramural air in a young adult man with large and small bowel injury. **A**, Multislice spiral CT images show multiple bubbles of free intraperitoneal air (*white arrowheads*) and pericolonic fat infiltration (*curved arrows*). Right colonic wall is thickened with intramural air (*black arrowhead*). Subtle amount of oral contrast extravasation (*arrows*) is also seen. **B**, CT images show in left mid abdomen multiple loops of proximal small bowel (*arrows*) wall thickening and free intraperitoneal fluid (*curved arrows*) between bowel loops. At surgery proximal small bowel and right colonic perforation were repaired.

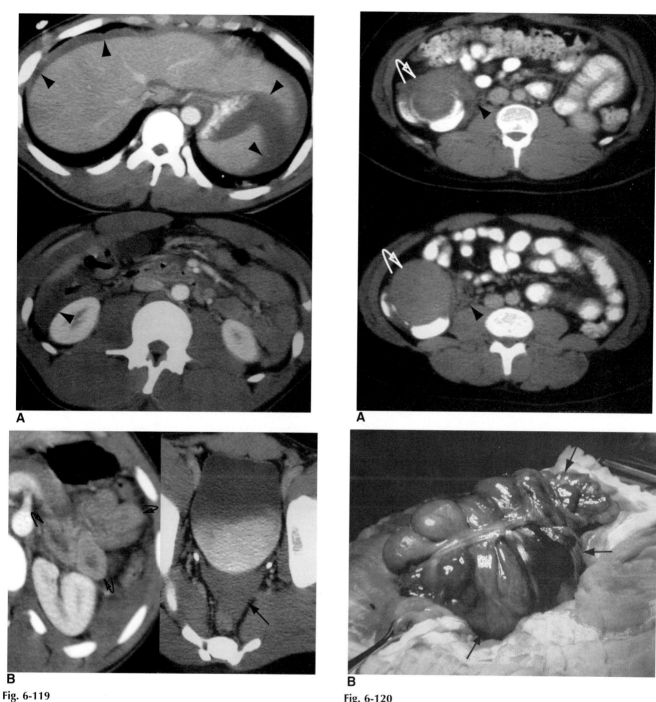

Fig. 6-119

Moderate amount of free intraperitoneal blood with full-thickness bowel injury in 19-year-old man admitted after motor vehicle collision. **A,** Multislice helical CT images show moderate amount of free intraperitoneal fluid (*arrowheads*) around liver, spleen, and in right paracolic gutter. No solid organ injury is seen. **B,** CT images in mid abdomen and pelvis show some thick-walled small bowel (*curved arrows*) and intraperitoneal fluid (*arrow*) in pelvis. At celiotomy transected small bowel was repaired.

Fig. 6-120

Ascending colon wall hematoma in a patient after industrial accident. A beam fell on patient's abdomen. The patient had minimal abdominal pain and no tenderness on clinical examination. **A,** Helical CT images show a large focal colonic wall hematoma (*curved arrows*) with mass effect on colonic contrast material. Infiltration of pericolonic fat (*arrowheads*) is also seen. **B,** Intraoperative photograph shows extent of colonic wall hematoma. A right hemicolectomy was performed.

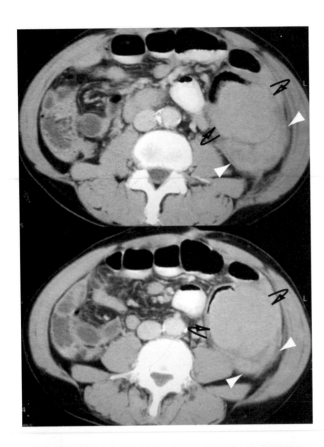

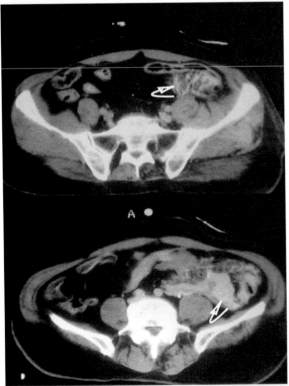

Fig. 6-121
Descending colon wall hematoma in a 57-year-old man who sustained blunt trauma while receiving anticoagulant therapy. Helical CT images show a large descending colonic wall hematoma (*curved arrows*) causing mass effect on colonic air column. Retrocolonic hematoma (*arrowheads*) is also seen within fat. At surgery a large colonic hematoma was found in descending colon with extrusion of hematoma into retrocecal fat. A left hemicolectomy was performed.

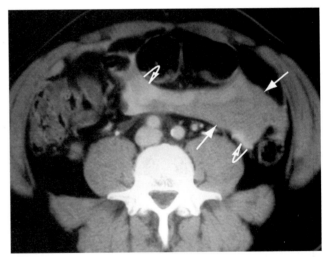

Fig. 6-122
Active bleeding in mesentery in patient admitted after blunt force trauma. Helical CT images show active bleeding (*curved arrows*) in mesentery in left iliac fossa. At surgery, after control of hemorrhage, devascularized small bowel was resected.

Fig. 6-123
Active bleeding in mesenteric leaves of a 40-year-old man admitted after blunt trauma. Helical CT images show large amount of blood (*arrows*) in mesentery with areas of active bleeding (*curved arrows*) similar in density to intravenous contrast material seen within aorta and IVC. These findings were confirmed at celiotomy.

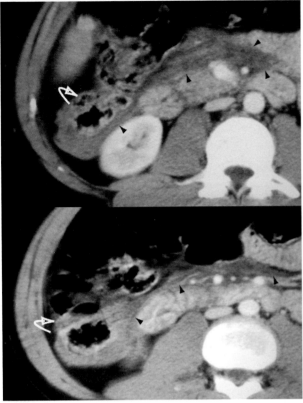

Fig. 6-124
Mesenteric injury with bowel wall thickening. Helical CT images show pericolonic mesenteric contusion (*arrowheads*) and ascending colon (*curved arrow*) wall thickening. At surgery a tear of both layers of colonic mesocolon was repaired.

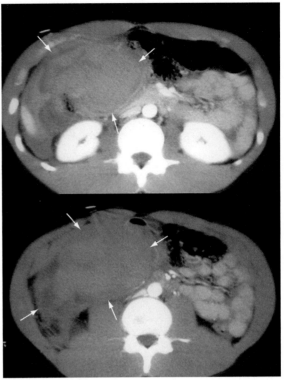

Fig. 6-126
Large mesenteric hematoma in a 17-year-old man admitted after blunt injury. Helical CT images show a large right mesenteric hematoma (*arrows*) with displacement of bowel to left side of abdomen. No associate bowel wall thickening is seen.

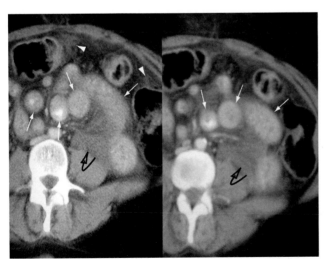

Fig. 6-125
Mesenteric injury with bowel wall thickening. Contiguous helical CT images show a mesenteric contusion (*curved arrows*) extending adjacent to thick-walled small bowel loops (*arrows*) in left mid abdomen. Other areas of mesenteric fat infiltration (*arrowheads*) are also seen.

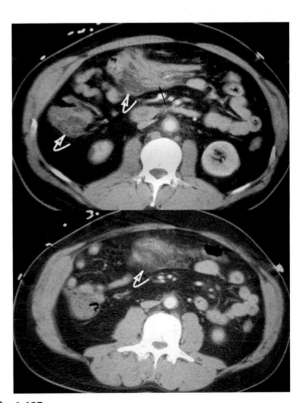

Fig. 6-127
Mesenteric hematoma and infiltration (other images shown in Fig. 6-7). Multislice CT images show multiple areas of mesenteric injury including mesenteric contusions or infiltration of mesenteric fat (*curved arrows*) and a mesenteric hematoma (*arrow*).

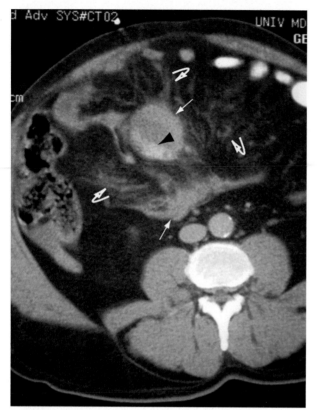

Fig. 6-128

Mesenteric injury in a 57-year-old man admitted after blunt trauma. Helical CT image shows two areas of mesenteric hematoma (*arrows*). Active bleeding (*arrowhead*) is seen within anterior mesenteric hematoma. Areas of mesenteric infiltration or contusion (*curved arrow*) are also seen. These findings were confirmed at celiotomy .

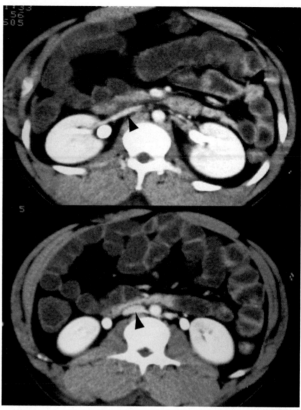

Fig. 6-129

Shock-bowel. Conventional CT images show multiple fluid-filled small bowel loops with wall enhancement, collapsed IVC (*arrowheads*), dense renal parenchyma enhancement, and a small diameter abdominal aorta. This constellation of CT findings results from hypovolemia and hypoperfusion.

to discuss the radiologic and clinical findings on an individual patient basis as the trauma surgeon and trauma radiologist plan management, which may include serial physical examination, a follow-up CT in 4 to 6 hours, DPL, or laparoscopy.

Traumatic Lumbar Hernia. Traumatic abdominal wall hernias have been historically diagnosed with laparotomy. Traumatic lumbar hernias occur through weaknesses in the posterolateral abdominal wall, either through the Grynfeltt-Lesshaft triangle or the Petit triangle.[396-398] The Petit triangle is formed inferiorly by the iliac crest, the external oblique muscle anteriorly, and the latissimus dorsi muscle posteriorly. The Grynfeltt-Lesshaft triangle is formed by the twelfth rib superiorly, internal oblique muscle anteriorly, and erector spinae muscle posteriorly.

Deceleration forces acting on the abdominal wall from improper use of three-point restraint or seat belt use are

the mechanism proposed in the literature for this injury.[399-401] Delays in diagnosis of traumatic lumbar hernias are common because hernias are easily overlooked, as the force that is required to disrupt the abdominal wall musculature is sufficient to create additional visceral injuries that draw the attention at the time of injury.

Killen et al.[396] reported 15 patients with blunt traumatic lumbar hernia; 14 of these hernias occurred through Petit's triangle. Herniation of retroperitoneal fat was seen in nine patients; two patients had herniation of both colon and small bowel; and three patients had herniation of the colon alone (Figs. 6-136 and 6-137). Associate injuries were seen in nine of the fifteen patients. Only one patient had clinical signs of the hernia. Five of the patients underwent exploratory laparotomy for their injuries, and three of the lumbar hernias were confirmed and repaired at surgery. The lumbar hernia was initially missed at laparotomy in one patient.

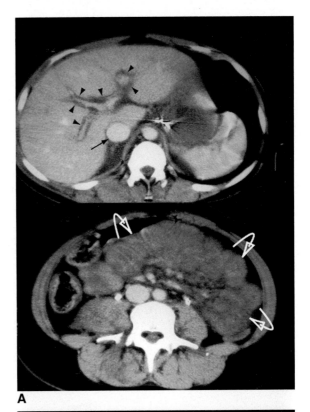

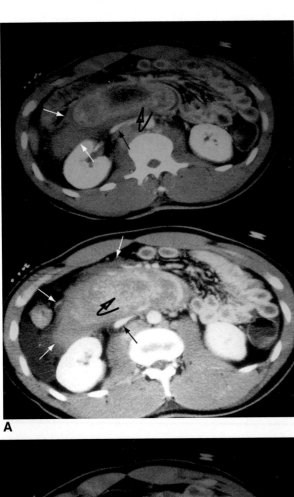

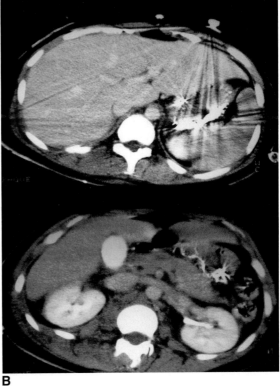

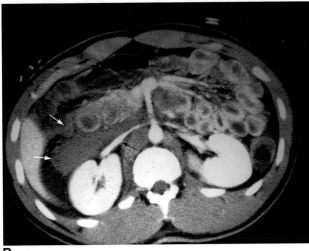

Fig. 6-130
Concurrent bowel injury and shock bowel in a man crushed by a handlebar across upper abdomen. **A** and **B**, Conventional CT images show a periduodenal and retroperitoneal hematoma (*white arrows*) with disruption of third part of duodenum (*curved arrows*). The IVC (*black arrows*) is flat. Multiple fluid-filled small bowel loops with wall enhancement are seen. The renal parenchyma is dense from hypoperfusion.

Fig. 6-131
Increased central venous pressure. **A**, Admission helical CT images show periportal lymphedema (*arrowheads*), a markedly distended IVC (*arrow*), and diffuse bowel wall edema predominantly involving small bowel (*curved arrows*). **B**, Follow-up CT images 36 hours after admission CT show resolution of CT findings related to expansion of venous volume. Small bowel wall edema has resolved. No free intraperitoneal air, focal bowel wall thickening, or free intraperitoneal fluid was seen. (From Chamrova Z, Shanmuganathan K, Mirvis SE, et al: *Emerg Radiol* 1:85, 1994.)

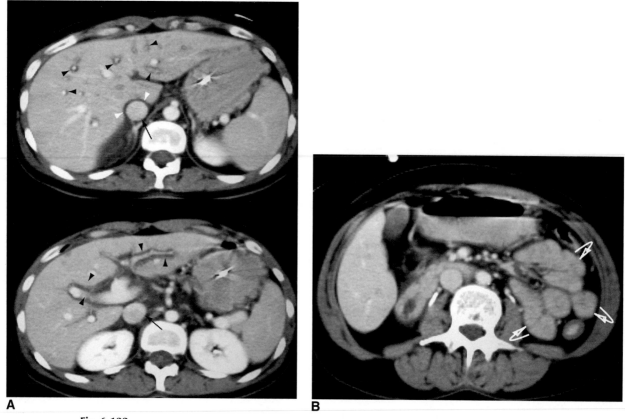

Fig. 6-132
Increased central venous pressure. **A** and **B**, Admission conventional CT images show periportal lymphedema (*black arrowheads*), a markedly distended IVC (*arrows*), and fluid (*white arrowheads*) around IVC. Diffuse small bowel wall edema (*curved arrows*) is also seen from venous volume overexpansion.

Subsequently this patient developed bowel obstruction 1 week later from herniation sigmoid colon and ileum.

CONCLUSION

Diagnostic imaging technology has advanced considerably during the past two decades. During this period conventional CT was replaced by single-slice helical CT, followed by multislice spiral CT. This has revolutionized cross-sectional imaging in trauma radiology. CT has become the imaging modality of choice to evaluate blunt trauma patients. Volumetric imaging with spiral CT has been a major factor for nonoperative management of solid organ injuries.

Most trauma centers in the United States have state-of-the-art single-slice or multislice spiral CT scanner suites in close proximity to the patient admitting area with facilities to monitor and maintain patient physiologic support. Now more than ever, newer versatile multislice CT protocols allow imaging not only of the abdomen and pelvis but also of multiple anatomic regions within a shorter period of time. This enables faster patient treatment in a busy trauma center. These new imaging protocols create exceptionally high resolution images in the axial plane and also allow multiplanar and 3-dimensional reformatted images, helping to improve detection of injuries. Diagnosis of hemorrhage and vascular injuries has been revolutionized by these techniques' helping to select patients for angiography and transcatheter embolization. Future advances in the multislice spiral CT technology, allowing more than four images per gantry rotation, will help the trauma radiologist to further exploit the technology's true potential.

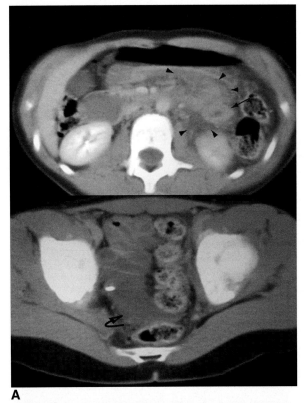

A

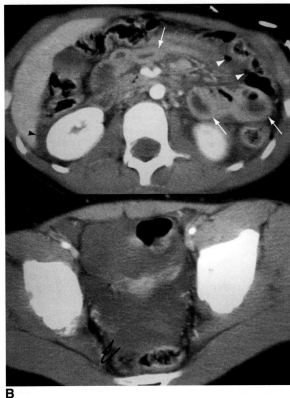

B

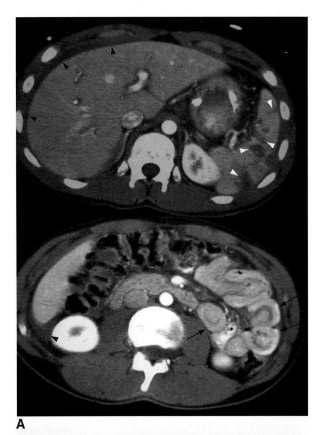

A

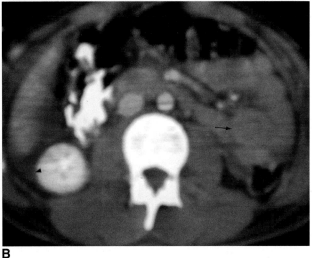

B

Fig. 6-133

Transmural bowel injury in an adult man admitted with minimal abdominal pain after a motor vehicle collision. **A,** Admission helical CT images show focal jejunal wall thickening (*arrow*) and adjacent mesenteric contusion (*arrowheads*); free intraperitoneal fluid (*curved arrow*) is seen in pelvis. **B,** Routine follow-up multislice spiral CT performed when patient had only minimal abdominal pain shows increase in the extent of focal jejunal wall thickening (*arrows*) and free intraperitoneal fluid (*curved arrows*) in pelvis. Free intraperitoneal air (*white arrowheads*) and free fluid in Morison's pouch (*black arrowheads*) are new findings. At celiotomy a transmural jejunal injury was repaired.

Fig. 6-134

Resolution of bowel wall contusion on follow-up CT in a 16-year-old blunt trauma patient. **A,** Admission multislice CT images show a grade IV splenic injury (*white arrowheads*) and loops of proximal small bowel with bowel wall thickening (*arrows*). Free intraperitoneal fluid (*black arrowheads*) is seen around liver and in right upper abdomen. No free intraperitoneal air is seen. Splenic and bowel injury were managed nonoperatively. **B,** Follow-up CT to assess bowel injury shows only a single loop of thick-walled small bowel (*arrow*). Intraperitoneal fluid (*arrowhead*) is less than observed on CT in right upper abdomen. Patient was successfully managed nonoperatively.

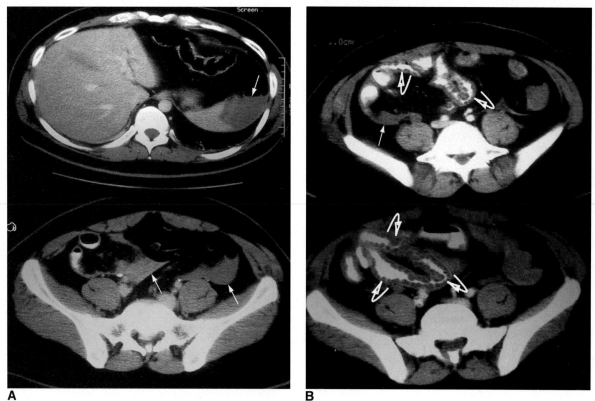

Fig. 6-135
Mesenteric injury resulting in bowel infarction on follow-up CT. **A,** Admission helical CT images show intraperitoneal fluid (*arrows*) adjacent to spleen and within mesentery of iliac fossa region. Highest density fluid is seen in right iliac fossa. No bowel wall thickening or free intraperitoneal air was seen. **B,** Follow-up CT obtained for persistent abdominal pain shows thick-walled terminal ileum (*curved arrows*), showing evidence of "thumbprinting" and minimal free intraperitoneal fluid (*arrow*). At surgery infarcted distal ileum was resected.

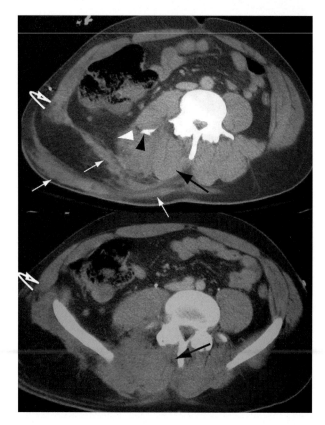

Fig. 6-136
Traumatic lumbar hernia in a 37-year-old man admitted after right-side abdominal trauma. Helical CT images show soft tissue contusion (*white arrows*) of right flank, right paraspinal muscle hematoma (*black arrows*), and avulsion (*curved arrows*) of right anterior abdominal wall muscle from its attachment to iliac crest leading to a lumbar hernia with retroperitoneal fat herniation (*white arrowhead*). Fracture of a right transverse process (*black arrowhead*) is also seen.

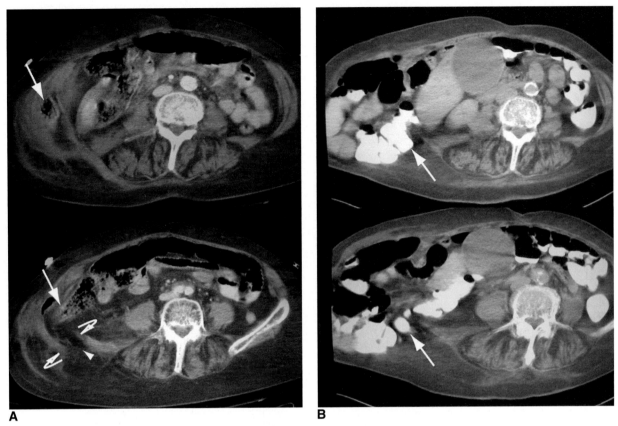

Fig. 6-137
Delayed presentation of a traumatic lumbar hernia in a 74-year-old woman. **A**, Admission helical CT images show avulsion of right abdominal wall muscle (*curved arrows*) with herniation of retroperitoneal fat (*arrowhead*) and colon (*arrows*) into a lumbar hernia in Petit's triangle. The colon is seen herniating between layers of anterior abdominal wall muscles. This hernia was not clinically confirmed or repaired on initial admission. **B**, Follow-up CT performed for a right flank mass 5 weeks after initial trauma shows a large lumbar hernia containing both large and small bowel (*arrows*). This hernia was surgically repaired.

REFERENCES

1. National Safety Council: *Injury facts*, Itasca, Ill., 2000 ed.
2. U.S. Department of Transportation, National Highway Traffic Safety Administration, 2000.
3. U.S. Department of Transportation: *Traffic safety facts*, Washington, DC, 1999.
4. Jones TK, Walsh JW, Maull KI: Diagnostic imaging in blunt trauma of the abdomen, *Surg Gynecol Obstet* 157:389, 1983.
5. Fabian TC, Mangiante EC, White TJ, et al: A prospective study of 91 patients undergoing computed tomography and peritoneal lavage following blunt abdominal trauma, *J Trauma* 26:602, 1986.
6. Bain M, Kirby RM, Tiwari P, et al: Survey of abdominal ultrasound and diagnostic peritoneal lavage for suspected intra-abdominal injury following blunt trauma, *Injury* 29:65, 1998.
7. Davis RJ, Morrison AL, Perkins SE, et al: Ultrasound: impact on diagnostic peritoneal lavage, abdominal computed tomography, and resident training, *Am Surg* 65:555, 1999.
8. Peitzman AB, Makaroun MS, Slasky BS, et al: Prospective study of computed tomography in initial management of blunt abdominal trauma, *J Trauma* 26:585, 1986.
9. McLellan BA, Hanna SS, Montoya DR, et al: Analysis of peritoneal lavage parameters in blunt abdominal trauma, *J Trauma* 25:393, 1985.
10. Swann IJ, Allister CA, Lewis HJ, et al: The value of peritoneal lavage in the assessment of patients with stab wounds of the abdomen and lower chest, *J R Coll Surg Edinb* 31:40, 1986.
11. Mackersie RC, Tiwary AD, Shackford SR, et al: Intra-abdominal injury following blunt trauma: identifying high risk patients using objective factors, *Arch Surg* 124:809, 1991.
12. Rodriguez A, DuPriest RW, Shantney CM: Recognition of intraabdominal injury in blunt trauma victims, *Am Surg* 48:456, 1982.
13. Patcher HL, Guth AA, Hofstetter SR, et al: Changing patterns in the management of splenic trauma: the impact on nonoperative management, *Ann Surg* 227:708, 1998.
14. Cogbill TH, Moore EE, Jurkovich GJ, et al: Nonoperative management of blunt splenic trauma: a multicenter experience, *J Trauma* 29:1312, 1989.
15. Nix JA, Costanza M, Daley BJ, et al: Outcome of the current management of splenic injuries, *J Trauma* 50:835, 2001.
16. Scafani SJA, Shafton GW, Scalea TM, et al: Nonoperative salvage of computed tomography-diagnosed splenic injuries: utilization of angiography for triage and embolization for hemostasis, *J Trauma* 39:818, 1995.
17. Mirvis SE, Shanmuganathan K: Abdominal computed tomography in blunt abdominal trauma, *Semin Roentgenol* 27:150, 1992.

18. Smith JS, Wengrovitz MA, DeLong BS: Prospective validation of criteria, including age, for safe, nonsurgical management of the ruptured spleen, *J Trauma* 33:363, 1992.

19. Croce MA, Fabian TC, Menke PG, et al: Nonoperative management of blunt hepatic trauma is the treatment of choice for hemodynamically stable patients: results of a prospective trial, *Ann Surg* 221:774, 1995.

20. Carrillo EH, Spain DA, Wohlmann CD, et al: Interventional techniques are useful adjunct in nonoperative management of hepatic injuries, *J Trauma* 46:619, 1999.

21. Sherman HF, Savage BA, Jones LM, et al: Nonoperative management of blunt hepatic injuries safe at any grade? *J Trauma* 37:616, 1994.

22. Rutledge R: The increasing frequency of nonoperative management of patients with liver and splenic injury, *Adv Surg* 30:385, 1997.

23. Sartorelli KH, Frumiento C, Rogers FB, et al: Nonoperative management of hepatic, splenic, and renal injuries in adults with multiple injuries, *J Trauma* 49:56, 2000.

24. Byrne RV: Diagnostic abdominal tap, *West J Surg* 64:369, 1956.

25. Morton JH, Hinshaw JR, Morton JJ: Blunt trauma to the abdomen, *Ann Surg* 145:699, 1957.

26. Root HD, Hauser CW, McKinley CR, et al: Diagnostic peritoneal lavage, *Surgery* 57:633, 1965.

27. Hodgson NF, Stewart TC, Girotti MJ: Open or closed diagnostic peritoneal lavage for abdominal trauma? a meta-analysis, *J Trauma* 48:1091, 2000.

28. Velmahos GC, Demitriades D, Stewart M, et al: Open versus closed diagnostic peritoneal lavage: a comparison on safety, rapidity, efficacy, *J R Coll Surg Edinb* 235, 1998.

29. Nagy KK, Roberts RR, Joseph KT, et al: Experience with over 2500 diagnostic peritoneal lavages, *Injury* 30:479, 2000.

30. Hennemann PL, Marx JA, Moore EE, et al: Diagnostic peritoneal lavage: accuracy in predicting necessary laparotomy following blunt and penetrating trauma, *J Trauma* 30:1345, 1990.

31. Lazarus HM, Nelson JA: A technique for peritoneal lavage without risk or complications, *Surg Gynecol Obstet* 149:889, 1979.

32. Fischer RP, Berverlin BC, Engrav LH, et al: Diagnostic peritoneal lavage: fourteen years and 2586 patients later, *Am J Surg* 136:701, 1978.

33. Ochsner MG, Herr D, Drucker W, et al: A modified Seldinger technique for peritoneal lavage in trauma patients who are obese, *Surg Gynecol Obstet* 173:158, 1991.

34. Menedez C, Gubler KD, Maier RV: Diagnostic accuracy of peritoneal lavage in patients with pelvic fractures, *Arch Surg* 129:477, 1994.

35. Cue JI, Miller FB, Cryer HM, et al: A prospective, randomized comparison between open and closed peritoneal lavage techniques, *J Trauma* 30:880, 1990.

36. Wilson WR, Schwartz TH, Pilcher DB: A prospective randomized trial of Lazarus-Nelson vs. the standard peritoneal dialysis catheter for peritoneal lavage in blunt trauma, *J Trauma* 27:1177, 1987.

37. Powell DC, Bevins BA, Bell RM: Diagnostic peritoneal lavage, *Surg Gynecol Obstet* 155:257, 1982.

38. Parvin S, Smith DE, Asher M, et al: Effectiveness of peritoneal lavage in blunt trauma, *Ann Surg* 181:255, 1975.

39. Kearney PA Jr, Vahey T, Burney RE, et al: Computed tomography and diagnostic peritoneal lavage in blunt abdominal trauma, *Arch Surg* 124:344, 1989.

40. Fabian TC, Croce MA: Abdominal trauma including indications for celiotomy. In Mattox KL, Feliciano DV, Moore EE, eds: *Trauma*, ed 4, New York, 2000, McGraw-Hill.

41. Hubbard SG, Bivins BA, Sachatello, et al: Diagnostic errors with peritoneal lavage in patients with pelvic fractures, *Arch Surg* 114:844, 1979.

42. Gilliand MG, Ward RE, Flynn TC, et al: Peritoneal lavage and angiography in the management of patients with pelvic fractures, *Am J Surg* 144:744, 1982.

43. Federle MP: Comparative value of computed tomography in the evaluation of trauma, *Emerg Med Rep* 4:147, 1983.

44. Kane NM, Dorfman GS, Cronan JJ, et al: Efficacy of CT following peritoneal lavage in abdominal trauma, *J Comput Assist Tomogr* 11:998, 1987.

45. Toombs BD, Lester RG, Ben-Menachem YB, et al: Computed tomography in blunt trauma, *Radiol Clin North Am* 19:17, 1981.

46. Freeman T, Fischer RP: The inadequacy of peritoneal lavage in diagnosing acute diaphragmatic rupture, *J Trauma* 16:538, 1976.

47. Hawkins ML, Bailey RL Jr, Carraway RP: Is diagnostic peritoneal lavage for blunt trauma obsolete? *Am Surg* 56:96, 1990.

48. Gelman R, Mirvis SE, Gens D: Diaphragmatic rupture due to blunt trauma: imaging assessment in 50 patients, *AJR Am J Roentgenol* 156:51, 1991.

49. Hawkins ML, Scofield WM, Carraway RP, et al: Diagnostic peritoneal lavage in blunt trauma, *South Med J* 81:255, 1988.

50. Akhrass R, Yaffe MB: Pancreatic trauma: a ten year multi-institutional experience, *Am Surg* 63:598, 1997.

51. Ballard RB, Badellino MM, Eynon A, et al: Blunt duodenal rupture: a 6-year statewide experience, *J Trauma* 43:229, 1997.

52. Orwig DS, Jeffrey RB Jr: Case report: CT of false-negative peritoneal lavage following blunt abdominal trauma, *J Comput Assist Tomogr* 11:1079, 1987.

53. Sullivan KR, Nelson MJ, Tandberg D: Incremental analysis of diagnostic peritoneal lavage fluid in adult abdominal trauma, *Am J Emerg Med* 15:277, 1997.

54. Sweeney JF, Bischof AE, McAllister EW, et al: Diagnostic peritoneal lavage: volume of lavage effluent needed for accurate determination of a negative lavage, *Injury* 25:659, 1994.

55. Perry JF, DeMeules JE, Root HD: Diagnostic peritoneal lavage in blunt abdominal trauma, *Surg Gynecol Obstet* 131:742, 1970.

56. Deepak V, Horan P, Obeid FN, et al: The importance of the WBC count in peritoneal lavage, *JAMA* 249:636, 1983.

57. Alyono D, Perry JF Jr: Value of quantitative cell count and amylase activity of peritoneal lavage fluid, *J Trauma* 21:345, 1981.

58. Jacobs DG, Angus L, Rodriguez A, et al: Peritoneal lavage white count: a reassessment, *J Trauma* 30:607, 1990.

59. Fang JF, Chen RJ, Lin BC: Cell count ratio: new criterion of diagnostic peritoneal lavage for detection of hollow organ perforation, *J Trauma* 45:540, 1998.

60. McAnena OJ, Marx JA, Moore EE: Peritoneal lavage enzyme determination following blunt and penetrating abdominal trauma, *J Trauma* 31:1161, 1991.

61. Jaffin JH, Ochsner MG, Cole FJ, et al: Alkaline phosphatase levels in diagnostic peritoneal lavage fluid as a predictor of hollow visceral injury, *J Trauma* 34:829, 1993.

62. Marx JA, Moore EE, Jorden RC, et al: Limitations of computed tomography in evaluation of acute abdominal trauma: a prospective comparison with diagnostic peritoneal lavage, *J Trauma* 25:933, 1985.

63. Tso P, Rodriguez A, Cooper C, et al: Sonography in blunt abdominal trauma: a preliminary progress report, *J Trauma* 33:39, 1992.

64. Lentz KA, McKenney MG, Nunez DB Jr, Martin L: Evaluation of blunt abdominal trauma: role for ultrasound, *J Ultrasound Med* 15:447, 1996.

65. Kretschmer KH, Bohndorf K, Pohlenz O: The role of sonography in abdominal trauma: the European experience, *Emerg Radiol* 4:62, 1997.

66. Bode PJ, van Vugt AB: Ultrasound in the diagnosis of injury, *Injury* 27:379, 1996.

67. Bode PJ, Niezen RA, Van Vugt AB, et al: Abdominal ultrasound as a reliable indicator for conclusive laparotomy in blunt abdominal trauma, *J Trauma* 34:27, 1993.

68. Chambers JA, Pilbrow WJ: Ultrasound in abdominal trauma: an alternative to peritoneal lavage, *Arch Emerg Med* 5:26, 1988.

69. Rozycki GS: Abdominal ultrasonography in trauma, *Surg Clin North Am* 75:175, 1995.

70. Glaser K, Tschemelitsch J, Klinger P, et al: Ultrasonography in the management of blunt abdominal and thoracic trauma, *Arch Surg* 129:743, 1994.

71. Goletti G, Ghiselli G, Lippolis PV, et al: The role of ultrasonography in blunt abdominal trauma: results in 200 consecutive cases, *J Trauma* 36:178, 1994.

72. Liu M, Lee CH, Peng FK: Prospective comparison of diagnostic peritoneal lavage, computed tomographic scanning, and ultrasonography of blunt abdominal trauma, *J Trauma* 35:267, 1993.

73. Huang MS, Liu M, Wu JK, et al: Ultrasonography for the evaluation of hemoperitoneum during resuscitation: a simple scoring system, *J Trauma* 36:173, 1994.

74. Rothlin MA, Naf R, Amgwered M, et al: Ultrasound in blunt abdominal and thoracic trauma, *J Trauma* 34:488, 1993.

75. Fernandez L, McKenney MG, McKenney KL, et al: Ultrasound in blunt abdominal trauma. *J Trauma* 45:841, 1998.

76. McGahan JP, Richard JR: Blunt abdominal trauma: the role of emergent sonography and a review of the literature, *AJR Am J Roentgenol* 172:897, 1999.

77. Dolich MO, McKenney MG, Esteban JE, et al: 2,576 ultrasounds for blunt abdominal trauma, *J Trauma* 50:108, 2001.

78. McKenney KL, Nunez DB Jr, McKenney MG, et al: Sonography as the primary screening technique for blunt abdominal trauma: experience with 899 patients, *AJR Am J Roentgenol* 170:979, 1998.

79. McKenney KL, McKenney MG, Cohn SM, et al: Hemoperitoneum score helps determine need for therapeutic laparotomy, *J Trauma* 50:650, 2001.

80. Boulanger BR, McLellan BA, Brenneman FD, et al: Prospective evidence of the superiority of a sonography based algorithm in the assessment of blunt abdominal injury, *J Trauma* 47:632, 1999.

81. Goodwin H, Holmes JF, Wisner DH: Abdominal ultrasound examination in pregnant blunt trauma patient, *J Trauma* 50:689, 2001.

82. Boulanger BR, McLellan BA, Brenneman FD, et al: Emergent abdominal sonography as a screening test in a new diagnostic algorithm for blunt trauma, *J Trauma* 40:867, 1996.

83. Gruessner R, Mentges B, Duber CH, et al: Sonography versus peritoneal lavage in blunt abdominal trauma, *J Trauma* 29:242, 1989.

84. McKenney M, Lentz K, Nunez D, et al: Can ultrasound replace diagnostic peritoneal lavage in the assessment of blunt trauma? *J Trauma* 37:439, 1994.

85. Rozycki GS, Ballard RB, Feliciano DV, et al: Surgeon-performed ultrasound for the assessment of truncal injuries: lesson learned from 1540 patients, *Ann Surg* 228:557, 1998.

86. Bode PJ, Edwards MJR, Kurit MC, et al: Sonography in a clinical algorithm for early evaluation of 1671 patients with blunt abdominal trauma, *AJR Am J Roentgenol* 172:905, 1999.

87. Pearl WS, Todd KH: Ultrasonography for initial evaluation of blunt abdominal trauma: a review of prospective trials, *Ann Emerg Med* 27:353, 1996.

88. McGahan JP, Rose J, Coates TL, et al: Use of ultrasonography in the patient with acute abdominal trauma, *J Ultrasound Med* 16:653, 1997.

89. Chiu WC, Cushing BM, Rodriguez A, et al: Abdominal injuries without hemoperitoneum: a potential limitation of focused abdominal sonography for trauma, *J Trauma* 42:817, 1997.

90. Sherbourn CD, Shanmuganathan K, Mirvis SE, et al: Visceral injury without hemoperitoneum: a limitation of screening abdominal sonography for trauma, *Emerg Radiol* 4:301, 1997.

91. Shanmuganathan K, Mirvis SE, Sherbourn CD, et al: Hemoperitoneum as the sole indicator of abdominal visceral injuries: a potential limitation of screening abdominal US for trauma, *Radiology* 212:423, 1999.

92. Ballard RB, Rozycki GS, Newman PG, et al: An algorithm to reduce the incidence of false-negative FAST examinations in patients at high risk for occult injury: focused assessment for the sonographic of the trauma patient, *J Am Coll Surg* 189:145, 1999.

93. Coley BD, Mutabagani KH, Martin LC, et al: Focused abdominal sonography for trauma (FAST) in children with blunt abdominal trauma, *J Trauma* 48:902, 2000.

94. Beny EC, Lim-dunham JE, Landrum O, et al: Abdominal sonography in examination of children with blunt abdominal trauma, *AJR Am J Roentgenol* 176:1613, 2000.

95. Oschner MG, Knudson MM, Patcher HL, et al: Significance of minimal or no free intraperitoneal fluid visible on CT scan associated with blunt liver and splenic injuries: a multicentric analysis, *J Trauma* 49:505, 2000.

96. Emery KH, McAneney CM, Racaido JM, et al: Absent peritoneal fluid on screening trauma ultrasonography in children: a prospective comparison with computed tomography, *J Pediatr Surg* 36:565, 2001.

97. Brown MA, Casola G, Sirlin CB, et al: Importance of evaluating organ parenchyma during screening abdominal ultrasonography after blunt trauma, *J Ultrasound Med* 20:577, 2001.

98. Ma JO, Kefer MP, Stevison KF, et al: Operative versus nonoperative management of blunt abdominal trauma: role of ultrasound measured intraperitoneal fluid levels, *Am J Emerg Med* 19:284, 2001.

99. Holmes JF, Brant WE, Bond WF, et al: Emergency department ultrasonography in the evaluation of hypotensive and normotensive children with blunt abdominal trauma, *J Pediatr Surg* 36:968, 2001.

100. McKenney KL. Ultrasound of blunt abdominal trauma, *Radiol Clin North Am* 37:879, 1999.

101. Rozycki GS, Ochsner G, Feliciano DV, et al: Early detection hemoperitoneum by ultrasound examination of the right upper quadrant: a multicenter study, *J Trauma* 45:878, 1998.

102. Branney SW, Wolfe RE, Moore EE, et al: Quantitative sensitivity of ultrasound in detecting free intraperitoneal fluid, *J Trauma* 39:375, 1995.

103. Paajanen H, Lathti P, Nordback I: Sensitivity of transabdominal ultrasonography in detecting intraperitoneal fluid in humans, *Eur Radiol* 9:1423, 1999.

104. Richards JR, McGahan JP, Jones CD, et al: Ultrasound detection of blunt splenic injury, *Injury* 32:95, 2001.

105. Kuligowska E, Barish MA, Soto JA, et al: Real time ultrasound versus spiral computed tomography in evaluation of blunt abdominal trauma (abstract), *J Ultrasound Med* 27:353, 1996.

106. Siniluoto TM, Pavivansalo MJ, Lanning FP, et al: Ultrasonography in traumatic splenic rupture, *Clin Radiol* 46:391, 1992.

107. Wong JJ, Shanmuganathan K, Chiu WC, et al: Sonography compared to CT in the detection and grading of liver injuries. Presented at ARRS, San Francisco, 1998.

108. Richards JR, McGahan JP, Pali MJ, et al: Sonographic detection of blunt hepatic trauma: hemoperitoneum and parenchymal patterns of injury, *J Trauma* 47:1092, 1999.

109. Yoshii H, Sato M, Yamamoto S, et al: Usefulness and limitations of ultrasonography in the initial evaluation of blunt abdominal trauma, *J Trauma* 45:45, 1998.

110. Knudson M, Maull KI: Nonoperative management of solid organ injuries, *Surg Clin North Am* 79:1357, 1999.

111. Kemmeter PR, Hoedema RE, Foote JA: Concomitant blunt enteric injuries with injuries of the liver and spleen: a dilemma for trauma surgeons, *Am Surg* 67:221, 2001.

112. Shackford SR, Roger FB, Osler TM, et al: Focused abdominal sonogram for trauma: the learning curve of nonradiologist clinicians in detecting hemoperitoneum, *J Trauma* 46:553, 1999.

113. Buzzas GR, Kern SJ, Smith RS, et al: A comparison of sonographic examination for trauma performed by surgeons and radiologist, *J Trauma* 44:604, 1998.

114. Rozycki GS, Oschner MG, Schmith JA, et al: A prospective study of surgeon-performed ultrasound as the primary adjuvant modality for injured patient assessment, *J Trauma* 39:492, 1995.

115. Rozycki GS, Ochsner MG, Jaffin JH, Champion HR: Prospective evaluation of surgeons' use of ultrasound in the evaluation of trauma patients, *J Trauma* 34:516, 1993.

116. Cushing BM, Chiu WC: Credentialing for the ultrasonographic evaluation of trauma patients, *Trauma Q* 13:205, 1997.

117. Scalea TM, Rodriguze A, Chiu WC, et al: Focused assessment with sonography for trauma (FAST): results from an international consensus conference, *J Trauma* 46:466, 1999.

118. Federle MP, Crass RA, Jefferey RB, et al: Computed tomography in blunt abdominal trauma, *Arch Surg* 117:645, 1982.

119. Fuchs WA, Robotti G: The diagnostic impact of computed tomography in blunt abdominal trauma, *Clin Radiol* 34:261, 1983.

120. Taylor CR, Degutis L, Burns R, et al: Computed tomography in the initial evaluation of hemodynamically stable patients with blunt abdominal trauma: impact of severity of injury scale and technical factors on efficacy, *J Trauma* 44:893, 1998.

121. Jhirad R, Boone D: Computed tomography for evaluation of blunt abdominal trauma in the low-volume nondesignated trauma center: the procedure of choice? *J Trauma* 45:64, 1998.

122. Livingston DH, Lavery RF, Passannante MR, et al: Admission or observation is not necessary after a negative abdominal computed tomographic scan in patients with suspected blunt abdominal trauma: results of a prospective, multi-institutional trial, *J Trauma* 44:273, 1998.

123. Jeffery RB, Cardoza JD, Olcott EW: Detection of active abdominal arterial hemorrhage: value of dynamic contrast-enhanced CT, *AJR Am J Roentgenol* 156:65, 1991.

124. Federle MP: Computed tomography in blunt abdominal trauma, *Radiol Clin North Am* 21:461, 1983.

125. Jeffery RB, Federle MP, Walls S: Value of computed tomography in detecting occult intestinal perforation, *J Comput Assist Tomogr* 7:825, 1983.

126. Federle MP, Goldberg HI, Kaiser JA, et al: Evaluation of trauma by computed tomography, *Radiology* 138:637, 1981.

127. Navarrete-Navarro P, Vazquez G, Bosch JM, et al: Computed tomography vs clinical and multidisciplinary procedure for early evaluation of severe abdominal and chest trauma, *Intensive Care Med* 22:208, 1996.

128. Mirvis SE, Whitley NO, Gens DR: Blunt splenic trauma in adults: CT-based classification and correlation with prognosis and treatment, *Radiology* 171:33, 1989.

129. Mirvis SE, Whitley NO, Vainwright JR, et al: Blunt hepatic trauma in adults: CT-based classification and correlation with prognosis and treatment, *Radiology* 171:27, 1989.

130. Shanmuganathan K, Mirvis SE, Sover ER: Value of contrast-enhanced CT in detecting active hemorrhage in patients with blunt abdominal or pelvic trauma, *AJR Am J Roentgenol* 161:65, 1993.

131. Jacobs LM: The effect of prospective reimbursement on trauma patients, *Bull Am Coll Surg* 70:17, 1985.

132. MacKenzie EJ, Morris JA, Smith GS, et al: Acute hospital cost of trauma in the United States: implications for regionalized trauma system of care, *J Trauma* 30:1087, 1990.

133. Nastanski F, Cohen A, Lush SP, et al: The role of oral contrast administration immediately before the computed tomographic evaluation of the blunt trauma victim, *Injury* 32:545, 2001.

134. Shankar KR, Lloyd DA, Kitteringham L, Carty HM: Oral contrast with computed tomography in the evaluation of blunt abdominal trauma in children, *Br J Surg* 86:1073, 1999.

135. Clancy TV, Ragozzino MW, Ramshaw D, et al: Oral contrast is not necessary in the evaluation of blunt abdominal trauma by computed tomography, *Am J Surg* 166:680-684, 1993.

136. Stafford RE, McGonigal MD, Weigelt JA, et al: Oral contrast solution and computed tomography for blunt abdominal trauma: a randomized study, *Arch Surg* 134:622-626, June 1999.

137. Federle MP, Yagan N, Peitzman AB, et al: Abdominal trauma: use of oral contrast material for CT is safe, *Radiology* 205:91, 1997.

138. Federle MP, Peitzman A, Krugh J. Use of oral contrast material in abdominal trauma CT scans: is it dangerous? *J Trauma* 38:51, 1995.

139. Shanmuganathan K, Mirvis SE, Reaney SM: Pictorial review: CT appearance of contrast medium extravasation associated with injury sustained from blunt abdominal trauma, *Clin Radiol* 50:182, 1995.

140. Orwig D, Federle MP: Localized clotted blood as evidence of visceral trauma on CT: the sentinel clot sign, *AJR Am J Roentgenol* 153:747, 1989.

141. Mirvis SE, Rodrigous A: Abdominal and pelvic trauma. In Mirvis SE, Young WR, eds: *Imaging in trauma and critical care*, Baltimore, 1992, Williams & Wilkins.

142. Livingston DH, Lavery RF, Passannante MR, et al: Free fluid on abdominal computed tomography without solid organ injury after blunt abdominal injury does not mandate celiotomy, *Am J Surg* 182:6, 2001.

143. Harris HW, Morabito DJ, Mackersie RC, et al: Leukocytosis and free fluid are important indicators of isolated intestinal injury after blunt trauma, *J Trauma* 46:656, 1999.

144. Brasel KJ, Olson CJ, Stafford RE, et al: Incidence and significance of free fluid on abdominal computed tomographic scan in blunt trauma, *J Trauma* 44:889, 1998.

145. Cunningham MA, Tyroch AH, Kaups KL, Davis JW: Does free fluid on abdominal computed tomographic scan after blunt trauma require laparotomy? *J Trauma* 44:599, 1998.

146. Hulka L, Mullins RJ, Leanardo V, et al: Significance of peritoneal fluid as an isolated finding on abdominal computed tomographic scan in pediatric trauma patients, *J Trauma* 44:1069, 1998.

147. Levine CD, Patel UJ, Waschberg RH, et al: CT in patients with blunt abdominal trauma: clinical significance of intraperitoneal fluid detected on a scan with otherwise normal findings, *AJR Am J Roentgenol* 164:1381, 1995.

148. Sirlin CB, Casola G, Brown MA, et al: Use of blunt abdominal trauma: importance of free pelvic fluid in women of reproductive age, *Radiology* 219:229, 2001.

149. Shackford SR, Molin M: Management of splenic injuries, *Surg Clin North Am* 70:595, 1990.

150. Morris DH, Bullock FD: Importance of the spleen in resistance to infection, *Ann Surg* 70:513, 1919.

151. King H, Shumacker HB: Splenic studies, *Ann Surg* 136:239, 1952.

152. Eichner ER: Splenic function: normal, too much and too little, *Am J Med* 66:311, 1979.

153. Green JB, Shackford SR, Sise MJ, et al: Late complications in adults following splenectomy for trauma: a prospective analysis of 144 patients, *J Trauma* 116:651, 1986.

154. Pimpl W, Dapunt O, Kaindl H, et al: Incidence of septic and thromboembolic related deaths after splenectomy in adults, *Br J Surg* 76:517, 1989.

155. Davis KA, Fabian TC, Corce MA, et al: Improved success in non-operative management of blunt splenic injury: embolization of splenic artery pseudoaneurysm, *J Trauma* 44:1008, 1998.

156. Shanmuganathan K, Mirvis SE, Boyd-Kranis R, et al: Nonsurgical management of blunt splenic injury: use of CT criteria to select patients for splenic arteriography and potential endovascular therapy, *Radiology* 217:75, October 2000.

157. Brasel KJ, DeLisle CM, Olson CJ, Borgstrom DC: Splenic injury: trends in evaluation and management, *J Trauma* 4:283, 1998.

158. Archer LP, Rogers FB, Shackford SR: Selective nonoperative management of liver and splenic injuries in neurologically impaired adult patients, *Arch Surg* 131:309, 1996.

159. Federle MP, Goldberg HH, Kaiser JA, et al: Evaluation of abdominal trauma by computed tomography, *Radiology* 138:637, 1981.

160. Fischer RP, Miller-Crotchett P, Reed RL II: Gastrointestinal disruption: the hazard of nonoperative management in adults with blunt abdominal injuries, *J Trauma* 28:1445, 1988.

161. Federle MP, Griffiths B, Minage H, Jeffrey RB: Splenic trauma: evaluation with CT, *Radiology* 162:69, 1987.

162. Morrell DG, Chang FC, Helmer SD: Changing trends in the management of splenic injuries, Am J Surg 170:686, 1995.

163. Malangoni MA, Cue JI, Fallat ME, et al: Evaluation of splenic injury by computed tomography and its impact on treatment, Ann Surg 211:592, 1990.

164. Becker CD, Spring P, Glattli A, Schweizer W: Blunt splenic trauma in adults: can CT findings be used to determine the need for surgery? AJR Am J Roentgenol 162:343, 1994.

165. Starnes S, Klein P, Magagna L, et al: Computed tomographic grading is useful in the selection of patients for nonoperative management of blunt injury to the spleen, Am Surg 64:743, 1998.

166. Downey EC, Shackford SR, Fridlund PH, et al: Long-term depressed immunity in patients splenectomized for trauma, J Trauma 27:661, 1987.

167. Najjar VA, Nishioka K: Tuftsin: a natural phagocytosis stimulating peptide, Nature 228:672, 1970.

168. Kohn JS, Clark DE, Isler RJ, et al: Is computed tomographic grading of splenic injury useful in the management of blunt trauma? J Trauma 36:385, 1994.

169. Moore EE, Cogbill TH, Jurkovich GJ, et al: Organ injury scaling: spleen and liver (1994 revision), J Trauma 38:323, 1995.

170. Becker CD, Mentha G, Terrier F: Blunt abdominal trauma in adults: role of CT in the diagnosis and management of visceral injuries, Eur Radiol 8:553, 1998.

171. Shapiro MJ, Krausz C, Durham RM, et al: Overuse of splenic scoring and computed tomography, J Trauma 47:651, 1999.

172. Sutyak JP, Chiu WC, D'Ameilo LF, et al: Computed tomography is inaccurate in estimating the severity of adult splenic injury, J Trauma 39:514, 1995.

173. Moore EE, Shackford SR, Patcher HL, et al: Organ injury scale: spleen, liver, and kidney, J Trauma 29:1664, 1989.

174. Moore EE, Cogbill TH, Malangoni MA, et al: Organ injury scale II: pancreas, duodenum, small bowel, colon, and rectum, J Trauma 30:1427, 1990.

175. Buntain WL, Gould HR, Maull KI: Predictability of splenic salvage by computed tomography, J Trauma 28:24, 1987.

176. Sclafani SJA, Weisberg A, Scalea TM, et al: Blunt splenic injuries: nonsurgical treatment with CT, arteriography, and transcatheter arterial embolization of the splenic artery, Radiology 161:189, 1991.

177. Hagiwara A, Yukioka T, Ohta S, et al: Nonsurgical management of patients with blunt splenic artery: efficacy of transcatheter arterial embolization, AJR Am J Roentgenol 167:159, 1996.

178. Federle MP, Courcoulas AP, Powell M, et al: Blunt splenic injury in adults: clinical and CT criteria for management, with emphasis on active extravasation, Radiology 206:137, 1998.

179. Gavant ML, Schurr M, Flick PA, et al: Predicting clinical outcome of nonsurgical management of blunt splenic injury: using CT to reveal abnormalities in the splenic vasculature, AJR Am J Roentgenol 168:207, 1997.

180. Upddhyaya P, Simpson JS: Splenic trauma in children, Surg Gynecol Obstet 126:781, 1968.

181. Wesson DE, Filler RM, Ein SH, et al: Ruptured spleen—when to operate? J Pediatr Surg 16:324, 1981.

182. Pearl RH, Wesson DE, Spence LJ, et al: Splenic injury: a five year update with improved results and changing criteria for conservative management, J Pediatr Surg 24:428, 1989.

183. Feliciano PD, Mullins RJ, Trunckey DD, et al: A decision analysis of traumatic splenic injuries, J Trauma 33:340, 1992.

184. Demetriades D, Vandenbossche P, Ritz M, et al: Non-therapeutic operations for penetrating trauma: early morbidity and mortality, Br J Surg 80:860, 1993.

185. Fakhry SM, Brownstein M, Watts DD, et al: Relatively short diagnostic delays (<8 hours) produce morbidity and mortality in blunt small bowel injury: an analysis of time to operative intervention in 198 patients from a multicenter experience, J Trauma 48:408, 2000.

186. Renz BM, Feliciano DV: Unnecessary laparotomy for trauma: a prospective study of morbidity, J Trauma 38:350, 1995.

187. Weigelt JA, Kingman RG: Complications of negative laparotomy for trauma, Am J Surg 156:544, 1988.

188. Rappaport W, McIntyre KE Jr, Carmona R: The management of splenic trauma in the adult patient with blunt multiple injuries, Surg Gynecol Obstet 170:204, March 1990.

189. Patcher HL, Spence FC, Hofstetter SR, et al: Experience with selective operative and nonoperative treatment of splenic injuries in 193 patients, Ann Surg 211:583, 1990.

190. Shackford SR, Molin M: Management of splenic injuries, Surg Clin of North Am 70:595, 1990.

191. Velmahos GC, Chan LS, Kamel E, et al: Nonoperative management of splenic injuries: have we gone too far? Arch Surg 135:674, 2000.

192. Bee TK, Corce MA, Miller PR, et al: Failure of splenic nonoperative management: is the glass half empty or half full? J Trauma 50:230, 2001.

193. Myers JG, Dent DL, Stewart RM, et al: Blunt splenic injuries: dedicated trauma surgeons can achieve a high rate of nonoperative success in patients of all ages, J Trauma 48:801, 2000.

194. Krause KR, Howell GA, Bair HA, et al: Nonoperative management of blunt splenic injury in adults 55 years and older: a twenty-year experience, Am Surg 66:636, 2000.

195. Smith SJ, Wengrovitz MA, DeLong BS: Prospective validation of criteria, including age, for safe, nonsurgical management of the ruptured spleen, J Trauma 33:363, 1992.

196. Mirvis SE: Role of CT in diagnosis and management of splenic injury, Applied Radiol, April 2000, p 7.

197. Peitzman AB, Heil B, Rivera L, et al: Blunt splenic injury in adults: multi-institutional study of the Eastern Association for the Surgery of Trauma, J Trauma 49:177, 2000.

198. Godley CD, Warren RL, Sheridan RL, et al: Nonoperative management of blunt splenic injury in adults: age over 55 years as a powerful indicator for failure, J Am Coll Surg 183:133, 1996.

199. Cocanour CS, Moore FA, Ware DN, et al: Age should not be a consideration for nonoperative management of blunt splenic injury, J Trauma 48:606, April 2000.

200. Gaunt WT, McCarthy MC, Lambert CS, et al: Traditional criteria for observation of splenic trauma should be challenged, Am Surg 65:689, July 1999.

201. Krause KR, Howells GA, Bair HA, et al: Nonoperative management of blunt splenic injury in adults 55 years and older: a twenty-year experience, Am Surg 66:636, July 2000.

202. Starnes S, Klein P, Magagna L, et al: Computed tomographic grading is useful in the selection of patients for nonoperative management of blunt injury to the spleen, Am Surg 64:743, 1998.

203. Scatamacchia SA, Raptopoulos V, Fink MP, Silva WE: Splenic trauma in adults: impact of CT grading on management, Radiology 171:725, 1989.

204. Longo WE, Baker CC, McMillen MA, et al: Nonoperative management of adult blunt splenic trauma: criteria for successful outcome, Ann Surg 210:626, November 1989.

205. Fischer RP, Miller-Crotchett P, Reed RL: Gastrointestinal disruption: the hazard of nonoperative management in adults with blunt abdominal injury, J Trauma 28:1445, 1988.

206. Archer LP, Rogers FB, Shackford SR: Selective nonoperative management of liver and splenic injuries in neurologically impaired adult patients, Arch Surg 131:309, 1996.

207. Rosai J: Ackerman's surgical pathology, ed 8 St Louis, 1996, Mosby.

208. Hiraide A, Yamamoto H, Yahata K, et al: Delayed rupture of the spleen caused by an intrasplenic pseudoaneurysm following blunt trauma: case report, J Trauma 36:743, 1994.

209. Omert LA, Salyer D, Dunham M, et al: Implications of the "contrast blush" finding on computed tomographic scan of spleen in trauma, *J Trauma* 51:272, 2001.

210. Lewis D, Mirvis SE, Shanmuganathan K: Segmental renal infarcts, *Emerg Radiol* 3:236, 1996.

211. Uecker J, Pickette C, Dunn E: The role of follow-up radiographic studies in nonoperative management of splenic trauma, *Am Surg* 67:22, 2001.

212. Thaemert BC, Cogbill TH, Lambert PJ: Nonoperative management of splenic injuries: are follow-up computed tomographic scans of any value? *J Trauma* 43:748, 1997.

213. Federle MP: Splenic trauma: is follow-up CT of value? *Radiology* 194:23, 1995.

214. Lawson DL, Jacobson JA, Spizarny DL, et al: Splenic trauma: value of follow-up CT, *Radiology* 197:97, 1995.

215. Chiarugi M, Goletti O, Pucciarelli M, et al: Post-traumatic intrasplenic pseudoaneurysm successfully managed by embolization, *Injury* 26:705, 1995.

216. Baron BJ, Scalea TM, Sclafani SJA, et al: Nonoperative management of blunt abdominal trauma: the role of sequential diagnostic peritoneal lavage, computed tomography, and angiography, *Ann Emerg Med* 22:1556, 1993.

217. Schurr MJ, Fabian TC, Gavant M, et al: Management of blunt splenic trauma: computed tomographic contrast blush predicts failure of nonoperative management, *J Trauma* 39:507, 1995.

218. Killeen KL, Shanmuganathan K, Boyd-Kranis R, et al: CT findings after embolization for blunt splenic trauma, *J Vasc Interv Radiol* 12:209, 2001.

219. Haney PJ, Whitley NO, Brotman S, et al: Liver injury and complications in postoperative trauma patients: CT evaluation, *AJR Am J Roentgenol* 139:271, 1982.

220. Patcher HL, Spencer FC, Hofstetter SR. Management of juxta venous injuries without an arterial caval shunt: preliminary clinical observations, *Surgery* 99:569, 1986.

221. Feliciano DV, Mattox KL, Jordan GL, et al: Management of 1000 consecutive cases of hepatic trauma (1979-1984), *Ann Surg* 204:438, 1986.

222. Asensio JA, Demetriades D, Chahwan S, et al: Approach to the management of complex hepatic injuries, *J Trauma* 48:66, 2000.

223. Cogbill TH, Moore EE, Jurkovich GJ, et al: Severe hepatic trauma: a multi-center experience with 1,335 liver injuries, *J Trauma.* 28:1433, October 1988.

224. Pachter HL, Feliciano DV: Complex hepatic injuries, *Surg Clin North Am* 76:763, August 1996.

225. Denton JR, Moore EE, Cordwell DM: Multimodality treatment for grade V hepatic injuries: perihepatic packing, arterial embolization, and venous stenting, *J Trauma* 42:964, 1997.

226. Ciraulo DL, Luk S, Palter M, et al: Selective hepatic arterial embolization of grade IV and V blunt hepatic injuries: an extension of resuscitation in the nonoperative management of traumatic hepatic injuries, *J Trauma* 45:353, August 1998.

227. Chen RJ, Fang JF, Lin BC, et al: Factors determining operative mortality of grade V blunt hepatic trauma, *J Trauma* 49:886, 2000.

228. Becker CD, Mentha G, Terrier F: Blunt abdominal trauma in adults: role of CT in the diagnosis and management of visceral injuries. 1. Liver and spleen, *Eur Radiol* 8:553, 1998.

229. Jeffrey RB Jr, Olcott EW: Imaging of blunt hepatic trauma, *Radiol Clin North Am* 29:1299, November 1991.

230. Pachter HL, Hofstetter SR: The current status of nonoperative management of adult blunt hepatic injuries, *Am J Surg* 169:442, April 1995.

231. Goff CD, Gilbert CM: Nonoperative management of blunt hepatic trauma, *Am Surg* 61:66, January 1995.

232. Young JS, Meredith JW: Nonoperative management of blunt hepatic injuries: current concepts, *Surg Annu* 27:71, 1995.

233. Poletti PA, Mirvis SE, Shanmuganathan K, et al: CT criteria for management of blunt liver trauma: correlation with angiographic and surgical findings, *Radiology* 216:418, August 2000.

234. Couinaud C: *Le foie: etudes anatomiques et chirurgicales,* Paris, 1957, Masson.

235. Williams PL, Warwick R, Dyson M, Bannister LH: Abdominal viscera. In *Gray's anatomy,* ed 37, Edinburgh, 1989, Churchill Livingstone.

236. Knudson MM, Lim RC Jr, Oakes DD, et al: Nonoperative management of blunt liver injuries in adults: the need for continued surveillance, *J Trauma* 30:1494, 1990.

237. Goff CD, Gilbert CM: Nonoperative management of blunt hepatic trauma, *Am Surg* 61:66, 1994.

238. Hiatt JR, Harrier DH, Koenig BV, Ransom KJ: Nonoperative management of major blunt liver injury with hemoperitoneum, *Arch Surg* 125:101, 1990.

239. Sherman HF, Savage BA, Jones LM, et al: Nonoperative management of blunt hepatic injuries at any grade? *J Trauma* 37:616, 1994.

240. Federico JA, Horner WR, Clark DE, et al: Blunt hepatic trauma nonoperative management in adults, *Arch Surg* 125:905, 1990.

241. Meyer AA, Crass RA, Lim RC, et al: Selective nonoperative management of blunt liver injury using computed tomography, *Arch Surg* 120:550, 1985.

242. Trauma Committee, Canadian Association of Pediatric Surgeons: Canadian Association of Pediatric Surgeons: liver trauma study, *J Pediatr Surg* 24:1035, 1989.

243. Brasel KJ, DeLisle CM, Olson CJ, et al: Trends in the management of hepatic injury, *Am J Surg* 174:674, 1997.

244. Holland MJ, Little JM: Non-operative management of blunt liver injuries, *Br J Surg* 78:968, 1991.

245. Meredith JW, Young JS, Bowling J, et al: Nonoperative management of blunt hepatic trauma: the exception or the rule? *J Trauma* 36:529, April 1994.

246. Patcher HL, Knudson MM, Esrig B, et al: Status of nonoperative management of blunt hepatic injuries in 1995: a multicenter experience with 404 patients, *J Trauma* 40:31, 1996.

247. Rutledge R: The increasing frequency of nonoperative management of patients with liver and spleen injury, *Adv Surg* 30:385, 1996.

248. Hagiwara A, Yukioka T, Ohta S, et al: Nonsurgical management of patients with blunt hepatic injury: efficacy of transcatheter arterial embolization, *AJR Am J Roentgenol* 169:1151, 1997.

249. Sugimoto K, Horiik S, Hirata M, et al: The role of angiography in the assessment of blunt liver injury, *Injury* 25:283, 1994.

250. Wagner WH, Lundell C, Donovan A: Percutaneous angiographic embolization for hepatic arterial hemorrhage, *Arch Surg* 120:1241, 1985.

251. McClelland RN, Shiers GT: Management of liver trauma in 259 consecutive patients, *Postgrad Med* 48:200, 1970.

252. Rouhana SW: Biomechanics of abdominal trauma. In Nahum AM, Melvin JW, eds: *Accidental injuries biomechanics and prevention,* New York, 1993, Springer-Verlag.

253. Mirvis SE, Dunham CM: Abdominal/pelvic trauma. In Mirvis SE, Young JWR, eds: *Imaging in trauma and critical care,* Baltimore, 1992, Williams & Wilkins.

254. Becker CD, Gal I, Baer HU, et al: Blunt hepatic trauma in adults: correlation of CT injury grading with outcome, *Radiology* 201:215, October 1996.

255. Brick SH, Taylor GA, Potter BM, Eichelberger MR: Hepatic and splenic injury in children: role of CT in the decision for laparotomy, *Radiology* 165:643, 1987.

256. Bulas DI, Eichelberger MR, Sivit CJ, et al: Hepatic injury from blunt trauma in children: follow up evaluation with CT, *AJR Am J Roentgenol* 160:347, 1993.

257. Gay SB, Sistrom CL: Computed tomographic evaluation of blunt abdominal trauma, *Radiol Clin North Am* 30:367, 1992.

258. Markert DJ, Shanmuganathan K, Mirvis SE, et al: Budd-Chiari syndrome resulting from intrahepatic IVC compression secondary to blunt hepatic trauma, *Clin Radiol* 52:384, 1997.

259. Geis WP, Schulz KA, Giacchino JL, et al: The fate of unruptured intrahepatic hematomas, *Surgery* 90:689,1981.

260. Savolaine ER, Grecos GP, Howard J, et al: Evolution of CT findings in hepatic hematoma, *J Comput Assist Tomogr* 9:1090, 1985.

261. Patten RM, Spear RP, Vincent LM, et al: Traumatic lacerations of the liver limited to the bare area: CT findings in 25 patients, *AJR Am J Roentgenol* 160:1019, 1993.

262. Beal SL: Fatal hepatic hemorrhage: an unresolved problem in the management of complex liver injuries, *J Trauma* 30:163, 1990.

263. Burch JM, Feliciano DV, Mattox KL: The atriocaval shunt facts and fiction, *Ann Surg* 207:555, 1988.

264. Ochsner MG, Jaffin JH, Golocovsky M, Jones RC: Major hepatic trauma, *Surg Clin North Am* 73:337, 1992.

265. Ciresi KF, Lim RC Jr: Hepatic vein and retrohepatic vena caval injury, *World J Surg* 14:472, 1990.

266. Weber S, Murphy MM, Pitzer ME, et al: Management of retrohepatic venous injuries with atrial caval shunts, *AORN J* 64:376, 1996.

267. Fang JF, Chen RJ, Wong YC, et al: Pooling of contrast material on computed tomography mandates aggressive management of blunt hepatic injury, *Am J Surg* 176:315, October 1998.

268. Fang JF, Chen RJ, Wong YC, et al: Classification and treatment of pooling of contrast material on computed tomographic scan of blunt hepatic trauma, *J Trauma* 49:1083, 2000.

269. Schwartz RA, Teitelbaum GP, Katz MD, et al: Effectiveness of transcatheter embolization in the control of hepatic vascular injuries, *J Vasc Interv Radiol* 4:359, 1993.

270. Pain JA, Heaton ND, Karani JB, et al: Selective arterial embolization for hepatic trauma, *Ann R Coll Surg Edin* 73:189, 1991.

271. Rubin BE, Katzen BT: Selective hepatic artery embolization to control massive hepatic hemorrhage after trauma, *AJR Am J Roentgenol* 129:253, 1977.

272. Hashimoto S, Hiramatsu K, Ido K, et al: Expanding role of emergency embolization in the management of severe blunt hepatic trauma, *Cardiovasc Intervent Radiol* 13:193, 1990.

273. Carrillo EH, Spain DA, Wohltmann CD, et al: Interventional techniques are useful adjuncts in nonoperative management of hepatic injuries, *J Trauma* 46:619, April 1999.

274. Macrander SJ, Lawson TL, Foley WD, et al: Periportal tracking in hepatic trauma: CT features, *J Comput Assist Tomogr* 13:952, 1989.

275. Yokota J, Sugimoto T: Clinical significance of periportal tracking on computed tomographic scan in patients with blunt liver trauma, *Am Surg* 168:247, 1994.

276. Shanmuganathan K, Mirvis SE, Amerosa M: Periportal low density on CT in patients with blunt trauma: association with elevated venous pressure, *AJR Am J Roentgenol* 160:279, 1992.

277. Patrick EL, Turner BI, Atkinson GO, et al: Pediatric blunt abdominal trauma: periportal tracking at CT, *Radiology* 183:689, 1992.

278. Soderstrom CS, Maekawa K, Dupriest RW, Dowley RA Jr: Gallbladder injuries resulting from blunt abdominal trauma: an experience and review, *Ann Surg* 193:60, 1981.

279. Ball DS, Friedman AC, Radecki PD, et al: Avulsed gallbladder: CT appearance, *J Comput Assist Tomogr* 12:538, 1988.

280. Brickley HD, Kaplan A, Freeark RJ, et al: Immediate and delayed rupture of the extrahepatic biliary tract following blunt abdominal trauma, *Am J Surg* 100:107, 1960.

281. Erb RE, Mirvis SE, Shanmuganathan K: Gallbladder injury secondary to blunt trauma: CT findings, *J Comput Assist Tomogr* 18:778, 1994.

282. Hall ER, Howard JM, Jordan GL, et al: Traumatic injuries of the gallbladder, *Ann Surg* 72:520, 1956.

283. Oldham KT, Guice KS, Ryckman F, et al: Blunt liver injury in childhood: evolution of therapy and current perspective, *Surgery* 100:542, 1986.

284. Pirola RC, Davis AE: Effects of ethyl alcohol on sphincteric resistance at the choledocho-duodenal junction in man, *Gut* 9:557, 1968.

285. Smith SW, Hastings TN: Traumatic rupture of the gallbladder, *Ann Surg* 139:517,1956.

286. Burgess P, Fulton RL: Gallbladder and extrahepatic biliary duct injury following abdominal trauma, *Injury* 23:413, 1992.

287. Scaglione M, Rossi G, Pinto F, et al: Gallbladder blunt trauma: comparison between radiologic and anatomo-surgical findings, *Radiol Med (Torino)* 96:592, 1998.

288. McNabeny WK, Rudek R, Pemberton LB: The significance of gallbladder trauma, *J Emerg Med* 8:277, 1990.

289. Sharma O: Blunt gallbladder injuries: presentation of twenty-two cases with review of the literature, *J Trauma* 39:576, 1995.

290. Esensten M, Ralls PW, Colletti P, et al: Posttraumatic intrahepatic biloma: sonographic diagnosis, *AJR Am J Roentgenol* 140:303, 1983.

291. Feliciano DV: Biliary injuries as a result of blunt and penetrating trauma, *Surg Clin North Am* 74:897, August 1994.

292. Rydell WB Jr: Complete transection of the common bile duct due to blunt abdominal trauma, *Arch Surg* 100:724, 1970.

293. Sugiyama M, Atomi Y, Matsuoka T, et al: Endoscopic biliary stenting for treatment of persistent biliary fistula after blunt hepatic injury, *Gastrointest Endosc* 51:42, 2000.

294. Hollands MJ, Little JM: Post-traumatic bile fistulae, *J Trauma* 31:117, 1991.

295. Sugimoto K, Asari Y, Sakaguchi T, et al: Endoscopic retrograde cholangiography in the nonsurgical management of blunt liver injury, *J Trauma* 35:192, 1993.

296. Scioscia PJ, Dillon PW, Cilley RE, et al: Endoscopic sphincterotomy in the management of posttraumatic biliary fistula, *J Pediatr Surg* 29:3, 1994.

297. Moser JJ, Schweizer W, Czerniak A, et al: Segmental bile duct injury after blunt abdominal trauma: a difficult diagnosis, *Hepatogastroenterology*, 42:103, 1995.

298. Charters CA: Intrahepatic bile duct rupture following blunt abdominal trauma, *Arch Surg* 113:873, 1978.

299. D'Amours SK, Simon RK, Scadamore CH, et al: Major intrahepatic bile duct injuries detected after laparotomy: selective nonoperative management *J Trauma* 50:480, 2001.

300. Fletcher WS, Mahnke DE, Dunphy JE: Complete division of the common bile duct due to blunt trauma, *J Trauma* 1:87, 1961.

301. Davis KA, Brody JM, Cioffi WG: Computed tomography in blunt hepatic trauma, *Arch Surg* 131:255, 1996.

302. Byone RP, Bell RM, Miles WS, et al: Complications of nonoperative management of blunt hepatic injuries, *J Trauma* 32:308, 1992.

303. Olsen WR: Late complications of central liver injuries, *Surgery* 92:733, 1982.

304. Abramson SJ, Berdon WE, Kaufman RA, Ruzal-Shapiro C: Hepatic parenchymal and subcapsular gas after hepatic laceration caused by blunt abdominal trauma, *AJR Am J Roentgenol* 153:1031, 1989.

305. Howdieshell TR, Purvis J, Bates WB, et al: Biloma and biliary fistula following hepatorrhaphy for liver trauma: incidence, natural history, and management, *Am Surg* 61:165, 1995.

306. Weissmann HS, Byun KJC, Freeman LM: Role of Tc-99m IDA scintigraphy in the evaluation of hepatobiliary trauma, *Semin Nucl Med* 13:199, 1985.

307. Barker SL, Fromm D: Bile peritonitis following expectant management of liver fracture, *NY State J Med* 87:565, 1987.

308. De Becker A, Fierens H, De Schepper A, et al: Diagnosis and nonsurgical management of bile leak complicated by biloma after blunt liver injury: report of two cases, *Eur Radiol* 8:1619, 1998.

309. Esensten M, Ralls PW, Colletti P, et al: Posttraumatic intrahepatic biloma: sonographic diagnosis, *AJR Am J Roentgenol* 140:303, 1983.

310. Schmidt B, Bhatt GM, Abo MN: Management of post-traumatic vascular malformations of the liver by catheter embolization, *Am J Surg* 140:332, 1980.

311. Bulas DI, Eichelberger MR, Sivit CJ, et al: Hepatic injury from blunt trauma in children: follow-up evaluation with CT, *AJR Am J Roentgenol* 160:347, 1993.

312. Karp MP, Cooney DR, Pros GA, et al: The nonoperative management of pediatric hepatic trauma, *J Pediatr Surg* 18:512, 1983.

313. Allins A, Ho T, Nguyen TH, et al: Limited value of routine follow-up CT scans in nonoperative management of blunt liver and splenic injury, *Am Surg* 62:883, 1996.

314. Northrup WF, Simmons RL: Pancreatic trauma: a review, *Surgery* 71:27, 1972.

315. Freeman CP: Isolated pancreatic damage following seat belt injury, *Injury* 16:478, 1985.

316. Stone HH, Fabian TC, Satiani B, et al: Experiences in the management of pancreatic trauma, *J Trauma* 21:257, 1981.

317. Jones RC: Management of pancreatic trauma, *Am J Surg* 150:698, 1985.

318. Wilson RH, Moorehead RJ: Current management of trauma to the pancreas, *Br J Surg* 78:1196, 1991.

319. Hendel R, Rusnak CH: Management of pancreatic trauma, *Can J Surg* 28:359, 1985.

320. Nilsson E, Norrby S, Skullman S, et al: Pancreatic trauma in a defined population, *Acta Chir Scand* 152:647, 1986.

321. Canty TG Sr, Weinman D: Management of pancreatic duct injuries in children, *J Trauma* 50:1001, 2001.

322. Jones WG II, Reilly DM, Barie PS: Pancreatic injuries diagnosis, treatment, *AORN J* 53:917, 1991.

323. Craig MH, Talton DS, Hauser CJ, et al: Pancreatic injuries from blunt trauma, *Am Surg* 61:125, 1995.

324. Bradley EL III, Young PR, Chang MC, et al: Diagnosis and initial management of blunt pancreatic trauma, *Ann Surg* 227:861, 1997.

325. Patton JH, Lyden SP, Croce MA, et al: Pancreatic trauma: a simplified management and guideline, *J Trauma* 43:234, 1997.

326. Glancy KE: Review of pancreatic trauma, *West J Med* 151:45, 1989.

327. Barkin JS, Ferstenberg RM, Panullo W, et al: Endoscopic retrograde cholangiopancreatography in pancreatic trauma, *Gastrointest Endosc* 34:102, 1988.

328. Feliciano DV, Martin TD, Cruse PA: Management of combine pancreaticoduodenal injuries, *Ann Surg* 205:673, 1987.

329. Tal AP, Wilson RF: A pattern of sever blunt trauma to the region of pancreas, *Surg Gynecol Obstet* 118:773, 1964.

330. Lucas CE: Diagnosis and treatment of pancreatic and duodenal injury, *Surg Clin North Am* 57:49, 1977.

331. Horst HM, Bivins BA: Pancreatic transection: a concept of evolving injury, *Arch Surg* 124:1093, 1989.

332. Craig MH, Talton DS, Hauser CJ, et al: Pancreatic injuries from blunt trauma, *Am Surg* 61:125, 1995.

333. Donovan AJ, Turrill F, Berne CJ: Injuries of the pancreas from blunt trauma, *Surg Clin North Am* 52:649, 1972.

334. Bouwman DL, Weaver DW, Walt AJ Serum amylase and its isoenzymes: a clarification of their implications in trauma, *J Trauma* 24:573, 1984.

335. Jeffrey RB Jr, Federele MP, Crass RA: Computed tomography of pancreatic trauma, *Radiology* 147:491, 1983.

336. Cogbill TH, Moore EM Kashuk JL: Changing trends in the management of pancreatic trauma, *Arch Surg* 117:722, 1982.

337. Ryan S, Sandler S, Trenhaile S, et al: Pancreatic enzyme elevation after blunt trauma, *Surgery* 116:622, 1994.

338. Takishima T, Sugimoto K, Hirata M, et al: Serum amylase level on admission in the diagnosis of blunt injury to the pancreas, *Ann Surg* 226:70, 1997.

339. Akhrass R, Yaffe MB, Brandt CP, et al: Pancreatic trauma: a ten-year multi-institutional experience, *Am Surg* 63:598, July 1997.

340. Cook DE, Walsh JW, Vick CW, Brewer WH: Upper abdominal trauma: pitfalls in CT diagnosis, *Radiology* 159:65, 1986.

341. Bigattini D, Boverie JH, Dondelinger RF: CT of blunt trauma of the pancreas in adults, *Eur Radiol* 9:244, 1999.

342. Akhrass R, Kim K, Brandt C: Computed tomography: an unreliable indicator of pancreatic trauma, *Am Surg* 62:647, 1996.

343. Patel SV, Spencer JA, El-Hasani S, et al: Imaging of pancreatic trauma, *Br J Radiol* 71:985, 1998.

344. Lane MJ, Mindelzun RE, Sandhu JS, et al: CT diagnosis of blunt pancreatic trauma: importance of detecting fluid between the pancreas and the splenic vein, *AJR Am J Roentgenol* 163:833, 1994.

345. Lane MJ, Mindelzun RE, Jeffrey RB: Diagnosis of pancreatic injury after blunt abdominal trauma, *Semin Ultrasound CT MR* 17:177, 1996.

346. Dodds WJ, Taylor AJ, Erickson SJ, et al: Traumatic fracture of the pancreas: CT characteristics, *J Comput Assist Tomogr* 14:375, 1990.

347. Procacci C, Grazaiani R, Bigego E, et al: Blunt pancreatic trauma: role of CT, *Acta Radiol* 38:543, 1997.

348. Wong YC, Wang LJ, Lin BC, et al: CT grading of blunt pancreatic injuries: prediction of ductal disruption and surgical correlation, *J Comput Assist Tomogr* 21:246, 1997.

349. Jeffrey RB, Laing FC, Wing VW: Ultrasound in acute pancreatic trauma, *Gastrointest Radiol* 11:44, 1986.

350. Whittwell AW, Gomez GA, Byers P, et al: Blunt pancreatic trauma: prospective evaluation of early endoscopic retrograde pancreatography, *South Med J* 82:586, 1989.

351. Barkin JS, Frestenberg RM, Panullo W, et al: Endoscopic retrograde cholangiopancreatography in pancreatic trauma, *Gastrointest Endosc* 34:102, 1988.

352. Chandler C, Waxman K: Demonstration of pancreatic ductal integrity by endoscopic retrograde pancreatography allows conservative surgical management, *J Trauma* 40:466, 1996.

353. Canty TG Sr, Weinman D: Treatment of pancreatic duct disruption in children by an endoscopically placed stent, *J Pediatr Surg* 36:345, 2001.

354. Clements RH, Reisser JR: Urgent endoscopic retrograde pancreatography in the stable trauma patient, *Am Surg* 62:446, 1996.

355. Chamrova Z, Shanmuganathan K, Mirvis SE, et al: Retroperitoneal fluid resulting from rapid intravascular resuscitation in trauma: CT mimic of retroperitoneal injury, *Emerg Radiol* 1:85, 1994.

356. Nirula R, Velmahos GC, Demetriades D: Magnetic resonance cholangiopancreatography in pancreatic trauma: a new diagnostic modality? *J Trauma* 47:585, 1999.

357. Ward J, Charmers AG, Larvi AJ, et al: T2-weighted and dynamic enhanced MRI in acute pancreatitis: comparison with contrast enhanced CT, *Clin Radiol* 52:109, 1996.

358. Fulcher AS, Turner MA, Yelon JA, et al: Magnetic resonance cholangiopancreatography (MRCP) in the assessment of pancreatic ductal trauma and its sequelae: preliminary findings, *J Trauma* 48:1001, 2000.

359. Soto JA, Alverez O, Munera F, et al: Traumatic disruption of the pancreatic duct: diagnosis with MR pancreatography, *AJR Am J Roentgenol* 176:175, 2001.

360. Fulcher AS, Turner MA, Capps GW, et al: Half-Fourier RARE MR cholangiopancreatography in 300 subjects, *Radiology* 207:21, 1998.

361. Sica GT, Braver J, Cooney MJ, et al: Comparison of endoscopic retrograde cholangiopancreatography with MR cholangiopancreatography in patients with pancreatitis, *Radiology* 203:605, 1999.

362. Sherman S, Lehman GA: ERCP- and endoscopic sphincterotomy–induced pancreatitis, *Pancreas* 6:350, 1991.

363. Soto JA, Yucel EK, Barish MA, et al: MR cholangiopancreatography after unsuccessful ERCP, *Radiology* 199:91, 1996.

364. Doctor N, Dooley JS, Davidson BR: Assessment of pancreatic duct damage following trauma: is endoscopic retrograde cholan-

giopancreatography the gold standard? *Postgrad Med J* 71:116, 1995.

365. Huckfeldt R, Agee C, Nichols WK, et al: Nonoperative treatment of traumatic pancreatic duct disruption using an endoscopically placed stent, *J Trauma* 41:143, 1996.

366. Harrell DJ, Vitale GC, Larson GM: Selective role for endoscopic retrograde cholangiopancreatography in abdominal trauma, *Surg Endosc* 12:400, 1998.

367. Takishima T, Horiike S, Sugimoto K, et al: Role of repeat computed tomography after emergency endoscopic retrograde pancreatography in the diagnosis of traumatic injury to pancreatic ducts, *J Trauma* 40:253, 1996.

368. Kim HS, Lee DK, Kim IW, et al: The role of endoscopic retrograde pancreatography in the treatment of traumatic pancreatic duct injury, *Gastrointest Endosc* 54:49, 2001.

369. Moore JB, Moore EE: Changing trends in the management of combined pancreatoduodenal injuries, *World J Surg* 8:791, 1984.

370. Timberlake G: Blunt pancreatic trauma: experience at a rural referral, *Am Surg* 63:282, 1997.

371. Carr ND, Cairns SJ, Lees WR, et al: Late complications of pancreatic trauma, *Br J Surg* 76:1244, 1989.

372. Lewis G, Krige JE, Bornman PC, et al: Traumatic pancreatic pseudocyst, *Br J Surg* 80:89, 1993.

373. Rizzo MJ, Federle MP, Griffiths BG: Bowel and mesenteric injury following blunt abdominal trauma: evaluation with CT, *Radiology* 173:143, 1989.

374. Donohue J, Crass R, Trunkey D: Management of duodenal and small intestinal injury, *World J Surg* 9:904, 1985.

375. Burney RE, Mueller GL, Coon WW, et al: Diagnosis of isolated small bowel injury, *Ann Emerg Med* 12:71, 1983.

376. Donohue JH, Federle MP, Griffiths BG, et al: Computed tomography in the diagnosis of blunt intestinal and mesenteric injuries, *J Trauma* 27:11, 1987.

377. Mirvis SE, Gens DR, Shanmuganathan K: Rupture of the bowel after blunt abdominal trauma: diagnosis with CT, *AJR Am J Roentgenol* 159:1217, 1992.

378. Sherck JP, Oakes DD: Intestinal injuries missed by computed tomography, *J Trauma* 30:1, 1990.

379. Meyer DM, Thal ER, Weigert JA, et al: Evaluation of computed tomography and diagnostic peritoneal lavage in blunt abdominal trauma, *J Trauma* 29:1168, 1989.

380. Malhotra AK, Fabian TC, Katsis SB, et al: Blunt bowel and mesenteric injuries: the role of screening computed tomography, *J Trauma* 48:991, 2000.

381. Killeen KL, Shanmuganathan K, Poletti PA, et al: Helical computed tomography of bowel and mesenteric injuries, *J Trauma* 51:26, 2001.

382. Janzen DL, Zwirewich CV, Breen DJ, et al: Diagnostic accuracy of helical CT for detection of blunt bowel and mesenteric injuries, *Clin Radiol* 53:193, 1998.

383. Dowe MF, Shanmuganathan K, Mirvis SE, et al: CT findings of mesenteric injury after blunt trauma: implications for surgical intervention, *AJR Am J Roentgenol* 168:425, 1997.

384. Breen DJ, Janzen DL, Zwirewich CV, et al: Blunt bowel and mesenteric injury: diagnostic performance of CT signs, *J Comput Assist Tomogr* 21:706, 1997.

385. Sivit CJ, Eichelberger MR, Taylor GA: CT in children with rupture of the bowel caused by blunt trauma: diagnostic efficacy and comparison with hypoperfusion complex, *AJR Am J Roentgenol* 163:1195, 1994.

386. Otomo Y, Henmi H, Mashiko K, et al: New diagnostic peritoneal lavage criteria for diagnosis of intestinal injury, *J Trauma* 44:991, 1998.

387. Fang J, Chen R, Lin B, et al: Small bowel perforation: is urgent surgery necessary? *J Trauma* 47:515, 1999.

388. Mirvis SE, Shanmuganathan K, Erb R: Diffuse small bowel ischemia in hypotensive adults after blunt trauma (shock bowel): CT findings and clinical significance, *AJR Am J Roentgenol* 163:1375, 1994.

389. Sivit CJ, Taylor GA, Bulas DI, et al: Posttraumatic shock in children: CT findings associated with hemodynamic instability, *Radiology* 182:723, 1992.

390. Sherbourne CD, Mirvis SE: Computed tomographic diagnosis of bowel and mesenteric injuries after blunt abdominal trauma, *Contemp Diagn Radiol* 20:1, 1997.

391. Bulkley GB, Kvietys PR, Parks DA, et al: Relationship of blood flow and oxygen consumption to ischemic injury in the canine small intestine, *Gastroenterology* 89:852, 1985.

392. Butela ST, Federle MP, Chang PJ, et al: Performance of CT in detection of bowel injury, *AJR Am J Roentgenol* 176:129, 2001.

393. Allen GS, Moore FA, Cox CS, et al: Hollow visceral injury and blunt trauma, *J Trauma* 45:69, 1998.

394. Neugebauer H, Wallenboeck E, Hungerford M: Seventy cases of injuries of small intestine caused by blunt abdominal trauma: a retrospective study from 1970 to 1994, *J Trauma* 46:116, 1999.

395. Cantry TG Sr, Cantry TG, Brown C: Injuries of the gastrointestinal tract from blunt trauma in children: a 12-year experience at a designated pediatric trauma center, *J Trauma* 46:234, 1999.

396. Killeen KL, Girard S, DeMeo JH, et al: Using CT to diagnose traumatic lumbar hernia, *AJR Am J Roentgenol* 174:1413, 2000.

397. Faro SH, Racette CD, Lally JF, et al: Traumatic lumbar hernia: CT diagnosis, *AJR Am J Roentgenol* 154:757, 1990.

398. Baker ME, Weinerth JL, Andriani RT, et al: Lumbar hernia: diagnosis by CT, *AJR Am J Roentgenol* 148:565, 1987.

399. Payne DD, Resnicoff SA, States JD, et al: Seat-belt abdominal wall muscular avulsion, *J Trauma* 13:262, 1973.

400. McCarthy MC, Lemmon GW: Traumatic lumbar hernia: a seat belt injury, *J Trauma* 40:121, 1996.

401. Damsechen DD, Landercasper J, Cogbill TH, et al: Acute traumatic abdominal hernia: case report, *J Trauma* 36:273, 1994.

7   Injuries to the Urinary System and Retroperitoneum

Stuart E. Mirvis

This chapter considers imaging findings related to blunt injury of the urinary system. The focus is on acute traumatic injury but also considers, where appropriate, iatrogenic injury and complications arising from urinary system injury. In recent years computed tomography (CT) has become the primary diagnostic tool for the rapid and accurate assessment of acute traumatic urinary tract trauma, substantially replacing both intravenous pyelography and nuclear scintigraphy. As such, the CT appearances of various traumatic urinary system injuries will be emphasized. In certain situations other modalities, including intravenous urography, retrograde nephrography, sonography, renal nuclear scintigraphy, renal angiography, and renal MRI, are still required, and their use is discussed where applicable.

During the past decade diagnostic imaging, particularly CT, has provided information that is valuable for the "staging" of urinary system trauma, likely improving decision making regarding optimal patient management. Interventional radiology has increasingly been used to manage vascular renal injury and complications of renal injury, often avoiding the need for surgical exploration. The use of diagnostic and therapeutic radiology in the management of urinary tract injury is also emphasized in this section.

IMAGING RENAL INJURY
Clinical Aspects

Renal injury is common, occurring in 8% to 10% of all cases of blunt and penetrating abdominal injury.[1] The clinical indications to perform imaging evaluation of the urinary system are controversial and depend on the overall hemodynamic status of the patient, other injuries sustained, location of blunt injury, and other imaging studies required. Patients who are hemodynamically unstable and cannot be rapidly resuscitated are usually taken directly to surgery. A rapid intravenous pyelogram (IVP) can be performed in the admission area but is probably best obtained in the operating room once hemodynamic stability is achieved. This single radiograph will allow visualization of both kidneys, if functional, and detect the majority of major renal parenchymal injury.[2] Minor renal parenchymal lacerations and contusions may not be detected by a screening IVP but are unlikely to have major clinical ramifications.

The value of the presence of hematuria as an indicator of significant renal injury has been debated, but a consensus appears to be developing. Hardeman et al.[3] found that 21 of 25 patients (84%) presenting with gross hematuria after trauma had documented renal injury from blunt force trauma. Microscopic hematuria without hypotension is very *unlikely* to be associated with major renal injury. Miller and McAninch[4] reviewed 1588 blunt trauma patients who had presented without hematuria or shock on admission. Only three had significant renal injuries, and all were diagnosed at laparotomy indicated for other reasons.[4] Among this population were 515 patients who had no renal imaging evaluation at all, and none had delayed problems related to renal injury. A combination of four series, including 2873 blunt trauma patients with microscopic hematuria but without shock on admission, reported only 10 patients with significant renal injuries, most of which were detected at laparotomy performed for other indications.[4] Alternatively, these authors reported that 78 of 422 patients admitted with gross hematuria or microscopic hematuria with shock had grades II to V renal injuries (Table 7-1), of which 34 required repair.[4] However, in the pediatric trauma population, Stein et al.[5] reported CT results of 412 patients and stated that microscopic hematuria without hypotension *could* be associated with significant renal injuries and recommended CT for gross and microscopic hematuria. Finally, a normal urinalysis does not exclude renal artery avulsion and in one series[6] was reported in up to 24% of patients with major renal artery occlusion.

At the University of Maryland Shock Trauma Center (UMSTC), it is not customary to obtain an imaging evaluation of the urinary system for microscopic hematuria in hemodynamically stable patients with blunt injury (almost exclusively adult trauma victims). Given this complex relationship between hematuria and possible renal injury, decisions regarding imaging evaluation are still controversial. Several other clinical factors should also be considered and are reflected in the imaging guidelines utilized at UMSTC, as listed in Table 7-2.

CT Technique for Renal Trauma

In general, the kidneys and proximal collecting systems are evaluated as part of the abdominal CT study without special protocols. Currently, UMSTC uses a quad detector Philips 8000 Mx (Philips Medical Systems, Best, Netherlands). The urinary tract is imaged as part of the routine abdominal-pelvic CT for trauma, using 2.5-mm image slice thickness. Because of the rapid scanning capability, imaging of the kidneys typically shows only renal cortical enhancement without contrast excretion into the collecting system (Fig. 7-1). To adequately assess renal function and to detect renal contrast extravasation, delayed images through the urinary tract are mandatory. Typically, this follow-up study is delayed for 1 to 2 minutes, as the first image series is immediately available for review to detect any urgent conditions. Early arterial-phase CT images through the kidneys demonstrate perfu-

Table 7-1	
American Association for the Surgery of Trauma Renal Injury Grading Scale	
AAST Injury Grade	**Description**
I	Renal contusion or subcapsular hematoma with intact capsule
II	Superficial cortical laceration that does not involve the deep renal medulla or collecting system or nonexpanding perinephric hematoma
III	Deep laceration(s) with or without urinary extravasation
IV	Lacerations extending into the collecting system with contained urine leak
V	Shattered kidney, renal vascular pedicle injury, devascularized kidney

From Santucci RA, McAninch JW, Safir M, et al: *J Trauma* 50:195, 2001.

Table 7-2	
Indications for Renal Imaging in Acute Trauma	
Indication	**Imaging Study**
Penetrating flank and back trauma	Chest, abdominal-pelvic CT with IV, oral, and rectal contrast
Gross hematuria—hemodynamically stable or resuscitated	Abdominal-pelvic CT with oral and IV contrast
Hemodynamically unstable—requiring emergency surgery	Intraoperative IVP when stabilized
Hemodynamically stable with microscopic hematuria but no other indication for abdominal-pelvic CT	Observation for resolution of hematuria
Hemodynamically stable with microscopic hematuria but other indications for abdominal-pelvic CT (positive abdominal examination, decreasing hematocrit, indeterminate result of peritoneal lavage or abdominal sonography, unreliable physical examination)	Abdominal-pelvic CT with oral and IV contrast
Hemodynamically stable with or without microscopic hematuria, with evidence of major flank impact as lower posterior rib or lumbar transverse process fracture, major contusion of flank soft tissues	Abdominal-pelvic CT with oral and IV contrast

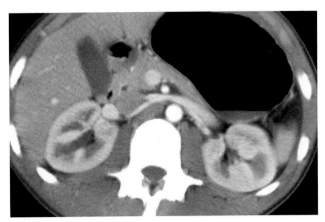

Fig. 7-1
Early arterial phase of multislice CT shows bright cortical enhancement only with marked contrast against low-attenuation medullary areas.

sion and active bleeding, while the delayed renal images provide more information about extent of parenchymal injury and collecting system integrity. As noted subsequently, this CT study should not be considered to provide an adequate basis for CT cystography if the urinary drainage catheter has been clamped prior to the CT, although bladder injuries frequently are diagnosed in this manner.

Although renal sonography can be used in the acute setting to identify renal injury, it does not appear to be highly sensitive. Perry et al.[7] reported three cases of major renal injury that were missed by sonography and highlighted CT as the initial study of choice. Similarly, McGahan et al.[8] described results of renal sonography in 32 patients with documented renal trauma. Most patients with renal injury did not display free intraperitoneal fluid (an indirect sign of injury), and only 8 of 37 total injuries (22%) were directly seen on dedicated renal sonography. A positive sonogram was more likely with higher grades of renal injury, but a negative renal sonogram had a very low negative predictive value.[8]

CT Grading of Renal Injury and Implications for Management

The management of renal injury largely depends on extent of injury combined with overall patient status. CT provides an excellent technique to assess renal parenchymal integrity and function, urinary excretion, extent of perinephric or perirenal hematoma, and ongoing renal bleeding. The American Association for the Surgery of Trauma (AAST) has devised a renal injury severity score based on surgical observations, as described in Table 7-1, which correlates with likely outcomes for management of renal trauma.[9]

This classification is useful to predict which patients are likely to be successfully managed nonoperatively

(grades I and II) and those that will likely or definitely require operative or nonoperative intervention (grades IV and V). There are several types of pathology diagnosed by CT that are not included in this grading scale. A useful CT grading scale should mimic the surgical classification whenever possible to ensure accurate and consistent communication. Table 7-3 describes the renal injury grading scale in use at UMSTC, including observations that may be unique to contrast-enhanced spiral CT imaging.

CT of Minor Renal Injury. Most renal injuries are minor (75% to 98%), represented by CT grades I and II, and are successfully treated without intervention[10] (Figs. 7-2 and 7-3). Contusions are visualized as ill-defined low-attenuation areas with irregular margins (Fig. 7-4). They may appear as regions with a striated nephrogram pattern because of differential blood flow through the

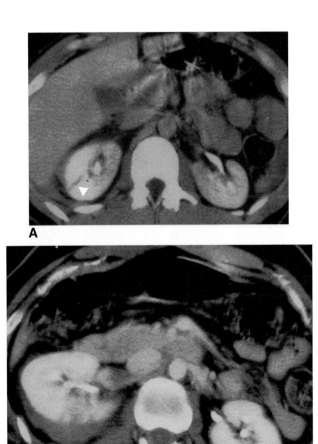

Fig. 7-2
Minor renal injury. **A,** A small superficial cortical laceration is present (*arrowhead*). Note minimal perinephric and pararenal hemorrhage. **B,** Posterior perinephric hematoma with small superficial cortical lacerations. (**B** from Mirvis SE, Hastings G, Scalea TM: Diagnostic imaging, angiography, and interventional radiology in the trauma patient. In Mattox KL, Feliciano DL, Moore EE, eds: *Trauma,* ed 4, New York, 2000, McGraw-Hill.)

Table 7-3
Contrast-Enhanced Spiral CT Grading of Blunt Renal Injury

Injury Grade	Description or CT Finding
I	Superficial laceration(s) involving cortex
	Renal contusion(s)
	<1-cm subcapsular hematoma
	Perinephric hematoma not filling Gerota's space and no active bleeding
	Segmental renal infarction
II	Renal laceration extending to medulla with intact collecting system
	>1-cm subcapsular hematoma without delayed renal function
	Stable perinephric hematoma without active bleeding confined to nondistended perinephric space
III	Laceration extending into collecting system with urine extravasation limited to retroperitoneum
	Perinephric hematoma distending perinephric space or extending into pararenal spaces without active bleeding
	Renal split (2 fragments) with >50% viable parenchyma
	Subcapsular hematoma causing delayed renal urine excretion
IV	Fragmentation (3 or more segments) of the kidney (usually partially devitalized with large perinephric hematoma)
	Devascularization >50% of renal parenchyma
	Renal vascular pedicle injury
	Active bleeding or pseudoaneurysm
	Extravasation of urine into peritoneal cavity or extensive extravasation
	Subcapsular hematoma compromising renal perfusion
	Pelvis or ureteropelvic junction tear

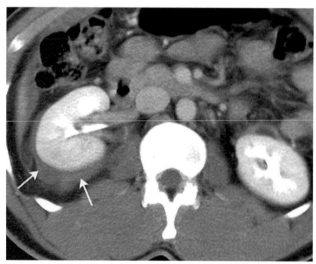

Fig. 7-3
Minor renal injury. Small perinephric hematoma (*arrows*).

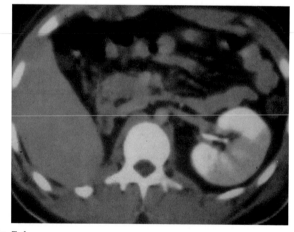

Fig. 7-4
Renal contusion. Single hypertrophic left kidney shows differential contrast flow with areas of diminished density in midportion, suggesting edema that slows perfusion in this area.

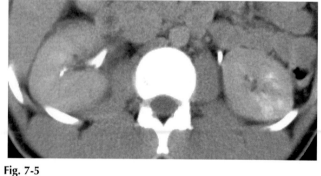

Fig. 7-5
Renal contrast intravasation. Areas of leaked contrast persist into excretory phase of left kidney, indicating injury to intraparenchymal collecting system.

contused area or may demonstrate focal areas of renal parenchymal extravasation on delayed noncontrast CT studies[11] (Fig. 7-5). The lesions usually resolve during follow-up imaging.

Segmental renal infarcts are relatively common in blunt renal trauma and result from stretching and subsequent occlusion of an accessory renal artery, extra- or intrarenal artery branch vessel, or capsular artery.[12] These infarcts appear as sharply demarcated wedge-shaped areas of very low attenuation, typically involving the renal pole(s) (Figs. 7-6 and 7-7). Associated major renal injuries may or may not accompany segmental renal

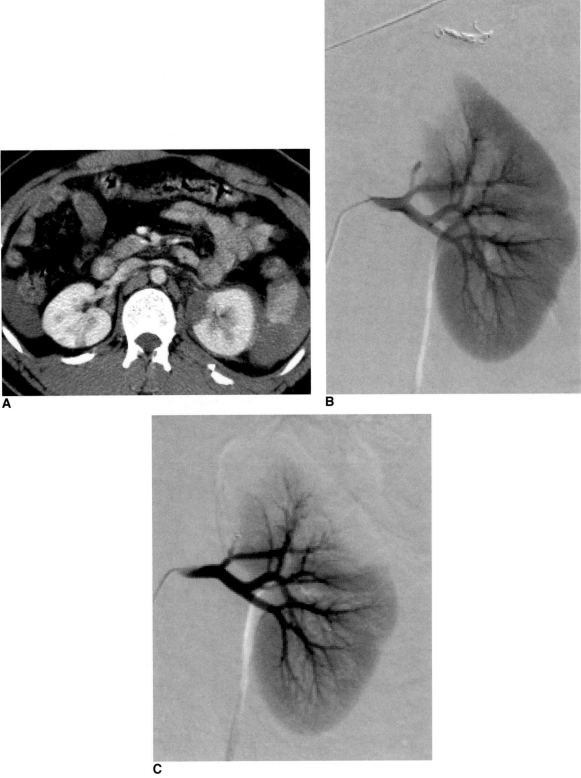

Fig. 7-6
Segmental renal infarct. **A**, A sharply delineated wedge of nonperfusion in the anterior left upper kidney represents infarcted segment. Note posterior splenic infarct and anterior pole laceration. **B**, Arteriogram shows occlusion of segmental renal artery to upper pole. **C**, Arteriogram after coil embolization of renal artery.

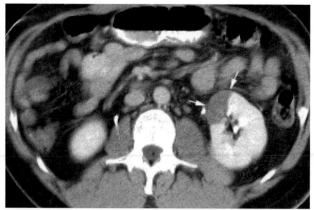

Fig. 7-7
Segmental renal infarct. CT shows well-defined wedge-shaped low-attenuation region in left upper pole (*arrowheads*). No other renal or perinephric injury is seen.

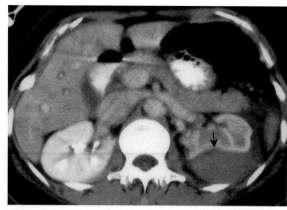

Fig. 7-9
Subcapsular renal hematoma. High-density clot in subcapsular space of left kidney compresses adjacent parenchyma. There is minimal perinephric hemorrhage.

infarction. While renal arteriography will demonstrate the injured vessel and embolization can be performed, in general, specific angiographic confirmation and treatment *are not* warranted if the segmental infarct appears as an isolated renal injury.[11,12]

Subcapsular renal hematomas are rare because of the difficulty in separating the renal capsule from the cortex, particularly in older adults. When these hematomas do occur, they are typically limited in extent by the renal capsule and assume a convex shape, indenting the renal parenchyma (Figs. 7-8 and 7-9). Some delay in renal perfusion is typically seen with these injuries, secondary to increased resistance to arterial perfusion. In most cases the injury will resolve without specific treatment, although signs of acute or delayed onset of hypertension

from renal parenchymal compression (Page kidney) should be sought. Large subcapsular hematomas could theoretically compress the kidney to or near systolic-level pressures, preventing perfusion and requiring surgical release of renal tamponade.

CT of Major Renal Injury. More significant renal injuries, such as CT grade III, may or may not require intervention by angiography or surgery. These injuries include renal fractures extending into the renal collecting system with a urine leak contained by Gerota's fascia or a large perinephric hematoma distending Gerota's fascia that shows no CT evidence of active bleeding and is stable on follow-up CT (Figs. 7-10 to 7-12). This finding indicates a significant amount of hemorrhage has

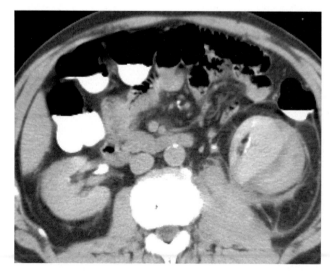

Fig. 7-8
Subcapsular renal hematoma. Hemorrhage into left subcapsular space of left kidney produces marked compression of the adjacent parenchyma.

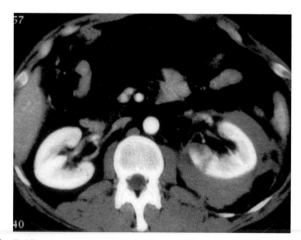

Fig. 7-10
Major renal injury. Deep left renal lacerations extend into medullary region. Perirenal hematoma is confined to but distends Gerota's fascia, and there is no active bleeding. Injury corresponds to CT grade III.

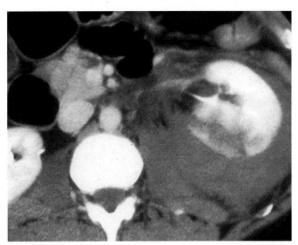

Fig. 7-11
Major renal injury. Deep left posterior laceration that fractured the kidney into two viable segments shows large, nonbleeding perinephric hematoma distending the perinephric space. Grade III. (From Mirvis SE, Hastings G, Scalea TM: Diagnostic imaging, angiography, and interventional radiology in the trauma patient. In Mattox KL, Feliciano DL, Moore EE, eds: *Trauma,* ed 4, New York, 2000, McGraw-Hill.)

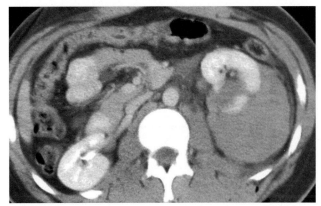

Fig. 7-12
Major renal injury. Deep left renal laceration that fractures viable parenchyma. A large perinephric hematoma is confined to but distends Gerota's fascia. Injury corresponds to CT grade III.

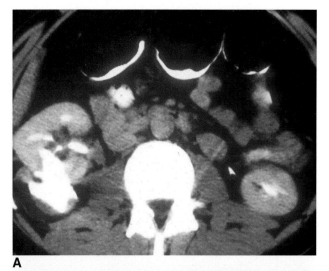

A

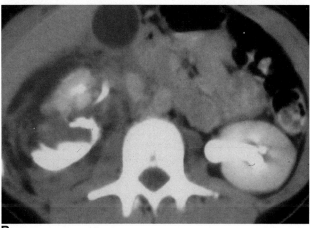

B

Fig. 7-13
Urinomas. **A** and **B**, Collections of opacified urine fill urinoma posterior to right kidney. Both kidneys have normal antegrade flow. These injuries resolved without intervention. (From Mirvis SE, Shanmuganathan K, Killeen KL: Injuries to the genitourinary tract. In Grainger RG, Allison DJ, Adam A, Dixon AK, eds: *Grainger & Allison's diagnostic radiology,* ed 4, Edinburgh, 2001, Churchill Livingstone.)

occurred, most likely from a renal arterial origin. The management of contained urine extravasation in a hemodynamically stable blunt trauma patient without definite need for renal bed exploration has evolved from surgical inspection and repair to observation.[13,14] At UMSTC, urinomas are observed and usually resolve over time without complications (Figs. 7-13 and 7-14), particularly if there is unimpeded antegrade flow of urine. Dependent urinomas may rarely become infected because of urine stasis and are managed by percutaneous catheter drainage if needed. Collecting system leaks that persist may be treated more efficiently with the addition of nephrostomy or double-J ureteral catheterization to min-

imize pressure at the injured region. On occasion, surgical repair is required, particularly for extensive injuries.

The treatment of large perinephric or pararenal hemorrhages resulting from renal trauma or growth of hematoma over time is dependent upon clinical presentation and course, associated injuries, and required treatment. Patients who are hemodynamically stable, with evidence of major perirenal hemorrhage but without a clear indication for laparotomy, can undergo selective renal angiography with distal embolization of bleeding sites to maximize preservation of viable renal tissue (see Chapter 12). Patients who are unstable, display a rapidly falling hematocrit, or have clear indications for emergent

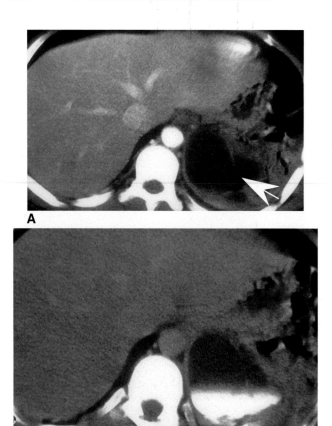

A

B

Fig. 7-14
Delayed appearance of urinoma. **A,** Fluid collection observed superior to left kidney of low attenuation (*arrowhead*). **B,** Delayed scan shows opacified urine filling collection.

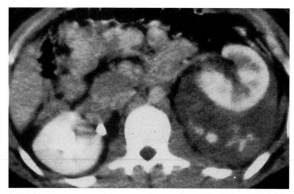

Fig. 7-15
Catastrophic renal injury. A large perinephric hematoma displaces the left kidney anteriorly. Focal areas of increased density within the hematoma are due to active arterial bleeding that presents before opacification of the collecting system. Distinction of bleeding from contrast leak can be made by time of appearance of the density in relation to renal opacification and connection to the collecting system.

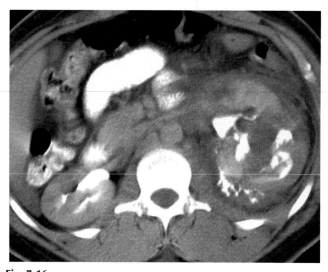

Fig. 7-16
Catastrophic renal injury. Left kidney is fragmented. Multiple foci of increased density are noted but are seen at high density during collecting system opacification when arterial bleeding should be decreasing in density. These represent collecting system leaks due to severe disruption and renal fragmentation.

surgery will have renal hemorrhage managed by direct surgical methods. While the nephrectomy rate may be higher for patients with major renal injury treated by open surgery than for those treated nonoperatively, such patients may also tend to have more severe injuries at the outset.[14]

CT of Catastrophic Renal Injury. Injuries included in CT grade IV will require intervention by angiography and/or surgery. These include major renal pedicle injuries (renal artery or vein), CT finding of fragmentation of the kidney associated with segmental devascularization and typically large perinephric and pararenal hematoma, renal arterial bleeding or pseudoaneurysm as detected by CT, renal pelvis disruption, and urinary leak into the peritoneal space (Figs. 7-15 to 7-21).

In blunt force trauma the kidneys are displaced outward toward the lateral aspect of the retroperitoneum. This motion stretches the renal arterial intima beyond its elastic limit, leading to disruption. Some time later, clotting begins to form on and around the disrupted intima, leading to partial or complete renal artery occlusion. The artery usually occludes between the proximal and middle

one-third of the vessel (Fig. 7-22). It is quite common for the nonperfused kidney and surrounding tissue to appear otherwise intact. The diagnosis is usually quite apparent using contrast-enhanced spiral CT because of lack of renal opacification and diminished renal size, as well as the potential for peripheral renal cortical enhancement from collateral vessels (Figs. 7-23 to 7-25). Spiral CT can usually confirm the diagnosis, based on axial renal images and CT angiography.[15] Renal angiography is not needed to establish the diagnosis and should not be performed for this reason: although angiography

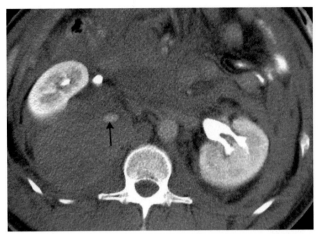

Fig. 7-17
Catastrophic renal injury. The posterior pole of the left kidney is disrupted. Contrast extravasates into the perinephric hematoma (*arrow*) and does not connect with the collecting system, indicating probable arterial hemorrhage. Some hemorrhage extends into the anterior pararenal space.

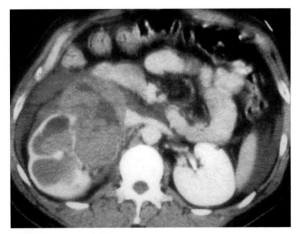

Fig. 7-19
Ruptured renal pelvis. The patient has an underlying congenital ureteropelvic junction obstruction, and the collecting system ruptured with blunt impact. Clot fills the collecting system and perinephric space. There is free intraperitoneal fluid in the paracolic gutters.

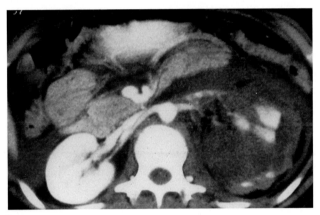

Fig. 7-18
Catastrophic renal injury. The left kidney is macerated with probable proximal occlusion of the left main renal artery. Some focal areas of enhancement may represent arterial collateral bleeding or viable islands of renal parenchyma. Hemorrhage extends into the anterior pararenal space, displacing the pancreatic tail. Free intraperitoneal fluid is seen in the right paracolic space.

can map the precise vascular anatomy, the time required to obtain this study will surely contribute to the further lowering of an already extremely low renal salvage rate. There is potential to place a renal arterial stent to gain patency through the injured renal artery if the required interventional radiologic skill is available. Further studies are needed to assess the potential of arterial stenting in this acute trauma setting.[16] In most cases renal revascularization must be accomplished within 2 hours of injury, but delayed attempts at renal revascularization can be successful many hours to days after injury,

depending on collateral renal blood supply and the completeness of renal artery occlusion.[17] An unusual sign described with renal artery occlusion on the right side is passive reflux of contrast material injected into the inferior vena cava (IVC) into the right renal vein.[18] The CT study shows what appears to be the renal collecting system filling without renal parenchymal opacification. In fact, the contrast is opacifying the renal veins, and the kidney is without arterial inflow (Fig. 7-26). Bilateral renal artery occlusion is quite rare, with about 14 cases reported worldwide.[19] This injury can be very difficult to diagnose when both kidneys either do not enhance or enhance poorly to a symmetric degree. The kidneys will appear less dense than would be anticipated based on the density of the adjacent aorta or proximal renal arteries (Fig. 7-27).

In the clinical setting, main renal vein disruption appears to be less common than main renal artery injury. This injury can produce extensive perinephric bleeding, but because of lower venous pressure this is likely to be limited by the retroperitoneum (Fig. 7-28). Occlusion of the renal vein will lead to a delayed and progressively dense nephrogram because of high venous outflow resistance.

Ongoing bleeding into the kidney or surrounding tissue appears as patchy, dense contrast material surrounded by less dense, clotted blood. Often the hemorrhage is apparent, since the arterial extravasation appears before there is opacification of the renal collecting system (see Figs. 7-15, 7-17, 7-20, and 7-21). Extravasated arterial contrast typically measures greater than 80 H and is typically within 10 H of an adjacent artery.[20] In stable patients, bleeding sites can be confirmed

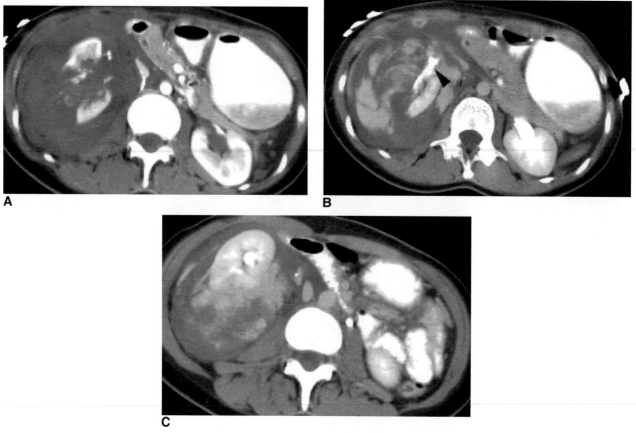

Fig. 7-20
Catastrophic renal injury. **A,** The left kidney is split, and there are three probable foci of active bleeding. A large hematoma extends to the anterior abdominal wall. The IVC is compressed by the hematoma. **B,** Delayed image shows multiple areas of high density within the perinephric hematoma, representing diffusion of extravasated arterial contrast. A collecting system leak also appears (*arrowhead*). **C,** A substantial portion of the upper half of the injured kidney remains intact.

by selective renal angiography and embolized with Gelfoam pledgets followed by coils (Fig. 7-29).

Injury to the renal pelvis most likely results from hyperextension, with secondary overstretching of the pelvis.[21] The injury manifests as gross contrast (urine) extravasation near the ureteropelvic junction (UPJ) (Figs. 7-30 to 7-32). In the author's experience the involved kidney is typically intact, with limited or no parenchymal dysfunction. The injury can be missed on helical CT if the scan traverses the kidneys prior to contrast appearing in the renal pelvis (see Fig. 7-30). Also, extravasation of contrast-enhanced urine into the anterior pararenal space could mimic a duodenal rupture with leakage of oral contrast. When there is evidence of a renal pelvic injury, visualization of the distal ureter indicates that only a partial disruption exists. Partial disruptions can be managed with transureteral catheter stenting, while larger or complete disruptions require operative repair.

The dilated renal pelvis resulting from congenital or acquired urinary outflow obstruction is at increased risk for rupture from a given traumatic impact[22] (Fig. 7-33; see also Fig. 7-19).

Occasionally, contrast material arising from an extraperitoneal bladder rupture can track up into the perinephric and pararenal spaces, mimicking a contrast leak of renal origin. The renal parenchyma should, however, appear intact, and the contrast can be followed on sequential images to the bladder disruption (Fig. 7-34).

Severe fragmentation of the renal parenchyma is usually a surgical lesion, although in occasional cases a nonoperative course, supplemented by renal angiography and percutaneous drainage, is possible, particularly if the surrounding perinephric hematoma is stable and there is limited or no urine extravasation. In most cases nephrectomy will be required. On occasion considerable restoration of renal anatomy and function can be seen after

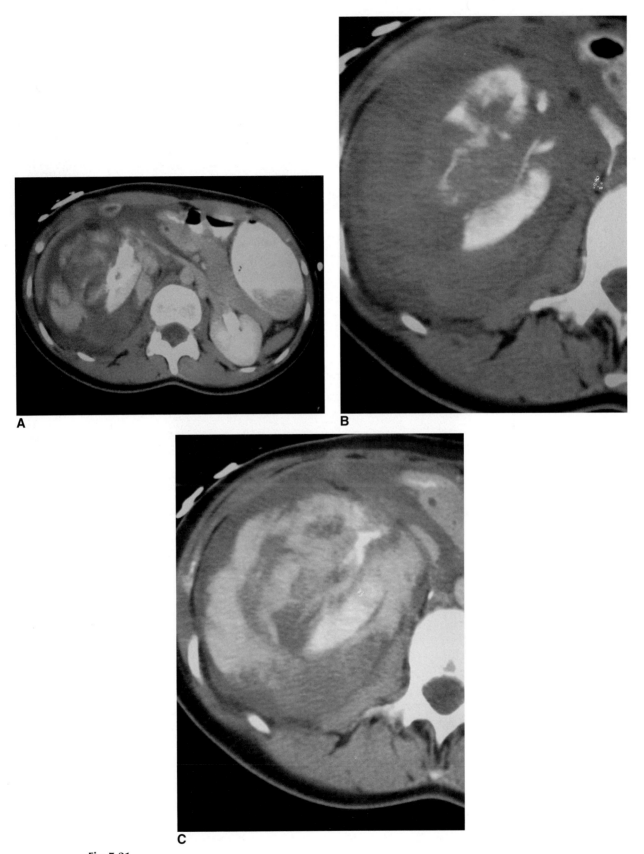

Fig. 7-21
Catastrophic renal injury. **A** to **C**, CT images show marked fragmentation of the right kidney with extensive surrounding perinephric and anterior pararenal hematoma. There is no definite active bleeding or iodinated urine leak.

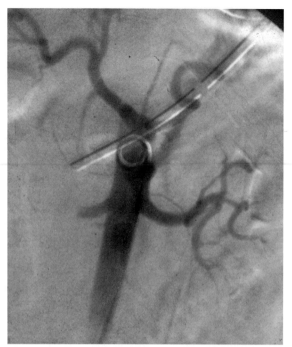

Fig. 7-22
Renal artery occlusion. The single renal artery to the right kidney is occluded in its proximal one-third, which is typical for main renal arterial injuries.

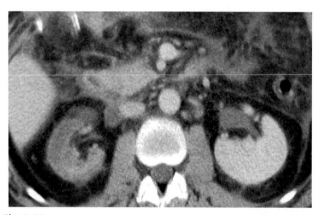

Fig. 7-23
Renal artery occlusion. The right kidney appears smaller than the left and shows enhancement of only the peripheral cortex. The left kidney enhances normally. There is minimal fluid adjacent to the IVC but no other evidence of right renal parenchymal injury. Stranding of the mesentery may be due to pancreatitis or primary mesentery injury.

nonoperative treatment of renal fragmentation. When there is a minimal amount of renal function contributed by the injured kidney or there is clinical concern of ongoing blood loss, then nephrectomy is the appropriate choice. Management decisions concerning renal injuries must consider the presence and viability of remaining renal parenchyma, should nephrectomy be required.

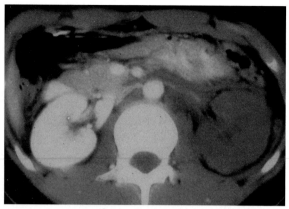

Fig. 7-24
Renal artery occlusion. The left kidney is normal in size and appears intact but is completely nonenhancing.

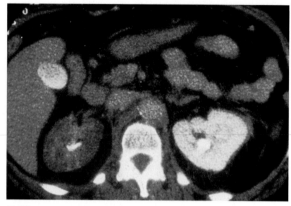

Fig. 7-25
Renal artery occlusion. The right kidney is nonenhancing but contains a small amount of contrast in the collecting system. In this case a small portion of the kidney was supplied by an accessory renal artery (not shown) and permitted some function.

Intervention in Renal Injury. Percutaneous methods have become increasingly valuable in permitting nonoperative management of major renal injuries. As previously noted, percutaneously placed catheters can assist in draining persistent urinomas or perinephric abscesses. When there is acute or delayed hemorrhage from a branch of the renal artery, embolization can stop bleeding and avoid much of the parenchymal loss associated with partial or total nephrectomy (see Fig. 7-29) (see Chapter 12). An 82% to 88% success rate for renal artery branch embolization has been reported in three series.[22-24] Care must be taken to be as selective as possible, since nontargeted embolization will reduce viable parenchyma. Renal injuries managed by interventional techniques may require combined vascular and nonvascular interventions. Recurrent renal hemorrhage is often successfully treated with repeat embolization.[22,24,25] When there is a flow-limiting injury to the main renal

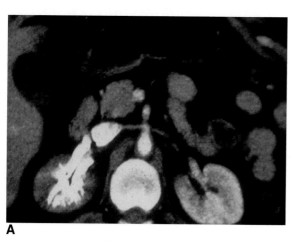
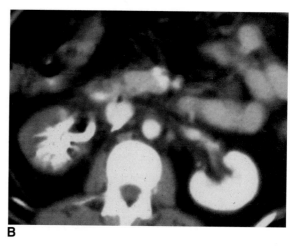

A **B**

Fig. 7-26
Renal artery occlusion, atypical CT presentation. **A** and **B**, Contrast was injected into the IVC. The right kidney demonstrates contrast centrally but no cortical-medullary enhancement. The contrast actually opacifies the renal veins by retrograde filling, since the right renal artery is occluded and the renal venous pressure is lower than injection pressure and central venous pressure. (From Mirvis SE, Shanmuganathan K, Killeen KL: Injuries to the genitourinary tract. In Grainger RG, Allison DJ, Adam A, Dixon AK, eds: *Grainger & Allison's diagnostic radiology*, ed 4, Edinburgh, 2001, Churchill Livingstone.)

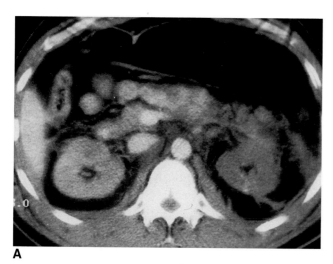
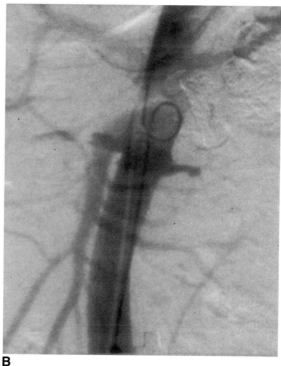

A **B**

Fig. 7-27
Bilateral renal artery occlusion (personal watercraft accident). **A**, Neither kidney demonstrates parenchymal enhancement despite the bright aorta, IVC, liver, and superior mesenteric vein. **B**, Arteriogram shows proximal occlusion of both renal arteries. (From Mirvis SE, Shanmuganathan K, Killeen KL: Injuries to the genitourinary tract. In Grainger RG, Allison DJ, Adam A, Dixon AK, eds: *Grainger & Allison's diagnostic radiology*, ed 4, Edinburgh, 2001, Churchill Livingstone.)

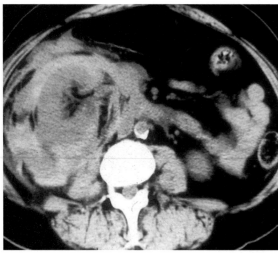

Fig. 7-28
Renal vein avulsion. The right kidney is surrounded by blotted and liquid blood and is displaced anteriorly and laterally. The renal parenchyma appears intact. A main renal vein avulsion was found and repaired surgically.

artery, angioplasty or stenting may be helpful in unusual cases if logistics permit implementation before irreversible ischemic damage develops.[26] As indicated before, assuming total occlusion, this procedure would probably need to take place within 2 hours of injury. Renal artery pseudoaneurysms can rarely result from blunt trauma (Fig. 7-35) but are most likely the result of penetrating injury.[27] These injuries may be asymptomatic for years after injury and present with delayed rupture.

URETERAL INJURY

Ureteral injury associated with blunt injury typically occurs at the ureteropelvic junction.[28] Hyperextension, with overstretching of the ureter or compression of the ureter against lumbar transverse processes, is the likely mechanism of injury. Ureteral injury can range from contusion to partial tear to complete disruption. In cases of blunt trauma the diagnosis is usually suspected on the basis of CT findings showing contrast material accumulating in the inferior medial perinephric space[29] (see Figs. 7-30 to 7-32). It is important that CT images be obtained in the *excretory phase* of contrast excretion to visualize the collecting system and ureter. Rarely the ureter distal to the UPJ can be injured as a result of blunt trauma forces because of either stretching or puncture by bone fragments (Figs. 7-36 and 7-37). Mulligan et al.[30] described five adult patients with UPJ disruption, three of whom had a negative initial helical CT and a delay in diagnosis of more than 24 hours. All three missed diagnoses were the result of scanning the kidneys in the preexcretory phase because of absent or very subtle contrast extravasa-

tion. The integrity of the ureter can be assessed by determination of whether iodinated urine is seen in the ureter below the level of injury, indicating a partial disruption that may be amenable to ureteral stenting rather than open repair. Retrograde pyelography can be used to document the site and extent of ureteral disruption, especially when findings of IVP or CT are uncertain. On rare occasions, renal nuclear scintigraphy has been used to detect urine extravasation, but this was primarily before the advent of fast conventional or spiral CT.

Ureteric injury occurs iatrogenically in 0.4% to 2.5% of patients undergoing gynecologic surgery for nonmalignant conditions.[31] Conditions that increase the likelihood of iatrogenic ureteral injury include hemorrhage, endometriosis, uterine enlargement, cancer, and adhesions. When the injury is recognized at the time of surgery, immediate repair can be performed. In many cases the injury remains unrecognized, and patients present with fever, loin pain, fistula formation, or signs of infection or obstruction. Once the diagnosis is suspected, it is best confirmed by retrograde pyelography to establish location and extent of injury.

BLADDER INJURY
Diagnostic Technique

About 70% of patients with traumatic bladder injury have sustained concurrent fractures of the pelvis. The severity of the pelvic injury roughly correlates with the likelihood of bladder and urethral injury.[11] Urinary bladder rupture occurs in 5% to 10% of patients who sustain pelvic fracture.[6] Hematuria, typically gross, almost always accompanies significant bladder injury.[32,33] A cystogram or CT cystography must be performed on all patients with gross hematuria associated with pelvic fractures.[11,32]

Cystography is performed after urethral injury has been excluded and retrograde bladder catheterization is safe. To reliably diagnose bladder injury, sufficient distension must be obtained to initiate detrusor muscle contraction. Instillation of less than 250 ml of iodinated contrast material can produce a falsely negative cystogram because of inadequate distension. At UMSTC, 350 to 400 ml of 30% contrast medium is instilled. Typically, scout, full-bladder, and postvoid pelvic radiographs are obtained. If it is highly likely that a bladder injury exists, based on extent of pelvic fracture, instillation of an initial 100 ml of contrast is followed by anteroposterior (AP) pelvic radiography to avoid extensive extravasation of contrast that could increase artifacts if selective pelvic angiography and embolization are required. If no injury is seen, the recommendation is to instill the remaining contrast and obtain full-bladder and postvoid studies. If a question of minimal extravasation exists, a bladder washout with normal saline can be per-

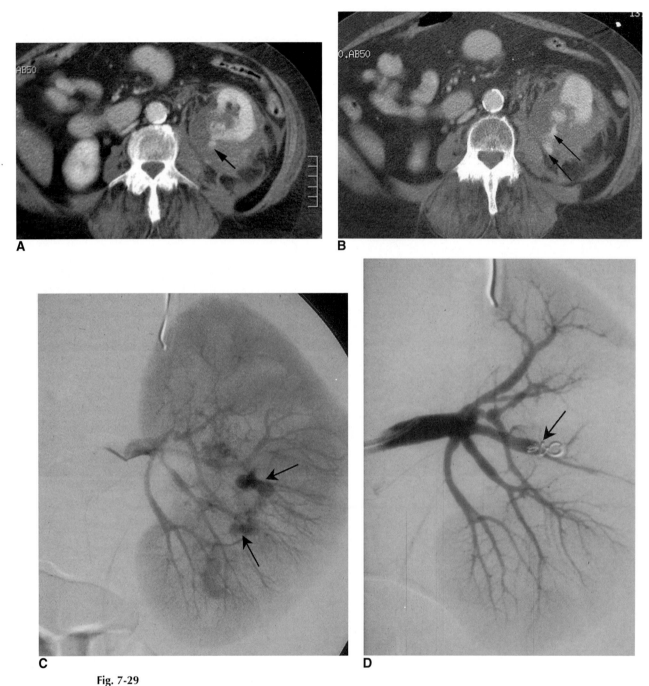

Fig. 7-29
CT of renal arterial bleed. **A** and **B**, CT reveals pool of bright contrast (*arrows*) within hematoma surrounding left kidney. The contrast blush appears in the angiographic phase before there is excretion of urine into the collecting system. **C**, Selective right renal angiogram shows contrast extravasation from midportion of kidney with tracking above and below (*arrows*). **D**, Bleeding is arrested after selective coil embolization (*arrow*) with preservation of superior and inferior polar perfusion. (**C** and **D** from Mirvis SE, Shanmuganathan K, Killeen KL: Injuries to the genitourinary tract. In Grainger RG, Allison DJ, Adam A, Dixon AK, eds: *Grainger & Allison's diagnostic radiology*, ed 4, Edinburgh, 2001, Churchill Livingstone.)

formed to localize any contrast remaining after voiding.[32] If pelvic angiography is contemplated for ongoing hemorrhage, cystography should await completion of that procedure. An "on-the-angio-table" cystogram can be conveniently performed in the angiographic suite, using fluoroscopy and radiography upon completion of the arteriogram.

Lis and Cohen[34] have advocated the use of CT scan cystography for patients with pelvic fractures already undergoing pelvic CT study. These authors used a drip

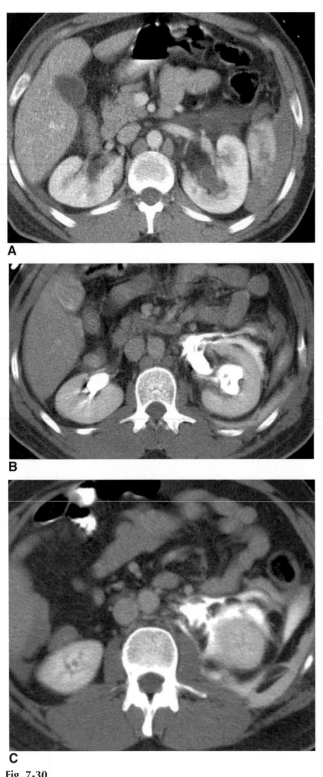

Fig. 7-30
CT of ureteropelvic junction (UPJ) injury. **A**, CT in the arterial phase shows hemorrhage in the anterior pararenal space, splenic lacera- tion, and perisplenic hemorrhage. **B** and **C**, Delayed images show extravasation of contrast into the anteromedial perinephric space and around the ureter, indicating UPJ disruption. Note importance of obtaining the delayed image during excretory phase.

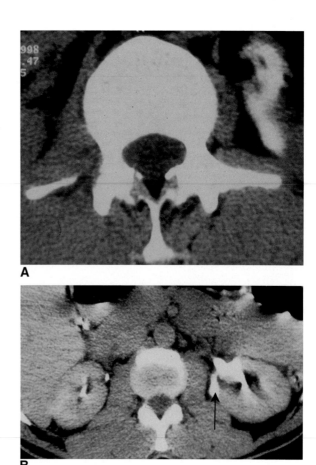

Fig. 7-31
CT of ureteropelvic junction (UPJ) injury. **A**, CT of lumbar spine revealed unexpected contrast pool adjacent to left paraspinal area along with a right transverse process fracture. **B**, A repeat abdomi- nal-pelvic CT showed contrast leak from area of UPJ (*arrow*) that was not detected on admission CT of this area.

bladder infusion of 4.4% contrast material up to 350 ml unless limited by detrusor contraction. After contrast instillation the pelvis was scanned at 10-mm sections with a full bladder and after voiding or catheter drainage. The authors suggested that the method was more accu- rate than standard cystography for detection of bladder injuries and eliminated the extra time required for that study.

A standard CT scan with intravenous contrast bolus and a clamped bladder catheter is *not reliable* to exclude bladder injury.[11] Haas et al.[35] reviewed results of spiral CT and standard cystography in 15 patients with sus- pected bladder injury. Retrograde cystography accurately diagnosed and classified the injury in all patients, while CT was successful in only 9 of 15 patients (60%).[35] Kane et al.[36] advocated a delay in CT scanning of the pelvis for 15 to 30 minutes, with a clamped in-dwelling catheter to permit adequate distension of the bladder. This approach

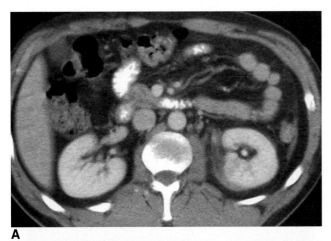

A

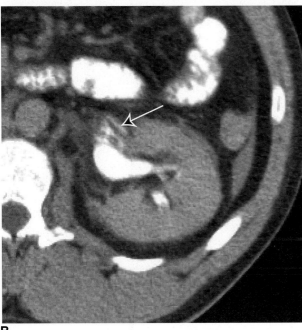

B

Fig. 7-32
A, CT of ureteropelvic junction (UPJ) injury. **B,** CT demonstrates typical pattern of contrast leak from UPJ region *(arrow)* in the anteromedial perinephric space and along the proximal ureter.

appears rather time-consuming for a busy trauma-emergency center and still cannot be relied upon to predictably produce adequate bladder distension.

Classification of Bladder Injury

Intraperitoneal bladder rupture (IBR) usually occurs at the anatomically weak bladder dome and results from blunt impact to a full bladder or transmission of hydraulic pressure waves in a partially filled bladder. IBR accounts for 10% to 20% of all bladder ruptures.[11] IBR is recognized radiographically or with CT by free intraperitoneal contrast outlining the peritoneal recesses and

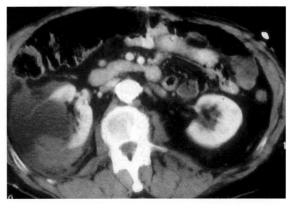

Fig. 7-33 CT of renal cyst rupture. Large ruptured right renal cyst demonstrates intracystic and perinephric hemorrhage.

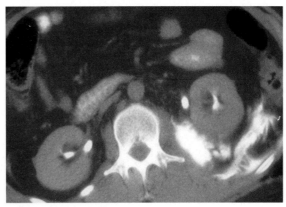

Fig. 7-34
CT of pseudo renal injury. CT shows perinephric contrast material with anterior displacement of the left kidney. The appearance suggests injury of renal origin (collecting system), but the kidney appears intact. Actually contrast has tracked up through the retroperitoneum from an extraperitoneal bladder rupture.

bowel loops (Figs. 7-38 and 7-39). Leak of opacified urine into the vagina (posterior fornix) can mimic IBR into the pelvis (Fig. 7-40). IBR requires surgical repair. On CT, spillage of iodinated contrast into the peritoneal cavity can mimic bowel rupture with oral contrast leak or even hemorrhage into the peritoneal cavity. In many cases a clear demarcation in CT density is seen between urine extravasated before and after contrast enhancement. Also, dense urinary contrast can obscure intraperitoneal blood or intestinal contents, diminishing overall diagnostic accuracy of abdominal pelvic CT for trauma.

Extraperitoneal bladder rupture (EBR) creates a streaky appearance as it dissects through adjacent fascial planes into the anterior prevesical space of Retzius, anterior abdominal wall, inguinal region and upper thigh, the lateral paravesical space, and the presacral space (Fig. 7-41). If there is a concurrent disruption of the urogenital

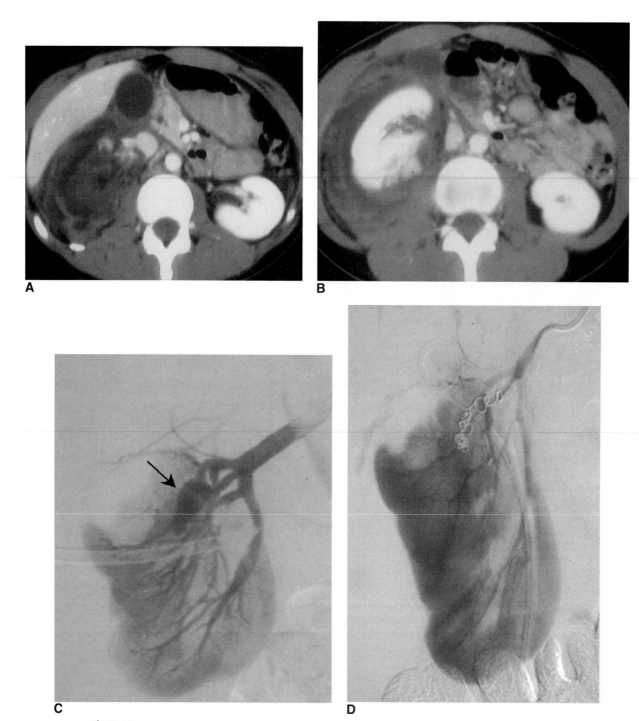

Fig. 7-35
Grade III renal injury with pseudoaneurysm. **A** and **B**, Images show devascularized right upper pole and perinephric hemorrhage. There is no active bleeding or urine leak. **C**, One week after injury the patient had increasing right flank pain and a fall in hematocrit. A repeat CT showed a much larger perinephric hematoma. Selective renal angiogram shows a pseudoaneurysm arising from a proximal segmental renal artery (*arrow*). **D**, After coil embolization the pseudoaneurysm is obliterated, with persisting flow to remaining viable kidney.

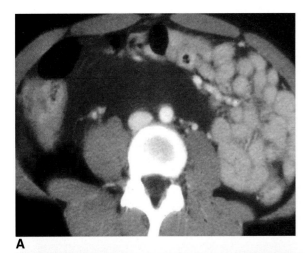

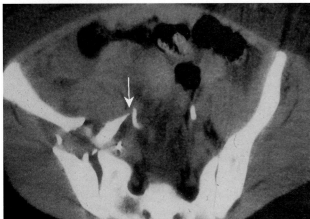

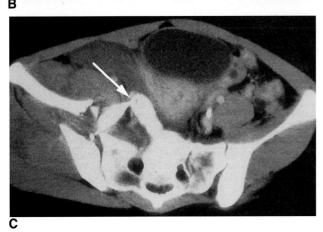

Fig. 7-36
CT of ureteral perforation. **A**, CT shows a large low-attenuation retroperitoneal fluid collection in a patient with a major displaced pelvic fracture. **B**, Repeat CT shows a bone spicule adjacent to the lower right ureter (*arrow*). **C**, Delayed scan through the same area demonstrates accumulation of contrast material (*arrow*) at site of bone spicule, indicating ureteral perforation. Collection on initial CT represented nonopacified urine in the retroperitoneum. (From Mirvis SE, Shanmuganathan K, Killeen KL: Injuries to the genitourinary tract. In Grainger RG, Allison DJ, Adam A, Dixon AK, eds: *Grainger & Allison's diagnostic radiology*, ed 4, Edinburgh, 2001, Churchill Livingstone.)

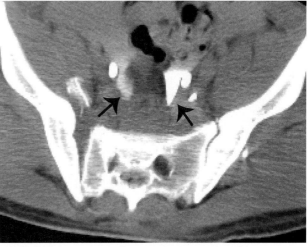

Fig. 7-37
Blunt ureteral injury. CT through pelvis shows contrast leak from both distal ureters (*arrows*) in a blunt trauma patient. There is focal arterial extravasation adjacent to a major right sacroiliac diastasis. (From Mirvis SE, Shanmuganathan K, Killeen KL: Injuries to the genitourinary tract. In Grainger RG, Allison DJ, Adam A, Dixon AK, eds: *Grainger & Allison's diagnostic radiology*, ed 4, Edinburgh, 2001, Churchill Livingstone.)

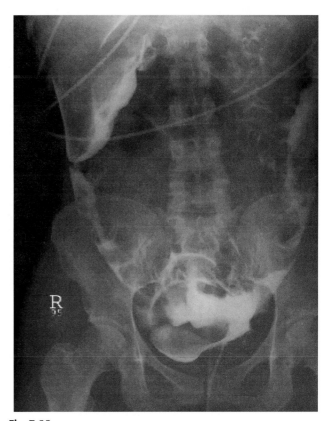

Fig. 7-38
Intraperitoneal bladder rupture. Postvoid study obtained after a cystogram shows extensive leak of contrast into the smooth intraperitoneal recesses throughout the abdomen.

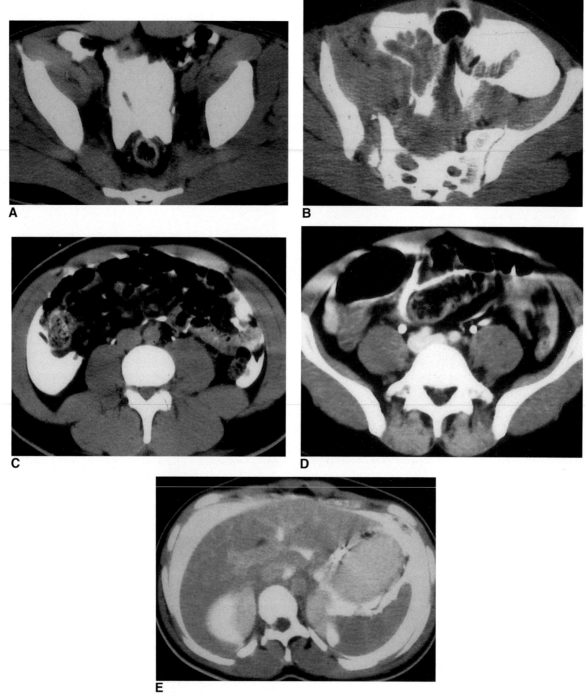

Fig. 7-39
CT of intraperitoneal bladder rupture. **A** to **E**, Contrast leaking from the bladder fills a variety of intraperitoneal recesses. (**D** from Shanmuganathan K, Mirvis SE, Reaney SM: *Clin Radiol* 50:186, 1995.)

diaphragm (posterior urethra) and bladder base, contrast can extend into the perineum and scrotum. CT can often directly demonstrate the exact site of bladder wall disruption (Fig. 7-42). Most cases of EBR are treated with bladder drainage, either transurethral or suprapubic, but large tears may require surgical repair. Urine leak from

the base of the bladder may be confused with a concurrent posterior urethral injury (Table 7-4).

Rarely, the bladder can be entrapped in a displaced pelvic fracture, requiring open reduction and repair[37] (Figs. 7-43 and 7-44). The bladder on cystogram has a distorted shape and is in proximity to an adjacent dis-

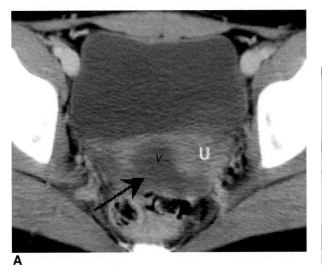

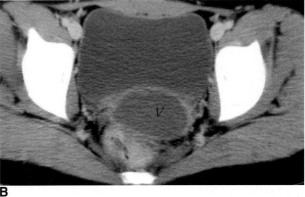

Fig. 7-40
A and **B**, Fluid (blood or urine) accumulating in vaginal canal (*arrow*), mimicking intraperitoneal fluid. *U*, Uterus; *V*, vaginal canal.

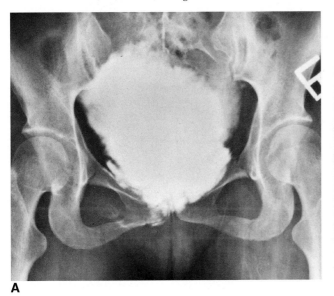

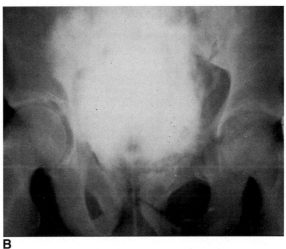

Fig. 7-41
Extraperitoneal bladder rupture. **A** and **B**, Two cystograms demonstrating typical "streaky" appearance of opacified urine leaking into the potential extraperitoneal spaces around the bladder. (Note arrowhead in **A**.)

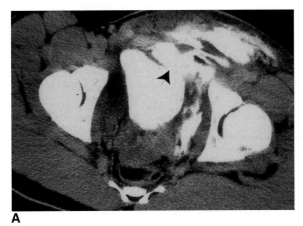

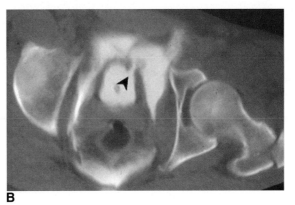

Fig. 7-42
CT demonstrating site of bladder tear. **A** and **B**, Focal tears are demonstrated in the left anterolateral bladder wall (*arrowheads*). (From Shanmuganathan K, Mirvis SE, Reaney SM: *Clin Radiol* 50:186, 1995.)

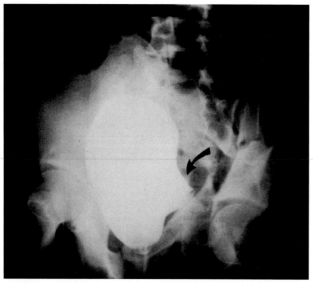

Fig. 7-43
Bladder wall is entrapped by displaced pelvic fracture (*curved arrow*), as demonstrated on cystogram. (From Mirvis SE: *Clin Imaging* 13:269, 1989.)

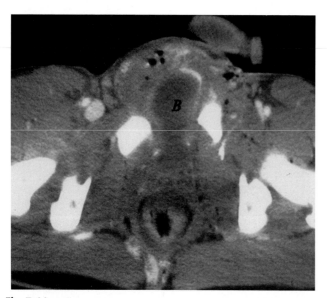

Fig. 7-44
CT of herniated bladder. Image shows displacement of bladder (*B*) through diastasis of pubic symphysis with surrounding extravesical hematoma.

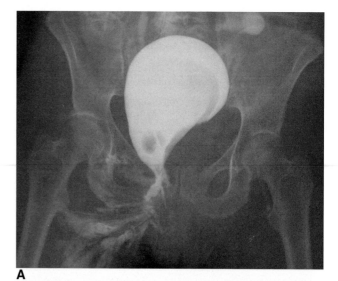

A

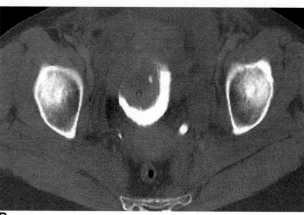

B

Fig. 7-45
Paravesical hemorrhage. **A**, Cystogram obtained on patient with pelvic fractures after blunt trauma shows mass effect on left side of bladder, indicating hematoma. There is contrast extravasation below the urogenital diaphragm. **B**, CT shows diffuse extent of pelvic hematoma with significant space of Retzius involvement and intravesical hematoma.

These injuries are rarely of clinical importance. Intravesical blood clots may result from traumatic injury to the urinary tract. Clots arising from the ureteral orifices are most likely due to renal or ureteral injury rather than direct bladder injury (Figs. 7-45 and 7-46).

URETHRAL INJURY

Urethral injuries occur in about 10% of major pelvic fracture cases and typically involve the proximal (posterior) portion. Most urethral injuries occur in men but have been described in women, particularly with major peritoneal soft tissue and vaginal injury.[38] In males, urethral injury is suspected by blood at the urethral meatus, inability to void, elevation of the prostate on digital rectal examination, or perineal swelling or hematoma.[11]

placed or diastatic fracture. Cystography can reveal the presence of pelvic hematomas by displacement of the bladder, but CT scan provides this information with greater accuracy, indicating the site and extent of other pelvic injuries and, in many cases, the location of pelvic arterial injury.[20] Mucosal lacerations and bladder wall contusions may produce hematuria but are unlikely to cause significant abnormalities by CT or cystography.

Table 7-4
Classification of Urethral Injuries

Colapinto and McCallum		Goldman and Sandler
Grade I	Posterior urethral stretched but intact (Fig. 7-47)	Same
Grade II	Posterior urethral tear above intact urogenital diaphragm (Fig. 7-48)	Partial or complete posterior urethral tear above intact urogenital diaphragm (UGD)
Grade III	Posterior urethral tear with extravasation through torn UGD (Fig. 7-49)	Partial or complete tear of combined anterior and posterior urethra with torn UGD
Grade IV	—	Bladder neck injury with extension to the urethra (Fig. 7-50)
Grade IV-A	—	Injury to bladder base with extravasation simulating type 4 (pseudo type 4) (Fig. 7-51)
Grade V	—	Anterior urethral injury (Fig. 7-52)

Imaging assessment of the urethra should precede cystography, which should not be performed until after pelvic arteriography if indicated. A retrograde urethrogram is performed using 30 ml of 60% contrast material via a Foley balloon catheter positioned in the distal urethra and inflated with 2 ml of saline. Ideally, the study should be conducted using fluoroscopy but is most typically performed using oblique radiographs obtained with the shaft of the penis perpendicular to the femur to visualize the full extent of the urethra.[34]

Classically, urethral injuries have been described using the Colapinto and McCallum classification[39] but more recently have been reclassified by Goldman and Sandler into a unified anatomic-mechanical classification.[40] Table 7-4 compares the two classification systems (Figs. 7-47 to 7-52).

Anterior urethral injury is encountered less frequently in cases of blunt trauma than in cases involving iatrogenic or penetrating trauma. The bulbous urethra may be injured from crushing between the impacting body object and inferior symphysis pubis.

The extent of contrast leak from anterior urethral injury may be limited to the corporal bodies if Buck's fascia remains intact (see Fig. 7-52) or may spread extensively through the scrotum, perineum, and anterior abdominal wall if Buck's fascia is disrupted.

SCROTAL INJURY

Injury to the testis may occur from penetrating wounds, direct impact of high-velocity objects against the testis, or compression of the testis against the pubic arch and impacting object. Clinical assessment of extent and type of scrotal injury is difficult, particularly for distinction between uncomplicated hematocele, a collection of blood within the tunica vaginalis, and testicular rupture.[11] The distinction is vital because a ruptured testis can be

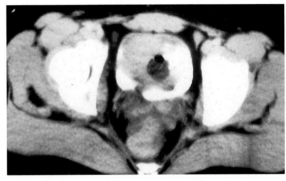

Fig. 7-46
Intravesical hematoma arising from right ureteral orifice indicates hemorrhage is most likely of right renal origin.

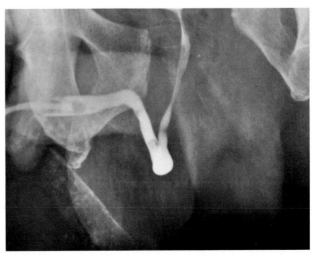

Fig. 7-47
Type 1 urethral injury. Cystoureterogram shows marked diastasis of the pubic symphysis with superior displacement of the left hemipelvis. The prostatic and membranous portions of the urethra are stretched with elevation of the bladder. No contrast extravasation is seen.

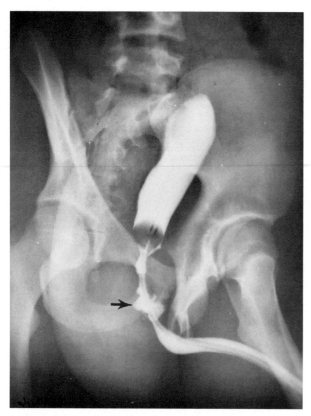

Fig. 7-48
Type 2 urethral tear. Cystourethrogram obtained in oblique projection reveals focal tear at the level of the membranous portion (*arrow*) but no evidence of contrast leak below the urogenital diaphragm. The bladder is elongated, suggesting compression from both sides due to pelvic hematoma.

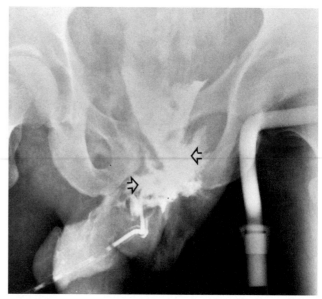

Fig. 7-50
Bladder neck injury with posterior urethral extension (*open arrows*). (From Mirvis SE, Shanmuganathan K, Killeen KL: Injuries to the genitourinary tract. In Grainger RG, Allison DJ, Adam A, Dixon AK, eds: *Grainger & Allison's diagnostic radiology*, ed 4, Edinburgh, 2001, Churchill Livingstone.)

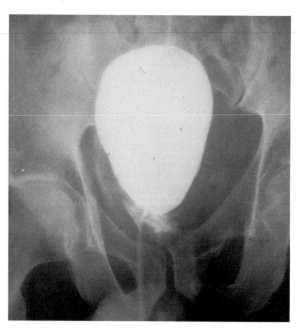

Fig. 7-51
Injury to bladder base, with extraperitoneal extravasation, simulating bladder neck-posterior urethral injury (pseudo type 4 of Goldman and Sandler).

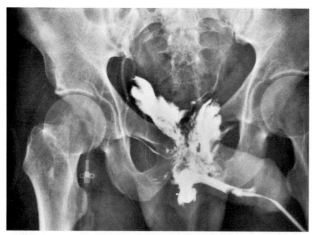

Fig. 7-49
Type 3 urethral tear. Anteroposterior view from cystogram shows severe symphysis pubis diastasis and marked diastasis of the right sacroiliac joint with vertical displacement of the right hemipelvis. A portion of the right sacral ala is avulsed. Contrast extravasation below the urogenital diaphragm is seen. The tear arises from either the posterior urethra or the vesicourethral junction.

salvaged in 90% of patients if repaired within 72 hours, but the salvage rate decreases to 55% after this period.[41] Failure to promptly diagnose testicular rupture can result in atrophy, abscess formation, and chronic pain.

Sonography is the imaging modality of choice in the setting of acute scrotal trauma and is performed with 5- or

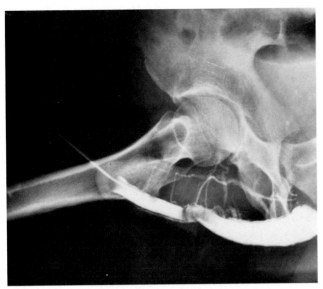

Fig. 7-52
Anterior urethral injury. A retrograde urethrogram demonstrates extravasation of contrast into the corpora cavernosum at the level of the midpenile urethra after a direct impact. There is uptake of contrast into draining veins but confinement within Buck's fascia.

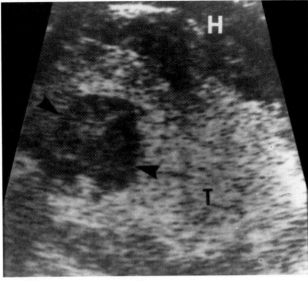

Fig. 7-54
Testicular contusion and hematocele. Sonogram of testicle (T) obtained following blunt trauma shows an area of decreased echogenicity (*arrowheads*) believed to represent contusion or hematoma. A mildly echogenic fluid collection (*H*) surrounds the testicle, compatible with a hematocele.

7.5-MHz transducers. A scrotal hematoma appears as an echogenic collection between the tunica dartos and tunica vaginalis or in the scrotal septum. The hemorrhage becomes more sonolucent over time. A hydrocele is a liquefied hematoma or serous collection between the layers of the tunica vaginalis (Fig. 7-53). Sonographically, a hydrocele is an echolucent fluid collection around the testis. A hematocele is a complex collection seen between the leaves of the tunica vaginalis, which can mimic testicular rupture[42] (Figs. 7-54 and 7-55). The hematocele is usually managed medically but can be surgically evacuated.[43]

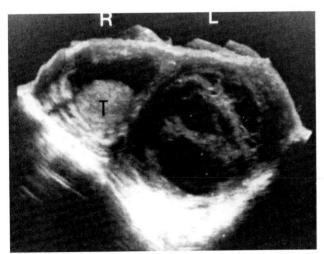

Fig. 7-53
Testicular rupture and hydrocele. Sonogram of scrotum obtained after blunt trauma reveals complex disruption of left testicular parenchyma (rupture) and a hydrocele surrounding the right testis (*T*).

Testicular rupture implies tearing of the tunica albuginea, with extrusion of testicular parenchyma into the scrotal sac. The margins of the testis are poorly defined, and the echogenicity of the testis is heterogeneous (see Figs. 7-53 and 7-55). Jeffrey et al. were able to diagnose testicular rupture correctly in 11 of 12 patients by using sonography but found recognition of a fracture plane difficult.[42] Laceration, fragmentation, intratesticular hematoma, and infarction usually accompany testicular rupture (see Figs. 7-53 and 7-55). A testicular contusion appears as a focal region of heterogeneous echo pattern within the background uniform echo pattern of the testicular parenchyma (see Figs. 7-54 and 7-55).

Trauma to the testis can also result in testicular dislocation or torsion. Dislocation is typically into the inguinal canal and may be detected by CT or sonography (Fig. 7-56). Torsion may be difficult to distinguish from rupture with infarction or a large scrotal hematoma, and sonography or nuclear medicine perfusion scanning may be utilized (see Chapter 13).

RETROPERITONEAL INJURY
Adrenal Injury

Adrenal injury, once believed to be rare following blunt torso trauma, has been more frequently reported with the increased use of CT screening of patients sustaining blunt force abdominal trauma.[44-47] Burks et al.[45] reported findings of adrenal injury in 20 of 1120 patients (2%) undergoing CT for blunt force injury. In CT studies of pediatric

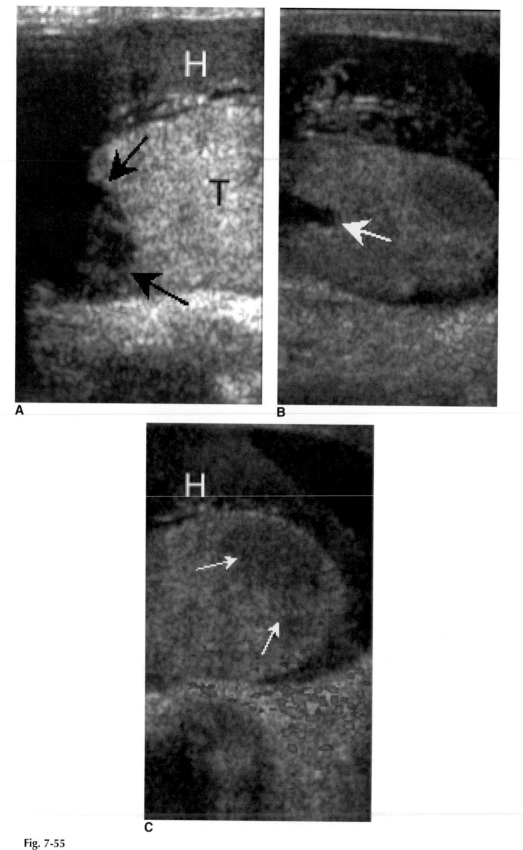

Fig. 7-55
Sonography of testicular injuries. **A**, Posttrauma sonogram shows tear from pole of testis (*T*) (*arrows*) and hematocele (*H*). **B**, Linear laceration of same testis (*white arrow*). **C**, Opposite testis shows area of lower echogenicity in pole consistent with contusion (*arrows*). Note surrounding hydrohematocele (*H*).

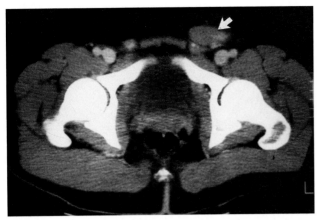

Fig. 7-56
Traumatic dislocation of testis. CT image through the pelvis of man injured in motorcycle accident shows an abnormal soft tissue mass in the left inguinal ring (*arrow*). The patient had sustained direct impact to the scrotum. The testis could be palpated in the inguinal ring. There was a history of a right orchiopexy.

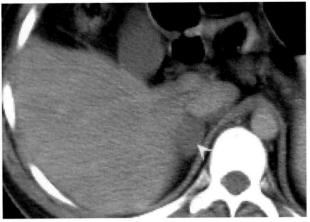

Fig. 7-58
CT shows an oval-shaped enlarged right adrenal gland, consistent with an adrenal hematoma (*arrowhead*).

blunt trauma, the injury was seen in 1% to 5% of patients.[44,46] In most cases the injury is unilateral and involves the right gland, but it can also occur on the left side or be bilateral.[45,47] Usually there is no clinical clue to the presence of the injury, but rarely in the subacute posttrauma period, adrenal insufficiency may develop with bilateral gland injury.[45]

The most common mechanism of injury appears to be compression of the right adrenal gland between the posteromedial right lobe of the liver and the spine. It is not uncommon for concurrent hepatic contusions to be present in the posteromedial right lobe among patients with right adrenal injury (Fig. 7-57). Other mechanisms that have been postulated to cause or contribute to adrenal

gland injury include increased intra-adrenal venous pressure transmitted through valveless adrenal veins from the inferior vena cava at impact and shearing forces between the cortical and medullary portions either tearing penetrating vessels or occurring at such a point where vessels perforate the adrenal capsule.[45]

In most cases of adrenal injury, as seen on contrast-enhanced CT, hemorrhage appears to arise in the medullary portion of the gland and expand uniformly outward. The gland typically assumes an oval to arrowhead appearance[45,47] (Figs. 7-57 to 7-60). Usually some portion of the enhancing adrenal cortex is visible in the periphery. Stranding of the periadrenal fat with hemorrhage is commonly seen and was present in 60% of patients described by Burks et al.[45] Thickening of the

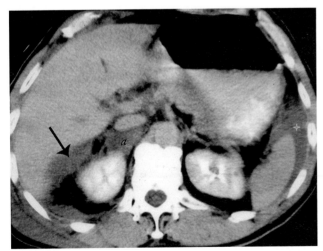

Fig. 7-57
CT shows adrenal hematoma (*a*) with right medial liver contusion (*arrow*). Note perisplenic hemorrhage. There is slight compression of the inferior vena cava.

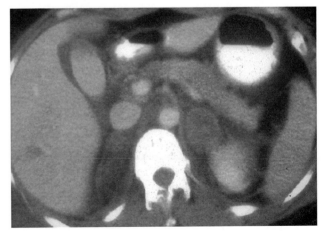

Fig. 7-59
CT shows bilateral oval-shaped adrenal glands, compatible with adrenal hematomas. Note the higher density adrenal cortex stretched around the periphery.

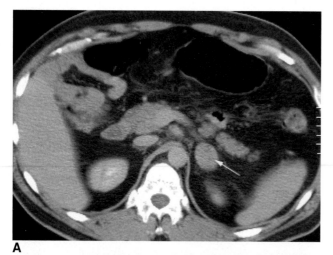

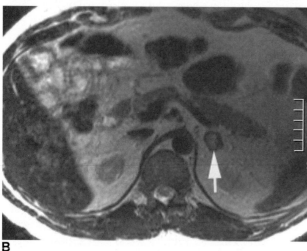

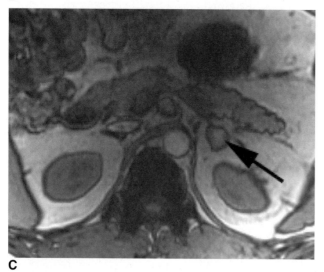

Fig. 7-60
Follow-up CT of adrenal hematoma without other injury. **A**, Oval-shaped left adrenal mass noted in blunt trauma patient (arrow). No other evidence of injury seen. **B** and **C**, Gradient echo in-phase (a) and out-of-phase (b) MRI, done as part of study to characterize lesion at 1 month, shows decrease in size of high-signal mass (arrows) and no evidence of significant fat content, consistent with relatively stable hematoma.

diaphragmatic crura or diaphragm by hemorrhage ipsilateral to the adrenal injury is present in 40% to 61% of cases.[45,47] If there is any concern that the adrenal mass may not be of traumatic origin, a delayed CT at 6 to 8 weeks can show resolution of an adrenal hematoma (see Fig. 7-60).

Adrenal injury is a strong predictor for the presence of other abdominal injuries, seen in 50% to 61% of patients, and thoracic injury, seen in 44% to 67% of patients.[44,47] Delayed complications, such as infection or delayed bleeding, occur rarely from adrenal injury.[45] Active bleeding of adrenal origin can occur, which is more frequently detected with faster CT systems and better contrast bolus timing, and can be a source of continual blood loss.

Hyperintense enhancement of the normally shaped adrenal gland has been described as an element of the hypoperfusion complex seen in children and includes a small aorta and IVC as well as intense enhancement of the kidneys, pancreas, aorta, IVC, bowel wall, and mesentery.[48]

Retroperitoneal Hematoma

The identification, quantification, and stability of retroperitoneal hematoma(s) (RPH) following blunt or penetrating trauma are crucial in detecting the site(s) of potentially significant but often clinically occult blood loss and in planning management. The location of RPH within the total clinical setting in terms of mechanism of injury, clinical stability, and associated injuries is a major factor determining the most appropriate management.[49] The clinically unstable patient will be investigated immediately by surgery, although interventional angiography may be utilized subsequently to supplement control of hemorrhage. In general, hemodynamically stable patients with evidence of an expanding or actively bleeding RPH, recognized by direct visualization, angiography, or CT, will require intervention by endovascular or surgical means. Similarly, in the setting of penetrating injury, the risk for vascular injury is higher than that in the blunt force trauma setting, increasing the need for angiographic or surgical investigation.

Goins et al.[50] reported an incidence of RPH of 2.9% of blunt abdominal trauma admissions to UMSTC. Porter et al.[51] reported that RPH was present in 12% of 466 stable patients having abdominal CT for blunt trauma. Most RPH results from blunt trauma (67% to 80%) rather than from penetrating trauma (20% to 33%). The kidney is the most commonly injured organ seen in association with RPH.[51] Feliciano has emphasized the importance of the location of RPH in the decision whether to surgically investigate. The location was described by use of zones of the anatomy,[52] and more recently this description has been modified by using more focal localization.[49] Zone I involves injuries in the upper to mid central retroperitoneum and is the least common location (Fig. 7-61).

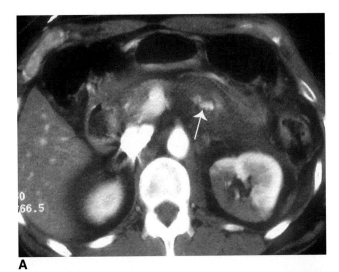

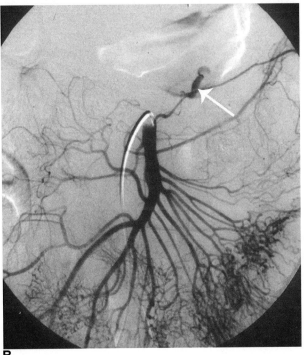

Fig. 7-61
Zone 1 retroperitoneal hematoma. **A,** CT shows a hematoma primarily in the left anterior pararenal space, with focus of active bleeding (*arrow*). **B,** Superior mesenteric angiogram shows bleeding site arising from first branch (*arrow*). This branch was embolization with cessation of bleeding (not shown).

Zone II RPH refers to the flank or lateral retroperitoneum and constitutes the second most common site (Fig. 7-62; see also Figs. 7-11, 7-15 to 7-21, 7-28, and 7-29). Zone III includes pelvic RPH and is the most frequently affected location (Fig. 7-63). Feliciano[49] further divides some of these areas, based upon mechanism of injury and suggested management.

In blunt trauma, pelvic RPH should not be investigated surgically because of the risk for detamponade of bleeding, inaccessibility to bleeding sites, and lack of control of hemorrhage with occlusion of both internal iliac arteries.[49] Internal iliac ligation excludes subsequent angiographic embolization. Potential indications to explore this hematoma in blunt injury include pelvic RPH combined with major intraperitoneal injuries; expanding, ruptured, or pulsatile pelvic hematoma at surgery; major pelvic arterial injury; exsanguinating pelvic bleeding; or bleeding into a peritoneal wound.[49] In most patients, pelvic RPH is controlled by external pelvic fixation or other means to reduce pelvic volume and embolization. RPH in the *supracolic* midline is surgically investigated, given the association with major vascular injury. *Inframesocolic* RPH is also explored to exclude lumbar artery etiology. RPH in the lateral paraduodenal area and portal areas also requires investigation to exclude vascular, biliary tree, and duodenal injury. RPH in the lateral pericolonic region and retrohepatic region can typically be managed without surgery if shown to be stable at surgery or by CT. Feliciano notes that most sites of RPH resulting from penetrating trauma are explored (except the lateral perirenal areas when the kidney is "reasonably intact," as documented by CT or other studies). Experience with CT has shown high accuracy in assessment of organ injury occurring in the general setting of penetrating back and flank trauma.[53-56]

The determination of site of RPH thus is clearly of major importance for optimal management. In addition, the concurrent presence of other injuries, especially involving the intraperitoneal space, strongly influences initial management choices. Obviously, an exsanguinating splenic hemorrhage or full-thickness bowel injury must take priority over a stable retroperitoneal hematoma. Other nonabdominal-pelvic injuries, including those within the cranium and thorax, must, of course, also be considered. Thus detailed knowledge about injury in both intra- and retroperitoneal spaces, as well as in the head, neck, and chest, may often be required first in order to establish treatment priorities.

As discussed fully in Chapter 6, the best study or combination of studies to achieve this purpose is controversial and perhaps varies for different clinical settings. Clearly, however, state-of-the-art multidetector CT is fully capable of simultaneously imaging the intraperitoneal and retroperitoneal compartments as well as the abdominal-pelvic skeleton in one rapid pass, requiring less than 30 seconds while maintaining high spatial resolution and minimal artifact. The head, neck (spine), and chest can be evaluated at the same setting, as indicated by the clinical survey. The decision whether to use CT as the principle screening test for blunt and selected cases of penetrating trauma depends upon the hemodynamic state of the patient, proximity to the full resuscitative resources of the trauma admission area, the physiologic support and monitoring capacity in the CT suite, and the

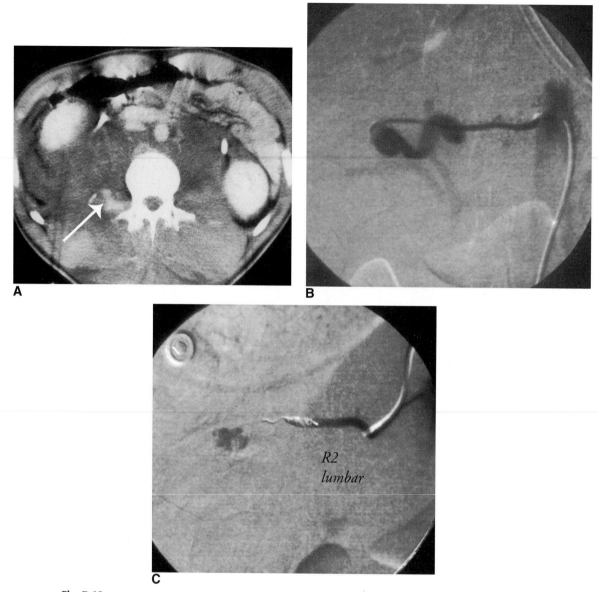

Fig. 7-62
Zone 2 retroperitoneal hematoma. **A**, A large retroperitoneal hematoma involves the posterior pararenal space bilateral but extends along the right lower flank. The right kidney is displaced anteriorly. There is a site of active bleeding arising near the lumbar artery (*arrow*). **B**, Selective second right lumbar arteriogram demonstrates a torn vessel that was subsequently embolized with coils, arresting hemorrhage shown in **C**.

speed of image availability for review.[57] The availability and experience of the interpreting physician(s) are, in many respects, the most important factors in this consideration, since the imaging information is only as good as its timely interpretation. Although the plain abdominal and pelvic AP radiographs can provide information suggesting the presence of RPH, as reflected in areas of uniform increased density or more usually by mass effect on adjacent visceral structures, they are relatively insensitive and nonspecific and have been substantially abandoned

for this purpose. CT is highly accurate in identifying the hematoma and determining its extent, likely origin, and stability. Cerva et al.[20] have shown that helical CT can demonstrate the site of active bleeding in pelvic RPH as a guide to the need for and site of embolization. CT can identify other sites of RPH and active bleeding, indicating the likely vascular origins and providing a map for surgical or angiographic investigation. The location of the hematoma, as previously noted, has direct influence on the decision to explore the hematoma and adjacent vas-

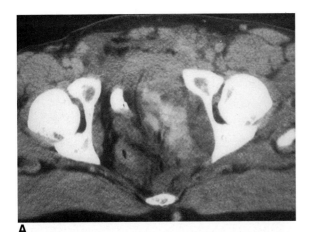

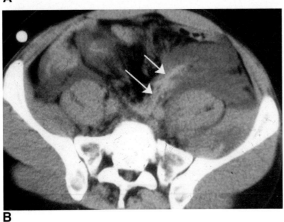

Fig. 7-63
Zone 3 retroperitoneal (pelvic) hematoma. **A,** Left lateral pelvic hematoma with active bleeding. **B,** Active bleeding into left pelvic hematoma overlying iliopsoas muscle. Bleeding within left iliopsoas is also noted (*arrows*).

culature. Serial CT can be used to document stability or expansion of RPH, a factor that will also influence management.

The presence of a *focal* retroperitoneal hematoma may act as a "sentinel clot"[58] for a particular organ, such as the colon or duodenum. RPH frequently extends beyond the confines of the pelvic retroperitoneum into the perirenal or pararenal spaces and may suggest injury in these areas where none exists. Tracking the hematoma on successive images and carefully examining the adjacent extrapelvic organs should help in this determination. It is also important to recognize that in actively bleeding patients, extravasated contrast may appear at some distance from its vessel of origin, particularly if the scan occurs late in the equilibrium phase of the contrast bolus or beyond. Scanning in the early arterial phase is needed to reveal the actual source of bleeding.

On several occasions in the author's experience the presence of thickening or hemorrhage along the anterior Gerota's fascia or lateral conal fascia has been an indirect CT marker for significant injury to adjacent organs, such

as the colon or pancreas. When this fascial thickening sign is observed on the initial posttrauma CT, careful clinical and repeat CT follow-up is recommended.

Injury to the Inferior Vena Cava and Abdominal Aorta

Injury to the inferior vena cava is usually the result of penetrating injury.[59] Mortality from IVC injury is high (39%) and is related to both the failure to recognize the injury and the difficulty in surgical repair.[60-62] Higher mortality is seen among patients with IVC injury from blunt trauma, a suprarenal location of injury, shock on admission, free hemorrhage into the peritoneal cavity, and a number of concurrent vascular injuries.[59-62] Blunt IVC injury is typically related to decelerating trauma and is seen in conjunction with blunt hepatic trauma. Shearing forces can also tear the IVC in a suprahepatic and intrapericardial location.[63]

Few studies have described imaging findings of IVC injury. Parke et al.[64] noted CT findings of RPH with a pericaval epicenter, irregularity of the caval contour (Fig. 7-64), and contrast extravasation from the IVC. Radin[65] described hypoattenuation in the pericaval and perihepatic vein region, "hepatic venous tracking," in a single child with liver and caval injury. The specificity of this finding for IVC or major hepatic vein injury is unknown. Compression of the IVC and hepatic veins by intrahepatic or subcapsular liver hematoma can result in a Budd-Chiari–type syndrome, with a large quantity of ascites and direct visualization of IVC and hepatic vein compression[66] (Fig. 7-65).

Abdominal aorta injury (AAI) usually results from penetrating trauma and is managed by surgical inspection if there is any question of abdominal aortic involvement. Such patients may be studied angiographically prior to surgery. Rarely, CT may show a direct vascular injury, periaortic hematoma, or extravasation due to penetrating injury when this is not clinically considered likely (Fig. 7-66). Blunt force AAI is quite rare, with Fontaine[67] reporting 55 cases in the literature between 1953 and 1997. Patients with AAI from blunt trauma frequently are wearing lap belts without shoulder restraints and have a common association with distractive injuries of the thoracic or lumbar spine (Chance pattern)[67-69] (Fig. 7-67). The diagnosis may be suspected in cases where there is decreased or absent femoral pulse amplitude or in any blunt trauma patient with a Chance mechanism of thoracolumbar spine fracture. Injury most likely results from distractive force applied to the abdominal aorta at the point of osseous injury. A spectrum of aortic injuries occurs, including intimal flaps, pseudoaneurysm, partial or complete aortic thrombosis, and full-thickness circumferential laceration.[69] Lesions can present in an acute or chronic state.[70] According to Lock,[71] most blunt

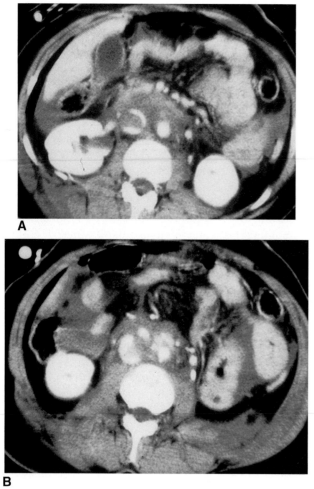

Fig. 7-64

CT of IVC tear. **A**, A clot is seen within the IVC (*arrow*) with hemorrhage surrounding the IVC and aorta. **B**, On a more caudal image there is hematoma and multifocal areas of contrast extravasation surrounding the abdominal aorta and IVC in blunt trauma victim. Free fluid is seen in the peritoneal cavity, and there is proximal small bowel contusion. The aorta was intact at surgery, but the IVC was torn.

force AAI (71%) occurs at the level of the inferior mesenteric or renal artery, with 27% mortality. The diagnosis can certainly be established with contrast-enhanced abdominal CT by direct visualization of aortic injury and should be suspected in any patient with periaortic hematoma,[68,70] particularly in association with thoracic or lumbar Chance-type fractures.

CONCLUSION

The retroperitoneum offers a potential space for the accumulation of large amounts of hemorrhage, and injury in this space can remain occult to clinical assessment and radiographic imaging. The utility of sonography in this area has not been established. For these reasons, contrast-

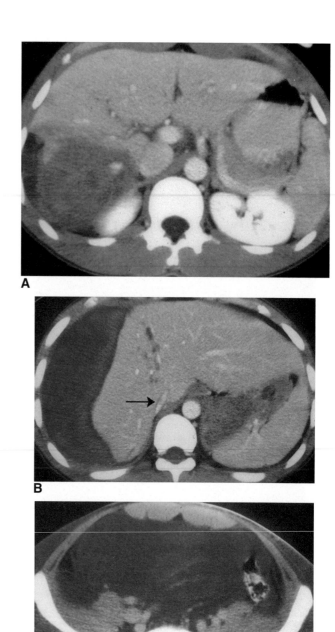

Fig. 7-65

IVC compression by hepatic hematoma (Posttraumatic Budd-Chiari Syndrome). **A**, CT image obtained in a pugilist injured in an officially sanctioned boxing match demonstrates a right posterior hepatic hematoma with active focus of bleeding with extension to subcapsular space. **B**, Follow-up study 1 week after injury shows a larger low-attenuation subcapsular collection that has extended from the original injury. The IVC is compressed (*arrow*) because of mass effect. **C**, The peritoneal cavity has filled with ascites resulting from near occlusion of the IVC. (From Markert DJ, Shanmuganathan K, Mirvis SE, et al: *Clin Radiol* 52:384, 1997.)

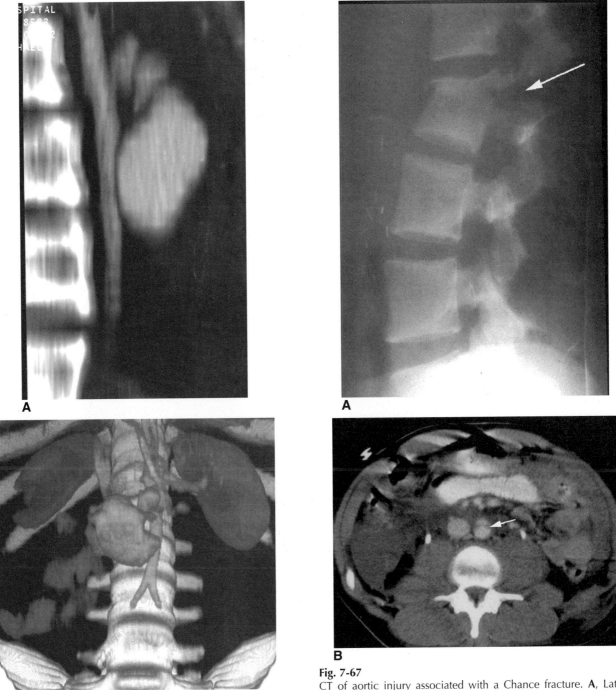

Fig. 7-66
Aortic knife wound. **A,** Sagittal MPR CT image of adult male assault victim, who was thought to have a superficial abdominal knife wound, shows a large contrast leak from the abdomen aorta. **B,** Three-dimensional surface rendering dramatically illustrates extent of bleeding. (From Bernstein MP, Mirvis SE: *Emerg Radiol* 8:45, 2001.)

Fig. 7-67
CT of aortic injury associated with a Chance fracture. **A,** Lateral lumbar spine study shows a Chance fracture of L2 (*arrow*). Surgical clips seen anterior to lumbar spine. **B,** Preoperative CT of abdomen shows an intimal flap (*arrow*) across abdominal aortic lumen. In addition there is peritoneal free fluid, bowel wall thickening, and periaortic/pericaval retroperitoneal fluid. (From Reaney SM, Parker M, Mirvis SE, et al: *Clin Radiol* 50:836, 1995.)

enhanced CT is the best available study to evaluate the retroperitoneum for hemorrhage and the presence and extent of urinary tract injury from both blunt and penetrating trauma. Clues to the presence of injuries to the retroperitoneal portions of the duodenum and colon may be appreciated as small amounts of focal retroperitoneal gas bubbles or focal adjacent retroperitoneal hematomas. In trauma patients exhibiting a decreasing hematocrit of unknown etiology, CT is mandated to assess the retroperitoneal spaces.

REFERENCES

1. Brower P, Paul J, Brosman SA: Urinary tract abnormalities presenting as a result of blunt abdominal trauma, *J Trauma* 18:719, 1978.
2. Roberts RA, Belitsky P, Lannon SG, et al: Conservative management of renal lacerations in blunt trauma, *Can J Surg* 30:253, 1987.
3. Hardeman SW, Husmann DA, Chinn HK, et al: Blunt urinary tract trauma: identifying those patients who require radiological diagnostic studies, *J Urol* 1380:99, 1987.
4. Miller KS, McAninch JW: Radiographic assessment of renal trauma: our 15-year experience, *J Urol* 154:352, 1995.
5. Stein JP, Kaji DM, Eastham J, et al: Blunt renal trauma in the pediatric population: indications for radiographic evaluation, *Urology* 44:406, 1994.
6. Carlton CE: Injuries of the kidney and ureter. In Harrison RF, Giles GR, Perlmutter AD, eds: *Campbell's urology*, Philadelphia, 1978, WB Saunders.
7. Perry MJ, Porte ME, Urwin GH: Limitations of ultrasound evaluation in acute closed renal trauma, *J R Coll Surg Edinb* 42:420, 1997.
8. McGahan JP, Richards JR, Jones CD, et al: Use of ultrasonography in the patient with acute renal trauma, *J Ultrasound Med* 18:207, 1999.
9. Santucci RA, McAninch JW, Safir M, et al: Validation of the American Association for the Surgery of Trauma organ injury severity scale for the kidney, *J Trauma* 50:195, 2001.
10. Thomason RB, Julian JS, Mostellar HC, et al: Microscopic hematuria after blunt trauma. Is pyelography necessary? *Am Surg* 55:145, 1989.
11. Mirvis SE: Trauma. In Novelline RA, ed: Advances in uroradiology. II. *Radiol Clin North Am* 34:1225, 1996.
12. Lewis DR, Mirvis SE: Segmental renal artery infarction following blunt abdominal trauma: clinical appearance and appropriate management, *Emergency Radiology* 3:236, 1996.
13. Cheng DL, Lazan D, Stone N: Conservative treatment of type III renal trauma, *J Trauma* 36:491, 1994.
14. Robert MN, Drianno N, Muir G, et al: Management of major blunt renal lacerations: surgical or nonoperative approach? *Eur Urol* 30:335, 1996.
15. Nunez D Jr, Becerra JL, Fuentes D, et al: Traumatic occlusion of the renal artery: helical CT diagnosis, *AJR Am J Roentgenol* 167:777, 1996.
16. Villas PA, Cohen G, Putnam SG, et al: Wallstent placement in a renal artery after blunt abdominal trauma, *J Trauma* 46:1137, 1999.
17. Hoffmann RM, Stieper KW, Johnson RW, et al: Renal ischemic tolerance, *Arch Surg* 109:550, 1974.
18. Cain MP, Matsomoto JM, Husmann DA: Retrograde filling of the renal vein on computerized tomography for blunt renal trauma: an indicator of renal artery injury, *J Urol* 153:1247, 1995.
19. Klink BK, Sutherin S, Heyes P, et al: Traumatic bilateral renal artery thrombosis diagnosed by computed tomography with successful revascularization: case report, *J Trauma* 32:259, 1992.
20. Cerva DS Jr, Mirvis SE, Shanmuganathan K, et al: Detection of bleeding in patients with major pelvic fractures: value of contrast-enhanced CT, *AJR Am J Roentgenol* 166:131, 1996.
21. Templeton PA, Mirvis SE, Whitley NO: Traumatic avulsion of the ureter: computed tomography correlation, *J Comput Tomogr* 12:159, 1988.
22. Huang Y, Zhu Z: Massive hydronephrosis associated with traumatic rupture, *Injury* 28:505, 1997.
23. Heyns CF, van Vollenhoven P: Increasing role of angiography and segmental artery embolization in the management of renal stab wounds, *J Urol* 147:1231, 1992.
24. Uflacker R, Paolini RM, Lima S: Management of traumatic hematuria by selective renal artery embolization, *J Urol* 132:662, 1984.
25. Corr P, Hacking G: Embolization in traumatic intrarenal vascular injuries, *Clin Radiol* 43:262, 1991.
26. Whigham CJ Jr, Bodenhamer JR, Miller JK: Use of the Palmaz stent in primary treatment of renal artery intimal injury secondary to blunt trauma, *J Vasc Interv Radiol* 6:175, 1995.
27. Jebara VA, El Rassi I, Achouh PE, et al: Renal artery pseudoaneurysm after blunt abdominal trauma, *J Vasc Surg* 27:362, 1998.
28. Whitesides E, Kozlowski DL: Ureteral injury from blunt abdominal trauma: case report, *J Trauma* 36:745, 1994.
29. Kawashima A, Sandler CM, Corriere JN Jr, et al: Ureteropelvic junction injuries secondary to blunt abdominal trauma, *Radiology* 205:487, 1997.
30. Mulligan JM, Caggianos I, Collins JP, et al: Ureteropelvic junction disruption secondary to blunt trauma: excretory phase imaging (delayed films) should help prevent a missed diagnosis, *J Urol* 159:67, 1998.
31. Drake MJ, Noble JG: Ureteric trauma in gynecologic surgery, *Int Urogynecol J Pelvic Floor Dysfunct* 9:108, 1998.
32. Sclafani SJ, Becker JA: Radiologic diagnosis of extrarenal genitourinary trauma, *Urol Radiol* 7:201, 1985.
33. Spirnak JP: Pelvic fracture and injury to the lower urinary tract, *Surg Clin North Am* 68:1057, 1988.
34. Lis LE, Cohen AJ: CT cystography in the evaluation of bladder trauma, *J Comput Assist Tomogr* 14:386, 1990.
35. Haas CA, Brown SL, Spirnak JP: Limitations of routine spiral computerized tomography in the evaluation of bladder trauma, *J Urol* 162:51, 1999.
36. Kane NM, Francis IR, Ellis JH: The value of CT in the detection of bladder and posterior urethral injuries, *AJR Am J Roentgenol* 153:1243, 1989.
37. Wright DG, Taitsman L, Laughlin RT: Pelvic and bladder trauma: a case report and subject review, *J Orthop Trauma* 10:351, 1996.
38. Ahmed S, Neel KF: Urethral injury in girls with fractured pelvis following blunt abdominal trauma, *Br J Urol* 78:450, 1996.
39. Colapinto V, McCallum RW: Injury to the male posterior urethra in fractured pelvis: a new classification, *J Urol* 118:575, 1977.
40. Goldman SM, Sandler CM, Corriere JN Jr, et al: Blunt urethral trauma: a unified, anatomic mechanical classification, *J Urol* 157:85, 1997.
41. Krone KD, Carroll BA: Scrotal ultrasound, *Radiol Clin North Am* 23:121, 1985.
42. Jeffrey RB, Laing FC, Hricak H, et al: Sonography of testicular trauma, *AJR Am J Roentgenol* 141:993, 1983.
43. Patil MG, Onuora VC: The value of ultrasound in the evaluation of patients with blunt scrotal trauma, *Injury* 25:177, 1994.
44. Schwarz M, Horev G, Freud E, et al: Traumatic adrenal injury in children, *Isr Med Assoc J* 2:132, 2000.
45. Burks DW, Mirvis SE, Shanmuganathan K: Acute adrenal injury after blunt abdominal trauma: CT findings, *AJR Am J Roentgenol* 158:503, 1992.
46. Luchtman M, Breitgand A: Traumatic adrenal hemorrhage in children: an indicator of visceral injury, *Pediatr Surg Int* 16:586, 2000.
47. Sivit CJ, Ingram JD, Taylor GA, et al: Posttraumatic adrenal hemorrhage in children: CT findings in 34 patients, *AJR Am J Roentgenol* 158:1299, 1992.
48. O'Hara SM, Donnelly LF: Intense contrast enhancement of the adrenal glands: another abdominal CT finding associated with hypoperfusion complex in children, *AJR Am J Roentgenol* 173:995, 1999.

49. Feliciano DV: Management of traumatic retroperitoneal hematoma, *Ann Surg* 211:109, 1990.

50. Goins WA, Rodriguez A, Lewis J, et al: Retroperitoneal hematoma after blunt trauma, *Surg Gynecol Obstet* 174:281, 1992.

51. Porter JM, Singh Y: Value of computed tomography in the evaluation of retroperitoneal organ injury in blunt abdominal trauma, *Am J Emerg Med* 16:225, 1998.

52. Kudsk KA, Sheldon GF: Retroperitoneal hematoma. In Blaisdell FW, Trunkey DD, eds: *Abdominal trauma*, New York, 1982, Thieme-Stratton.

53. Federle MP, Brown TR, McAninch JW: Penetrating renal trauma: CT evaluation. *J Comput Assist Tomogr* 11:1026, 1987.

54. Boyle EM Jr, Maier RV, Salazar JD, et al: Diagnosis of injuries after stab wounds to the back and flank, *J Trauma* 42:260, 1997.

55. Himmelman RG, Martin M, Gilkey S, et al: Triple-contrast CT scans in penetrating back and flank trauma, *J Trauma* 31:852, 1992.

56. Phillips T, Sclafani SJ, Goldstein A, et al: Use of contrast-enhanced CT enema in the management of penetrating trauma to the flank and back, *J Trauma* 26:593, 1986.

57. Mirvis SE, Hastings G, Scalea TM: Diagnostic imaging, angiography, and interventional radiology in the trauma patient. In Mattox KL, Feliciano DV, Moore EE, eds: *Trauma*, ed 4, New York, 2000, McGraw-Hill.

58. Orwig D, Federle MP: Localized clotted blood as evidence of visceral trauma on CT: the sentinel clot sign, *AJR Am J Roentgenol* 153:747, 1989.

59. Coimbra R, Santos PE, Caffaro RA, et al: Inferior vena cava trauma: analysis of 36 cases, *Rev Assoc Med Bras* 39:229, 1993.

60. Leppaniemi AK, Savolainen HO, Salo JA: Traumatic inferior vena caval injuries, *Scand J Thorac Cardiovasc Surg* 28:103, 1994.

61. Degiannis E, Velmahos GC, Levy RD, et al: Penetrating injuries of the abdominal inferior vena cava, *Ann R Coll Surg Engl* 78:485, 1996.

62. van de Wal HJ, Draaisma JM, Vincent JG, et al: Rupture of the supradiaphragmatic inferior vena cava by blunt decelerating trauma: case report, *J Trauma* 30:111, 1990.

63. Fey GL, Deren MM, Wesolek JH: Intrapericardial caval injury due to blunt trauma, *Conn Med* 63:259, 1999.

64. Parke CE, Stanley RJ, Berlin AJ: Infrarenal vena caval injury following blunt trauma: CT findings, *J Comput Assist Tomogr* 17:154, 1993.

65. Radin DR: Liver trauma and transection of the inferior vena cava: sentinel contrast sign and hepatic perivenous tracking, *Acta Radiol* 33:255, 1992.

66. Markert DJ, Shanmuganathan K, Mirvis SE, et al: Budd-Chiari syndrome resulting from intrahepatic IVC compression secondary to blunt hepatic trauma, *Clin Radiol* 52:384, 1997.

67. Fontaine AB, Nicholls SC, Borsa JJ, et al: Seat belt aorta: endovascular management with a stent-graft, *J Endovasc Ther* 8:83, 2001.

68. Reaney SM, Parker MS, Mirvis SE, et al: Abdominal aortic injury associated with transverse lumbar spine fracture—imaging findings, *Clin Radiol* 50:834, 1995.

69. Inaba K, Kirkpatrick AW, Finkelstein J, et al: Blunt abdominal aortic trauma in association with thoracolumbar spine fractures, *Injury* 32:201, 2001.

70. Naude GP, Back M, Perry MO, et al: Blunt disruption of the abdominal aorta: report of a case and review of the literature, *J Vasc Surg* 250:931, 1997.

71. Lock JS, Huffman AD, Johnson RC: Blunt trauma to the abdominal aorta, *J Trauma* 27:674, 1987.

8 Thoracic and Lumbar Spine Trauma

Stacy E. Smith

Imaging of the spine in trauma patients requires knowledge of the underlying anatomy of the thoracic lumbar spine as well as of the various forces of injury that act on this region and their resultant radiographic appearances. The forces of injury include compression, flexion, extension, torsion, and shear, all of which can occur alone or in combination and will be discussed in detail in this chapter. In addition, with the increased accessibility to computed tomography (CT) and magnetic resonance imaging (MRI) in emergent trauma centers the evaluation of not only the ossific structures but also the adjacent soft tissues, spinal cord, and cauda equina is invaluable in these often diagnostically challenging patients.

Although the cervical spine is the most commonly imaged portion of the spinal column in trauma patients, thoracic and lumbar spine fractures make up a significant percentage of injuries, most frequently as the result of falls, jumps, airplane crashes, automobile accidents, and winter sport injuries. Thoracic spine fractures account for 20% of all spinal fractures with 10% of these having associated spinal cord injuries.[1-4] The majority of the fractures in the thoracic and lumbar spine in adults occur at the thoracolumbar junction via flexion and axial loading (the most common forces in thoracic spine injuries). Sixty percent of fractures occur between T12 and L2, and 90% occur between T11 and L4.[5-7] The increased susceptibility to injury is most likely secondary to the transitional nature of the thoracolumbar junction with (1) its alteration of spinal curvature from kyphotic to lordotic, (2) loss of the stabilizing rib cage and its associated inter-costal muscle support inferior to T12, and finally (3) the change in orientation of articular facet joints from thoracic coronal to lumbar sagittal plane.[8-10]

Of the thoracic lumbar fractures, the burst fracture is one of the most significant, with 65% associated with neurologic deficit.[11] Multilevel nonspecific spinal fractures occur in 5% to 20% of adult cases, with 4% being noncontiguous.[1,12,13] Mid and upper thoracic spine fractures are most commonly associated with a second fracture at the thoracolumbar junction or in the cervical spine.[12] Thoracolumbar fractures are rarely associated with secondary fractures of L4 or L5, or of the cervical spine. In children, the majority of fractures occur at T4, T5, and L2 levels. Multiple contiguous fractures occur more commonly in children than in adults.

Given the close proximity of the adjacent paraspinal (soft tissues, ligaments, muscle, and neurovascular bundles), intrathoracic, and intraperitoneal structures, in combination with the associated large forces required to injure the thoracolumbar spine, injury to other organ systems is not uncommon. Other organ systems are injured in 50% of cases, with one additional organ system involved in 30% of these cases, two additional systems in 10% to 20%, and three additional organ systems in 5% of cases.[14] Such injuries include rib fractures, lung contusions, and hemo- or pneumothoraces, all of which are commonly seen in association with displaced thoracic spine fractures. Other associated skeletal injuries can be present in 20% of cases, the most common being calcaneal fractures and vertical shear fractures of the pelvis in association with crush fractures of the spine.[7,15]

Our institution has also described a case report of a rare esophageal perforation injury secondary to thoracic spine fracture dislocation.[16] Other rare reports of secondary injury include a posttraumatic compressive subarachnoid cyst, pneumocephalus associated with thoracic vertebral fracture and secondary subarachnoid pleural fistula, and a traumatic aortic injury secondary to an "osseous pinch" mechanism between the anterior surfaces of the thoracic spine and the anterior bony complex (manubrium, clavicle, and first rib) in a compression injury of the thorax.[17-19]

ANATOMIC CONSIDERATIONS

To understand the types of thoracolumbar fracture patterns and to delineate stable versus unstable fractures, one must first have an understanding of the basic anatomy of the thoracic and lumbar spine. The typical vertebral body consists of the anterior body and the adjoining posterior vertebral arch composed of two pedicles and two paired laminae (Fig. 8-1). The bilateral laminae join posteriorly to form the spinous process at each level. Transverse processes project bilaterally from the posterior vertebral body. Four ossific extensions from the lamina/pedicle junction form the facet or apophyseal joints (synovial joints with a fibrous capsule) that are important in determining the range and direction of vertebral column motion and are involved in weight bearing. Fibrocartilaginous intervertebral discs, composed of both the central nucleus pulposus and peripheral annulus fibrosus, are present between the vertebral bodies and comprise the majority of the weight-bearing function. The configuration of the discs differs depending on the location within the vertebral column. The discs are taller ventrally than dorsally in the lumbar spine (similar to the cervical spine) with increasing thickness from L1 to L4, with L4 being the largest disc (Fig. 8-2). Alternatively, the discs are approximately of equal height anteriorly and posteriorly throughout the thoracic spine.

Ligaments include the anterior longitudinal ligament, posterior longitudinal ligament, ligamentum flavum, intraspinous ligaments, supraspinous ligaments, and lateral longitudinal ligament (Fig. 8-3). The posterior longitudinal ligament is centrally located behind the vertebral body and disc spaces and joins with the fibers of the annulus fibrosus, yet is separated from the posterior vertebral body by a venous plexus. The anterior longitudinal ligament is wider and stronger than the narrow centrally located posterior longitudinal ligament. The ligamentum flavum is a thick, paired ligament extending between the lamina of adjacent vertebrae that blends with the articular capsules of the facet joints.

The spinal canal and cord anatomy should also be reviewed. The spinal cord and its meningeal covering extend to the L1/2 disc space in the adult and the L2/3 level in the newborn. The spinal cord terminates at the conus medullaris with the filum terminale continuing distally, eventually blending in with the posterior ligament and sacral canal. The dural sac envelops both structures to the S2 level. Extradural fat and epidural venous plexus fill the potential space between the bony canal and the dura mater. The vertebral canal is smaller in the thoracic spine than the lumbar spine secondary to the large size of the thoracic cord, giving rise to little residual capacity for adaptation to injuries and hematomas impinging on the spinal cord at this level.

SPINAL INSTABILITY

Determination of spinal instability is crucial. Several concepts of instability are described in the literature.[20-23] These can, however, be simplified into two components: mechanical stability and neurologic stability.[24] A mechanically unstable spine is one that can progressively deform under physiologic stress. A neurologically unstable spine has the potential to increase an incomplete injury or produce a new deficit. Acute and chronic instability can occur. In the acute sense, an unstable injury is one that risks neurologic injury. In the chronic setting, an injury fails to heal or demonstrates increasing deformity, or there is increased mobility at the injured level with or without neurologic deficit. The chronically unstable patients are therefore the most difficult to assess initially by radiographic criteria.[25]

Radiographic signs of instability in the thoracolumbar spine include displaced vertebrae, widening of the facet joints or interspinous and interpedicular spaces, and perched or dislocated facet joints, as well as vertebral compression greater than 50% and disc narrowing. These injuries produce enough derangement to allow for abnormal motion at the site of injury. CT can be of benefit in further evaluation of these injuries.

The stability or instability of a spinal injury is best evaluated by using the functional three-column anatomical model of the spine as described in the sagittal plane by Denis (Fig. 8-4).[24-26] Denis, McAfee et al., and Ferguson and Allen have described several models,[6,24,26,27] but the following model by Denis is the most workable classification system to date.

The spine is divided into anterior, middle, and posterior columns. The anterior column consists of the anterior longitudinal ligament and the anterior two thirds of the vertebral body and annulus fibrosus. The middle column is composed of the posterior longitudinal ligament, the posterior one third of the vertebral body, and the posterior one third of the annulus fibrosus. The posterior column is formed by the posterior arch, articular processes, and the posterior ligamentous complex, the latter of which is largely responsible for spinal stability. The posterior ligamentous complex is composed of the supraspinous and intraspinous ligaments (which connect the posterior arches of the vertebral bodies), the liga-

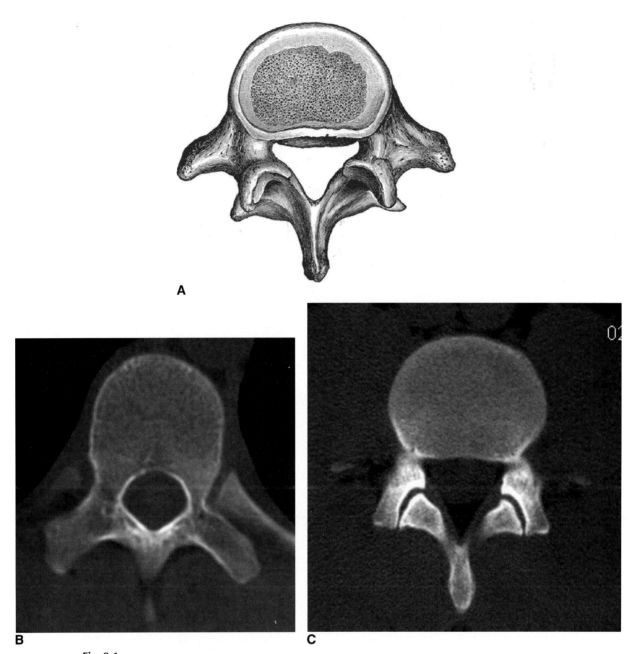

Fig. 8-1
A, Anatomic drawing of normal lumbar vertebral body. **B**, CT image of a normal thoracic vertebral body at level of pedicles. **C**, CT image of a normal lumbar vertebral body at level of facet joints. The lumbar spinal canal is somewhat more capacious.

mentum flava, and the capsular ligaments of the articular pillars. Although Holdsworth believed the posterior column was the key to stability, we now consider the integrity of the middle column of Denis's classification system to be crucial to spinal stability.[15,28] Columnar involvement can be delineated as one-, two-, or three-column injuries. Disruption of the middle column makes the injury unstable. This is depicted best on CT imaging with sagittal reconstruction images. Vertebral displacement and increased interpedicular distance implies disruption of all three columns, the latter finding visualized

in unstable burst fractures. Facet subluxation or dislocation is secondary to injury of the posterior longitudinal ligament and annulus fibrosus and is diagnosed by the "naked facet" sign on CT.[29]

IMAGING EVALUATION
Radiography

Anteroposterior (AP) and lateral (centered at L2/L3 for the lumbar spine) radiographs are still the initial method of investigating the thoracolumbar spine in the

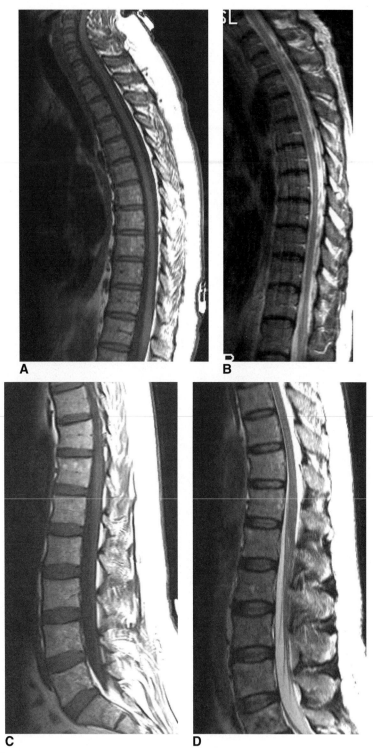

Fig. 8-2
T1-weighted (**A**) and T2-weighted (**B**) sagittal MR sequences of a normal thoracic vertebral column. T1-weighted (**C**) and T2-weighted (**D**) sagittal MR sequences of a normal lumbar vertebral column. Note the difference in size and shape of the discs in lumbar spine as compared with the thoracic spine.

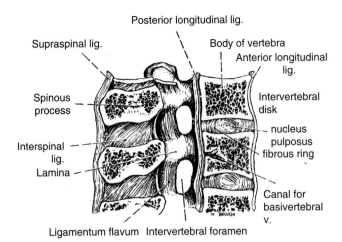

Fig. 8-3
Diagrammatic representation of the ligamentous anatomy of the thoracolumbar spine.(From Woodburne RT: *Essentials of human anatomy*, ed 5, New York, 1973, Oxford University.)

traumatized patient. Patients are divided into two groups prior to imaging: first, the mildly injured without neurological symptoms, alert and able to cooperate, and second, the more severely injured and often unconscious with multisystem trauma. The lateral view is replaced with a cross table lateral view in the severely injured patient so as to decrease patient movement. The lateral views are positive in 70% to 90% of cases.[30,31] Oblique views of the lumbar spine and coned down views of the lateral L5/S1 junction are often used.

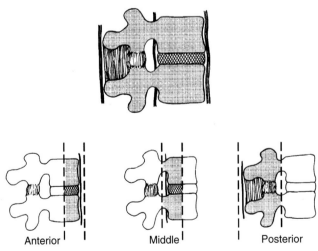

Fig. 8-4
Denis's three column model of the spine. The anterior column is made up of the anterior longitudinal ligament and anterior two thirds of vertebral body and annulus fibrosus. The middle column is made up of the posterior longitudinal ligament, the posterior annulus fibrosis, and the posterior aspect of the vertebral body and disc. The posterior column comprises the posterior arch, articular processes, and the posterior ligamentous complex (supraspinous and intraspinous ligaments, ligamentum flava, and capsular ligaments of articular pillars).(From Garfin SR, Blair B, Eismont FJ, Abitbol J: Thoracic and upper lumbar spine injuries. In Browner BD, Levine AL, Jupiter JB, Trafton PG, eds: *Skeletal trauma*, ed 2, Philadelphia, 1998, WB Saunders.)

Computed Tomography

CT is now indispensable as an adjunct to plain film examination in evaluating spinal trauma. Indications for CT include presence or suggestion of vertebral body fracture on plain film or a discrepancy between radiographic findings and neurologic status. Neurologic deficits occur in 40% of thoracolumbar injuries, and radiographs often underestimate both the ossific and soft tissue damage.[32] At our institution the new multislice CT scanners provide axial images as thin as 1.5 mm through the area of interest as localized on and tailored by the initial radiographic findings. Some advantages of CT are (1) the optimal axial assessment of vertebral injuries and associated soft tissue injuries, (2) the ability to provide sagittal and coronal reconstructions or even three-dimensional reconstruction for further assessment of fracture displacements both anteriorly and within the spinal canal, and (3) more accurate assessment of specific columnar involvement in order to determine stability without having to change patient position, which can be critical in multitrauma patients. The additional planes are extremely useful in seat belt injuries, particularly those with associated horizontal Chance fractures, which can be difficult to visualize on axial images alone. CT can also be enhanced with intravenous or intrathecal contrast material for assessment of soft tissue injury or cord compression respectively.[33] The increased use and accessibility of MRI has markedly decreased the need for invasive CT myelography in larger centers.

Magnetic Resonance Imaging

MRI, with its multiplanar capability, increased spatial and soft tissue contrast resolution, and noninvasive nature, is now being used more frequently in our institution for assessment of, most importantly, spinal cord injuries, as well as other soft tissue injuries, such as paraspinal injuries (epidural hematoma), ligament disruption, and posttraumatic disc herniations. Indications for MRI include those patients with incomplete neurologic deficits, neurologic deficits without radiographic abnormalities (central cord syndrome), or incongruity of neurologic deficit and traumatic radiographic findings.[34] Posttraumatic spinal cord lesions can occur without skeletal, discal, or ligamentous abnormalities.[35]

A spinal phased-array coil is used for improved resolution. Both sagittal and axial T1- and T2-weighted sequences are provided for full assessment of anatomy and abnormalities in two orthogonal planes. Coronal sequences can be added if necessary. Other sequences used within the spine are gradient echo sagittal sequences for assessment of posttraumatic blood within the cord and fast STIR sagittal sequences for assessing ligamentous injury with changes of hemorrhage and edema.[36]

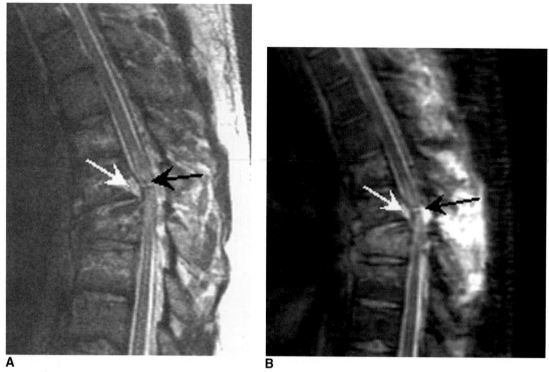

Fig. 8-5
MRI of thoracolumbar spine injury. **A**, Mid thoracic burst fracture demonstrates focal kyphosis and retropulsion of a mid thoracic vertebral body. T2-weighted sequence indicates a hematoma (*white arrow*) lifting the posterior longitudinal ligament and compressing the anterior thoracic spinal cord. Increased cord signal spanning a level above and below the compression site represents contusion. Focal low signal at the center of the edema at the impact site is blood (*black arrow*). **B**, An inversion recovery sequence shows contusion (edema) in at least four adjacent vertebrae above and below the focal kyphosis. Cord edema and hemorrhage (*black arrow*) are better seen than on T2-weighted study. The subligamentous hematoma (*white arrow*) compressing the cord is noted.

Three patterns of cord injury are noted on MRI images: (1) contusion or edema, (2) hemorrhage, and (3) mixed central hemorrhage and peripheral edema (Fig. 8-5). Differentiation of edema from hemorrhage within the spinal cord in the acute stages is clinically important, as the literature has shown that patients demonstrating edema have significant neurologic improvement as compared to those with cord hemorrhage.[37,38] Acute cord hemorrhage is seen as central hypointensity on T1-weighted images. In later stages, this area or hemorrhage demonstrates central hypointensity with a peripheral rim of hyperintensity on T2-weighted images (see

Fig. 8-5). The signal intensity of blood on MRI sequences depends on the chronicity of the hemorrhage, and the sequence from acute to chronic hemorrhage is summarized in Table 8-1.[39] These changes are related to the changes in oxygenation of hemoglobin over time. Focal hyperintense signal on T2-weighted images with hypointensity or isointensity signal on T1-weighted images suggests spinal cord edema and contusion, with similar signal intensity noted in ligamentous and paravertebral edema. Mixed signal represents edema and hemorrhage. Gradient echo sequences also can be useful in detecting or confirming hemorrhage secondary to its blooming effects.

Table 8-1
Cord Hemorrhage: Signal Intensity on MRI

Age	Blood Products	T1 Signal	T2 Signal
Hyperacute (0 to 1 day)	Oxyhemoglobin/serum	Isointense	Bright
Acute (1 to 3 days)	Deoxyhemoglobin	Isointense	Dark
Early subacute (4 to 7 days)	Intracellular methemoglobin	Bright	Dark
Late subacute (>7 days)	Extracellular methemoglobin	Bright	Bright
Chronic (>2 weeks)	Hemosiderin	Dark	Dark

Complete transection of the cord can be delineated by transverse hemorrhage between the segments, with or without enlargement of the cord.

In the chronic stages, progressive neurologic deterioration can develop secondary to posttraumatic syringomyelia, for which MRI is now the procedure of choice for diagnosis (Fig. 8-6). Other sequelae of trauma identified on MRI include myelomalacia, intramedullary cysts, infarction, or syrinx.

Ligaments are normally of low signal intensity (dark) on all pulse sequences on MRI. High signal intensity edema and hemorrhage in and around an injured ligament is noted on STIR images (see Fig. 8-5), with discontinuity of the ligament noted with complete rupture. Thickening and intrasubstance high signal intensity is noted in partial ligament tears. Imaging should be done within the first 3 days of injury before edema has the chance to resolve if present. Traumatic disc extrusions are important to exclude before surgical intervention to prevent progressive neurologic deficits. Nerve roots can be strained or avulsed, and leakage of intraspinal fluid may provide a clue to a nerve avulsion site. A contused nerve demonstrates high signal intensity and enlargement of the nerve on T2-weighted sequences.[36] Epidural hematomas are also well demonstrated by MRI (Fig. 8-7).

Traumatic disc extrusions have more serious implications within the cervical spine, but can present in the thoracic or lumbar spine. T2-weighted images demonstrate higher signal intensity than usual within the injured disc if hemorrhage is present, often with decreased disc height. Signal is isointense to a normal disc if no hemorrhage is present. The abnormal configuration, bulge, or displacement of the disc is important in diagnosis in this latter case.

MRI is much less sensitive than CT for ossific fractures and therefore should not be used as a replacement examination for CT. It is, however, very sensitive for marrow and soft tissue edema and hemorrhage in trabecular bone that can suggest an area of vertebral body fracture not initially identified on CT imaging (Fig. 8-8).

Despite MRI's many advantages, contraindications to it include pacemakers, cerebral aneurysm clips, incompatible life support systems, and halo devices. Newer technologic advances such as MRI-compatible titanium devices and other MRI-compatible metals are increasing the accessibility of this modality. Despite its high resolution for soft tissues, one disadvantage of MRI is its lack of high resolution of osseous anatomy in comparison with CT imaging as described above.

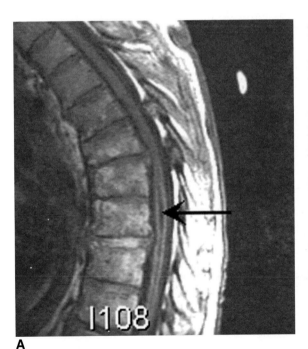

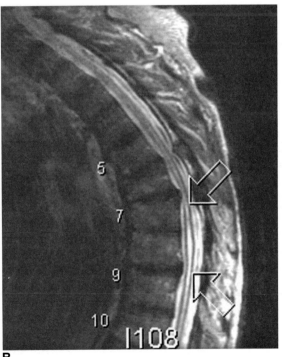

A   B

Fig. 8-6
MRI of traumatic syrinx. **A,** Sagittal T1-weighted MR image of patient with prior history of thoracic spine trauma. Central low signal syrinx is noted within the mid thoracic cord. **B,** Sagittal T2-weighted MR image demonstrating increased signal intensity within the focal cord syrinx.

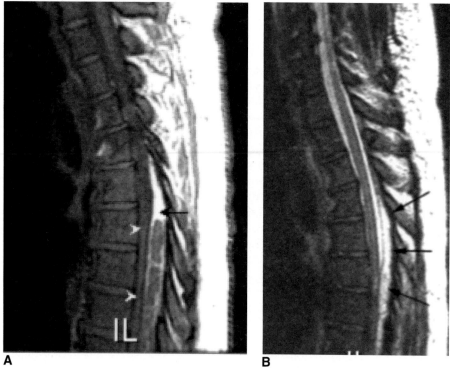

Fig. 8-7
MRI of epidural hematoma. **A**, T1-weighted sequence demonstrates a mixed signal posterior thoracic epidural hematoma (*arrow*). The spinal cord is compressed by the hematoma (*white arrowheads*). **B**, T2-weighted sequence shows epidural hematoma (*arrows*) as region of bright signal. The low signal dura separates epidural and subdural spaces.

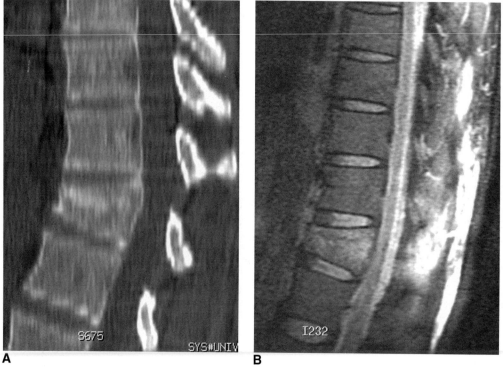

Fig. 8-8
A, Sagittal reconstructed CT image of a T12 Chance fracture demonstrating the horizontal fracture line and deformity of the vertebral body. **B**, Sagittal T2-weighted MR image of the same patient is more sensitive for detecting the associated bone marrow edema and soft tissue hemorrhage within the anterior and posterior soft tissues and ligaments at the T12 level.

SIGNS OF TRAUMA (PLAIN RADIOGRAPHS)

The "ABCs" of spinal assessment in trauma as described by Daffner include Alignment, Bone integrity, Cartilage (joint) spaces, and Soft tissues.[2] Disruption or subluxation of the posterior vertebral line or of the spinolaminar line, in addition to the findings summarized in Box 8-1, are radiographic indications of malalignment. Joint space or cartilage abnormality is suspected when any of the radiographic findings in Box 8-2 are present. Cortical buckling, disruption of anterior or posterior vertebral cortices, anterior wedging, or fractures depict disruption of bone integrity (Box 8-3). A discrepancy of greater than 2 mm between the anterior and posterior height of the vertebral body indicates a fracture, except at T11-L1, where this variant can exist normally. A 50% discrepancy is always abnormal and suggests serious ligamentous damage. Soft tissue disruption is suspected with loss of the psoas margin, widening of the paraspinal soft tissues (Fig. 8-9), deviation of the airway within the upper thoracic spine, and vacuum disc phenomenon. Other soft tissue signs resulting from fractures of the upper thoracic vertebrae are left apical capping, paravertebral hematoma, and mediastinal widening (in 80%) on radiographs. Other ancillary findings in thoracic spine injuries are rib fractures, pleural fluid (hemothorax), and sternal fractures.

Foreign bodies such as glass, metal, or bullet fragments should be noted on initial radiographs. Positioning of these bodies over or near the region of the neural canal or paraspinal soft tissues should lead to further investigation with CT imaging to better delineate the foreign body's location and proximity to the spinal cord, as well as associated bone and soft tissue trauma, as a possible preoper-

---

Box 8-1
Signs of Malalignment

Disruption of posterior vertebral line or spinolaminar line
Kyphosis
Scoliosis
Spinous process rotation
Loss of lumbar lordosis
Widened interpedicular spaces

Box 8-2
Cartilage/Joint Space Integrity

Facet joint widening
Narrowed intervertebral disc spaces
Widening disc spaces
Widening of the spinous processes

Box 8-3
Bone Integrity Loss

Cortical buckling
Disruption of anterior or posterior vertebral cortices
Anterior wedging deformity
Fractures

---

ative roadmap (Fig. 8-10).[40] It is important to remove metallic foreign bodies from the spinal canal, as myelopathy results in a high percentage of cases with delayed myelopathy reported as long as 36 years following initial injury.[41-43] MRI is contraindicated in patients with bullet fragments or metal fragments near the spinal cord or vascular structures, because magnetic forces cause increased motion of metal objects within the body.

CLASSIFICATION OF FRACTURES

Spinal injuries can be classified as either major or minor.[5,24,26] Minor injuries include fractures of the transverse or spinous process, pars interarticularis, and isolated fractures of the articular process. These rarely cause neurologic symptoms and are considered stable. Major fractures have often been classified into three categories: anterior compression, burst fractures, and fracture-dislocations. This chapter includes these categories, but will expand the classification according to the mechanism of injury (Box 8-4). Each of the types of major thoracolumbar fractures will be discussed along with their associated injuries and typical columnar involvement. As described previously, the most common type of thoracolumbar fracture is the hyperflexion injury, usually secondary to motor vehicle accidents.

Flexion Injuries

Hyperflexion Compression Injuries. The prototype of this category is the anterior wedge compression fracture that accounts for 48% of thoracic and lumbar spine fractures.[26] Flexion injuries in the thoracolumbar spine display failure of the anterior column under compressive forces, similar to that seen in the cervical spine, with associated mild to moderate distraction posteriorly. The anterior compressive force is greatest, owing to the short distance from the central nucleus pulposus (axis of flexion) to the anterior rather than posterior elements of the vertebra, hence the characteristic "anterior wedge" compression fracture deformity. Depression of the anterior column is usually less than 50% of total vertebral body height and is usually most prominent at the superior end plate (Fig. 8-11).

The thoracolumbar junction poses some difficulty in diagnosing these injuries, as there is naturally a subtle

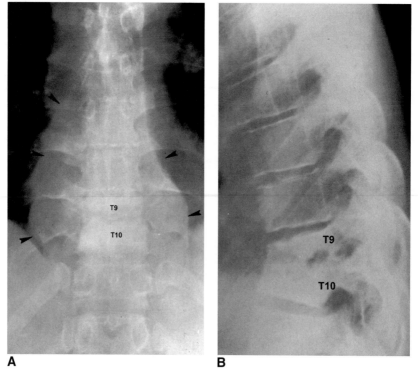

Fig. 8-9
Compression fracture. **A**, Anteroposterior (AP) view of the lower thoracic spine demonstrates a large paraspinous soft tissue mass (*arrowheads*) indicating hematoma. **B**, The lateral view demonstrates greater than 50% loss of height of T9, most marked at the anterior aspect, consistent with a severe wedge compression fracture. T10 demonstrates less severe compression deformity.

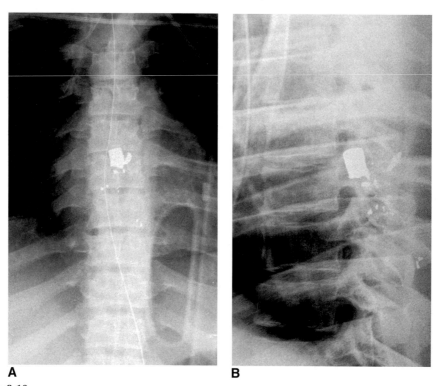

Fig. 8-10
Ballistic injury to spine. **A**, AP radiograph of the thoracic spine demonstrates focal bullet fragment over the upper thoracic spine. **B**, Lateral radiograph confirms that the bullet projects posteriorly within the thorax overlying the spinal column.

Continued

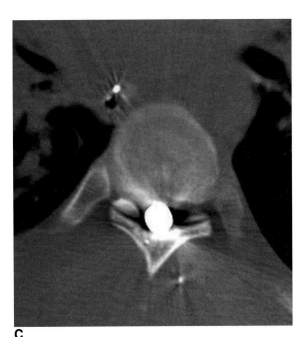
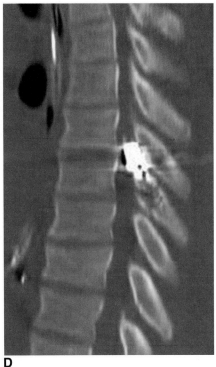

Fig. 8-10, cont'd
Axial (**C**) and sagittal (**D**) multiplanar reconstruction CT images further localize the position of the bullet within the spinal canal with associated bullet fragments involving the posterior elements at two vertebral levels.

shortening of the anterior height of the vertebral bodies at this location in comparison to the posterior height. Murphey et al. describe a rule they have found helpful: A fracture is present only if the end plates are unequally wedged anteriorly or there is isolated wedging of one end plate (usually superiorly).[44] Radiographic findings (other than loss of anterior height) include increased kyphosis or scoliosis and paravertebral soft tissue swelling. Paraspinal soft tissue swelling can mimic traumatic aortic rupture in the upper and mid thoracic regions.[45] Additional findings include endplate buckling, impaction of the anterosuperior vertebral corner, eburnation adjacent to the end plate, and in more severe cases, disc space narrowing.[46] Occasionally a vertebral endplate fracture may be present, but this is more common in osteoporotic vertebral bodies.[47]

In simple hyperflexion compression (stage 1) injuries, the posterior ligaments are not typically ruptured, interpedicular distance and posterior elements are normal (without posterior element distraction), and the middle column is intact (Fig. 8-12). They therefore are typically considered to be stable injuries, with infrequent neuro-

logic sequelae. Even if there is neurological involvement, 80% of these injuries are incomplete, and most improve dramatically without intervention.[27]

An injury with lateral compression forces may produce lateral wedging of the vertebral body (Figs. 8-13 and 8-14). This type of injury is commonly the result of automobile accidents and is seen in 48% of thoracolumbar fractures.[26] It occurs most frequently at L1, L2, and T12 in adults, becoming increasingly more common with age as the rate of osteopenia increases, with involvement at T4, T5, and L2 most commonly seen in children. This injury is stable, though it has been reported to have a slightly poorer prognosis than the simple anterior wedge fracture.[7,48] Some degree of paraspinal soft tissue swelling is usually present (Fig. 8-14).

If the compressive forces in combination with the hyperflexion are too great, further distraction of the posterior elements can occur, manifest as widening of the interspinous distance on radiographs, with associated ligamentous injury posteriorly (Fig. 8-15). There is usually greater than 50% loss of the anterior vertebral body height present in these instances, and subluxation or

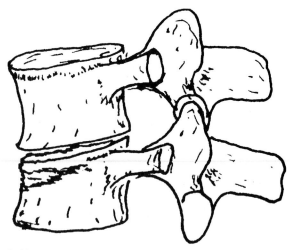

Fig. 8-11
Diagrammatic illustration of a hyperflexion (wedge) fracture of the spine. Wedging of the involved vertebral body involves only the anterior aspect. There is no loss of height of the posterior vertebral body.

dislocation of the facet joints may occur. Neurologic injuries are more common with this more severe type of injury. CT is of benefit in evaluation of these anterior compression fractures in order to exclude extension of the fracture into the posterior cortex (middle column) because this will have an effect on the surgical management. If no posterior cortical involvement is present, cortical rods can be applied to the laminae of the surrounding vertebra, causing distraction on the anterior vertebral body, using the intact posterior cortex as a fulcrum. Involvement of the posterior cortex will preclude this type of treatment, which would only worsen the vertebral compression. Distraction rods must be used in this latter case. Involvement of the posterior cortex is rare in hyperflexion compression injuries, but reports of posterior comminution of the fracture with protrusion of the fracture fragments and disruption of the middle column are noted (Fig. 8-16). These resemble the burst fracture; however, the burst fracture is secondary to pure axial loading rather than hyperflexion and compression. Ferguson and Allen found that the posterior height was maintained or greater than adjacent vertebral bodies in the hyperflexion compression variant of this injury that argues against a pure crush injury or burst fracture.[27] Axial CT with sagittal reformations is required to determine the size, number, and position of fragments and degree of involvement of the spinal canal.

Flexion-Distraction Injuries

Several variants are noted in this category, the most common being that of the "seat belt type injury" or sudden deceleration injury, which has become increasingly more common with the increasing use of seat belts in moving vehicles.[14,26,27,49] These injuries make up about 5% of spinal injuries.[24] They represent disruption of both the posterior and middle columns under tension and distraction.[50] The fulcrum of force is located more anteriorly, within the abdominal wall rather than the vertebral column, as the upper body is thrown forward in hyperflexion while the body below the belt is restrained.

The typical horizontal cleavage forces of seat belt injuries can disrupt osseous components, ligamentous components, or both, with distraction forces acting initially on either the posterior bony neural arch or the posterior ligamentous complex. Three types of seat belt injuries have been described.[50]

The first pattern of horizontal fracture involves the neural arch (spinous process, laminae, and pedicles) extending anteriorly to involve the posterior superior aspect of the vertebral body. The posterior ligaments remain intact. This is what has been called the Chance fracture (type 1), which is usually isolated to one level, the most common location being L1-L3.[51] Two adjacent

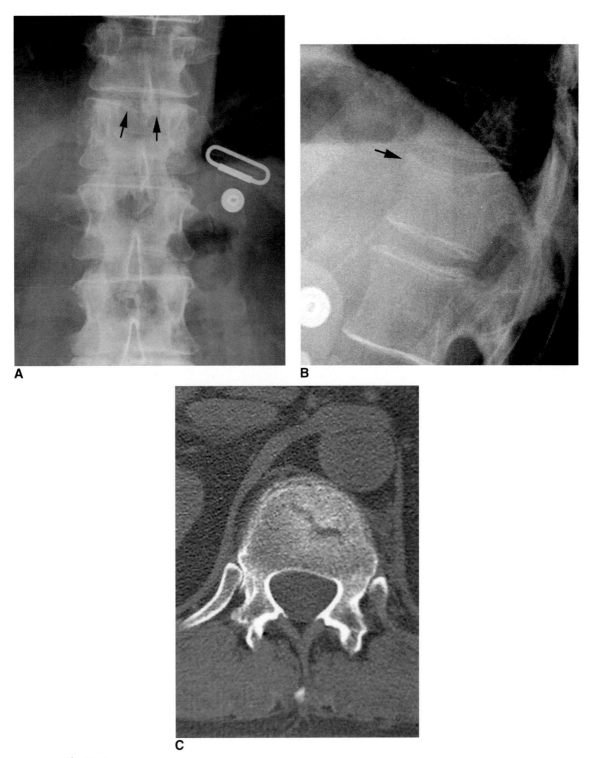

Fig. 8-12
A, AP radiograph of a simple wedge compression fracture of T12 thoracic vertebral body demonstrates subtle depression of the superior endplate (*arrows*) without increased interpedicular distance. **B**, Subtle anterior compression (*arrow*) without posterior element distraction is noted on the lateral radiograph. **C**, Anterior fracture is better visualized on the axial CT image and confirms the lack of posterior element and middle column involvement.

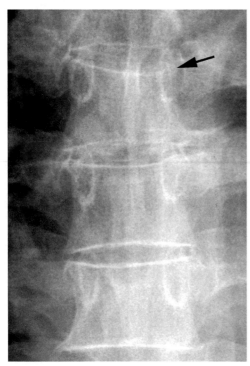

Fig. 8-13
AP view of left lateral compression fracture of the T5 vertebral body with asymmetric decreased height on the left (*arrow*).

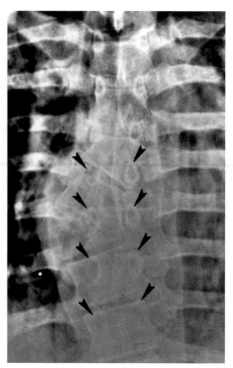

Fig. 8-14
Lateral compression fracture. AP thoracic spine radiograph shows massive lateral flexion of T7 on T8, with a gross crush fracture of the left side of T8. The fact that throughout the injury the pedicles are in the correct alignment (*arrowheads*) indicates significant disruption of the vertebral bodies, not just at T7 but also at T6, where the vertebral body is separated from its pedicles.

levels may be involved. In severe variations, the horizontal fracture can extend through the vertebral body (horizontal splitting fracture) (Fig. 8-17). The fracture is best viewed on the lateral radiograph with horizontal fractures anteriorly and posteriorly. However, the posterior elements are often difficult to discern on the lateral view. The AP study is crucial with regard to the posterior elements with horizontal clefts in the pedicles and spinous processes and lack of overlap between the vertebral body and posterior elements (known as the "empty vertebral body" sign) caused by elevation of the posterior elements (see Fig. 8-17). Minimal mild anterior vertebral body wedging may be present, but the anterior longitudinal ligament remains intact, and the anterior column is regarded as uninvolved (Fig. 8-18).

The second type of horizontal injury initially disrupts the posterior ligament (supraspinous and interspinous ligament), with fracture beginning at the junction of the lamina and spinous process without disruption of the posterior ossific spinous process. The fracture extends to the posterior vertebral body as the Chance fracture does, with varying involvement of the anterior structures. This is known as the Smith fracture (type 2)[52] (Fig. 8-19). The force may continue anteriorly and rupture the ligamentum flavum, joint capsule, posterior longitudinal ligament, and the intervertebral disc. Widening of the interspinous processes is noted on the lateral radiograph,

with possible avulsion of the posteroinferior corner of the vertebral body. Facet distraction can be present.

While CT is recommended for assessment of the bone and associated intraabdominal injuries, both these injuries are difficult to assess on axial slices secondary to the horizontal plane of injury. The disappearing laminae sign on axial CT slices provides a clue to the presence of a horizontal fracture through the laminae with associated diastasis.[53] Sagittal and coronal reconstruction images are essential for complete evaluation. The intact spinous process on the sagittal reconstruction images in a Smith fracture with associated widening of the interspinous processes is helpful in differentiating between the two types of injuries described. A third variant (type 3) exists where there is involvement of the posterior elements on one side only, secondary to an associated rotational force. Dislocations can rarely occur without a fracture.

Approximately half of patients who sustain seat belt types of spinal injuries have associated major intraabdominal injuries, such as hollow viscous or visceral lacerations, hematomas, and solid organ contusions. Smith et al.[52] described abdominal and neurologic injuries in approximately 20% of cases. In one study, 20% of patients had bowel injury, 21% had lumbar spine

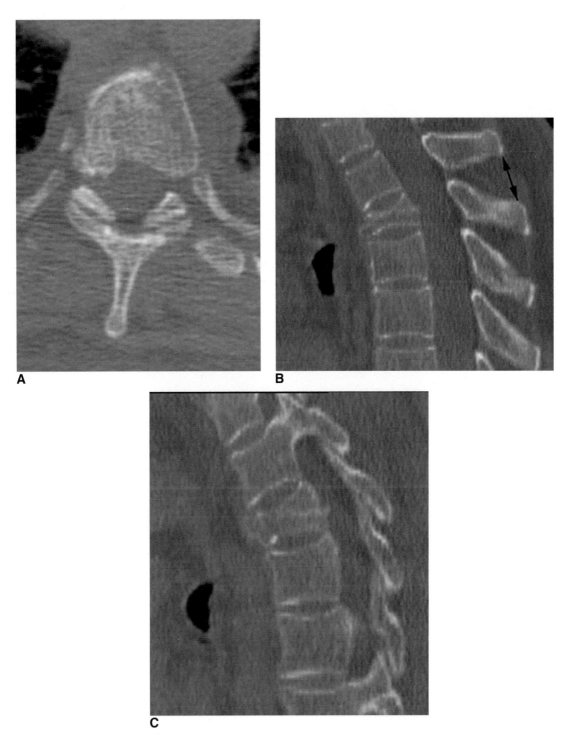

Fig. 8-15
Compression fracture. **A**, Axial CT image of moderately severe anterior compression fracture. Sagittal multiplanar reconstruction images (**B** and **C**) depict anterior compression of the vertebral body, subtle loss of posterior height, and mild interspinous widening (*double-headed arrow*), the latter suggesting ligamentous injury.

injuries, 2% had bladder laceration, and 8% had both spine and hollow viscous injuries.[54] Children with lap belt injuries often have linear ecchymosis across their lower abdomen and should be further evaluated for associated intraabdominal injuries and spinal injuries.[55]

Garrett and Braunstein[56] coined the term "seat belt syndrome" to describe an association of injuries found in massive deceleration injuries to passengers wearing seat belts. As well as the seat belt fracture of the spine, injuries to the spinal cord or cauda equina; rupture of the spleen,

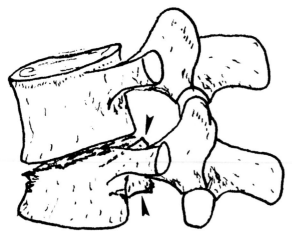

Fig. 8-16
Diagrammatic illustration of severe hyperflexion injury. There is marked compression of the anterior vertebral body; however, in this case there is also involvement of the dorsal aspect of the vertebral body. A fragment of the superior dorsal aspect has been "rotated" into the spinal canal (*arrowheads*) and would be expected to compromise the contents of the canal.

pancreas, and second or third part of the duodenum; tears of the small bowel; rupture of the musculature of the abdominal wall; and abrasions of the abdominal wall at the location of the seat belt impact may be seen. Rupture of the gravid uterus and circumferential laceration of the serosa of the sigmoid colon have been reported, as has, more commonly, perforation of the cecum secondary to traction on the fixed cecum.[57]

The other major type of flexion-distraction injury is one in which the middle and posterior columns are disrupted by tension and the annulus fibrosus is torn, allowing for subluxation, a finding not seen in the Chance or Smith fractures. Two thirds of patients with this subluxation component have neurologic symptoms, in contrast to only 20% of those with seat belt injury variants.[24,52] All flexion-distraction injuries are unstable.

Bilateral facet dislocation, when pure in nature, is secondary to hyperflexion with some distraction without axial loading, similar to the mechanism in the cervical spine (Figs. 8-20 and 8-21). This injury is rare in the thoracolumbar spine, however.[58] Significant ligamentous injury occurs if compression is also present, and compression fractures of the subjacent vertebra may be seen. Fractures of the articular processes may occur. Ligamentous injury can involve the posterior ligamentous groups, capsular ligaments, posterior longitudinal ligament, and most likely the anterior longitudinal ligament, which creates the potential for spinal instability.

Flexion-Rotation Injuries

In this type of injury, the posterior ligaments are ruptured, the superior articular process fractures, and the middle column fails[26] (Fig. 8-22). The anterior column may fail in rotation, giving rise to wedging deformity of the vertebral body. The anterior longitudinal ligament is stripped from the bone along with other ligaments secondary to the rotational component. The thoracolumbar junction is involved in the majority of cases, owing to the transition in the facet joints.[48]

The rotational force can affect the disc or the vertebral body.[24] If it courses through the disc, subluxation or dislocation of the vertebral body on the one below is noted with compression of the vertebral body below. If it involves the vertebral body, the superior portion of the body is fractured horizontally ("slice fracture"), and this upper body fracture fragment, along with the spine above, subluxes with respect to the lower fragment. Displacement of a fracture of the superior articular process and widening of the interspinous distance are seen radiographically, both signaling rotation. The posterior vertebral height is normal on the lateral view. Radiographically, this injury may look similar to the unilateral locked facet injury of the cervical spine. Unilateral facet dislocation rarely occurs in the thoracic lumbar spine; however, the mechanism is similar to that of the cervical spine's being secondary to flexion rotation without axial loading, with the rotational forces heavily outweighing the flexion component (Fig. 8-23).

On the AP view, the spinous process may be rotated to the side of the involvement and fracture, though the superior endplate may be present. Asymmetric disc space narrowing can be present on the AP view and is confirmed on the lateral view. Sagittal CT reconstruction images help to detect the slice fracture through the vertebral body, with axial images helpful for articular process fractures. Fractures of ribs, facets (may be dislocated), lamina, and transverse processes are often present in conjunction with this type of injury. Neurologic deficit approaches 70%.[46,48]

Axial Loading (Vertical Compression)

Burst fractures are the predominant vertical compression injuries of the spine and account for 14% of spinal injuries.[24,26] They occur most commonly from T4 to L5, with half occurring at L1[59,60] (Figs. 8-24 to 8-28). Two burst fractures, either contiguous or noncontiguous, occur in less than 10% of cases.[61] Atlas et al.'s series also demonstrated an incidence of separate associated spinal injuries of greater than 40%, leading to the recommendation that radiographs of the entire spine be performed when a burst fracture is detected.[61] The injury usually occurs following a fall or jump from a considerable height, accounting for the severe axial load on the spine when the person lands, either on the feet or buttocks.[62] As a result, there is a high association with calcaneal fractures (Lover's fractures) and vertical shear injuries of the

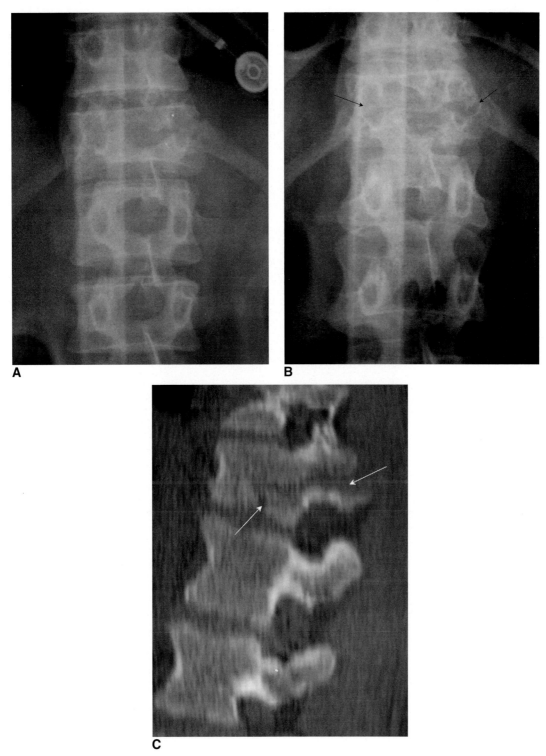

Fig. 8-17
Chance fracture of L1. AP lumbar spine without (**A**) and with (**B**) arrows depicts the empty vertebral body sign caused by horizontal fractures with resultant clefts (*arrows*) through the pedicles and spinous processes. **C**, Sagittal MPR CT image of the lumbar spine allows clear visualization of the horizontal fracture through the posterior vertebral body, pedicles, and spinous process (*arrows*).

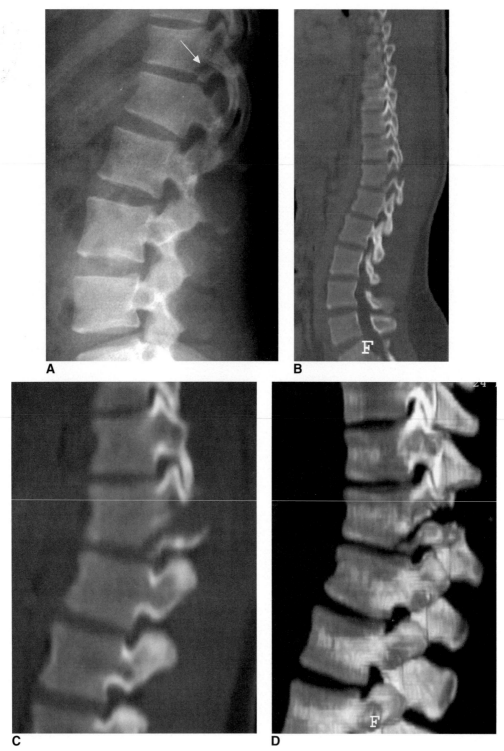

Fig. 8-18
Chance fracture of T12. **A**, Lateral lumbar radiograph in blunt trauma patient shows an oblique fracture traversing the posterior inferior corner of T12. **B**, Reformatted thoracolumbar sagittal CT and close-up view (**C**) demonstrate that the fracture crosses the articular pillars. A mild focal kyphosis is at T12-L1. **D**, Volume-rendered image nicely depicts fracture plane and also suggests mild compression of L1 endplate.

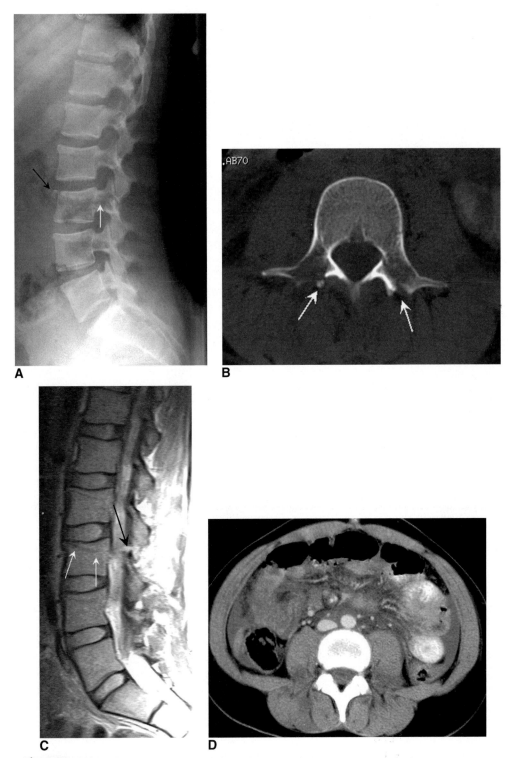

Fig. 8-19

Seat belt (Smith) fracture of L3. **A**, Lateral radiograph demonstrates a horizontal fracture crossing the superior aspect of the L3 pedicles and body (*arrows*). **B**, Axial CT shows fractures involving the posterior articular masses (*arrows*), but sparing the spinous process and laminae. **C**, Proton density MRI shows a tear of the ligamentum flavum at L2-L3 (*black arrow*). Fracture across the vertebral body is also seen as line of decreased signal within the brighter marrow signal (*white arrows*). **D**, Axial abdominal CT shows retroperitoneal fluid around the aorta and inferior vena cava, intraperitoneal fluid, and mesenteric edema. Bowel and mesenteric injuries can occur with flexion-distraction injuries and should be carefully sought.

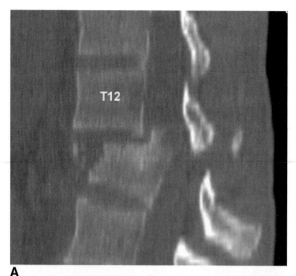

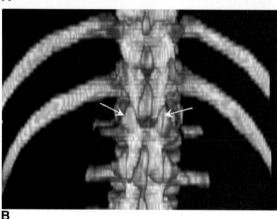

Fig. 8-20
Bilateral facet dislocation. **A**, Sagittal MPR CT shows anterior dislocation of T12 on L1 extending over 40% of the AP vertebral body diameter of L1. There is anterior compression of the L1 body and anterior displacement of the T12 spinous process relative to L1. **B**, Surface-rendered CT image from posterior perspective shows inferior T12 facets displaced anterior to L1 superior facets (*arrows*), indicating dislocation. Note widening of intraspinous distance accompanying dislocation.

pelvis, and these additional injuries should be excluded with calcaneal and pelvic radiographs.

Both the anterior and middle columns fail in this type of injury, making this an unstable fracture with neurologic deficits seen in half of the cases.[26,27] The driving downward force on the vertebral body causes herniation of the nucleus pulposus into the vertebral body below, leading ultimately to an internal explosion or bursting of the vertebral body, hence the name "burst fracture."[61] This causes severe comminution of the body (most commonly the superior half) with fracture of one or both endplates (the superior being the most common). The posterior vertebral body line is disrupted; loss of posterior vertebral body height occurs; and fragments from the posterior aspect of the vertebral body are typically retropulsed into the spinal canal. Fragments usually originate from the posterior superior corner, but inferior origins have been noted. The presence of a retropulsed fragment is almost always pathognomonic of an axial loading injury.[63]

Characteristic radiographic findings include a vertical vertebral fracture, anterior wedging, widened interpedicular distance, vertical fractures at the spinolaminar junction, and loss of posterior vertebral height. Obliteration of the posterior margin occurs in 12% of burst fractures.[60] Curiously, however, despite the retropulsed fragments, the posterior longitudinal ligament is usually intact. CT is notably helpful in these cases to evaluate the size and position of retropulsed fragments and the degree of involvement of the spinal canal, posterior margins, and posterior elements (articular pillars, pedicles, and laminae), the latter of which can be missed on plain radiographs.

While initially it was felt that posttraumatic disruption or narrowing of the spinal canal correlated with the severity of neurologic impairment, Trafton and others have found that the percentage of neural canal narrowing in the upper thoracic spine or in the lower lumbar spine found in initial CT evaluation does not necessarily correlate with the degree of clinical neurologic symptoms.[64,65] This is particularly true within the lumbar spine, where the dimensions of the canal are widest.[66-68] The cauda equina alone occupies the spinal canal at and caudad to the second lumbar level and, unlike the case in spinal cord or conus medullaris, neurologic dysfunction in this area simulates a peripheral nerve injury with the potential for spontaneous recovery. Only within the thoracolumbar junction did Trafton et al. find that burst fractures with a 50% decrease in midsagittal diameter secondary to retropulsed fragments or fractures of the lamina had a significant risk of neurologic involvement. Whether the neurologic injury was due to mechanical narrowing versus the initial large force of the injury is not certain, and postsurgical recovery may be secondary to stabilization rather than decompression.[64] Long-term studies are ensuing.

CT imaging can help preoperatively to determine the difficulty of the fracture fragment reduction and the rotational component of the fragment. Compression rods cannot be used if the posterior margin is not intact, and distraction rods are the treatment of choice. Postoperative CT assessment of the fracture and fragment reduction is most useful because the most common reason for Harrington rod distraction instrumentation failure is retained residual ossific fragments in the canal.[69] MRI is useful in assessing the direct effects of the retropulsed fragment on the cord.

Of note, several recent reports showed no neurologic deterioration in nonoperatively managed patients versus operatively treated patients with L2-5 burst fractures in

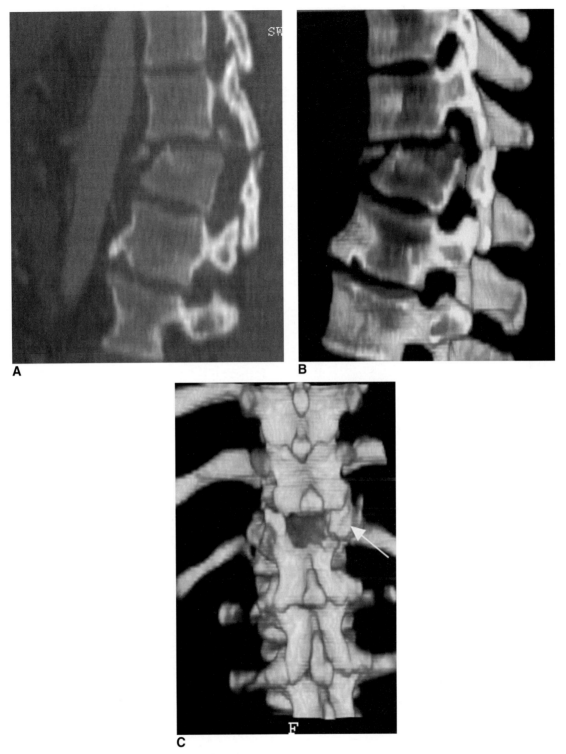

Fig. 8-21
Bilateral facet fracture-dislocation. **A,** Sagittal CT reformation shows fracture-dislocation of T11 on T12 with compression of the anterior superior endplate of T12 and perching of the articular process tips. T11 is anteriorly displaced on T12, and there is a fracture of a facet. **B,** Volumetric lateral view shows same findings. **C,** A volumetric posterior view shows marked widening between T11 and T12 spinous processes with visualization of T12 body between them. A fracture, most likely arising from the right superior T12 articular process (*arrow*), is also seen.

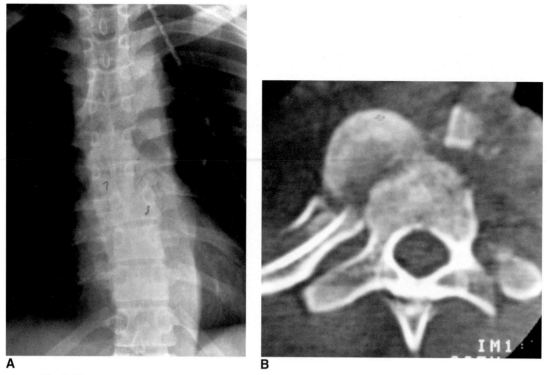

A   **B**

Fig. 8-22
Flexion-rotation injury. **A**, AP radiograph demonstrates obvious lateral displacement of T7 with respect to T8. The vertebral bodies also overlie each other, indicating a degree of impaction. **B**, Axial CT image demonstrates overlapping of the vertebral bodies of T7 and T8 with impacted fractures of both vertebrae.

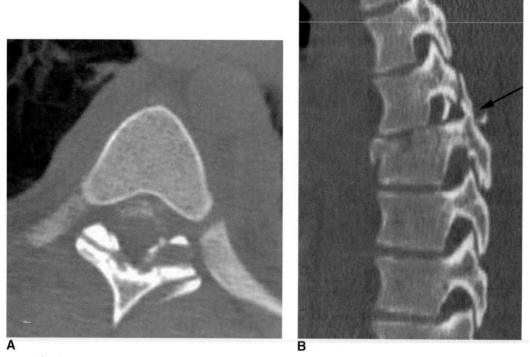

A   **B**

Fig. 8-23
Perched unilateral facet lock. **A**, Axial CT demonstrates the "naked facet" sign at T6-T7 with disruption of the left facet joint. **B**, Sagittal reformatted image reveals fracture of the superior T7 vertebral body with associated left unilateral perched facets (*black arrow*) with fracture also noted within the inferior T6 facet.

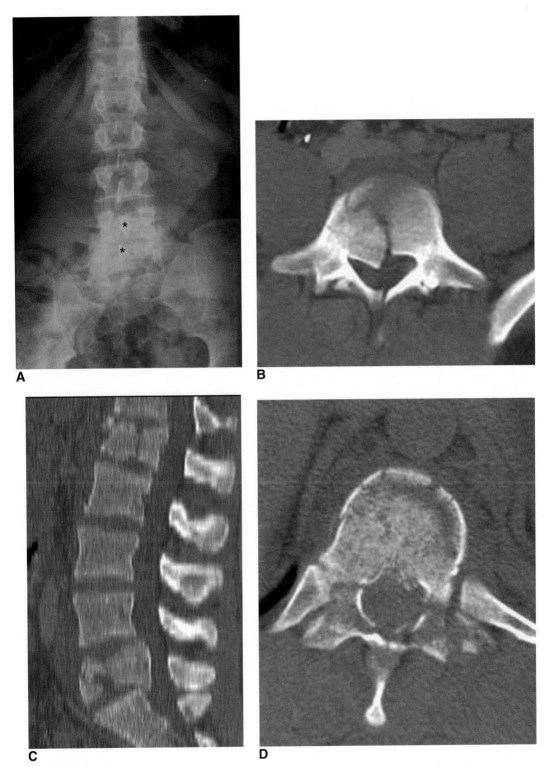

Fig. 8-24
Burst fracture of L5. **A,** AP radiograph with right deviation of the spinous process of L5 with respect to the proximal levels (*asterisks*). **B,** Axial CT image of L5 showing fracture extending through the entire vertebral body with cortical discrepancy posteriorly and prominent encroachment on the anterior spinal canal. **C,** Sagittal CT image depicting the prominent posterior retropulsion of the vertebral body at L5 in keeping with a burst fracture. A T12 vertebral body fracture is also noted. **D,** Axial CT of T12 confirms a second burst fracture in this patient with fragmentation of the vertebral body and also involving the middle column, making this fracture unstable.

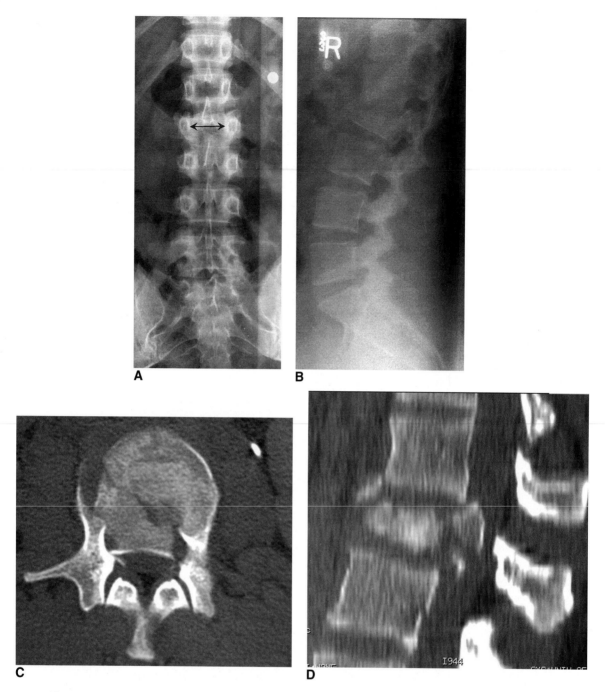

Fig. 8-25
Burst fracture. **A**, AP thoracolumbar radiograph shows loss of height of L2 body and increased inter-pedicle distance (*two-headed arrow*). **B**, Lateral radiograph of region shows loss of height of ante-rior and posterior aspect of L2. **C**, Axial CT image reveals large retropulsed bone fragment and laminar junction fracture. The right facet joint appears diastatic. **D**, Sagittal reformation confirms marked extent of retropulsion and canal compromise.

long-term follow-up if there was no neurologic deficit or only a partial single nerve root paralysis noted initially.[70-74]

One specific group of vehicular injuries, particularly motorcycle injuries, deserves discussion here. Motorcycle injuries are unique in that the majority of them involve the thoracic spine and are secondary to an axial loading compression type of injury or possibly a flexion injury. The victims are usually catapulted over the handlebars and hit the kyphotic curvature of the thoracic spine on a solid object, most commonly involving T4-T7.[75] Approximately 5% of motorcycle accident victims have

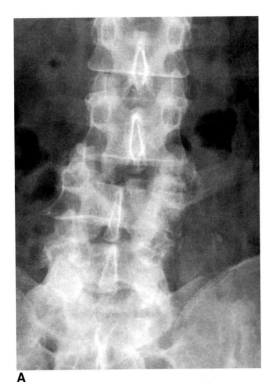

A

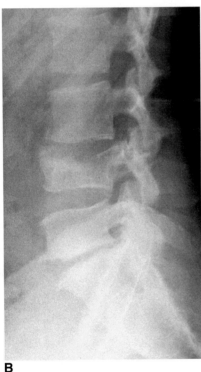

B

Fig. 8-26
Burst fracture. **A**, Frontal lumbar spine radiograph shows marked height loss of L4 and rotation of L3 in relation to L4 and L5 as indicated by offset of spinous processes. **B**, Uniform L4 height loss anteriorly and posteriorly is shown in lateral radiograph.

thoracic spine injuries.[76] Daffner et al. recommend that all motorcyclists who have sustained severe trauma be examined with an overpenetrated film of the upper thoracic region, as this region is often difficult to visualize on

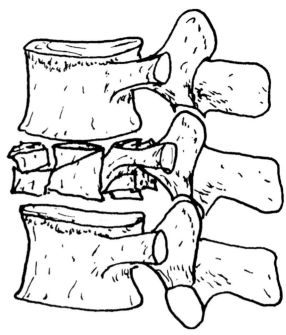

Fig. 8-27
Diagrammatic illustration of a burst fracture, the complete fragmentation of the vertebral body with loss of height of both the anterior and posterior elements.

standard thoracic radiographs. If any discrepancy is noted, CT scanning or even MRI may be of benefit.

Fracture-Dislocations

Fracture-dislocations represent 16% of all spinal fractures and 20% of all major fractures in Denis's study. They are considered the most unstable of the spinal injuries, with disruption of all three spinal columns and associated neurologic deficits in 75% of them, making this category the most clinically significant.[24] Combinations of compression, tension, rotation, and shear forces lead to this type of injury, with flexion-distraction, flexion rotation, and shear injuries also contributing to this category.

The hallmark of the fracture-dislocation injury is displacement or subluxation of one vertebral body with respect to another on AP or lateral radiographs.[26] An associated fracture is present in almost all cases (Figs. 8-29 to 8-31).

Most injuries of this type arise from a force directed to the dorsal aspect of the spine.[77] Flexion-distraction injuries, including the typical seat belt injury, have already been discussed in this chapter. The most severe type demonstrates subluxation of the vertebral bodies secondary to disruption of the middle and posterior columns by tension and disruption of the anterior column with tearing of the annulus fibrosus, consistent with fracture-dislocation injury.

Although CT scanning is not always required to diagnose a fracture-dislocation, it is optimal for evaluating

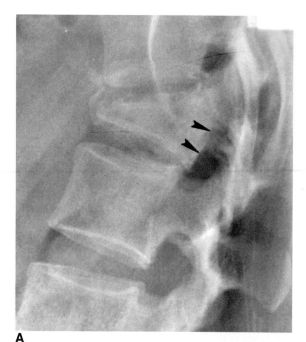

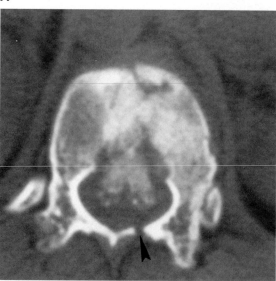

A

Fig. 8-28
A, Lateral radiograph of the lumbar spine indicates a compression fracture of L1 due to hyperflexion associated with axial loading. The majority of the loss of height has occurred anteriorly, indicating hyperflexion. However, obvious bulging of the posterior vertebral cortex (*arrowheads*) indicates involvement of the middle column. **B,** CT scan confirms the finding and indicates a more extensive involvement of the spinal canal than may be appreciated on the plain film. Also, a fracture of the left lamina (*arrowhead*) indicates that axial compression occurred, in contrast to wedge compression fractures, where the posterior elements are spared.

displacement of the vertebral bodies and spinal canal involvement and for detecting facet involvement, particularly the dislocated articular processes, which can be recognized by the "naked facet" sign on axial images.[29,78] While common in the cervical spine, locked facets are rare in the thoracic and lumbar spine.[15,30,79,80] Three

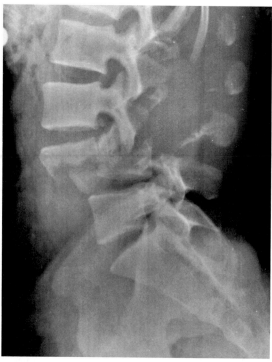

Fig. 8-29
Lateral lumbar radiograph demonstrates severe hyperextension fracture-dislocation. The L4 body has sheared off horizontally with anterior displacement of the superior portion. The spinous processes of L1, L2, and L3 are fractured and markedly displaced posteriorly. The superior articular facets of L4 are fractured and anteriorly displaced.

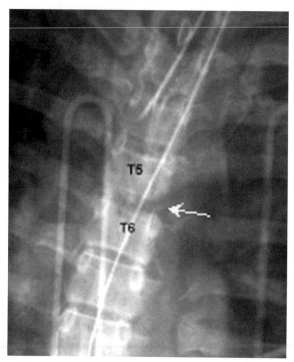

Fig. 8-30
Fracture-dislocation of T5 with respect to T6 on AP radiograph with left lateral widening of the interposing disc space. Note fracture-dislocation of the left posteromedial ribs as well.

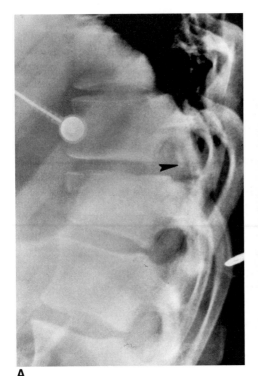

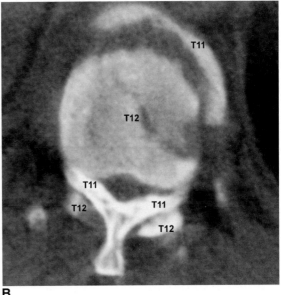

Fig. 8-31
Facet fracture-dislocation. **A,** Lateral radiograph demonstrates a hyperflexion wedge fracture of T12. The body of T11 has been displaced anteriorly, with an area of bone density representing the inferior articular facets of T11, superior to the pedicles of T12 (*arrowhead*). This indicates facet fracture-dislocation. **B,** Axial CT scan demonstrates a fracture through the anterolateral aspect of T12, with the anterior rim of T11 lying anterior to T12, giving rise to the "double rim" sign. The spinous process and laminae of T12 are also displaced anteriorly overlying the spinal canal in this image lying anterior to the superior articular facets of T12.

patterns of facet abnormalities that have been reported with thoracic fracture dislocations as well as flexion rotation injuries are (1) anteriorly locked facets (inferior facets of the upper segments are anterior to the superior facets of the lower vertebral body segment), (2) laterally locked facets, and (3) superiorly locked facets. Although the displacement/subluxation of the vertebral bodies is more difficult to detect on axial images than sagittal images, the "double rim" sign depicting the vertebral body overlap on the axial images has proven useful[78] (see Fig. 8-31). The normal pattern of the articular processes must be understood in order to interpret the axial images correctly. Normally the superior articular facets are directed posteromedially and have a concave articular surface, with the inferior articular facets directed anterolaterally with a convex articular surface. Any disruption of this pattern is suggestive of a facet abnormality. Sagittal reconstruction images allow assessment of the degree of vertebral body displacement and the "slice fracture" of a flexion rotation injury and can again determine the degree of canal compromise. In some cases,

however, CT may not be able to be performed because the patient is too unstable or cannot be moved acutely.

Traumatic spondylopelvic dissociation is a very rare and severe type of fracture dislocation, with only three case reports noted in the literature.[81] This injury involves complete displacement of the lumbar spine into the pelvis and is an extremely challenging management situation. CT imaging and three-dimensional reconstruction provide optimal imaging in preparation for surgical management.[82]

Shearing (Translational) Injuries

Pure shear injuries cause axially oriented fractures of the articular pillars together with sagittal dislocation, though in the lumbar spine, lateral shearing can occur with lateral displacement of the vertebral body. The majority of these injuries are due to a force causing straight displacement anteriorly or posteriorly. In both types of injury, all three columns are disrupted, including the anterior longitudinal ligament, and neurologic compromise is frequent, the most common deficit being paraplegia.[24] The most common cause of these injuries is horizontal impaction from a falling object.

In posteroanterior shear injury, the most superior segment subluxes and sustains fractures of the posterior arch and spinous process with an associated fracture of the superior articular processes of the vertebral body below (Figs. 8-32 to 8-34). Occasionally, the lower vertebra is displaced anteriorly.[77] In anteroposterior translation injury, all ligaments rupture and the segment above dislocates posteriorly. Its superior facet may lock the anterior vertebrae, and either no fracture or an isolated fracture of the spinous process can be present.[24]

Hyperextension Injuries

Hyperextension or whiplash type injuries to the thoracolumbar spine are extremely rare, but can occur if a patient falls and hyperextends over an object, or if there is lack of seat protection to the mid lower spine in automobile injuries. The resultant deformity is the exact opposite of that seen in the hyperflexion injuries, with posterior compression and anterior distraction (Figs. 8-35 to 8-37). Rarely, sprain injury to the anterior longitudinal ligament can occur with associated widening of the anterior disc space, similar to that seen in the cervical spine. Posterior arch fractures were noted in hyperextension injuries in one study, but disruption of the anterior longitudinal ligament could not be shown with pure hyperextension injuries. Roaf[58] believes that rotary motion is required for ligament disruption. Dorsal blows to the back can give rise to hyperextension injuries, with posterior subluxation superior to the focus of injury. Of note, ankylosing spondylitis can predispose patients to this type of injury with just mild trauma (Fig. 8-38) (see Special Considerations).

Radiographic findings in hyperextension injury and fracture include widening of the anterior disc space, retrolisthesis, posterior arch fractures due to compressive forces, and a triangular avulsion fracture fragment, usually from the anterosuperior vertebral body. In severe cases, this type of fracture anterior placement of fragments resembles the hangman fracture of C2 and is associated with significant neurologic injury.

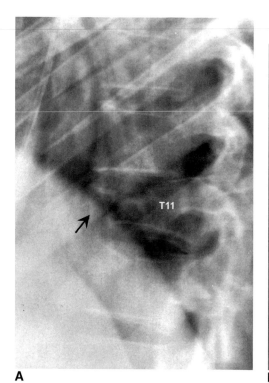
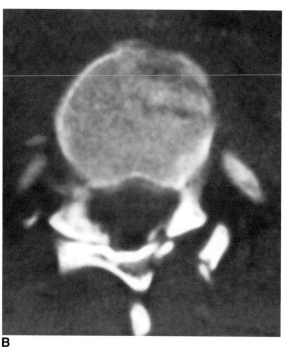

A   **B**

Fig. 8-32
Shearing injury with some axial compression. **A,** Radiograph demonstrates loss of height of the T11 vertebral body with anterior displacement of the anterior fragment (*arrow*). A mild compression injury of T12 is also present. Significant anterior displacement of T10 with respect to T11 is seen. **B,** Axial CT image through the inferior aspect of the T11 vertebral body demonstrates the fracture of the anterior aspect. Fractures are also seen through the posterior elements, indicating posterior injury, with disruption of the facet joint on the left. This indicates that there was a rotational component to the shearing forces.

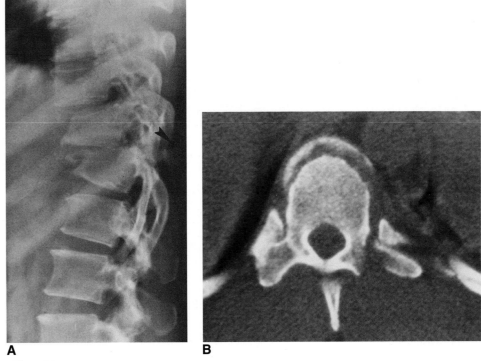

Fig. 8-33

Shearing injury. **A,** Radiograph demonstrates wedge compression fractures of T11 and T12 with significant anterior subluxation of T10 on T11 and T11 on T12. This implies facet dislocation, most likely related to significant bony injury. A horizontal shear fracture of the spinous process of T11 is also present (*arrowhead*). **B,** CT image of T12 indicates the anterior rim of T12 is in the same plane (double rim sign). A coronal oriented fracture runs through the transverse process of T12 on the left, and the fractured spinous process of T11 is also slightly malaligned.

Transverse Process Fractures of the Lumbar Spine

While these have classically been categorized as one of the minor injuries of the spine, recent studies have shown that a statistically significant association exists between transverse process fractures and abdominal injury.[83] Fractures of the transverse process result from direct blunt trauma, violent lateral flexion-extension forces, avulsion of the psoas muscle, or Malgaigne fractures of the pelvis.[84,85] Abdominal visceral injuries were present in association with transverse process fractures in 21% of patients in one series.[86] Often subtle transverse process fractures are overlooked on conventional radiographs. The presence of such a fracture should be an indication for CT imaging diagnosis of patients with blunt abdominal trauma, to exclude associated genitourinary, hepatic, splenic, or bowel injuries.[86]

SPECIAL CONSIDERATIONS
Multiplicity of Sites of Spinal Injury

As described above, attention to the entire spine is required in certain multiple trauma victims in order to confidently exclude or confirm secondary injuries. In par-

ticular, the following guidelines have proven useful: (1) if a primary injury at C5-7 is found, thoracic and lumbar radiographs should be performed, as there is a high association with secondary injury at T12 or in the lumbar spine; (2) primary injury at T2-4 is often associated with a secondary injury in the cervical spine, and (3) a primary injury at T12-L2 is associated with secondary injury at L4-5, and lumbar radiographs are required.[1,2]

Mimics

Scheuermann's Disease. Old healed Scheuermann's disease should not be confused with acute multiple wedge compression fractures. Scheuermann's disease is an uncommon process consisting of nonspecific depression of the endplates of at least four continuous mid thoracic vertebral bodies, and is more commonly seen in adolescent males (Fig. 8-39). Acute fractures should have more acute angulation on radiographs and CT sagittal images, but if there is need for differentiation and there are no prior radiographs for comparison, three-phase bone scan can be useful, showing increased technetium-99m uptake in the acute fracture setting and showing no uptake in the patient with Scheuermann's disease.[28]

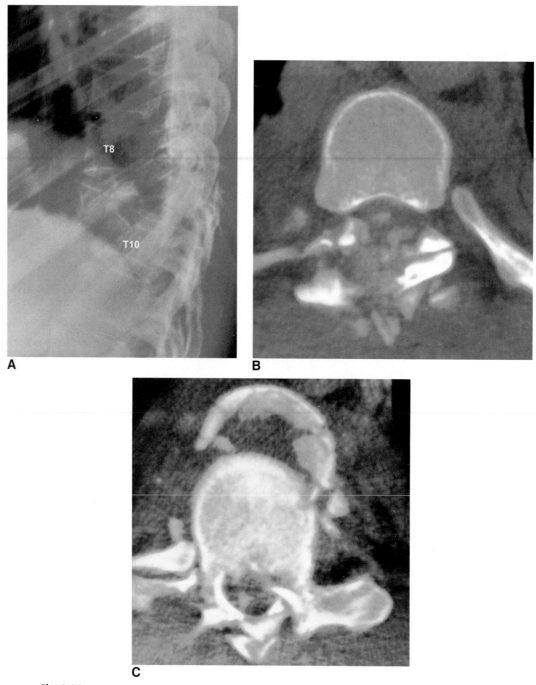

Fig. 8-34
Shearing injury. **A**, Lateral radiograph of the lower thoracic spine demonstrates impaction and anterior displacement of T9 with respect to T10. **B**, CT scan demonstrates gross disruption of the posterior elements, with fragmentation and displacement of multiple fragments into the spinal canal. **C**, CT scan taken at the T9-T10 junction demonstrates the anterior rim of the comminuted T9 vertebral body lying anterior to T10. Again considerable disruption of the posterior elements of T10 is present with fragmentation and displacement of fragments into the spinal canal.

Scoliosis. Scoliosis may contribute to anatomic variations on the axial CT images of the spine, and apparent double rim sign should not be confused with a shear injury in this case. Correlation with thoracic and lumbar spine radiographs is paramount in order to analyze the curvature and assess the CT findings in light of the variation in vertebral body positioning. In addition, underlying congenital malformations of the spine may have unusual appearances on axial CT scans, and correlation with prior radiographs as well as sagittal and coronal

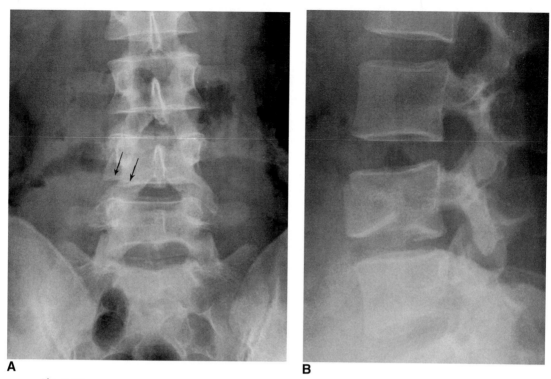

Fig. 8-35
Hyperextension injury L4. **A**, AP radiograph shows cortical discrepancy at the right central inferior endplate of L4 (*arrows*). **B**, Minimally displaced anteroinferior vertebral body fracture of L4 is confirmed on the lateral radiograph.

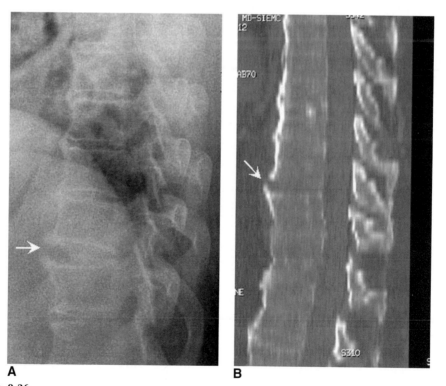

Fig. 8-36
Hyperextension injury. **A**, Lateral radiograph of low thoracic region shows anterior opening of T11-T12 anterior disc space (*arrow*), suggesting extension sprain. **B**, Sagittal reformatted image confirms this impression (*arrow*).

Continued

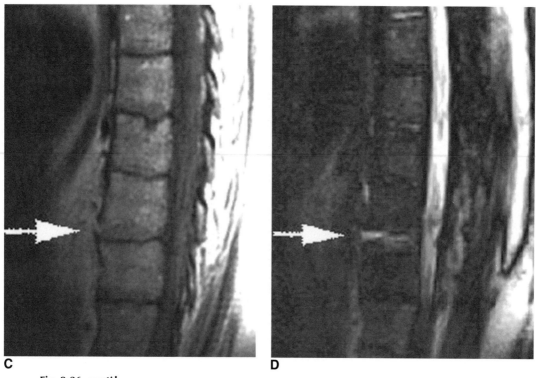

C

D

Fig. 8-36, cont'd,
C, T1-weighted sagittal MR sequence confirms interruption of the anterior longitudinal ligament (*arrow*). **D,** Inversion recovery MR sequence indicates edema or hemorrhage in disc space (*arrow*).

reconstruction images is important to distinguish between the underlying congenital fusion or absence of a particular structure and true superimposed trauma.

Kummel's Disease. It is important not to confuse acute posttraumatic wedge compression fractures with the syndrome of delayed posttraumatic vertebral collapse known as Kummel's disease.[87] While poorly understood, this is a progressive disease, felt by most to be secondary to avascular necrosis of the endplates of the vertebral bodies, causing an anterior wedge deformity at multiple levels. It is most common within the thoracic spine. Patients are usually osteopenic, can have intravertebral vacuum phenomenon, and many patients have a long history of corticosteroid use, the latter two of which further support the etiologic theory of osteonecrosis. MRI may be of benefit to exclude acute fracture and associated soft tissue changes in order to confirm the diagnosis.

Schmorl Nodes. These shallow concavities within the superior and inferior endplates of vertebral bodies are of questionable clinical significance and are fairly common in the older patient. They should not be confused with acute compression fractures or cortical fractures of the vertebral column. They are most common in the lower thoracic and upper lumbar spine. Herniation of a portion

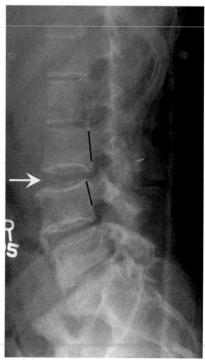

Fig. 8-37
Hyperextension-subluxation. Lateral radiograph of lumbar spine shows posterior displacement of L3 with respect to L4 (*arrow*). Black lines denote posterior cortical margin of vertebral body.

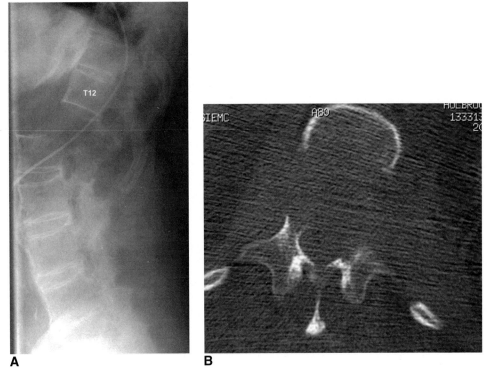

Fig. 8-38
Hyperextension-dislocation. **A**, Lateral thoracolumbar radiograph shows severe hyperextension-dislocation at T12-L1 in a patient with underlying spinal fusion secondary to ankylosing spondylitis. **B**, Axial CT image shows fracture through the superior endplate of L1 and marked vertebral body displacement with surrounding hematoma.

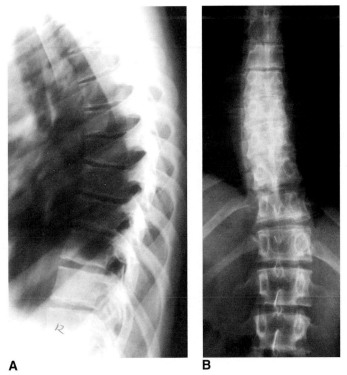

Fig. 8-39
Scheuermann's disease. **A** and **B**, Lateral radiographs of 17-year-old male with typical anterior wedge deformity of at least four thoracic vertebral bodies, with resultant moderate kyphosis not unexpected considering the patient's age. This is more commonly found in males.

of the disc (nucleus pulposus) through the cartilaginous and osseous portions of the adjacent vertebral body (vertebral spongiosa) occurs at focal areas of weakness caused by defects in chondrification in the early stages of spinal development. With time, reactive sclerosis forms around the herniated cartilage nodule that allows it to be visible on CT images and radiographs (Fig. 8-40). Schmorl nodes are most commonly central within the disc and vertebral body, but can be eccentric. The appearance is diagnostic on MRI, with postgadolinium enhancement around the Schmorl node.

Preexisting Spinal Conditions Predisposed to Trauma

Ankylosing Spondylitis. Patients with ankylosing spondylitis have a certain predisposition for serious injury to the spine. Prominent syndesmophyte formation throughout the spine is present with eventual fusion of multiple adjacent vertebral bodies. This process, in conjunction with multilevel disc space calcification/ossification, gives rise to the typical "bamboo spine" appearance and rigidity that are characteristic of this disease. Biomechanical alterations then predispose these patients to serious spinal injury, even after a minor injury such as a sin-

gle fall.[88] It has been hypothesized that the neutral plane for bending stress is displaced in the ankylosed spine from its normal location near the nucleus pulposus, giving rise to the altered biomechanics described above. The application of a bending force then causes failure in tension and the development of a shearing force through bone, similar to a seat belt type injury.[89] Compressive forces have not been found to play a significant role in the spinal injuries in this group of patients. Fractures through the ossified disc spaces or vertebral body have been seen in more than 50% of some series and can occur within all regions of the spine[89,90] (Figs. 8-41 to 8-43). Simultaneous cervical and thoracic injuries have been described.[91] A pseudoarthrosis develops at the site of injury and places the patient at risk for further vertebral body displacement and subluxation with incremental soft tissue and cord injuries. Fractures of the ankylosed spine are therefore considered unstable fractures.

While the need for surgical intervention is recognized in severe complicated instances, the literature emphasizes the need for conservative management if possible, as mortality rates are much lower (25%) than in those with surgical intervention (50%).[89,90,92] In particular, the latter category often only shows minimal neurologic improvement postsurgery. Epidural hemorrhage is unique to this patient population in the shock trauma

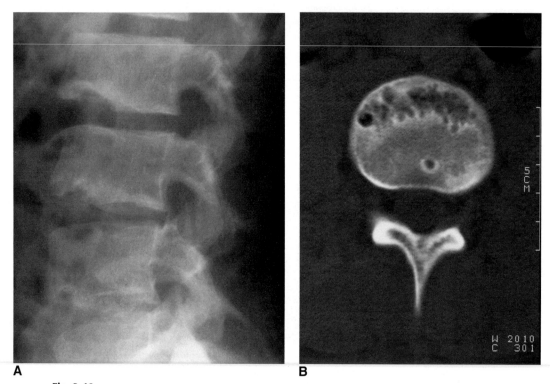

A   **B**

Fig. 8-40
Schmorl nodes. Lateral radiograph (**A**) and sagittal CT (**B**) of the lumbar spine. Well-defined concave defects within the superior and inferior endplates of the lumbar vertebral bodies are noted–most prominent at L2 and L3. These are a normal variant and are not to be confused with fractures.

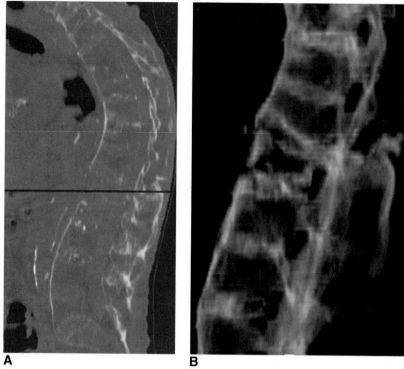

Fig. 8-41
Hyperextension injury in ankylosing spondylitis. **A**, Sagittal reformatted CT image of an elderly man with long-standing ankylosing spondylitis shows marked thoracic kyphosis and severe osteoporosis. A fracture plane crosses obliquely through the L1-L2 level. **B**, Volume-rendered 3-D CT image shows tear across L1-L2 discs space and possible injury to L2-L3 as well.

setting, and as this is considered a progressive neurologic lesion, neurologic decompression is recommended in these cases, though this is more of a serious complication within the cervical spine. MRI is of critical importance in detecting and diagnosing this complication in order to triage the patient for the operating room rather than conservative management. Radiographs should give the initial diagnosis of underlying ankylosing spondylitis, and MRI is then recommended for assessment of the ligaments, soft tissues, and cord as soon as possible. In Brant's series, both of his cases of thoracic spine fractures developed an anterior cord syndrome, but both survived. Death secondary to spinal injury in ankylosing spondylitis patients is most common in the cervical rather than thoracic and lumbar spines and is usually secondary to respiratory complications (13% to 17%).

Diffuse Idiopathic Skeletal Hyperostosis. Diffuse idiopathic skeletal hyperostosis (DISH) is described as undulating flowing thick vertical ossification anterior to the vertebral bodies, extending over at least 3 to 4 disc spaces bridging the involved vertebral body levels. This solid ossification gives rise to a partially ankylosed spine. Traumatic disruption of the anterior ossification can give rise to altered biomechanics much as in ankylosing

spondylitis and result in subluxation, ligament stripping, or disc space injury, or spinal cord involvement may occur. Israel et al. describe a case of postsurgical hyperextension T9-10 thoracic spine fracture-dislocation and paraplegia in a woman with DISH after being placed in the typical hyperextended axially rotated position for retroperitoneal surgery.[93] Presurgical assessment of the spine in patients undergoing surgery in this position is now recommended.

Pathologic Fracture. Care should be taken in the trauma setting to not overlook possible pathologic causes for fracture or soft tissue hemorrhage or mass. This is particularly important in the elderly population with a higher incidence of neoplastic disease who have pathologic fractures secondary to primary or metastatic disease (Figs. 8-44 and 8-45). Inappropriate cause and effect should alert the clinician to the possibility of underlying pathology.

CONCLUSION

Despite the increased access to and number of technologic advances used in diagnostic evaluation of the traumatized patient, plain radiographs remain the initial

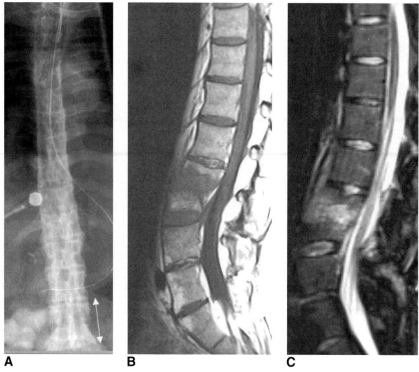

Fig. 8-42
Ankylosing spondylitis. **A,** Frontal lumbar radiograph shows apparent increased height of the L3 vertebral body (*two-headed arrow*). T1-weighted (**B**) and T2-weighted (**C**) sagittal MR images show disruption across L3 body with distraction of major fragments.

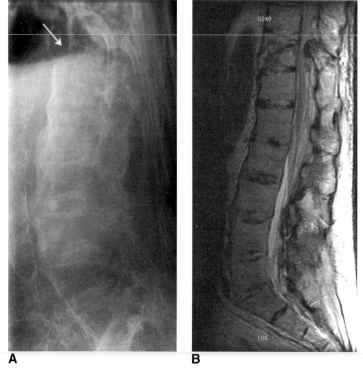

Fig. 8-43
Ankylosing spondylitis. **A,** Lateral lumbar radiograph demonstrates extension injury at T11-T12 in a patient with ankylosing spondylitis. **B,** Sagittal T2-weighted MR image shows oblique fracture line across T11.

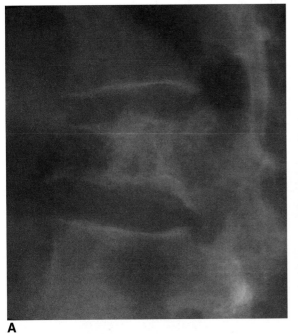
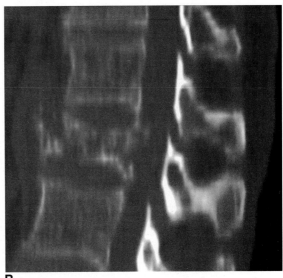

A   B

Fig. 8-44
Pathologic fracture. **A,** Lateral thoracolumbar radiograph reveals loss of height in L1 throughout length of the body. **B,** A sagittal CT reformation shows significant loss of mineral content and height. Fracture was secondary to plasmacytoma.

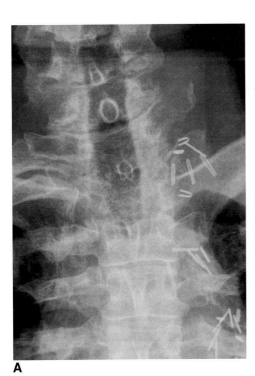
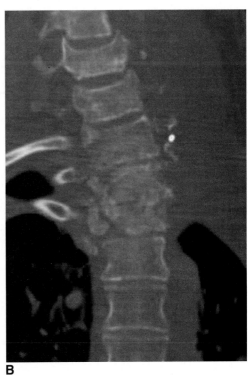

A   B

Fig. 8-45
Pathologic fracture of T2. **A,** AP radiograph of the cervical thoracic junction reveals surgical clips about the T2 level with irregular appearance and lack of normal cortical margins at this level and at the adjacent T3 superior endplate. **B,** Coronal reformatted CT image demonstrates the degree of fragmentation and loss of normal bone structure with associated curvature of the spine and soft tissue swelling.

Continued

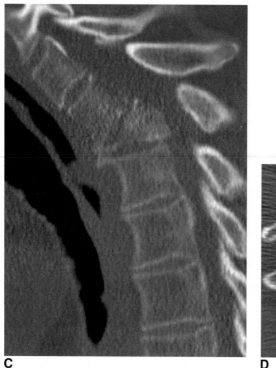
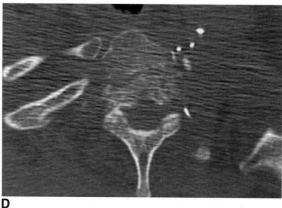

Fig. 8-45, cont'd,
C, Sagittal CT depicts the marked posterior kyphosis at the affected level. **D,** Axial CT of T2 shows loss of cortical margins and soft tissue interface, in keeping with diffuse metastatic disease of bone with associated collapse.

screening method of choice in the examination of thoracolumbar spine trauma in most cases. CT is the most commonly used advanced modality with its superior depiction of ossific injuries and reconstruction and 3D capabilities. Both CT and MRI are indicated on a case-by-case basis according to the clinical scenario and the initial findings on the radiographic study, or as suggested by incongruity between the initial neurologic symptoms and radiographic findings. MRI, with its multiplanar capability, higher spatial resolution, and soft tissue resolution capacity, is now more commonly used in our trauma center to evaluate most importantly the spinal cord, as well as the discs, nerves, and vessels in severely injured patients.

Accurate and timely detection of bone, joint, soft tissue, and neurovascular abnormalities, as well as possible associated intrathoracic or intraabdominal injuries, is critical in these patients. Delineation of stable from unstable spinal injuries by the above-described imaging modalities is paramount in order to provide directed urgent clinical care and/or specific surgical intervention, not only to alleviate the initial injury but to prevent further injuries or complications in these often multitraumatized patients.

REFERENCES

1. Calenoff L, Chessare JW, Rogers LF, et al: Multiple level spinal injuries: importance of early recognition, *AJR* 130:665, 1978.
2. Daffner RH: *Imaging of vertebral trauma*, Rockville, Md, 1988, Aspen Publications.
3. Jefferson G: Discussion on spinal injuries, *Proc R Society Med* 8:625, 1927.
4. Harkonen M, Kataja M, Lepisto P, et al: Fractures of the thoracic spine: clinical and radiologic results in 98 patients, *Arch Orthop Trauma Surg* 94:179, 1979.
5. Meyer, S: Thoracic spine trauma, *Semin Roentgenol* 27:254, 1992.
6. McAfee PC, Yuan HA, Frederickson BE, et al: The value of computed tomography in thoracolumbar fractures, *J Bone Joint Surg Am* 65:461, 1983.
7. Nicoll EA: Fractures of the dorsolumbar spine, *J Bone Joint Surg* 31B:376, 1949.
8. Kaye, JJ, Nance EP: Thoracic and lumbar spine trauma, *Radiol Clin North Am* 28:361, 1990.
9. Angtuaco EJC, Binet EF: Radiology of thoracic and lumbar fractures, *Clin Orthop* 189:43, 1984.
10. Keene JS: Radiographic evaluation of thoracolumbar fractures, *Clin Orthop* 189:58, 1984.
11. Faerber EM, Wolpert SM, Sist RM: Computed tomography of spinal fractures, *J Comput Assist Tomogr* 3:657,1979.
12. Post MJD, Green BA: The use of computed tomography in spinal trauma, *Radiol Clin North Am* 21:327, 1983.
13. Griffith HB, Gleave JRW, Taylor RG: Changing patterns of fracture of the dorsal and lumbar spine, *Br Med J* 1:891, 1966.

14. Gumley G, Taylor TKF, Ryan MD: Distraction fractures of the lumbar spine, *J Bone Joint Surg* 64B:520,1982.

15. Holdsworth FW: Fractures, dislocations and fracture dislocations of the spine, *J Bone Joint Surg Am* 52:1534, 1970.

16. Maroney MJ, Mirvis SE, Shanmuganathan K: Esophageal occlusion caused by thoracic spine fracture or dislocation: CT diagnosis, *AJR Am J Roentgenol* 167:714, 1996.

17. Coffin CM, Weill A, Miaux Y, et al: Posttraumatic spinal subarachnoid cyst, *Eur Radiol* 6:523, 1996.

18. Uemura K, Meguro K, Matsumura A: Pneumocephalus associated with fracture of the thoracic spine: a case report, *Br J Neurosurg* 11:253, 1997.

19. Cohen AM, Crass JR, Thomas HA, et al: CT evidence for the "osseous pinch" mechanism of traumatic aortic injury, *AJR Am J Roentgenol* 159:271, 1992.

20. Jacobs R, Asher M, Snider R: Thoracolumbar spine injuries, *Spine* 5:463, 1980.

21. Posner I, White A, Edwards W, et al: A biomechanical analysis of the clinical stability of the lumbar and lumbosacral spine, *Spine* 7:374, 1982.

22. McAfee PC, Yuan HA, Lasada NA: The unstable burst fracture, *Spine* 7:365, 1982.

23. Roberts JB, Curtiss PH: Stability of the thoracic and lumbar spine in traumatic paraplegia following fracture or fracture-dislocation, *J Bone Joint Surg Am* 52:1115, 1970.

24. Denis F: The three column spine and its significance in the classification of acute thoracolumbar spinal injuries, *Spine* 8:817, 1983.

25. Rockwood CA Jr, Green DP: *Fractures in adults*, vol 2, Philadelphia, 1984, JB Lippincott.

26. Denis F: Spinal instability as defined by the three column spine concept in acute spinal trauma, *Clin Orthop* 189:65, 1984.

27. Ferguson RL, Allen BL Jr: A mechanistic classification of thoracolumbar spine fractures, *Clin Orthop* 189:77, 1984.

28. El-Khoury GY, Moore TE, Kathol MH: Radiology of the thoracic spine, *Clin Neurosurg* 38:261, 1992.

29. O'Callaghan JP, Ullrich CG, Yuan HA, et al: CT of facet distraction in flexion injuries of the thoracolumbar spine: the "naked" facet, *AJR Am J Roentgenol* 134:563, 1980.

30. Berquist TH: *Imaging of orthopedic trauma and surgery*, Philadelphia, 1966, WB Saunders.

31. Gehweiler JA Jr, Osborne RL Jr, Becker RF: *The radiology of vertebral trauma*, Philadelphia, 1980, WB Saunders.

32. Brant-Zawadzki M, Jeffrey RB Jr, Minagi H, et al: High resolution CT of thoracolumbar fractures, *AJNR* 3:69, 1982.

33. Dalinka MK, Boorstein JM, Zlatkin MB: Computed tomography of musculoskeletal trauma, *Radiol Clin North Am* 27:933, 1989.

34. Slucky AV, Potter HG: Use of magnetic resonance imaging in spinal trauma: indications techniques, and utility, *J Am Assoc Orthop Surg* 6:134, 1998.

35. Paleologos TS, Fratzoglou MM, Papadopoulou SS, et al: Posttraumatic spinal cord lesions without skeletal or discal and ligamentous abnormalities: the role of MR imaging, *J Spinal Disord* 11:346, 1998.

36. Helms CA, Kaplan PA, Dussault R, et al: How to image the spine. In *Musculoskeletal MRI*, Philadelphia, 2001, WB Saunders.

37. Kulkarni MV, McArdle CB, Kopanicky D, et al: Acute spinal cord injury: MR imaging at 1.5 T, *Radiology* 164:837, 1987.

38. Hackney DB, Asato R, Sci DM, et al: Hemorrhage and edema in acute spinal cord compression: demonstration by MR imaging, *Radiology* 161:387, 1986.

39. Bradley WG Jr: MR appearance of hemorrhage in the brain, *Radiology* 189:15, 1993.

40. Plumley TF, Kilocoyne RF, Mack LA: Computed tomography in evaluation of gunshot wounds of the spine, *J Comput Assist Tomogr* 7:310, 1983.

41. Myers P: Open injuries of the spine and spinal cord, missile wounds and shell fragments, *Proc Veterans Adm Spinal Cord Inj Conf* 19:157, 1973.

42. Yashon D: Missile injuries of the spinal cord, *Proc Veterans Adm Spinal Cord Inj Conf* 19:160, 1973.

43. Jones FD, Woosley RE: Delayed myelopathy secondary to retained intraspinal metallic fragment: case report, *J Neurosurg* 55:979, 1981.

44. Murphey MD, Batnitzky S, Bramble JM: Diagnostic imaging of spinal trauma, *Radiol Clin North Am* 27:855, 1989.

45. Dennis LN, Rogers LF: Superior mediastinal widening from spine fractures mimicking aortic ruptures on chest radiographs, *AJR Am J Roentgenol* 152:27, 1989.

46. Berquist TH: *Imaging of orthopedic trauma*, ed 2, New York, 1992, Raven Press.

47. DeSmet AA, Robinson RG, Johnson BE, Luhert BP: Spinal compression fractures in osteoporotic women: patterns and relationship to kyphosis, *Radiology* 166:497, 1988.

48. Bradford DS, Thompson RC: Fractures and dislocations of the spine: indications for surgical intervention, *Minn Med* 59:711, 1976.

49. Dehner JR: Seat belt injuries of the spine and abdomen, *AJR Am J Roentgenol* 111:833, 1971.

50. Rogers LF: The roentgenographic appearances of transverse or Chance fractures of the spine: the seat belt fracture, *AJR Am J Roentgenol* 111:844, 1971.

51. Chance CQ: Note on a type of flexion fracture of the spine, *Br J Radiol* 21:452, 1948.

52. Smith WS, Kaufer H: Patterns and mechanisms of lumbar injuries associated with lap seat belts, *J Bone Joint Surg Am* 51:239, 1969.

53. Kricun ME, Kricun R: Fractures of the lumbar spine, *Semin Roentgenol* 27:262, 1992.

54. Sivit CJ, Taylor GA, Newman KD, et al: Safety-belt injuries in children with lap-belt ecchymosis: CT findings in 61 patients, *AJR Am J Roentgenol* 157:111, 1991.

55. Reid AB, Letts RM, Black GB:. Pediatric Chance fractures: association with intraabdominal injuries and seat belt use, *J Trauma* 30:384, 1990.

56. Garrett JW, Braunstein PW: Seat belt syndrome, *J Trauma* 2:220, 1962.

57. Rennie W, Mitchell N: Flexion distraction fractures of the thoracolumbar spine, *J Bone Joint Surg Am* 55:386,1973.

58. Roaf R: A study of the mechanics of spinal injuries, *J Bone Joint Surg Br* 42:810, 1960.

59. Rogers LF: *Radiology of skeletal trauma*, vol 1, New York, 1982, Churchill Livingston.

60. Daffner RH, Deeb ZL, Rothfus WE: The posterior vertebral body line: importance in the detection of burst fractures, *AJR Am J Roentgenol* 148:93,1987.

61. Atlas WS, Regenbogen V, Rogers LF, et al: The radiographic characterization of burst fractures of the spine, *AJR Am J Roentgenol* 147:575,1986.

62. Smith GR, Northrop CH, Loop JW: Jumper's fractures: patterns of thoraco-lumbar spine injuries associated with vertical plunges: a review of 38 cases, *Radiology* 122:657, 1977.

63. Guerra J Jr, Garfin SR, Resnick D: Vertebral burst fractures: CT analysis of the retropulsed fragment, *Radiology* 153:769, 1984.

64. Trafton PG, Boyd CA Jr: Computed tomography of thoracic and lumbar spine injuries, *J Trauma* 24:506, 1984.

65. Keene JS: Significance of acute posttraumatic bony encroachment of neural canal, *Spine* 14:799, 1989.

66. Braakman R, Fontijne WP, Zeegers R, et al: Neurological deficit in injuries of the thoracic and lumbar spine: a consecutive series of 70 patients, *Acta Neurochir (Wien)* 111:11, 1991.

67. Finn CA, Stauffer ES: Burst fracture of the fifth lumbar vertebra, *J Bone Joint Surg Am* 74:398, 1992.

68. Keene JS, Fischer SP, Vanderby R, et al: Significance of acute posttraumatic bony encroachment of the neural canal, *Spine* 14:799, 1989.

69. Golimbu C, Firooznia H, Rafii M, et al: Computed tomography of thoracic and lumbar spine fractures that have been treated with Harrington instrumentation, *Radiology* 151:731,1984.

70. Andreychik DA, Alander DH, Senica KM, Stauffer ES: Burst fractures of the second through fifth lumbar vertebrae, *J Bone Joint Surg* 78:1156, 1996.

71. Weinstein JN, Collalto P, Lehmann TR: Thoracolumbar "burst" fractures treated conservatively: a long term follow up, *Spine* 13:33, 1988.

72. Chan DP, Seng NK, Kaan KT: Nonoperative treatment in burst fractures of the lumbar spine (L2-L5) without neurologic deficits, *Spine* 18:320, 1993.

73. Mumford J, Weinstein JN, Spratt KF, Goel VK: Thoracolumbar burst fractures: the clinical efficacy and outcome of nonoperative management, *Spine* 18:955, 1993.

74. An HS, Simpson JM, Ebraheim NA, et al: Low lumbar burst fractures: comparison between conservative and surgical treatments, *Orthopedics* 15:367,1992.

75. Daffner RH, Deeb ZL, Rothfus WE: Thoracic fractures and dislocations in motorcyclists, *Skeletal Radiol* 16:280, 1987.

76. Kupferschmid JP, Weaver NL, Raves JJ, et al: Thoracic spine injuries in victims of motorcycle accidents, *J Trauma* 29:592, 1989.

77. DeOliveira JC: A new type of fracture-dislocation of the thoracolumbar spine, *J Bone Joint Surg Am* 60:481, 1978.

78. Manaster BJ, Osborn AG: CT patterns of facet fracture dislocation in the thoracolumbar region, *AJR Am J Roentgenol* 148:335, 1987.

79. Gellad FE, Lavine AM, Joslyh JN, et al: Pure thoracolumbar facet dislocation: clinical features and CT appearance, *Radiology* 161:505, 1986.

80. Sharafuddin MF, Hitchon PW, el-Khoury GY, Dyst GN: Locked facets in the thoracic spine: report of three cases and a review, *J Spinal Disord* 3:255, 1990.

81. Bents RT, France JC, Glover JM, Kaylor KL: Traumatic spondylopelvic dissociation: a case report and literature review, *Spine* 21:1814, 1996.

82. Van Savage JG, Dahners LE, Renner JB, Baker CB: Fracture-dislocation of the lumbosacral spine: case report and review of the literature, *J Trauma* 33:779, 1992.

83. Patten RM, Gunberg SR, Brandenburger DK: Frequency and importance of transverse process fractures in the lumbar vertebra at helical abdominal CT in patients with trauma, *Radiology* 215:831, 2000.

84. Pathria M: Physical injury, spine. In Resnick D, ed: *Diagnosis of bone and joint disorders*, ed 3, Philadelphia, 1995, WB Saunders.

85. Krueger MA, Green DA, Hoyt D, Garfin SR: Overlooked spine injuries associated with lumbar transverse process fractures, *Clin Orthop* 327:191, 1996.

86. Sturm JT, Perry JF: Injuries associated with the transverse processes of the thoracic and lumbar vertebrae, *J Trauma* 24:597, 1984.

87. Brower AC, Downey EF Jr: Kummel disease: report of a case with serial radiographs, *Radiology* 141:363, 1981.

88. Gelman MI, Umber JS: Fractures of the thoracolumbar spine in ankylosing spondylitis, *AJR Am J Roentgenol* 130:485, 1978.

89. Graham B, Van Peteghem K: Fractures of the spine in ankylosing spondylitis: diagnosis, treatment, and complications, *Spine* 14:803, 1989.

90. Weinstein PR, Karpman RR, Gall EP, Pitt M: Spinal cord injury, spinal fracture, and spinal stenosis in ankylosing spondylitis, *J Neurosurg* 57:609, 1982.

91. Osgood C, Abassy M, Matthews T: Multiple spine fractures in ankylosing spondylitis, *J Trauma* 15:163, 1975.

92. Hunter T, Dubo HI: Spinal fractures complicating ankylosing spondylitis, *Arthritis Rheum* 26:751, 1983.

93. Israel Z, Mosheiff R, Gross E, et al: Hyperextension fracture-dislocation of the thoracic spine with paraplegia in a patient with diffuse idiopathic skeletal hyperostosis, *J Spinal Disord* 7:455, 1994.

9 Pelvic and Acetabular Fractures

Charles S. Resnik

High-speed injuries to the pelvis have become commonplace. Young et al.[1] reported that more than 300 patients with pelvic fractures were seen in less than 3 years at the University of Maryland Shock Trauma Center, and the center now sees more than 300 pelvic and acetabular fractures yearly. Prompt recognition of the specific pattern of fractures allows early and accurate pelvic stabilization, often contributing to reduced blood loss and increased likelihood of survival.[2]

A useful classification of pelvic fractures takes into consideration the direction of force that created the injury. This allows the orthopedic surgeon to determine the correct counterforce that needs to be applied with an external fixation frame. Although computed tomography (CT) provides exquisite detail of virtually all pelvic fractures, many hospitals and trauma centers are not ideally equipped to obtain pelvic CT in the minutes after a patient arrives, particularly if the patient has sustained severe trauma to multiple sites, including thoracic and spinal injuries that demand immediate attention. On the other hand, plain radiographic imaging of the pelvis is easily performed immediately in conjunction with chest and cervical spine radiographs. It has also been shown that conventional radiographic examination is sufficient to identify virtually all *clinically important* pelvic fractures and dislocations.[3] Therefore, the most practical classification system is based on fracture patterns visualized on a single anteroposterior (AP) radiograph of the pelvis.

If the clinical situation allows, supplemental radiographs in different positions can be used to provide additional information. For most pelvic fractures, inlet (obtained with the patient supine and the X-ray beam angled approximately 45 degrees toward the feet) and outlet (obtained with the patient supine and the X-ray beam angled approximately 45 degrees toward the head) views allow excellent visualization of both anterior and posterior injuries.[4] The inlet view is useful for demonstrating anterior or posterior displacement of fracture fragments and often provides the best view of pubic fractures that are oriented horizontally or coronally. The inlet view is also helpful in demonstrating disruption of sacral arcuate lines due to a crush fracture (Fig. 9-1). The outlet view is useful for demonstrating cephalad or caudad displacement of fracture fragments; this view is also good for showing extension of sacral fractures into neural foramina (Fig. 9-2).

If an acetabular fracture is present, additional Judet (45-degree oblique) views can aid in accurate classification.[5] CT can be obtained once the patient is stabilized for more detailed evaluation, including detection of intraarticular fracture fragments that can be difficult to see on conventional radiographs.[6,7]

PERTINENT PELVIC ANATOMY

The bony pelvis consists of the midline posterior sacrum and two lateral components made up of the ilium, the ischium, and the pubis. These three independent bony structures are joined together into a stable ring by a series of supporting ligaments (Fig. 9-3). The symphysis pubis is surrounded by a fibrous capsule anteriorly, with additional support provided by the superior pubic and arcuate pubic ligaments. However, the stability of the pelvic ring is dependent almost entirely on the ligaments bridging the sacroiliac joints and those connecting the sacrum to the ischium inferiorly.

The interosseous sacroiliac ligament is a very strong, short ligament that unites the tuberosities of the ilium and sacrum. The posterior sacroiliac ligament consists of short fibers coursing obliquely from the posterior superior and posterior inferior iliac spines to the ridge of the sacrum, as well as longer fibers coursing more inferiorly that intermingle with the sacrotuberous ligament. The anterior sacroiliac ligament connects the anterior surface of the sacrum to the anterior ilium.

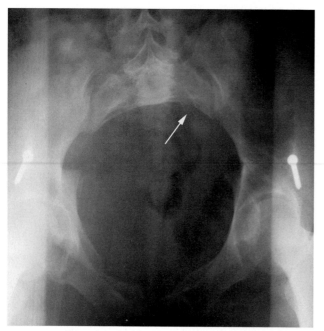

Fig. 9-1
Inlet view of the pelvis shows a typical crush fracture of the left sacrum (*arrow*). There are also bilateral pubic rami fractures and malalignment of the right sacroiliac joint.

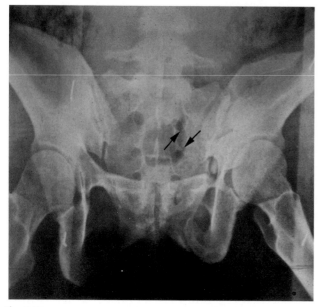

Fig. 9-2
Outlet view of the pelvis shows vertically oriented fractures of the left superior and inferior pubic rami, an oblique fracture of the left ilium, and a fracture of the left sacrum extending into neural foramina (*arrows*). There is cephalad displacement of the left hemipelvis.

Structures that help support the pelvic floor include the sacrotuberous and sacrospinous ligaments. The strong sacrotuberous ligament originates from the lateral border of the sacrum, intermingles with fibers of the pos-

terior sacroiliac ligament, and extends to the ischial tuberosity. The sacrospinous ligament also arises from the lateral border of the sacrum and courses deep to the sacrotuberous ligament to attach to the ischial spine. Additional pelvic stability is provided by the iliolumbar ligaments connecting the fifth lumbar transverse processes to the superior border of the iliac bones, as well as the lateral lumbosacral ligaments.

Several major arterial branches are vulnerable to direct injury, owing to their intimate relationship to the bones of the pelvis. These include the superior gluteal artery as it passes through the sciatic notch; the median sacral, lateral sacral, and iliolumbar arteries as they course in proximity to the sacrum; and the pudendal, obturator, and vesical branches as they course along the anterior and lateral walls of the pelvis. Diastasis of the sacroiliac joint may also be associated with direct injury to the internal iliac artery.[8]

The urinary bladder and urethra are also vulnerable to injury, particularly when there is diastasis of the symphysis pubis or fractures of the pubic rami. In men, the posterior urethra and the membranous urethra are relatively fixed structures as they course up to and through the urogenital diaphragm, accounting for the higher prevalence of urethral injury than that which occurs in women, where the urethra is shorter and more mobile.

Neurologic damage is observed more frequently with injury to posterior pelvic structures. Fractures of the sacrum often involve the neural foramina, with direct injury to exiting nerve roots. The sciatic nerve exits the pelvis between the inferior margin of the piriformis muscle and the ischial border of the greater sciatic notch, and the pudendal, superior gluteal, inferior gluteal, obturator internus, and posterior femoral cutaneous nerves all course in proximity to the greater sciatic notch. Finally, the perforating cutaneous nerve, which supplies the skin of the lower buttock, pierces the sacrotuberous ligament and is thus vulnerable to posterior pelvic injury.

CLASSIFICATION OF PELVIC INJURIES

Over the past 3 to 4 decades, numerous descriptions and classifications of pelvic injuries have appeared in the medical literature.[1,2,4,9-23] Many of these systems attempt to differentiate stable from unstable injuries. Stable injuries have been reported to include "single" fractures of the pelvic ring, isolated fractures of the iliac wing (Duverney fracture), "straddle" fractures of the pubic rami, "chip" or avulsion fractures, and isolated acetabular fractures. Unstable fractures are described as disruption of the pelvic ring at more than one site, with specific emphasis on sacral or sacroiliac complex disruption. This includes Malgaigne ("bucket handle") fractures, with fractures of superior and inferior pubic rami plus a posterior pelvic fracture, and "open book" injuries, with

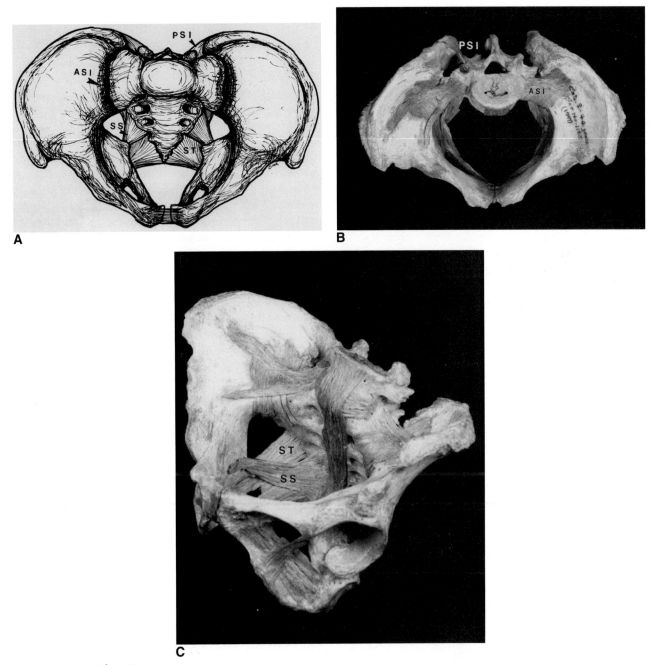

Fig. 9-3
Pelvic ligaments. **A**, Drawing illustrates posterior sacroiliac (*PSI*), anterior sacroiliac (*ASI*), sacrotuberous (*ST*), and sacrospinous (*SS*) ligaments. **B**, Anatomic specimen, cephalocaudad view, shows posterior sacroiliac (*PSI*) and anterior sacroiliac (*ASI*) ligaments. **C**, Anatomic specimen, oblique view, shows sacrotuberous (*ST*) and sacrospinous (*SS*) ligaments.

diastasis of the symphysis pubis and one or both sacroiliac joints.

While grossly displaced fractures present no problem in determining instability, it must be stressed that overall stability of the pelvis is entirely dependent on the sup-porting ligaments.[9] Disruption of the anterior ligaments at the symphysis pubis has been shown to allow separation of the symphysis only up to 2.5 cm as long as the posterior ligaments remain intact.[20] With disruption of the anterior sacroiliac, sacrospinous, and sacrotuberous ligaments, the symphysis may separate to a greater degree, and further disruption of the posterior sacroiliac ligament creates complete pelvic instability. While "single" fractures have been used in some classification systems,[24,25] such fractures have been shown to include a second site of pelvic ring injury in almost all cases, making this classification unreliable.[13] Other classification systems have been based on various combinations of sacroiliac joint and symphysis disruption,[17] interruption of major lines of weight transmission,[10] or anterior versus posterior fractures.[16]

The development of external fixation as the primary method of treatment for pelvic injuries created the need for a classification system based on the force vectors that caused the injury.[4,15,20,26,27] Subsequent refinement of this concept has produced a classification system that provides the orthopedic surgeon with the information necessary to apply the most appropriate corrective forces.[1,22] This system divides pelvic injuries into three distinct mechanisms: anteroposterior compression, lateral compression, and vertical shear.[28]

Anteroposterior Compression Injuries

AP compression injuries are the result of forces applied in the sagittal plane from the front to the back or from the back to the front. This occurs most frequently in motor vehicle collisions. The resulting injuries that begin in the anterior pelvis and progress to the posterior pelvis can be divided into three basic types, dependent on the severity of the causative force.

Type I AP compression injuries include either disruption of the ligaments of the symphysis pubis or vertically oriented fractures of the superior and inferior pubic rami on one or both sides. This vertical orientation is an important distinguishing feature from the fractures that occur in lateral compression injuries, which are oriented horizontally or coronally (Fig. 9-4). Type I injuries do not produce pelvic instability, since the posterior ligaments remain intact. When present, diastasis of the symphysis pubis will be 2.5 cm or less.

Type II AP compression injuries add disruption of the sacrospinous, sacrotuberous, and anterior sacroiliac ligaments. This allows diastasis of the symphysis pubis greater than 2.5 cm, as well as diastasis of the anterior aspect of one or both sacroiliac joints (Fig. 9-5). External rotation of the iliac bones creates an "open book" appearance.

Type III AP compression injuries include all of the features of type I and type II plus disruption of all of the sacroiliac ligaments, allowing complete separation of the iliac wing from the sacrum and hence complete pelvic instability (Fig. 9-6). In rare instances, a small fracture fragment may be separated from the lateral aspect of the sacrum because of avulsion of the origin of the sacrospinous and sacrotuberous ligaments (Fig. 9-7).

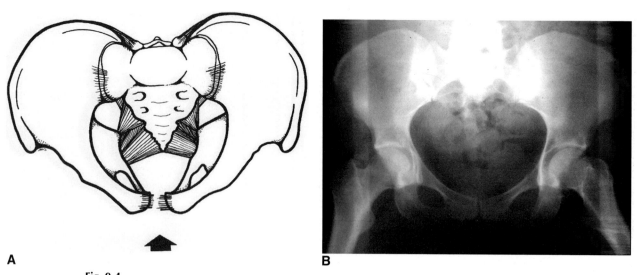

A **B**

Fig. 9-4
Type I AP compression injury. **A,** Drawing illustrates disruption of pubic ligaments, with all posterior ligaments intact. **B,** AP radiograph shows vertically oriented fractures of the left superior and inferior pubic rami.

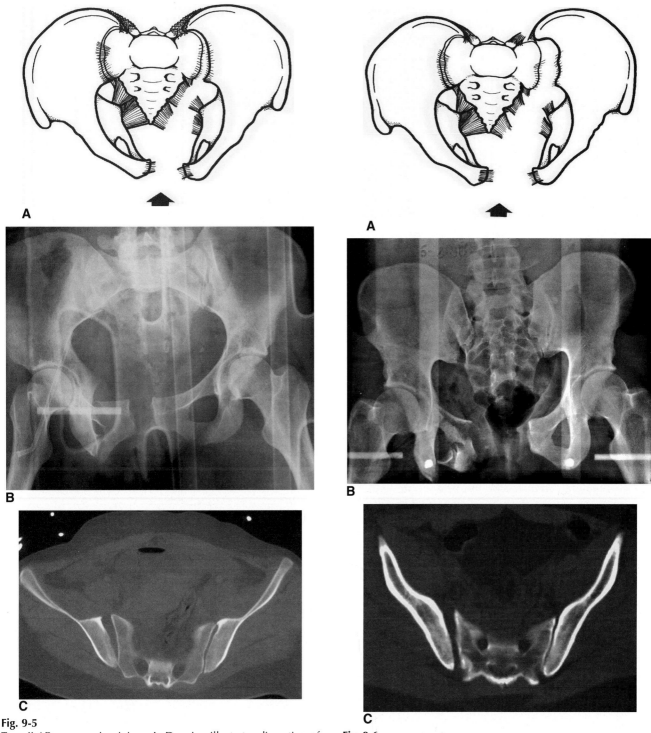

Fig. 9-5
Type II AP compression injury. **A**, Drawing illustrates disruption of pubic, sacrotuberous, sacrospinous, and anterior sacroiliac ligaments. **B**, AP radiograph shows vertically oriented fractures of the right superior and inferior pubic rami, diastasis of the symphysis pubis, and widening of the right sacroiliac joint. There is also a fracture of the left acetabulum. No sacral fracture is present. **C**, Axial CT section shows characteristic widening of the anterior aspect of the right sacroiliac joint.

Fig. 9-6
Type III AP compression injury. **A**, Drawing illustrates disruption of pubic, sacrotuberous, sacrospinous, anterior sacroiliac, and posterior sacroiliac ligaments. **B**, AP radiograph shows diastasis of the symphysis pubis, fractures of the right superior and inferior pubic rami, and widening of the right sacroiliac joint. **C**, Axial CT section shows widening of the right sacroiliac joint anteriorly and posteriorly.

Surprisingly, sacral fractures of any kind are seen in less than 10% of AP compression injuries, another distinguishing feature from lateral compression injuries. However, a fracture that has been reported to accompany more than 50% of injuries of this type involves the posterior wall of the acetabulum.[22] This most commonly occurs in a motor vehicle collision where the knee strikes the dashboard. The force is transmitted along the flexed femur, causing posterior dislocation of the femoral head. This is different from the central acetabular fracture that occurs in lateral compression injuries.

Lateral Compression Injuries

Lateral compression injuries are the result of impact forces applied to the side of the pelvis. Such forces of injury are more common than any other pelvic injury mechanism.[22,23] As with AP compression injuries, lateral compression injuries may be divided into three basic types that depend both on the severity of the causative force and on the location from which it is applied, either posterolateral or anterolateral.

Type I lateral compression injuries are the most common and the least severe. The force is applied laterally from the mid to posterior aspect of the pelvis, creating an impaction (crush) fracture of the sacrum in up to 90% of cases. There are also horizontally or coronally oriented fractures of the pubic rami, unilateral or bilateral, in almost 100% of cases (Fig. 9-8). This injury does not cause pelvic instability.

Type II lateral compression injuries occur with the force being applied to the side of the pelvis more anteriorly. This causes internal rotation of the anterior hemipelvis and external rotation of the posterior hemipelvis, with the pivot point along the anterior aspect of the sacroiliac joint. In most instances, this leads to dis-

ruption of the ipsilateral posterior sacroiliac ligament and widening of the posterior sacroiliac joint, in addition to a crush fracture of the sacrum and horizontal pubic rami fractures (type IIA) (Fig. 9-9). In about 20% of cases, there is an oblique fracture of the ipsilateral iliac wing instead of disruption of the posterior sacroiliac ligament (type IIB) (Fig. 9-10). These injuries are unstable to compressive forces and are therefore corrected by application of external fixation to counter the internal rotation injury force.

Type III lateral compression injuries also occur because of forces applied to the anterior aspect of the side of the pelvis. However, the severity of the force is greater, leading to external rotation of the contralateral hemipelvis in addition to internal rotation of the ipsilateral hemipelvis, often due to the patient being "rolled over" by a heavy object (Fig. 9-11). This causes disruption of the contralateral sacrospinous, sacrotuberous, and

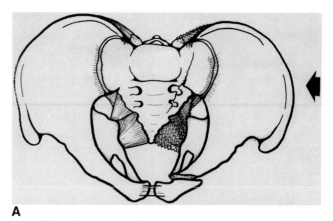

A

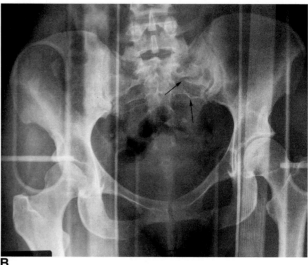

B

Fig. 9-8
Type I lateral compression injury. **A**, Drawing illustrates a horizontally oriented pubic fracture and a sacral crush fracture. **B**, AP radiograph shows a horizontally oriented fracture of the left inferior pubic ramus and a crush fracture of the left sacrum characterized by subtle disruption of arcuate lines (*arrows*).

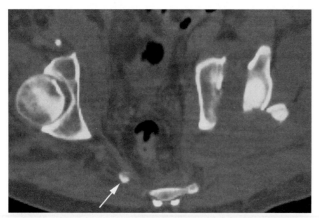

Fig. 9-7
Axial CT section shows a small fracture fragment separated from the lateral aspect of the right side of the sacrum because of avulsion of the origin of the sacrospinous and sacrotuberous ligaments (*arrow*). There is also a fracture of the left acetabulum.

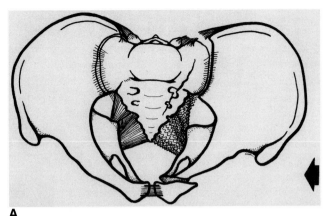

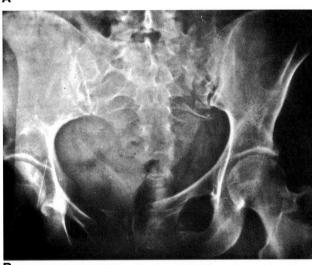

Fig. 9-9
Type IIA lateral compression injury. **A,** Drawing illustrates a horizontally oriented pubic fracture, a sacral crush fracture, and disruption of the posterior sacroiliac ligament. **B,** AP radiograph shows horizontal fractures of the pubic rami, a crush fracture of the left sacrum, and widening of the posterior aspect of the left sacroiliac joint.

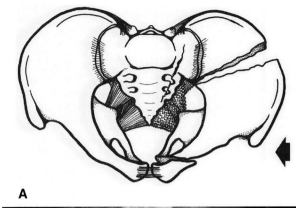

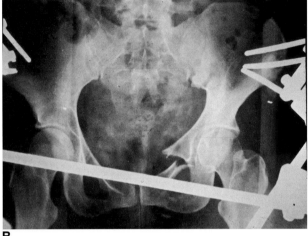

Fig. 9-10
Type IIB lateral compression injury. **A,** Drawing illustrates a horizontally oriented pubic fracture, a sacral crush fracture, and an oblique iliac fracture. **B,** AP radiograph shows a horizontal fracture of the left superior pubic ramus and an oblique fracture of the left iliac wing.

anterior sacroiliac ligaments. Thus the ipsilateral side has the appearance of a type II lateral compression injury, while the contralateral side has the appearance of an AP compression injury (Fig. 9-12). This has been called the "windswept pelvis"[23] (Fig. 9-13). As with type II injuries, the ipsilateral posterior injury may be disruption of the posterior sacroiliac ligament (type IIIA) or an oblique fracture of the iliac wing (type IIIB).

The characteristic fractures that accompany lateral compression injuries are horizontal fractures of the pubic rami and a crush fracture of the sacrum. The latter can be very subtle on pelvic radiographs, and careful attention must be paid to the integrity of all of the sacral arcuate lines. In some patients, there may be a fracture of the central aspect of the ipsilateral acetabulum, another differentiating feature from AP compression injuries where acetabular fractures involve the posterior wall.

Vertical Shear Injuries

Vertical shear injuries occur in patients who fall from a height or those who are struck on the head or back with a heavy object. This is the least common mechanism of pelvic injury. There may be disruption of the symphysis pubis and sacroiliac joint(s), as well as various combinations of pubic, iliac, and sacral fractures. When present, pubic fractures are vertically oriented, similar to AP compression injuries. However, there will often be cephalad or caudad displacement of one portion of the pelvis as opposed to anterior or posterior displacement in AP compression injuries (Fig. 9-14). This may be seen best on the outlet view radiograph. Most vertical shear injuries are grossly unstable.

Complex Fracture Patterns and Radiographic Analysis

In some instances, fracture patterns do not correspond to the basic AP compression, lateral compression, or vertical

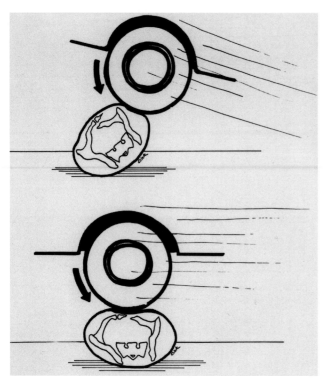

Fig. 9-11
Drawing illustrates "roll over" mechanism of type III lateral compression injury, with internal rotation of the ipsilateral hemipelvis and external rotation of the contralateral hemipelvis.

shear injuries. Complex or combination injuries must be analyzed carefully to determine fracture patterns and thus appropriate external fixation forces. Therefore, a thorough understanding of the classification system previously described allows recognition of most, if not all, pelvic injuries. When an "isolated" pubic fracture is initially observed, it must be determined to be vertical or horizontal. If horizontal, indicating a lateral compression injury, the sacral arcuate lines must be carefully assessed for a fracture that is likely present. If the pubic fracture is vertical, the AP, inlet, and outlet views must be observed for either anterior/posterior displacement, indicating an AP compression injury, or cephalad/caudad displacement, indicating a vertical shear injury. In all instances, the sacroiliac joints must be assessed for diastasis anteriorly, posteriorly, or both. Finally, acetabular fractures must be categorized into those that involve the posterior wall (AP compression injuries) and those that involve the central acetabulum (lateral compression injuries) (Table 9-1).

ACETABULAR FRACTURES

Classification of acetabular fractures is actually much more complex than that of posterior wall and central fractures.[29-31] In fact, the most widely used classification divides acetabular fractures into 10 distinct types.[5,32-35]

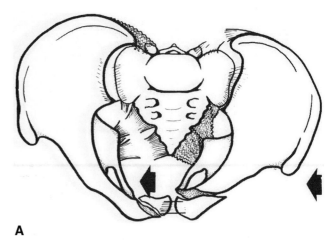

A

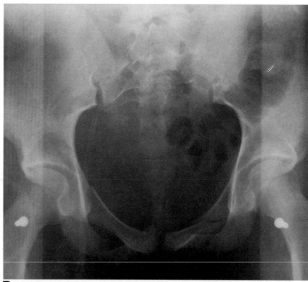

B

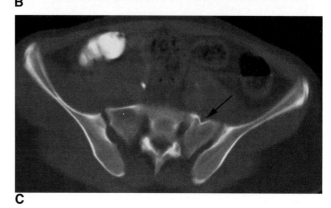

C

Fig. 9-12
Type IIIA lateral compression injury. **A,** Drawing illustrates an ipsilateral horizontally oriented pubic fracture and disruption of the posterior sacroiliac ligament, along with a contralateral oblique pubic fracture and disruption of sacrotuberous, sacrospinous, and anterior sacroiliac ligaments. **B,** AP radiograph shows a horizontal fracture of the left superior pubic ramus, minimal diastasis of the symphysis pubis, a crush fracture of the left sacrum, a fracture of the right medial pubis, vertically oriented fractures of the right superior and inferior pubic rami, and widening of the right sacroiliac joint (same patient as Fig. 9-1). **C,** Axial CT section shows the typical crush fracture of the left anterior sacrum (*arrow*) and widening of the right sacroiliac joint.

Table 9-1
Characteristic Features Differentiating Anteroposterior Compression Injuries from Lateral Compression Injuries

	Anteroposterior Compression	Lateral Compression
Pubic rami fractures	Vertical	Horizontal
Symphysis diastasis	Types II and III	Type III
Sacral fracture	4%	88% (crush)
Sacroiliac diastasis		
Anterior	Types II and III	—
Posterior	Type III	Types IIA and IIIA
Contralateral	Variable	Type III
Acetabular fracture	Posterior	Central

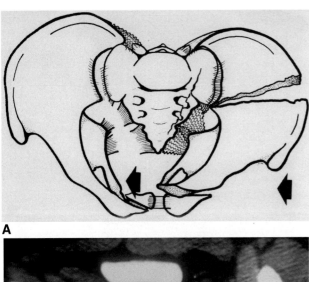

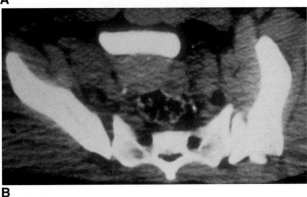

Fig. 9-13
Type IIIB lateral compression injury. **A**, Drawing illustrates an ipsilateral horizontally oriented pubic fracture, a sacral crush fracture, and an oblique iliac fracture, along with a contralateral oblique pubic fracture and disruption of sacrotuberous, sacrospinous, and anterior sacroiliac ligaments. **B**, Axial CT section shows a fracture of the left ilium, with internal rotation and widening of the anterior aspect of the right sacroiliac joint, creating a "windswept pelvis."

Five of these are elementary fractures with a single fracture line (anterior column, posterior column, anterior wall, posterior wall, and transverse), and five are combinations of these, termed "associated" fractures (both column, posterior column with posterior wall, anterior

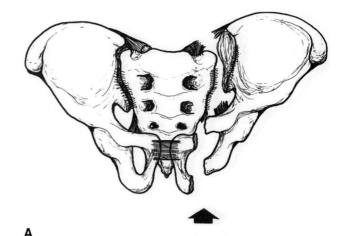

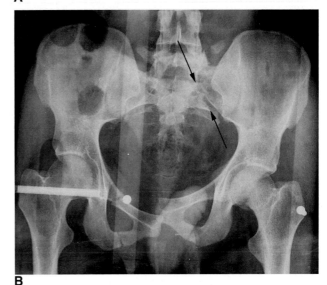

Fig. 9-14
Vertical shear injury. **A**, Drawing illustrates vertically oriented pubic fractures and disruption of sacrospinous, anterior sacroiliac, and posterior sacroiliac ligaments. **B**, AP radiograph shows a vertically oriented fracture of the left sacrum (*arrows*) and L5 transverse process with cephalad displacement of the left hemipelvis. There are also undisplaced fractures of the right superior and inferior pubic rami.

column with posterior hemitransverse, transverse with posterior wall, and T-shaped). Correct classification of acetabular fractures is important to the orthopedic surgeon in order to determine the most practical surgical approach.

Anatomically, the acetabulum may be divided into anterior and posterior columns, anterior and posterior walls (also called "lip" or "rim"), and a central quadrilateral plate. The larger anterior column comprises the anterior aspect of the ilium along with the lateral aspect of the superior pubic ramus. Thus disruption of the iliopubic (iliopectineal) line on pelvic radiographs indicates a fracture involving the anterior column and/or the anterior wall. Also, fractures of the iliac wing indicate anterior column involvement. The posterior column comprises the junction of the ilium and ischium. Thus disruption of the ilioischial line on pelvic radiographs indicates a fracture involving the posterior column and/or the posterior wall. Fractures of the obturator ring are also important to identify radiographically, since almost all column fractures extend into the ring and all ring fractures indicate involvement of the anterior column and/or the posterior column.

The most common acetabular fractures are posterior wall, transverse with posterior wall, and both column fractures. Together, these fracture types comprise approximately two-thirds of all acetabular fractures.[32,35] Adding transverse and T-shaped fractures to these three types accounts for up to 90% of acetabular fractures.[32] All 10 types of acetabular fractures can be differentiated by observation of the integrity of five radiographic landmarks: the iliopectineal line, the ilioischial line, the iliac wing, the obturator ring, and the posterior acetabular wall.

An elementary posterior wall fracture is the only acetabular fracture that does not disrupt one or both of the iliopectineal and ilioischial lines (Fig. 9-15). However, a fracture classified as a posterior wall fracture may occasionally disrupt the ilioischial line. This is still differentiated from a posterior column fracture, which would include disruption of both the ilioischial line and the obturator ring. While the elementary posterior column fracture does not involve the posterior wall, the associated posterior column with posterior wall fracture does.

An elementary anterior wall fracture includes disruption of the iliopectineal line and a fracture extending to the iliac wing. An elementary anterior column fracture includes both of these features plus disruption of the obturator ring (Fig. 9-16). The associated anterior column with posterior hemitransverse fracture is similar to the anterior wall fracture with disruption of the iliopectineal line and fracture of the iliac wing, but there is additional disruption of the ilioischial line. This fracture type is the only "column" fracture that may not disrupt the obturator ring.

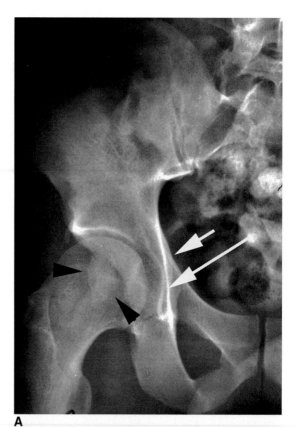

A

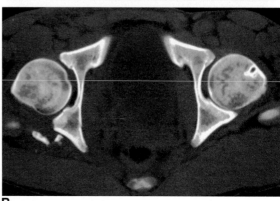

B

Fig. 9-15
Posterior wall acetabular fracture. **A,** AP radiograph shows a fracture fragment of the right posterior acetabular wall (*arrowheads*). Iliopectineal (*short arrow*) and ilioischial (*long arrow*) lines are intact. **B,** Axial CT section shows fracture fragments separated from the right posterior acetabular wall.

There are three additional transverse-type fractures. The elementary transverse fracture disrupts both the iliopectineal and ilioischial lines and divides the acetabulum into superior and inferior halves. On CT, the fracture line may be observed to extend from anterior to posterior, as opposed to column fractures, which are in a medial to lateral orientation. The associated transverse

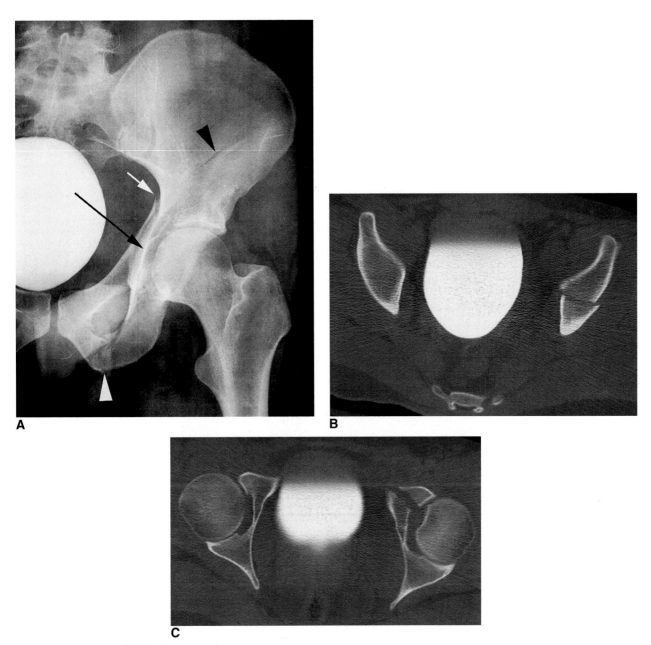

Fig. 9-16
Anterior column acetabular fracture. **A,** AP radiograph shows a left acetabular fracture with disruption of the iliopectineal line (*white arrow*). There are also fractures of the iliac wing and the obturator ring (*arrowheads*). The ilioischial line (*black arrow*) is intact. **B,** Axial CT section shows a fracture of the acetabular roof/iliac wing in a medial to lateral orientation, characteristic of a column fracture. **C,** Axial CT section 3.5 cm caudal to **B** shows the continuation of the fracture into the anterior column.

with posterior wall fracture is in fact similar to the anterior column (wall) with posterior hemitransverse fracture, with the more complex portion of the fracture located posteriorly instead of anteriorly (Fig. 9-17). The T-shaped fracture could be considered as an associated transverse with posterior column fracture, which includes

disruption of the iliopectineal line, the ilioischial line, and the obturator ring.

Finally, the both column fracture includes disruption of the iliopectineal line, the ilioischial line, and the obturator ring and a fracture of the iliac wing. This combination separates the anterior column from the posterior

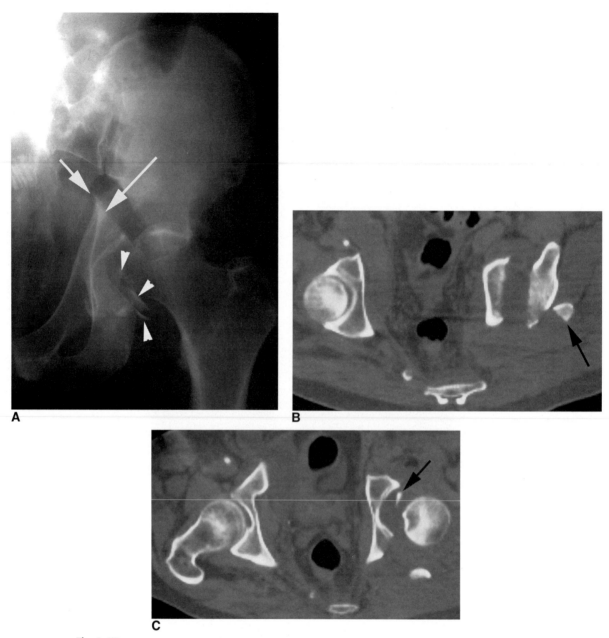

Fig. 9-17
Transverse with posterior wall acetabular fracture (same patient as Fig. 9-7). **A**, AP radiograph shows a left acetabular fracture with disruption of the iliopectineal (*short arrow*) and ilioischial (*long arrow*) lines. The femoral head is dislocated from the acetabular roof, and there are several intraarticular fracture fragments (*arrowheads*). **B**, Axial CT section through the acetabular roof shows the fracture line in an anterior to posterior orientation, characteristic of a transverse fracture. There is also a fragment separated from the posterior wall (*arrow*). **C**, Axial CT section 2 cm caudal to **B** shows two additional posterior wall fragments, one of which is intraarticular (*arrow*).

column and separates both columns from the posterior iliac fragment, thus detaching the acetabulum completely from the axial skeleton. The posterior iliac fragment can be observed to terminate inferiorly as a spur, which differentiates this type of fracture from all other acetabular fractures (Fig. 9-18).

In summary, the 10 different types of acetabular fractures can be differentiated by careful attention to five distinct radiograph features[32,33] (Table 9-2). As with all pelvic injuries, correct classification aids the orthopedic surgeon in establishing the most efficacious approach to definitive fixation.

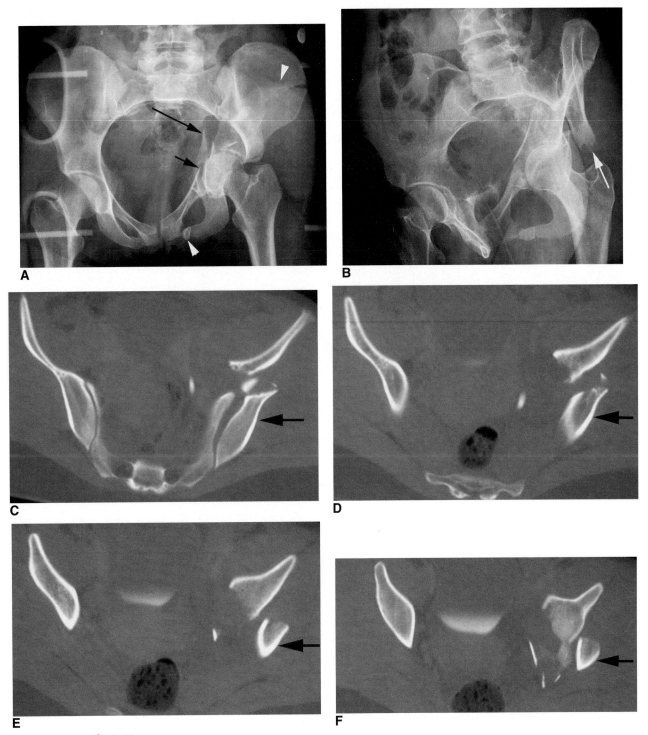

Fig. 9-18

Both column acetabular fracture. **A,** AP radiograph shows a left acetabular fracture with disruption of the iliopectineal (*short arrow*) and ilioischial (*long arrow*) lines. There are also fractures of the iliac wing and the obturator ring (*arrowheads*). **B,** Oblique radiograph shows the posterior iliac fragment terminating inferiorly as a spur (*arrow*). **C** to **I,** Axial CT sections at 1-cm intervals show a comminuted fracture of the acetabular roof/iliac wing in a medial to lateral orientation, with continuation of the fracture into the anterior and posterior columns. The posterior iliac fragment can be observed to terminate inferiorly (*arrows* in **C** to **G**), corresponding to the spur in **B.**

Continued

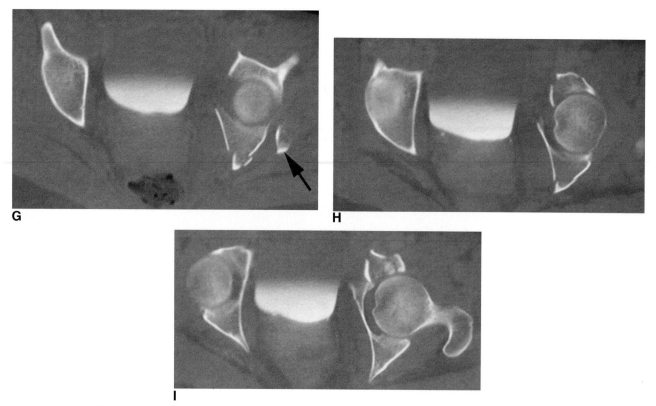

Fig. 9-18, Cont'd
For legend see p.571

Table 9-2
Radiographic Features of 10 Distinct Acetabular Fracture Types

Fracture Type	Iliopectineal Line Disruption	Ilioischial Line Disruption	Obturator Ring Disruption	Iliac Wing Fracture	Posterior Wall Fracture
Posterior wall	-	±	-	-	+
Posterior column	-	+	+	-	-
Posterior column with posterior wall	-	+	+	-	+
Anterior wall	+	-	-	±	-
Anterior column	+	-	+	+	-
Anterior column with posterior hemitransverse	+	+	±	+	-
Transverse	+	+	-	-	-
Transverse with posterior wall	+	+	-	-	+
T-shaped	+	+	+	-	-
Both column	+	+	+	+	-

Modified from Brandser EA, El-Khoury GY, Marsh JL: *Emerg Radiol* 2:18, 1995.

REFERENCES

1. Young JWR, Burgess AR, Brumback RJ, et al: Pelvic fractures: value of plain radiography in early assessment and management, *Radiology* 160:445, 1986.
2. Burgess AR, Eastridge BJ, Young JWR, et al: Pelvic ring disruptions: effective classification system and treatment protocols, *J Trauma* 30:1, 1990.
3. Resnik CS, Stackhouse DJ, Shanmuganathan K, et al: Diagnosis of pelvic fractures in patients with acute pelvic trauma: efficacy of plain radiographs, *AJR Am J Roentgenol* 158:109, 1992.
4. Pennal GF, Tile M, Waddell JP, et al: Pelvic disruption: assessment and classification, *Clin Orthop* 151:12, 1980.
5. Judet R, Judet J, Letournel E: Fractures of the acetabulum: classification and surgical approaches for open reduction, *J Bone Joint Surg [Am]* 46:1615, 1964.
6. Gilula LA, Murphy WA, Tailor CC, et al: Computed tomography of the osseous pelvis, *Radiology* 132:107, 1979.
7. Harley JD, Mack LA, Winquist RA: CT of acetabular fractures: comparison with conventional radiography, *AJR Am J Roentgenol* 138:413, 1982.
8. Smith K, Ben-Menachem Y, Duke JH, et al: The superior gluteal: an artery at risk in blunt pelvic trauma, *J Trauma* 16:273, 1976.
9. Bucholz RW: The pathological analog of Malgaigne fracture dislocations of the pelvis, *J Bone Joint Surg [Am]* 63:400, 1981.
10. Conolly WB, Hedberg EA: Observations on fractures of the pelvis, *J Trauma* 9:106, 1969.
11. Dunn AW, Morris MD: Fractures and dislocations of the pelvis, *J Bone Joint Surg [Am]* 50:1639, 1968.
12. Edeiken-Monroe BS, Browner BD, Jackson H: The role of standard roentgenograms in the evaluation of instability of pelvic ring disruption, *Clin Orthop* 240:63, 1989.
13. Gertzbein SD, Chenoweth DR: Occult injuries of the pelvic ring, *Clin Orthop* 128:202, 1977.
14. Holdsworth TW: Dislocation and fracture dislocation of the pelvis, *J Bone Joint Surg [Br]* 30:461, 1972.
15. Huittinen VM, Slatis P: Fractures of the pelvis: trauma mechanism, types of injury and principles of treatment, *Acta Chir Scand* 138:563, 1972.
16. Looser KG, Crombie HD: Pelvic fractures: an anatomic guide to severity of injury: review of 100 cases, *Am J Surg* 132:638, 1976.
17. Monahan PRW, Taylor RG: Dislocation and fracture dislocation of the pelvis, *Injury* 6:325, 1975.
18. Reynolds BM, Balsano A, Reynolds FX: Pelvic fractures, *J Trauma* 13:1011, 1973.
19. Thaggard A, Mark TS, Carlson V: Fractures and dislocations of the bony pelvis and hip, *Semin Roentgenol* 13:117, 1978.
20. Tile M: *Fractures of the pelvis and acetabulum*, Baltimore, 1986, Williams & Wilkins.
21. Trunkey DD, Chapman MW, Lim RC, et al: Management of pelvic fractures in blunt trauma injury, *J Trauma* 24:912, 1974.
22. Young JWR, Burgess AR: *Radiologic management of pelvic ring fractures*, Baltimore, 1987, Urban & Schwartzenberg.
23. Young JWR, Burgess AR, Brumbach RJ, et al: Lateral compression fractures of the pelvis: the importance of plain radiographs in the diagnosis and surgical management, *Skeletal Radiol* 15:103, 1986.
24. Kane WJ: Fractures of the pelvis. In Rockwood CA, Green DD, eds: *Fractures in adults*, ed 2, Philadelphia, 1984, Lippincott.
25. Rothenberger DA, Fischer RP, Strare R, et al: The mortality associated with pelvic fractures, *Surgery* 84:356, 1978.
26. Mears DC, Freddie HF: Modern concepts of external fixation of the pelvis, *Clin Orthop* 151:65, 1980.
27. Wild JJ, Hanson GW, Tullos HS: Unstable fractures of the pelvis treated by external fixation, *J Bone Joint Surg [Am]* 64:1010, 1982.
28. Young JWR, Resnik CS: Fracture of the pelvis: current concepts of classification, *AJR Am J Roentgenol* 155:1169, 1990.
29. Dunn AW, Russo CL: Central acetabular fractures, *J Trauma* 13:695, 1973.
30. Eichenholtz AN, Stark R: Central acetabular fractures, *J Bone Joint Surg [Am]* 46:695, 1964.
31. Lansinger O: Fractures of the acetabulum: a clinical, radiological and experimental study, *Acta Orthop Scand* 165:1, 1977.
32. Brandser EA, El-Khoury GY, Marsh JL: Acetabular fractures: a systematic approach to classification, *Emerg Radiol* 2:18, 1995.
33. Brandser E, Marsh JL: Acetabular fractures: easier classification with a systematic approach, *AJR Am J Roentgenol* 171:1217, 1998.
34. Letournel E: Acetabulum fractures: classification and management, *Clin Orthop* 151:81, 1980.
35. Potok PS, Hopper KD, Umlauf MJ: Fractures of the acetabulum: imaging, classification, and understanding, *Radiographics* 15:7, 1995.

10 Extremity Trauma

Michael Mulligan

Extremity injuries that occur in patients who have sustained major trauma are, by necessity, attended to only after other life-threatening injuries to the head, chest, abdomen, and pelvis are addressed. Injuries to the limbs are noted during the initial evaluation, and major deformities and dislocations are reduced as soon as is practical. High-quality radiographs in standard positions, with the standard number of views,[1] should be obtained whenever possible. Most extremity injuries are not threatening to life or limb, but they are a major source of morbidity and many require prolonged rehabilitation. This chapter is not intended to be a comprehensive review of all extremity trauma; rather, the intent is to review the common injuries suffered by adult patients who are treated at major trauma centers.

TERMINOLOGY

The type of fracture line (transverse, oblique, spiral) should be delineated and should correspond with the reported mechanism of injury, although in patients with high-energy trauma, the mechanism of injury is often complex. Standard terms for fracture description include displacement, distraction, angulation, and comminution. Fractures are comminuted whenever there are more than two fracture fragments. Segmental fractures are comminuted with two or more fracture lines at different levels along the shaft of the bone resulting in separation of a segment of the shaft. Gas within the soft tissues next to a fracture site or an adjacent laceration is a sign of an open fracture. Open fractures are considered surgical emergencies.

Orthopedic surgeons frequently use eponyms and classification schemes for many fractures. Although an accurate description of the fracture is the primary goal of the radiologist, familiarity with the common eponyms and favored classification schemes certainly aids communication and rapport.

UPPER LIMB INJURIES
Shoulder Region

Scapula and Clavicle. Isolated fractures of the scapula are uncommon. Scapula fractures are usually the result of high-energy trauma, most often due to motor vehicle accidents (MVAs).[2] Patients with scapula fractures usually have multiple additional orthopedic injuries (Fig. 10-1), including ipsilateral rib and clavicle fractures, and acromioclavicular (AC) separations.[3] Computed tomography (CT) usually is requested if extension to the articular surface of the glenoid is a consideration (Fig. 10-2). Distracted fractures of the clavicle should raise concern for scapulothoracic dissociation (STD). Wide separation of the AC joint or sternoclavicular joint also may indicate STD. Patients with STD may need emergent angiography and surgery.[4,5] Isolated AC joint injuries are not uncommon, especially after MVA. Injuries of the AC joint can be very subtle or overt. One must remember the normal measurements for the various spaces in the shoulder region. The AC joint averages 3 to 4 mm in width, the acromiohumeral space should not be less than 6 mm, and the coracoclavicular distance should not exceed 12 mm. Grade I AC joint injuries are not apparent radiographically; there is only point tenderness. Grade II injuries show abnormal widening of the AC joint but have a normal coracoclavicular space. Grade III injuries show widening of both the AC joint and the coracoclavicular space (Fig. 10-3). Standard orthopedic textbooks describe additional grades IV, V, and VI injuries based on marked superior, posterior, or inferior displacement of the clavicle.

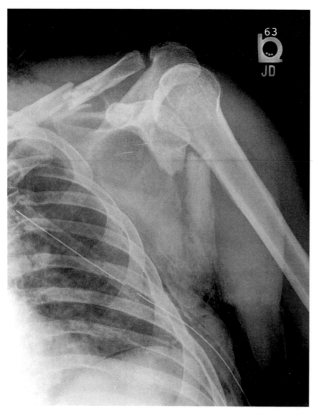

Fig. 10-1
Radiograph of a 40-year-old man involved in motorcycle accident. Anteroposterior view of shoulder shows fractures of the scapula, clavicle, and ribs.

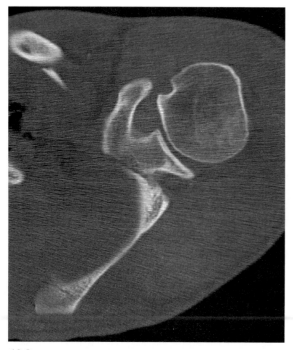

Fig. 10-2
Same patient as Fig. 10-1. Axial CT section shows no extension of fracture lines to glenoid articular surface.

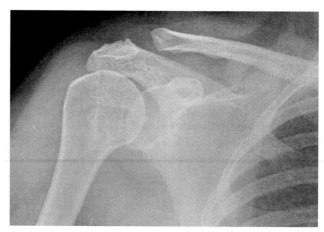

Fig. 10-3
Radiograph of a 60-year-old man after seizure and fall. Anteroposterior view of shoulder shows marked widening of acromioclavicular joint and abnormal widening of coracoclavicular space, indicating grade III acromioclavicular separation.

Humerus. Standard anterior or posterior dislocations of the humeral head may be encountered, but complex fracture dislocations are the more challenging injuries diagnostically (Fig. 10-4). CT often is obtained for comminuted fractures of the surgical neck and humeral head, to look for so-called head-splitting fractures that extend to the articular surface (Fig. 10-5). Multislice axial CT acquisition with coronal reformation is the preferred technique[6] at the University of Maryland Shock Trauma Center (UMSTC). Table 10-1 shows our current multislice CT protocols. Although the Neer classification of proximal humeral fractures has fallen out of favor, the position and number of fracture fragments are still important.

Humeral shaft fractures are not a diagnostic challenge but, depending on their location along the shaft, there may be associated injuries of the radial nerve or brachial artery (Fig. 10-6). Fortunately, vascular injuries are uncommon and neurologic injuries usually are transient.

Elbow Region

Intercondylar fractures of the distal humerus usually are described as T or Y shaped (Fig. 10-7). About 90% of distal humeral fractures extend to the joint surface, so the intraarticular fracture line should be sought carefully. The surgical technique for reduction and fixation usually includes an olecranon osteotomy. This osteotomy should not be confused with a fracture on follow-up studies (Fig. 10-8).

Elbow dislocations are most often posterior or posterolateral (Fig. 10-9). There may or may not be associated fractures of the distal humerus, proximal radius, or proximal ulna. The combination of radial head dislocation with fracture of the proximal ulna shaft is known as a Monteggia fracture (Fig. 10-10). The direction of radial

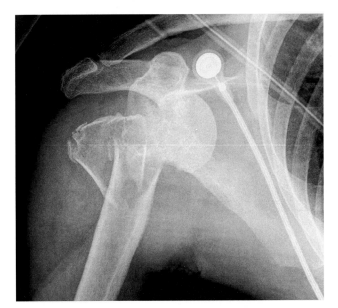

Fig. 10-4
Radiograph of a 48-year-old man who was struck by a vehicle. Anteroposterior view of shoulder shows fracture and dislocation, with humeral head dislocated anteriorly underneath the coracoid.

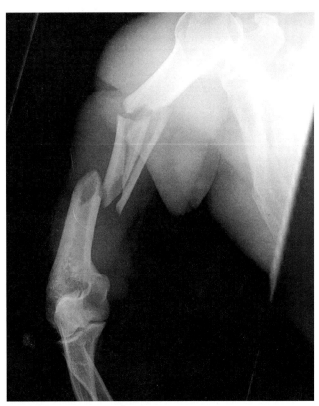

Fig. 10-6
Initial anteroposterior radiograph of a 41-year-old man involved in motorcycle crash shows comminuted, segmental fracture of humeral shaft with significant displacement and angulation.

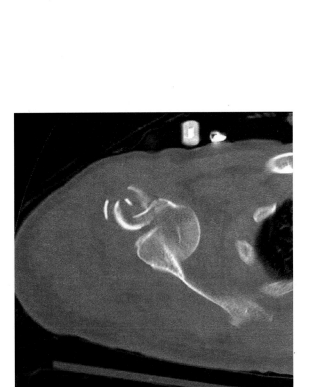

Fig. 10-5
Same patient as Fig. 10-4. Axial CT shows humeral fracture dislocation but no extension of fracture line into the humeral head articular surface.

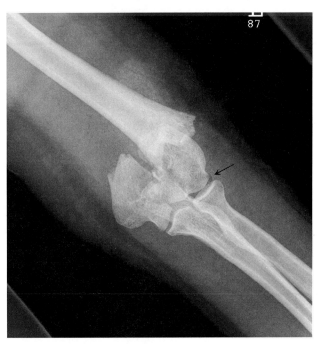

Fig. 10-7
Initial anteroposterior radiograph of a 30-year-old woman after motorcycle crash shows comminuted T-type fracture of distal humerus, with extension to midpoint of trochlear articular surface (*arrow*). Note small gas bubble in joint (*arrow*) indicating an open injury.

Table 10-1
Imaging Parameters for Musculoskeletal Multislice CT Protocols

Protocol	Slice Width (mm) Thickness	Increment (mm) or Interval*	Pitch	FOV (cm)	kV(p)	mAs	Resolution	Position
Shoulder—								
Small/average	2.0	1.0	0.875	25	140	250+	St	Other arm over head
Large	2.5	1.3	0.625		140	350+	St	
Elbow	1.0	0.5	0.775	20	140	200	High	Arm over head, elbow bent
Wrist and hand	0.5	0.2	0.875	10	140	190	UH	Arm over head, palm up
Hip—								
Small/average	2.0	1.0	0.625	25	140	250	St	45° oblique
Large	2.5	1.5	0.625	25	140	300+	St	
Knee	0.5/1.0	0.2/0.6	0.875	10	140	200+	High	—
Ankle and foot	0.5	0.2	0.675	10	140	200	High	—
Small joints, limited hardware	0.5	0.3	0.625	10	140	200	High	—
Large joints, large hardware	2.5	1.0	0.625	25	140	350+	St	—

Modified from Buckwalter KA, Rydberg J, Kopecky KK, et al: *AJR Am J Roentgenol* 176:979, 2001. (Phillips Mx 8000 CT scanner)

*Reconstruction interval.

FOV, Field of view; *kV(p)*, kilovolt (peak); *mAs*, milliamperes; *St*, standard; *UH*, ultrahigh.

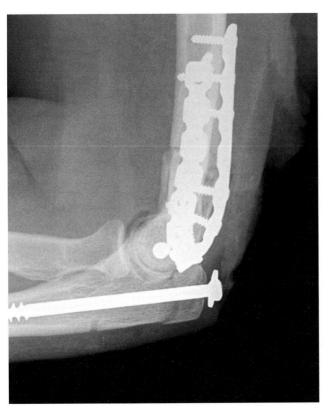

Fig. 10-8
Same patient as Fig. 10-7. Postoperative lateral radiograph shows olecranon osteotomy stabilized with lag screw. Osteotomy was done for surgical exposure.

head dislocation (anterior, posterior, or lateral) determines if it is a type I, II, or III Monteggia fracture. Type IV has an additional fracture of the proximal radius.

Forearm, Wrist, and Hand

Forearm fractures usually are not difficult to diagnose. If there is a midshaft fracture of one of the forearm bones, there is usually a fracture or dislocation of the other one as well, because they act as equal axial load-bearing struts (Fig. 10-11), although solitary fractures of the distal ulna shaft (nightstick fractures) are seen frequently because of the transverse force vector (Fig. 10-12). In a study done at the author's center, 114 of 119 consecutive patients with forearm injuries had double (both bone) injury.[7] One type of double injury that may be difficult to recognize is the Galeazzi "fracture." This is a combination of distal radius shaft fracture and dislocation of the ulna at the distal radioulnar joint (DRUJ). The subluxation or dislocation of the ulna may be difficult to recognize (Fig. 10-13). CT of both wrists (DRUJs) in the neutral, pronated, and supinated positions is usually diagnostic.[8] Both bone fractures are treated most often with side plate and screw fixation devices. These fractures are difficult to immobilize with just a cast, because the strong supinator muscle is very proximal in the forearm and the strong pronator muscle (pronator quadratus) is far distal. Another type of injury is the Essex-Lopresti fracture-dislocation, which

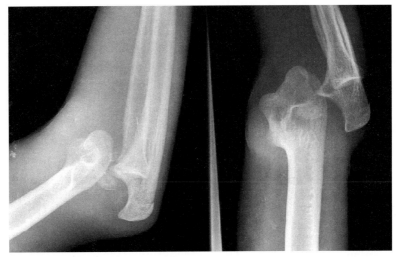

Fig. 10-9
Radiograph of a 56-year-old woman after motor vehicle accident. Lateral radiograph shows open elbow fracture and dislocation, with comminuted fracture of olecranon and anterior dislocation of radius and ulna.

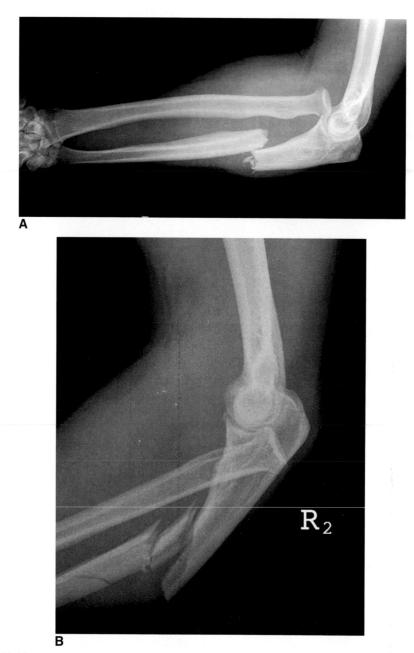

Fig. 10-10
A, Initial lateral radiograph of a 38-year-old man after motor vehicle accident shows type I Monteggia fracture, with anterior dislocation of radius and fracture of proximal ulna. **B**, A 53-year-old man after motor vehicle accident. Lateral radiograph shows type II Monteggia fracture, with posterior dislocation of radius and fracture of ulna.

is a combination of radial head fracture and DRUJ disruption.

The entire gamut of wrist and hand injuries may be encountered including simple Colles-type fractures, scaphoid fractures, complex carpal disruptions, and metacarpal or phalangeal fractures. Colles fractures, by definition, are transverse fractures of the metaphysis of the distal radius with dorsal displacement and angulation of the distal fragment. The fractures may be comminuted, and it is important to look for and describe any extension of fracture lines into either the radiocarpal joint surface or the DRUJ surface (Fig. 10-14). A Smith

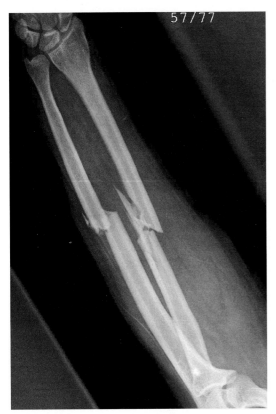

Fig. 10-11
Simple both-bone forearm fracture.

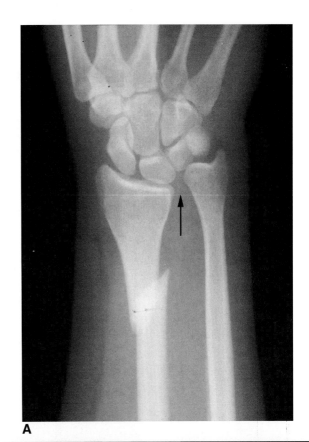

A

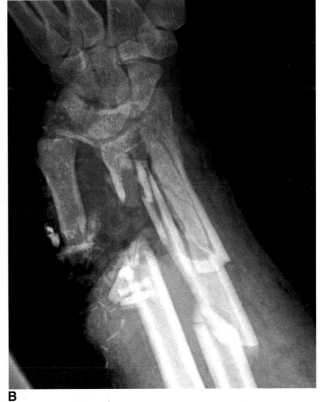

B

Fig. 10-13
A, A 20-year man after motorcycle crash. Posteroanterior radiograph shows Galeazzi injury with disruption of distal radioulnar joint (*arrow*) and distal radius fracture. **B**, Initial radiograph of a 43-year-old man after rollover motor vehicle accident shows open forearm fractures of radius and ulna with severe comminution. There is also disruption of the distal radioulnar joint.

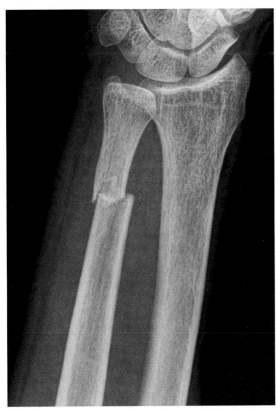

Fig. 10-12
Nightstick fracture. Anteroposterior radiograph of a 70-year-old man who was assaulted shows minimally displaced transverse fracture of distal ulna.

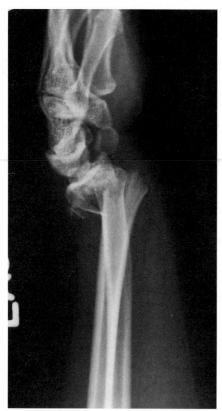

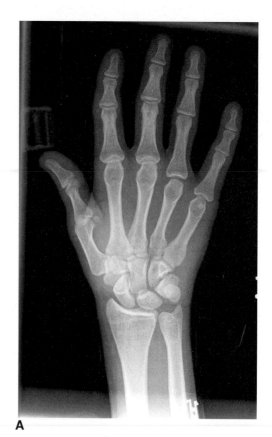

A

Fig. 10-14
Lateral radiograph demonstrates severe dorsal displacement and angulation of a distal radius fragment following fracture. There is also a less obvious fracture of the distal ulna.

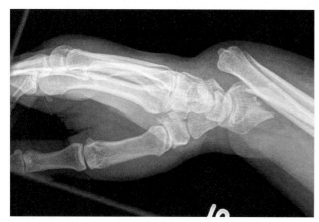

Fig. 10-15
Lateral radiograph of a 42-year-old woman after a motorcycle crash shows a Smith fracture with full shaft-width volar displacement of distal fragment.

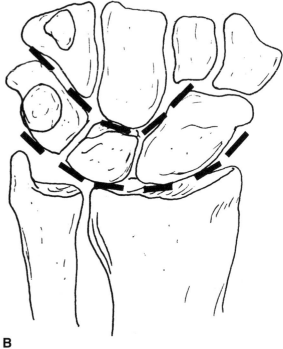

B

Fig. 10-16
An 18-year-old man after motorcycle crash. **A**, Posteroanterior radiograph shows normal carpal bone alignment. **B**, Drawing of normal carpal arcs.

fracture is the opposite of a Colles fracture. Therefore, there is volar displacement and angulation of the distal fragment (Fig. 10-15). Barton fracture involves only the dorsal or volar lip of the distal radius articular surface.

Displacements of the carpal bones can be assessed in a fashion similar to assessment of the cervical spine, because a series of arcuate lines (carpal arcs) indicates normal or abnormal positioning (Fig. 10-16). The carpal arcs are evaluated using the standard posteroanterior (PA) radiograph.[9] When the carpal arcs are disrupted, a perilunate dislocation or scapholunate dissociation is likely. Although the terms *perilunate dislocation* and *lunate dislocation* are still useful descriptors of the radiographic appearance, it is thought now that these two seemingly different injuries are the result of the same mechanism of injury. These injuries are due to falls on the outstretched hand or axial loading forces and result in disruptions of the volar and dorsal carpal ligaments. The carpal bones usually assume the pattern of a perilunate dislocation (Fig. 10-17).

Occasionally, as the carpus is reduced, the lunate assumes a volar position and gives rise to the radiographic picture of a lunate dislocation (Fig. 10-18). Fractures of the scaphoid are seen commonly in association with perilunate dislocations, giving rise to the term *transscaphoid perilunate fracture dislocation.*

The complication of osteonecrosis associated with fractures of the scaphoid is well known to radiologists. This diagnosis is difficult to make by conventional radiography, because increased density does not always indicate osteonecrosis. The tenuous blood supply to the proximal pole may result in a "pseudoosteonecrosis" during the early hyperemic phase of healing, with the surrounding carpal bones and distal pole of the scaphoid showing hyperemic osteoporotic changes. The proximal pole of the scaphoid maintains its preinjury bone density, because it does not "see" the same hyperemia as the remainder of the carpus. Fig. 10-19 shows a case of pseudoosteonecrosis of the proximal pole of the

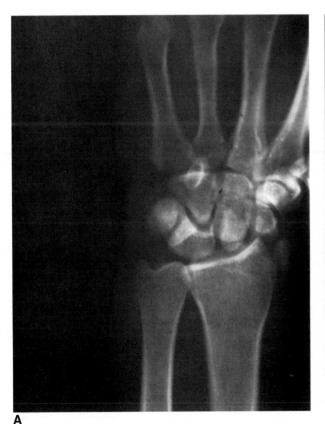

A

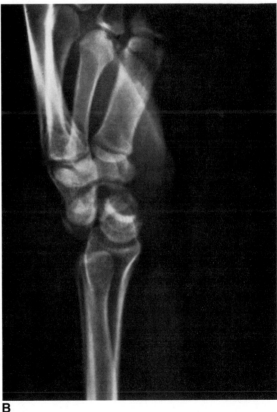

B

Fig. 10-17
Anteroposterior (**A**) and lateral (**B**) radiographs show transscaphoid perilunate fracture dislocation. Carpal arcs are disrupted on the posteroanterior view; lateral view shows posterior displacement of capitate, with lunate maintaining its normal position.

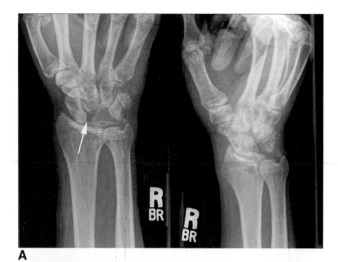

A

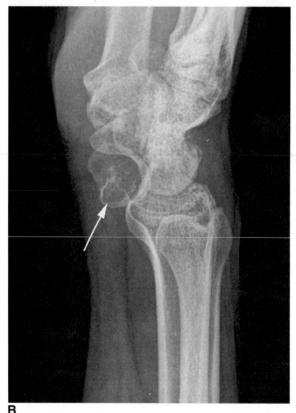

B

Fig. 10-18
A 52-year-old man after motor vehicle accident. **A**, Posteroanterior radiograph shows abnormal carpal arcs (**A** and **B**) and abnormal carpal alignment, with widening of scapholunate space and so-called pie-shaped lunate (*arrow*). **B**, Lateral radiograph shows volar displacement of lunate (*arrow*). Capitate is still aligned with distal radius.

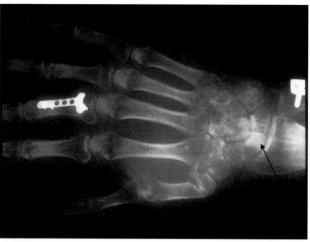

Fig. 10-19
Posteroanterior radiograph shows marked increased density in proximal pole of scaphoid (*arrow*), but patient did not have a scaphoid fracture. Note multiple fractures elsewhere in the hand.

LOWER LIMB INJURIES
Femoral Fractures

Femoral head and neck fractures are discussed in Chapter 9 in the context of pelvic fractures.

Intertrochanteric and Subtrochanteric Fractures. Intertrochanteric fractures extend obliquely from the greater trochanter to the lesser trochanter, separating the femoral head and neck segment from the femoral shaft. Fragments of either the greater trochanter or lesser trochanter also may be present. The fracture pattern then may result in two, three, or four "parts" of the femur separated from each other. This gives rise to the simple description (classification) of intertrochanteric fractures as two-, three-, or four-part fractures (Fig. 10-20). Subtrochanteric fractures involve the most proximal portion of the femoral shaft and may extend into the lesser trochanter (Fig. 10-21). The subtrochanteric region of the femur is the part below the greater trochanter and is defined as the 3 or 4 inches of the femur extending distally from the proximal edge of the lesser trochanter. Intertrochanteric and subtrochanteric fractures require different types of fixation, so the distinction is important and the type of fracture should be determined clearly. MR imaging is considered the best method of searching for proximal femur fractures that are radiographically occult (Fig. 10-22). The MR imaging protocol at UMSTC includes axial and coronal plane imaging with T1-weighted and inversion recovery sequences.

Femoral Shaft Fractures. Femoral shaft fractures usually are comminuted in high-energy trauma patients. They may be segmented, or there may be one or more

scaphoid in a patient with multiple hand injuries but no scaphoid fracture. Magnetic resonance (MR) imaging with intravenous contrast is the preferred method for evaluation of suspected scaphoid osteonecrosis.[10]

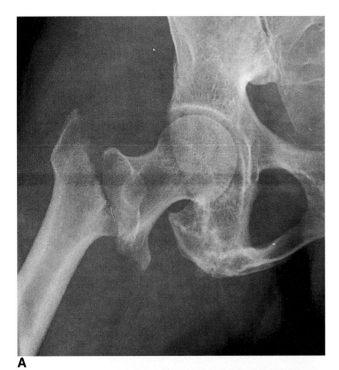

A

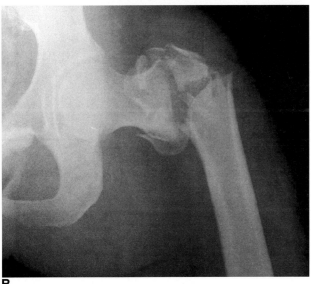

B

Fig. 10-20
A, Anteroposterior radiograph of this 44-year-old woman after a motor vehicle accident shows a two-part intertrochanteric fracture. Note old fracture of right ischium and inferior pubic ramus. **B**, A 42-year-old female pedestrian struck by vehicle. Anteroposterior radiograph shows four-part intertrochanteric fracture, with moderate comminution and coxa vara.

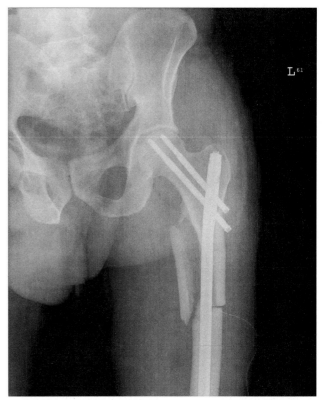

Fig. 10-21
Anteroposterior radiograph of a 51-year-old woman after motor vehicle accident shows subtrochanteric fracture.

so-called wedge or butterfly fragments (Fig. 10-23). It is important to understand that patients with severely comminuted fractures of the femoral shaft or distal femur also may have severely comminuted fractures of the proximal tibia or tibial shaft. One injury may mask the other initially, so the patient must be examined carefully (Fig. 10-24). Femoral shaft fractures often are treated with an

intramedullary rod or nail. The standard method of placement was to begin at the level of the greater trochanter and pass the rod distally (antegrade placement). The rod or nail also can be passed beginning at the intercondylar notch of the distal femur and proceeding proximally across the fracture site (retrograde placement).[11] Retrograde nailing has been reported as better for controlling distal femoral shaft fractures.[12]

Supracondylar and Intercondylar Fractures. Fractures of the distal femoral metaphysis may be transverse, separating the shaft from the condyles, but in high-energy trauma there is frequently extension of a fracture line into one or both condyles or the intercondylar notch, similar to that of the T- or Y-shaped fractures of the distal humerus (Fig. 10-25). Extension into one of the condyles usually means that the articular surface is involved. Involvement of the articular surface may be very subtle on initial anteroposterior and lateral radiographs. Oblique views can be helpful, but CT often is needed to acquire this important information (Fig. 10-26). CT also helps to identify the Hoffa fracture in supracondylar injuries. This is an additional coronal plane fracture that usually involves the lateral femoral condyle.[13] Isolated fractures involving either the medial or lateral femoral condyle are unusual.

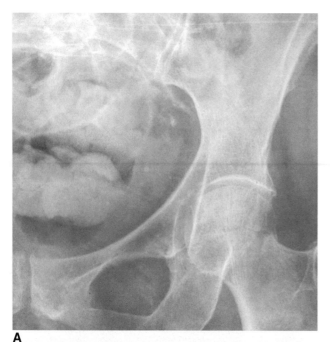

A

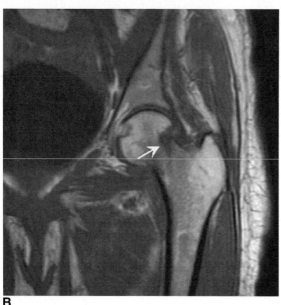

B

Fig. 10-22
A, An 81-year-old woman who fell. Initial anteroposterior radiograph shows apparent disruption of femoral neck cortex, suspicious for fracture. **B**, Coronal T1-weighted MR image shows linear low signal intensity area in femoral neck (*arrow*) diagnostic of fracture.

Knee Joint Dislocation

Knee joint dislocations can be limb threatening if there is damage to the popliteal artery. Popliteal artery injury has been reported in 16% to 80% of knee dislocations.[14] Nerve injuries are less common and usually are transient. Arterial injuries are more common, because the artery is fixed in its position above and below the joint. Above the joint, the artery is tethered as it passes through the adduc-

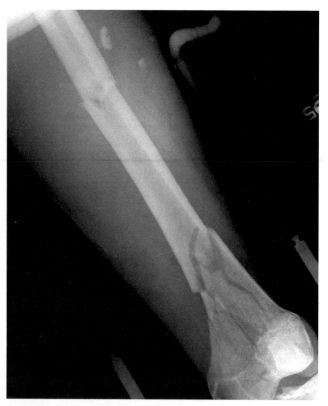

Fig. 10-23
A 39-year-old man after motor vehicle accident. Anteroposterior radiograph shows segmental femoral shaft fracture, with proximal and distal fractures isolating a segment of the midshaft.

tor canal, and below the joint the artery is fixed by its bifurcation or trifurcation. Knee dislocations are considered surgical emergencies[15] and must be evaluated quickly both clinically and radiologically. If there is a vascular injury, the limb salvage rate is 80% or greater when the injury is repaired within 8 hours. If the vascular injury repair is not done within 8 hours, the limb salvage rate is only 14%.[16] At UMSTC, when no pulses are detectable on initial evaluation, the patient is taken to the operating room and a single-injection angiogram is performed to determine the level of the vascular injury. If pulses are detectable on initial evaluation, a complete angiogram is done in the radiology angiographic suite to look for intimal tears or other signs of vascular injury as soon as the patient is stable enough to be transferred. CT angiography or MR angiography may have a role for vascular injury evaluation in the near future.

Anterior dislocations of the tibia (Fig. 10-27) are more common than posterior dislocations, and anterior dislocations are associated more often with popliteal artery injuries. Neither fractures of the femoral condyles or tibial plateau are seen commonly in association with knee dislocation. Soft tissue injuries are extensive in patients

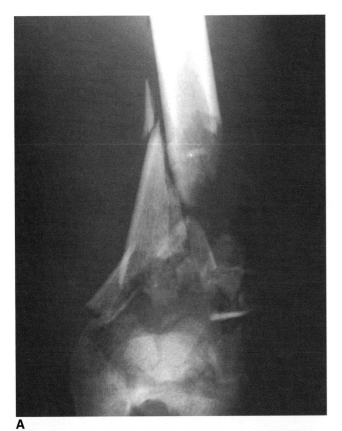

A

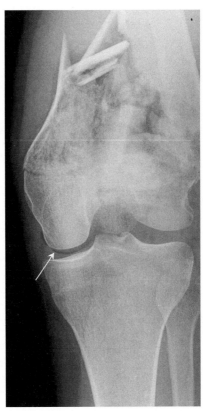

Fig. 10-25
A 38-year-old woman after motor vehicle accident. Anteroposterior radiograph shows severely comminuted fracture of distal femur. Extension to joint in intercondylar notch is subtle. Note gas in joint indicating that this is an open fracture (*arrow*).

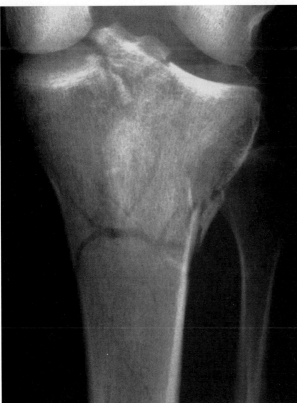

B

Fig. 10-24
A, Anteroposterior radiograph of a 26-year-old woman after motor vehicle accident shows severely comminuted, intraarticular fracture of distal femur. **B**, Anteroposterior radiograph shows severely comminuted fracture of proximal tibia, with extension through tibial plateau.

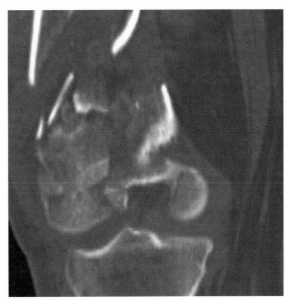

Fig. 10-26
Same patient as Fig. 10-25. Coronal CT reconstruction from multislice axial acquisition shows fracture line extending to joint.

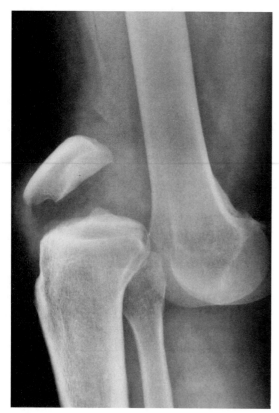

Fig. 10-27
Lateral radiograph of a 29-year-old man after motorcycle crash shows anterior dislocation of tibia. No fractures are noted.

with knee dislocation. The rule of thumb is that three of the four major ligament complexes (anterior cruciate, posterior cruciate, medial collateral, lateral collateral) will be injured in a patient with a knee dislocation. MR imaging is an excellent way to determine the extent of soft tissue injury, but it is not often done during the immediate posttrauma period (Fig. 10-28).

Tibial Plateau Fractures

Fractures of the tibial plateau are very common in patients who have sustained high-energy trauma. Segond fractures are seemingly insignificant avulsions of the lateral margin of the tibial plateau, but they are almost always associated with complete tears of the anterior cruciate ligament (Fig. 10-29). If a fat-fluid level (lipohemarthrosis) is evident on the initial cross-table lateral radiograph, then an intraarticular fracture probably is present and most commonly will involve the tibial plateau (Fig. 10-30). The Schatzker classification[17] is currently in use at UMSTC. It describes six types of tibial plateau fractures (Fig. 10-31). The first three types

describe lateral tibial plateau fractures. Type I is a simple split fracture, type II is a combination split-depression, and type III is a simple depression fracture. Type IV is any fracture of the medial tibial plateau. Type V is a fracture involving both the medial and lateral aspects of the tibial plateau. Type VI fractures have an additional metaphyseal component that results in separation of the tibial plateau from the shaft of the tibia. Any depression of the articular surface equal to the normal cartilage thickness of that articular surface is considered clinically significant.[18] Because the normal cartilage thickness of the tibial plateau is about 3 mm, any depression of 3 mm or more is significant. CT almost always is obtained at the UMSTC to define the full extent of the fracture and to look for gaps or depressions in the articular surface. MR imaging can be done to show associated soft tissue injuries and is considered as accurate as CT or conventional tomography for defining fracture extent.[19,20] Meniscal injuries requiring surgery were reported in 47% of patients in one series.[21]

Tibial plateau fractures are often the result of a valgus stress mechanism. This accounts for statements in the literature that 85% of tibial plateau fractures involve the lateral aspect of the plateau. The same proportionate involvement also is seen in high-energy trauma patients, with unpublished statistics from UMSTC showing 89% of 250 tibial plateau fractures involving the lateral side. Tibial plateau fractures usually are treated with lateral buttress plate and screw fixation devices.

Tibia and Fibula Shaft Fractures

Musculoskeletal injuries below the knee, specifically the lower leg, ankle, and foot, account for much of the morbidity in patients who survive high-energy trauma accidents (Dr. Andrew Burgess, personal communication, 2001.) Car safety design features over the last 10 years have improved greatly the protection of the head and torso and, therefore, the survivability of severe accidents. Safety features for the lower legs and feet are being developed.

Uncomplicated, closed fractures of the tibia have an average healing time of 6 months. Most tibia and fibula shaft fractures from high-energy trauma are comminuted, with a resultant increase in healing time. Delayed unions and nonunions are not uncommon.[22]

Classification schemes for tibia shaft fractures are numerous, but the Gustilo-Anderson (GA) system[23] has important clinical features and is the one favored at the UMSTC. It combines soft tissue and bone injury information. A GA type I fracture has no soft tissue injury or a clean laceration less than 1 cm in length, with a simple

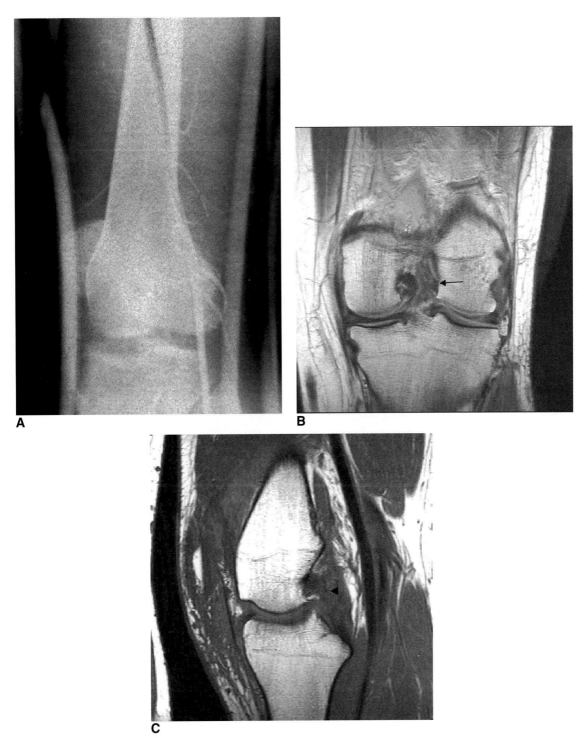

Fig. 10-28
Same patient as Fig. 10-27. **A**, Film from angiogram shows normal popliteal artery. **B** and **C**, MR images show tears of the anterior cruciate ligament (*arrow*), posterior cruciate ligament (*arrowhead*), medial collateral ligament, and lateral meniscus.

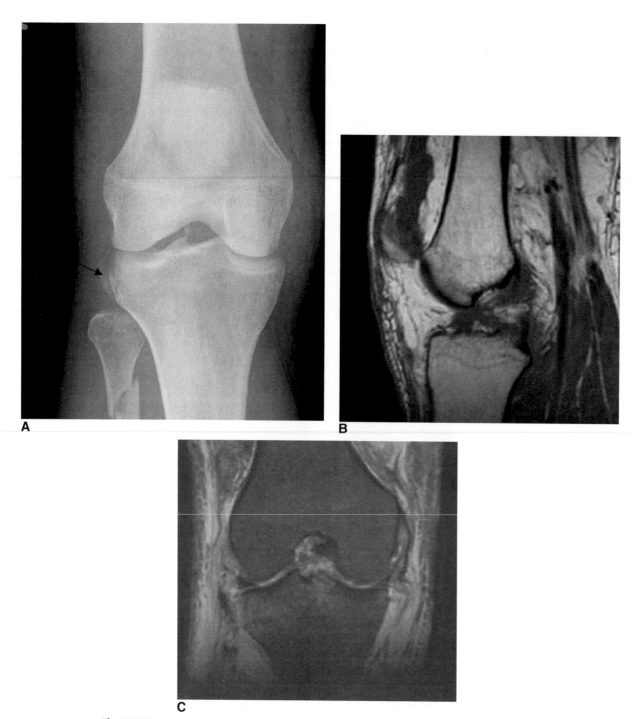

Fig. 10-29
A 39-year-old male pedestrian struck by a vehicle. **A,** Anteroposterior radiograph of the right knee shows Segond-type fracture at lateral edge of tibial plateau (*arrow*). **B,** Sagittal T1-weighted MR image shows complete midsubstance tear of anterior cruciate ligament. **C,** Coronal inversion recovery MR image shows Segond fracture fragment and absence of the anterior cruciate ligament. Patient also had a tear of the medial collateral ligament and popliteus.

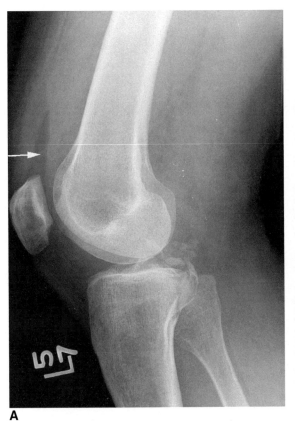
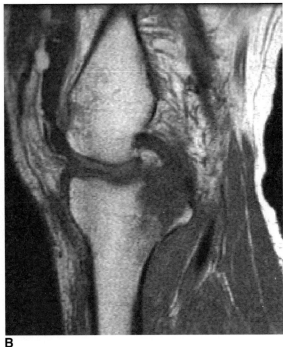

Fig. 10-30
A, Cross-table lateral radiograph shows several fracture fragments along posterior margin of tibia in a 43-year-old man after a motor vehicle accident. Note lipohemarthrosis with fat-fluid level (*arrow*).
B, Sagittal MRI shows avulsion of posterior cruciate ligament.

fracture of the tibia shaft (the type of fibula shaft fracture is not considered). A GA type II fracture has a soft tissue wound greater than 1 cm, with a minimally comminuted tibia shaft fracture. A GA type III fracture has a severe crush fracture and extensive soft tissue injury or vascular injury that will require grafting. Approximately two thirds of the open tibia fractures seen at the UMSTC are GA type III (Fig. 10-32). Because the nature of the soft tissue injury may not be evident on the radiographs, it is difficult for the radiologist to use this system. However, the radiologist should realize that the extent of soft tissue injury is critically important to the orthopedic surgeon. Comminuted tibia shaft fractures are treated with intramedullary rods or nails or with external fixators. The ideal method of treatment is controversial.[24,25] Intramedullary rods or nails are combined with "locking screws" in most cases. If fracture healing is delayed, one set of locking screws may be removed to "dynamize" the set-up in an attempt to cause further impaction of fracture fragments and, thus, promote healing. If dynamiza-

tion does not result in further healing, bone grafting is usually the next step. If a fibula shaft fracture is present, it often will heal before the tibia shaft fracture does. The healed fibula fracture may then act as a strut that "holds" the tibia fracture apart and delays healing of the tibia fracture. Partial resection of the fibula may be done to promote healing of the tibia fracture.

Lower leg injuries differ from forearm injuries with respect to double fractures or fracture-dislocation combinations. The tibia and fibula are not equal load-bearing struts like the radius and ulna; therefore, it is not uncommon to have a fracture of the tibia without a fracture (Fig. 10-33) or dislocation of the fibula.[26]

Ankle Fractures and Dislocations

The usual types of "twisted ankle" fractures may be seen in patients after high-energy trauma, but comminution or other foot and ankle injuries often result in complex injuries. The usual types of twisted ankle fractures are

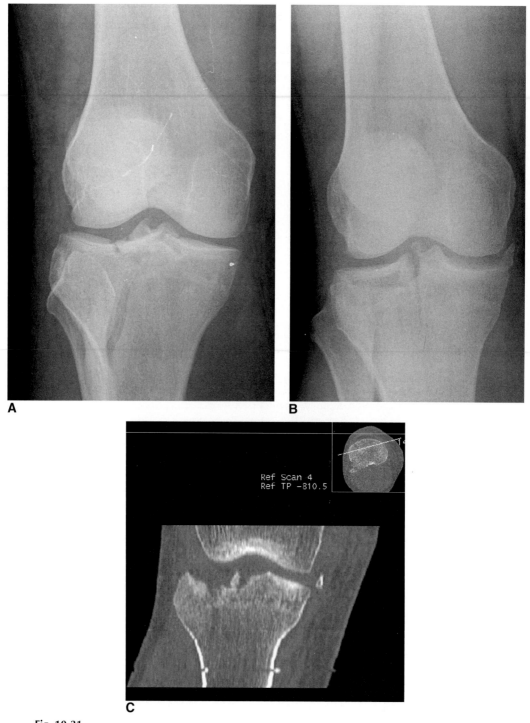

Fig. 10-31
Schatzker-type tibial plateau fractures. **A**, Type I simple split fracture. Anteroposterior radiograph (**B**) and CT (**C**) of type II split-depression fracture.

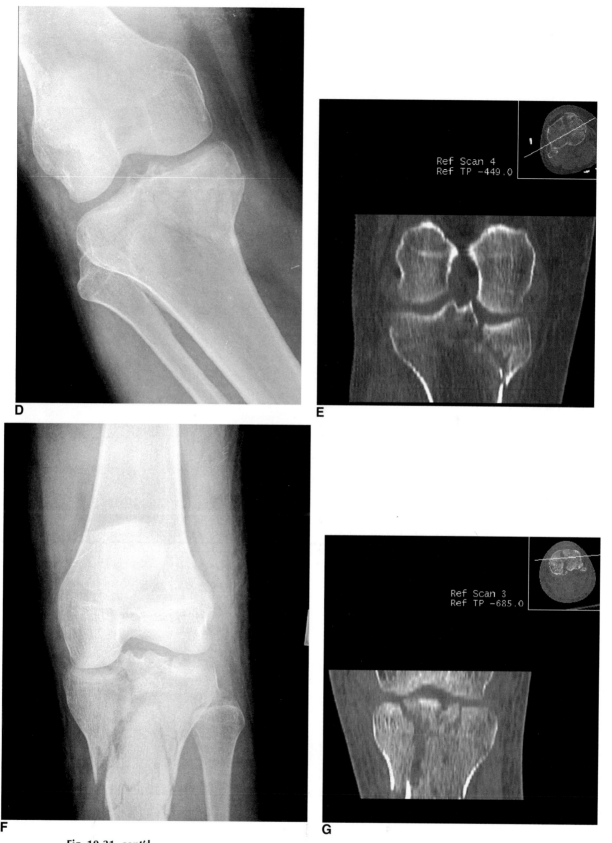

Fig. 10-31, cont'd
Anteroposterior radiograph (**D**) and CT (**E**) of type IV medial plateau fracture. Anteroposterior radiograph (**F**) and CT (**G**) of type V fracture showing both medial and lateral fractures.

Continued

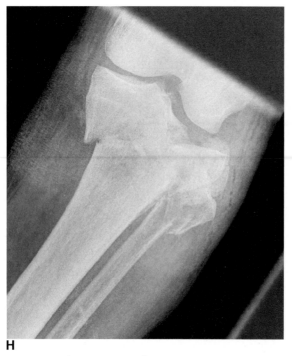

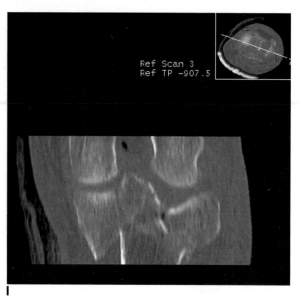

Fig. 10-31, cont'd
Radiograph (**H**) and CT (**I**) of type VI fracture showing metaphyseal component. (Type III—simple depression not shown.)

summarized in Fig. 10-34 and Table 10-2. The classification scheme of Lauge-Hansen is favored by radiologists, because it emphasizes a search method to identify all the possible fractures or ligament injuries (Fig. 10-35). The Danis-Weber (AO) classification scheme is nearly identical but is favored by orthopedists, because it emphasizes the need for surgery with certain fracture types.[27]

Pilon fractures are common with high-energy trauma. A pilon (pylon) fracture is any fracture that involves the horizontal portion of the distal tibia articular surface.[28] This surface is referred to as the plafond. Pilon is an architectural term that describes a stone archway. The ankle mortise, especially the plafond, has been likened to the architectural archway, thus the term *pilon fracture*. CT often is needed to determine the degree of comminution (Fig. 10-36). In one study, the CT information led to a change in the operative plan for 64% of patients.[29] Coronal and sagittal multiplanar reformation should be done to check for depression of fracture fragments or

	Fibula Fracture Location	Fracture Type/ Orientation	Radiograph Projection	Syndesmosis	Treatment for Fibula Fracture
SA (Weber A)	Below joint line	Transverse	AP	Intact	Closed reduction
SE (Weber B)	At joint line	Oblique/spiral	Lateral	Intact	Closed reduction
PA (Weber C1)	Just above syndesmosis	Oblique ML	AP	Disrupted	Surgical
PE (Weber C2)	Well above syndesmosis	Oblique AP	AP/lateral	Disrupted	Surgical

Table 10-2
Important Characteristics of Lauge-Hansen and Weber-Type Fractures

Modified from Mulligan ME: *Radiologist* 5:130, 1998.

AP, Anteroposterior; *ML*, mediolateral; *PA*, pronation-abduction; *PE*, pronation external rotation; *SA*, supination adduction; *SE*, supination external rotation.

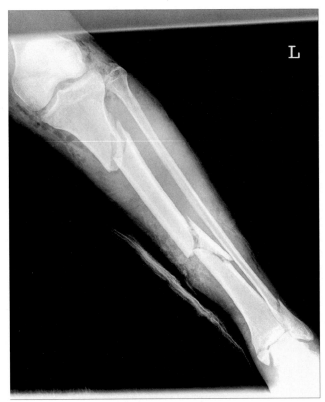

Fig. 10-32
A 53-year-old male pedestrian struck by vehicle. Anteroposterior radiograph shows open, segmental, comminuted tibia shaft fracture, Gustilo-Anderson type III. Note fractures of medial and lateral malleoli, as well.

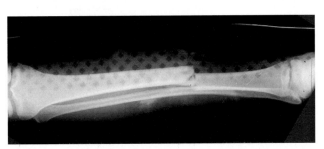

Fig. 10-33
Anteroposterior radiograph of a 16-year-old male pedestrian struck by a vehicle shows comminuted fracture of distal tibia with displacement of one half of shaft width but no fracture of fibula. Fibula is slightly bowed.

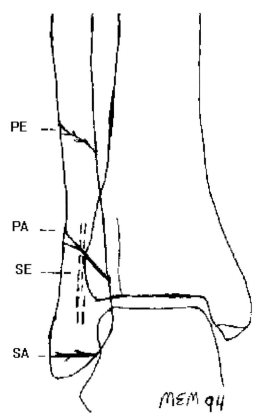

Fig. 10-34
Summary diagram of fibula fracture types. Lauge-Hansen supination adduction (SA or Weber A) is low transverse. Lauge-Hansen supination external rotation (SE or Weber B) is shown as dashed lines extending to tibiotalar joint line. Lauge-Hansen pronation abduction (PA or Weber C1) is oblique, just above level of tibiofibular syndesmosis. Lauge-Hansen pronation external rotation (PE or Weber C2) is several centimeters above joint line and may be as high as the midshaft of the fibula.

gaps of the articular surface. Isotropic multislice CT techniques have been described.[6] If multislice CT equipment is not available, direct axial and coronal imaging with thin overlapping sections should be done. Then, if the patient cannot be positioned for direct coronal sections, the thin overlapping axial sections should provide for adequate coronal and sagittal reconstructions. Any depression of the articular surface that measures more than 2 to 3 mm usually is considered significant, because that would represent a full-cartilage thickness in this location.

Ankle (talar) dislocations are usually posterior or posterolateral and are associated frequently with fractures of the malleoli. Subtalar and talonavicular dislocations also may be seen. In patients with subtalar dislocation, CT was reported to show additional injuries in all of the patients in one series. The new information resulted in a treatment change for nearly one half (44%) of the patients.[30]

Talar neck fractures are classified using the Hawkins system.[31] A Hawkins type 1 fracture is a nondisplaced fracture of the talar neck (Fig. 10-37). The risk of osteonecrosis of the talar dome, in these cases, is less than 10%. A Hawkins type 2 fracture is displaced slightly, with subluxation or dislocation of the subtalar joint but a normal tibiotalar joint. These cases have about a 40% chance of osteonecrosis. Hawkins type 3 fractures are displaced, with dislocation of the body of the talus from both the tibiotalar and subtalar joints (Fig. 10-38). The incidence of osteonecrosis is about 90%. The Canale-Kelly modification[32] of the Hawkins scheme includes a type 4 fracture that has an incidence of osteonecrosis that approaches 100%. The talar dome fragment is extruded, and the talar head is subluxed or dislocated at the talon-avicular joint (Fig. 10-39). The risk of osteonecrosis is high, because the major blood supply to the talus enters in the neck along the inferior surface. As in the wrist, with scaphoid fractures, it is the proximal fracture fragment that undergoes osteonecrosis. Posttraumatic osteoarthritis has been reported in more than 90% of patients who have displaced talar fractures.[33]

The calcaneus is the most commonly fractured tarsal bone in general trauma patients. In high-energy trauma, the fractures usually are comminuted with extension to the articular surfaces, most importantly to the posterior facet of the subtalar joint. If the patient has fallen from a significant height there may be associated compression fracture(s) in the spine. Additional fractures in the same leg or the opposite leg are seen with about the same frequency (10% to 15%) as an associated spine fracture. Subtle calcaneal fractures may be suspected by noticing a decrease in calcaneal height and in the Boehler angle on the lateral radiograph (Fig. 10-40). Boehler angle normally should not be less than 25 degrees. The amount of calcaneal flattening, quantified by the initial measurement of the Boehler angle, may have prognostic significance, with a poor outcome reported for patients with an initial angle of zero degrees or less.[34] Operative results also deteriorate as the number of articular fragments increases.[35]

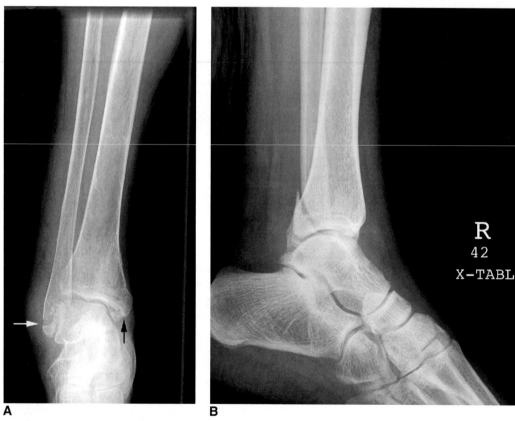

A   **B**

Fig. 10-35
Ankle fracture cases. **A**, Supination adduction (Weber A) (*arrow*) stage 2. Note low transverse fibula fracture (stage 1) and subtle fracture of medial malleolus (stage 2). **B**, Supination external rotation (Weber B) stage 2. Note short oblique distal fibula fracture (stage 2) extending to level of tibiotalar joint line. Stage 1 (not visible) is disruption of anterior inferior tibiofibular ligament. Stage 3 (posterior malleolar fracture) and stage 4 (medial malleolar fracture) not present in this patient.

Continued

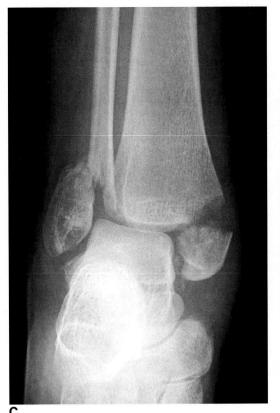

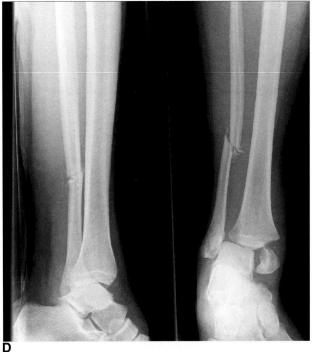

Fig. 10-35, cont'd
C, Posteroanterior (Weber C1) stage 3. Note transverse fracture of medial malleolus (stage 1) and oblique fracture of distal fibula (stage 3) that is just above level of the syndesmosis. There is lateral subluxation of the talus. Stage 2 (injury of the tibiofibular ligaments) is not visible. **D**, Pronation external rotation (Weber C2) stage 3. Note transverse fracture of medial malleolus (stage 1), widening of tibiofibular syndesmosis (stage 2), and high fibula fracture (stage 3). Stage 4 injury (fracture of posterior malleolus) was not present in this patient.

CT examinations are done with multislice technique, direct axial and coronal sectioning, or axial sectioning with MPR. Orthopedic surgeons at the UMSTC usually do not request sagittal plane imaging. On the axial or long-axis images of the calcaneus, the radiologist should assess the extent of comminution of the medial and lateral walls and extension to the calcaneocuboid joint surface (Fig. 10-41). The position of the peroneal tendons should be noted, because fracture fragments can entrap them. The coronal or short axis images are used to evaluate the subtalar joint surfaces (see Fig. 10-41). Comminution of the posterior facet and any depression or gap along the articular surface should be noted. The size of the sustentacular fracture fragment is important to the orthopedic surgeon. Extension to the articu-lar surfaces of the middle or anterior facet should be noted.

There are several classification schemes for calcaneal fractures, but none is universally accepted. The Sanders system[35] appears to address most of the important factors but is not complex enough to cover all fracture types encountered.

Midfoot and Forefoot Injuries

Isolated fractures of the other tarsal bones are infrequent. In high-energy trauma, they often are associated with subluxations or dislocations. The most important dislocations are the Chopart and Lisfranc types. A Chopart dislocation separates the talocalcaneal unit

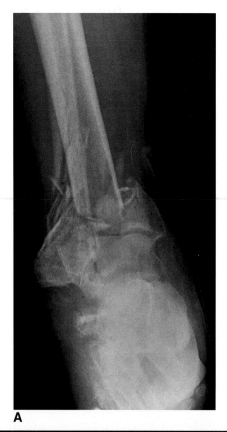

A

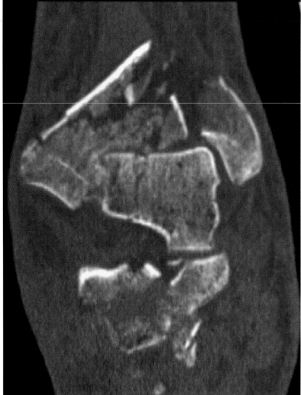

B

Fig. 10-36
Pilon fracture. **A**, Anteroposterior radiograph of a 66-year-old woman after a motor vehicle accident shows severely comminuted distal tibia and fibula fractures, with extension to articular surface of tibia. **B**, Coronal CT reconstruction shows articular surface involvement of distal tibia, as well as fracture of the talus and calcaneus.

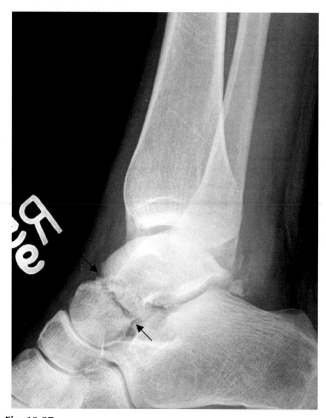

Fig. 10-37
A 43-year-old woman after motor vehicle accident. Lateral radiograph shows nondisplaced talar neck fracture (*arrows*) (Hawkins I).

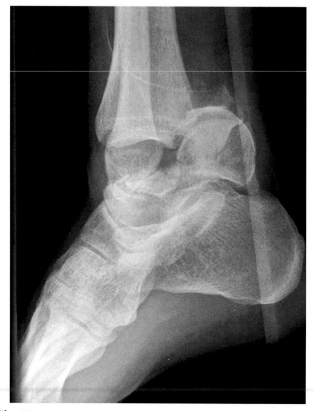

Fig. 10-38
Lateral radiograph of a 22-year-old woman after motor vehicle accident shows talar neck fracture, with complete dislocation of the body of the talus. Note normal relationship of talar head to navicular (Hawkins III).

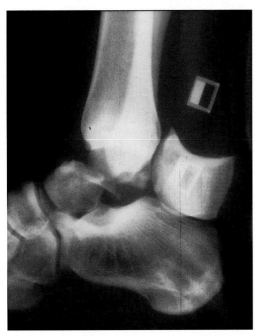

Fig. 10-39
Lateral radiograph of this 50-year-old woman after a motor vehicle accident shows talar fracture with marked subluxation of talar head and talar body (Hawkins IV).

from the navicular and cuboid (Fig. 10-42). The Lisfranc injury occurs at the tarsometatarsal junction. There are two major types of Lisfranc injury, homolateral and divergent (Fig. 10-43). In the homolateral type, all of the involved metatarsals are subluxed or dislocated laterally. In the divergent type, the first metatarsal is subluxed or dislocated medially with the other metatarsals subluxed or dislocated laterally. Lateral radiographs may show dorsal subluxations or dislocations of the metatarsals. CT or MR images may be done for further assessment.[36] With MR imaging, the Lisfranc ligament, itself, can be evaluated directly (Fig. 10-44). This may be necessary in subtle cases when the initial radiographic evaluations are inconclusive. Careful evaluation of the tarsometatarsal alignment on the initial radiographs usually results in a confident diagnosis.[37] The bases of the second and third metatarsals should align perfectly with the medial edges of their respective cuneiforms. Any misalignment at these joints is indicative of a Lisfranc injury (Fig. 10-45).

PENETRATING ORTHOPEDIC INJURIES

Penetrating injuries from gunshots and knives, unfortunately, are seen frequently at major urban trauma

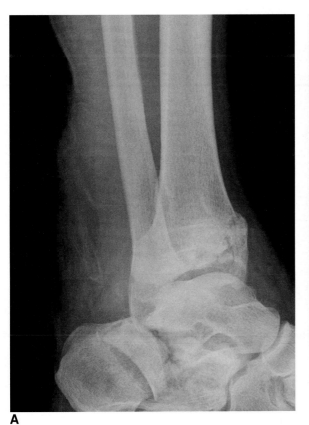

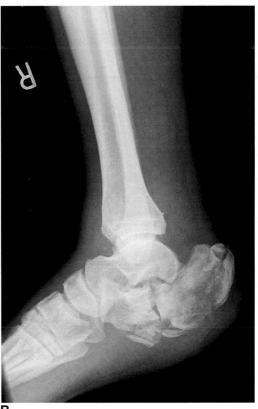

A   B

Fig. 10-40
A, Lateral radiograph shows calcaneal fracture with loss of height resulting in abnormal Boehler angle. **B**, Lateral radiograph shows calcaneal fracture with severe impaction resulting in a negative Boehler angle.

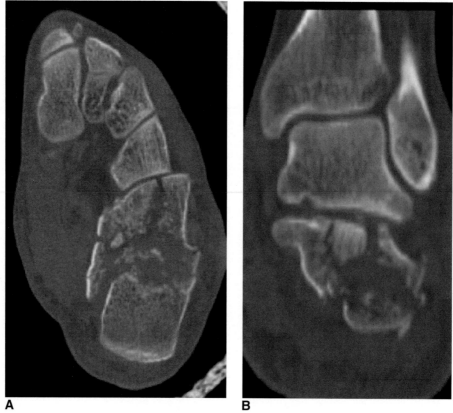

Fig. 10-41
A 37-year-old man fell 20 feet from a tree. **A**, Axial (long axis) CT section shows extension to calcaneocuboid joint. Note comminution of medial and lateral walls and perched peroneal tendons. **B**, Coronal (short axis) CT section shows involvement of posterior and middle facets of subtalar joint.

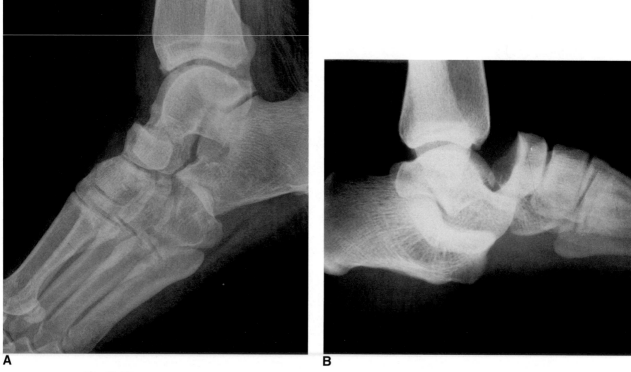

Fig. 10-42
Chopart injuries. **A**, Lateral radiograph shows dislocation at talonavicular and calcaneocuboid joints without fracture. **B**, A 38-year-old man after motorcycle crash. Lateral radiograph shows overlapping of talonavicular and calcaneocuboid joints, indicating Chopart injury.

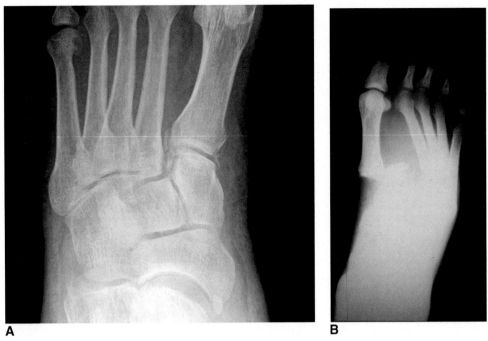

A **B**

Fig. 10-43
Lisfranc injuries. **A,** Posteroanterior radiograph shows lateral subluxations of tarsometatarsal joints (homolateral type). **B,** Posteroanterior radiograph shows medial dislocation of first tarsometatarsal joint with lateral subluxations of other tarsometatarsal joints (divergent type).

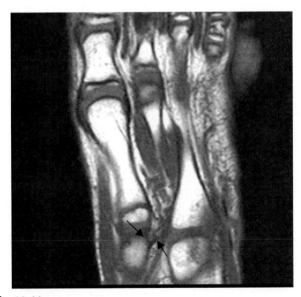

Fig. 10-44
Axial T1-weighted MR image shows intact Lisfranc ligament extending between lateral edge of medial cuneiform and base of second metatarsal (*arrows*).

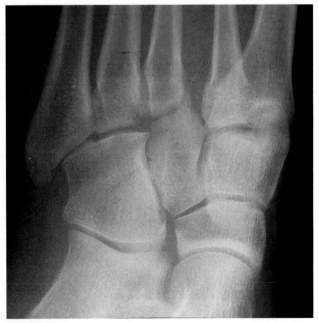

Fig. 10-45
Lisfranc injury. This 52-year-old man fell 40 feet. Posteroanterior radiograph shows subtle offset of third tarsometatarsal joint and small fracture fragments at base of first metatarsal. Note calcaneal fracture as well.

centers. Other projectiles or penetrating items also are encountered from time to time (Fig. 10-46). High-velocity weapons, like other causes of high-energy trauma, cause severely comminuted fractures with extensive soft tissue injury (Fig. 10-47). Low-velocity weapons may result in no fracture or only minimal fracture when the bullet hits the bone (Fig. 10-48). Shotgun injuries are distinguished by multiple similar-sized pellets (Fig. 10-49).

Regardless of the type of weapon or projectile that causes the injury, angiography may be needed to look for arterial injuries, especially when there is an expanding hematoma.

If gas is seen in the joint space near the site of a penetrating injury, contamination of the joint is assumed. Stabbing injuries sometimes result in small-chip fracture fragments along the edges of the osseous structures.

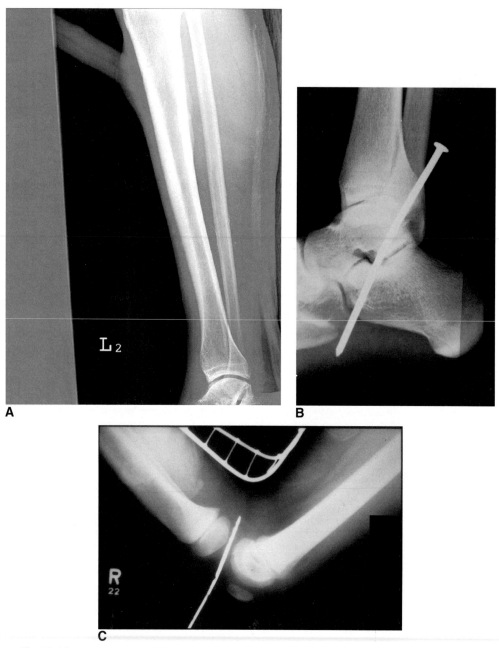

Fig. 10-46
Penetrating injuries. **A**, Lateral radiograph of a 43-year-old man after bicycle accident shows tree branch embedded in soft tissues of proximal leg. **B**, A 38-year-old woman. Lateral radiograph shows nail with tip embedded in calcaneus. **C**, Lateral radiograph of an 8-year-old boy shows mattress spring embedded in knee joint.

Continued

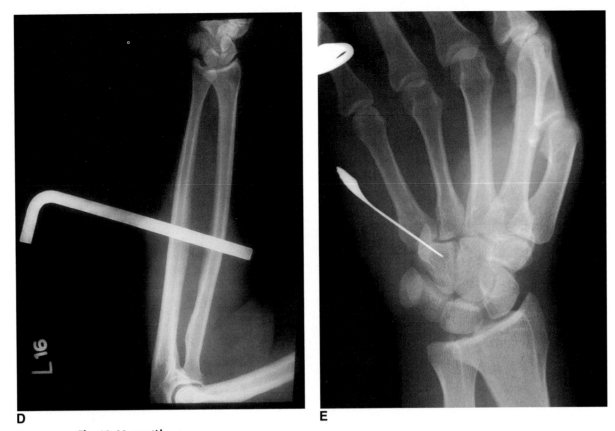

Fig. 10-46, cont'd
D, A 25-year-old man after motor vehicle accident. Anteroposterior radiograph shows Allen wrench embedded in soft tissues of forearm. **E**, Posteroanterior radiograph shows knife blade embedded in hamate.

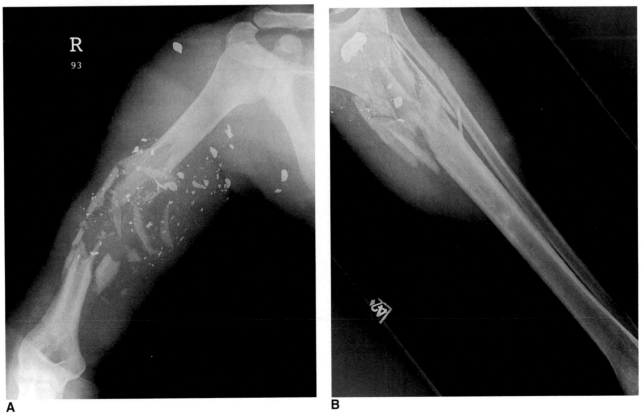

Fig. 10-47
High-velocity gunshot injuries. **A**, A 20-year-old man suffered a severely comminuted gunshot fracture of humerus. **B**, A 22-year-old man with a severely comminuted gunshot fracture of tibia.

Continued

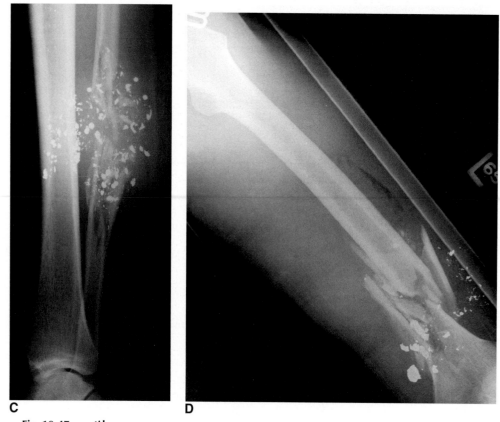

C **D**

Fig. 10-47, cont'd
C, Severely comminuted gunshot fracture of fibula in a 31-year-old man. **D**, Gunshot wound with comminution to femur.

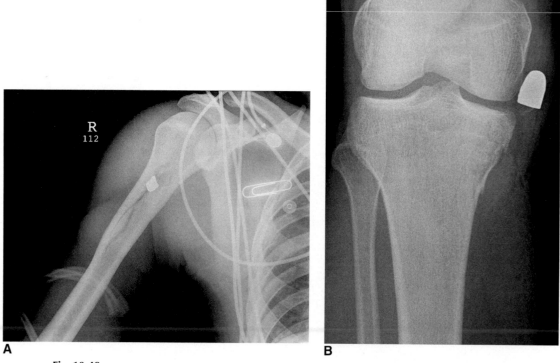

A **B**

Fig. 10-48
Low-velocity gunshot injuries. **A**, An 18-year-old man with a nondisplaced gunshot fracture of humerus. **B** and **C**, Anteroposterior and lateral radiographs of a 20-year-old man show a nondeformed bullet adjacent to medial femoral condyle. Note subtle fracture of medial tibial plateau and gas in joint.

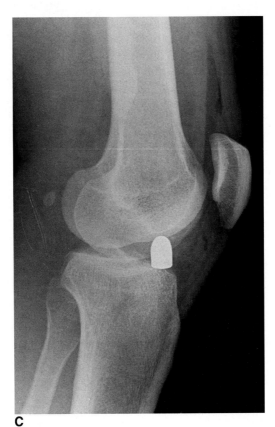

Fig. 10-48, cont'd
For legend see opposite page.

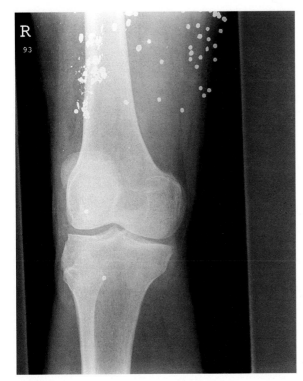

Fig. 10-49
Shotgun injury of lower leg.

Forensic information can be gleaned from the size, type, and number of bullet fragments but is beyond the scope of this chapter.[38-40]

REFERENCES

1. Brandser EA, Berbaum KS, Dorfman DD, et al: Contribution of individual projections alone and in combination for radiographic detection of ankle fractures, *AJR Am J Roentgenol* 174:1691, 2000.

2. Imatani RJ: Fractures of the scapula: a review of 53 fractures, *J Trauma* 15:473, 1975.

3. Harris RD, Harris JH Jr: The prevalence and significance of missed scapular fractures in blunt chest trauma, *AJR Am J Roentgenol* 151:747, 1988.

4. Rubenstein JD, Ebraheim NA, Kellam JF: Traumatic scapulothoracic dissociation, *Radiology* 157:297, 1985.

5. Sheafor DH, Mirvis SE: Scapulothoracic dissociation: report of five cases and review of the literature, *Emerg Radiol* 2:279, 1995.

6. Buckwalter KA, Rydberg J, Kopecky KK, et al: Musculoskeletal imaging with multislice CT, *AJR Am J Roentgenol* 176:979, 2001.

7. Goldberg HD, Young JWR, Reiner BI, et al: Double injuries of the forearm: a common occurrence, *Radiology* 185:223, 1992.

8. Nakamura R, Horii E, Imaeda T, Nakao E: Criteria for diagnosing distal radioulnar joint subluxation by computed tomography, *Skeletal Radiol* 25:649, 1996.

9. Gilula LA: Carpal injuries: analytic approach and case exercises, *AJR Am J Roentgenol* 133:503, 1979.

10. Cerezal L, Abascal F, Canga A, et al: Usefulness of gadolinium-enhanced MR imaging in the evaluation of the vascularity of scaphoid nonunions, *AJR Am J Roentgenol* 174:141, 2000.

11. Ricci WM, Bellabarba C, Evanoff B, et al: Retrograde versus antegrade nailing of femoral shaft fractures, *J Orthop Trauma* 15:161, 2001.

12. Leggon RE, Feldmann DD: Retrograde femoral nailing: a focus on the knee, *Am J Knee Surg* 14:109, 2001.

13. Baker BJ, Escobedo EM, Nork SE, Henley MB: Hoffa fracture: a common association with high-energy supracondylar fractures of the distal femur, *AJR Am J Roentgenol* 178:994, 2002.

14. Kendall RW, Taylor DC, Salvian AJ, O'Brien PJ: The role of arteriography in assessing vascular injuries associated with dislocations of the knee, *J Trauma* 35:875, 1993.

15. Wascher DC: High-velocity knee dislocation with vascular injury: treatment principles, *Clin Sports Med* 19:457, 2000.

16. Meyers MH, Moore TM, Harvey JP: Follow-up notes on articles previously published in the journal: traumatic dislocation of the knee joint, *J Bone Joint Surg Am* 57:430, 1975.

17. Schatzker J, McBroom R, Bruce D: The tibial plateau fracture: the Toronto experience, *Clin Orthop* 138:94, 1979.

18. Tscherne H, Lobenhoffer P: Tibial plateau fractures: management and expected results, *Clin Orthop* 292:87, 1993.

19. Kode L, Lieberman JM, Motta AO, et al: Evaluation of tibial plateau fractures: efficacy of MR imaging compared with CT, *AJR Am J Roentgenol* 163:141, 1994.

20. Barrow BA, Fajman WA, Parker LM, et al: Tibial plateau fractures: evaluation with MR imaging, *Radiographics* 14:553, 1994.

21. Vangsness CT, Ghaderi B, Hohl M, Moore TM: Arthroscopy of meniscal injuries with tibial plateau fractures, *J Bone Joint Surg Br* 76:488, 1994.

22. Oni OOA, Hui A, Gregg PJ: The healing of closed tibial shaft fractures, *J Bone Joint Surg Br* 70:787, 1988.

23. Gustilo RB, Mendoza RM, Williams DN: Problems in the management of type III (severe) open fractures: a new classification of type III open fractures, *J Trauma* 24:742, 1984.

24. Khalily C, Behnke S, Seligson D: Treatment of closed tibia shaft fractures, *J Orthop Trauma* 14:577, 2000.

25. Bhandari M, Guyatt GH, Swiontkowski MF, Schemitsch EH: Treatment of open fractures of the shaft of the tibia, *J Bone Joint Surg Br* 83:62, 2001.

26. Tschopp O, Stern RE: Bilateral fracture of the tibial shaft with intact fibulae, *Am J Orthop* 30:341, 2001.

27. Mulligan ME: Ankle fracture classifications clarified, *Radiologist* 5:127, 1998.

28. Helfet DL, Koval K, Pappas J, et al: Intraarticular "pilon" fracture of the tibia, *Clin Orthop Rel Res* 298:221, 1994.

29. Tornetta P, Gorup J: Axial computed tomography of pilon fractures, *Clin Orthop* 323:273, 1996.

30. Bibbo C, Lin SS, Abidi N, et al: Missed and associated injuries after subtalar dislocation: the role of CT, *Foot Ankle Int* 22:324, 2001.

31. Hawkins L: Fractures of the neck of the talus, *J Bone Joint Surg Am* 52:991, 1970.

32. Canale ST, Kelly FB: Fractures of the neck of the talus, *J Bone Joint Surg Am* 60:143, 1978.

33. Fortin PT, Balazsy JE: Talus fractures: evaluation and treatment, *J Am Acad Orthop Surg* 9:114, 2001.

34. Loucks C, Buckley R: Bohler's angle: correlation with outcome in displaced intra-articular calcaneal fractures, *J Orthop Trauma* 13:554, 1999.

35. Sanders R, Fortin P, DiPasquale T, Walling A: Operative treatment in 120 displaced intraarticular calcaneal fractures, *Clin Orthop* 290:87, 1993.

36. Preidler KW, Brossmann J, Daenen B, et al: MR imaging of the tarsometatarsal joint: analysis of injuries in 11 patients, *AJR Am J Roentgenol* 167:1217, 1996.

37. Norfray JF, Geline RA, Steinberg RI, et al: Subtleties of Lisfranc fracture-dislocations, *AJR Am J Roentgenol* 137:1151, 1981.

38. Wilson AJ: Gunshot injuries: what does a radiologist need to know? *Radiographics* 19:1358, 1999.

39. Hollerman JJ, Fackler ML, Coldwell DM, Ben-Menachem Y: Gunshot wounds. 2. Radiology, *AJR Am J Roentgenol* 155:691, 1990.

40. Messmer JM, Fierro MF: Radiologic forensic investigation of fatal gunshot wounds, *Radiographics* 6:457, 1986.

11 Angiography and Interventional Radiology in Trauma

Geoffrey S. Hastings

The use of angiography and interventional radiology (IR) in trauma is constantly changing and expanding. Computed tomography (CT), ultrasound, and other non-invasive modalities continually replace angiography in diagnosis, often providing more definitive information in the process. Meanwhile, the use of percutaneous image-guided interventions in the trauma patient is ever increasing so that, on balance, the interventional radiologist is more closely involved in the care of the trauma patient than ever before. This chapter will focus on trauma-related issues outside the head and neck, where the interventional radiologist has an important established or emerging role.

GENERAL COMMENTS
Personnel

Because of the emergent nature of trauma, prompt availability of the IR team and quick, decisive performance of appropriate therapeutic procedures are of paramount importance. An experienced or fellowship-trained interventionist is essential. A radiologic technologist who can anticipate or respond quickly to the equipment needs of the interventionist during the case is extremely helpful. Nurses who are familiar with trauma and able to provide proper physiologic monitoring and communicate the changing needs of the patient to the interventionist are indispensable, also. Coordination of efforts between referring clinicians and the IR team, with appropriate prioritization of which injuries need to be addressed first, is crucial. A hemodynamically unstable patient can test any or all of these elements; speed and simplicity are the keys to success.

Equipment

Angiographic equipment does not need to be state-of-the-art, but it should be in good working order and capable of at least 3 frames per second. Digital subtraction arteriography is very helpful, because it saves so much time. A C-arm also saves time and minimizes the need to move the injured patient. The angiographic room ideally should be located close to the emergency ward and operating rooms and be large enough to accommodate the additional ventilation, monitoring, and resuscitation equipment that tend to accompany the trauma patient. Disposable equipment should include the standard needles, catheters, and guide wires. Microcatheters (sub-3 French catheters introduced coaxially through the lumen of a standard catheter) are not absolutely essential but allow more precise localization and management of hemorrhage with less damage to tissue that is not targeted. Basic embolic materials, such as gelatin sponge (Gelfoam, Upjohn, Kalamazoo, MI), macrocoils (0.035- to 0.038-inch diameter), and microcoils (0.018-inch), should be readily available and familiar to radiologists and technologists, alike. Balloon occlusion catheters can be lifesaving when used to temporize bleeding from a large vessel that cannot be sacrificed.

Major Findings of Arterial Trauma

Much of IR in trauma concerns control of arterial hemorrhage, so it is important to recognize its four major radiographic findings. These findings may be seen in isolation or, more commonly, in combination with one another. Extravasation (Fig. 11-1) is the first and most familiar sign of arterial hemorrhage, seen as pooling of contrast that persists after venous washout. Occasionally, a subtraction artifact will masquerade as extravasation, but this can be sorted out by performing fluoroscopy over the area immediately after the run has finished. The second sign of hemorrhage is pseudoaneurysm (Fig. 11-2). Seen as an outpouching from the artery that may retain contrast briefly, this finding indicates a vessel rupture that is contained, frequently by only a thin layer of adventitia. It is a "smoking gun" of prior extravasation that heralds a potentially devastating hemorrhage if left untreated. The third sign of arterial injury is arteriovenous fistula (AVF) (Fig. 11-3) that represents simultaneous injury of an adjacent artery and vein, allowing the injured artery to decompress into the vein. But this explanation typically tells only part of the story, because there is frequently hemorrhage outside the vein that often forms enough of a hematoma to narrow the lumen of the vein. Because of the potential for ongoing hemorrhage or late development of symptoms from excessive flow, it is generally best to manage this in a manner similar to the other findings of arterial hemorrhage. Abrupt termination (Fig. 11-4) is the fourth and trickiest sign of arterial hemorrhage. It is easy to miss, especially when hidden in the midst of a territory with

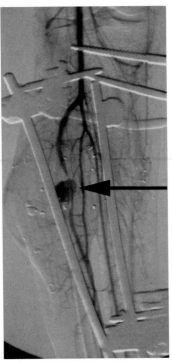

Fig. 11-2
Pseudoaneurysm. *Arrow* indicates outpouching arising from the anterior tibial artery. This patient received a gunshot wound to the leg, which was managed with debridement and external fixation. Weeks later he developed a pulsatile mass in this area, managed by placement of coils in the anterior tibial artery distal and proximal to the pseudoaneurysm. (From Mattox KL, Feliciano DV, Moore EE, eds: *Trauma*, ed 4, New York, 2000, McGraw-Hill.)

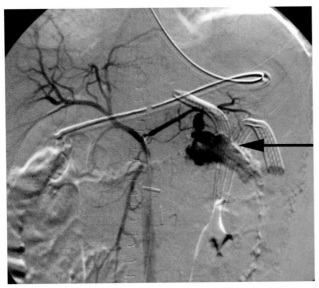

Fig. 11-1
Extravasation. *Arrow* indicates extravascular puddle of contrast arising from the splenic artery in the vicinity of surgical drains. This patient was the victim of a stab wound to the abdomen. The surgeon was unable to control bleeding due to difficult posterior retroperitoneal exposure. Bleeding was subsequently halted with coil embolization.

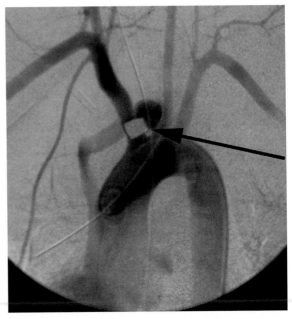

Fig. 11-3
Arteriovenous fistula. Note simultaneous opacification of great vessels and central veins. *Arrow* indicates bullet lodged in the mediastinum causing a direct communication between the brachiocephalic artery and vein. Managed by surgical interposition graft.

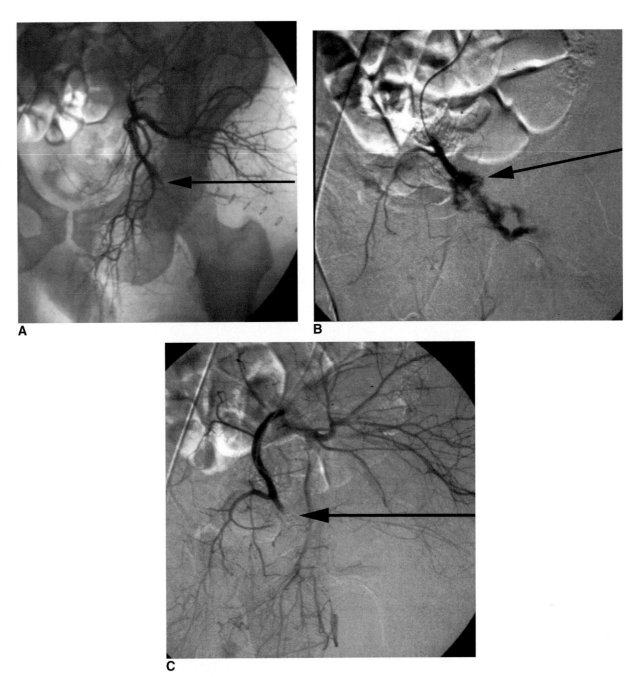

Fig. 11-4
Abrupt termination. **A,** Catheter tip in left internal iliac artery; *arrow* indicates abrupt termination of left inferior gluteal artery. **B,** As noted in the text, this finding carries a differential diagnosis, but its true nature is revealed upon selective injection of the inferior gluteal artery, whereupon there is extravasation of contrast indicated by the *arrow*. **C,** Appearance after embolization with coils, which can be seen faintly where indicated by the *arrow*.

complex or unpredictable branching, such as the pelvis, liver, or spleen. Moreover, abrupt termination is a finding that carries a differential diagnosis that includes both hemorrhagic lesions (such as vessel avulsion or spasm related to downstream hemorrhage), occlusive ones (such as traumatic dissection, embolization), and simple spasm. The clinical picture or a more selective angiogram typically gives clues to the real nature of the lesion. If in doubt in a trauma setting, it generally is best to manage this as a

hemorrhagic lesion. Venous and capillary hemorrhage can be very significant but generally are quite difficult to diagnose or manage percutaneously.

Endovascular Control of Hemorrhage: Tools of the Trade

The principal means by which the interventional radiologist controls hemorrhage is intentional transcatheter occlusion of a bleeding artery, or embolization. The goal of embolization is to stop bleeding completely from the injured artery without causing end-organ ischemia or allowing embolic material to go to a nontarget area. The consequences of nontarget embolization (NTE) vary with territory, which weighs into risk-versus-benefit decision making whenever embolotherapy is considered. In the central nervous system, NTE can be devastating; in the kidney, NTE simply results in more parenchymal loss; in the liver or spleen, most NTE is well tolerated; and in the pelvis, some NTE is desirable to prevent back-bleeding from collateral vessels. Whenever it is possible to gain access to the vessel both proximal and distal to the injury, such as in many pseudoaneurysms and AVFs, embolization should be carried out in both places, bridging the lesion and, thus, preventing back-bleeding from collateral vessels.

There are multiple options for embolic materials, each with its own characteristics of size, durability, and cost as detailed in Table 11-1. Small particles (rarely used in trauma) travel distally within the arterial tree, occluding small branches and leaving little opportunity for collateral flow. Thus, the risk of back-bleeding is low but the risk of ischemia is high. Conversely, large materials, such as coils, occlude proximally and are equivalent to surgical ligation, with little risk of ischemia but often a substantial risk of back-bleeding. Coils are useful when the injury involves a larger arterial branch, when the catheter has been negotiated distally enough that there is little

potential for collateral flow, or to "top off" and add durability to an embolization done primarily with temporary, small, or intermediate-size particles. Intermediate-size materials, such as Gelfoam, provide a good balance of characteristics and are often the agents of choice in trauma. Gelfoam can be delivered either as individual 2- to 3-mm pledgets, or more quickly and conveniently as slurry. Slurry is made by cutting the material into small chunks, placing these in a syringe, drawing up contrast material, and sloshing the mixture back and forth between two syringes through a stopcock until a thin paste is formed. Permanent occlusion is typically not necessary for durability in trauma. Materials that degrade over days to weeks work well, because the arterial injury generally will heal before recanalization. Cost is seldom considered in the heat of the moment, but it is helpful to use less expensive materials, because substantial quantities often are required to achieve the desired result. Gelfoam and metallic coils suffice for most trauma situations (Fig. 11-5).

Coils of 0.035- or 0.038-inch caliber or Gelfoam can be delivered through any standard angiographic catheter of appropriate inner diameter and not made of polyurethane. If the desired position cannot be achieved with a standard catheter, a flexible microcatheter can be placed coaxially through the standard catheter and negotiated into a more selective position, as shown in Fig. 11-6. This allows more precise embolization, but the additional time required may not be acceptable with an

Table 1-1
Comparison of Embolic Materials

Material	Size	Durability	Cost	Comments
Gelfoam	Intermediate	Temporary	Low	Agent of choice for most VIR in trauma; can use individual 2- to 3-mm pledgets or (more easily) make slurry
Coils	Large to intermediate	Permanent	Low to intermediate	Available in variety of sizes and shapes, often fiber-coated for increased thrombogenicity; macrocoils (0.035- or 0.038-inch) or microcoils (0.018-inch) are delivered by pushing through catheter with guide wire; very useful in trauma
Autologous clot	Intermediate	Temporary	Free	Oldest agent, always available
Detachable balloons	Large	Permanent	High	Useful in head and neck and where very precise placement and avoiding distal embolization while vessel clots are necessary; can bridge AVFs and pseudoaneurysms; finicky; not all FDA approved
Polyvinyl alcohol particles	Intermediate to small	Permanent	Intermediate	Manufactured by shaving a block of polyvinyl alcohol plastic and sorting the shavings by size; limited applicability in trauma
Cyanoacrylate glue	N/A	Permanent	Very high	High cost without properties to justify its use in most trauma settings

VIR, Venous interventional radiology; *AVFs,* arteriovenous fistulas; *FDA,* Food and Drug Administration; *N/A,* not available.

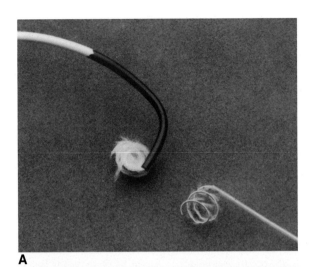

A

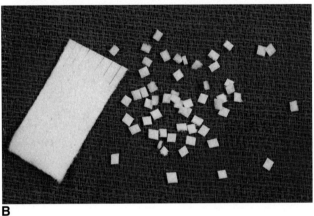

B

Fig. 11-5
Coils and Gelfoam, the mainstays of embolization in trauma. **A,** Two types of coils: macrocoils on the left measure 0.035 or 0.038 inch and are introduced via a conventional angiographic catheter. Microcoils on the right are introduced via a microcatheter that is used with a 0.014- to 0.018-inch guide wire. **B,** Gelfoam comes packaged in a small, thick sheet. After dicing, it can be used in one of two ways. Individual cubes can be injected as pledgets straight through the catheter. Alternatively, the cubes can be tamped down in a syringe, combined with contrast, and mixed into a slurry by passing it vigorously between two syringes. This slurry is injected until hemostasis is achieved. (From Mattox KL, Feliciano DV, Moore EE, eds: *Trauma,* ed 4, New York, 2000, McGraw-Hill.)

unstable patient. It is important to remember that the ability of almost all embolic materials to halt blood flow relies on the body's ability to make clot. When there is excessive blood loss or hypothermia, clotting ability may be impaired. Faced with this scenario, it is advisable to pack the artery as full as possible with embolic materials to cause a mechanical blockade, while simultaneously correcting coagulopathy and thrombocytopenia with appropriate blood products.

Occlusive lesions also occur in trauma patients. Spasm is very common and typically manifests as a segmental or beaded narrowing but can cause complete occlusion. Intimal injury can cause an appearance of

minimal luminal irregularity, with or without a visible flap, or may cause flow-limiting narrowing or even complete occlusion. Thrombus may form at an area of vascular injury and embolize downstream. Occasionally, ballistic fragments may enter a vessel and embolize to a remote location and cause ischemic symptoms there. Additionally, preexisting atherosclerotic occlusive disease can affect management planning.

Although much less common than embolization, angioplasty and endovascular stent or stent-graft placement can be useful in trauma—for both occlusive and hemorrhagic lesions. Stents and stent-grafts typically are reserved for situations in which preservation of flow is critical and surgical exposure is difficult or hazardous or the patient is particularly fragile. Such devices have been used in the thoracic aorta,[1-8] abdominal aorta,[9-13] and femoral,[14,15] subclavian,[16-24] innominate,[25,26] carotid,[27] and vertebral injuries.[28] These devices have been used mostly in acute injuries, but also in subacute[6] and chronic[4,6] situations, mostly for hemorrhagic lesions and less frequently for occlusive ones.[2,13] Success rates have been very high, but long-term follow-up is lacking. Stenoses and occlusions have occurred months after stent-graft placement,[6,21,23,29] more frequently with polyester than with polytetrafluoroethylene (PTFE). However, these results should be interpreted with caution, because most are case reports and small series; prospective clinical trials are ongoing.

THORAX

Traumatic rupture of the aorta (TRA) results when rapid chest deceleration and compression induces sufficient torsional and shearing forces at the junction of fixed and mobile segments of the aorta to cause a laceration and subsequent rupture.[30] Seventy percent result from motor vehicle crashes, with the remainder due to falls, blast injury, or other mechanisms. The injury is rapidly fatal in approximately 80% to 90% of victims, but the majority who survive the initial event can be managed successfully with prompt diagnosis and appropriate therapy.[31] The natural history of TRA without surgical repair is unclear. Older data obtained before definitive antemortem diagnosis was routinely available indicate a progressive increase in mortality from 32% after 24 hours to 90% within 4 months.[32] However, recent management algorithms have shown excellent outcomes in series that include patients in whom repair was deferred until stabilization of associated injuries or not performed at all.[33,34]

TRA occurs in three anatomic areas. The most common is the proximal descending aorta, accounting for approximately 80% (Fig. 11-7). This entity has a range of appearances, some examples of which are shown in Fig. 11-8. Rupture of the ascending aorta (Fig. 11-9) accounts for approximately 20% in autopsy series. Because it was

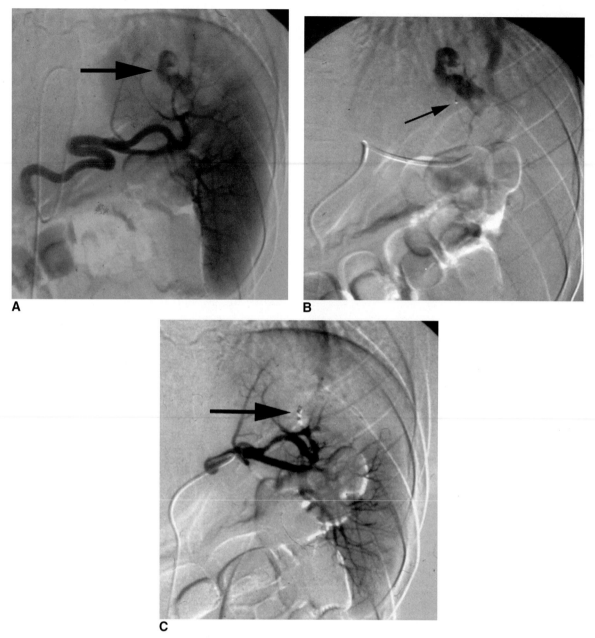

Fig. 11-6
Microcatheters allow more precise embolization, sparing nontarget normal parenchyma. **A**, Approximately 1 week after splenic trauma, a pseudoaneurysm developed, indicated by an *arrow* on an image from a splenic arteriogram. Advancing a conventional diagnostic catheter into the injured branch would be difficult or impossible, but a flexible microcatheter can be introduced coaxially within the conventional catheter and negotiated over a micro guide wire as superselectively as desired. **B**, The radiopaque dot at the end of the microcatheter is indicated by an arrow. **C**, After embolization with microcoils (*arrow*), flow to the pseudoaneurysm is halted, sacrificing only the tiniest amount of viable splenic parenchyma.

almost invariably fatal, rupture of the ascending aorta was essentially absent from the surgical literature before the 1990s. Since then, however, there is a growing number of reports of survivors of ascending TRA with subsequently successful surgical repair.[35-45] It has been speculated that this observation may be "due to a change in trauma mechanics (i.e., speed limits, seat belts, air bags), an improvement in diagnostic tools or both."[43] The least common site of TRA is the diaphragmatic hiatus.[46] Less than one half of patients with TRA have physical findings to suggest the diagnosis, and one third have no external evidence of trauma. Thus, diagnosis begins with clinical suspicion in a patient with an appropriate mechanism of injury and proceeds with imaging.

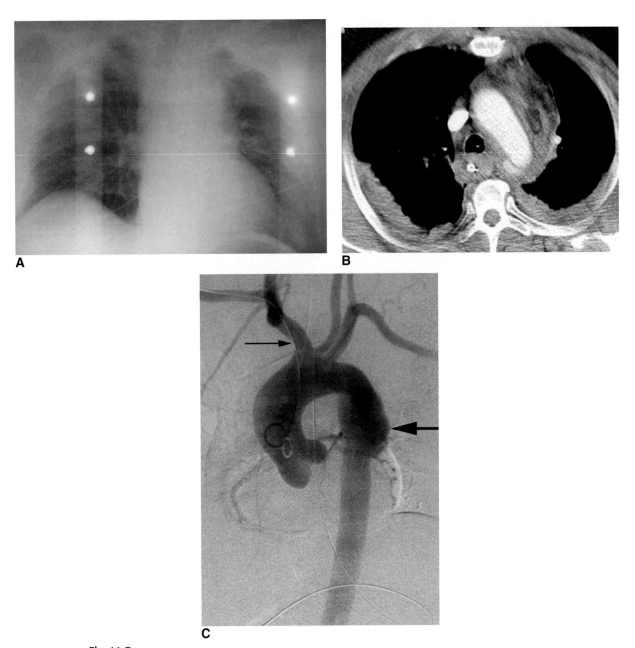

Fig. 11-7
Traumatic rupture of the aorta. **A,** Chest radiograph of victim of motor vehicle crash demonstrates findings suspicious for aortic trauma including wide, indistinct mediastinum. **B,** Chest CT demonstrates findings of mediastinal hemorrhage, with *arrow* indicating an abnormal contrast collection outside the main aortic lumen. **C,** *Large arrow* indicates pseudoaneurysm due to rupture of the proximal descending aorta. This patient had markedly diminished femoral pulses, a result of pseudocoarctation or compression of the aortic lumen by the pseudoaneurysm and surrounding tissues, necessitating a right axillary approach for the aortogram. *Small arrow* indicates angiographic catheter. (Courtesy Shelley Marder, MD.)

Imaging begins with a chest radiograph and then proceeds to a more definitive diagnostic modality, namely aortography or spiral CT. Specific chest radiograph and CT findings of TRA are discussed elsewhere in this text (Chapter 5), but it is worth noting that one in nine patients whose chest radiographs demonstrate suspicious findings will have a final diagnosis of TRA.[31] However, patients with suspected *ascending* TRA should be approached with greater caution, because it is estimated that the mediastinal silhouette is normal in 43% of patients with ascending aortic rupture.[37] Until recent years, aortography was considered the only standard way

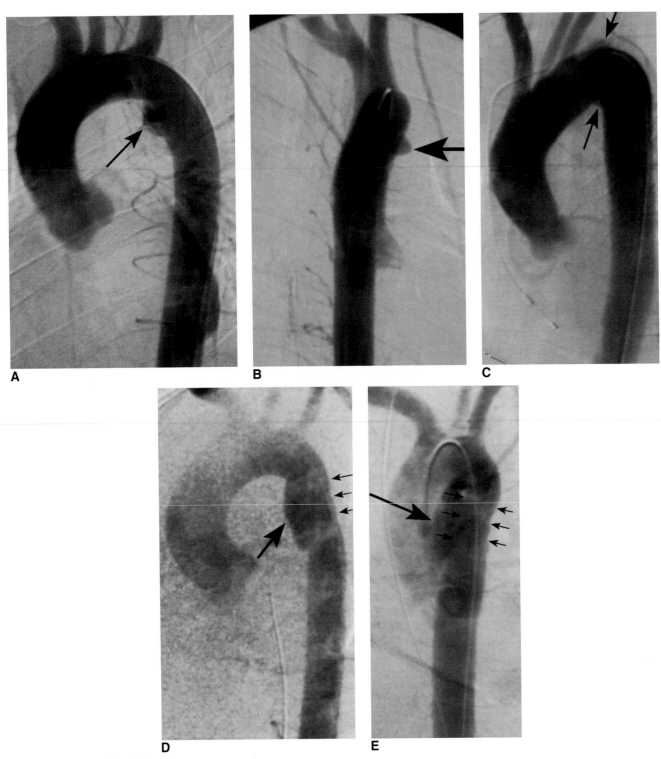

Fig. 11-8
Range of appearances of traumatic rupture of the proximal descending thoracic aorta. **A,** Classic appearance of a pseudoaneurysm (*arrow*) along the inside curve of the proximal descending thoracic aorta in left anterior oblique projection. **B,** Same patient as (**A**), right anterior oblique projection, with focal pseudoaneurysm again indicated by *arrow.* **C,** Elderly patient with nearly circumferential pseudoaneurysm indicated by *arrows.* **D** and **E,** The pseudoaneurysm of traumatic rupture of the aorta can narrow the adjacent lumen. *Large arrows* indicate the pseudoaneurysm, and *small arrows* show the narrowed adjacent lumen. (**A** from Mattox KL, Feliciano DV, Moore EE, eds: *Trauma,* ed 4, New York, 2000, McGraw-Hill.)

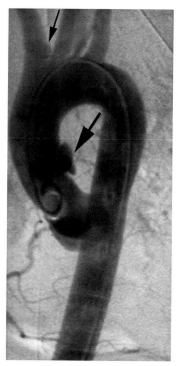

Fig. 11-9

Ascending aortic rupture. *Large arrow* indicates point of aortic injury, and *small arrow* indicates an associated brachiocephalic artery pseudoaneurysm. As noted in the text, decades ago such injuries were reported almost exclusively in autopsy series but are appearing with increasing frequency in surgical and imaging series for unclear reasons. Not uncommonly, chest radiographs on such patients will lack the mediastinal findings that trigger further workup.

to evaluate TRA, but it has been replaced by spiral CT in most cases in a growing number of centers. CT has the advantage that it is noninvasive, usually more rapidly available than angiography, and yields a wealth of information about associated injuries. Transesophageal echo (TEE) has been used by some in an effort to provide a diagnosis without moving the patient[39,42,43] but is best considered investigational, because there are concerns regarding the ability of TEE to adequately evaluate the ascending aorta and great vessels.[43] In centers where spiral CT for TRA is well established, negative findings ends the workup, and a definitely positive CT result often provides enough information for surgical planning. Aortography is reserved for cases in which CT findings are equivocal or there is uncertainty regarding specific anatomic findings crucial to surgical planning, such as great vessel involvement.

Thoracic aortography is accomplished by inserting a pigtail catheter with multiple side holes into the ascending aorta. This usually is done via a femoral approach, but an upper extremity approach can be advantageous for pseudocoarctation (narrowing of the aorta due to compression from surrounding pseudoaneurysm; see

Figs. 11-7 and 11-8) or other cause of diminished femoral pulses. Using intraarterial digital subtraction angiography, a 2-second contrast injection is filmed at 3 or more exposures per second. The contrast volume necessary for adequate opacification varies from one patient to another. High-quality images usually can be obtained with a standard 20 ml per second for a 40-ml total injection (higher for cut film), others (especially young healthy males) may require as much as 50 ml per second for a total of 100 ml, so that a 6- or 7-French catheter may be needed instead of the usual 5-French catheter. Bilateral oblique projections generally suffice for diagnosis, but ambiguous findings should be clarified with additional views or repositioning the catheter to the level of the left subclavian artery, or both.

Normally, the thoracic aortic contour is smooth and regular throughout. The pseudoaneurysm of TRA appears as an abrupt, often angulated and irregular outpouching that most commonly is located along the anteromedial wall of the proximal descending aorta. The outpouching may be localized, multilobular, or circumferential and sleevelike (see Figs. 11-7 and 11-8). A flap seen as a curvilinear lucency may be identified between the normal lumen and the pseudoaneurysm. Although distinguishing between TRA and a normal study result is usually straightforward, there are diagnostic pitfalls. The most common cause for confusion is called a *ductus bump* (Fig. 11-10), a smoothly contoured, symmetric bulge along the anteromedial surface of the proximal descending aorta in the region of the embryonic ductus arteriosus. Its most important distinguishing features are the obtuse angle its margins make with the adjacent aorta and the absence of retained contrast after the aorta has washed out. With increasing size and angulation, this entity is known as a *ductus diverticulum*, and in rare cases it cannot be distinguished angiographically from TRA.[31] Another pitfall, an ulcerated plaque (Fig. 11-11), is seen as an acutely angulated, irregular outpouching from the aorta. It generally occurs in older individuals with surrounding luminal irregularity typical of atherosclerotic disease. Helpful features are that the caliber of the aorta at the level of the ulcerated plaque is usually normal or enlarged, whereas the lumen at the level of a TRA may be narrowed by compression. Also, ulcerated plaques may occur anywhere in the aorta, whereas TRA typically occurs in the first few centimeters of the descending aorta. Correlation with CT frequently will eliminate any persistent uncertainty. Chronic TRAs can have a variety of appearances, which cannot always be distinguished from acute TRAs.[31] But the distinction is not always important. When the trauma is remote, most advocate surgical repair, but others advocate observation by repeat CT in asymptomatic, densely calcified aneurysms.[47]

As the use of angiography in the diagnosis of TRA diminishes with the advent of spiral CT, the role of IR in

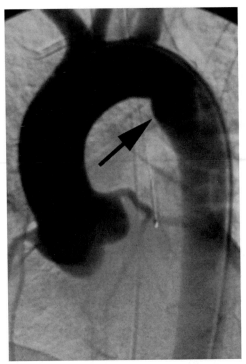

Fig. 11-10
Ductus bump. This normal variant is seen as a smooth, anteromedial bulge in the proximal descending thoracic aorta indicated by the *arrow*. Note that the angle formed between this bulge and the adjacent aorta is obtuse, whereas a rupture tends to form an acute angle. In real time, this segment of the aorta washes out at the same rate as the remainder of the aorta, as opposed to an aortic rupture which often retains contrast for a short time. (From Mattox KL, Feliciano DV, Moore EE, eds: *Trauma,* ed 4, New York, 2000, McGraw-Hill.)

endovascular repair of TRA, such as that seen in Fig. 11-12, is reported increasingly.[1-8] The potential advantages of endovascular over open surgical repair include lowered incidence of postoperative paraplegia and the ability to treat patients for TRA earlier in their hospital course, before fully managing associated injuries. Procedural success rates have been very high, with complications being mostly relatively minor and easily managed. Intermediate-term follow-up has also been favorable. To date, these reports have consisted of case reports and small case series with a variety of devices and should, therefore, be interpreted with caution. Within the next few years, reports of ongoing prospective clinical trials should become available, yielding a more credible assessment of this emerging technology.

ABDOMEN

The current status of angiography and IR in abdominal trauma exemplifies its evolving role in trauma. In diagnosis, angiography has been replaced largely by CT,[31] but there is increasing use of embolization as an alternative or supplement to operative control of hemorrhage or traditional nonoperative management.

Identifying three different scenarios will help in understanding this.

1. Embolization may be used as up-front management in hemodynamically stable or unstable patients with arterial injuries when surgery is less likely to have a favorable outcome. A classic example of this is a patient with pelvic fractures (discussed in the next section); this approach has shown promise, also, in high-grade liver injuries.

2. Embolization often is very effective when arterial hemorrhage cannot be controlled with operative maneuvers. Patients sometimes are referred on an emergency basis direct from the operating room, with arterial injuries deep within hepatic parenchyma which are difficult to localize and ligate.

3. Embolization also can be used to augment nonoperative management of hemodynamically stable patients with solid organ injuries, an area that has received considerable attention in recent years. As opposed to traditional nonoperative management in which a patient with a known solid organ injury is observed closely with rapid availability of diagnostic (usually CT) and treatment (usually surgical) modalities in case of deterioration, this augmented nonoperative management seeks to identify patients with arterial injuries early and manage them with embolization.

Several difficult issues arise in the course of such a pursuit, including the following:

1. Because arteriography is expensive and invasive it is desirable to have screening criteria to select those most likely to have an arterial injury. What screening modality and findings should be used, and how predictive are they?

2. How reliable is angiography for detecting arterial injury?

3. How much does this preemptive embolization improve outcomes? This last question is particularly difficult, because a reliable answer can come only from a prospective, randomized trial of a sort that would be difficult to justify or carry out in the acute trauma setting.

Spleen

At one time, splenectomy was performed routinely for significant splenic trauma, but "the traditional view of the spleen as an expendable organ is no longer tenable"[48] because splenectomy increases the risk of septic morbidity and mortality.[49,50] Because of this view, several strategies have been developed to salvage splenic function. These have included nonoperative management, splenorrhaphy[51] and, when splenectomy is unavoidable, heterotopic splenic autotransplantation.[52] The interventional radiologist has added splenic artery embolization to this

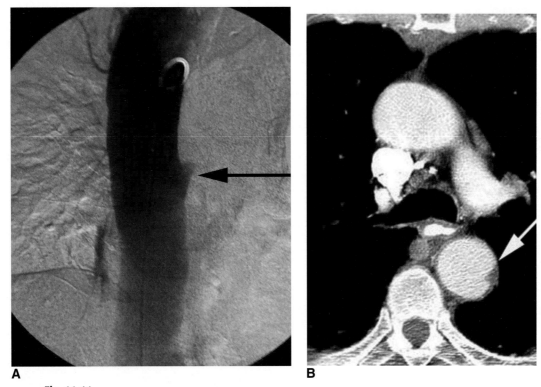

Fig. 11-11

Ulcerated plaque. **A,** *Arrow* indicates an outpouching of the lumen of the descending aorta. Characteristics that help distinguish this from an aortic rupture are (1) location in the middescending thoracic aorta as opposed to the proximal descending aorta where ruptures usually occur, (2) the adjacent aorta is normal to wide in caliber, as opposed to the situation with aortic rupture where the adjacent aorta is frequently narrowed by the pseudoaneurysm, and (3) the remainder of the aorta (not shown) has marked irregularity and tortuosity characteristic of atherosclerotic degeneration in this elderly individual. **B,** CT scan at corresponding level indicates focal plaque with outpouching and contour irregularity *(arrow)* accounting for the abnormality seen on angiography. Higher cuts (not shown) demonstrate more extensive plaque or mural thrombus. (Courtesy Shelley Marder, MD.)

armamentarium. Embolization generally is reserved for hemodynamically stable patients, with the intention of augmenting the number of patients who can be successfully managed nonoperatively. The following two methods have emerged: (1) coil embolization of the proximal splenic artery,[53,54] which decreases arterial pressure in the spleen but allows continued perfusion through collateral vessels, and (2) super-selective microcatheter embolization of the bleeding branch, preferred at the author's institution (Fig. 11-13). In recent series, nonoperative management has been successful in 60% to 91% without embolization[55-57] and 93% to 97% with embolization.[53,54,58]

In recent years, attention has been focused on the screening role for CT and CT angiography for signs indicating need for formal arteriography and potential intervention. A prospective analysis[58] demonstrated that, although grade of splenic injury by CT correlates with the likelihood of arterial injury, CT findings of contrast extravasation or pseudoaneurysm are better predictors (sensitivity 81%, specificity 84%, positive and negative predictive values of 92% and 65%, respectively). There were also small numbers of false-negative results with arteriography (perhaps due to missed abrupt termination, tamponade from subcapsular hematoma, spasm, or venous injuries) and patients who experienced subsequent hemorrhage despite an initially successful embolization. Although the goal of splenic preservation is to avoid septic complications, these still occur rarely, with a splenic abscess seen in 1 of 80 patients after splenic embolizations performed in a parallel study by the same group.[59] Moreover, the question of how much good is done by embolization in this situation can still be estimated only by comparison with older series of traditional nonoperative management. Thus, much more is known now than was known 5 years ago regarding

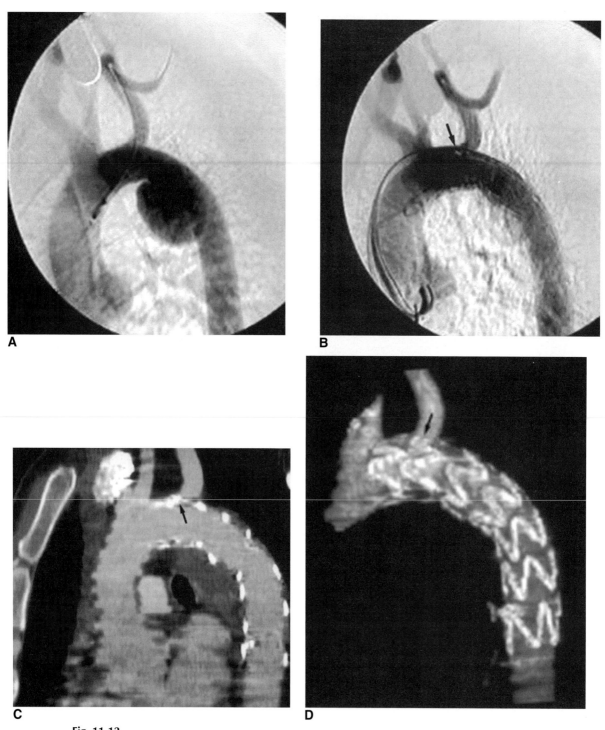

Fig. 11-12

Stent graft for treatment of traumatic aortic injury. **A,** Angiogram of a 35-year-old man who sustained blunt trauma shows an aortic pseudoaneurysm arising from the proximal descending thoracic aorta. **B,** After placement of an aortic stent graft in the aortic isthmus, the aneurysm appears excluded and the left subclavian remains patent. Multiplanar reformation (**C**) and volume-rendered image (**D**) indicate thrombosis of the pseudoaneurysm and patent left subclavian. Markers (*arrows*) indicate point of Dacron coverage. (From Fattori R, Napoli G, Lovato L, et al: AJR Am J Roentgenol 179:603, 2002.)

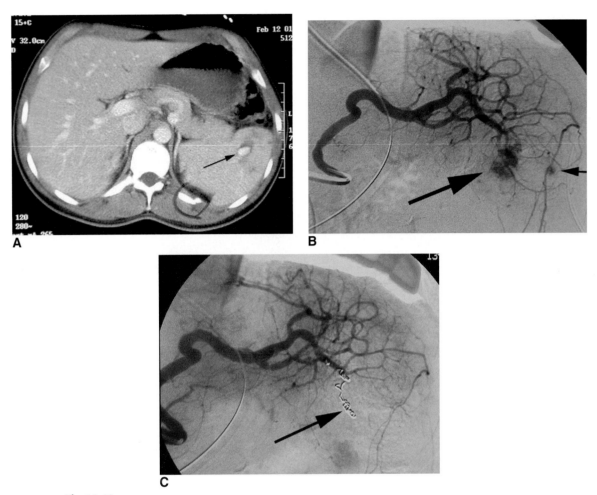

Fig. 11-13
Splenic laceration with arterial injury. **A,** *Arrow* shows rounded area of contrast density on CT, suspicious for pseudoaneurysm. **B,** *Large arrow* shows pseudoaneurysm arising from lower pole branch of splenic artery corresponding with CT scan. *Small arrow* indicates a second, smaller area of similar abnormality more laterally. **C,** After super-selective embolization (*arrows* show coils), pseudoaneurysms no longer fill.

IR-augmented nonoperative management of splenic trauma, but some uncertainty persists. Although this diagnostic and therapeutic methodology appears to be beneficial on the whole, there is enough imperfection in existing diagnostic and management modalities to urge a cautious approach for each patient.

Liver

Nonoperative management is used with increasing frequency for hepatic injuries, just as with the spleen.[60,61] But, unlike the spleen, the liver cannot be considered an expendable organ, so there is a longer history of embolotherapy as an adjunct to surgical management for hemorrhage related to liver trauma, and it has been used not only in hemodynamically stable patients but also in

unstable ones. Earlier reports of embolotherapy for liver trauma involve situations in which an injured artery is in an inaccessible area and surgery is unable to control it, or hemorrhage occurs as a delayed complication.[62-64] Later reports concern use of embolotherapy to augment nonoperative management of stable patients or as up-front treatment for hemodynamically unstable patients with high-grade liver injuries.[65-67] Because of the dual blood supply of the liver, super-selective hepatic arterial embolization can be done essentially without risk of ischemia. When the injury involves a large branch or small branches cannot be reached due to spasm or tortuous anatomy, lobar or proper hepatic artery embolization with medium-sized or large particles (Fig. 11-14) is generally safe, as well. Gallbladder infarction has been reported as a complication with smaller particles.[68-70]

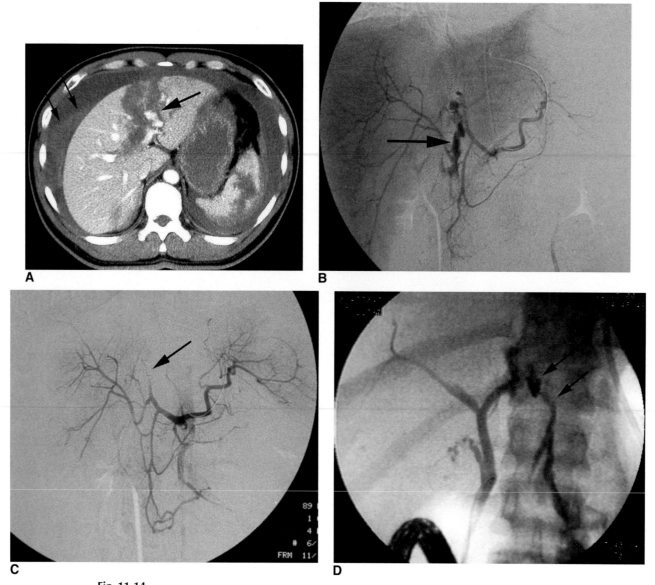

Fig. 11-14
Liver laceration with arterial and biliary injury. **A**, CT image shows deep liver laceration extending to the hilum with abnormal contrast collection (*larger arrow*), peritoneal fluid (some of which has higher density compatible with fresh blood, shown by *smaller arrows*), and associated splenic laceration. **B**, Arteriogram shows gross extravasation from the left hepatic artery (*arrow*). **C**, After embolization (*arrow* indicates faintly seen microcoils), flow in and extravasation from the left hepatic artery is halted. **D**, Endoscopic retrograde cholangiopancreatography several days later demonstrates injury to left hepatic duct with extravasation of contrast (*arrows*). Biliary injury was initially managed with stent, but ultimately the patient underwent semi-elective left hepatic lobe resection. (From Yang EY, Marder SR, Hastings G, Knudsen MM: *J Trauma* 52:982, 2002.)

Technical success rates in most series have been quite high. Clinical outcomes tend to parallel the grade of injury. Higher-grade injuries more frequently require multimodal management and have higher rates of mortality; some of this may be due to increased association with significant venous injuries.[71]

Bile leak and infectious complications are more common with high-grade liver injuries (see Fig. 11-14), so that drainage procedures commonly are needed in this group. Catheter drainage is usually successful in managing postoperative abscess, biloma,[72-74] and occasionally bilhemia.[75] More severe biliary injuries may require endoscopic or percutaneous stent placement or surgery.[76,77]

Kidney

Embolization is an effective means of halting hemorrhage from an injured renal artery branch (Fig. 11-15), achieving success rates of 82% to 88% in three series.[78-80] Not only

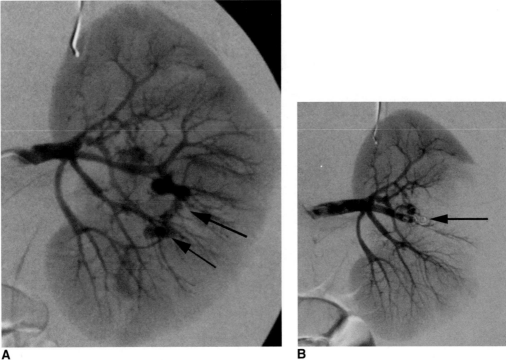

Fig. 11-15
Kidney laceration with arterial extravasation. CT scans (not shown) on this patient showed laceration of the left kidney, with worsening hemorrhage over the course of 1 to 2 hours. **A,** Arteriogram
demonstrates extravasation of contrast from an interpolar branch (*arrows*). **B,** After selective
embolization (*arrow* shows coils), the extravasation is no longer seen, with loss of flow to corresponding amount of renal parenchyma.

does this method have the advantage of being minimally
invasive, it also avoids much of the parenchymal loss associated with partial or total nephrectomy. There is very little
risk of back-bleeding from collateral vessels in the kidney,
so that embolization should be as super-selective as possible to preserve the maximum amount of viable
parenchyma. Hypertension and other complications are
very rare.[78-80] Recurrent hemorrhage can often be managed
successfully with repeat embolization.[79,80] Because lacerations of the kidney may involve the collecting system, renal
injuries managed by IR may require combined vascular
and nonvascular interventions (such as nephrostomy or
ureteral stent placement).

When there is a flow-limiting injury to the main renal
artery, angioplasty or stenting can be considered as
options for management, but it is unusual that logistics
permit them to be done before warm ischemia has taken
its toll.[81] With total occlusions, this would probably need
to take place within 1 to 2 hours of injury, a period that
almost always has elapsed before the patient has been
transported from the scene, resuscitated, and diagnosed,
leaving little or no time for arterial catheterization. In the
less common situation of a partially occluding flap

(Fig. 11-16), endovascular intervention is a more practical option.

Other Areas of the Abdomen

Occasionally, a lumbar artery will be the source of significant hemorrhage. This may be managed with embolization with a high rate of success.[82-84] With intercostal and
upper lumbar arteries, one must be careful not to inadvertently embolize branches to the spinal cord. Traumatic
rupture or dissection of the aorta in the abdomen is
much less common than in the thorax, but is seen occasionally and has been managed successfully by stent-graft
placement.[9-13]

PELVIS

Most pelvic hemorrhage in the trauma setting is secondary to blunt force with associated fractures, but penetrating mechanisms also are seen. Bony or venous
hemorrhage may resolve with conservative management
or immobilization by fixation, but arterial hemorrhage is
best managed by embolization. When arterial bleeding

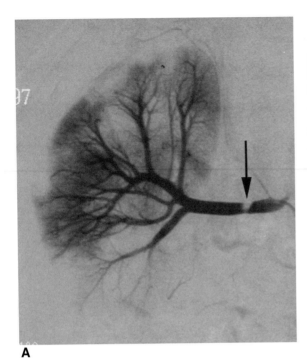

A

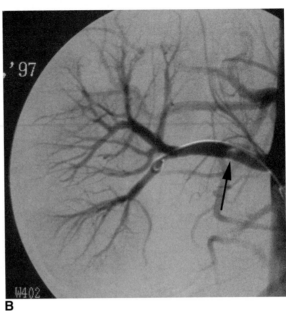

B

Fig. 11-16
Focal dissection of the renal artery. CT scan on this young female trauma victim showed markedly diminished flow to the right kidney. **A,** Selective arteriogram shows focal narrowing of the mid–renal artery (*arrow*). Aortogram (not shown) confirmed marked asymmetry of flow. **B,** Appearance following balloon angioplasty of right renal artery. Lumen diameter is much improved in the narrowed area (*arrow*). Nonselective aortogram and CT scan (not shown) showed restoration of symmetric flow to the two kidneys. This case is unusual in that the patient had a focal stenosis. In the more common situation of complete occlusion, warm ischemia time almost always has exceeded the 1- to 2-hour limit beyond which damage is irreversible.

is present, it almost always arises from the internal iliac territory. Embolotherapy has proved to be more effective than surgical ligation for two reasons as follows: (1) it can occlude broadly and peripherally enough to avoid back-bleeding from the rich network of collateral vessels in the pelvis and (2) it does not sacrifice the tamponade effect of an intact abdominal wall.[85] The risk of infection is also lower with embolization than with surgery.[31] Success rates of embolization are high (87% to 100%), with a very low incidence of complications, but mortality remains relatively high due to the severity and multiplicity of injuries in these patients.[86-88]

An earlier pattern of doing angiography only on patients whose hemodynamics fail to stabilize after external fixation has given way in many centers to early CT, with the need for angiography based on findings suspicious for arterial injury. CT has the additional advantage of demonstrating the presence or absence of potential sources of hemorrhage elsewhere in the abdomen and often helps localize the bleeding branch within the pelvis.[89]

It is advantageous to gain access to the femoral artery contralateral to the arterial lesion seen on CT, because catheter manipulations in the hypogastric territory are easier that way. However, ipsilateral femoral or upper extremity approaches can be used, if necessary. Angiography proceeds from a nonselective pelvic arteriogram to selective bilateral internal iliac arteriograms. The site of hemorrhage should be catheterized and embolized at a relatively selective level (Fig. 11-17) without wasting valuable time. If super-selective catheterization is difficult or impossible, especially if the patient is unstable, less selective embolization such as the entirety of both internal iliac arteries can be lifesaving and rarely results in ischemic problems.[90] In fact, many interventional radiologists advocate embolization of additional nearby branches within the pelvis, both ipsilaterally and contralaterally, to avoid late recurrent bleeding via collateral vessels. Gelfoam is the agent of choice in most instances (slurry is particularly convenient and effective) and can be followed by coil placement to add permanence. After embolization, a nonselective pelvic

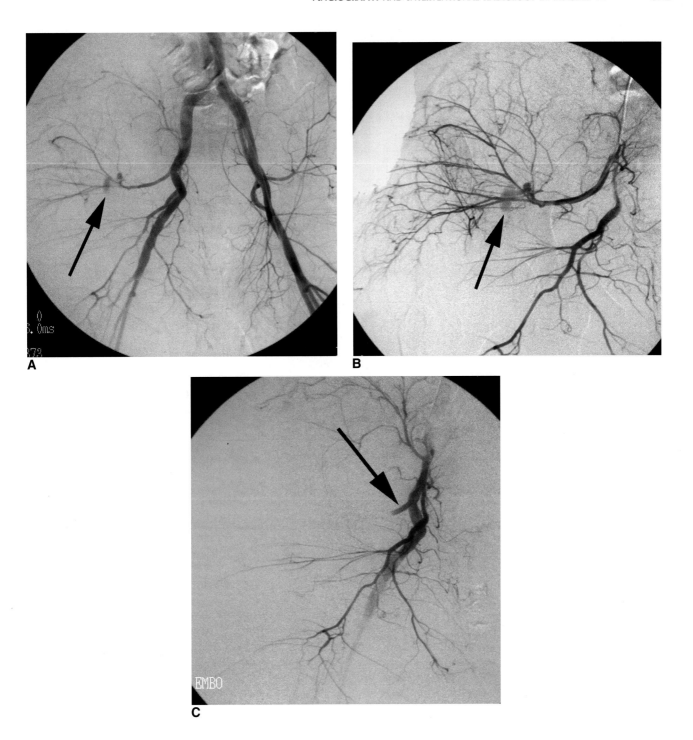

Fig. 11-17
Pelvic fracture with injury of superior gluteal artery. **A,** Nonselective pelvic arteriogram in a patient with a nearby vertical fracture of the iliac wing shows pseudoaneurysm of superior gluteal artery (*arrow*). **B,** Right internal iliac arteriogram confirms this finding (*arrow*). **C,** Appearance after gelatin sponge slurry embolization of superior gluteal artery. Now only the stump of the superior gluteal artery is seen (*arrow*), and there is no more filling of the pseudoaneurysm. The anterior division remains intact, and the patient remained stable.

arteriogram should be repeated to look for less common sources of pelvic hemorrhage such as external iliac branches, lumbar, or contralateral internal iliac branches.

It is worthwhile to note several pitfalls with this technique:

1. A persistent blush frequently is seen at the base of the penis in the absence of injury. Misinterpretation of this can lead to unnecessary bilateral internal pudendal artery embolization, with attendant potential for iatrogenic impotence.

2. Spasm may mask the true source of hemorrhage, only to require repeat angiography several days later for recurrent bleeding. Review of the initial study often shows that an absent or abruptly terminating branch was missed at the time of original interpretation, underscoring the need for detailed accounting of all of the expected branches of the internal iliac arteries bilaterally. As elsewhere, an abruptly terminating vessel in a patient who shows clinical signs of bleeding should be embolized.

3. Small branches of the external iliac artery, such as the symphyseal branch of the inferior epigastric artery or variant obturator artery, sometimes can be responsible for hemorrhage and often are picked up only on the "completion" postembolization nonselective pelvic arteriogram (Fig. 11-18).

4. Bleeding may appear to be coming from just one side, but after unilateral embolization it may reappear, supplied by the corresponding contralateral branch.

EXTREMITIES

The necessity and timing of angiographic evaluation of trauma to the arteries of the extremities is evolving and controversial. To understand this, it is helpful to discuss mechanisms of injury, severity of physical findings, and historical perspective. Interventions such as embolization and stent or stent-graft placement have a limited, but growing, role.

Proximity is a concept that arises when considering penetrating trauma to the extremities. Gunshot can injure vessels either by direct contact or by means of a blast effect, which is transmitted through tissues when a ballistic fragment passes close to the vessel. Stabbing lacks the potential for blast effect, so this exact concept of proximity does not apply. However, some consider stab wounds close to major vessels *proximity injuries,* because the precise path of a stab wound cannot be determined by physical findings (Fig. 11-19). Blunt trauma injures arteries by means of crush, stretch, shearing, torsion, or laceration on a fracture fragment; proximity simply does not apply here. Certain blunt injuries are associated more commonly with vascular trauma than others. For instance, it is estimated that up to 40% of posterior knee dislocations result in popliteal artery injury, an injury with a substantial risk of limb loss

especially if unrecognized.[91] Bleeding, swelling, or reperfusion may cause vascular compromise by means of a compartment syndrome, regardless of the original mechanism.

To determine the need for and timing of arteriography in extremity trauma, it is useful to think of the physical findings of vascular trauma to the extremities in three categories. (1) Patients with "unequivocal evidence of arterial injury [in whom] operative approach is established easily by the mechanism and site of injury"[92] or who are hemodynamically unstable, have other evidence of significant active hemorrhage, or suffer from severe ischemia require emergent surgical exploration without the delay of preoperative arteriography. (2) Patients with an extremity injury accompanied by hard physical findings suspicious for vascular injury, but who are stable, generally are studied with urgent angiography. This establishes the presence or absence of injury and provides information about its nature and severity, as well as the status of inflow and outflow vessels. Most practitioners, but not all,[93] use urgent arteriography to assess the need for and to help in planning surgery in these patients. The exact physical findings that should trigger an urgent arteriogram are a subject of some debate. Traditionally, "hard" signs of vascular injury have been defined as bruit, loss of pulses, limb ischemia, active bleeding, expanding hematoma, or history of pulsatile bleeding.[94] But other findings, such as neurologic deficits, decrease in minimum ankle–brachial index, fractures associated with gunshot wounds, multiple pellet (i.e., shotgun) injuries, and other "soft" findings, increase the likelihood of significant arterial injury.[94-96] Depending on the series and the criteria used, 41% to 76% of such patients with physical findings suspicious for vascular injury will have positive arteriogram results.[95-98] (3) Patients with proximity injuries are a more controversial group, an understanding of which is aided by a brief historical discussion.

During the Korean War, the problem of proximity injuries was evident, and a practice of mandatory surgical exploration of these patients developed to avoid missing vascular injuries without associated physical findings.[99] Using this method, avoiding missed injuries resulted in many negative exploration findings with attendant morbidity.[100] Arteriography then emerged as a reliable but quicker, safer, and less expensive alternative.[100,101] As experience with angiography mounted, it has become evident that the likelihood of a positive study result is low in this group (3.6% to 19%) and that most of the lesions do not require surgical or endovascular intervention.[94,95,98,102,103] Critics of arteriography for proximity injury cite its expense and invasiveness, stating "the great majority of these injuries heal spontaneously with few sequelae," so that "routine arteriography for proximity alone may be of minimal clinical benefit and an inefficient use of medical resources."[95] Proponents of angiography point out that some such patients will have delayed

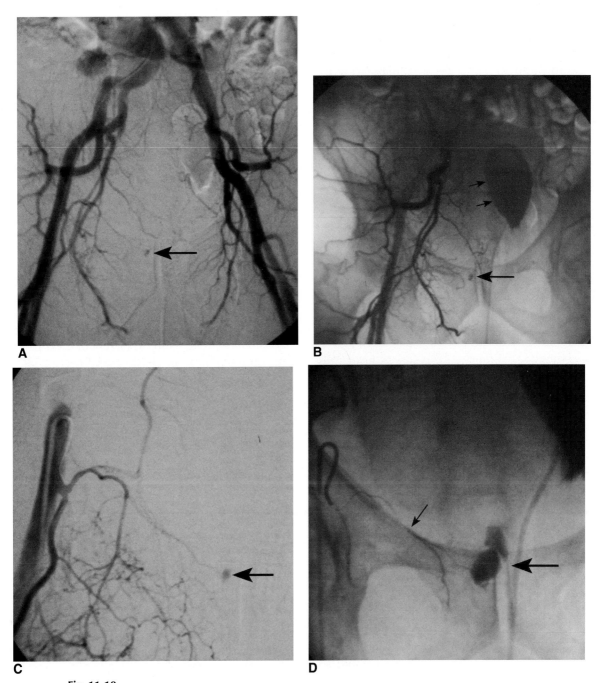

Fig. 11-18
Pelvic fracture with bleeding from external iliac artery branch; value of postembolization arteri-ogram in an 80-year-old bicycle-versus-automobile crash victim. **A,** Flush pelvic arteriogram shows extravasation of contrast overlying the right pubis *(arrow)*. **B,** Selective internal iliac arteriogram shows persistent extravasation *(large arrow)*, but note that there is opacification of the external iliac, as well. Leftward displacement of bladder *(small arrows)* attests to the size of the growing pelvic hematoma. After embolization of the internal iliac artery, a repeat flush pelvic arteriogram (not shown) demonstrated persistent extravasation over the right pubis. **C,** Inferior epigastric arteriogram shows persistent extravasation *(arrow)* from a symphyseal branch. **D,** Using a microcatheter (tip is indicated by *small arrow*), extravasation was confirmed *(large arrow)* and embolization performed using Gelfoam slurry followed by microcoil placement. Postembolization arteriogram (not shown) showed extravasation was finally gone.

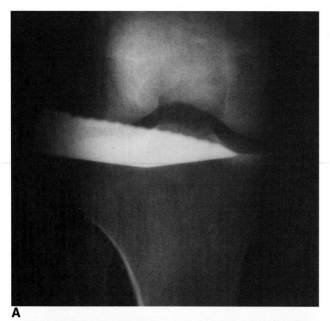

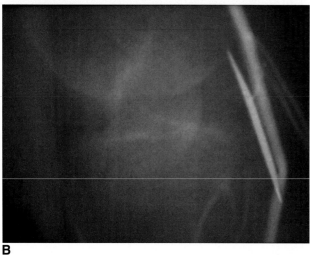

Fig. 11-19

Stab wound to knee. This patient arrived in the emergency department with the blade of a knife broken off inside the knee. Pulses and neurologic examination were normal. **A**, Frontal radiograph demonstrates knife blade in knee. Lateral film showed the blade was located posteriorly in the popliteal fossa. Note that the sharp, serrated edge is oriented superiorly. **B**, Knife blade tents the popliteal artery, but there is no arterial injury because the edge that abuts the artery is the dull one. During surgery, the knife was removed uneventfully without the need for full surgical exposure. This case demonstrates how stab wounds can stretch the definition of proximity injury. Although stab wounds lack blast effect to fit the classic definition of proximity injury, the path of a knife is uncertain, even in a case like this on which the knife was left in place.

clinical manifestations, indicating that "the problem with this group is that they are unreliable...they do not come back for follow-up, so you have to resolve the problem initially: do they have an injury or not?"[95] Ultimately, this dispute may be resolved by using a cheaper and less

invasive mode of assessment, such as duplex ultrasonographic or CT angiography. It is estimated that arteriography in this setting is cost effective only "if major occult injuries equal or exceed 1%."[104] Duplex sonography showed 100% sensitivity and 100% specificity for traumatic arterial injury in two series[105,106] but only 50% sensitivity in another.[107] Duplex study can also be quite valuable for assessment of venous injuries. Helical CT has shown sensitivity and specificity from 90% to 100% in assessment of trauma to the large arteries of the extremities.[108] Thus, the workup of these patients varies from one institution to another and one patient to another. Arteriography for these patients is not emergent and can be done within 24 hours as part of the routine schedule, provided the patient is observed in-hospital during the interim.[31,109,110]

Lesions seen in the extremities are like those seen elsewhere in angiography of trauma. Hemorrhagic lesions include extravasation, pseudoaneurysm, AVF, and abrupt termination. Occlusive lesions run the gamut from non–flow-limiting minor intimal irregularity or segmental narrowing of spasm or adjacent swelling, which are best left alone, to significant stenoses or frank occlusions that often require revascularization. In elderly patients, arteriography frequently demonstrates existing atherosclerotic disease that may be important in planning therapy.

Most small and intermediate-size bleeding branches can be managed effectively by embolization (Fig. 11-20), postponing surgery until the patient is stabilized or obviating surgery altogether.[111] Ischemic complications are rare, owing to collateral circulation that sometimes can be a source of back-bleeding. Because of this, embolization of pseudoaneurysm and AVFs should be done both proximal and distal to the lesion, if possible. Larger vessels with hemorrhagic or occlusive lesions typically require an intervention that preserves flow. Because of the superior durability of surgery and the often young age of these patients, bypass is typically the procedure of choice, but certain circumstances such as regions with difficult access like the shoulder, a contaminated operative field, and patients who need to be stabilized so that other more pressing injuries can be addressed may tip the balance in favor of endovascular management. Accordingly, there have been case reports and small series of stents and stent-grafts for hemorrhagic and occlusive lesions in femoral,[14,15] subclavian,[16-24] and innominate[25,26] arteries with very high rates of procedural success but some problems with late development of stenosis or occlusion.

VENOUS THROMBOEMBOLIC DISEASE

Venous thromboembolic disease is a significant cause of morbidity and mortality in trauma patients. It is largely preventable by the use of ultrasonographic surveillance

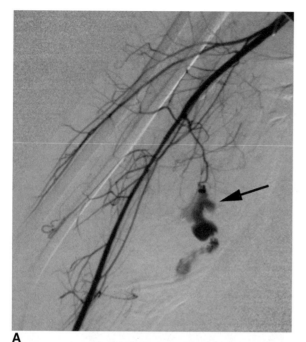

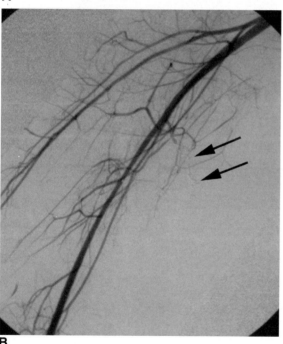

Fig. 11-20

Stab wound to arm with arterial hemorrhage. **A,** Arteriogram in this patient referred for pulsatile hemorrhage demonstrates extravasation (*arrow*) from small muscular branch of the brachial artery. **B,** After placement of microcoils super selectively (faintly seen, indicated by *arrows*), extravasation has stopped. (From Mattox KL, Feliciano DV, Moore EE, eds: *Trauma*, ed 4, New York, 2000, McGraw-Hill.)

and prophylaxis in high-risk groups, reducing pulmonary embolism (PE) and PE-related death from 6% and 4% to zero in a typical study.[112] In the absence of contraindications, prophylaxis consists of subcutaneous heparin, enoxaparin, serial compression devices, or a

combination. However, these prophylactic measures are not feasible or safe for many of the patients at highest risk (such as those with spinal cord injury, pelvic fracture, multiple lower extremity fracture, venous injuries in abdomen or pelvis or both). A large proportion of significant deep vein thrombosis (DVT) is in the pelvis,[113] where ultrasonographic surveillance is of little or no use. These factors have led to the prophylactic use of inferior vena cava filters (VCF) in these high-risk patients who cannot tolerate anticoagulation.[114-120]

When a DVT or PE is identified in a trauma patient with a contraindication to anticoagulation, the decision to place a VCF is straightforward; prophylactic use is a subject of some controversy. Most reports concerning the prophylactic use of VCF indicate a significant reduction in the incidence of nonfatal and fatal PE.[114-119] Complication rates are low, with the incidence of inferior vena cava (IVC) and insertion site thrombosis being lower with prophylactic indication than in typical patients with DVT or PE as an indication.[121] However, all of these reports are based on comparison with historical controls, and none is a prospective, randomized trial. Furthermore, some reports have shown no benefit to the use of VCF in this situation,[122,123] with concerns over cost effectiveness, the safety of transporting critically ill patients to the radiology suite, and long-term effect of filters when placed in young trauma victims looming large in the minds of some. Accordingly, a recent practitioner survey shows widely varying practices regarding the use of VCF but indicates that use would increase if some of these issues, such as the permanent nature of VCF, were to change.[124]

Many of these issues are being addressed with recent technologic advances. Early reports of removable VCFs have been favorable.[125,126] There are a growing number of reports of VCF placement at the bedside.[127-136] Many of these have shown a substantial reduction in patient charges when compared with VCF placement in the radiology suite or the operating room (OR).[127,131,134] Also touted is the elimination of the perceived danger of patient transport, but none of these reports comparing outcomes of bedside placement with IR or OR placement documents the supposedly dangerous nature of patient transport—a situation that is unavoidable for most IR and OR procedures. Moreover, ultrasound-guided bedside VCF placement has shown a substantial number of technical failures and complications.[128,134] Venographically guided bedside placement has shown a better technical success record[129-131,133,135,136] and allows visualization of important findings typically missed by ultrasound, which require major alterations in VCF placement technique, such as duplicated IVC,[137] megacava,[138] or IVC clot. Unfortunately, the availability of high-quality venography at the bedside is far from universal, so that bedside placement that is as safe and

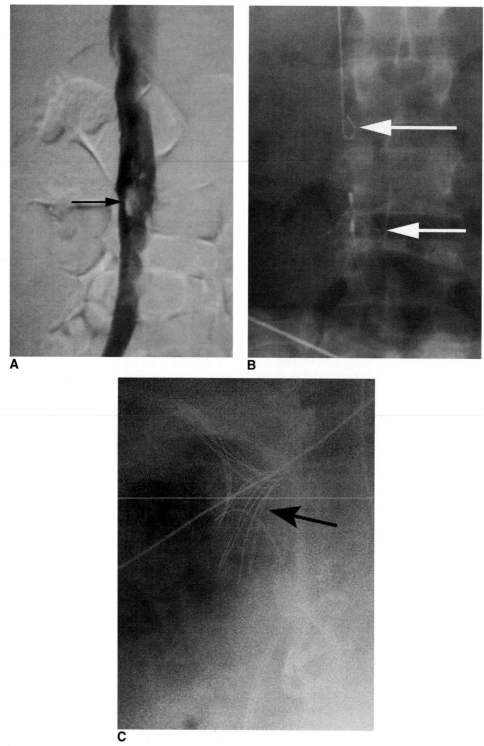

Fig. 11-21

Inferior vena cava filters. **A**, Inferior vena cava filter in trauma patient has trapped a clot (indicated by *arrow*), serving its intended purpose and preventing pulmonary embolism. **B**, Despite their beneficial effects, filters can cause problems when the wire used for central venous catheter placement (*long arrow*) comes in contact with a filter (*short arrow*), whereupon they can become entangled and possibly result in filter dislodgement as shown by the arrow in (**C**).

efficacious as that done in the radiology suite may require a different methodology, such as intravascular ultrasound.[139,140]

In a busy trauma center, awareness of VCFs is important, because they occasionally may entrap J-shaped guide wires during central venous catheter placement (Fig. 11-21), sometimes leading to filter dislodgement. Interventional radiologists can be indispensable in the (often challenging) safe removal of entrapped guide wires and for repositioning or removing displaced VCFs.[141-146] Interventional radiologists should also assume some responsibility for educating clinicians who place central lines, especially at critical times such as the beginning of the academic year, when many less-experienced physicians arrive.

SUMMARY

The interventional radiologist plays an important role in angiographic diagnosis and endovascular and other percutaneous treatment of the trauma patient. There is a trend toward less use of angiography for diagnosis and an expanding role in treatment. Still, arteriography is an indispensable tool for demonstrating the exact location, extent, and nature of arterial damage. Embolotherapy is effective in controlling hemorrhage in a wide variety of trauma situations. Stents, especially covered ones, can repair damage to larger arteries, where preservation or restoration of flow is critical and operative repair is undesirable. Image-guided catheter drainage is useful for abscesses, leaks, and other abnormal fluid collections that frequently occur during the hospital course of severe trauma victims. Inferior VCF placement is an important tool for the prevention of PE, a significant cause of morbidity and mortality in trauma victims. To optimize patient care, the interventional radiologist must be readily available at all times and work in close coordination with the trauma team to provide expeditious treatment in situations that typically do not tolerate delay.

REFERENCES

1. Ruchat P, Capasso P, Chollet-Rivier M, et al: Endovascular treatment of aortic rupture by blunt chest trauma, J Cardiovasc Surg 42:77, 2001.
2. Lagattola N, Matson M, Self G, et al: Traumatic rupture of the aortic arch treated by stent grafting, Eur J Vasc Endovasc Surg 17:84, 1999.
3. Desshpande A, Mossop P, Gurry J, et al: Treatment of traumatic false aneurysm of the thoracic aorta with endoluminal grafts, J Endovasc Surg 5:120, 1998.
4. Kato N, Dake MD, Miller DC, et al: Traumatic thoracic aortic aneurysm; treatment with endovascular stent-grafts, Radiology 205:657, 1997.
5. Semba CP, Kato N, Kee ST, et al: Acute rupture of the descending thoracic aorta: repair with use of endovascular stent-grafts, J Vasc Interv Radiol 8:337, 1997.
6. Rousseau H, Soula P, Perreault P, et al: Delayed treatment of traumatic rupture of the thoracic aorta with endoluminal covered stent, Circulation 101:E96, 2000.
7. Avrahami R, Noyman Levine M, et al: Treatment of traumatic false aneurysm of the thoracic aorta with stent graft, Harefuah 140:483, 2001.
8. Fujikawa T, Yukioka T, Ishimaru S, et al: Endovascular stent grafting for the treatment of blunt thoracic aortic injury, J Trauma 50:223, 2001.
9. Fontaine AB, Nicholls SC, Borsa JJ, et al: Seat belt aorta: endovascular management with a stent-graft, J Endovasc Ther 8:83, 2001.
10. Scharrer-Pamler R, Gorich J, Orend KH, et al: Emergent endoluminal repair of delayed abdominal aortic rupture after blunt trauma, J Endovasc Surg 5:134, 1998.
11. White R, Donayre C, Walot I, et al: Endograft repair of an aortic pseudoaneurysm following gunshot wound injury: impact of imaging on diagnosis and planning of intervention, J Endovasc Surg 4:352, 1997.
12. Michaels AJ, Gerndt SJ, Taheri PA, et al: Blunt force injury of the abdominal aorta, J Trauma 41:105, 1996.
13. Marty-Ane CH, Alric P, Prudhomme M, et al: Intravascular stenting of traumatic abdominal aortic dissection, J Vasc Surg 23:156, 1996.
14. Sharma S, Bhargava B, Mahapatra M, Malhotra R: Pseudoaneurysm of the superficial femoral artery following accidental trauma: result of treatment by percutaneous stent-graft placement, Eur Radiol 9:422, 1999.
15. Uflacker R, Elliott BM: Percutaneous endoluminal stent-graft repair of an old traumatic femoral arteriovenous fistula, Cardiovasc Intervent Radiol 19:120, 1996.
16. Stecco K, Meier A, Seiver A, et al: Endovascular stent-graft placement for treatment of traumatic penetrating subclavian artery injury, J Trauma 48:948, 2000.
17. Ohki T, Veith FJ, Kraas C, et al: Endovascular therapy for upper extremity injury, Semin Vasc Surg 11:106, 1998.
18. Pfammatter T, Kunzli A, Hilfiker PR, et al: Relief of subclavian venous and brachial plexus compression syndrome caused by traumatic subclavian artery aneurysm by means of transluminal stent-grafting, J Trauma 45:972, 1998.
19. Patel AV, Marin ML, Veith FJ, Kerr A, Sanchez LA: Endovascular graft repair of penetrating subclavian artery injuries, J Endovasc Surg 3:382, 1996.
20. Tyagi S, Rao BH, Arora R: Transfemoral placement of an endovascular stent-graft for a traumatic subclavian arteriovenous fistula, Indian Heart J 50:443, 1998.
21. Szeimies U, Kueffer G, Stoeckelhuber B, Steckmeier B: Successful exclusion of subclavian aneurysms with covered nitinol stents, Cardiovasc Intervent Radiol 22:86, 1999.
22. Watelet J, Clavier E, Reix T, et al: Traumatic subclavian artery pseudoaneurysm: periprocedural salvage of failed stent-graft exclusion using coil embolization, J Endovasc Ther 8:197, 2001.
23. Hilfiker PR, Razavi MK, Kee ST, et al: Stent-graft therapy for subclavian artery aneurysms and fistulas: single-center mid-term results, J Vasc Interv Radiol 11:578, 2000.
24. d'Othee BJ, Rousseau H, Otal P, Joffre F: Noncovered stent placement in a blunt traumatic injury of the right subclavian artery, Cardiovasc Intervent Radiol 22:424, 1999.
25. Axisa BM, Loftus IM, Fishwick G, et al: Endovascular repair of an innominate artery false aneurysm following blunt trauma, J Endovasc Ther 7:245, 2000.
26. Ruebben A, Merlo M, Verri A, et al: Combined surgical and endovascular treatment of a traumatic pseudo-aneurysm of the brachiocephalic trunk with anatomical anomaly, J Cardiovasc Surg 38:173, 1997.
27. Simionato F, Righi C, Melissano G, et al: Stent-graft treatment of a common carotid artery pseudoaneurysm, J Endovasc Ther 7:136, 2000.
28. Waldman DL, Barquist E, Poynton FG, Numaguchi Y: Stent graft of a traumatic vertebral artery injury: case report, J Trauma 44:1094, 1998.

29. Parodi JC, Schonholz C, Ferreira LM, Bergan J: Endovascular stent-graft treatment of traumatic arterial lesions, *Ann Vasc Surg* 13:121, 1999.

30. Shkrum MJ, McClafferty KJ, Green RN, et al: Mechanisms of aortic injury in fatalities occurring in motor vehicle collisions, *J Forensic Sci* 44:44, 1999.

31. Pais SO: Assessment of vascular trauma. In Mirvis SE, Young JWR, eds: *Imaging in trauma and critical care*, Baltimore, 1992, Williams & Wilkins.

32. Parmley LF, Mattinly TW, Manion WC, Janke EJ: Non-penetrating traumatic injury of the aorta, *Circulation* 17:1086, 1958.

33. Pate JW, Gavant ML, Weiman DS, Fabian TC: Traumatic rupture of the aortic isthmus: program of selective management, *World J Surg* 23:59, 1999.

34. Galli R, Pacini D, Di Bartolomeo R, et al: Surgical indications and timing of repair of traumatic ruptures of the thoracic aorta, *Ann Thorac Surg* 65:461, 1998.

35. Iannettoni MD, McCurry KR, Rodriguez JL, et al: Simultaneous traumatic ascending and descending thoracic aortic rupture, *Ann Thorac Surg* 57:481, 1994.

36. Prater SP, Leya FS, McKiernan TL: Post traumatic pseudoaneurysm of the ascending aorta—an incidental finding two decades later, *Clin Cardiol* 17:566, 1994.

37. Symbas PJ, Horsley WS, Symbas PN: Rupture of the ascending aorta caused by blunt trauma, *Ann Thorac Surg* 66:113, 1998.

38. Lancey RA, Davliakos GP, Vander Salm TJ: Simultaneous repair of multiple traumatic aortic tears, *Ann Thorac Surg* 60:1120, 1995.

39. Catoire P, Bonnet F, Delaunay L, et al: Traumatic laceration of the ascending aorta detected by transesophageal echocardiography, *Ann Emerg Med* 23:356, 1994.

40. Ahrar K, Smith DC, Bansal RC, et al: Angiography in blunt thoracic aortic injury, *J Trauma* 42:665, 1997.

41. Bouchart F, Bessou JP, Tabley A, et al: Acute traumatic rupture of the thoracic aorta and its branches: results of surgical management, *Ann Chir* 126:201, 2001.

42. West O, Vanderbush E, Anagnostopoulos CE: Traumatic rupture of the aortic valve and ascending aorta diagnosed by transesophageal echocardiography, *J Cardiovasc Surg* 40:671, 1999.

43. von Segesser LK, Fischer A, Vogt P, Turina M: Diagnosis and management of blunt great vessel trauma, *J Card Surg* 12(suppl 2):181, 1997.

44. Dunn JA, Williams MG: Occult ascending aortic rupture in the presence of an air bag, *Ann Thorac Surg* 62:577, 1996.

45. French BG, Hughes CF: Post-traumatic chronic false aneurysm of the ascending aorta with long-term survival, *Aust N Z J Surg* 64:284, 1994.

46. Murakami R, Tajima H, Ichikawa K, et al: Acute traumatic injury of the distal descending aorta associated with thoracic spine injury, *Eur Radiol* 8:60, 1998.

47. Katsumata T, Shinfeld A, Westaby S: Operation for chronic traumatic aortic aneurysm: when and how? *Ann Thorac Surg* 66:774, 1998.

48. O'Connor GS, Geelhoed GW: Splenic trauma and salvage, *Am Surgeon* 52:456, 1986.

49. Sekikawa T, Shatney CH: Septic sequelae after splenectomy for trauma in adults, *Am J Surg* 145:667, 1983.

50. Chadwick SJ, Huizinga WK, Baker LW: Management of splenic trauma: the Durban experience, *Br J Surg* 72:634, 1985.

51. Weinstein ME, Govin GG, Rice CL, Virgilio RW: Splenorrhaphy for splenic trauma, *J Trauma* 19:692, 1979.

52. Tricarico A, Sicoli F, Calise F, et al: Conservative treatment in splenic trauma, *J R Coll Surg Edinb* 38:145, 1993.

53. Sclafani SJ, Shaftan GW, Scalea TM, et al: Nonoperative salvage of computed tomography–diagnosed splenic injuries: utilization of angiography for triage and embolization for hemostasis, *J Trauma* 39:818, 1995.

54. Hagiwara A, Yukioka T, Ohta S, et al: Nonsurgical management of patients with blunt splenic injury: efficacy of transcatheter arterial embolization, *AJR Am J Roentgenol* 167:159, 1996.

55. Alidria-Ezati I: A review of non-operative treatment of splenic trauma, *Trop Doct* 25:112, 1995.

56. Federle MP, Courcoulas AP, Powell M, et al: Blunt splenic injury in adults: clinical and CT criteria for management, with emphasis on active extravasation, *Radiology* 206:137, 1998.

57. Morse MA, Garcia VF: Selective nonoperative management of pediatric blunt splenic trauma: risk for missed associated injuries, *J Pediatr Surg* 29:23, 1994.

58. Shanmuganathan K, Mirvis SE, Boyd-Kranis R, et al: Nonsurgical management of blunt splenic injury: use of CT criteria to select patients for splenic angiography and potential endovascular therapy, *Radiology* 217:75, 2000.

59. Killeen KL, Shanmuganathan K, Boyd-Kranis R, et al: CT findings after embolization for blunt splenic trauma, *J Vasc Interv Radiol* 12:209, 2001.

60. Archer LP, Rogers FB, Shackford SR: Selective nonoperative management of liver and spleen injuries in neurologically impaired adult patients, *Arch Surg* 131:309, 1996.

61. Carles J, Dubuisson V, Duows C, et al: Traitement conservateur des traumatismes hepatiques: prise en charge et evolution. [Conservative treatment of hepatic injuries: management and course.] *Chirurgie* 120:444, 1994-1995.

62. Fandrich BL, Gnanadev DA, Jaecks R, Boyle W: Selective hepatic artery embolization as an adjunct to liver packing in severe hepatic trauma: case report, *J Trauma* 29:1716, 1989.

63. Pain JA, Heaton ND, Karani JB, Howard ER: Selective arterial embolization for hepatic trauma, *Ann R Coll Surg Engl* 73:189, 1991.

64. De Toma G, Mingoli A, Modini C, et al: The value of angiography and selective hepatic artery embolization for continuous bleeding after surgery in liver trauma; case reports, *J Trauma* 37:508, 1994.

65. Ciraulo DL, Luk S, Palter M, et al: Selective hepatic arterial embolization of grade IV and V blunt hepatic injuries: and extension of resuscitation in the nonoperative management of traumatic hepatic injuries, *J Trauma* 45:353, 1998.

66. Hagiwara A, Yukioka T, Ohta S, et al: Nonsurgical management of patients with blunt hepatic injury: efficacy of transcatheter arterial embolization, *AJR Am J Roentgenol* 169:1151, 1997.

67. Hashimoto S, Hiramatsu K, Ido K, et al: Expanding role of emergency embolization in the management of severe blunt hepatic trauma, *Cardiovasc Intervent Radiol* 13:193, 1990.

68. Kuroda C, Iwasaki M, Tanaka T, et al: Gallbladder infarction following hepatic transcatheter arterial embolization: angiographic study, *Radiology* 149:85, 1983.

69. Takayasu K, Moriyama N, Muramatsu Y, et al: Gallbladder infarction after hepatic artery embolization, *AJR Am J Roentgenol* 144:135, 1985.

70. Simons RK, Sinanan MN, Coldwell DM: Gangrenous cholecystitis as a complication of hepatic artery embolization: case report, *Surgery* 112:106, 1992.

71. Poletti PA, Mirvis SE, Shanmuganathan K, et al: CT criteria for management of blunt liver trauma: correlation with angiographic and surgical findings, *Radiology* 216:418, 2000.

72. Sheldon GF, Rutledge R: Hepatic trauma, *Adv Surg* 22:179, 1989.

73. Feliciano DV: Surgery for liver trauma, *Surg Clin North Am* 69:273, 1989.

74. Howdieshell TR, Purvis J, Bates WB, Teeslink CR: Biloma and biliary fistula following hepatorrhaphy for liver trauma: incidence, natural history, and management, *Am Surgeon* 61:165, 1995.

75. Blum U, Buitrago-Tellez C, el Seif M, Wimmer B: Posttraumatic bilhemia: conservative management by percutaneous drainage, *Cardiovasc Intervent Radiol* 16:55, 1993.

76. Carrillo EH, Spain DA, Wohltmann CD, et al: Interventional techniques are useful adjuncts in nonoperative management of hepatic injuries, J Trauma 46:619, 1999.

77. D'Amours SK, Simons RK, Scudamore CH, et al: Major intrahepatic bile duct injuries detected after laparotomy: selective nonoperative management, J Trauma 50:480, 2001.

78. Heyns CF, van Vollenhoven P: Increasing role of angiography and segmental artery embolization in the management of renal stab wounds, J Urol 147:1231, 1992.

79. Uflacker R, Paolini RM, Lima S: Management of traumatic hematuria by selective renal artery embolization, J Urol 132:662, 1984.

80. Corr P, Hacking G: Embolization in traumatic intrarenal vascular injuries, Clin Radiol 43:262, 1991.

81. Whigham CJ Jr, Bodenhamer JR, Miller JK: Use of the Palmaz stent in primary treatment of renal artery intimal injury secondary to blunt trauma, J Vasc Interv Radiol 6:175, 1995.

82. Haydu P, Chang J, Knox G, Nealon TF Jr: Transcatheter arterial embolization of a traumatic lumbar artery false aneurysm, Surgery 84:288, 1978.

83. Sclafani SJ, Florence LO, Phillips TF, et al: Lumbar arterial injury: radiologic diagnosis and management, Radiology 165:709, 1987.

84. Armstrong NN, Zarvon NP, Sproat IA, Schurr MJ: Lumbar artery hemorrhage: unusual cause of shock treated by angiographic embolization, J Trauma 42:544, 1997.

85. van Urk H, Perlberger RR, Muller H: Selective arterial embolization for control of traumatic pelvic hemorrhage, Surgery 83:133, 1978.

86. Panetta T, Sclafani SJ, Goldstein AS, Phillips TF: Percutaneous transcatheter embolization for arterial trauma, J Vasc Surg 2:54, 1985.

87. Yellin AE, Lundell CJ, Finck EJ: Diagnosis and control of posttraumatic pelvic hemorrhage: transcatheter angiographic embolization techniques, Arch Surg 118:1378, 1983.

88. Matalon TS, Athanasoulis CA, Margolies MN, et al: Hemorrhage with pelvic fractures: efficacy of transcatheter embolization, AJR Am J Roentgenol 133:859, 1979.

89. Cerva DS, Mirvis SE, Shanmuganathan K, et al: Detection of bleeding in patients with major pelvic fractures: value of contrast enhanced CT, AJR Am J Roentgenol 166:131, 1996.

90. Velhamos GC, Chahwan S, Hanks SE, et al: Angiographic embolization of bilateral internal iliac arteries to control life-threatening hemorrhage after blunt trauma to the pelvis, Am Surgeon 66:858, 2000.

91. Applebaum R, Yellin AE, Weaver FA, et al: Role of routine arteriography in blunt lower extremity trauma, Am J Surg 160:221, 1990.

92. Bandyk DF: Vascular injury associated with extremity trauma, Clin Orthop 318:117, 1995.

93. Anderson RJ, Hobson RW, Padberg FT, et al: Penetrating extremity trauma: identification of patients at high-risk requiring arteriography, J Vasc Surg 11:544, 1990.

94. Kaufman JA, Parker JE, Gillespie DL, et al: Arteriography for proximity of injury in penetrating extremity trauma, J Vasc Interv Radiol 3:719, 1992.

95. Gahtan V, Bramson RT, Norman J: The role of emergent arteriography in penetrating limb trauma, Am Surgeon 60:123, 1994.

96. Weaver FA, Yellin AE, Bauer M, et al: Is arterial proximity a valid indication for arteriography in penetrating extremity trauma? Arch Surg 125:1256, 1990.

97. McCorkell SJ, Harley JD, Morishima MS, Cummings DK: Indications for angiography in extremity trauma, AJR Am J Roentgenol 145:1245, 1985.

98. Hartling RP, McGahan JP, Blaisdaell FW, Lindfors KK: Stab wounds to the extremities: indications for angiography, Radiology 162:465, 1987.

99. Inui FK, Shannon J, Howard JM: Arterial injuries in the Korean conflict (experiences with 111 consecutive injuries), Surgery 37:850, 1955.

100. Geuder JW, Hobson RW, Padberg FT, et al: The role of contrast arteriography in suspected arterial injuries of the extremities, Am Surgeon 51:89, 1985.

101. Snyder WH, Thal ER, Bridges RA, et al: The validity of normal arteriography in penetrating trauma, Arch Surg 113:424, 1978.

102. King TA, Perse JA, Marmen C, Darvin HI: Utility of arteriography in penetrating extremity injuries, Am J Surg 162:163, 1991.

103. Reid JDS, Weigelt JA, Thal ER, Hugh F: Assessment of proximity of a wound to major vascular structures as an indication for arteriography, Arch Surg 123:942, 1988.

104. Keen JD, Dunne PM, Keen RR, Langer BG: Proximity arteriography; cost-effectiveness in asymptomatic penetrating extremity trauma, J Vasc Interv Radiol 12:813, 2001.

105. Fry WR, Smith RS, Sayers DV, et al: The success of duplex ultrasonographic scanning in diagnosis of extremity vascular proximity trauma, Arch Surg 128:1368, 1993.

106. Knudson MM, Lewis FR, Atkinson K, Neuhaus A: The role of duplex ultrasound arterial imaging in patients with penetrating extremity trauma, Arch Surg 128:1033, 1993.

107. Bergstein JM, Blair JF, Edwards J, et al: Pitfalls in the use of color flow duplex ultrasound for screening of suspected arterial injuries in penetrated extremities, J Trauma 33:395, 1992.

108. Soto JA, Munera F, Cardoso N, et al: Diagnostic performance of helical CT angiography in trauma to large arteries of the extremities, J Comput Assist Tomogr 23:188, 1999.

109. Frykberg ER, Crump JM, Vines FS, et al: A reassessment of the role of arteriography in penetrating proximity extremity trauma: a prospective study, J Trauma 29:1041, 1989.

110. Lipchick EO, Kaebnick HW, Beres JJ, Towne JB: The role of arteriography in acute penetrating trauma to the extremities, Cardiovasc Intervent Radiol 10:202, 1987.

111. Fisher RG, Ben-Menachem Y: Interventional radiology in appendicular skeletal trauma, Radiol Clin North Am 25:1203, 1987.

112. Khansarinia S, Dennis JW, Veldenz HC, et al: Prophylactic Greenfield filter placement in selected high-risk trauma patients, J Vasc Surg 22:231, 1995.

113. Spritzer CE, Arata MA, Freed KS: Isolated pelvic deep venous thrombosis: relative frequency as detected with MR imaging, Radiology 219:521, 2001.

114. Rosenthal D, McKinsey JF, Levy AM, et al: Use of the Greenfield filter in patients with major trauma, Cardiovasc Surg 2:52, 1994.

115. Leach TA, Pastena JA, Swan KG, et al: Surgical prophylaxis for pulmonary embolism, Am Surgeon 60:292, 1994.

116. Gosin JS, Graham AM, Ciocca RG, Hammond JS: Efficacy of prophylactic vena cava filters in high-risk trauma patients, Ann Vasc Surg 11:100, 1997.

117. Rogers FB, Shackford SR, Ricci MA, et al: Prophylactic vena cava filter insertion in selected high-risk orthopaedic trauma patients, J Orthop Trauma 11:267, 1997.

118. Langan EM, Miller RS, Casey WJ, et al: Prophylactic inferior vena cava filters in trauma patients at high risk: follow-up examination and risk/benefit assessment, J Vasc Surg 30:484, 1999.

119. Wojcik R, Cipolle MD, Fearen I, et al: Long-term follow-up of trauma patients with a vena caval filter, J Trauma 49:839, 2000.

120. Rogers FB, Strindberg G, Shackford SR, et al: Five-year follow-up of prophylactic vena cava filters in high-risk trauma patients, Arch Surg 133:406, 1998.

121. Aswad MA, Sandager GP, Pais SO, et al: Early duplex scan evaluation of four vena caval interruption devices, J Vasc Surg 24:809, 1996.

122. Spain DA, Richarson JD, Polk HC, et al: Venous thromboembolism in the high-risk trauma patient: do risks justify aggressive screening and prophylaxis? J Trauma 42:463, 1997.

123. McMurtry AL, Owings JT, Anderson JT, et al: Increased use of prophylactic vena cava filters in trauma patients failed to decrease

overall incidence of pulmonary embolism, *J Am Coll Surg* 189:314, 1999.

124. Quirke TE, Ritota PC, Swan KG: Inferior vena caval filter use in U.S. trauma centers: a practitioner survey, *J Trauma* 43:333, 1997.

125. Millward SF, Bhargava A, Awuino J, et al: Gunther Tulip filter: preliminary clinical experience with retrieval, *J Vasc Interv Radiol* 11:75, 2000.

126. Vos LD, Tielbeek AV, Bom EP, et al: The Gunther temporary inferior vena cava filter for short-term protection against pulmonary embolism, *Cardiovasc Intervent Radiol* 20:91, 1997.

127. Sato DT, Robinson KD, Gregory RT, et al: Duplex directed caval filter insertion in multi-trauma and critically ill patients, *Ann Vasc Surg* 13:365, 1999.

128. Benjamin ME, Sandager GP, Cohn EJ, et al: Duplex ultrasound insertion of inferior vena cava filters in multitrauma patients, *Am J Surg* 178:92, 1999.

129. Sing RF, Jacobs DG, Heniford BT: Bedside insertion of inferior vena cava filters in the intensive care unit, *J Am Coll Surg* 192:570, 2001.

130. Sing RF, Cicci CK, Lequire MH, Stackhouse DJ: Bedside carbon dioxide cavagrams for inferior vena cava filters: preliminary results, *J Vasc Surg* 32:144, 2000.

131. Tola JC, Holtzman R, Lottenberg L: Bedside placement of inferior vena cava filters in the intensive care unit, *Am Surgeon* 65:833, 1999.

132. Rose SC, Kinney TB, Valji K, Winchell RJ: Placement of inferior vena caval filters in the intensive care unit, *J Vasc Interv Radiol* 8:61, 1997.

133. Sing RF, Stackhouse DJ, Cicci CK, Le Quire MH: Bedside carbon dioxide (CO_2) preinsertion cavagram for inferior vena cava filter placement: case report, *J Trauma* 47:1140, 1999.

134. Nunn CR, Neuzil D, Naslund T, et al: Cost-effective method for bedside insertion of vena caval filters in trauma patients, *J Trauma* 44:419, 1998.

135. Sing RF, Cicci CK, Smith CH, Messick WJ: Bedside insertion of inferior vena cava filters in the intensive care unit, *J Trauma* 47:1104, 1999.

136. Sing RF, Stackhouse DJ, Jacobs DG, Heniford BT: Safety and accuracy of bedside carbon dioxide cavography for insertion of inferior vena cava filters in the intensive care unit, *J Am Coll Surg* 192:168, 2001.

137. Putnam SG, Ball D, Cohen GS: Placement of bilateral Simon Nitinol filters for an inferior vena caval duplication through a single groin access, *J Vasc Interv Radiol* 10:431, 1999.

138. Baron HC, Klapholz A, Nagy AA, Wayne M: Bilateral iliac vein filter deployment in a patient with megacava, *Ann Vasc Surg* 13:634, 1999.

139. Bonn J, Liu JB, Exhelman DJ, et al: Intravascular ultrasound as an alternative to positive contrast vena cavography prior to filter placement, *J Vasc Interv Radiol* 10:834, 1999.

140. Oppat WF, Chiou AC, Mastamura JS: Intravascular ultrasound-guided vena cava filter placement, *J Endovasc Surg* 6:285, 1999.

141. Sing RF, Adrales G, Baek S, Kelley MJ: Guidewire incidents with inferior vena cava filters, *J Am Osteopath Assoc* 101:231, 2001.

142. Barraco RD, Scalea TM: Dislodgment of inferior vena cava filters during central line placement: case report, *J Trauma* 48:140, 2000.

143. Yegul TN, Bonilla SM, Goodwin SC, et al: Retrieval of a Greenfield IVC filter displaced to the right brachiocephalic vein, *Cardiovasc Intervent Radiol* 23:403, 2000.

144. Goldberg ME, Principato RE, Diamond SM, et al: Entrapment of an exchange wire by an inferior vena caval filter: a technique for removal, *J Clin Anesth* 11:609, 1999.

145. Ellis PK, Deutsch LS, Kidney DD: Interventional radiological retrieval of a guide-wire entrapped in a Greenfield filter—treatment of an avoidable complication of central venous access procedure, *Clin Radiol* 55:238, 2000.

146. Hastings GS, Chughtai S, Radack DM, Santilli JG: Repositioning the 12-F over-the-wire Greenfield filter, *J Vasc Interv Radiol* 11:1207, 2000.

12 Imaging of Penetrating Trauma to the Torso and Chest

K. Shanmuganathan and Thomas M. Scalea

The number of patients admitted with penetrating injuries to urban trauma centers throughout the United States has steadily increased.[1,2] The second leading cause of injury-related death in the United States is firearms.[3] It is estimated that for every firearm death, three to five other nonfatal firearm injuries occur.[4] Firearm-related injuries have become a major public health problem, having a devastating impact on American society with substantial emotional and financial cost. This chapter will review the role of imaging in evaluating patients admitted with penetrating injuries to the chest and abdomen and the influence of imaging findings on management.

BALLISTICS

A missile exits the barrel of a weapon with significant kinetic energy. The kinetic energy of the bullet depends on its mass and velocity (related to the amount of gunpowder that drives it forward) by the relationship $KE = mass/2 \times velocity^2$. Military weapons and hunting rifles are high-energy weapons and have a muzzle velocity greater than 1000 ft/sec. Most civilian gunshot wounds result from medium-energy handguns, with a muzzle velocity less than 1000 ft/sec.

The extent of tissue damage caused by a projectile is more severe if the missile has high energy, yaws early in its path through tissue, is large in mass, hits bone (forming secondary missiles), expands, deforms, or fragments when it strikes tissue.[5,6] A permanent cavity results from the missile crushing the tissues it transits. Temporary cavitation results several milliseconds following the passage of the bullet through the tissues from stretching. The temporary cavity may enlarge from 20 to 25 times the diameter of the bullet fired from high-energy weapons. Severe damage results from the temporary cavity formation in fluid-filled organs such as the bladder or heart and organs that contain less elastic tissue and have a dense parenchyma such as the liver (Fig. 12-1), kidney, and brain.[7] More elastic tissue, such as lung parenchyma (Figs. 12-2 and 12-3) or muscle, is able to stretch and remodel, resisting severe damage from the temporary cavity. The temporary cavity formed with medium-energy weapons (handgun) is insignificant and does not contribute to the amount of tissue damage in far- or intermediate-range civilian gunshot wounds. However, at close range a shotgun traditionally used for hunting behaves as a high-energy weapon. Hand-driven, low-energy weapons, such as a knife or ice pick, cause tissue damage only with their sharp cutting edge or point.

PENETRATING INJURIES TO THE TORSO
Mechanism of Injury

Most stab wounds are caused by knives, but they may also result from other sharp objects or instruments. Only two thirds of patients with a stab to the anterior abdominal wall have peritoneal penetration.[8-10] These low-energy injuries cause significant peritoneal injuries in approximately 50% of patients. Only one quarter to one third of patients with stab wounds to the anterior abdomen require laparotomy. Unlike stab wounds, gunshot wounds result in peritoneal penetration in 85% of abdominal gunshot wounds, and 80% of these patients have significant organ injury.[8-12] Moore et al.[11] used a penetrating trauma index score to predict the severity of

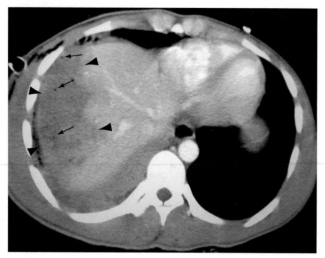

Fig. 12-1
Severe liver injury from temporary cavity formation. Axial CT image shows parenchymal contusion and hematoma (*arrowheads*) in dome of right lobe of liver along the bullet track outlined by air (*arrows*) from temporary cavity formation.

injury and risk of complications that occur following penetrating injuries. In this study gunshot wounds were associated more often with a higher injury score (>25) and complication rate than stab wounds because bullets have greater kinetic energy and travel further through the body. A high penetrating trauma injury index, as is typical of gunshot wounds, is associated with a higher likelihood of overtly positive clinical signs, such as peritoneal signs, and means fewer, if any, further investigations are needed to confirm peritoneal violation.[13,14]

Mandatory Laparotomy

Before the mid-1960s it was believed that routine exploration for penetrating torso injuries would reduce mortality by 12% to 27% compared with expectant management. This concept arose from military experience since World War I.[3,6,8,15-18] However, if such an approach were applied to all *civilian* penetrating injuries, 15% to 20% of gunshot wounds and 35% to 53% of stab wounds

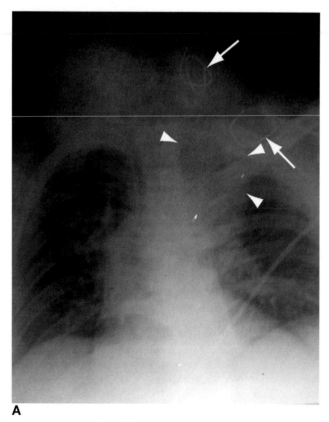

A

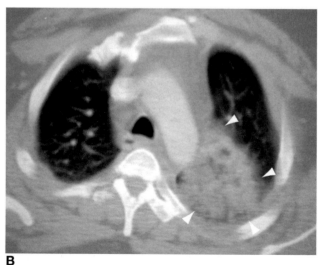

B

Fig. 12-2
Temporary cavity formation away from bullet track. **A,** Anteroposterior radiograph of chest shows entry and exit sites marked by clips (*arrows*) on skin surface. Increased density (*arrowheads*) seen in left upper lobe represents lung contusion. **B,** CT image confirms pulmonary contusion (*arrowheads*) in left upper lobe occurring without bullet penetrating left hemithorax, because of temporary cavitation in lung that is adjacent to the bullet track.

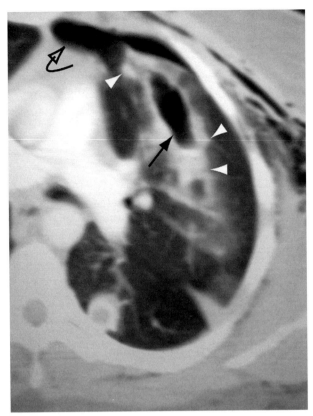

Fig. 12-3
Lung injury from gunshot wound to chest. CT image shows a post-traumatic pneumatocele (traumatic lung cyst) (*arrow*) surrounded by contused lung (*arrowheads*). A small anterior pneumothorax (*curved arrow*) is also seen.

to the torso would lead to an unnecessary (nontherapeutic) laparotomy.

Some proponents of mandatory laparotomy base their beliefs on unproven assertions that intraabdominal injury cannot be diagnosed short of exploration. They also believe clinical examination is often unreliable in patients with serious injuries, that a delay in diagnosis of these penetrating injuries will result in unacceptably high morbidity and mortality, and that nontherapeutic laparotomies are rarely associated with morbidity.[14,15,17,19-23]

Urgent laparotomy is the standard of care in the United States for patients who are hemodynamically unstable after sustaining gunshot or stab wounds or who have overt clinical signs of peritonitis. The availability of new surgical concepts and techniques, sophisticated new radiologic technology, use of antibiotics, and recognition of the potential morbidity and increased hospital costs associated with laparotomy have challenged the dictum of mandatory exploration of the abdomen in the civilian setting. The optimum diagnostic workup to assess potential peritoneal violation for hemodynamically stable patients with penetrating trauma is controversial.

Selective Conservative Management

In the past three decades, evidence of visceral injury has replaced simple peritoneal violation as the indication for abdominal exploration.[13-15,17,18,20,22] In the United States, this policy is more often applied to stab wounds than gunshot wounds in stable patients.[8,14,24] Ideally a selective conservative approach should reduce the number of negative and nontherapeutic laparotomies without increasing the number, morbidity, or mortality of missed or delayed diagnoses of serious injuries.

The optimal method of excluding peritoneal violation or significant visceral injury in hemodynamically stable patients with equivocal peritoneal signs following penetrating injury to the torso (defined by the area between the internipple line and upper third of the thigh) is controversial. The basic approaches currently available include observation with serial physical examinations, local wound exploration, diagnostic peritoneal lavage (DPL), abdominal ultrasound, computed tomography, and diagnostic laparoscopy. The anatomic location of the entry wound and the local practice at a given trauma center may dictate the management approach selected.

Anatomic Regions

The torso is divided into five anatomic regions (Fig. 12-4) to categorize site of injury:
1. The *thoracoabdominal* area, defined by the internipple line superiorly, costal margins extended posteriorly to inferior tip of the scapula inferiorly.
2. The *anterior abdomen,* defined by the costal margins superiorly, anterior axillary lines laterally, inguinal ligaments and symphysis pubis inferiorly.
3. The *flank,* defined by the anterior and posterior axillary line (tip of the scapula superiorly and iliac crests inferiorly) and from the costal margin to the iliac crest.
4. The *back,* defined by the tips of the scapula superiorly and iliac crests inferiorly.
5. The *pelvis,* defined by the iliac crests and inguinal ligaments superiorly and upper thirds of the thighs inferiorly.

MANAGEMENT APPROACHES
Observation

Of patients with penetrating injury to the anterior abdomen or back, 34% to 72% are hemodynamically stable without overt signs of peritonitis, and may be candidates for observation. Numerous studies have demonstrated that the practice of observation with serial physical examination (ideally performed by the same examiner) can be accomplished safely, thereby reducing

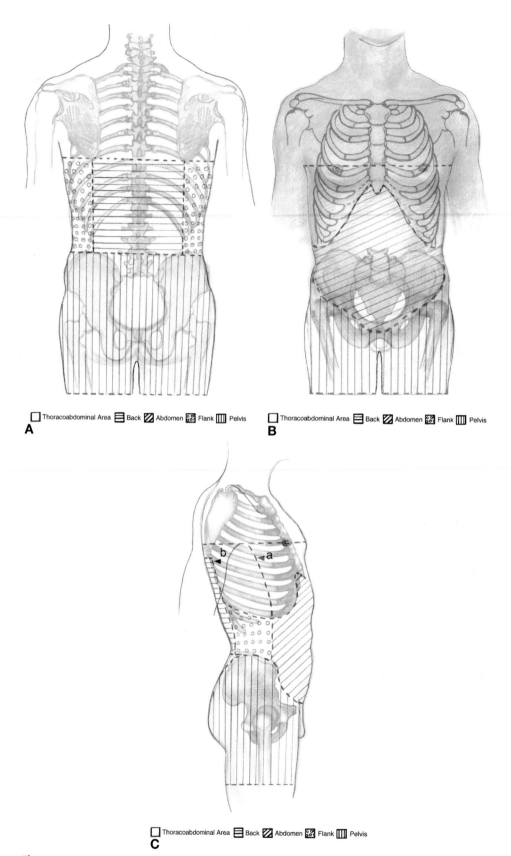

Fig. 12-4
Anatomic regions of torso. **A** to **C,** Thoracoabdominal area (*blank*), back (*horizontal lines*), abdomen (*diagonal lines*), flank (*dots*), pelvis (*vertical lines*). *a,* Anterior axillary line. *b,* Posterior axillary line. (From Shanmuganathan K, Mirvis SE, Chiu W, et al: *AJR Am J Roentgenol* 177:1247, 2001.)

the number of nontherapeutic laparotomies.* Although the majority of these studies investigated abdominal stab wounds, in the appropriate clinical setting this practice may also be applied to gunshot wounds.[14,17] Two studies also included patients who were observed even with evidence of free intraperitoneal air on radiographs and/or evisceration of omentum or bowel without signs of peritonitis.[14,22] Missed injuries requiring subsequent surgical exploration occurred in 4% to 6% of patients in the observation group with an average delay in treatment ranging from 3 hours to 5 days. Compared with mandatory laparotomy, this management approach reduced a nontherapeutic laparotomy rate of 53% down to 3% to 8% in some series.

One disadvantage of observation with serial examination is the need for admission to the hospital for up to 72 hours because a significant amount of time may be needed for clinical signs of peritonitis to develop after perforation, especially if the injury involves the retroperitoneal colon or duodenum. In a busy trauma center or in a small community hospital, staff may not be available to perform frequent examinations. This limits the number of patients that can be observed. Physical examination may be unreliable, and it may be difficult to elucidate signs of peritonitis in patients with associated severe head or spinal cord injuries, intoxication with alcohol or drugs, or other distracting injury.

Local Wound Exploration and DPL

Local wound exploration and DPL are both used to evaluate abdominal trauma. Root et al. initially found DPL to be a useful method of evaluating patients with intraperitoneal injury following blunt trauma.[30] This technique has been extended to evaluate hemodynamically stable patients without peritonitis who are at risk for penetration of the peritoneum.[13,20,24,25,31-38] The peritoneal tap is considered positive if gross blood, feces, bile, or food material is aspirated through the catheter placed within the peritoneal cavity.[13,31,36,38] A negative peritoneal tap is followed by a peritoneal lavage performed through the same catheter by using 1 liter of normal saline, and the lavage effluent is sent for analysis. Box 12-1 shows the criteria used at the authors' trauma center for a positive DPL in penetrating torso trauma. Local wound exploration is generally performed in the admission area under local anesthesia and sterile conditions. If the peritoneum has not been violated, the exploration site is closed and the patient can be discharged from the hospital. If there is penetration of the peritoneum or if wound exploration is equivocal for peritoneal violation, DPL may then be performed to evaluate for intraperitoneal injuries.

Many studies have been performed to discern the optimal technique for DPL and to establish the peritoneal lavage red blood cell (RBC) count that is an appropriate trigger for exploration.[13,20,24,25,31-38] Some of these studies have been summarized in Table 12-1. Currently the number of RBCs per cubic milliliter sufficient to perform surgical exploration ranges from 1000 to $100,000/mm^3$ and varies among trauma centers and according to mechanism of injury. The technique is highly sensitive when based on low RBC counts and highly specific using high RBC counts.

One limitation of DPL is a lack of consensus among surgeons regarding the definition of a positive RBC count. Significant injuries to the diaphragm and small bowel may occur with minimal hemorrhage and can be associated with a falsely negative DPL. The inability to define the anatomic source of hemorrhage or severity of

*References 1, 14, 17, 18, 22, 25-29.

Box 12-1
Criteria for Positive DPL

Aspiration of gross blood
Red blood cell count ≥10,000
White blood cell count ≥500
Presence of bile
Presence of feces
Presence of food material

Table 12-1
Sensitivity and Specificity of Peritoneal Lavage RBC Count for Detecting Intraperitoneal Injury

Study	Mechanism of Injury	No. Patients	Sensitivity (%)	Specificity (%)	Technique	RBC
Feliciano[31]	SW	500	96.3	88.2	LWE, DPL	50,000
Kelemen[32]	GSW	44	100	71.4	DPL	100,000
Muckart[38]	SW	121	76	75	DPL	100,000
			94	75	DPL	50,000
			100	0	DPL	5,000
Goldberg[36]	SW	29	69	—	LWE, DPL	20,000

injury by DPL may increase the rate of nontherapeutic laparotomies in nonbleeding solid visceral injuries. Because DPL does not survey the retroperitoneum, it is unreliable in evaluating retroperitoneal organ injury and should not be used as the sole technique in the evaluation of patients with penetrating injuries to the flank and back.[29,39,40] Local wound exploration may be difficult in obese patients, patients with thick back muscles, or in the presence of a large, actively bleeding abdominal wall hematoma.[8,41]

To improve the patient flow, busy trauma centers prefer local wound exploration and DPL to observation with serial physical examination in order to triage patients with penetrating torso injury. Unlike serial physical examination, which warrants admission of a large number of patients for up to 3 days, wound exploration and DPL can immediately eliminate patients who need not be observed.[13,31,34] Intraperitoneal injuries in asymptomatic patients are also diagnosed much more acutely. This approach eliminates the risk of potential morbidity and mortality associated with a delay in injury diagnosis.

Computed Tomography

Penetrating trauma to the flank and back in asymptomatic patients is rarely associated with injury to critical retroperitoneal viscera, because these organs are well-protected by ribs, the spine, and the large back and paraspinal muscles.[39,40] Patients with isolated retroperitoneal injuries emanating from these two distinct anatomic locations may not show overt clinical signs or symptoms and DPL does not evaluate them well.

The excellent sensitivity (89% to 100%), negative predictive value, accuracy (92% to 96%), and low associated nontherapeutic laparotomy rate (2.3%) of triple-contrast CT have made it a popular triage technique for posterior penetrating wounds.[40,42-46] Injuries to the colon are more likely to occur with posterior penetrating trauma. Most authors have emphasized the importance of routine use of rectal contrast material to opacify the entire colon, demonstrate contrast extravasation, and enhance the ability to diagnose subtle colonic injuries.[40,42,43] Oral and intravenous contrast are also used routinely to optimize the detection of injuries to the intraperitoneal bowel, solid organs, mesentery, retroperitoneal genitourinary system, and duodenum. Triple-contrast CT results may be classified into negative, minor or low-risk injuries, and major or high-risk injuries.[40,43] Patients with minor or low-risk injuries (small retroperitoneal hematoma or minor renal injury) are generally managed conservatively. Patients with major injuries are managed with surgery or angiography.

Intraperitoneal injuries are incurred by 58% of patients with penetrating trauma to the back or flank. Combined intraperitoneal and retroperitoneal injuries may occur in 16% of these patients.[39] Because of concerns about the ability to diagnose hollow viscus injury by CT, DPL has been used as an adjunct to CT to diagnose these potentially associated intraperitoneal injuries in some studies.

Recent retrospective studies have also found CT to be accurate in determining trajectory and peritoneal violation in hemodynamically stable patients with gunshot wounds with a potential peritoneal trajectory elsewhere in the torso.[47,48] In a retrospective study performed by Ginzberg et al.,[48] triple-contrast CT was used as the initial screening tool to evaluate for peritoneal violation and to minimize nontherapeutic laparotomies. The study included 83 stable patients admitted following gunshot wounds to the torso. Forty-five patients incurred gunshot wounds to the flank, and 38 patients to the abdomen.[48] Patients with equivocal CT for peritoneal violation underwent cavitary endoscopy to verify CT findings. No injuries were missed in the 53 patients with negative CT results who were observed for 23 hours. Fifteen patients had evidence of peritoneal violation or liver injury. CT had a specificity of 54%, negative predictive value of 100%, and overall accuracy of 71% for the abdominal wounds and a specificity of 98%, negative predictive value of 100%, and overall accuracy of 98% for flank wounds. In a retrospective study performed over a 6-year period, Grossman et al.[47] used CT to determine trajectory and to exclude intraperitoneal injury in 37 patients following transabdominal or transpelvic gunshot wounds without clinical or radiographic evidence of peritoneal penetration. CT showed the trajectory to be extraperitoneal in 20 patients and intraperitoneal in 17 patients. Eight therapeutic laparotomies were performed in the patients who underwent exploration. No complications from missed injuries were reported in the 20 patients with negative CT results. Both these studies concluded that CT was safe and effective as an initial screening tool to evaluate for peritoneal violation in hemodynamically stable patients with torso gunshot wounds.

The authors have performed a prospective study to evaluate the role of triple-contrast spiral CT in hemodynamically stable patients with penetrating trauma for determining both peritoneal violation and need for laparotomy.[49] The study included 104 patients: 44 suffered gunshot wounds (16 multiple wounds), 48 were stabbed (7 multiple wounds), and 2 were impaled. The entry site was in the thoracoabdominal region in 40% (42/104), the pelvis in 20% (21/104), the abdomen in 17% (18/104), the flank in 13% (13/104), and the back in 11% (11/104). None of the patients had radiographic or clinical indication for immediate laparotomy. A positive CT was defined as evidence of peritoneal violation (free intraperitoneal air, fluid, intraperitoneal contrast extravasation, or visceral injury) or injury to the retroperitoneal colon, major vessel, or urinary tract. Patients with a positive CT, excluding selected patients with isolated liver injury or free fluid, underwent laparotomy. Patients with a negative CT were observed for 12 hours.

CT studies were positive in 34% (35/104) of the patients and negative in 66% (69/104). Among those with a negative CT, 67 of 69 (97%) were managed nonoperatively without missed injuries. Laparotomy was performed in 63% (22/35) of the patients with a positive CT. Of these, 86% (19/22) were therapeutic, 9% (2/22) nontherapeutic, and 5% (1/22) negative. Nine patients with isolated hepatic injuries were successfully managed without laparotomy. Similar results have been reported by Renz et al.[50] in a prospective study of seven stable patients sustaining right thoracoabdominal gunshot wounds, in which CT helped select patients with isolated liver injury for successful nonoperative management.

In the authors' study, triple-contrast spiral CT was a highly accurate means of excluding peritoneal violation in hemodynamically stable patients with penetrating torso trauma. Among patients with peritoneal violation, spiral CT was also accurate in predicting the need for laparotomy and in verifying isolated liver injury, allowing nonoperative management for patients with penetration limited to the right upper quadrant. CT had 100% (19/19) sensitivity, 96% (69/72) specificity, 100% (69/69) negative predictive value, and 97% (101/104) accuracy in predicting the need for laparotomy. Currently, in our busy level I trauma center, triple-contrast spiral CT is being used as a safe and reliable technique to triage stable patients with penetrating injuries to the torso in whom there are no clinical or radiographic signs of peritoneal violation.

Diagnostic Laparoscopy

Laparoscopy enables direct visualization of the peritoneum and the intraperitoneal viscera in order to diagnose peritoneal violation and evaluate potential organ injury. Although gasless laparoscopy can be performed to avoid the potentially serious complication of carbon dioxide pneumoperitoneum (gas embolism, tension pneumothorax, hypercarbia), most studies performed to triage hemodynamically stable patients with penetrating injuries used conventional laparoscopy under general anesthesia.[51-59] These studies recommend the conversion of the diagnostic laparoscopy to a laparotomy in the presence of peritoneal violation, major organ injury, or significant hematoma.[52-59] Patients with no peritoneal penetration or with nonbleeding solid organ injuries may be observed or discharged. Studies show that though laparoscopy still carries a 17% to 20% rate of nontherapeutic laparotomy and 17% negative laparotomy rates, laparoscopy has been found to prevent unnecessary laparotomies in 34% to 60% of patients,

with a concurrent reduction in hospitalization duration and costs.[52-59]

The strength of diagnostic laparoscopy appears to be in the evaluation of patients with penetrating injuries to the thoracoabdominal area.[51] Local wound exploration is unreliable and associated with the risk of creating a pneumothorax in this region. Laparoscopy reduces the number of nontherapeutic laparotomies as compared with DPL that may be performed among the subset of patients with minor splenic and liver injuries that have stopped bleeding by the time of surgery. Laparoscopy has been shown to be optimally suited to evaluate the diaphragm for injuries in asymptomatic patients with less than 10,000 RBC/mm³ in the DPL effluent.[52,60,61]

The limitations of laparoscopy include the need for general anesthesia and inadequate visualization of the retroperitoneum. Laparoscopy may also miss gastrointestinal injuries. Ivatory et al.[52] reported diagnostic laparoscopy had a sensitivity of 18% for diagnosing bowel injury following penetrating trauma to the abdomen. In this study, only two patients with bowel injury were diagnosed by laparoscopy. Ten additional bowel injuries were identified only during laparotomy. Thoracic injuries needing surgical intervention may also be missed with laparoscopy.

Tension pneumothorax may develop during laparoscopy in patients with diaphragm injury, and special precaution should be taken to avoid this complication. One major contraindication for laparoscopy is a history of multiple adhesions. Laparoscopy is also contraindicated for patients with elevated intracranial pressure who may suffer adverse effects from the insufflation of carbon dioxide.[52] A significant cost savings will be gained only if laparoscopy is performed under local anesthesia.[52,53,57]

Ultrasound

There has been little enthusiasm to embrace ultrasound as an initial screening study to evaluate patients with penetrating trauma to the torso.[1,62,63] Although ultrasound can demonstrate free intraperitoneal fluid in blunt trauma patients, these results have not been reproduced in patients suffering penetrating injuries to the abdomen. In a prospective study at the authors' trauma center performed by Udobi et al.[62] to determine the role of ultrasound in penetrating abdominal trauma, the overall sensitivity of focused assessment of sonography for trauma (FAST) to detect free fluid in the peritoneal cavity was 47%. Sonography was only used to detect free fluid in the perisplenic, perihepatic, pelvic, and pericardial spaces. Nine patients with a negative FAST had hemoperitoneum. A significant number of patients with negative FAST studies had serious abdominal injuries requiring surgical repair, including liver (n=4), small bowel (n=4), diaphragm (n=3), colon (n=3), and stomach (n=1). A positive FAST was a strong predictor of intraabdominal injury (specificity, 94%; positive predictive value, 90%). Thus, a positive FAST should prompt immediate exploration.

In a prospective study of 74 patients with penetrating injuries to the abdomen, thoracoabdominal area, and thorax, Rozycki et al. reported false-negative ultrasound examinations in 10 patients with intraperitoneal injuries requiring surgical intervention.[63] Both studies concluded that ultrasound cannot be used to exclude injury after penetrating trauma and that additional studies should be performed to diagnose occult injuries. Ultrasound has also been used to examine wound tracks to determine peritoneal or pleural violation.[64] In a pilot study using a 7-MHz ultrasound probe, an accurate evaluation of the wound track was performed in 21 stable patients with tangential penetrating injuries to the abdomen. Ultrasound demonstrated peritoneal penetration in three patients that was confirmed at surgery. However, the ultrasound findings did not factor in further diagnostic or therapeutic management decisions.

Imaging of Penetrating Torso Trauma

Radiography. Radiographs are the initial imaging modality performed to localize a bullet and to evaluate for peritoneal violation.[65] To determine the missile caliber from radiographs the bullets should be seen on two views with no deformity, and the degree of magnification should be taken into account.[65] Localization of a bullet or penetrating foreign body calls for two radiographs obtained at 90° or tomographic images (Figs. 12-5 and 12-6). Occasionally these two views may not be able to accurately localize the exact site of the penetrating object (Figs. 12-7 to 12-9). It is extremely risky to determine the course of a penetrating object using radiographs by extrapolating a straight line between the entry and exit wounds or between the bullet and the entry site. Missiles do not take the shortest path between two points, because the victim may have been in motion when injured and missiles change course when traveling through dense tissue[66,67] (Fig. 12-10).

At the authors' trauma center routine views include a chest radiograph and two views (anteroposterior and lateral projections) of the abdomen usually taken without moving the patient. Chest radiographs should be routinely obtained in all patients with penetrating trauma to the torso, because upper abdominal and thoracoabdominal penetrating injuries are associated with thoracic pathology and radiographs are needed to assess for pneumoperitoneum. If feasible, chest radiographs should be obtained in the erect position to increase sensitivity for the detection of pneumoperitoneum. These three views help in the evaluation of peritoneal penetration and localize the penetrating object. Localized views may be required in obese patients or regions of dense structure, such as the pelvis, to localize the penetrating object or evaluate for fractures. Radiographic findings of peritoneal violation include an intraperitoneal bullet or penetrating object (see Fig. 12-5), pneumoperitoneum (Figs. 12-11 and 12-12), and free intraperitoneal fluid. Displacement of intraperitoneal organs by hematomas may help to localize the site and extent of injury. Abdominal and chest radiographs have a low sensitivity and lack specificity for intraabdominal injuries[62,68] (see Figs. 12-7 to 12-9). A study performed by Udobi et al.[62] to evaluate the role of ultrasound in penetrating abdominal trauma reported that erect chest radiographs were positive for pneumoperitoneum in only two (18%) of 11 patients with surgically proven intestinal perforation. The erect chest radiographs were not an adjunct to FAST in this study.

Computed Tomography. CT is the imaging modality of choice to evaluate patients who are hemodynamically stable following blunt trauma, and it has been shown during the last two decades[69-73] to be increasingly accurate in diagnosing solid organ and hollow viscus injury. In the setting of penetrating trauma, CT is both far more sensitive and more specific than radiography in identifying injuries to organs along wound tracks.[40,42-44,47-50,65] At the University of Maryland Shock Trauma Center (UMSTC), hemodynamically stable patients with penetrating injuries to the torso without radiographic or clinical signs of peritonitis are evaluated for peritoneal violation and intraperitoneal and retroperitoneal injuries using triple-contrast multislice spiral CT.

Technique. Triple-contrast spiral CT scans are obtained from the internipple line to the symphysis pubis following administration of intravenous, rectal, and oral contrast material. The CT parameters used at our institution for conventional, helical, and multislice spiral CT and for administration of intravenous contrast material are shown in Table 12-2. Currently, we use only multislice spiral CT to image our trauma patients. A total volume of 600 ml of 2% sodium diatrizoate (Hypaque sodium, Nycomed, Inc., Princeton, NJ) oral contrast material is administered 30 minutes before and immediately before initiation of the scan. An enema of 1 to 1.5 L of 2% sodium diatrizoate is also administered on the CT table to opacify the colon before scanning. Delayed images are obtained routinely about 3 minutes following injection of intravenous contrast material to evaluate the renal collecting system for injury.

Active Bleeding, Hemoperitoneum, and Free Fluid. CT is extremely sensitive in detecting even small quantities of free intraperitoneal fluid or hemoperitoneum.[74] Using density measurements of free intraperitoneal fluid seen

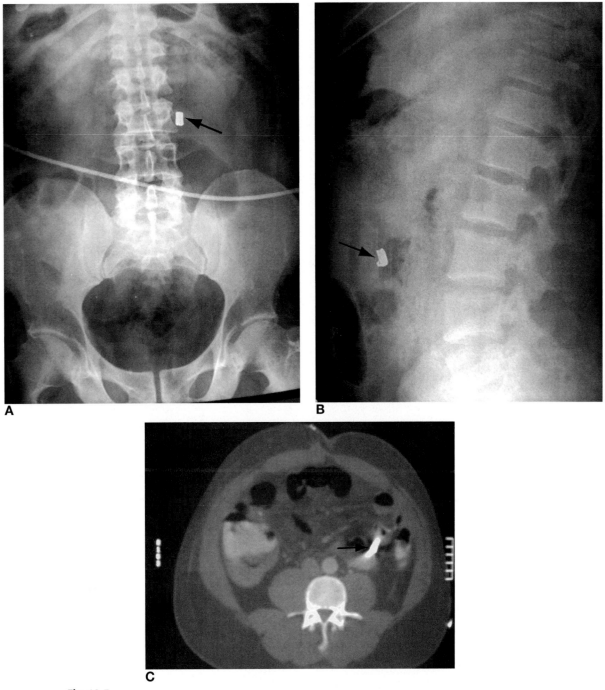

Fig. 12-5
Intraperitoneal bullet seen on radiographs in a 26-year-old man who was shot in the abdomen and lower chest. Anteroposterior (**A**) and cross-table lateral (**B**) views of abdomen show a bullet (*arrow*) within peritoneal cavity in left lower abdomen. **C**, CT image obtained following surgery to evaluate for an abscess confirms intraperitoneal location of bullet (*arrow*).

within the peritoneal cavity, CT is able to distinguish between free fluid, blood, hematoma, bile, and active bleeding[72,74,75] (Figs. 12-13 to 12-15). On contrast-enhanced CT scans free intraperitoneal fluid measures between 0 to 15 Hounsfield units (HU), free blood between 20 and 40 HU, clotted blood or hematoma

between 40 and 70 HU, and active bleeding within 10 HU of the density of intravenous contrast material seen within the adjacent major artery.[72,74]

The significant difference in the attenuation value of extravasated contrast material (range, 85 to 350 HU; mean, 132 HU) and hematoma (range, 40 to 70 HU;

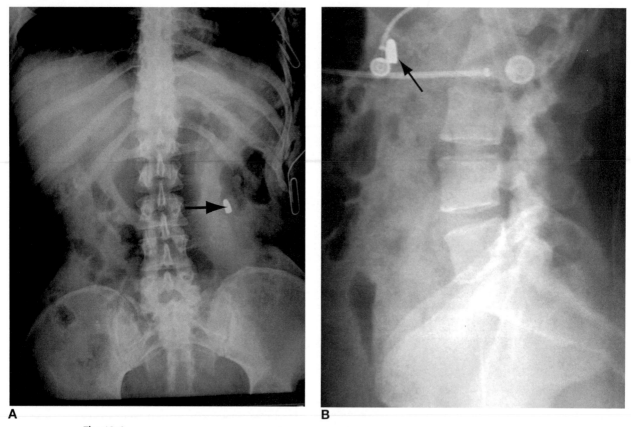

Fig. 12-6
Intraperitoneal bullet. Anteroposterior (**A**) and lateral (**B**) radiographs show a bullet (*arrow*) within the peritoneal cavity in the left mid abdomen. The entry site is marked by a paper clip. At surgery multiple small bowel injuries were repaired.

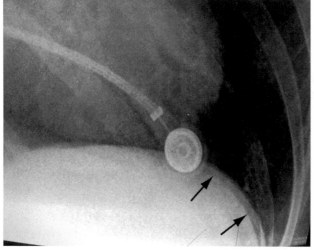

Fig. 12-7
Localized view of the left hemidiaphragm on admission chest radiograph shows curvilinear lucency (*arrows*) below the left diaphragm, suggestive of free intraperitoneal air. Free air was not detected on admission CT scan.

mean, 51 HU) is helpful in differentiating active bleeding from clotted blood.[72] This attenuation difference between clotted blood and active bleeding may often be appreciated on inspection and without need for measuring attenuation values using a region of interest (ROI). The extended areas that could be scanned precisely by multislice spiral CT during various phases (arterial, portal venous, and excretory) of intravenous contrast material administration help to better demonstrate ongoing hemorrhage than what can be demonstrated by single-slice spiral CT. On multislice CT ongoing hemorrhage may be seen as an increase in the amount of intravenous contrast material extravasated on images obtained in the identical anatomic region during arterial and delayed renal pyelogram (equilibrium) phases of contrast administration (Fig. 12-16). Clotted and liquid blood and fluid are typically hypodense compared with the contrast-enhanced parenchyma of solid organs (Fig. 12-14). Blood appears hyperdense compared with parenchyma

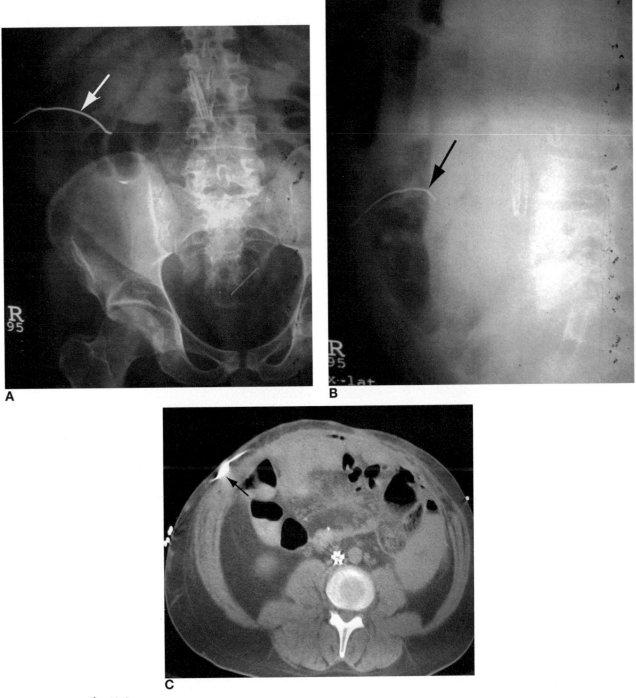

Fig. 12-8
Attempted impalement with a metallic wire by a patient from a mental institution. Anteroposterior (**A**) and lateral (**B**) views of abdomen show a metallic wire (*arrows*) with its tip in peritoneal cavity. **C**, CT image at the level of wire shows the wire (*arrow*) to be superficial to abdominal wall muscles.

on unenhanced CT (see Fig. 12-17). Blood or hematoma may appear isodense to suboptimally enhancing parenchyma, making it difficult to diagnose by CT. In order to avoid this pitfall, it is important to scan during peak parenchymal enhancement and to administer an adequate volume and concentration of intravenous contrast material. Bolus tracking techniques are helpful in optimizing scan initiation to achieve peak arterial enhancement without use of excessive contrast quantities. Administration of oral and rectal contrast material

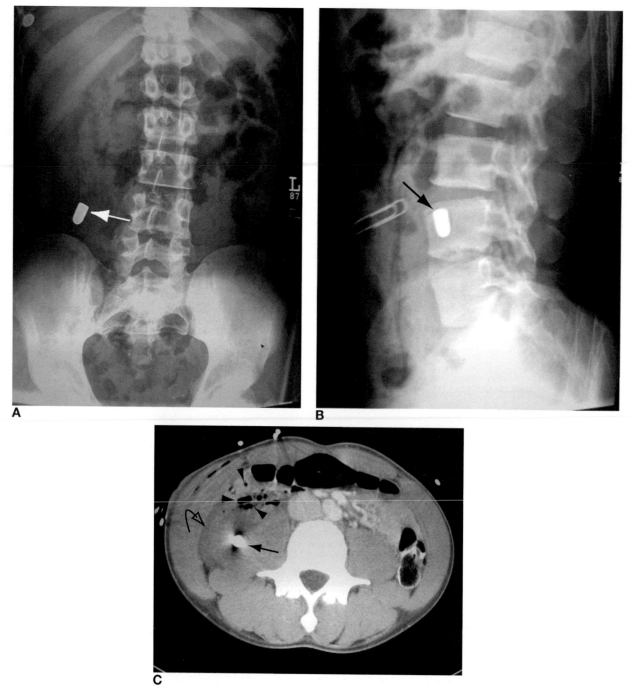

Fig. 12-9
Gunshot wound to the flank. Anteroposterior (**A**) and lateral (**B**) radiographs of the abdomen show a bullet (*arrow*) in the lateral right abdomen. No free intraperitoneal air is seen. Precise location of bullet (intraperitoneal or extraperitoneal) cannot be determined from these two films. **C**, CT image at the level of bullet (*arrow*) shows a moderate right psoas and small retroperitoneal hematoma (*curved arrow*). Retroperitoneal air is observed anterior to the psoas muscle (*arrowheads*). CT did not show peritoneal violation, and this was confirmed at surgery.

usually opacifies portions of the small bowel and most of the colon and helps to distinguish small quantities of intermesenteric blood, fluid, or hematoma from aggregated nonopacified bowel that can mimic these findings.

Small amounts of blood or free fluid are usually seen in the most gravity-dependent regions of the peritoneal cavity. In the supine position the most dependent region of the peritoneal cavity is the hepatorenal fossa (Morison's pouch) (Fig. 12-18). Other areas where free

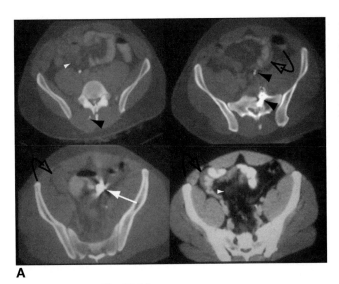

A

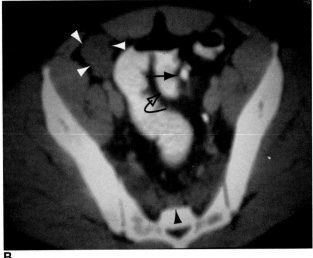

B

Fig. 12-10
Unpredictable ballistic track. Pelvic gunshot wound with peritoneal violation in a 20-year-old man. **A**, CT images through pelvis show bullet fragments, air, and blood along transsacral wound track (*black arrowheads*). Largest bullet fragment (*arrow*) is seen within the peritoneal cavity. Wound track extends to the sigmoid colon. Bullet has been deflected by sacrum and has not taken the shortest path between entry and final resting points. A mesenteric contusion (*white arrowheads*) and free intraperitoneal fluid (*curved arrow*) are also seen. **B**, CT image with window and level set to minimize streak artifact from bullet shows free intraperitoneal fluid (*white arrowheads*) with largest bullet fragment next to the sigmoid colon (*curved arrow*). Blood (*black arrowhead*) is seen anterior to sacrum. Sigmoid colon and adjacent mesenteric injury were confirmed at surgery. (From Shanmuganathan K, Mirvis SE, Chiu W, et al: *AJR Am J Roentgenol* 177:1247, 2001.)

fluid or blood is often seen in trauma patients are the pelvis adjacent to the bladder, paracolic gutters, and perihepatic and perisplenic spaces (Fig. 12-19). Careful inspection of these areas is necessary to identify small quantities of fluid or blood that may be the only CT sign of peritoneal violation suggesting a subtle or occult intraperitoneal visceral injury (see Fig. 12-18).

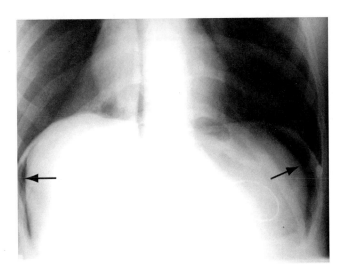

Fig. 12-11
Moderate pneumoperitoneum (*arrows*) on admission chest radiograph of patient with penetrating torso trauma

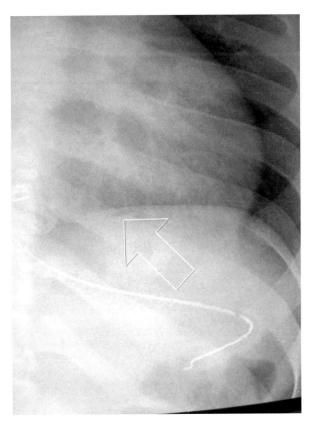

Fig. 12-12
Small amount of free intraperitoneal air (*arrow*) is seen under the left hemidiaphragm of patient with penetrating torso trauma

Table 12-2
Recommended CT Scan Techniques for Torso Trauma

	Volume of IV Contrast (ml)	Delay Rate (sec)*	Injection Speed (ml/sec)	Collimation	Table	Pitch
Conventional CT	150	20	1.5	10 mm	—	—
Single-slice spiral CT	150	60	3	8 mm	8 mm	1
Multislice spiral CT	150	70	3	2.5 mm × (4)†	10 mm	1

*Delay in initiation of scan from beginning of IV bolus.
†Number of slices obtained per rotation (0.8 sec)

By measuring the attenuation value of the free intraperitoneal blood in the peritoneal cavity following blunt trauma, Orwig and Fedrele[76] demonstrated that the highest density blood is seen adjacent to the injured organ. They referred to this as the "sentinel clot." In their study the "sentinel clot" sign was the only finding in 14% of 120 patients that indicated the source of hemorrhage. The current authors have also found this CT sign to be reliable and helpful in evaluating CT scans of patients with hemoperitoneum following penetrating trauma.

Performance of DPL can decrease the attenuation value of hemoperitoneum by dilution. Whenever DPL is performed before CT, this knowledge is required for accurate interpretation. At the UMSTC, any fluid that measures more than 10 HU after a pre-CT DPL is considered to contain admixed blood, and oral or rectal contrast material.[69] Density measurements should be obtained for all fluid collections identified by CT to help characterize their origin. Care should be taken to avoid volume averaging in assigning the ROI around the fluid.

The CT attenuation value of bile is usually below zero because of its high cholesterol content. Intraperitoneal or combined intraperitoneal and extraperitoneal bladder injuries can result in urine leaking into the peritoneal cavity. Unopacified urine is usually similar in density to fluid and measures between 0 and 15 HU. It can mimic free intraperitoneal fluid. However, on delayed images obtained during the renal excretory phase the density of urine may increase in value or be similar in attenuation values to urinary contrast material seen within the bladder as a result of admixing of extravasated urinary contrast material and unopacified urine within the peritoneal cavity.[77]

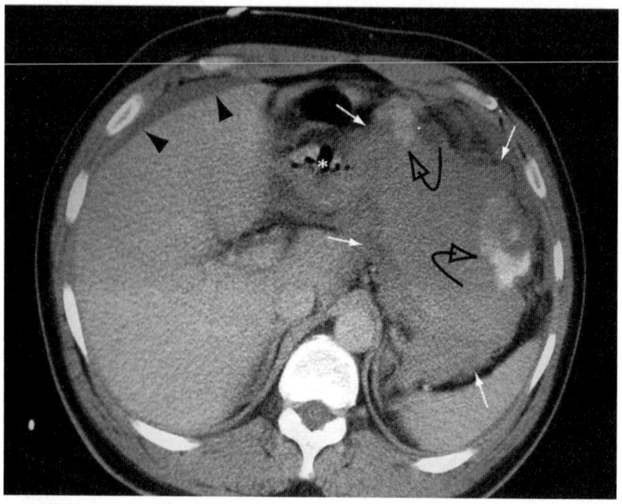

Fig. 12-13
CT appearance of free intraperitoneal blood. Stab wound to left thoracoabdominal region in a 23-year-old man. CT image through upper abdomen shows free intraperitoneal fluid anterior to the liver (*arrowheads*). A large amount of clotted blood (*arrows*) is seen in the lesser sac displacing the stomach (*asterisk*) anteriorly. Within the lesser sac hematoma is an area of active bleeding (*curved arrows*). A significant attenuation difference is seen between clotted blood and active bleeding. At surgery an actively bleeding vessel was seen along the posterior wall of the lesser sac and ligated. No injury to the stomach was noted.

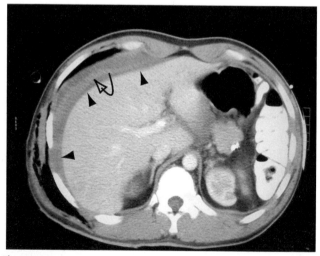

Fig. 12-14
CT appearance of clotted blood in a 34-year-old patient stabbed in the right thoracoabdominal region. CT image obtained through the liver shows free intraperitoneal (*arrowheads*) and clotted blood (*curved arrow*). Clotted blood is denser than free intraperitoneal blood.

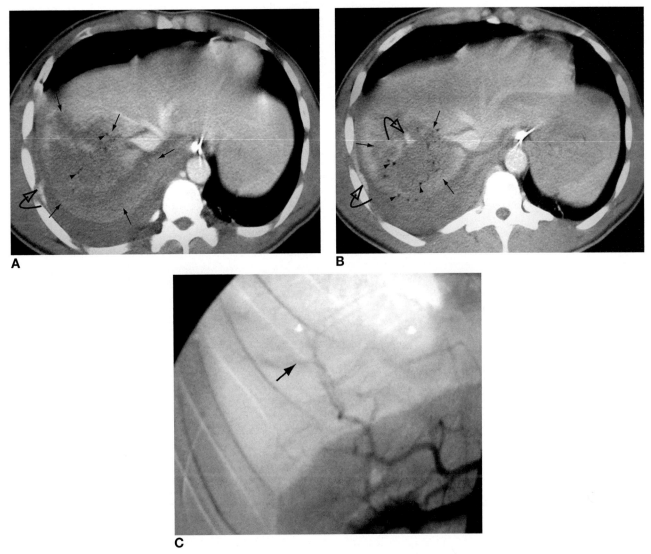

Fig. 12-15
Active bleeding into liver. This patient was shot in right thoracoabdominal region. **A** and **B**, CT images show an intraparenchymal hematoma (*arrows*) and air (*arrowheads*) in the dome of liver. Areas of high-density active bleeding (*curved arrows*) are seen within the right lobe and the right pleural space. The density of extravasated contrast material is similar in density to contrast material seen within inferior vena cava and abdominal aorta. Active bleeding from liver has entered pleural space through a tear in right hemidiaphragm. **C**, Active bleeding (*arrow*) is seen peripherally in liver and was embolized successfully.

Wound Track and Peritoneal Violation. The presence of air, hemorrhage, or bullet fragments along a wound track allows identification through CT of the bullet or knife trajectory. Usually bullet tracks are more easily delineated compared with low-energy stab wound tracks (Figs. 12-20 to 12-27). The greater the amount of hemorrhage (see Figs. 12-22 and 12-23), air, and metal fragments seen along gunshot wound tracks, the more clearly they are

demonstrated. Knife wound tracks may be subtle, and it is important to identify the wound track, its extension into the peritoneal cavity, and its relationship to abdominal viscera (see Fig. 12-26). Prior knowledge of the wound entry site with a radio-opaque marker and use of optimum CT windows and level (window = 550, level = 75) aid in identifying subtle wound tracks and localizing visceral injury sites.[49] CT should be considered positive for peritoneal violation in the presence of a wound track outlined by air, hemorrhage, or bullet fragments due to the missile or knife entering the peritoneal cavity (trajectory of missile or knife). It is important to review images on bone and lung window settings to determine the precise location of air bubbles seen along the wound track that are located adjacent to the peritoneum. Intraperitoneal free air or fluid, bullet fragments, visceral, mesenteric, or vascular injury are diagnostic CT findings of peritoneal violation (see Figs. 12-13, 12-14, 12-25, and 12-26).

In a prospective study performed at our institution to evaluate the role of triple-contrast CT for penetrating trauma to the torso, CT demonstrated peritoneal violation in 34% (35/104) of patients.[49] The most common CT finding in patients with peritoneal violation was intraperitoneal free fluid, found in 94% (33/35) and the only finding in 11% (4/35). Other CT signs useful to diagnose peritoneal violation included intraperitoneal visceral injury (Figs. 12-28 to 12-30) seen in 60% (21/35), and free intraperitoneal air (Fig. 12-31) seen in 43% (15/43). These two signs were more often associated

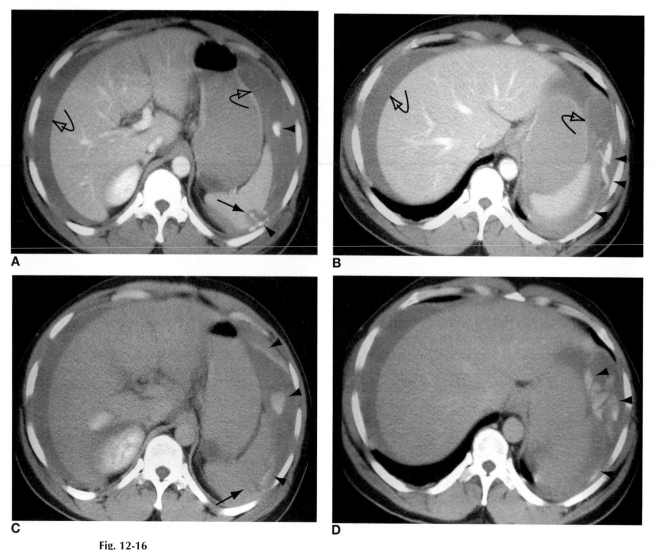

Fig. 12-16
Increasing amounts of active bleeding seen on multislice CT in a man stabbed in left upper quadrant. **A** and **B**, CT images obtained in portal venous phase shows an actively bleeding splenic laceration (*arrow*) with a large amount of free intraperitoneal blood (*curved arrows*). Active bleeding is seen in splenic parenchyma and peritoneal cavity (*arrowheads*). **C** and **D**, CT images obtained in renal excretory phase at the same level show increased intraperitoneal bleeding (*arrowheads*).

Continued

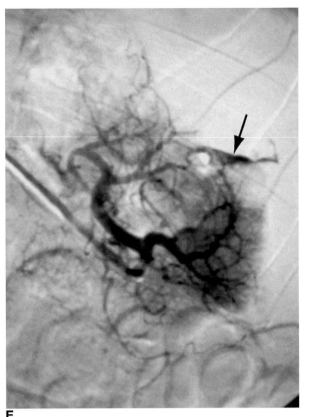

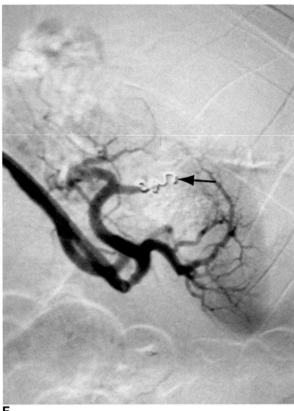

E **F**

Fig. 12-16, cont'd
E, Splenic angiogram shows an area of bleeding (arrow). **F,** Bleeding was successfully treated by distal transcatheter coil embolization *(arrow).*

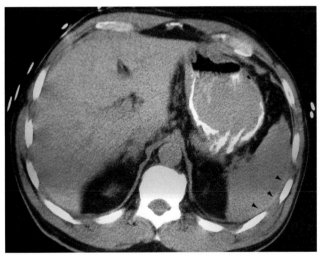

Fig. 12-17
Appearance of blood on unenhanced CT. Unenhanced CT image in region of spleen in a trauma patient shows a small amount of subcapsular blood *(arrowheads)*. Blood appears hyperdense compared with the splenic parenchyma.

with gunshot wounds than stab wounds. CT was negative for peritoneal violation in 66% (69/104) of study patients on initial evaluation, and 97% (67/69) of patients were managed nonoperatively without any late complications as a result of missed injuries. In this study, triple-contrast spiral CT was highly accurate for excluding peritoneal violation, and it reliably triaged select patients to nonoperative management.

Solid Organ Injury. The liver is the most commonly injured solid organ seen following penetrating trauma to the torso.* Injuries to the liver and spleen are seen more frequently following penetrating injuries to the thoracoabdominal region, upper abdomen, and flank. The three principal types of parenchymal injury that may be seen on CT are hematoma, laceration, and active bleeding.

Hematomas may be subcapsular or intraparenchymal (Fig. 12-32; see Figs. 12-1, 12-15, and 12-30). On contrast-

_____
*References 8, 17, 38, 49, 53, 78.

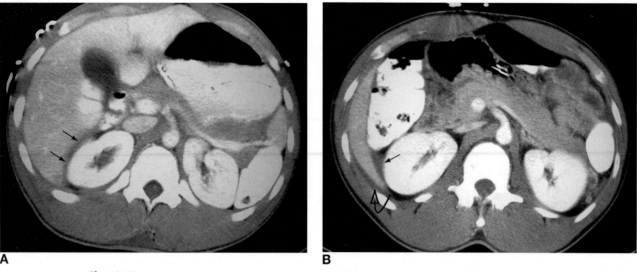

Fig. 12-18
Free intraperitoneal fluid in a 35-year-old man admitted following a gunshot wound. **A** and **B**, Two CT images of the upper abdomen show small amount of free fluid (*arrows*) in Morison's pouch and perihepatic (*curved arrow*) region.

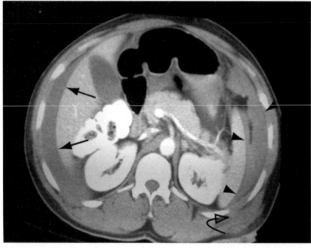

Fig. 12-19
"Sentinel clot" sign. CT image through the upper abdomen in a patient who was stabbed in the left flank shows higher density blood (*arrowheads*) adjacent to the spleen as compared with blood (*arrows*) seen adjacent to liver. Note a left flank soft tissue hematoma (*curved arrow*) from the stab wound.

enhanced CT, intraparenchymal hematomas are seen along the wound track as low-attenuation areas when compared with the normally enhancing parenchyma of the liver or spleen. Intraparenchymal hematomas seen along the wound track are usually larger following a high-energy gunshot wound, which generally causes more tissue damage than a stab wound (see Figs. 12-1, 12-15, 12-31, and 12-33). Subcapsular hematomas are seen as low-attenuation collections between the parenchyma and

Glisson's capsule. Subcapsular hematomas cause direct compression of the underlying normal parenchyma. This CT sign is helpful to differentiate a subcapsular hematoma from free intraperitoneal blood.

Subcapsular hematomas are less frequently seen or are smaller in size with penetrating injury than with blunt trauma. The penetrating object typically tears Glisson's capsule and allows decompression of the hematoma into the peritoneal cavity rather than into the subcapsular space. Subcapsular or parenchymal hematomas may also occur some distance away from the wound track without penetration of the solid organ. This is particularly true with high-energy injuries such as gunshot wounds. These hematomas usually result from the temporary cavity formation transmitted via high-energy missiles into dense parenchyma such as the liver and spleen.[7,67]

Lacerations occur along the wound track resulting from crushing of parenchyma. On contrast-enhanced CT acute lacerations are seen as linear low-attenuation areas, compared with the normal enhancing parenchyma (Fig. 12-33; see Figs. 12-16 and 12-32). CT helps to identify the relationship between lacerations and major vascular structures such as hepatic veins, the porta hepatis, intrahepatic inferior vena cava, and splenic hilum. These CT findings may help plan management and predict outcome. Poletti et al.[79] reported, in a review of 72 patients with blunt liver injury, that extension of liver lacerations into the region of one or more of the hepatic veins had a significant association with active bleeding and failed nonoperative management. While lacerations resulting from blunt trauma typically display

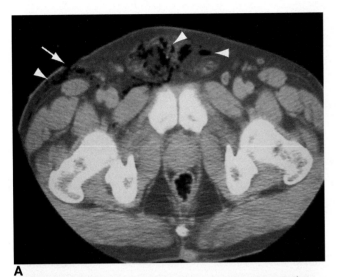

A

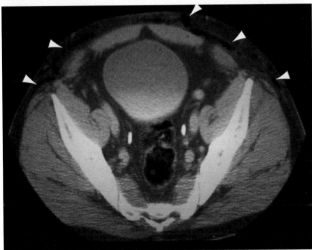

B

Fig. 12-20

A 41-year-old man impaled by metal spike in fall. **A** and **B**, low and mid pelvic images show an entry site in the right groin (*arrow*) with large amount of soft tissue air (*arrowheads*) in the anterior abdominal wall. No free intraperitoneal air or fluid is seen. Surgical debridement of the anterior abdominal wall wound track confirmed no evidence of peritoneal violation. (From Shanmuganathan K, Mirvis SE, Chiu W, et al: *AJR Am J Roentgenol* 177:1247, 2001.)

a multiple parallel or stellate pattern, such patterns do not occur from penetrating trauma. As a liver laceration heals, it enlarges, develops smooth margins, and assumes a round or oval shape (see Fig. 12-32).

Active hemorrhage (see Figs. 12-15, 12-16, and 12-32) resulting from penetrating injury is seen as an irregular high-density area of contrast extravasation surrounded by less dense hematoma, and usually increases in amount on delayed images using multislice spiral CT (see Fig. 12-16). Posttraumatic vascular injuries, such as pseudoaneurysms (Figs. 12-34 and 12-35), arteriovenous fistulas,

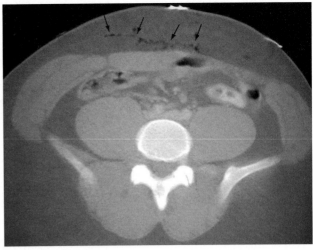

Fig. 12-21

Gunshot wound to the anterior abdomen. CT image through lower abdomen shows a bullet track outlined by air (*arrows*) within the anterior abdominal wall. No free intraperitoneal air is seen to indicate peritoneal violation. The patient was discharged following a short period of observation.

or portovenous fistulas are seen as well-defined areas of high density, similar in density seen within the adjacent vessels. Posttraumatic vascular lesions usually become less dense or "wash out" on multislice CT during the equilibrium phase images. Patients with active hemorrhage or posttraumatic vascular lesions require angiographic embolization or surgical treatment (see Figs. 12-15, 12-16, 12-30, 12-34, and 12-35).

Retrohepatic Vena Caval and Major Hepatic Vein Injury. Injuries to the major hepatic veins or retrohepatic inferior vena cava (IVC) (juxtahepatic venous injuries) are, fortunately, rarely seen following abdominal trauma.[80-83] However, up to 87% of all retrohepatic vena caval injuries result from penetrating trauma.[81,83] Unlike the 11% mortality rate reported in surgically managed penetrating hepatic injuries without involvement of the intrahepatic inferior vena cava, retrohepatic caval injuries are typically associated with a very high mortality (up to 90%).[80-83] In most series this high mortality has been attributed to excessive blood loss, coagulopathy resulting in delayed recognition of the injury, and difficulty in obtaining surgical exposure for repair.[81-83]

Retrohepatic IVC injuries should be suspected on CT on the basis of liver lacerations extending into the major hepatic veins or IVC, and/or profuse hemorrhage behind the right lobe of the liver into the lesser sac or near the posterior diaphragm. A combined therapeutic approach for high-grade liver lacerations with injury to the retrohepatic IVC may involve both the trauma surgeon and interventional radiologist. Initially the trauma surgeon controls the massive hemorrhage with temporary perihepatic packing. Recurrent hepatic parenchymal

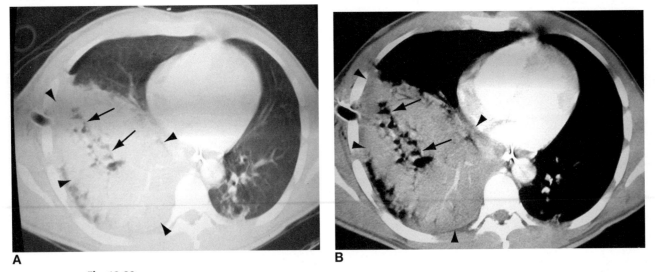

Fig. 12-22
Patient shot in right thoracoabdominal area. CT images in the lower chest—lung (**A**) and soft tissue (**B**) windows—show the bullet track outlined by lung lacerations (*arrows*) and contusions (*arrowheads*).

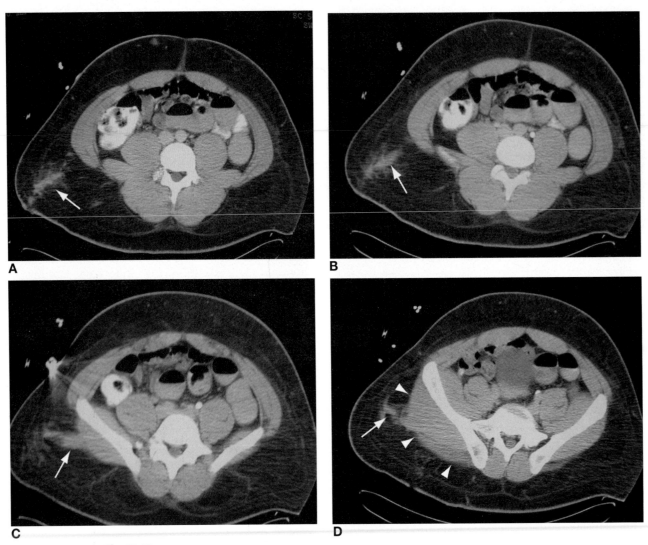

Fig. 12-23
Stab wound to the right pelvis. **A** to **D**, Four images through the pelvis show a wound track outlined by blood (*arrow*) extending from the skin to the right gluteal muscle. Enlargement of right gluteal muscle has resulted from hematoma (*arrowheads*).

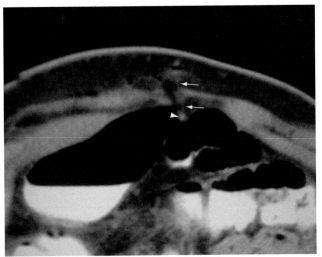

Fig. 12-24
Stab wound to the anterior abdomen in a 35-year-old man. CT image through the upper abdomen shows a knife track outlined by hemorrhage (*arrows*) extending to the stomach, indicating peritoneal violation. Infiltration of the mesentery (*arrowhead*) anterior to stomach and a defect in rectus sheath are also seen. At surgery peritoneal violation was confirmed and a small tear in the omentum was repaired.

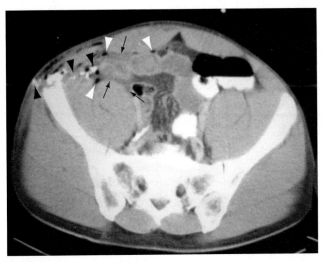

Fig. 12-25
Gunshot track outlined by bullet fragments in right pelvis. CT image shows bullet fragments (*black arrowheads*) along a wound track extending from the skin lateral to the anterior superior iliac spine into the peritoneal cavity. Free intraperitoneal air (*white arrowheads*) and fluid (*arrows*) are also seen.

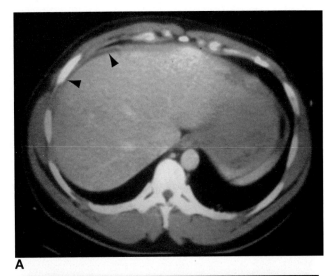

A

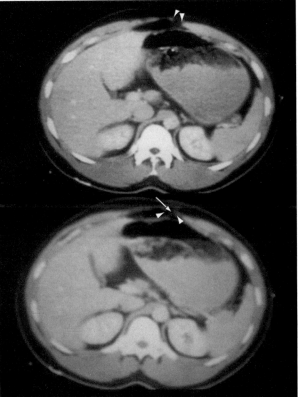

B

Fig. 12-26
Stab wound to the stomach of a 35-year-old man. **A**, CT image shows a small amount of free intraperitoneal fluid (*arrowheads*) anterior to liver. **B**, Two contiguous images show a defect (*arrowheads*) in the anterior abdominal wall with a wound track (*arrow*) extending up to the stomach. At surgery a perforation of the anterior gastric wall was repaired. (From Shanmuganathan K, Mirvis SE, Chiu W, et al: *AJR Am J Roentgenol* 177:1247, 2001.)

hemorrhage following liver packing may be successfully managed by using transcatheter embolization of the arterial sources of blood loss. Even bleeding from major hepatic veins potentially can be controlled by balloon occlusion or intravenous stent placement.[84]

Isolated Hepatic Injuries. The widespread availability of CT and its capacity to image both intra- and retroperi-

toneal viscera, identify injury morphology, and relate the injury to adjacent major vascular structures has been the basis for nonoperative management of isolated hepatic injuries in hemodynamically stable patients

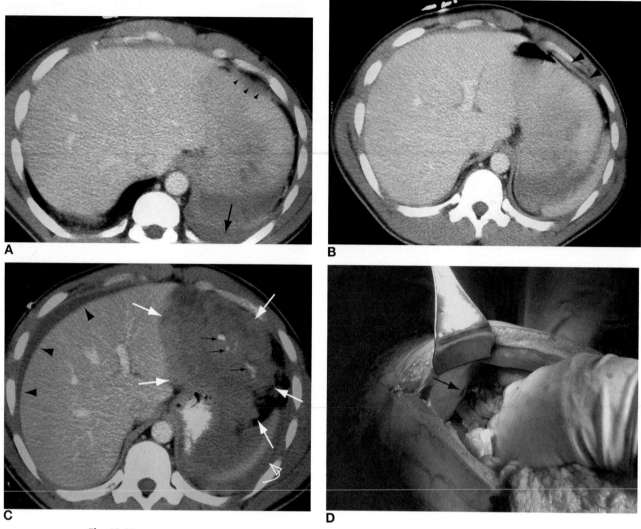

Fig. 12-27
Stab wound to left thoracoabdominal region. **A** and **B**, CT images through the upper abdomen show thickening of the left diaphragm (*arrowheads*) and a left hemothorax (*arrow*). No evidence of peritoneal violation is seen. **C**, Follow-up CT 18 hours after admission for abdominal pain and distention shows free intraperitoneal blood around liver (*arrowheads*) with mesenteric hematoma (*white arrows*) and active bleeding (*black arrows*) in the mesentery anterior to stomach. Perisplenic clot (*curved arrow*) is also seen. **D**, At surgery a mesenteric hematoma (*not shown*) and left hemidiaphragm injury (*arrow*) were identified.

without signs of peritonitis.[50,85-87] This concept has become the standard of care in blunt hepatic injuries.[87] The associated high incidence of bowel injury seen following penetrating trauma with peritoneal violation makes it difficult for many surgeons to observe these patients.[50] However, the large number of nontherapeutic laparotomies performed on patients with nonbleeding hepatic injuries following penetrating injuries to the right lower chest and thoracoabdominal region has led to the adoption of this nonsurgical approach in some centers.[49,50,88]

Prospective studies by Renz and Feliciano[50] and at the UMSTC have shown that CT aids in the selection of patients with apparent isolated liver injury for nonoperative management after right thoracoabdominal penetrating trauma.[49] Nonoperative management was successful in all seven patients managed by Renz and Feliciano[50] and all nine patients in the current authors' study.[49] None of the 16 patients needed laparotomy or developed delayed complications. In the study performed at the authors' center, angiography and embolization were used for three patients to treat hepatic hemorrhage shown by CT. Triple-contrast

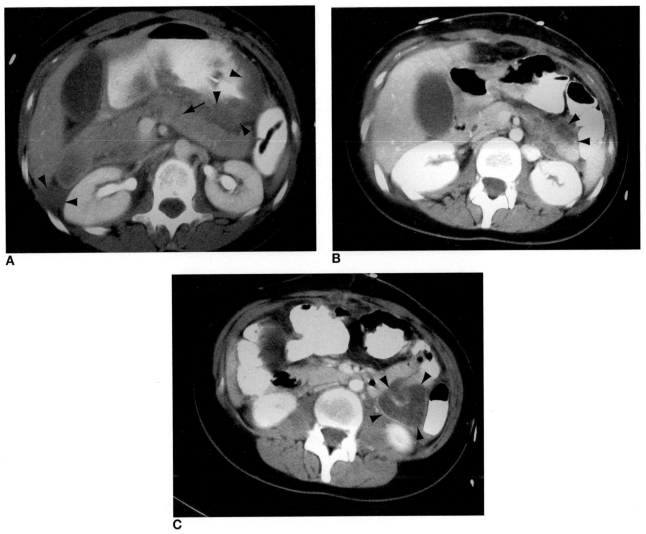

Fig. 12-28
Stab wound to the pancreas in a 37-year-old woman who sustained multiple stabs to abdomen and chest during robbery. **A**, CT image shows a transverse laceration (*arrow*) through the body of the pancreas. Free fluid (*arrowheads*) is seen in right paracolic gutter and lesser sac. **B** and **C**, Follow-up CT shows a peripancreatic fluid collection (*arrowheads*) inferior to pancreatic body as a complication of posttraumatic pancreatitis.

spiral CT provided the information necessary to attempt nonoperative management, including the ballistic trajectory, extent of liver injury, and perhaps most importantly exclusion of other injuries that would mandate celiotomy.

Bowel and Mesenteric Injuries. Hollow viscus injuries are the most common injury seen following all penetrating trauma.* These injuries may remain clinically occult for several hours. For the past decade concerns about the true sensitivity and specificity of CT in diagnosing bowel injury have limited the use of CT to evaluation of penetrating trauma to the back and flank. More recent retro-

spective and prospective studies have shown CT to be safe and reliable in detecting penetrating injuries of the entire torso.[47-49] Routine administration of oral and rectal contrast material is used to help opacify the bowel and increase CT sensitivity for detection of small amounts of intermesenteric fluid, mesenteric contusions, or infiltration of the mesenteric fat that may be the only evidence of bowel injury (see Fig. 12-26). Also, adequate bowel distention by gastrointestinal contrast material enhances the ability of CT to directly demonstrate bowel wall pathology. Specific CT findings of bowel or mesenteric injury in patients with penetrating trauma include extravasation of oral or colonic contrast material (Figs. 12-36 to 12-39), bowel wall thickening (Figs. 12-40 and

*References 1, 8, 18, 20, 53, 89.

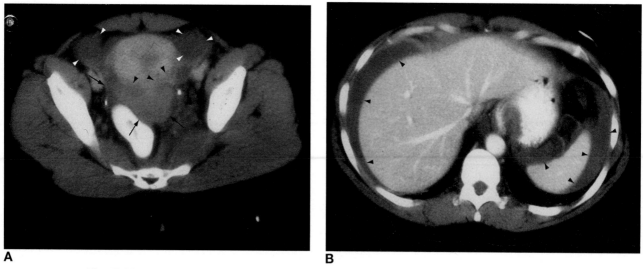

Fig. 12-29
Gunshot wound to the uterus in a 33-year-old patient with an entry site in right lower flank and a bullet in the left labia. **A,** CT image shows deformity of lower uterine segment (*black arrowheads*), free intraperitoneal blood (*white arrowheads*), and high-density clotted blood (*arrows*) adjacent to the uterus. **B,** CT image through the upper abdomen shows free intraperitoneal blood (*arrowheads*) around liver and spleen. At surgery, injury to the uterus and broad ligament were repaired. The highest density blood was seen adjacent to organ of injury.

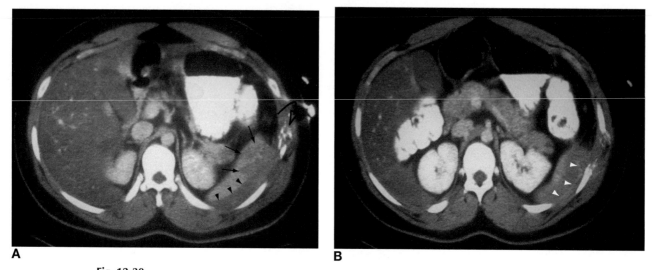

Fig. 12-30
Active bleeding in a 30-year-old man admitted following a gunshot wound to left thoracoabdominal region. **A** and **B,** Two axial CT images show a lower pole splenic hematoma (*arrows*) with active bleeding (*white arrowheads*) in perisplenic blood (*black arrowheads*). A left rib fracture (*curved arrow*) is also seen. (From Shanmuganathan K, Mirvis SE, Chiu W, et al: *AJR Am J Roentgenol* 177:1247, 2001.)

12-41), mesenteric bleeding (Figs. 12-42 and 12-43; see Fig. 12-27), discontinuity or defect in the bowel wall or focal mesenteric hematoma (see Figs. 12-10 and 12-42) or infiltration (Fig. 12-44). A wound track extending up to the wall of a hollow viscus (see Fig. 12-26) is also considered a CT sign of bowel injury.

The presence of pneumoperitoneum without evidence of a pneumothorax, pneumomediastinum, or retroperitoneal air decompressing into the peritoneal cavity is a specific CT finding of bowel injury and mandates surgery in *blunt* trauma. However, free air may be introduced into the intraperitoneal cavity by a bullet or knife during

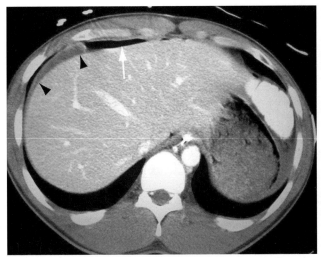

Fig. 12-31
Free intraperitoneal air. CT image through the upper abdomen in a patient with stab wounds to the abdomen shows pneumoperitoneum (*arrow*) and free intraperitoneal blood (*arrowheads*) around the liver, indicating peritoneal violation. This was surgically confirmed.

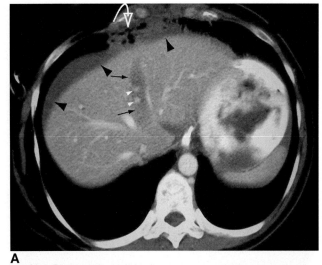

A

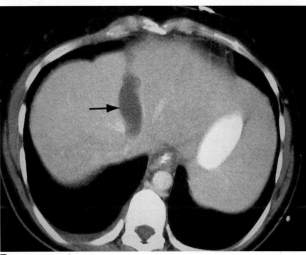

B

Fig. 12-32
Intraparenchymal liver hematoma and laceration in 37-year-old woman stabbed multiple times in the abdomen. **A**, CT image shows low-attenuation laceration/hematoma (*arrows*). An area of active bleeding (*white arrowheads*) is seen within the laceration/hematoma. Free intraperitoneal fluid (*black arrowheads*) and pneumoperitoneum (*curved arrow*) are also seen. **B**, Follow-up CT 6 weeks after admission shows enlargement of the liver injury (*arrow*) with rounded margins consistent with healing.

violation of the peritoneum. Therefore, pneumoperitoneum is a sign of peritoneal violation and should not be considered a specific CT finding of bowel injury in penetrating trauma. In penetrating trauma, free intraperitoneal blood may result from bleeding from an injury to the abdominal wall, peritoneal lining itself, or from extraperitoneal blood leaking through a defect caused by a wound track into the peritoneal cavity (Fig. 12-45). Free intraperitoneal fluid in the absence of solid organ injury should be considered a CT finding of *peritoneal violation* and not a specific finding of bowel injury. For these reasons, the inability to use the presence of *isolated* free intraperitoneal air or fluid as a diagnostic CT sign of bowel injury makes diagnosis of bowel injury far more challenging for the radiologist in the setting of penetrating trauma compared with blunt trauma (Fig. 12-46).

A prospective study to evaluate the role of triple-contrast CT in evaluating torso trauma performed at the authors' institution found 35 patients with peritoneal violation, of whom 37% (13/35) had bowel or mesenteric injury on CT.[49] A wound track extending adjacent to the injured bowel was the most common CT finding, seen in 69% (9/13) of patients with bowel injury. Other CT findings of bowel injury included bowel wall thickening in 54% (7/13) and oral or rectal contrast extravasation in 15% (2/13). All seven patients with bowel wall thickening had bowel injury that required intervention.

CT did not prospectively specifically localize the site of bowel injury in four patients. However, CT demonstrated peritoneal violation in all four, and in three of these showed a mesenteric injury adjacent to the bowel injury, the stomach (n=2) or the small bowel (n=1).

On retrospective review of the CT studies of these four patients, a wound track could be identified extending from the site of injury in the epigastrium to the stomach in two patients and bowel wall thickening was identified in the proximal jejunum corresponding to the operative findings in another patient. The fourth patient had no CT findings to suggest a bowel or mesenteric injury. A larger prospective CT study of penetrating trauma victims would help validate these observations and measure the sensitivity, specificity, and accuracy of triple-contrast

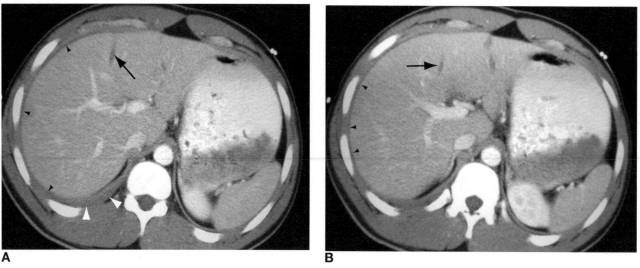

Fig. 12-33
Liver lacerations in a patient who was stabbed in the right upper abdomen. **A** and **B**, CT images show a low-attenuation laceration (*arrows*) in the anterior liver with free intraperitoneal fluid (*black arrowheads*) and a right hemothorax (*white arrowheads*).

spiral CT in specifically diagnosing bowel injury from penetrating trauma.

In the same study, mesenteric injuries were identified in 29% (10/35) of patients with peritoneal violation. CT findings of mesenteric injury included active bleeding (n=2), mesenteric contusion with adjacent bowel wall thickening (n=5), and isolated mesenteric contusion or infiltration of the mesenteric fat (n=3).[49] All five patients with active bleeding in the mesentery

or mesenteric contusion adjacent to thickened bowel wall had bowel or mesenteric injuries requiring surgical repair.

Urinary Tract Injuries. Contrast-enhanced CT has been clearly shown to be the imaging modality of choice to evaluate blunt trauma patients for urinary tract injuries.[90-97] Currently it is often used for penetrating trauma as well. Federle et al.[94] evaluated 27 consecutive patients with stab

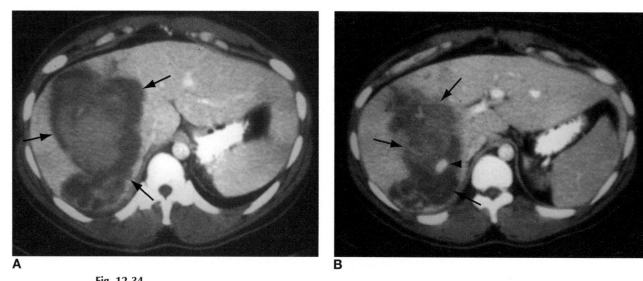

Fig. 12-34
Pseudoaneurysm of the liver in a man admitted following gunshot wound. **A** and **B**, CT images show a large mixed-density liver hematoma (*arrows*) involving both lobes. High-density hematoma indicates recent bleeding. A well-defined high-density area (*arrowhead*) seen within the hematoma represents a pseudoaneurysm.

Continued

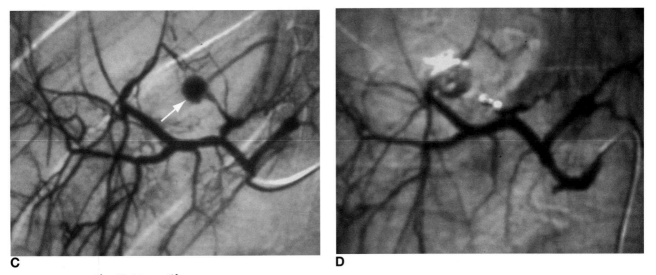

Fig. 12-34, cont'd
Preembolization (**C**) and postembolization (**D**) hepatic angiograms confirm a right hepatic artery branch pseudoaneurysm *(arrow)*. Transcatheter embolization of pseudoaneurysm was performed.

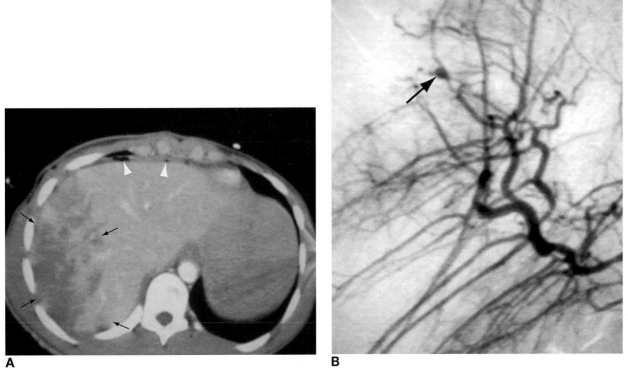

Fig. 12-35
Small pseudoaneurysm of hepatic branch vessel in a patient who was shot in the right thoracoabdominal region. **A**, CT image shows a large liver laceration and hematoma *(arrows)* in the lateral right lobe. A small amount of pneumoperitoneum *(arrowheads)* is also seen. **B**, Selective hepatic artery angiogram shows a small pseudoaneurysm *(arrow)* of distal branches of right hepatic artery.

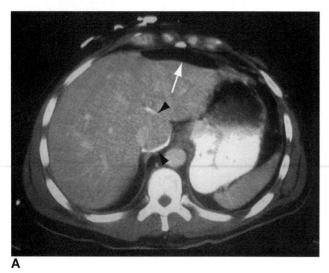

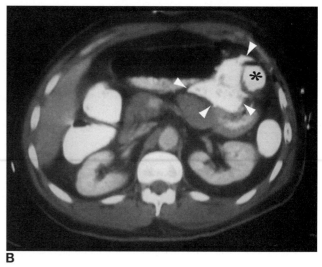

Fig. 12-36
Rectal contrast extravasation resulting from an anterior abdomen stab wound in a 39-year-old man. **A**, CT image shows pneumoperitoneum (*arrow*) anterior to the liver. Extravasation of contrast material (*arrowheads*) is seen adjacent to caudate lobe of liver and in the region of hepatoduodenal ligament. **B**, CT image shows extravasation of rectal contrast material (*arrowheads*) into the region of transverse mesocolon (*asterisk*). (From Shanmuganathan K, Mirvis SE, Chiu W, et al: *AJR Am J Roentgenol* 177:1247, 2001.)

wounds to the flank and back and compared CT and excretory urography. In many cases the findings of renal parenchymal injuries were indeterminate, underestimated, or overestimated by excretory urography. In this study excretory urography was not helpful in determining the extent of parenchymal injury in order to plan management.

Since there is no correlation between the magnitude of hematuria and extent of urinary tract injury, radiographic staging plays a major role in triaging patients for surgical or conservative management.[94-105] Conservative management of stable penetrating renal injuries has become the preferred therapeutic option. Studies report that more than half of the patients with renal parenchymal injuries can be treated nonoperatively based on radiologic, laboratory, and clinical criteria.[94,96,105] At the UMSTC, triple-contrast CT is used to determine the extent of renal

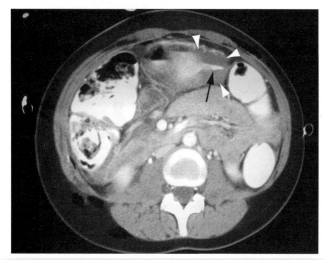

Fig. 12-37
Gastric contrast extravasation in a 37-year-old woman who sustained multiple stab wounds. CT image show gastric contrast material extravasating (*arrows*) into the lesser sac. Free fluid (*arrowheads*) is seen in lesser sac.

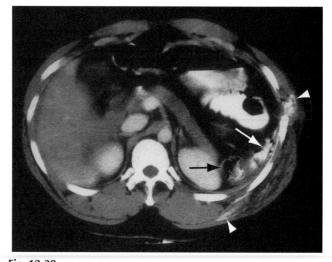

Fig. 12-38
Rectal contrast extravasation into peritoneum and wound track. CT images show rectal contrast extravasation from a descending colon injury (*black arrow*) into the peritoneal cavity (*white arrow*) and anterior abdominal wall along wound track (*arrowheads*).

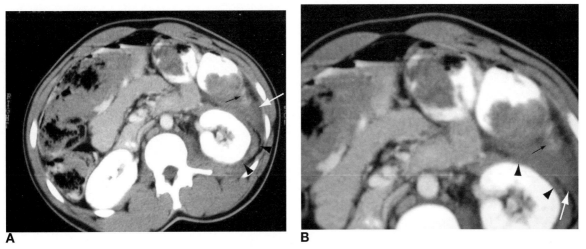

Fig. 12-39
A and **B**, CT images show a subtle amount of rectal contrast material extravasation (*black arrow*) adjacent to the colon. Free intraperitoneal blood (*white arrow*) and a small perinephric hematoma (*arrowheads*) are also seen. At surgery a colonic injury was repaired.

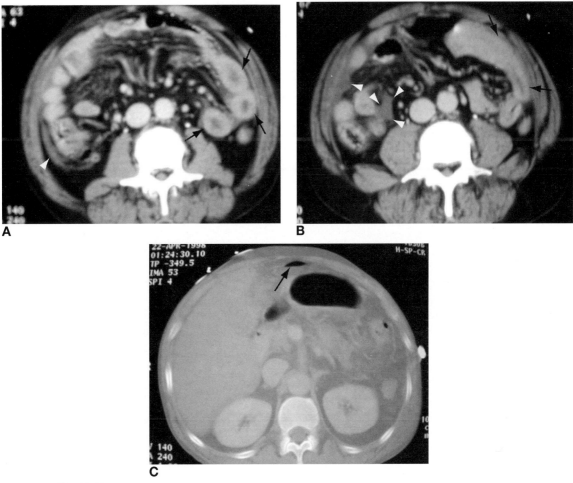

Fig. 12-40
Bowel wall thickening in a patient shot in the abdomen. **A** and **B**, CT images in mid abdomen show multiple loops of proximal small bowel with wall thickening (*arrows*) and free intraperitoneal fluid (*arrowheads*). **C**, CT image in upper abdomen shows pneumoperitoneum (*arrow*). Jejunal injury was repaired at surgery.

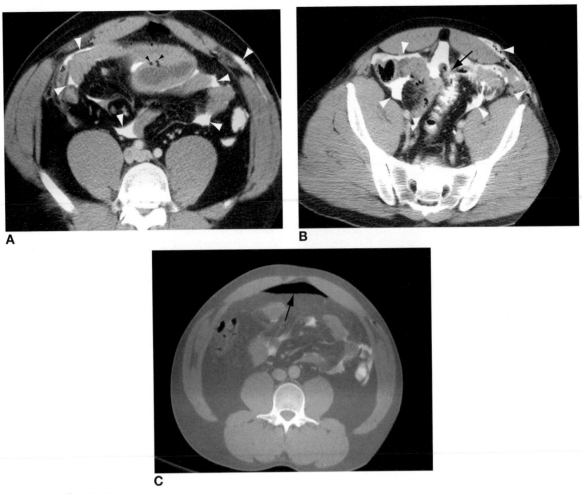

Fig. 12-41
Small bowel wall thickening and rectal contrast extravasation in a patient admitted following multiple gunshot wounds. **A** and **B**, CT images obtained in mid abdomen show thickening of small bowel wall and intramural air (*black arrowheads*). Rectal contrast extravasation (*white arrowheads*) is seen between mesenteric loops and the abdominal wall from a sigmoid injury (*arrow*). **C**, Pneumoperitoneum (*arrow*) is seen in the anterior abdomen. Both sigmoid and small bowel injuries were confirmed at surgery.

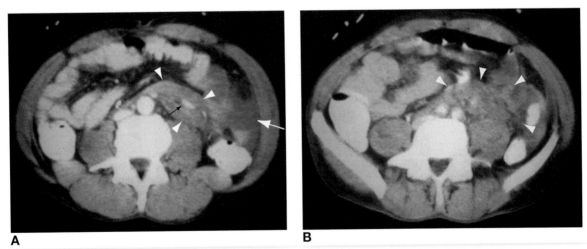

Fig. 12-42
Mesenteric hematoma with active bleeding in a 20-year-old woman. **A** and **B**, CT images show a left mesenteric hematoma (*arrowheads*) with active bleeding (*black arrow*). Free intraperitoneal fluid (*white arrow*) is seen in the left paracolic gutter. At surgery, mesenteric hematoma was confirmed and an injury to the inferior mesenteric artery was repaired.

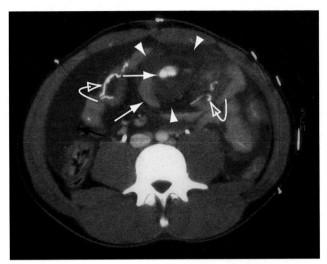

Fig. 12-43
Active bleeding in the mesentery. CT image obtained for hypotension following surgery for abdominal gunshot wound shows a large mesenteric hematoma (*arrowheads*) with active bleeding (*white arrows*) within the hematoma. Surgical staples (*curved arrows*) and free fluid (*black arrow*) are seen related to recent surgery. Repeat celiotomy revealed bleeding in mesentery.

parenchymal injury, as well as injuries to the renal vascular pedicle and collecting system, and the amount of perinephric hematoma.

"One Shot" Intravenous Pyelography (IVP). A "one-shot" IVP is a quick method of examining renal integrity in unstable patients with hematuria who require urgent surgical intervention. A single abdominal radiograph is obtained about 5 minutes after administration of 100 ml of 300 mg iodine/ml of intravenous contrast material. The study quality may be limited but can potentially provide information that may influence operative decisions. The one-shot IVP can identify major structural abnormalities of the renal parenchyma, as well as establish the presence of bilateral kidneys and their location. Other findings may include displacement of the kidneys or ureters by retroperitoneal hematoma, bilateral excretion of contrast material from the kidneys, and urinary contrast material extravasation into the intraperitoneal or retroperitoneal spaces.

A prospective study performed by Brennemann et al.[106] sought to determine the value of routine one-shot IVP performed preoperatively in 175 patients with suspicion of urinary tract trauma. The IVP influenced surgical therapy in only 3% (6/175) of these patients. If the indication for IVP were flank wounds with gross hematuria, this policy would lead to a 60% reduction in the number of routine IVPs performed.

Renal Injuries. Blunt trauma is the most common mechanism accounting for renal injuries, but there has been a steady increase in the incidence of penetrating renal injury with the rise in urban violence.[96] Stab wounds are the most common mechanism of penetrating trauma to the kidney. Common entry sites associated with renal injury are the flank, abdomen, and back.[96] In a review of 2245 patients presenting with renal trauma Miller et al.[98] demonstrated that a much greater proportion of the renal injuries resulting from penetrating trauma are major compared with those due to blunt trauma. Major renal injuries (grades II to V) were diagnosed in 67% (154/230) of patients with penetrating

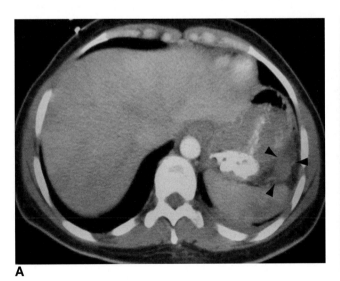

A

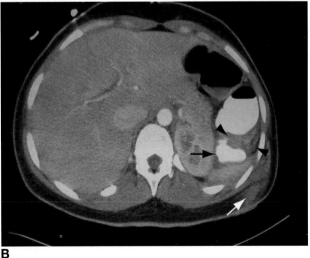

B

Fig. 12-44
Mesenteric infiltration in a patient stabbed in the thoracoabdominal region. **A** to **C**, CT images show infiltration (*arrowheads*) of pericolonic mesentery extending up to splenic flexure (*black arrow*). Soft tissue contusion (*white arrow*) is seen at the stab wound site.

Continued

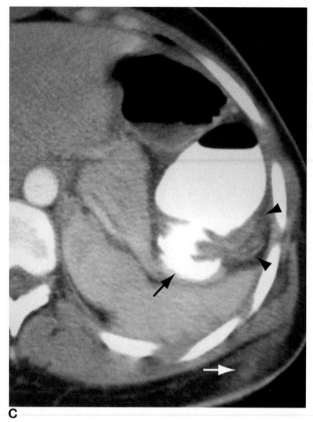

Fig. 12-44, cont'd
For legend see p. 663.

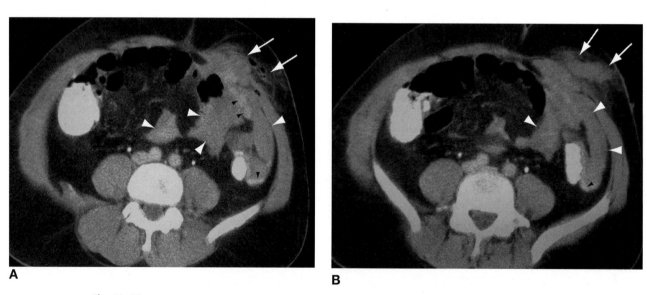

Fig. 12-45
Inferior epigastric artery bleeding into peritoneum through stab wound track. **A** and **B**, CT images show hemorrhage and air in a wound track (*arrows*) and free intraperitoneal and mesenteric blood (*white arrowheads*). Active bleeding (*black arrowheads*) is also seen at multiple sites. At surgery, bleeding from left inferior epigastric artery was controlled. No mesenteric or bowel injury was identified.

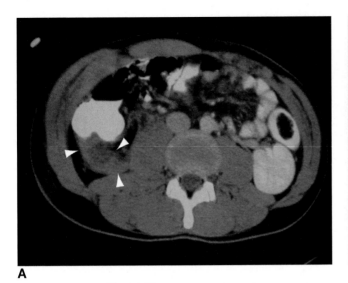
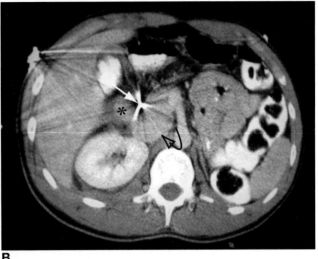

Fig. 12-46
Nontherapeutic laparotomy in a patient admitted following a shotgun wound to the right lower flank. **A**, CT image in the lower abdomen shows a retrocecal hematoma (*arrowheads*) in the region of ballistic entry site. **B**, CT image at level of pancreatic head shows a pellet (*arrow*) medial to the second part of the duodenum (*asterisk*) and adjacent to the pancreatic head (*curved arrow*). At surgery no significant injury needing repair was detected.

renal injuries and in only 4% (81/2,024) of patients with blunt renal injury. The amount of hematuria did not predict the injury severity, and 30% of renal stab wounds, 13% of renal gunshot wounds, and 21% of penetrating renal vascular injuries were not associated with hematuria on admission.[94-98] Associated injuries are seen in 61% to 81% of patients, including the liver (21%), bowel (25%), spleen (10%), and hemothorax or pneumothorax (19%).[95,96]

The renal parenchymal injury scaling system used at the UMSTC is based on the operative or CT findings shown in Tables 12-3 and 12-4, respectively.[107] The optimum radiologic evaluation of stable patients with grade II to grade V renal injuries is essential for the trauma surgeons and urologist to plan appropriate management.[98] Indications for renal exploration in penetrating trauma include persistent renal hemorrhage, pulsatile or expanding retroperitoneal hematoma, large devitalized renal parenchyma seen by imaging or at surgery, and incomplete clinical or radiographic staging.[95] Trauma centers attempting to manage penetrating renal injury patients nonoperatively should have facilities for bed rest, intensive monitoring, serial hematocrits, and transfusions as indicated for hypotension or decrease in hematocrit.

The most frequent CT findings seen following penetrating torso trauma include renal contusions, perinephric hematomas (Figs. 12-47 and 12-48), retroperitoneal hematoma (Fig. 12-49), and renal lacerations[94-96,98] (Figs. 12-50 and 12-51; see Fig. 12-48). The majority of these injuries can be safely managed without surgery. Miller et al.[98] reviewed the severity of renal injuries in 230 patients who had penetrating injuries. All 230 patients underwent radiologic evaluation, and 33% (76/230) were found to have renal contusions, 15% (35)

Table 12-3
Surgical Renal Injury Scaling System

Grade	Type	Description
I	Contusion	Microscopic or gross hematuria, urologic studies normal
	Hematoma	Subcapsular, nonexpanding, without parenchymal laceration
II	Hematoma	Nonexpanding perirenal hematoma confined to renal retroperitoneum
	Laceration	<1.0 cm parenchymal depth of renal cortex without urinary extravasation
III	Laceration	>1.0 cm parenchymal depth of renal cortex without collecting system rupture or urinary extravasation
IV	Laceration	Parenchymal laceration extending through renal cortex, medulla, and collecting system
	Vascular	Main renal artery or vein injury with contained hemorrhage
V	Laceration	Completely shattered kidney
	Vascular	Avulsion of renal hilum, devascularizing the kidney

Table 12-4
CT-Based Renal Injury Scaling System

Grade/Description	CT Findings

1
Brief medical
   description
	Superficial or cortical laceration
	Small perinephric hematoma confined
	   to Gerota's fascia without distention
	<1 cm subcapsular hematoma
	Segmental renal infarct
	Renal contusion

2
24-48 hours medical
   follow-up
	Deep laceration without involvement
	   of collecting system
	Perinephric hematoma confined to
	   Gerota's fascia
	Subcapsular +/– predischarge CT
	Hematoma >1 cm without delayed
	   renal excretion

3
Requires careful
   clinical and
   imaging
   follow-up
	Laceration into the collecting system
	   with urine leak confined to Gerota's
	   fascia
	Perinephric hematoma confined to
	   pararenal spaces without active
	   bleed or progression observation
	   and imaging follow-up
	Renal split (2 fragments) with greater
	   than 50% viable parenchyma
	Subcapsular hematoma with delayed
	   renal excretion

4
Requires intervention
	Laceration into collecting system with
	   contrast leak beyond Gerota's fascia
	Active bleeding-pseudoaneurysm
	Progression of hematoma on follow-
	   up CT
	Renal vascular pedicle injury
	Subcapsular hematoma without
	   renal excretion
	Pelvic or uretero-pelvic junction tear
	Renal fragmentation (>2 fragments) or
	   greater than 50% nonviable
	   parenchyma

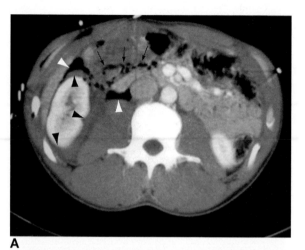

A

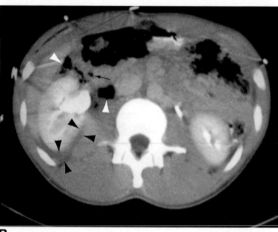

B

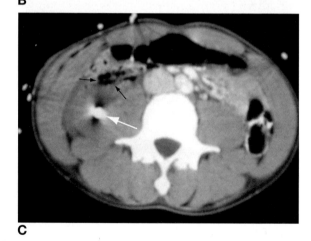

C

Fig. 12-47
Perinephric hematoma in a patient who was shot in the flank. **A** to **C**, CT images show a small right perinephric hematoma (*black arrowheads*) and free retroperitoneal (*white arrowheads*) and anterior pararenal air (*black arrows*) adjacent to right kidney. A bullet (*white arrow*) is seen more inferiorly in right retroperitoneum. Images obtained in excretory phase did not show urinary contrast extravasation. No duodenal injury was seen at surgery.

minor lacerations, 38% (88) major lacerations, 6% (13) vascular injuries, and 8% (18) both vascular injuries and lacerations.

Renal contusions are seen as focal or global low-attenuation areas compared with normal parenchyma. On delayed images these areas may be seen as hyperdense regions compared with normal parenchyma resulting from retained contrast material within injured renal tubules or parenchymal intravasation of urinary contrast material from the injured renal tubules. Renal contusions may result from a shock wave from a proximity high-energy gunshot wound without direct penetration of the

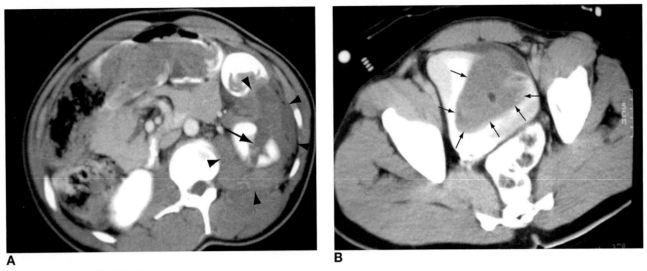

Fig. 12-48
Renal laceration and perinephric hematoma. **A**, CT image shows an inferior pole left renal laceration (*arrow*) with an associate moderate perinephric hematoma (*arrowheads*). **B**, CT image of bladder shows a large filling defect (*arrows*) as a result of hemorrhage from left renal laceration. No urinary contrast extravasation was seen on delayed images.

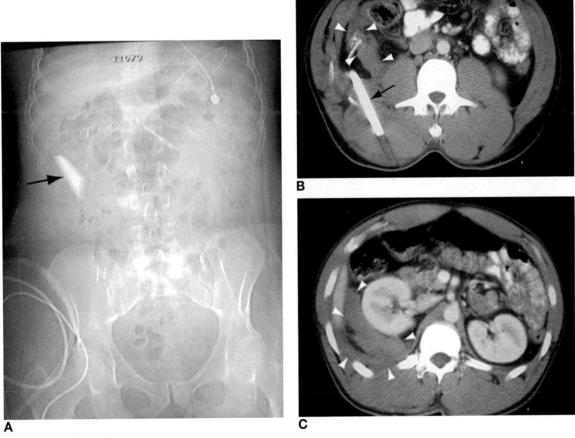

Fig. 12-49
Retroperitoneal hematoma in a man impaled by a large glass fragment. **A**, Scanogram of abdomen shows a large glass fragment (*arrow*) seen in the right flank. **B** and **C**, CT images show glass fragment (*arrow*) and a moderate-sized retroperitoneal hematoma (*arrowheads*) extending from right kidney to right iliac fossa with displacement of right kidney and colon medially.

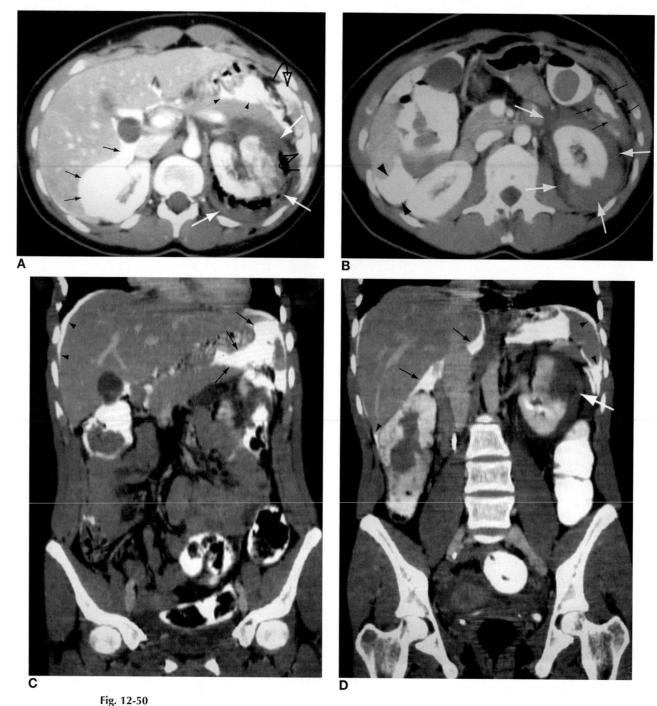

Fig. 12-50

Bowel and renal injury in 16-year-old woman who sustained a single gunshot wound to the left upper quadrant. **A**, CT image shows rectal contrast leak into lesser sac (*arrowheads*), Morison's pouch (*black arrow*), and peritoneum (*curved arrow*). A moderate-sized left renal injury with perinephric hematoma and air (*white arrows*) is seen. **B**, CT image shows thickening of the transverse colon (*black arrows*), free intraperitoneal rectal contrast leak (*arrowheads*), and a left perinephric hematoma (*white arrows*). **C** and **D**, Multiplanar reconstructed images show extent of rectal contrast extravasation into peritoneum (*arrowheads*), lesser sac (*black arrows*), with a left perinephric hematoma (*white arrow*).

Continued

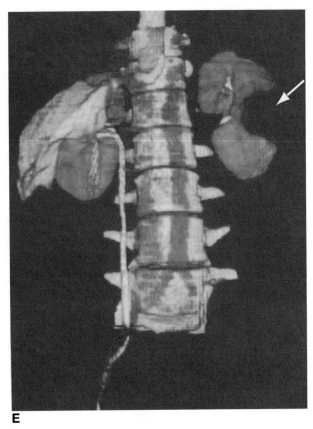

Fig. 12-50, cont'd
E, Four-dimensional CT image shows extent of renal injury along bullet track as a large defect in mid left renal parenchyma (*arrow*).

renal parenchyma. Perinephric hematomas are seen as hyperdense regions in the perinephric fat with no mass effect on the renal parenchyma (see Figs. 12-47, 12-48, 12-50, and 12-51). Compared with blunt trauma, subcapsular hematomas are less often seen following penetrating renal injuries. Subcapsular hematomas result from hemorrhage between the renal capsule and parenchyma and cause mass effect on the underlying normal parenchyma. This CT finding helps to distinguish a subcapsular hematoma from perinephric hematomas. Renal lacerations are seen as linear low-attenuation areas with normal adjacent parenchyma (see Figs. 12-48, 12-50, and 12-51). Compared with lacerations seen following blunt trauma, lacerations resulting from stab wounds tend to have well-defined margins and are more often associated with a perinephric hematoma (see Fig. 12-51).

Contrast-enhanced CT is much more sensitive than IVP in demonstrating urinary extravasation[91,94,96,108] (Fig. 12-52). Both the surgical and CT-based injury grading scales upgrade renal laceration from grade III to grade IV and from grade II to grade III respectively when associated with urinary extravasation. Delayed CT images

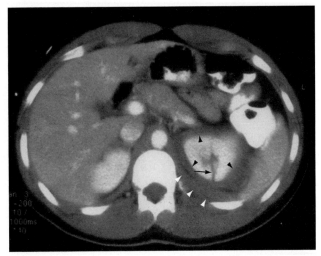

Fig. 12-51
Renal laceration in 23-year-old man who sustained multiple stab wounds. CT image shows a linear laceration in upper pole of right kidney (*arrow*) with a perinephric hematoma (*black arrowheads*) and a posterior pararenal hematoma (*white arrowheads*). No contrast leak was seen on excretory phase images (not shown) indicating this represents a minor renal injury.

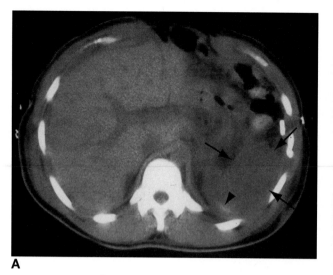

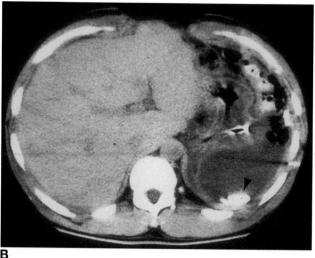

Fig. 12-52
Subtle amount of urinary contrast extravasation on delayed CT. Patient sustained multiple gunshot wounds to the abdomen. A splenectomy was performed with drainage of pancreatic and liver injuries. **A,** Delayed CT image shows fluid collection (*arrows*) in the splenectomy bed. A small amount of high-density material (*arrowhead*) is seen posteriorly in this collection. These findings suggest this collection could represent a urinoma. **B,** More delayed CT images through the same region show an increase in the amount of contrast extravasation (*arrowhead*). The density of the contrast material was similar to the urine seen within the collecting system (not shown), confirming the diagnosis of urinoma.

should be *routinely* obtained during the excretory phase after penetrating renal injuries when urinary contrast material is present within the collecting system (Fig. 12-53; see Fig. 12-52) to avoid missing this important injury as may occur when only arterial phase images are reviewed prior to excretion of iodinated contrast into the collecting system. CT can distinguish active hemorrhage, extravasated oral contrast material, and extravasated urinary contrast material.[77] Contrast opacified urine extravasates into the perinephric and anterior or posterior pararenal spaces and adjacent to the renal hilum, depending on the location of the collecting system disruption. Extravasated urine arising from the renal collecting system should be contiguous with the collecting system, similar in density to collecting system contrast, and not surrounded by a hematoma (see Fig. 12-53). Intravascular bleeding from renal penetrating injuries is typically surrounded by high-density clotted blood and is apparent in the early arterial phase prior to opacification of the renal collecting system.

Angiography with transcatheter embolization may help to manage active bleeding from penetrating renal injuries without surgical exploration among patients with CT evidence of persistent renal bleeding or expanding perirenal hematoma. Angiography and transcatheter embolization were demonstrated to be a safe and therapeutic technique by Eastham et al.[105] in 9 of the 11 stable patients who had renal stab wounds with renal branch vessel injuries including pseudoaneurysms (n=6), arteri-

ovenous fistulas (n=7), and active bleeding (n=3). Because surgical intervention for penetrating renal injuries often results in partial or occasionally total nephrectomy, there is an advantage to superselective angiographic techniques to identify the precise origin(s) of bleeding and the control of hemorrhage by transcatheter embolization with minimal loss of renal parenchyma.[105] Rapid availability and expertise for selecting angiographic treatment are paramount in considering this option.

Renal Pelvic and Ureteral Injuries. Renal pelvic and ureteral injuries are relatively rare following penetrating trauma and account for less than 1% of all urologic trauma.[99,102,103] The anatomic location and narrow caliber make the ureter less likely to be injured by external trauma. Penetrating trauma accounts for 84% of ureteral injuries.[109] Often these patients have multiple associated injuries, shock, and a high penetrating trauma index score.[99,101] Ideal management for penetrating ureteral injury is primary surgical repair. McGinty and Mendez[110] reported a 32% nephrectomy rate as a result of delayed diagnosis of ureteral injuries.

Findings of ureteral injury as demonstrated on IVP include deviation, dilation, or nonvisualization of the ureter. Up to 45% of patients with ureteral injury have no hematuria.[99,103] High-dose IVP with nephrotomography (Fig. 12-54) cannot be performed routinely in all patients and is often limited or incomplete. Presti et al.[99] reported

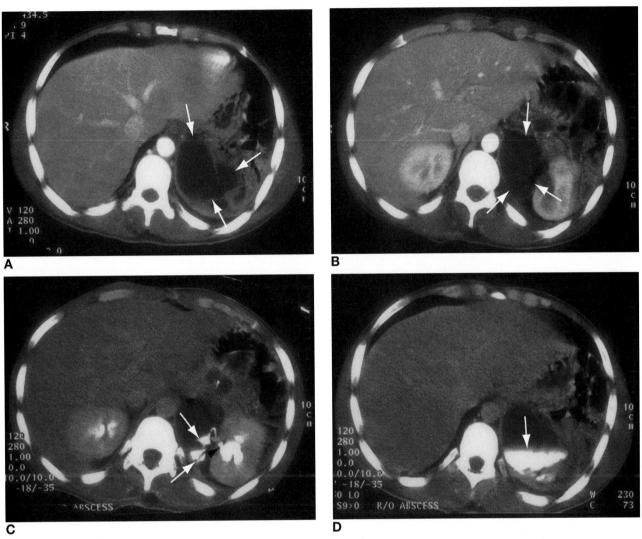

Fig. 12-53
Calyceal injury in a 23-year-old man who was shot in the back and had injuries to the spleen and pancreas requiring admission splenectomy. **A** and **B**, Portal venous phase CT images show a low-attenuation collection *(arrows)* medial and superior to upper pole of left kidney. These CT findings may represent a urinoma, pancreatic pseudocyst, or a resolving hematoma. **C** and **D**, Images obtained in excretory phase at same anatomic location show this collection represents a urinoma. Urinary contrast material *(arrows)* is seen leaking from an injured medial upper pole calyx *(arrowhead)* into urinoma.

that among 11 patients with penetrating ureteral injury in whom limited IVPs were performed on admission, the study was diagnostic for the injury in only two of them (18%). Brandes et al.[103] reported high-dose IVP was normal or nondiagnostic in nine patients with proven ureteral injury.

Contusion of the ureter may result from the blast effect of high-energy bullets passing in proximity to the ureter. The contusion may either resolve or progress to necrosis with potential for delayed urine extravasation.[111] Patients with ureteral contusion typically have hematuria, but a normal IVP.

The sensitivity and specificity of contrast-enhanced CT in demonstrating ureteral injuries are not known. CT is more sensitive than IVP in demonstrating urinary contrast extravasation.[77,90] Delayed images, during the excretory phase, are mandatory to demonstrate urinary contrast leak from a site of ureteral injury (Fig. 12-55). Direct CT signs of ureteral injury include extravasation of urinary contrast material from the ureter, normal excretion of contrast material from the ipsilateral kidney, and an intact calyceal system and renal pelvis.[112] Filling of the ureter distal to the injury is an important sign and may indicate a partial tear. CT signs suspicious for ureteral injury include a periureteral fluid collection or hematoma, a wound track seen extending into the region of the ureter, ureteral dilation proximal to the site of the wound track or hematoma, and ureteral wall thickening.

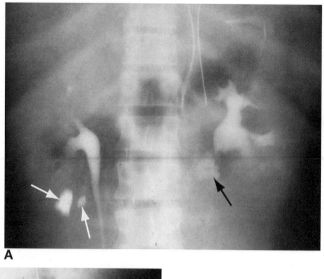

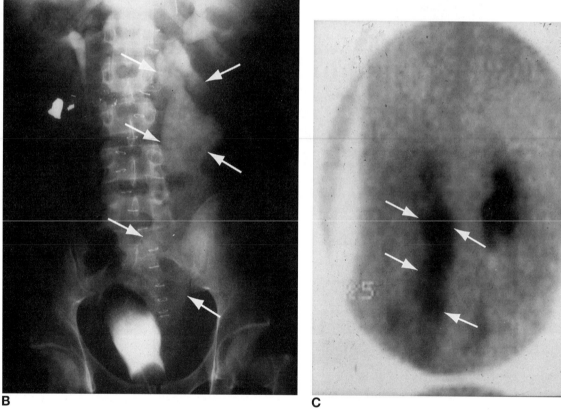

Fig. 12-54
Left ureteral injury in a 25-year-old man who was shot in the back. **A,** Tomogram obtained during an intravenous pyelourethrogram (IVU) shows extravasation of urinary contrast material (*black arrow*) from site of injury to the proximal left ureter. Bullet fragments (*white arrows*) are seen in right flank region. **B,** Delayed image in excretory phase shows a large extravasation (*arrows*) of urine into a large retroperitoneal urinoma. **C,** Posterior view of a technetium 99m–DTPA renogram also shows activity (*arrows*) within left retroperitoneal urinoma.

Bladder Injuries. From 25% to 43% of bladder injuries result from penetrating trauma.[113,114] The most frequent clinical findings seen following bladder injury include gross hematuria, abdominal tenderness, and shock. The lateral bladder wall is the most common location of rup-ture seen at surgery following penetrating trauma[113] (Fig. 12-56). The imaging modalities of choice to evaluate patients with clinical findings suggestive of bladder injury or wound proximity to the bladder are cystography with postdrainage radiographs or CT-cystography.[113-116]

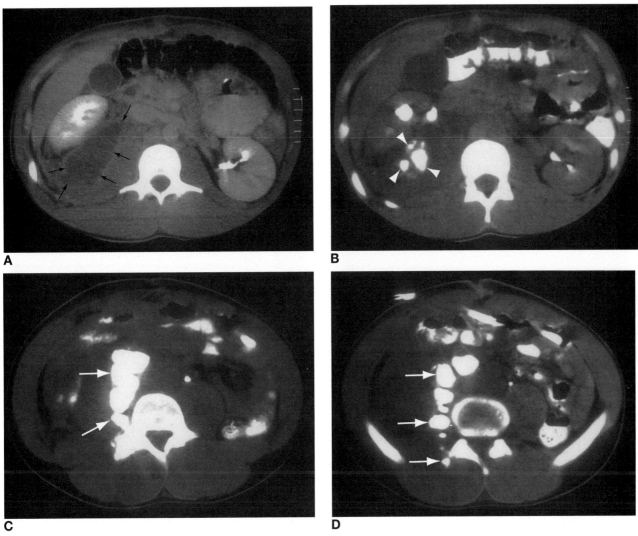

Fig. 12-55
Right ureteral injury following gunshot wound to back. **A**, CT scan at level of lower pole of right kidney shows a low-attenuation collection (*arrows*) displacing kidney anteriorly. **B**, CT scan about 3 minutes after IV contrast administration shows urinary contrast material (*arrowheads*) within right retroperitoneal urinoma. **C** and **D**, CT images through the lower abdomen show leak of urinary contrast material (*arrows*) from a right ureteric injury into urinoma along wound track.

Diaphragm Injuries. Studies are required to establish the role of CT in evaluating patients with penetrating injuries to the diaphragm. Patients with any penetrating injury to the thoracoabdominal area or radiographic or CT evidence of a wound trajectory in close proximity to the diaphragm are likely to have a diaphragmatic injury. Most penetrating diaphragmatic injuries are less than 2 cm in length and are diagnosed at surgical exploration, laparoscopy, or thoracoscopy via direct inspection.[117-119.]

Unlike the signs in patients with blunt trauma, the CT signs of these short diaphragm tears may be extremely subtle. Murray et al.[118] reported a 24% (26/110) incidence of occult diaphragm injuries diagnosed prospectively by laparoscopy in 110 stable patients with penetrating injuries to the thoracoabdominal region who had no clinical indication for celiotomy. In this study, the chest radiographs were normal in 62% (16/26) of the patients with diaphragm injury. A pneumothorax or hemothorax was demonstrated by chest radiography in 35% of patients with a diaphragm injury and in 24% of patients without. None of the patients with diaphragm injury had evidence of abdominal viscera herniating into the thoracic cavity.

Currently some trauma centers are attempting to use CT to diagnose intraperitoneal and retroperitoneal injuries in hemodynamically stable patients with penetrating trauma to the torso. It is important for the radiologist to be familiar with the CT signs of short tears in the diaphragm generally seen with penetrating injury. All patients with a penetrating injury track adjacent to the diaphragm should be considered to have potentially a diaphragm injury. Diagnostic CT signs of diaphragm injury included the CT "collar sign"(constriction of a herniating viscus at the diaphragmatic rent) (Fig. 12-57),

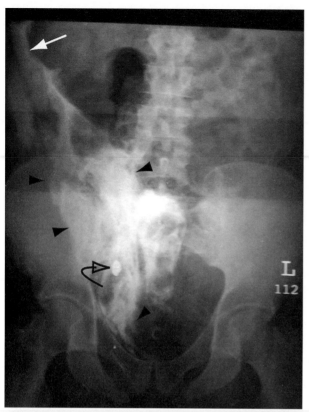

Fig. 12-56
Combined intraperitoneal and extraperitoneal bladder rupture in a patient shot in pelvis. A cystogram shows extraperitoneal (*arrowheads*) and intraperitoneal contrast material (*arrow*) extravasation from right lateral wall of the bladder. A bullet (*curved arrow*) is also seen in right pelvis.

herniation of abdominal content into the thoracic cavity through a diaphragmatic rent (Figs. 12-58 to 12-60), or the presence of injury on either side of the diaphragm in patients with single gunshot or stab wounds (Fig. 12-61). Some caution must be exercised for the latter finding, because ballistic injuries on one side of the diaphragm could conceivably injure the organ or structure on the other side through blast effect without direct penetration. CT findings suspicious for a diaphragm injury include a wound track extending adjacent to the diaphragm, diaphragm thickening as a result of hematoma or edema (see Fig. 12-27), and a defect in the continuity of the normal diaphragm or crus with adjacent hematoma or stranding of the adjacent fat. The latter represents the most specific finding for a direct traumatic diaphragm tear.

The authors reviewed CT findings in 19 patients with potential diaphragm injury with the wound track extending adjacent to the diaphragm.[49] The entry wound was thoracoabdominal in 79% (15/19) of the patients, abdominal in 11% (2), and through the back in 11% (2). The mechanism of injury included gunshot wounds in 63% (12) and stab wounds in 37% (7). The most common specific CT sign suggesting diaphragm injury in this study was organ injury on either side of the diaphragm, which was seen in 42% (8) of the patients. Herniation of abdominal fat through a diaphragm defect was seen in only one patient. CT findings were diagnostic in 47% (9) of the 19 patients. Other CT findings suggestive of a diaphragm injury include focal thickening of the diaphragm in 37% (7), and direct discontinuity of the diaphragm in 5% (1). The major limitation of this study was that the majority of patients with CT

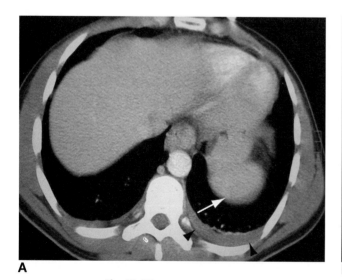

A

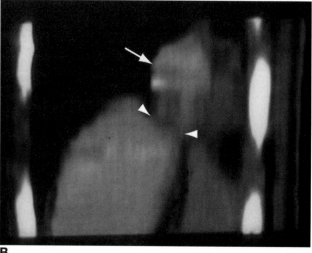

B

Fig. 12-57
"Collar sign" in 17-year-old who was admitted following multiple stab wounds to upper abdomen. Axial (**A**) and multiplanar (**B**) reformatted CT images show stomach (*arrow*) herniating into thoracic cavity. A small hemothorax (*black arrowheads*) is also seen. Focal constriction of the stomach (*white arrowheads*) is seen at site of diaphragmatic rent, creating the "collar sign."

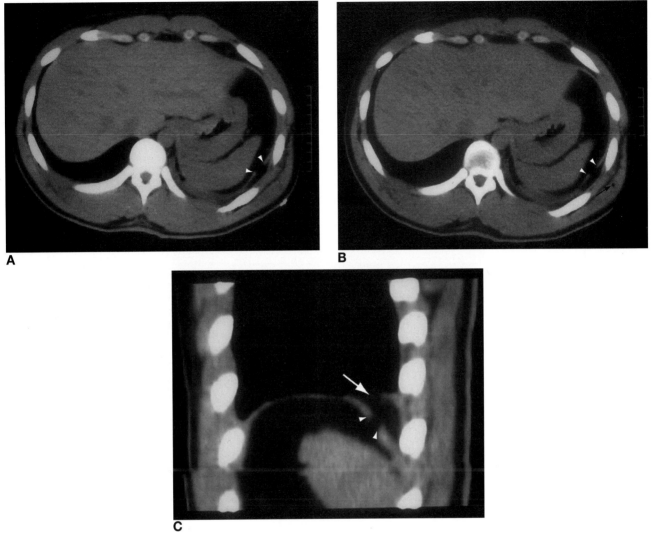

Fig. 12-58
Herniation of omental fat into the thorax and focal defect in diaphragm in a patient who was stabbed in left thoracoabdominal region. **A** and **B**, Contiguous CT images show a 1 cm defect (*arrowheads*) in left diaphragm. An air bubble (*arrow*) is seen within adjacent muscle along wound track. **C**, Multiplanar reformatted image through left hemidiaphragm shows herniation of abdominal fat (*arrow*) into thoracic cavity through diaphragmatic injury (*arrowheads*).

signs suggestive of a diaphragm injury were not definitively evaluated by thoracoscopy or surgery, so in many cases the CT result was unproven. Further prospective studies are needed to determine the sensitivity, specificity, and accuracy of various CT signs to diagnose diaphragm injury in penetrating trauma.

Imaging of Penetrating Chest Trauma

Approximately 4% to 15% of all trauma admissions to major trauma centers are attributed to penetrating thoracic injuries.[120] Most penetrating injuries to the chest are caused by knives or bullets from handguns.[121,122] The prehospital mortality from transmediastinal penetrating injuries may be as high as 86% for cardiac, 92% for thoracic vascular, and 11% for pulmonary vascular injuries.[120,123] Patients admitted to an emergency center with potential transmediastinal wounds or injury to the chest wall, pleura, and lungs that are symptomatic but physiologically stable require imaging studies to determine location and extent of injury.[120,122,124-128] Chest radiographs are the most common imaging study performed to evaluate these patients quickly (Figs. 12-62 and 12-63).

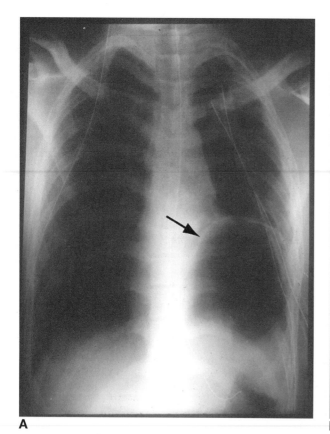

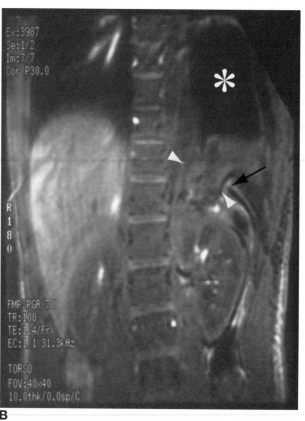

A   **B**

Fig. 12-59
Herniation of stomach through a dehiscence of diaphragmatic injury repaired following stab wound. **A**, Chest radiograph 3 days after surgery for repair of a left diaphragmatic injury due to a stab wound shows abnormal air (*arrow*) in left lower chest. **B**, Coronal MR scan shows abrupt termination of left diaphragm (*arrow*) with herniation of stomach (*asterisk*) into the thoracic cavity with a "collar sign" (*arrowheads*). At surgery stomach had herniated through a dehiscence of a prior diaphragmatic repair.

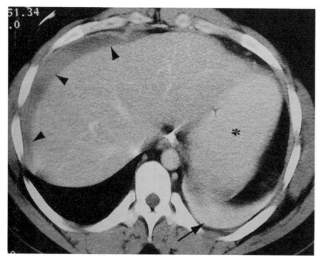

Fig. 12-60
Oral contrast extravasation into thoracic cavity through a left diaphragm injury in a 27-year-old man stabbed in left lower thoracoabdominal region. CT image through upper abdomen shows free intraperitoneal fluid (*arrowheads*) and a high-density left pleural effusion (*arrow*). Pleural effusion is similar in density to contrast seen within stomach.

Injury to Chest Wall, Pleura, and Lung. From 88% to 97% of patients admitted with penetrating injuries to the chest have noncardiac thoracic injuries to the chest wall, pleura, or lung.[120,129] Symptomatic patients sustain a hemopneumothorax in 41% to 45% of cases or a simple pneumothorax in 21% to 36% of cases.[129,130] Muckart et al.[130] performed a prospective study of 251 patients with penetrating pleural cavity. They reported that 83% of patients with hemopneumothorax required immediate intercostal tube drainage, and in 21% the initial hemopneumothorax worsens on follow-up. In this study, patients with isolated pneumothorax or hemothorax on admission chest radiographs were less likely to need an intercostal tube drain and were less likely to deteriorate on follow-up compared with patients with hemopneumothorax.

Asymptomatic stab wounds with normal admission chest radiographs may occur in up to 62% of patients admitted following civilian penetrating thoracic injuries.[131,132] Delayed complications are well recognized and occur in 8% to 12% of these patients as late as 48 hours to 5 days after injury.[120,122,128-130] Overall mortality in asymptomatic patients is 0.1% and results from

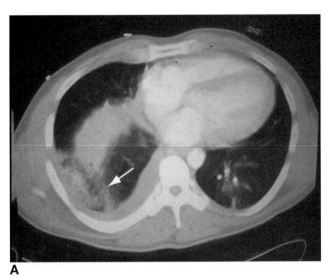
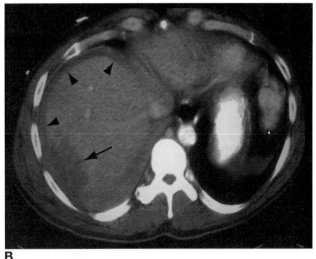

Fig. 12-61
Contiguous organ injury on either side of hemidiaphragm in a patient who sustained a single gunshot wound to right thoracoabdominal region. **A**, CT image shows pulmonary contusion in right lower lung. **B**, CT image through upper abdomen shows a right lobe liver laceration (*arrow*) with perihepatic intraperitoneal fluid (*arrowheads*). Presence of contiguous injuries on either side of hemidiaphragm suggests an injury to the right hemidiaphragm.

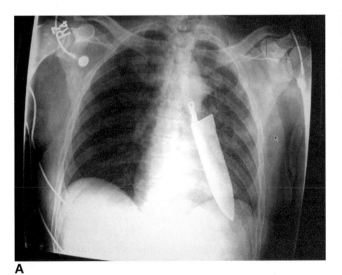
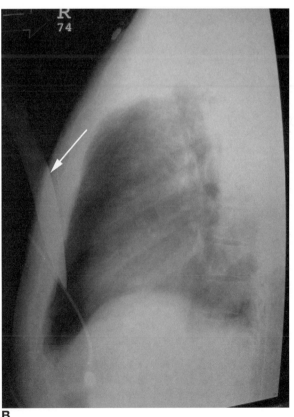

Fig. 12-62
Stab wound to left chest. Anteroposterior (**A**) and lateral (**B**) chest radiographs show a knife penetrating left chest wall with tip of knife in left pleural space (*arrow*).

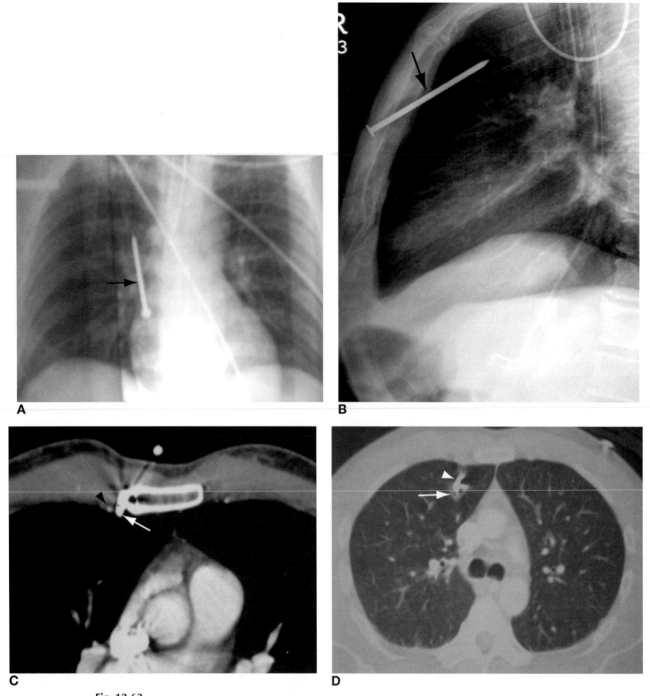

Fig. 12-63
Nail gun injury to chest. Anteroposterior (**A**) and lateral (**B**) chest radiographs show a nail (*arrows*) in right pleural space. **C,** CT image shows a nail entering right lung just medial to right internal mammary artery (*arrowhead*). **D,** CT image shows pulmonary contusion (*arrow*) around nail (*arrowhead*).

cardiac or major vascular injuries.[122] The appropriate length of time to observe these patients in a busy facility to identify those who will develop delayed complications is an ongoing controversy. Ordog et al.[122] performed a large prospective study of 4106 consecutive asympto-

matic penetrating chest injury patients without pneumothorax to less than 20% pneumothorax. Follow-up chest radiographs were obtained after 6 to 8 hours of observation. A delayed diagnosis of injuries was made in 13% (513/4016) of patients. Thoracostomy tubes were needed in 12% of patients with delayed onset of pneumothorax. The initial chest radiograph was 92.5% sensitive for injuries, but had only an 87% negative predictive value. This observation prevents immediate safe discharge of asymptomatic patients. However, the negative predictive value of chest radiographs for thoracic injury increased to 99.9% at 6 hours and allowed subsequent outpatient management.

Pneumothorax is a common injury following penetrating thoracic trauma. Prompt diagnosis, even of a small pneumothorax, is important, as significant respiratory and cardiovascular compromise may develop, especially for patients with impaired pulmonary function or if mechanical ventilation is instituted for patients with normal lung function.[139] Review of the literature indicates that small pneumothoraces are not initially recognized by clinical examination or by admission chest radiography in 30% to 50% of patients and are only diagnosed after thoracic CT.[133-139]

Hemothorax and Pleural Effusions. Pleural effusions that present after acute thoracic trauma are usually due to hemothorax (Fig. 12-64), and the majority of hemothoraces are managed by tube thoracostomy.[140] Hemothorax in penetrating trauma may be the result of injury to the visceral pleura, a laceration/contusion of lung parenchyma, or injury to the internal mammary, intercostal arteries, heart, or great vessels. When more than 1500 ml of blood accumulates in the pleural space, it is called a massive hemothorax (Figs. 12-65 and 12-66). Indications for thoracotomy include immediate removal of 1500 ml of blood from the pleural space, continuing hemorrhage resulting in a thoracostomy tube output of 200 ml/hour for 4 hours, or the need to completely evacuate large amounts of clotted blood from the pleural space.

Residual blood in the pleural space may trap significant amounts of normal lung with potential loss of lung function from the ensuing fibrothorax and adhesions. Clotted blood is an ideal nidus for secondary infection and development of empyema. To prevent or minimize these complications surgeons have started using minimally invasive surgical techniques, including thoracoscopy, to evacuate retained hemothorax.[141-143]

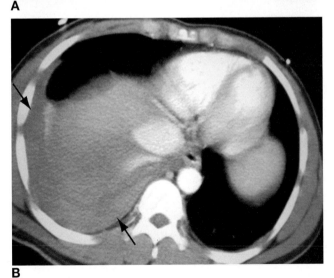

Fig. 12-64
Subpulmonic hemothorax in a patient with stab wound to right thoracoabdominal region. **A**, Admission anteroposterior radiograph shows elevation of lateral aspect (*arrow*) of right hemidiaphragm. **B**, CT image in lower chest region shows a small subpulmonic right hemothorax (*arrows*).

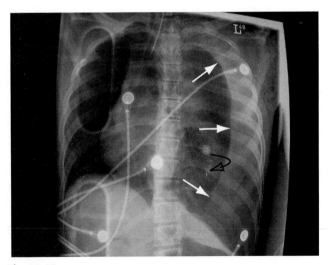

Fig. 12-65
Tension hemothorax in 18-year-old man shot in the left chest. Admission radiograph shows a large left hemothorax (*arrows*) with shift of mediastinum to contralateral side and depression of left diaphragm, indicating a tension hemothorax. Left lower lobe atelectasis and bullet fragments (*curved arrow*) in lower left chest are seen.

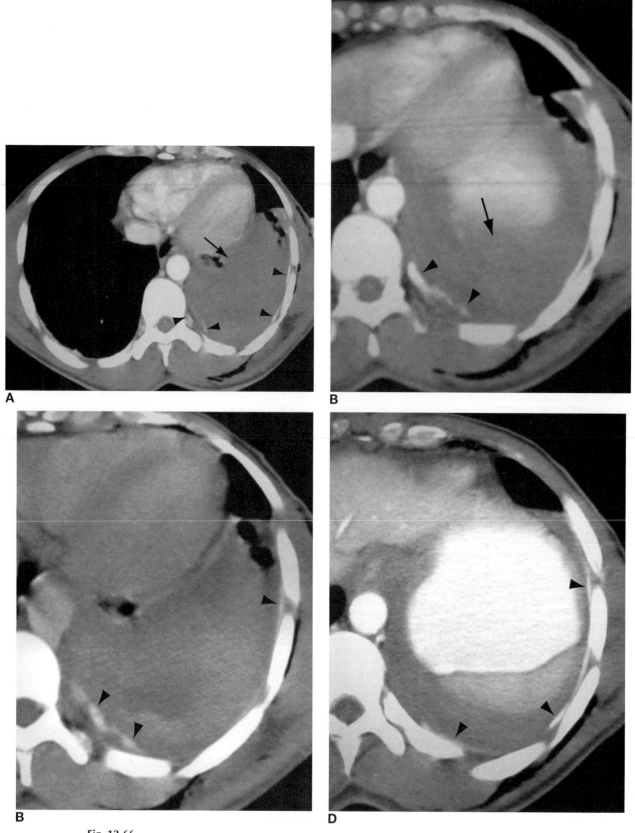

Fig. 12-66
Large hemothorax with active bleeding following stab wound to the left chest. **A** and **B**, Multislice CT images in lower chest region show a large mixed-density left hemothorax (*arrow*) with active bleeding (*arrowheads*). Compressive atelectasis noted as a result of large hemothorax. **C** and **D**, Delayed images obtained through the same region of lower chest reveal more intravenous contrast material (*arrowheads*) extravasation into left pleural space during the scan.

CT attenuation values may help delineate serous effusion (low attenuation) from hemothorax that has a CT density of 35 to 70 HU, depending on the degree of clot retraction (Fig. 12-67). Also, active hemorrhage into the pleural space occasionally can be delineated by spiral CT with power-injected intravenous contrast (see Fig. 12-66). The optimum time for thoracoscopy is between days 2 and 5 following injury, before clot organization and adhesion formation.[143] Although chest radiographs are the most frequently obtained imaging study to evaluate and follow patients with chest trauma and hemothoraces, they are unable to diagnose and precisely determine the amount of retained clotted blood in the thoracic cavity in order to plan its removal by thoracoscopy.[143] A prospective study performed by Velmahos et al.[143] to evaluate the accuracy of chest radiographs in determining the need for thoracoscopic evacuation of hemothorax showed the chest radiograph was insufficient to diagnose retained pleural blood. In this study chest radiographs identified only 10 of 20 patients diagnosed by CT with residual hemothorax of more than 300 ml volume. Seven of the patients thought to have intraparenchymal injury on chest radiographs showed they had retained hemothorax on CT. Overall the chest radiographs were incorrect in 48% of patients. CT was essential to assess the amount

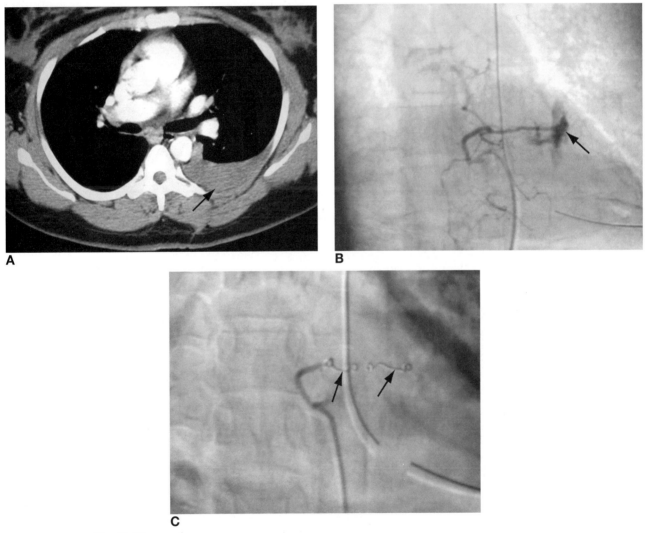

Fig. 12-67
Pleural space hemorrhage in a 30-year-old woman stabbed in left lower chest. **A,** Admission CT image shows a small high-density left hemothorax (*arrow*). **B,** Angiogram of left lower intercostal artery performed to evaluate for high output of blood from left chest tube shows active bleeding (*arrow*). **C,** Postembolization with coils (*arrows*) shows cessation of hemorrhage.

of residual hemothorax for triaging patients for thoracoscopy.

Bedside sonography has been used in the acute setting in some centers to confirm or exclude hemothorax.[144] Smaller quantities of pleural fluid may be detected on ultrasound compared with an erect chest radiograph. Pleural fluid or free blood in the pleura is seen as an anechoic area above the hyperechoic band representing the diaphragm. Blood or complex fluid collections reveal echogenic foci within the anechoic area. Clotted blood is more difficult to detect by ultrasound because it may be isoechoic with lung parenchyma, chest wall, and the mediastinum. A prospective study performed by Ma and Masteer[144] to determine the sensitivity, specificity, and accuracy of ultrasound examination compared with admission chest radiograph in detecting hemothorax reported an accuracy of sonography comparable to the chest radiograph. CT or tube thoracostomy was used as the gold standard to determine the presence of hemothorax. While sonography in experienced hands can assist in the rapid determination of the presence or absence of pleural fluid, in the authors' opinion it cannot replace chest radiographs in the initial evaluation of thoracic injuries. Chest radiographs should be routinely obtained without any delay in all patients to evaluate for pneumothorax, lung parenchymal, potential mediastinal, and osseous injuries.

Chylothorax is another of the etiologies of pleural fluid that should be considered in the setting of penetrating trauma. It results from interruption of the thoracic duct. The injury is suggested by low or negative pleural fluid attenuation values. Most thoracic duct injuries (88%) occur within the superior mediastinum at the junction on the thoracic duct and left subclavian vein in Porier's triangle and should be treated with early surgical intervention.[120] A bilious effusion is rare and results from concomitant laceration of the right hemidiaphragm and liver with formation of a biliary-pleural fistula[145] (Fig. 12-68).

Transmediastinal Wounds. Unlike injury to chest wall, pleura, and lung, penetrating transmediastinal wounds are associated with potential for injury to vital structures including the heart, great vessels, esophagus, and trachea.[120,124,125] Most civilian transmediastinal penetrating wounds warrant admission to a major emergency center, but do not warrant immediate surgery in the absence of obvious bleeding and maintenance of systolic blood pressure greater than 100 mm Hg.[124,125,146] A significant increase in morbidity and mortality is associated with delayed recognition of these injuries.[147-150]

Traditionally radiography, echocardiography, angiography, esophagoscopy, bronchoscopy, and contrast barium swallow are considered the optimum studies to evaluate for mediastinal vascular and aerodigestive injury. These multiple investigations often remove the patient from an environment of ideal clinical support and monitoring. CT is readily available in most institutions in the United States, and it is less expensive, less time-consuming, and less invasive than angiography and endoscopy.

Single or multislice spiral CT is optimally suited to visualize the individual mediastinal structures and can often demonstrate the trajectory of the objects penetrating into the thorax. Using newer multislice CT devices, mediastinal structures can be assessed at the peak of contrast enhancement, with minimal misregistration and motion artifact and with the possibility of excellent quality 2-D and 3-D image reconstruction (Figs. 12-69 to 12-72). When a thoracic wound track is *clearly shown* by

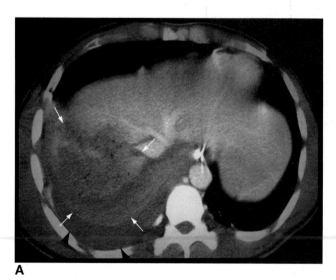

A

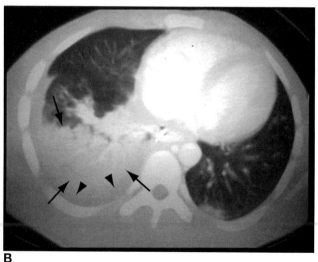

B

Fig. 12-68
For legend see opposite page.

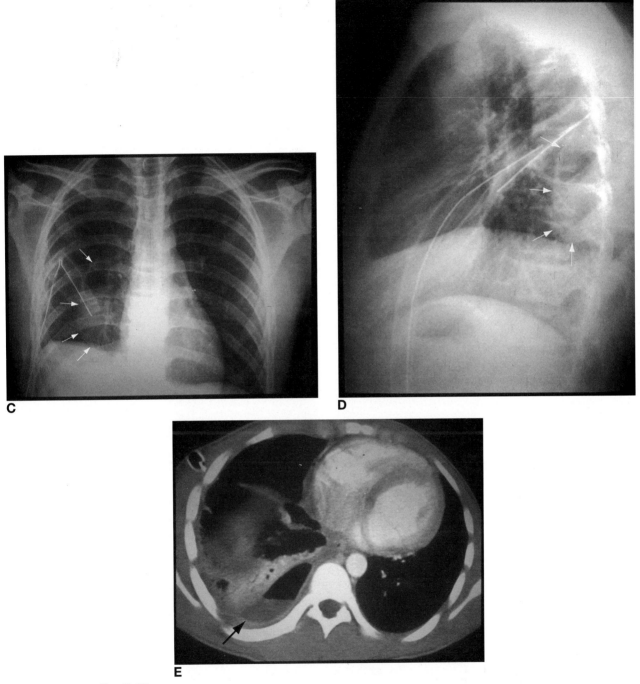

Fig. 12-68

Biliary-pleural fistula in a 16-year-old who sustained a single gunshot wound to the right thoracoabdominal region. **A** and **B**, Admission CT images show hematoma (*white arrows*) in posterior segment of right hepatic lobe. Right lower lobe parenchymal contusion (*black arrow*) and a small posterior effusion (*arrowheads*) are also seen. Contiguous injuries to liver and right lower lobe of lung indicate probable injury to the right hemidiaphragm. Anteroposterior (**C**) and lateral (**D**) follow-up chest radiographs show a fluid-containing cavity (*arrows*) in posterior right lower lobe. **E**, CT image of lower chest shows a cavity (*arrow*) with an air fluid level. Bile was aspirated under CT guidance from cavity in pleural space.

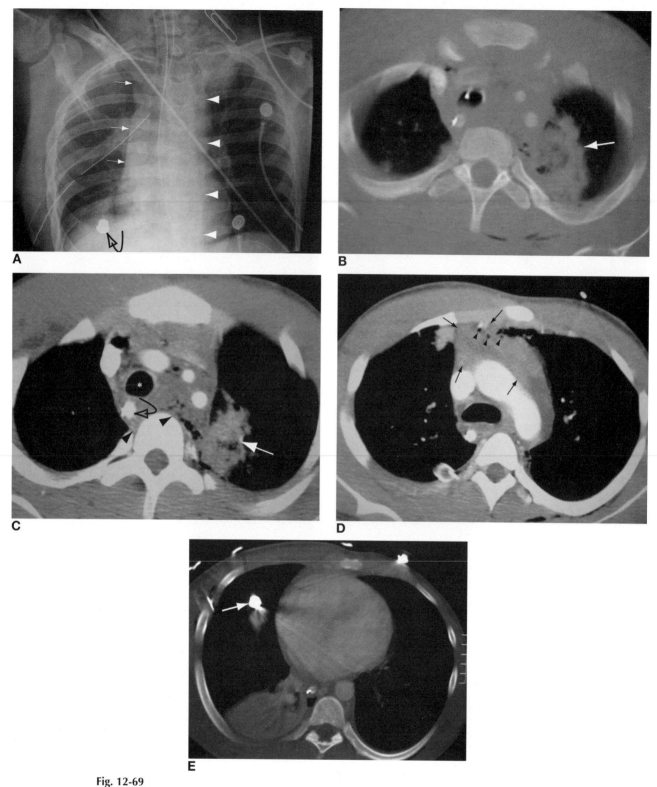

Fig. 12-69
Transmediastinal gunshot wound in a 26-year-old man. **A,** Admission radiograph shows the entry site marked by a paper clip in left supraclavicular region with a large bullet fragment (*curved arrow*) seen in lower right chest. Increased density is seen in the mediastinum with abnormal left paraspinal (*arrowheads*) and paratracheal (*arrows*) stripes. **B** and **C,** CT images in upper thorax show pulmonary contusion and laceration (*arrow*) in upper left chest. Mediastinal hematoma (*arrowheads*) displaces the tracheal (*asterisk*) and nasogastric tube (*curved arrow*) to right side. **D,** CT image lower in chest shows anterior mediastinal blood (*black arrows*) and mediastinal emphysema (*arrowheads*) **E,** Bullet resides in the middle lobe (*white arrow*). Angiography of the aorta, contrast swallow, and bronchoscopy were performed, but did not demonstrate a surgical lesion.

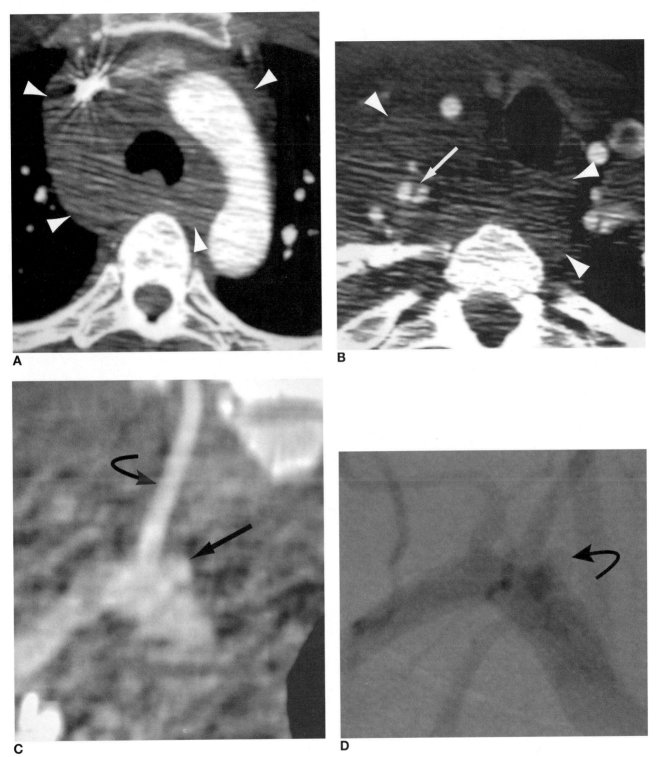

Fig. 12-70
Stab wound to upper chest and thoracic inlet with vascular injury. **A** and **B**, CT images show hemorrhage *(arrowheads)* in mediastinum and thoracic inlet with abnormal contour *(arrow)* of right subclavian artery. **C**, Multiplanar reformatted image shows a psedoaneurysm *(arrow)* at junction of right subclavian and vertebral artery *(curved arrow)*. **D**, Arteriogram confirms a small pseudoaneurysm *(curved arrow)* of right subclavian artery.

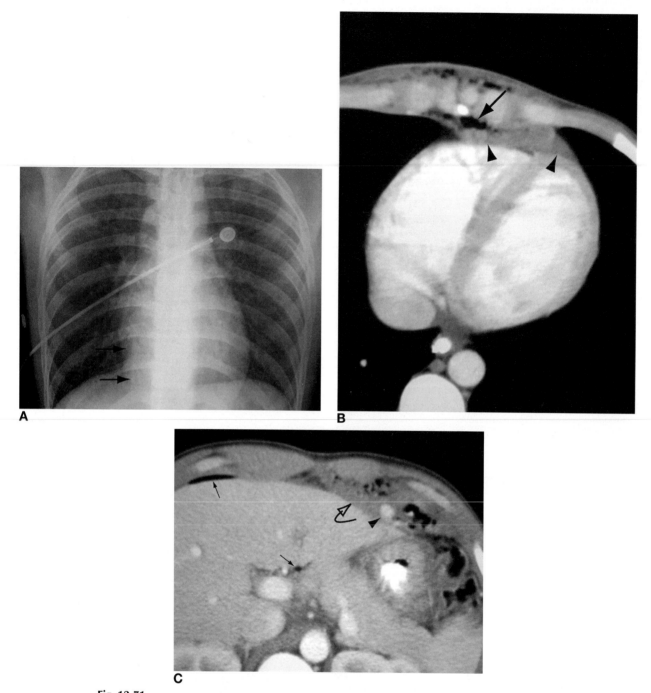

Fig. 12-71
Transmediastinal and peritoneal gunshot wound. **A,** Admission anteroposterior radiograph shows minimal increase in density (*arrow*) over right cardiophrenic angle. **B,** CT image in lower mediastinum shows anterior mediastinal blood (*arrowheads*) and air (*arrow*), indicating a transmediastinal trajectory. **C,** CT image shows active bleeding (*arrowhead*) in lower anterior mediastinum within a hematoma (*curved arrow*). Pneumoperitoneum (*arrows*) is also seen.

CT not to be in close proximity to vital mediastinal structures, the traditional workup of these patients may be deferred.[125] Hanpeter et al.[125] performed a prospective study using single-slice spiral CT to evaluate 25 patients with thoracic gunshot wounds potentially crossing the mediastinum as determined by chest radiographs and entry and exit sites. The routine workup of these patients would have required angiography, endoscopy, and contrast swallow. Proximity of the wound tract to the mediastinal vessels and esophagus required further diagnostic studies including angiography (n=8) and contrast swallow (n=9) in 12 patients. Thoracotomy was performed based on CT findings in one patient to remove a bullet lodged within the myocardium. Eleven

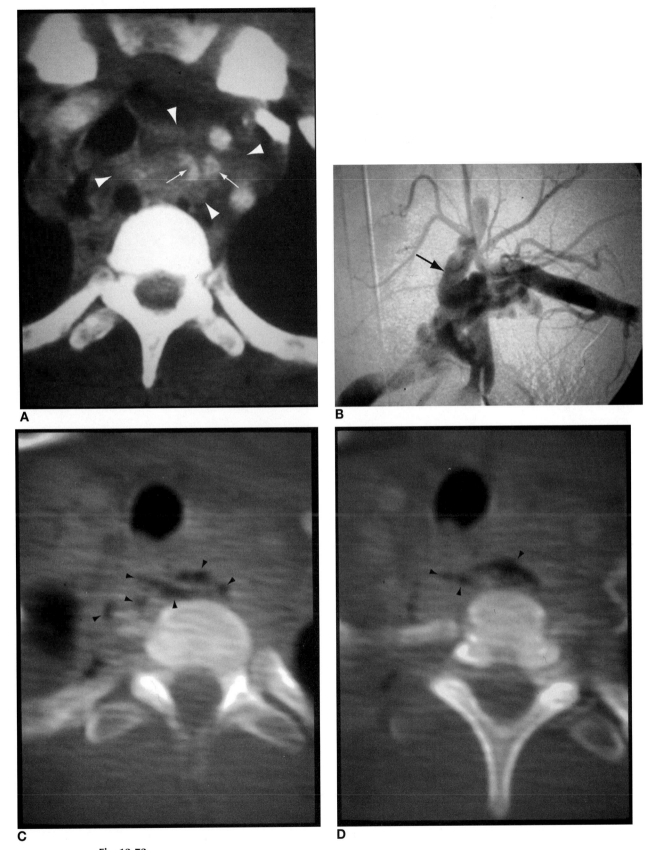

Fig. 12-72
Vascular and esophageal injuries in a patient with stab wound to lower neck and upper mediastinum.
A, CT image at thoracic inlet shows a mediastinal hematoma (*arrowheads*) with active bleeding
(*arrows*). **B**, Left subclavian artery angiogram shows an arteriovenous fistula with filling of the left jugular vein (*arrow*). **C** and **D**, CT images also show mediastinal air (*arrowheads*) adjacent to region of
esophagus.

Continued

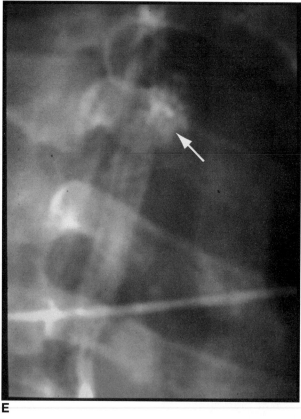

Fig. 12-72, cont'd
E, Contrast swallow shows oral contrast leak (*arrow*) from upper thoracic esophagus.

patients did not need any further diagnostic studies as CT demonstrated the wound track was well separated from the mediastinum. CT can provide accurate information to plan the appropriate workup in potential transmediastinal gunshot wounds. CT, in this clinical setting, can also reduce the number of invasive, time-consuming angiographic and endoscopic studies performed. Additional studies with larger numbers of patients may further delineate the role of newer multi-slice CT scanners for stable patients with transmediastinal gunshot wounds.

Tracheobronchial Injuries. Tracheobronchial injury (TBI) has been reported in 2.8% to 5.4 % of autopsy series of trauma victims and in 0.4% to 1.5% of clinical series of patients sustaining major trauma.[151-156] These injuries are relatively uncommon and often go unrecognized as a result of lack of visible external signs of injury. Early symptoms may be nonspecific and minimal, resulting in diagnosis only when late symptoms of TBI develop or at autopsy. Isolated tracheal injuries account for 25% of all TBIs.[154] TBI should be suspected in all patents with penetrating wounds of the chest or neck.[157] Penetrating trauma is less likely to injure the trachea (incidence of blunt trauma: penetrating trauma, 8:5) and generally involves the cervical trachea.[156] A retrospective review of tracheal injuries conducted for a 5-year period by Chen et al.[156] revealed that penetrating injuries most commonly involved the anterior aspect of the cervical trachea with injuries to the rings and the ligamentous portion between the tracheal cartilages. A higher incidence of associated esophageal and major vascular injuries (31%) is seen with penetrating TBI.[158]

The most common radiographic finding in TBI is air persistently leaking into the mediastinum and deep cervical soft tissue planes.[156,159] Up to 10% of patients with major airway injury have no radiographic findings in the immediate postinjury period.[160] Soft tissue and mediastinal emphysema is usually extensive, progressive, and not relieved by chest tube placement. Soft tissue air can dissect into the superficial and deep tissues of the neck, chest wall, and through the foramen of Bochdalek and Morgagni into the retroperitoneal and intraperitoneal space, potentially mimicking primary bowel injury. The disappearance of the extrapulmonary air does not exclude this injury.[153]

Pneumothorax is seldom seen following tracheal injuries and is more likely to be associated with distal bronchial tears.[153,156] Persistent pneumothorax and distal atelectasis from obstruction of a ruptured bronchus may occur. Rarely, the proximal end of the ruptured bronchus can be visualized on chest radiographs as a tapering air-filled structure referred to as the "bayonet" sign. Highly diagnostic but rarely seen is the "fallen lung" sign, in which the lung is detached from its mainstem bronchus and falls by gravity into the most dependent part of the thoracic cavity.[153,161] In such cases the hilum of the collapsed lung appears abnormally caudal in position. An extraluminal position of the endotracheal tube or balloon, or overexpansion of the balloon may be the earliest radiographic finding of tracheal injury.

CT has an overall sensitivity of 85% in detecting tracheal injury.[156] The capacity of single- or multislice CT to obtain volumetric data with less partial volume averaging and motion artifact can optimize reformatted coronal and sagittal images of the trachea and mainstem bronchi.[162,163] This could potentially help to delineate the airway injury site in cases with subacute or chronic presentation of airway injury. Compared to chest radiographs, a lesser quantity of mediastinal air is detected by conventional or spiral CT and may be the only sign of

tracheobronchial injury. Extrapulmonary air seen in direct contact with the trachea (paratracheal air) by CT among patients with pneumomediastinum is not pathognomonic for TBI.[156] Direct CT signs of airway injury include an overdistended endotracheal tube balloon (maximum transverse diameter measuring more than 2.8 cm) (Fig. 12-73), herniation of the endotracheal balloon outside the wall of the airway (Figs. 12-74 and 12-75), endotracheal tube projecting outside the airway (Fig. 12-76), fracture or deformity of the cartilaginous rings of the airway, and discontinuity of the airway wall.[156,164,165]

Bronchoscopy is the diagnostic modality of choice to confirm TBI, and early diagnosis is essential to obtain successful primary reanastomosis and optimal long-term results.[59,166-168] Although complete transection of the trachea is usually diagnosed soon after admission, partial tears of the trachea, and complete or partial tears of the bronchi may be detected only as late sequelae of TBI, including tracheal stenosis, tracheoesophageal fistula, empyema, mediastinitis, or bronchiectasis.

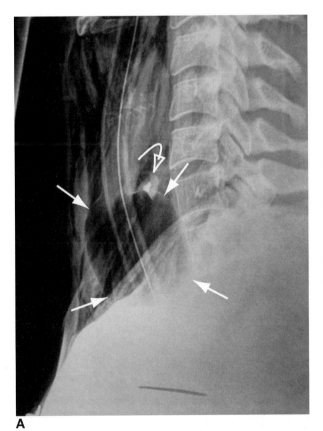

A

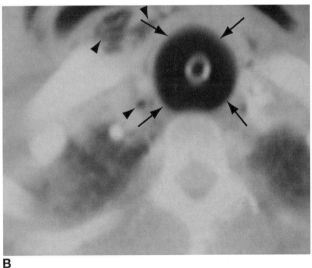

B

Fig. 12-73
Overdistended endotracheal tube balloon in a 35-year-old woman who underwent emergent endotracheal intubation (tracheal rupture). **A,** Lateral radiograph of cervical spine shows an overdistended endotracheal tube balloon (*arrows*) with deep cervical soft tissue air. A dislodged tooth (*curved arrow*) is also seen in the airway over balloon. **B,** CT image shows an overdistended endotracheal tube balloon (*arrows*) and soft tissue air (*arrowheads*) at level of thoracic inlet. Bronchoscopy revealed a long tear of the membranous trachea resulting from iatrogenic laceration of trachea by endotracheal tube introducer. (From Chen J, Shanmuganathan K, Mirvis SE, et al: *AJR Am J Roentgenol* 176:1273, 2001.)

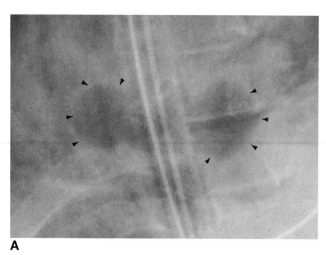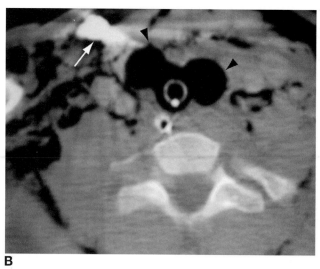

A **B**

Fig. 12-74
Herniation of endotracheal tube balloon through defect in tracheal wall in 15-year-old who sustained a gunshot wound to thoracic inlet region. Supine chest radiograph (**A**) and CT image (**B**) show herniation of endotracheal balloon (*arrowheads*) through bilateral injury sites in tracheal wall. A bullet (*arrow*) is seen in right thoracic inlet region. (From Chen J, Shanmuganathan K, Mirvis SE, et al: *AJR Am J Roentgenol* 176:1273, 2001.)

Esophageal Injury. All forms of trauma accounted for only 10% to 19% of esophageal perforations.[169,170] Isolated rupture of the esophagus is very uncommon, and most busy level I trauma centers may see between two to nine patients with penetrating esophageal injuries annually.[129,150,171-173] In any case of penetrating trauma that traverses the mediastinum, it is necessary to exclude esophageal injury. A large variation in the mechanism of penetrating esophageal injury (gunshot wounds versus

knife wounds) has been reported by different trauma centers in the literature.[120,142,174,175]

In a review of 77 patients with penetrating esophageal injuries, physical findings were only present in 34% of patients. A multicenter retrospective study performed by Asencio et al.[149] of 405 patients with penetrating esophageal injuries reported a longer length of hospital stay and a statistically significantly high incidence of morbidity in patients who underwent preoperative

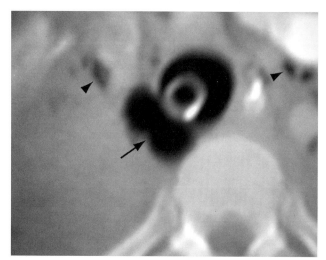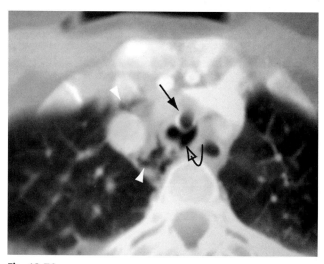

Fig. 12-75
Unilateral herniation of endotracheal balloon through injury site in trachea of a patient with transmediastinal gunshot wound. CT image shows herniation of endotracheal tube balloon (*arrow*) through injury site in right tracheal wall. Soft tissue air (*arrowheads*) is also seen.

Fig. 12-76
Endotracheal tube herniating outside tracheal wall. CT image shows endotracheal tube tip (*arrow*) outside wall of deformed trachea. At bronchoscopy a tracheal injury was seen. (From Chen J, Shanmuganathan K, Mirvis SE, et al: *AJR Am J Roentgenol* 176:1273, 2001.)

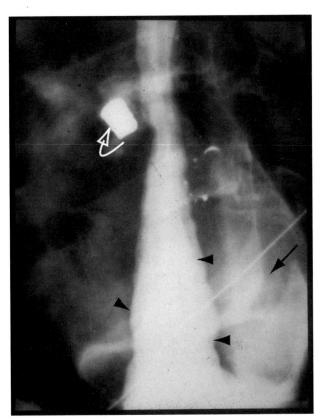

Fig. 12-77
Esophageal injury following transmediastinal gunshot wound. A contrast swallow shows oral contrast extravasation into mediastinum *(arrowheads)* and pericardial space *(arrow)*. A bullet fragment *(curved arrow)* is seen adjacent to the esophagus.

evaluation to identify injury versus those who went directly to surgery. Mortality was associated with delayed repair of esophageal injuries. The uncommon nature of this injury, lack of specific clinical signs or chest radiographic findings, and necessity for early diagnosis to avoid complications warrants a high index of clinical suspicion.

Most penetrating injuries that involve the cervical esophagus are associated with injuries to the respiratory tract (81%), central nervous system (23%), and vascular system (21%).[149] The most common presenting symptom is pain followed by fever, dyspnea, and crepitus.[173] Other signs and symptoms include dysphagia, odynophagia, hematemesis, stridor, abdominal tenderness, and a mediastinal "crunching" sound (Hamman's sign). The most frequent chest radiographic signs are cervical and mediastinal emphysema (60%) and left pleural effusion (66%).[172,176] Another radiographic sign of esophageal disruption is alteration of the mediastinal contour due to fluid leakage from the esophagus, associated mediastinal hemorrhage, or inflammatory reaction.

In the authors' practice, esophagography is the first study used to evaluate suspected esophageal injury (Fig. 12-77; see Fig. 12-72). Contrast esophagogram is performed first with water-soluble contrast, and if negative, with barium sulfate contrast. Fluoroscopic guidance is ideal, but if not possible because of the patient's overall condition, contrast can be instilled into the upper esophagus with chest radiographs performed during contrast injection of water-soluble contrast once the nasogastric tube position is verified. Contrast studies of the esophagus are about 57% to 100% sensitive in establishing a diagnosis of injury, with higher accuracy reported for thoracic esophageal than for cervical esophagus injuries.[142,169,172] The high average false-negative rate (21%) reported in the literature may be related to inability to obtain multiple projections to evaluate all the walls of the esophagus with barium sulfate.[175,177] Esophagoscopy has a similar diagnostic accuracy, but both studies together provide the best overall diagnostic accuracy. The role of CT scanning in the diagnosis of traumatic esophageal perforation is not established.[178] The demonstration of air bubbles in the mediastinum localized adjacent to the esophagus suggests esophageal perforation.

CONCLUSION

Selected emergency centers, including the authors', have used spiral CT to evaluate hemodynamically stable patients admitted after penetrating injuries to the torso and chest. Triple-contrast spiral CT is highly accurate in excluding peritoneal violation in patients with penetrating torso trauma who have no other indication for laparotomy. Patients with isolated liver injury can be selected using CT for nonoperative management. Chest CT has been used to attempt to verify the presence or absence of mediastinal involvement from penetrating thoracic trauma. Demonstration of a ballistic track that unequivocally *does not* involve the mediastinum avoids the need for evaluation of the esophagus, aorta, and mainstem bronchi. Knife wounds to the chest tend to have a less predictable course and are more likely to require mediastinal imaging assessment. If any doubt regarding the course of penetrating trauma exists, the mediastinal structures must be individually evaluated. Future studies will reveal what role advanced multislice CT scanning may play in replacing the current imaging regimen for penetrating torso and mediastinal trauma.

REFERENCES

1. Feliciano DV, Rozycki GS: The management of penetrating abdominal trauma, *Adv Surg* 28:1, 1995.
2. Schwab CW: Violence: American uncivil war: presidential address, sixth scientific assembly of the Eastern Association for the Surgery of Trauma, *J Trauma* 35:657, 1993.

3. The Violence Prevention Task Force of the Eastern Association for the Surgery of Trauma: Violence in America: a public health crisis—the role of firearms, *J Trauma* 38:163, 1995.

4. Annest JL, Mercy JA, Gibson DR, et al: National estimate of nonfatal firearm-related injuries: beyond the tip of the iceberg, *JAMA* 273:1749, 1995.

5. Hollerman JJ, Fackler ML, Coldwell DM, et al: Gunshot wounds. 1. Bullet, ballistics, and mechanism of injury, *AJR Am J Roentgenol* 155:685, 1990.

6. McSwain NE Jr: Kinematics of trauma. In Mattox KL, Feliciano DV, Moore EE, eds: *Trauma*, ed 4, New York, 2000, McGraw-Hill.

7. Ledgerwood AM: The wandering bullet, *Surg Clin North Am* 57:97, 1997.

8. Henneman PL: Penetrating abdominal trauma, *Emerg Med Clin North Am* 7:647, 1989.

9. Marx JA: Penetrating abdominal trauma, *Emerg Med Clin North Am* 11:125, 1993.

10. Hornyak SW, Shaftan GW: Value of "inconclusive lavage" in abdominal trauma management, *J Trauma* 19:329, 1979.

11. Moore EE, Dunn EL, Moore JB, et al: Penetrating abdominal trauma index, *J Trauma* 21:439, 1981.

12. McAlvanah MJ, Shaftan GW: Selective conservatism in penetrating abdominal wounds: a continuing reappraisal, *J Trauma* 18:206, 1978.

13. Thompson JS, Moore EE, Van Duzer-Moore S, et al: The evolution of abdominal stab wound management, *J Trauma* 20:478, 1980.

14. Demetriades D, Velmahos G, Cornwell E III, et al: Selective nonoperative management of gunshot wounds of the anterior abdomen, *Arch Surg* 132:178, 1997.

15. Nance ML, Nance FC: It is time we told the emperor about his clothes, *J Trauma* 40:185, 1996.

16. Moore EE, Moore JB, Van Duzer-Moore S, et al: Mandatory laparotomy for gunshot wounds penetrating the abdomen, *Am J Surg* 140:847, 1980.

17. Shafton GW: Indications for operation in abdominal trauma, *Am J Surg* 99:657, 1960.

18. Nance FC, Cohn I Jr: Surgical judgment in the management of stab wounds of the abdomen: a retrospective and prospective analysis based on a study of 600 stabbed patients, *Ann Surg* 170:569, 1969.

19. Welch CE: War wounds of the abdomen, *N Engl J Med* 237:156, 1947.

20. Feliciano DV, Burch JM, Spjut-Patrinely, et al: Abdominal gunshot wounds: an urban trauma center's experience with 300 consecutive patients, *Ann Surg* 208:362, 1988.

21. Renz BM, Feliciano DV: Unnecessary laparotomy for trauma: a prospective study of mortality, *J Trauma* 38:350, 1995.

22. Demetriades D, Rabinowitz B: Indications for operation in abdominal stab wounds: a prospective study of 651 patients, *Ann Surg* 203:129, 1987.

23. Bull JC, Mathewson C: Exploratory laparotomy in patients with penetrating wounds of the abdomen, *Am J Surg* 116:223, 1968.

24. McCarthy MC, Lowdermilk GA, Canal DF, et al: Prediction of injury caused by penetrating wounds to abdomen, flank, and back, *Arch Surg* 126:962, 1991.

25. Zubowski R, Nallathambi M, Ivatury R, et al: Selective conservatism in abdominal stab wounds: the efficacy of serial physical examination, *J Trauma* 28:1665, 1988.

26. Lee CW, Uddo JF, Nance FC: Surgical judgment in the management of abdominal stab wounds, *Ann Surg* 5:549, 1984.

27. Shorr M, Gottlieb MM, Webb K, et al: Selective management of abdominal stab wounds: importance of physical examination, *Arch Surg* 123:1141, 1988.

28. Shaftan GW: How we handle penetrating wounds to the abdomen, *Med Times* 104:60, 1976.

29. Demetriades D, Rabinowitz B, Sofiano C, et al: The management of penetrating injuries to the back-a prospective study of 230 patients, *Ann Surg* 207:72, 1988.

30. Root HD, Hauser CW, Mackinley CR, et al: Diagnostic peritoneal lavage, *Surgery* 57:633, 1965.

31. Feliciano DV, Bitondo CG, Steed G, et al: Five hundred open taps or lavages in patients with abdominal stab wounds, *Ann Surg* 147:772, 1984.

32. Keleman JJ, Martin RR, Obney JA, et al: Evaluation of peritoneal lavage in stable patients with peritoneal lavage, *Arch Surg* 132:909, 1997.

33. Thal ER, May RA, Beesinger D: Peritoneal lavage: its unreliability in gunshot wounds to the lower chest and abdomen, *Arch Surg* 115:430, 1980.

34. Oreskovich MR, Carrico J: Stab wounds to the anterior abdomen: analysis of a management plan using local wound exploration and quantitative peritoneal lavage, *Ann Surg* 198:412, 1983.

35. Galbraith TA, Oreskovich MR, Heimbach DM, et al: The role of peritoneal lavage in the management of stab wounds to the abdomen, *Am J Surg* 140:60, 1980.

36. Goldberg JH, Bernstine DM, Rodman GH Jr, et al: Selection of patients with abdominal stab wounds for laparotomy, *J Trauma* 22:476, 1982.

37. Taviloglu K, Guany K, Ertekin C, et al: Abdominal stab wounds: role of selective management, *Eur J Surg* 164:17, 1998.

38. Muckart DJ, McDonald MA: Unreliability of standard quantitative criteria in diagnostic peritoneal lavage performed for suspected penetrating abdominal stab wounds, *Am J Surg* 162:223, 1991.

39. Boyle EM, Maier RV, Salazar JD, et al: Diagnosis of injuries after stab wounds to back and flank, *J Trauma* 42:260, 1997.

40. Phillips T, Sclafani SA, Goldstein A, et al: Use of contrast-enhanced CT enema in the management of penetrating injuries trauma to the flank and back, *J Trauma* 26:593, 1986.

41. Rosemurgy AS, Albrink MH, Olson SM, et al: Abdominal stab wound protocol: prospective study documents applicability for widespread use, *Am Surg* 61:112, 1995.

42. Kirton OC, Wint D, Thrasher B, et al: Stab wounds to the back and flank in hemodynamically stable patients: a decision algorithm-based on contrast-enhanced computed tomography with colonic opacification, *Am J Surg* 173:189, 1997.

43. Maldjian PD, Zurlo JV, Sebastiano L: Role of abdominal computed tomography in the evaluation and management of stab wounds to the back and flank, *Emerg Radiol* 4:340, 1997.

44. Meyer DM, Thal E, Weigelt JA, et al: Role of abdominal CT in the evaluation of stab wounds to the back, *J Trauma* 29:1226, 1989.

45. Raptopoulos V: Abdominal trauma: emphasis on computed tomography, *Radiol Clin North Am* 32:969, 1994.

46. McAninch JW, Federle MP: Evaluation of renal injuries with computed tomography, *J Urol* 128:456, 1982.

47. Grossman MD, May AK, Schwab CW, et al: Determine anatomic injury with computed tomography in selected torso gunshot wounds, *J Trauma* 45:446, 1998.

48. Ginzburg E, Carrillo EH, Kopelman T, et al: The role of computed tomography in selective management of gunshot wounds to the abdomen and flank, *J Trauma* 45:1005, 1998.

49. Shanmuganathan K, Mirvis SE, Chiu W, et al: Value of triple-contrast spiral CT in penetrating torso trauma: a prospective study to determine peritoneal violation and the need for laparotomy, *AJR Am J Roentgenol* 177:1247, 2001.

50. Renz BM, Feliciano DV: Gunshot wounds to the right thoracoabdomen: a prospective study of nonoperative management, *J Trauma* 37:737, 1994.

51. Simon RJ, Ivatury RR: Current concepts in the use of cavitary endoscopy in the evaluation and treatment of blunt and penetrating truncal injuries, *Surg Clinic North Am* 75:157, 1995.

52. Ivatury RR, Simon RJ, Stahl WM: A critical evaluation of laparoscopy in penetrating abdominal trauma, *J Trauma* 34:822, 1993.

53. Fabian TC, Croce MA, Stewart RM, et al: A prospective analysis of diagnostic laparoscopy in trauma, *Ann Surg* 217:557, 1993.

54. Sosa JL, Baker M, Puente I, et al: Negative laparotomy in abdominal gunshot wounds: potential impact of laparoscopy, *J Trauma* 38:194, 1995.

55. Fernando HC, Alle KM, Chen J, et al: Triage by laparoscopy in patients with penetrating abdominal trauma, *Br J Surg* 81:384, 1994.

56. Ortega AE, Tang E, Froes ET, et al: Laparoscopic evaluation of penetrating thoracoabdominal traumatic injuries, *Surg Endosc* 10:19, 1996.

57. Guth AA, Patcher HL: Laparoscopy for penetrating thoracoabdominal trauma: pitfalls and promises, *JSLS* 2:123, 1998.

58. Marks JM, Youngelman DF, Berk T: Cost analysis of diagnostic laparoscopy vs. laparotomy in the evaluation of penetrating abdominal trauma, *Surg Endosc* 11:272, 1997.

59. DeMaria EJ, Dalton JM, Gore DC, et al: Complementary roles of laparoscopic abdominal exploration and diagnostic peritoneal lavage for evaluation of abdominal stab wounds: a prospective study, *JSLS* 10:131, 2000.

60. Ivatury RR, Simon RJ, Weksler B: Laparoscopy in the evaluation of the intrathoracic abdomen after penetrating injuries, *J Trauma* 35:101, 1992.

61. Salvino CK, Esposito TJ, Marshall WJ, et al: The role of diagnostic laparoscopy in the management of trauma: a preliminary assessment, *J Trauma* 34:506, 1993.

62. Udobi KF, Rodriguez A, Chiu WC, et al: Role of ultrasonography in penetrating abdominal trauma: a prospective clinical study, *J Trauma* 50:475, 2001.

63. Rozycki GS, Ochsner MG, Jaffin TH, et al: Prospective evaluation of surgeon's use of ultrasound in the evaluation of trauma patients, *J Trauma* 34:516, 1993.

64. Fry WR, Smith S, Schnider JJ, et al: Ultrasonographic examination of wound tract, *Arch Surg* 130:605, 1995.

65. Hollerman JJ, Fackler ML, Coldwell DM, et al: Gunshot wounds. 2. Radiology, *AJR Am J Roentgenol* 155:691, 1990.

66. Fabian TC, Corce MA: Abdominal trauma, including indications for celiotomy. In Mattox KL, Feliciano DV, Moore EE, eds: *Trauma*, ed 4, New York, 2000, McGraw-Hill.

67. Severance HW: Ballistic wounding, *Critical Decisions in Emergency Medicine* 13:7, 1999.

68. Jones TK, Walsh JW, Maull KI: Diagnostic imaging in blunt trauma of the abdomen, *Surg Gynecol Obstet* 157:389, 1983.

69. Mirvis SE, Rodriguez A: Abdominal and pelvic trauma. In Mirvis SE, Young JWR, eds: *Imaging in trauma and critical care*, Baltimore, 1992, Williams & Wilkins.

69a. Killeen KL, Mirvis SE, Shanmuganathan K, et al: Helical CT of diaphragmatic rupture caused by blunt trauma, *AJR Am J Roentgenol* 173:1612, 1999.

69b. Dowe MF, Shanmuganathan K, Mirvis SE, et al: CT findings of mesenteric injury after blunt trauma: implications for surgical intervention, *AJR Am J Roentgenol* 168:425, 1997.

69c. Killeen KL, Shanmuganathan K, Poletti PA, et al: Helical computed tomography of bowel and mesenteric injuries, *J Trauma* 51:26, 2001.

70. Federle MP, Crass RA, Jeffrey RB, et al: Computed tomography in blunt trauma, *Arch Surg* 117:645, 1982.

71. Mirvis SE, Gens DR, Shanmuganathan K: Rupture of bowel after blunt abdominal trauma: diagnosis with CT, *AJR Am J Roentgenol* 159:1217, 1992.

72. Shanmuganathan K, Mirvis SE, Solver ER: Value of contrast-enhanced CT to detect active hemorrhage in patients with blunt abdominal or pelvic trauma, *AJR Am J Roentgenol* 161:65, 1993.

73. Rizzo MJ, Federle MP, Griffiths BG: Bowel and mesenteric injury following blunt abdominal trauma: evaluation with CT, *Radiology* 173:413, 1989.

74. Federle MP, Goldberg HI, Kaiser JA, et al: Evaluation of trauma by computed tomography, *Radiology* 138:637, 1981.

75. Jeffrey RB, Cardoza JD, Olcott EW: Detection of active intra-abdominal arterial hemorrhage: value of dynamic contrast-enhanced CT, *AJR Am J Roentgenol* 156:725, 1991.

76. Orwig D, Federle MP: Localized clotted blood as evidence of visceral trauma on CT: the sentinal clot sign, *AJR Am J Roentgenol* 153:747, 1989.

77. Shanmuganathan K, Mirvis SE, Reaney SM: Pictorial review: CT appearance of contrast medium extravasation associated with injury sustained from blunt abdominal trauma, *Clin Radiol* 50:182, 1995.

78. Rossi P, Mullins, D, Thal E: Role of laparoscopy in the evaluation of abdominal trauma, *Am J Surg* 166:707, 1993.

79. Poletti PA, Mirvis SE, Shanmuganathan K, et al: Use of CT-criteria in the management of blunt liver trauma: correlation with angiographic and surgical findings, *Radiology* 216:418, 2000.

80. Feliciano DV, Jordan GL, Bitondo CG, et al: Management of 1000 consecutive cases of hepatic trauma (1979-1984), *Ann Surg* 204:438, 1986.

81. Burch JM, Feliciano DV, Mattox KL: The atriocaval shunt: facts and fiction, *Ann Surg* 204:555, 1988.

82. Hansen CJ, Bernardas C, West MA, et al: Abdominal vena caval injuries: outcome remains dismal, *Surgery* 128:572, 2000.

83. Khaneja SC, Pizzi WF, Barie PS, et al: Management of penetrating juxtahepatic inferior vena cava injuries under total vascular occlusion, *J Am Coll Surg* 184:469, 1997.

84. Denton JR, Moore EE, Cordwell DM: Multimodality treatment for grade V hepatic injuries: perihepatic packing, arterial embolization, and venous stenting, *J Trauma* 42:964, 1997.

85. Sherman HF, Savage BA, Jones LM, et al: Nonoperative management of blunt hepatic injuries: safe at any grade? *J Trauma* 37:616, 1994.

86. Meredith JW, Young JS, Bowling J, et al: Nonoperative management of blunt hepatic trauma: the exception or the rule? *J Trauma* 36:529, 1994.

87. Carrillo EH, Spain DA, Wohltmann CD, et al: Interventional techniques are useful adjuncts in nonoperative management of hepatic injuries, *J Trauma* 46:619, 1999.

88. Levine A, Grove P, Nance F: Surgical restraint in the management of hepatic injuries: a review of Charity Hospital experience, *J Trauma* 18:399, 1978.

89. Moore JB, Moore EE, Thompson JS: Abdominal injuries associated with penetrating trauma in the lower chest, *Am J Surg* 140:724, 1980.

90. Federle MP, Kaiser JA, McAninch JW, et al: The role of computed tomography in renal trauma, *Radiology* 141:455, 1987.

91. Mirvis SE, Gelman R: Imaging of acute renal trauma, *Contemporary Diagnostic Radiology* 15:1, 1992.

92. Guerriero WG, Carlton CE, Scott R, et al: Renal pedicle injuries, *J Trauma* 11:53, 1971.

93. Steinberg DL, Jeffrey RB, Federle MP, et al: The computerized tomography appearance of renal pedicle injury, *J Urol* 132:1163, 1984.

94. Federle MP, Brown TR, McAninch JW: Penetrating renal trauma: CT evaluation, *J Comput Assist Tomogr* 11:1026, 1987.

95. Wessells H, McAninch JW, Meyer A, et al: Criteria for nonoperative treatment of significant penetrating renal lacerations, *J Urol* 157:24, 1997.

96. Armenakas NA, Duckett CP, McAninch JW: Indications for nonoperative management of renal stab wounds, *J Urol* 161:768, 1999.

97. McAninch JW, Carroll PR, Armenakas NA, et al: Renal gunshot wounds: method of salvage and reconstruction, *J Trauma* 35:279, 1993.

98. Miller KS, McAninch JW: Radiographic assessment of renal trauma: our 15-year experience, *J Urol* 154:352, 1995.

99. Presti JC Jr, Carroll PR, McAninch JW: Ureteral and renal pelvic injuries from external trauma: diagnosis and management, *J Trauma* 29:370, 1989.

100. Ghali AMA, Malik EMA, Ibrahim AIA, et al: Ureteric injuries: diagnosis, management, and outcome, *J Trauma* 46:1508, 1999.

101. Velmahos GC, Degiannis E, Wells M, et al: Penetrating ureteral injuries: the impact of associate injuries on management, *Am Surg* 62:461, 1996.

102. Azimuddin K, Ivatury R, Poter J, et al: Penetrating ureteric injuries, *Injury* 29:363, 1998.

103. Brandes SB, Chelsky M, Buckman RF, et al: Ureteral injuries from penetrating trauma, *J Trauma* 36:766, 1994.

104. Medina D, Lavery R, Ross SE, Livingston DH: Ureteral trauma: preoperative studies neither predict injury nor prevent missed injuries, *J Am Coll Surg* 186:641, 1998.

105. Eastham JA, Wilson TG, Larsen DW, et al: Angiographic embolization of renal stab wounds, *J Urol* 148:268, 1992.

106. Brennemann NKK, Krosner KSM, Roberts FJJ, et al: Routine preoperative "one-shot" intravenous pyelography is not indicated in all patients with penetrating abdominal trauma, *J Am Coll Surg* 185:530, 1997.

107. Moore EE, Shackford SR, Patcher HL, et al: Organ injury scale: spleen, liver, and kidney, *J Trauma* 29:1664, 1989.

108. Nicolaisen GS, McAninch JW, Marshall GA, et al: Renal trauma: reevaluation of the indications for radiographic assessment, *J Urol* 133:183, 1985.

109. Carlton CE Jr, Scott R Jr, Guthire AG: The initial management of ureteral injuries: a report of 78 cases, *J Urol* 105:335, 1971.

110. McGinty DM, Mendez R: Traumatic ureteral injuries with delayed recognition, *J Urol* 10:115, 1977.

111. Cass AS: Ureteral contusion with gunshot wounds, *J Trauma* 24:59, 1984.

112. Templeton PA, Mirvis SE, Whitley NO: Traumatic avulsion of the ureter: computed tomographic correlation, *J Comput Assist Tomogr* 12:159, 1988.

113. Carroll PR, McAninch JW: Major bladder trauma: mechanism of injury and unified method of diagnosis and repair, *J Urol* 132:254, 1984.

114. Thomae KR, Kilambi NK, Poole GV: Method of urinary diversion in nonurethral traumatic bladder injuries: retrospective analysis of 70 cases, *Am Surg* 64:77, 1998.

115. Deck AJ, Shaves S, Talner L, et al: Computerized tomography cystography for the diagnosis of traumatic bladder rupture, *J Urol* 164:43, 2000.

116. Baniel J, Schein M: The management of penetrating trauma to the urinary tract, *J Am Coll Surg* 178:417, 1994.

117. Mueller CS, Pendravis RW: Traumatic injury of the diaphragm: report of seven cases and extensive literature review, *Emerg Radiol* 1:118, 1994.

118. Murray JA, Demetriades D, Asensio JA, et al: Occult injuries to the diaphragm: prospective evaluation of laparoscopy in penetrating injuries to the left lower chest, *J Am Coll Surg* 187:626, 1998.

119. Zantut LF, Ivatory RR, Smith S, et al: Diagnostic and therapeutic laparoscopy penetrating trauma: a multicentric experience, *J Trauma* 42:825, 1997.

120. Von Oppell UO, De Groot M: Penetrating thoracic injuries: what have we learned? *Thorac Cardiovasc Surg* 48:55, 2000.

121. Richardson JD, Spain DA: Injury to lung and pleura. In Mattox KL, Feliciano DV, Moore EE, eds: *Trauma*, ed 4, New York, 2000, McGraw-Hill.

122. Ordog GJ, Wasserberger J, Balasubramanium S, et al: Asymptomatic stab wounds of the chest, *J Trauma* 36:680, 1994.

123. Parmley LF, Mattingly TW, Manion WC: Penetrating wounds of the heart and aorta, *Circulation* 17:953, 1958.

124. Renz BM, Cava RA, Feliciano DV, et al: Transmediastinal gunshot wounds: a prospective study, *J Trauma* 48:416, 2000.

125. Hanpeter DE, Demetriades D, Asensio JA, et al: Helical computed tomographic scan in the evaluation of mediastinal gunshot wounds, *J Trauma* 49:689, 2000.

126. Cornwell EE, Kennedy F, Ayad IA, et al: Transmediastinal gunshot wounds: reconsideration of the role of aortography, *Arch Surg* 131:949, 1996.

127. Gasparri MG, Lorelli DR, Karlovich KA, et al: Physical examination plus chest radiography in penetrating periclavicular trauma: the appropriate trigger for angiography, *J Trauma* 49:1029, 2000.

128. Shatz DV, Pedraja J, Erbella J, et al: Efficacy of follow-up evaluation in penetrating thoracic injuries: 3- vs 6-hour radiographs of the chest, *J Emerg Med* 20:281, 2000.

129. Oparah SS, Mandal AK: Penetrating stab wounds to the chest: experience with 200 consecutive cases, *J Trauma* 16:868, 1976.

130. Muckart DJJ, Luvuno FM, Baker LW: Penetrating injuries of the pleural cavity, *Thorax* 39:789, 1984.

131. Kerr TM, Sood R, Buckman RF, et al: Prospective trial of the six-hour rule in stab wounds of the chest, *Surg Gynecol Obstet* 169:223, 1989.

132. Weiglet JA, Christian M, Aurbakken M, et al: Management of asymptomatic patients following stab wounds to the chest, *J Trauma* 22:291, 1982.

133. Tocino IM, Miller MH, Fairfax WR: Distribution of pneumothorax in supine and semi-recumbent critically ill patients, *AJR Am J Roentgenol* 144:901, 1985.

134. Wall SD, Federle MP, Jeffrey RB, et al: CT diagnosis of unsuspected pneumothorax after blunt trauma, *AJR Am J Roentgenol* 141:919, 1983.

135. Rhea JT, Novelline RA, Lawrason J, et al: The frequency and significance of thoracic injuries detected on abdominal CT scans in multiple trauma patients, *J Trauma* 29:502, 1989.

136. Rhea JT, van Sonnenburg E, McLoud TC: Basilar pneumothorax in the supine adult, *Radiology* 133:593, 1979.

137. Gordon R: Deep sulcus sign, *Radiology* 136:25, 1980.

138. Ziter FM, Westcott JL: Supine subpulmonary pneumothorax, *AJR Am J Roentgenol* 137:699, 1981.

139. Chiles C, Ravin CE: Radiographic recognition of pneumothorax in the intensive care unit, *Crit Care Med* 14:677, 1986.

140. Kish G, Kozloff L, Joseph WL, et al: Indications for early thoracotomy in the management of chest trauma, *Ann Thorac Surg* 22:23, 1976.

141. Meyer DM, Jessen ME, Wait MA, et al: Early evacuation of traumatic retained hemothoraces using thoracoscopy: a prospective randomized trial, *Ann Thorac Surg* 64:1396, 1997.

142. Heniford BT, Carillo EH, Spain DA, et al: The role of video-assisted thoracoscopy in the management of retained thoracic collections after trauma, *Ann Thorac Surg* 63:940, 1997.

143. Velmahos GC, Demetriades D, Chang L, et al: Predicting need for thoracoscopic evacuation of residual traumatic hemothorax: chest radiograph is insufficient, *J Trauma* 46:65, 1999.

144. Ma JO, Masteer JR: Trauma ultrasound examination versus chest radiograph in the detection of hemothorax, *Ann Emerg Med* 29:312, 1997.

145. Stark P: Pleura. In *Radiology of thoracic trauma.* Boston, 1993, Andover Medical Publishers.

146. Richardson JD, Flint LM, Snow NJ, et al: Management of transmediastinal gunshot wound, *Surgery* 90:671, 1981.

147. Peper WA, Obied FN, Horst HM, et al: Penetrating injuries of the mediastinum, *Am Surg* 52:359, 1986.

148. Asensio JA, Berne J, Demetriades D, et al: Penetrating esophageal injuries: time interval of safety for preoperative evaluation—how long is safe? *J Trauma* 43:319, 1997.

149. Asensio JA, Chahwan S, Forno W, et al: Penetrating esophageal injuries: multicentric study of the American Association for the Surgery of Trauma, *J Trauma* 50:289, 2001.

150. Hatzitheofilou C, Strahlendrof C, Charalambides D, et al: Penetrating external injuries of the oesophagus and pharynx, *Br J Surg* 80:1147, 1993.

151. Bertelsen S, Howitz P: Injuries of the trachea and bronchi, *Thorax* 27:188, 1972.

152. Barmada H, Gibbons JR: Tracheobroncheal injury in blunt and penetrating chest trauma, *Chest* 106:74, 1994.

153. Unger JM, Schuchmann GG, Grossman JE, et al: Tears of the trachea and main stem bronchi caused by blunt trauma: radiologic findings, *AJR Am J Roentgenol* 153:1175, 1989.

154. Mason AC, Mirvis SE, Templeton PA: Imaging of acute tracheobronchial injury: review of the literature, *Emerg Radiol* 1:250, 1994.

155. Lee RB: Traumatic injury of cervicothoracic trachea and major bronchi, *Chest Surg Clin N Am* 7:285, 1997.

156. Chen J, Shanmuganathan K, Mirvis SE, et al: Using CT to diagnose tracheal rupture, *AJR Am J Roentgenol* 176:1273, 2001.

157. Rossbach MM, Johnson SB, Gomez MA, et al: Management of major tracheobronchial injuries: a 28-year experience, *Ann Thorac Surg* 65:182, 1998.

158. Asensio JA, Valenziano CP, Falcone RE, et al: Management of penetrating neck injuries: the controversy surrounding zone II neck injuries, *Surg Clin North Am* 71:267, 1991.

159. Gaebler C, Mueller M, Schramm W, et al: Tracheobroncheal rupture in children, *Am J Emergency Medicine* 14:279, 1996.

160. Wiot JF: Tracheobronchial trauma, *Semin Roentgenol* 18:15, 1983.

161. Oh KS, Fleishner FG, Wyman SM: Characteristic pulmonary findings in traumatic complete transection of a main-stem bronchus, *Radiology* 92:371, 1969.

162. Wan YL, Tasi KT, Yeow KM, et al: CT findings of bronchial transection, *Am J Emergency Medicine* 15:176, 1997.

163. Naidich DP, Harkin TJ: Airway and lung: correlation of CT with fiberoptic bronchoscopy, *Radiology* 197:1, 1995.

164. Rollings RJ, Tocino I: Early radiographic signs of tracheal rupture, *AJR Am J Roentgenol* 148:695, 1987.

165. Starks P: Imaging of tracheobronchial injuries, *J Thorac Imaging* 10:206, 1995.

166. Huh J, Milliken JC, Chen JC: Management of tracheobronchial injuries following blunt and penetrating trauma, *Am Surg* 63:896, 1997.

167. Rossbach MM, Johnson SB, Gomez MA, et al: Management of major tracheobronchial injuries: a 28-year experience, *Ann Thorac Surg* 65:182, 1998.

168. Ramzy AI, Rodriguez A, Turney SZ: Management of major tracheobronchial ruptures in patients with multiple system trauma, *J Trauma* 28:1353, 1988.

169. Bladergroen MR, Lowe JE, Postlethwait RW: Diagnosis and recommended management of esophageal perforation and rupture, *Ann Thorac Surg* 42:235, 1986.

170. Jones WG II, Ginsberg RJ: Esophageal perforation: a continuing challenge, *Ann Thorac Surg* 53:534, 1992.

171. Maltby JD: The post-trauma chest film, *CRC Crit Rev Diagn Imaging* 14:1, 1980.

172. Van Moore A, Ravin CE, Putman CE: Radiologic evaluation of acute chest trauma, *CR Crit Rev Diagn Imaging* 19:89, 1983.

173. Nesbitt JC, Sawyer JL: Surgical management of esophageal perforation, *Am Surg* 53:183, 1987.

174. Demetriades D, Theodorous D, Cornwell E, et al: Transcervical gunshot injuries: mandatory operation is not necessary, *J Trauma* 40:758, 1996.

175. Defore WW Jr, Mattox KL, Hansen HA, et al: Surgical management of penetrating injuries of the esophagus, *Am J Surg* 134:734, 1977.

176. Kim-Deobald J, Kozarek RA: Esophageal perforation: an 8-year review of a multispecialty clinic's experience, *Am J Gastroenterol* 87:1112, 1992.

177. Popovsky J: Perforation of the esophagus from gunshot wounds, *J Trauma* 24:337, 1984.

178. LeBlang SD, Dolich MO: Imaging of penetrating thoracic trauma, *J Thorac Imaging* 15:128, 2000.

13 Nuclear Medicine Applications in Trauma and Critical Care Imaging

Lawrence E. Holder and Ismet Sarikaya

Nuclear medicine imaging techniques can be used in a variety of clinical situations involving critically injured trauma patients. However, when high-resolution fast computed tomography (CT) scanning is available, as is the case in most trauma centers and hospital emergency departments, the comprehensive multiple organ evaluations that fast CT provides relegates most nuclear medicine imaging to a secondary or tertiary modality for acute trauma care. The physiologic, rather than anatomic, basis of radionuclide studies often leads to their important role during the first hours or days after acute trauma for patients who often have distorted anatomy from injury or surgery or nonanatomically based problems. Early posttrauma imaging by nuclear medicine techniques may be advantageous in occasional circumstances, such as major allergy to intravenous contrast used for most CT studies in acute trauma, body weight exceeding table limits, technical difficulties using sonography also related to body habitus, or soft tissue air, among others.

The radionuclide studies most commonly used during the postacute period include brain flow imaging, hepatobiliary imaging, acute bleeding studies, bone imaging, ventilation and perfusion (V/Q) studies, and infection imaging. Radionuclide cisternography, myocardial perfusion imaging, peptide imaging for deep vein thrombosis, cardiac function imaging, avid infarct imaging for myocardial contusion, renal imaging, and brain perfusion single photon emission computed tomography (SPECT) have applications in trauma care, but are used less frequently.

Advances in all areas of imaging continue to increase the diagnostic choices available, and preferred diagnostic algorithms continue to change. For example, the evaluation of renal artery flow and parenchymal perfusion, once the total purview of nuclear imaging, now is performed in the acute setting in many centers using magnetic resonance (MR) angiography. In the subacute setting, however, technetium-99m (^{99m}Tc)-DTPA (diethylenetriamine pentaacetic acid) or ^{99m}Tc-MAG3 (mercaptoacetyltriglycine) should be considered, because these studies allow for evaluation of glomerular filtration rate or effective renal plasma flow, respectively, in addition to perfusion. Sulfur colloid imaging of the liver and spleen for detecting fracture or rupture, although superseded when CT is available, is still a valid technique.[1]

It is not the purpose of this brief chapter to review the principles of gamma camera imaging, nuclear medicine hardware, or data acquisition and processing software, for which information is available in standard texts.[2-4] Rather, the typical findings of the most frequently performed studies will be illustrated and the basic indications, technique, and diagnostic criteria discussed and some technical and interpretive pitfalls noted. Much of this experience has been discussed previously in greater detail for the nuclear medicine physician.[1] The interested reader is referred to that and other references for more information, particularly for less commonly performed studies.[5-9]

BRAIN PERFUSION IMAGING

Brain imaging in the acute setting is performed to confirm brain death. Sedation, drugs, and body temperature variations that can affect electroencephalographic analysis do not mask brain perfusion. According to the report of the Medical Consultants on the Diagnosis of Death to the President's Commission for the Study of Ethical Problems in Medicine and Biomedical and Behavioral Research, brain death is diagnosed by clinical examination and four-vessel intracranial contrast angiography, and it is confirmed by electroencephalographic and radionuclide brain imaging.[10]

Technique

With the patient supine and the head in neutral or slightly extended position, an anterior view is obtained after administration of 15 to 20 mCi (555 to 740 MBq) ^{99m}Tc-pertechnetate or ^{99m}Tc-HMPAO (hexamethylpropylene amine oxime) or ^{99m}Tc-ECD (ethylenediylbis cysteine diethylester [Neurolite]). The radiotracer is injected as a bolus, with imaging begun simultaneously, so that the earliest appearance of tracer in the neck arteries can be seen. A 1-second-per-image dynamic radionuclide angiogram (RNA) is acquired for 60 seconds, followed by an immediate 800k- to 1000k-count blood pool image. Lateral images usually are not necessary but can also be obtained. A dose of pertechnetate costs about 20 times less than a dose of the other tracers.

Interpretation Criteria

The normal cerebral RNA demonstrates perfusion through the anterior and middle cerebral arteries, creating the so-called *trident sign*. Perfusion of the cerebral hemispheres is symmetric and similar in intensity to scalp activity, which cannot be defined separately (Fig. 13-1). The immediate blood pool image confirms symmetric intracerebral activity (see Fig. 13-1). Brain death, or absent intracerebral perfusion, is manifested by absent perfusion through the anterior and middle cerebral vessels and absent intracerebral perfusion on both RNA and the blood pool images (Fig. 13-2). The latter image often documents absent sagittal sinus activity.[11] Because the sagittal sinus may drain both the internal and cerebral external circulations, its absence is seen often in brain death, but its presence is not diagnostic of normal intracerebral perfusion.

Positioning the patient with the head flexed should be avoided, because that position makes visualization of carotid perfusion difficult and obscures the sharp cutoff between the activity of carotid flow in the neck and the absence of intracranial carotid flow in brain death. Scalp bleeding or hematoma, with activity delivered by the external carotid circulation, can overlap and obscure the decreased parenchymal activity in the patient with brain death. In those situations, comparative lateral views are helpful to eliminate diagnostic uncertainty.[1] Some physicians, especially in centers that perform this study infrequently, prefer using ^{99m}Tc-HMPAO or ^{99m}Tc-ECD. These

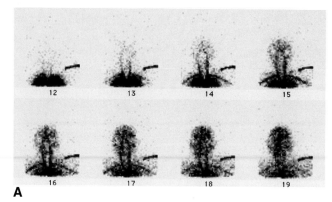

A

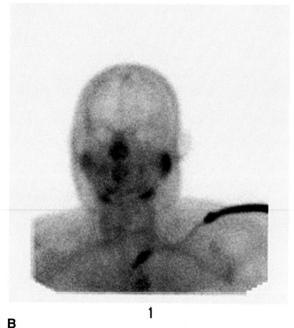

B

1

Fig. 13-1

Normal cerebral radionuclide angiogram and static blood pool image, after intravenous injection of ^{99m}Tc-pertechnatate. **A,** A 1-second-per-frame radionuclide angiogram demonstrates the trident representing normal perfusion through the anterior and middle cerebral arteries. Note the rapid appearance of intracerebral perfusion. **B,** Immediate anterior tissue phase or blood pool image demonstrates intracerebral perfusion, which appears just slightly less intense than the scalp activity. Incidental salivary gland activity is seen.

lipophilic tracers enter the brain and, after dissociating, remain trapped therein, producing increased prominence of perfused brain cells in the normal patient. Because of this tracer retention, the information obtained with RNA after bolus injection, although still potentially diagnostic, is less important for diagnostic certainty than it is when ^{99m}Tc-pertechnetate is used.

HEPATOBILIARY IMAGING

Hepatobiliary imaging (HBI) is performed most frequently in the subacute, often postoperative setting, when

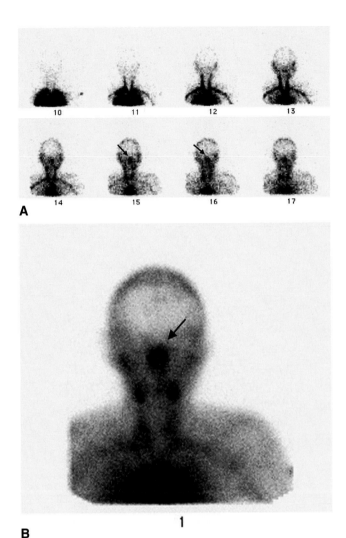

B

1

Fig. 13-2
Brain death. **A**, Cerebral radionuclide angiogram demonstrates lack of visualization of intracerebral vessels and the "hot nose" sign (*arrow*), which represents relatively increased perfusion through the external carotid system. **B**, Anterior blood pool or immediate tissue phase image demonstrates complete absence of intracerebral vascularity, with the "hot nose" sign again seen (*arrow*).

there is a question of abnormal drainage or a bile leak, or when an intrahepatic or perihepatic lesion is discovered on CT and information about its relationship to biliary system is desired.[1,12] During the in-hospital recovery period, hepatobiliary imaging is used, also, when acute cholecystitis, particularly of the acalculous type, is suspected (see Chapter 16). The biliary tract imaging properties of the iminodiacetic acid derivatives were discovered and developed by Loberg and his team[13] in the Division of Nuclear Medicine at the University of Maryland in 1976.

Technique

The standard HBI protocol for acute cholecystitis is modified slightly when hospitalized patients are suspected of having acute acalculous cholecystitis, abnormal bile drainage, or bile leakage. Although there is not universal agreement in the former case, especially in those patients with severe intercurrent illness or who have been receiving parenteral nutrition for more than 24 hours, we choose to pretreat with 0.02 µg/kg slow intravenous injection of cholecystokinin (CCK) over 2 to 2.5 minutes. This may empty a full gallbladder,[14,15] restore biliary tone, or shorten study time from 4 hours to 90 minutes.[14,16-18] If 45 to 60 minutes after injection, there has been liver clearance and there is extrahepatic duct activity but no gallbladder or bowel activity, 0.04 mg/kg intravenous morphine sulfate (MS) is given slowly over 3 minutes. This morphine augmentation should produce spasm in the sphincter of Oddi, raise biliary system pressure, and cause reflux of tracer into the gallbladder to overcome a "nonpathologic" obstruction, thus decreasing the false-positive result rate of hepatobiliary scintigraphy.

If the clinical concern is abnormal bile drainage or leak, CCK or MS may not be necessary. Especially important, however, before any injections are made or tracer given, is a full understanding of prior surgical procedures and resultant or presumed anatomic drainage, and a full review of prior imaging studies. Such knowledge not only helps during final interpretation, but also in positioning for initial imaging and in the choice of supplemental views, if needed. Two hours after injection, delayed imaging may be necessary to demonstrate small bilomas. At 10 to 15 minutes after CCK pretreatment, with the patient supine for an anterior view, bolus injection of 5 mCi of mebrofenin (Choletec) or disofenin (DISIDA) is made, with a 1-second-per-image RNA acquired for 60 seconds, followed by 118 30-second dynamic images. For possible acute cholecystitis, if the gallbladder is not visualized after 45 to 60 minutes, MS is given as long as there still is tracer in the liver and in the extrahepatic ducts, and 20 to 30 minutes of additional imaging at 30 seconds per image is obtained.[19] If the patient has moderate jaundice, 6 to 12 mCi of tracer is administered, and 10 to 15 mCi used with severe jaundice. Although concurrent treatment with MS *theoretically* increases biliary system pressures by sphincter of Oddi contraction or spasm, and might preclude obtaining an adequate imaging study, that has not been the author's experience. If there is any concern, 0.8 mg intravenous naloxone can reverse such spasm, with an effect that lasts for about 30 minutes per dose.

Interpretation Criteria

Liver clearance of tracer from the blood within 10 minutes, and intrahepatic and extrahepatic duct, gallbladder, and bowel activity visualization within 30 to 60 minutes is normal (Fig. 13-3). With or without pretreatment with CCK,

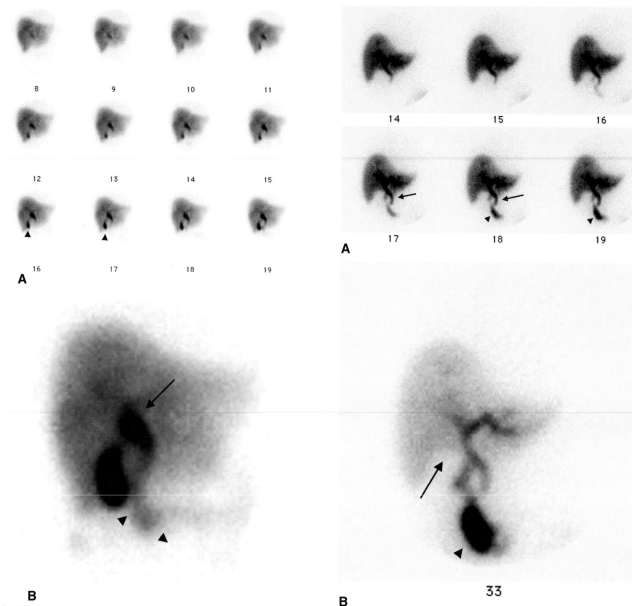

B

Fig. 13-3
Normal hepatobiliary imaging. **A**, Anterior view, 1-minute-per-frame dynamic sequence, selected images from minute 8 through minute 15 after injection. There is clearance of tracer into the liver, with visualization of right and left intrahepatic ducts and progressive filling of the gallbladder (*arrowheads*). **B**, Single image from end of sequence, 30 minutes after injection. The gallbladder has filled more completely, the common bile duct is seen (*arrow*), and the descending and horizontal portions of the duodenum are seen (*arrowheads*).

B   **33**

Fig. 13-4
Acute cholecystitis. **A**, Anterior view, selected images from dynamic sequence similar to Fig. 13-3, *A*. The common bile duct (*long arrows*) is seen entering the duodenum, with both antegrade and retrograde movement of tracer in the duodenum (*arrowheads*). There is no visualization of the gallbladder. **B**, Dynamic sequence performed after administration of morphine sulfate. Selected image obtained 20 minutes after administration. There is still no visualization of the gallbladder, with some relative photon deficiency in the gallbladder fossa region (*arrow*). More tracer has entered the duodenum and moved distally (*arrowhead*).

but certainly after MS augmentation, the gallbladder will not be visualized in patients with acute cholecystitis (Fig. 13-4). When there is no biliary clearance after good clearance from the blood, with no visualization of the intrahepatic or extrahepatic bile ducts after 1 hour, ascending cholangitis or common bile duct obstruction should be considered. It can be confirmed by finding a similar appearance on 4-hour postinjection images (Fig. 13-5).

Abnormal extrabiliary flow patterns, free-flowing bile leaks, or contained bilomas usually are seen within minutes after injection, although delayed images may be needed to confirm bile flow into a small collection seen on CT (Figs. 13-6 to 13-8). Cine mode display of dynamically acquired images is usually essential to localize the source of a leak. It is important to elucidate both the

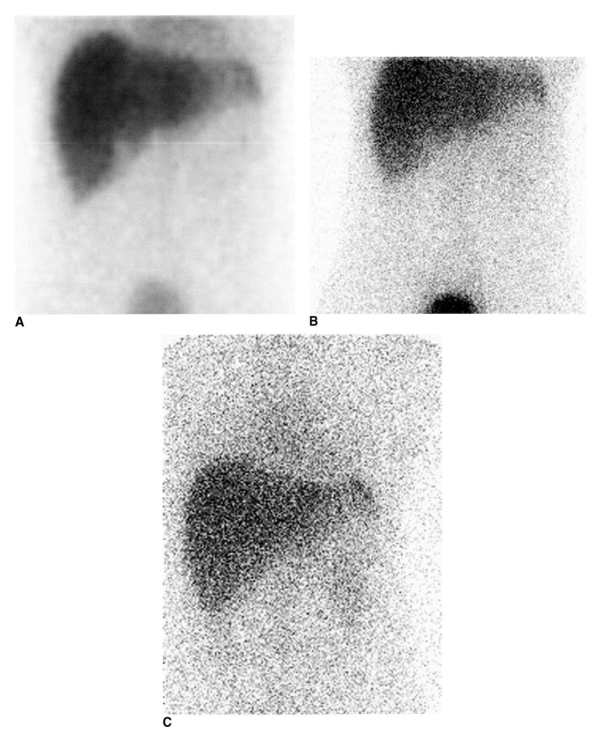

Fig. 13-5
Common bile duct obstruction. Single anterior images 1 hour (**A**), 2 hours (**B**), and 24 hours (**C**) after tracer administration. During the dynamic sequence there was prompt, but slightly decreased, tracer clearance from the blood as manifested by some continued tracer in the cardiac blood pool. There is no visualization on any of these images of intrahepatic or extrahepatic ducts, or gallbladder or bowel activity. Severe cholangitis can also have this pattern, usually with less tracer clearance from the blood and with a different clinical picture.

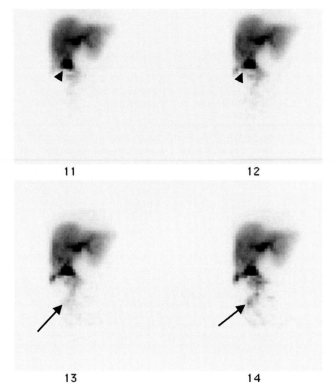

Fig. 13-6
Early, moderate-to-severe bile leak after trauma. Anterior view, 1-minute-per-frame dynamic sequence, selected images from minute 11 through minute 14 after injection. Intrahepatic duct activity is seen, with abnormal collection of tracer inferior to midportion of the right lobe (*arrowheads*), which shows progressive leakage into the peritoneum (*arrows*). There is no visualization of common duct or duodenum, suggesting that most of the drainage is moving through the abnormal pathway.

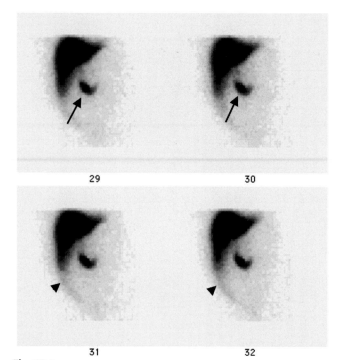

Fig. 13-7
Small biliary leak. Anterior view, 1-minute-per-frame dynamic sequence, selected images from minute 29 through minute 32 after injection. Although there is not good visualization of the intrahepatic ducts or common duct, the duodenum (*arrows*) was identified easily on the dynamic sequence. A small amount of tracer is seen tracking along the right lateral peritoneum (*arrowheads*), but the site of origin could not be determined. Note, however, that the greater amount of tracer is moving through the normal pathway.

dynamics of the flow and its pattern. For example, if most of the drainage follows a normal course, such a leak would more likely be observed than if most of the drainage was through an abnormal route (see Fig. 13-7), when drainage or operative diversion would become more likely.

ACUTE BLEEDING LOCALIZATION

Intraluminal gastrointestinal bleeding occurring in the subacute posttrauma patient is usually due to stress ulceration. Most often, endoscopic techniques are used to localize and directly manage the bleeding site(s). In some cases the site remains elusive, and the source may be identified by a radionuclide bleeding study.[20] Such localization can guide surgical management or angiographic diagnosis and management by interventional radiology. This study is done when patients demonstrate significant bleeding, with changes in vital signs, or if significant blood transfusion is required. A recent clinical[21] and technical review[22] emphasize the value of the ^{99m}Tc–red

blood cell (RBC) tracer using dynamic acquisition and cine mode display protocols. The on-line version of the latter reference provides Internet links to such dynamic images.

Technique

An anterior view with the patient supine, using the largest field-of-view camera available, allows for anatomic orientation and the opportunity to view as much of the region of suspected bleeding as possible. Ten milliliters of autologous RBCs labeled with 20 mCi (740 megabecquerels [MBq]) ^{99m}Tc using the commercially available UltraTag kit (Mallinckrodt Medical, St. Louis, Mo.), which provides 98% labeling efficiency, are injected as a bolus. A 1-second-per-image RNA is obtained for 60 seconds, followed by a 10-second-per-image dynamic acquisition for 1 hour. The latter is divided into four continuous 15-minute segments.[22] These dynamic images are usually essential for localizing the site of bleeding. Reframing into 30-second or 1-minute-per-frame images for increased spatial resolution to complement the temporal resolution acquisition is done often. In problem cases,

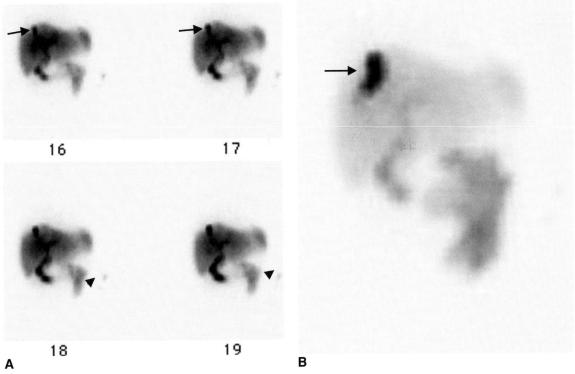

Fig. 13-8
Small biloma. **A,** Anterior view, 1-minute-per-frame dynamic sequence, selected images from minute 16 through minute 19 after injection. Almost concurrently with movement of tracer through intrahepatic ducts into the duodenum, there is focus of increasing tracer accumulation in relation to the dome of the right lobe (*arrows*). **B,** Single image 33 minutes after injection demonstrates further clearing from the normal liver and tracer movement into the jejunum (*arrowheads*), and continued retention of tracer in the biloma (*arrow*).

the study is reviewed directly on the monitor with the trauma surgeon and interventional radiologist, whose knowledge of the patient's anatomy and prior interventions is critical for diagnosis.

Interpretation Criteria

Any escape of blood from the intravascular space is abnormal. The purpose of the acute bleeding study is not just to confirm the clinical impression of bleeding but to localize accurately the active bleeding site. To that end, increasing intensity and movement of extravascular tracer must be seen directly during image (data) acquisition. Intraperitoneal pooling away from an extraluminal bleeding site and distant pooling or retrograde or antegrade movement from an intraluminal bleeding site can adversely affect site localization, and this was the major source of diagnostic error before introduction of the dynamic acquisition and viewing techniques (Fig. 13-9).

RADIONUCLIDE BONE IMAGING

Radionuclide bone imaging (RNBI) is used during the evaluation of acute skeletal trauma when the anatomic imaging examinations are technically limited, or in the subacute situation when known skeletal lesions do not explain potentially osseous pain after multisystem trauma.[23] Whole body imaging is also very valuable when battered child syndrome is suspected. Although MR imaging detects anatomic changes associated with fracture, nuclear medicine is still the only modality directly depicting increased bone turnover which, although less specific anatomically, is more specific physiologically.

Focal skeletal and soft tissue injury from acute thermal injury caused by heat, cold, or electrical energy can be evaluated with bone tracers and the demarcation of viable tissue ascertained before anatomic visible changes.[1] In the subacute time frame, sequelae of injury, including

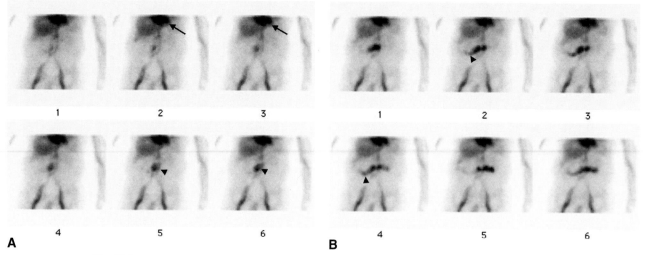

Fig. 13-9
Acute gastrointestinal bleeding. **A,** Anterior view, 1-minute-per-frame dynamic sequence, selected images from minute 1 through minute 6 after injection. Initial view demonstrates normal blood pool tracer localization in the heart (*arrows*), liver, aorta, and iliac veins. On the second and subsequent frames, increasing tracer accumulation is seen in the midabdomen (*arrowheads*). **B,** Selected images from dynamic sequence, minute 16 through minute 21 after injection. Antegrade movement to the left and retrograde movement to the right (*arrowheads*) were seen well on the movie mode display. Follow-up images confirmed a midtransverse colon bleed, in a segment located a little more inferiorly than usually seen.

heterotopic ossification (HO), reflex sympathetic dystrophy (RSD), and early osteomyelitis in violated bone, can be diagnosed in the absence of anatomic alteration when other imaging modalities are less sensitive.[24]

Technique

The standard imaging protocols for RNBI, including three-phase, whole body, and SPECT imaging, have been well described.[23] SPECT imaging, using a variety of alternative data acquisitions and processing protocols, allows adaptation to patients in pain or those with orthopedic hardware.[25] Imaging through cast material is accomplished easily, also. When possible, flow (RNA, radionuclide angiogram), blood pool (BP), and whole body imaging should be performed, because the increased vascularity depicted by the first two techniques often can aid in assessing underlying metabolism or inflammation. The whole body study detects unsuspected foci of abnormality in posttrauma patients unable to communicate adequately.

Interpretation Criteria

Although increased metabolic activity is a nonspecific finding, both focal and regional pattern recognition[23] often aid in establishing a specific diagnosis. Precise lesion characterization appropriately directs additional evaluation. To serve as examples, some specific lesions are described and illustrated below.

Acute Hip Fracture. Almost all hip fractures are detected immediately after trauma.[26] Very rarely, particularly in patients over 75 years old with osteoporosis, an impacted fracture will not immediately show increased tracer uptake, although changes on the RNA and BP images often will be seen. The RNA demonstrates curvilinear increased tracer activity, representing increased perfusion through the medial or lateral circumflex femoral artery. BP images show similar activity, representing the increased vascularity accompanying early repair. The delayed image appearance of subcapital, neck, and intertrochanteric fractures is typical[23] (Fig. 13-10).

Heterotopic Ossification. RNBI is ideal to detect the earliest development of hydroxyapatite crystals, well before increased density can be seen on radiographs or CT. HO often manifests as a fever of unknown origin. RNA and BP image findings may even be positive, with increased uptake corresponding to the HO, before positive delayed images. Oblique or orthogonal planar or SPECT images will separate the often intense abnormal increased uptake from the adjacent cortical activity[23] (Fig. 13-11). Sequential follow-up imaging of HO until the abnormal increased activity becomes normometabolic is used to determine when the lesion is mature.

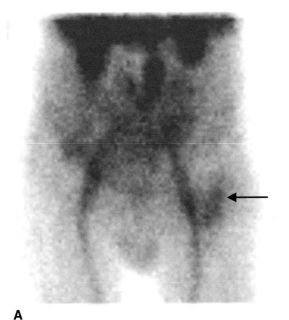

A

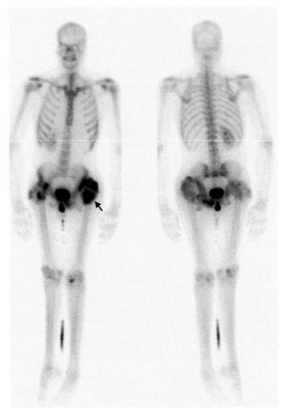

Fig. 13-11
Heterotopic ossification. Delayed whole body scan, anterior (*left*) and posterior (*right*) views. Intense tracer accumulation anterosuperiorly around the left hip (*arrow*) and medially around the right hip are more obvious on anterior view. The left kidney is absent.

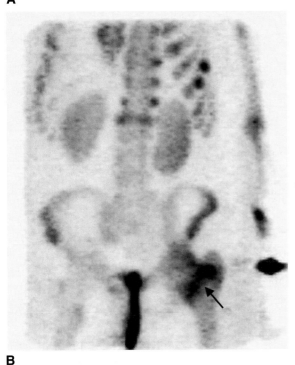

B

Fig. 13-10
Femoral neck fracture. **A,** Blood pool image, anterior view. Curvilinear increased uptake, representing increased relative vascularity in the distribution of the left medial or lateral circumflex femoral artery (*arrow*). **B,** Delayed scan. Single frame from 3-dimensional volumetric reconstruction from SPECT acquisition, slight left anterior oblique projection. Linear increased tracer accumulation at the femoral neck base (*arrow*) is typical appearance for a neck fracture. Rib and spine fractures are also present in this patient status after motor vehicle collision.

Reflex Sympathetic Dystrophy. Although RSD usually develops weeks to months after trauma, it can occur while the traumatized patient is still hospitalized. In that situation, the patient's musculoskeletal pain is out of proportion to that expected during the course of normal fracture or soft tissue healing. Only about 60% of patients will have radiographically demonstrable osteopenia. In the upper extremity, the typical pattern of RSD on delayed images consists of diffuse abnormal uptake throughout the wrist, metacarpals, and phalanges, with juxtaarticular accentuation[27,28] (Fig. 13-12). About one half of patients show increased perfusion on the RNA or BP portions of the three-phase bone scan. In the acute setting Lankford stage I, there is almost 100% sensitivity and specificity. In the lower extremity in adults, most authors describe a similar pattern[29] (Fig. 13-13). Some lower extremity pain syndromes have diffuse decreased activity and also have been called RSD.[30] The lower extremity sympathetic pain syndromes demonstrating decreased tracer on delayed images have recently been termed pseudodystrophy.[31] In children, RSD is not seen in the upper extremity. Because diffuse increased uptake can be seen in diabetic patients with foot infections, the specificity in the lower extremity is decreased when compared with the hand, although there is not usually any confusion when RSD is clinically suspected.

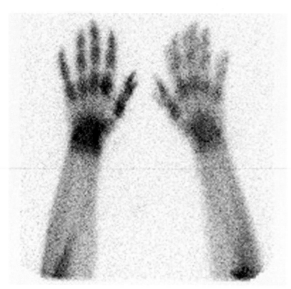

Fig. 13-12
Reflex sympathetic dystrophy, right hand and wrist. Delayed scan, palmar views. Intense increased tracer throughout the right wrist, metacarpals, and phalanges, with juxtaarticular accentuation.

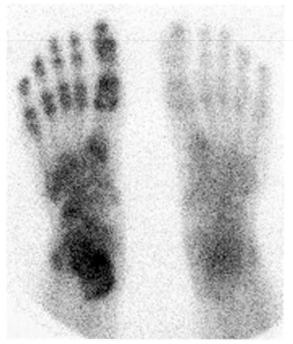

Fig. 13-13
Reflex sympathetic dystrophy, right foot. Delayed scan, plantar view. Intense increased tracer throughout the right hindfoot, midfoot, and forefoot, with juxtaarticular accentuation.

Thermal Injury. Necrotic or damaged tissue in a focal milieu of abnormal acid–base balance will be associated with abnormal precipitation of hydroxyapatite that will be detected with RNBI. Uptake associated with significant necrosis requiring debridement is usually more intense than uptake associated with mild damage, that the body will repair itself.[1,23] In frostbite, when tissue damage is often more global, the demarcation between viable and nonviable bone can be made easily on the delayed images, on which absent bone activity reflects a lack of even microcirculation.[1,23]

VENTILATION AND PERFUSION LUNG IMAGING

The emergence of fast and ultrafast CT imaging for the diagnosis of pulmonary embolism (PE) has not diminished the value of V/Q lung scanning to diagnose significant PE in the acute and subacute posttrauma setting. These especially included situations that preclude the injection of contrast, when the patient's condition precludes imaging in the CT scanner or when knowing the physiologic significance of an anatomic lesion is required. As this chapter is being written, advances in nuclear imaging with pulmonary SPECT are being investigated to increase both sensitivity and specificity; advances in CT imaging are occurring, also. Given this circumstance, it is anticipated that clinical algorithms will almost certainly undergo modification in the interval until publication.

Technique

Adjustments in well-established techniques for V/Q scanning[32,33] are often necessary when the patient is receiving ventilator assistance or is otherwise compromised. The timing and control of xenon gas delivery often requires assistance of respiratory therapy personnel. Specific care must be made during ^{99m}Tc-MAA (macroaggregated albumin) injection, especially with limited intravenous access.

Interpretation Criteria

Preliminary radiographs or CT scans are reviewed to determine if a lesion, such as pneumonia, pneumothorax, effusion, atelectasis, or rib fracture(s), is present that might satisfactorily explain the patient's signs or symptoms. Otherwise a V/Q scan can be done no matter how abnormal the lung fields appear. A normal perfusion study finding excludes PE. When there are parenchymal abnormalities present on CT or radiograph, the Prospective Investigation of Pulmonary Embolism Diagnosis (PIOPED) criteria for V/Q analysis do not hold, and any perfusion abnormality must be compared with the radiographic abnormality. Criteria are based on multiprojection planar images. Perfusion abnormalities smaller than the radiographic lesions reflect a low probability of PE, while perfusion abnormalities much larger than the radiographic abnormality reflect a high probability for PE (Fig. 13-14). It is logical to assume that, in

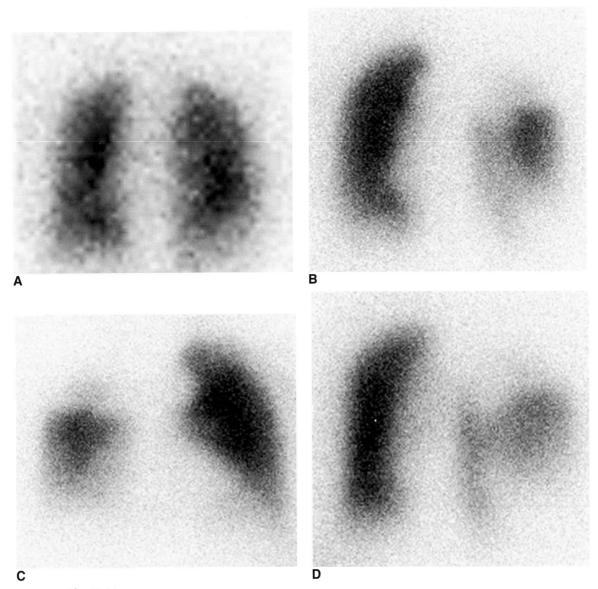

Fig. 13-14
Pulmonary emboli, high probability ventilation and perfusion lung scan. **A,** Ventilation scan. Equilibrium, posterior view. Normal distribution of xenon containing air. Slight right base decrease is secondary to diaphragm elevation. Perfusion scans in posterior (**B**), anterior (**C**), and (**D**). Right posterior oblique projections. Large segmental defects in upper and lower lobes.

the future, SPECT images will aid in defining segmental perfusion defects and increase the specificity in the intermediate group of patients with perfusion defects similar in size to the anatomic abnormalities. In the author's institution the fat embolism syndrome, which can manifest with confusion, hypoxia, and petechia, is extremely rare; the author has not encountered lung scans demonstrating subsegmental, segmental, or larger defects associated with this entity.

INFECTION IMAGING

Whole body infection imaging with indium-111 (^{111}In) or ^{99m}Tc-labeled white blood cells (WBCs) or gallium-67 (^{67}Ga) is performed not uncommonly in the multiple trauma or critical care patient for fever of unknown origin. Suspected focal sources of infection, such as abnormal fluid collections found on CT and not amenable to percutaneous drainage, a wound or scar, a dialysis graft, an intravenous access line or drain, or a healing fracture, are evaluated, also. Even in those circumstances, WBC imaging is performed to detect any unsuspected source for fever.

Technique

Each of the three available radiotracers has slightly different imaging protocols. ^{67}Ga, which has the advantage of not requiring blood handling for WBC labeling, is imaged at 4 to 6 hours and 24 to 48 hours after injection. ^{99m}Tc-WBCs are imaged at 30 minutes and 2 hours after injection (Figs. 13-15 and 13-16) and ^{111}In-WBCs 3 hours and 24 hours after injection (Fig. 13-17). The imaging characteristics of the ^{99m}Tc-WBCs provide the most pleasing images and, because there is no significant bowel excretion, is favored by many when an abdominal lesion is suspected.[34]

SPECT imaging always should be considered when ^{99m}Tc-WBCs or ^{67}Ga is used. For infection imaging, in particular, anatomic localization of lesions can be made by visually comparing or by registering or fusing the cross-sectional SPECT image sequence with CT or MR images, using software techniques which are available on most nuclear medicine computer systems. Also, there are several combined CT and SPECT units on the market for simultaneous acquisition of the CT and SPECT study, with absolute co-registration and fusion possible. Periorgan collections can be localized, also, using subsequent injections of ^{99m}Tc–sulfur colloid to delineate the liver and spleen, ^{99m}Tc-DMSA (dimercaptosuccinic acid) or ^{99m}Tc-GHA (glucoheptonate) to delineate the kidneys, and ^{99m}Tc-pertechnetate for outlining the stomach.

Interpretation Criteria

Abnormal foci of uptake must be separated from normal collections secondary to physiologic accumulation or excretion of the tracer. For example, labeled WBCs normally accumulate in the liver, spleen, and cardiac blood

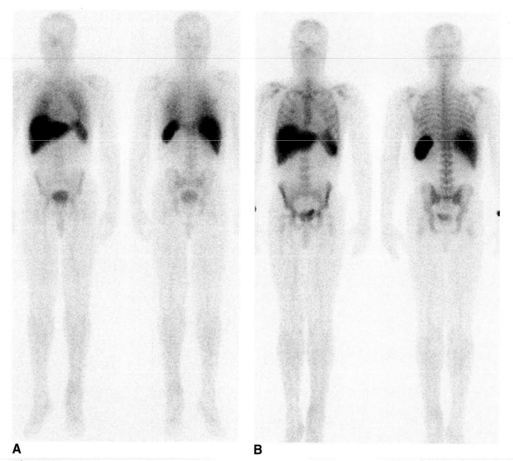

A　　　　　　　　　　　　　　**B**

Fig. 13-15
Normal ^{99m}Tc-white blood cell whole body scans. Anterior (*left*) and posterior (*right*). **A,** Taken 30 minutes after injection. Minimal lung activity, marked liver and spleen activity, some bladder and minimal marrow uptake. **B,** Taken 3 hours after injection. Liver, spleen, and bone marrow, and minimal bladder activity are normal. Injection site infiltration at right wrist.

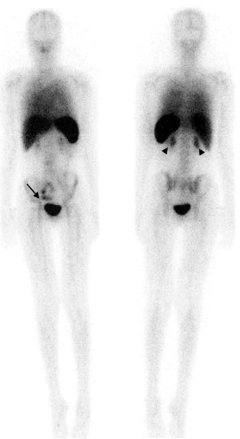

Fig. 13-16
Pelvic infection site, ^{99m}Tc-white blood cell whole body scans. Anterior (*left*) and posterior (*right*). Abnormal tracer in anterior right lower pelvis (*arrow*), projected above the bladder, was localized to distal small bowel on other views. Bilateral renal pelvic tracer is seen best on posterior views (*arrowheads*).

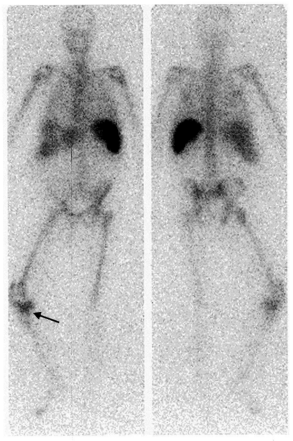

Fig. 13-17
Infection right knee. ^{111}In-white blood cell whole body scan 24 hours after injection. Asymmetric tracer accumulation (*arrow*).

pool (see Figs. 13-15 to 13-17), while ^{67}Ga can be seen in the liver, minimally in bone marrow, during the first 24 hours in the kidneys, and later in the bowel. Comparing the early and late images can be useful to help define normal activity.

OTHER INDICATIONS FOR RADIONUCLIDE IMAGING

Because nuclear medicine represents physiologic imaging, many questions can be answered using these techniques. The traumatologist, trauma radiologist, and clinical intensivist can utilize nuclear medicine as a problem-solving tool by communicating the need to the nuclear medicine physician or nuclear radiologist. The references at the end of this chapter have suggestions for further reading for many of the less common uses not covered in the chapter.

REFERENCES

1. Holder LE, Kelty NL, Tehan AM: Physiologic imaging in trauma care. In Freeman LM, ed: *Nuclear medicine annual 1996*, Philadelphia, 1996, Lippincott-Raven.
2. Wagner HN, Szabo Z, Buchanan J: *Principles of nuclear medicine*, ed 2, Philadelphia, 1995, WB Saunders.
3. Henkin RE, Boles MA, Dillehay GL, et al: *Nuclear medicine*, St Louis, 1996, CV Mosby.
4. Sandler MP, Coleman RE, Wacker FJT, et al: *Diagnostic nuclear medicine*, ed 3, Baltimore, 1996, Williams & Wilkins.
5. McKusick KA: The diagnosis of traumatic cerebrospinal fluid rhinorrhea, *J Nucl Med* 18:1234, 1977.
6. Holness R, Waxman K: Diagnosis of traumatic cardiac contusion utilizing single photon emission computed tomography, *Crit Care Med* 18:1, 1990.
7. Taillefer R, Therasse E, Turpin S, et al: Comparison of early and delayed scintigraphy with ^{99m}Tc-apcitide and correlation with contrast-enhanced venography in detection of acute deep vein thrombosis, *J Nucl Med* 40:2029, 1999.
8. Hellman RS, Collier BD: Single photon emission computed tomography: a clinical experience. In Freeman LM, ed: *Nuclear medicine annual 1987*, Philadelphia, 1987, Raven Press.
9. Ichise M, Chung DG, Wang P, et al: Technetium-99m-HMPAO SPECT, CT and MRI in the evaluation of patients with chronic traumatic brain injury: a correlation with neuropsychological performance, *J Nucl Med* 35:217, 1994.

10. Medical Consultants: Guidelines for the determination of death, *JAMA* 246:2184, 1981.
11. Lee VW, Hauck RM, Morrison MC, et al: Scintigraphic evaluation of brain death: significance of sagittal sinus visualization, *J Nucl Med* 28:1279, 1987.
12. Gartman DM, Zeman RK, Cahow CE, et al: The value of hepatobiliary scanning in complex trauma, *Radiology* 151:771, 1985.
13. Loberg M, Cooper M, Harvey E, et al: Development of new radiopharmaceuticals based on N-substitution of iminodiacetic acid, *J Nucl Med* 17:633, 1976.
14. Eikman EA, Cameron JL, Colman M, et al: A test for patency of the cystic duct in acute cholecystitis, *Ann Intern Med* 82:318, 1975.
15. Kim CK, Goyal M, San Pedro E, et al: The effect of CCK pretreatment on gallbladder visualization on delayed or morphine-augmented imaging (abst), *J Nucl Med* 36:74P, 1995.
16. Fink-Bennett D, Balon H, Robbins T, et al: Morphine-augmented cholescintigraphy: its efficacy in detecting acute cholecystitis, *J Nucl Med* 32:1231, 1991.
17. Freeman LM, Sugarman LA, Weissman HS: Role of cholecystokinetic agents in ^{99m}Tc-IDA cholescintigraphy, *Semin Nucl Med* 11:186, 1981.
18. Fig LM, Wahl RL, Stewart RE, et al: Morphine-augmented hepatobiliary scintigraphy in the severely ill: caution is in order, *Radiology* 175:467, 1990.
19. Chen CC, Holder LE, Maunoury C, et al: Morphine augmentation increases gallbladder visualization in patients pretreated with cholecystokinin, *J Nucl Med* 38:644, 1997.
20. Maurer AH: Cine scintigraphy of gastrointestinal bleeding, *Radiology* 187:877, 1993.
21. Passarell S, Holder LE, Hastings G: Life threatening hemorrhage of an unsuspected superficial circumflex iliac artery origin imaged with technetium-99m-labeled erythrocytes, *Clin Nucl Med* 25:427, 2000.
22. Holder LE: Radionuclide imaging in the evaluation of acute gastrointestinal bleeding, *Radiographics* 20:1153, 2000.
23. Holder LE, Fogelman I, Collier DC: *Atlas of planar and SPECT bone imaging,* ed 2, London, 2000, Martin Dunitz.
24. Fournier RS Holder LE: Reflex sympathetic dystrophy: diagnostic controversies, *Semin Nucl Med* 28:116, 1998.
25. Sarikaya I, Sarikaya A, Holder LE: The role of bone SPECT imaging, *Semin Nucl Med* 31:3, 2001.
26. Holder LE, Schwarz C, Wernicke PG, et al: Radionuclide bone imaging in the early detection of fractures of the proximal femur (hip): multifactorial analysis, *Radiology* 174:509, 1990.
27. MacKinnon SE, Holder LE: The use of three phase radionuclide bone scanning in the diagnosis of reflex sympathetic dystrophy, *J Hand Surg [Am]* 9:556, 1984.
28. Holder LE, MacKinnon SE: Reflex sympathetic dystrophy in the hand: strict clinical and scintigraphic criteria, *Radiology* 152:517, 1984.
29. Holder LE, Cole LA, Myerson M: Reflex sympathetic dystrophy in the foot: clinical and scintigraphic criteria, *Radiology* 184:531, 1992.
30. Intenzo, C, Kim S, Millin J, et al: Scintigraphic patterns of the reflex sympathetic dystrophy syndrome of the lower extremities, *Clin Nucl Med* 14:657, 1989.
31. Driessens M: Infrequent presentations of reflex sympathetic dystrophy and pseudodystrophy, *Hand Clin* 13:413, 1997.
32. The PIOPED investigators: Value of ventilation/perfusion scan in acute pulmonary embolism—results of the prospective investigation of pulmonary embolism diagnosis (PIOPED), *JAMA* 263:2753, 1990.
33. Alderson PO, Biello DR, Sacchariah KG, et al: Scintigraphic detection of pulmonary embolism in patients with obstructive lung disease, *Radiology* 138:661, 1981.
34. Datz FL: Abdominal abscess detection: gallium, ^{111}In-, and ^{99m}Tc-labeled leukocytes, and polyclonal and monoclonal antibodies, *Nucl Med Appl Trauma Crit Care Imaging.*

14 Special Considerations in the Pediatric Trauma Patient

Carlos J. Sivit

Prompt and accurate imaging diagnosis is essential in the initial evaluation of injured children. The imaging assessment of children after blunt and penetrating trauma provides valuable diagnostic information for the detection of thoracic, abdominal, pelvic, cranial, spinal, and skeletal injury. The radiologist plays a key role in the trauma team, delivering rapid and precise diagnoses. This chapter provides an overview of imaging in the acutely injured pediatric patient, emphasizing differences in injury type and appearance between children and adults.

THORACIC INJURY

The imaging evaluation of the thorax in children after blunt or penetrating trauma is a central feature of their acute assessment and management, because a reliable early clinical diagnosis of thoracic injury is often difficult. Chest radiography remains the primary method for the initial evaluation of thoracic injury. Computed tomography (CT) also plays an important role in the assessment of thoracic injury, because it often demonstrates abnormalities that are missed or underestimated with radiography.

Several important differences differentiate children from adults with thoracic injury. One important anatomic difference relates to the increased pliability of bony and cartilaginous structures in children. This results in bony injury, including rib fractures, occurring uncommonly even after significant thoracic injury. Another anatomic difference is the enhanced elasticity of great vessels of children, that results in aortic and great vessel injury occurring less frequently than in adults, even after severe injury.

An important physiologic difference in children when compared with adults is the smaller size of pulmonary blood vessels and the enhanced vasoconstrictive response in the pediatric population. Thus, bleeding stops spontaneously more frequently after injury in children than in adults. Conversely, children have a smaller circulating blood volume, resulting in greater physiologic derangement with a given amount of blood loss than would be seen in adults.

Technical Considerations

Imaging considerations that should be taken into account when evaluating the pediatric thorax with CT relate to the smaller patient size. These include using a smaller field of view, thinner collimation, decreased milliamperes (mA), and decreased amount of intravenous contrast. Common parameters include use of 4-mm collimation in children under 6 years of age and 8-mm collimation in children 6 years of age and older. Because the mA is the primary determinant of radiation dosage, it should be kept as low as possible. An mA of 65 in children under the age of 6 years, an mA of 100 in children 6 to 12 years of age, and an mA of 150 in children over 12 years of age are usual exposure settings. The intravenous contrast dosage should be based on patient weight, typically 2 ml/kg with a maximum of 120 ml.

Imaging Modalities

Chest radiography remains the primary screening modality for the evaluation of thoracic injury. Chest radiography is used to identify life-threatening injury (Fig. 14-1),

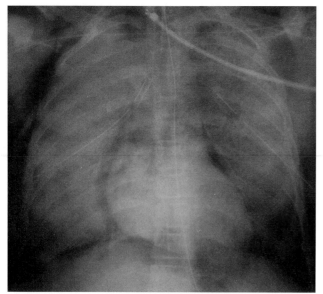

Fig. 14-1
Multifocal pulmonary contusion and pneumopericardium. Anteroposterior chest radiograph obtained in the resuscitation room demonstrates diffuse parenchymal air space disease indicative of multifocal pulmonary contusion and pneumopericardium.

to assess gas-exchange capability of the lungs and to localize tubes and catheters. Chest radiography in these patients typically is limited by patient positioning and by numerous external monitoring and support devices. An important limitation of chest radiography in injured children is that it lacks sensitivity for pleural and parenchymal injury, missing or underestimating over one third of such injuries[1,2] (Fig. 14-2). Additionally, radiography lacks specificity for mediastinal injury and provides imprecise localization of thoracostomy tubes.

CT provides improved detection and quantification of pleural, parenchymal, mediastinal, and chest wall injury.[1,2] It has greater specificity for the detection of mediastinal hemorrhage than chest radiography, and it provides more precise localization of thoracostomy tubes. Important limitations of CT are that it lacks specificity for esophageal, tracheal, and main bronchial injury. Additionally, it lacks sensitivity for cardiac injury.

Chest wall injury in children is uncommon. The bony and cartilaginous structures in children are relatively elastic and compliant. Therefore, significant pleural, parenchymal, and mediastinal injury often occurs without associated bony injury.[1,2] Because it takes a relatively large amount of force to produce a rib fracture, multiple fractures result from a great deal of kinetic energy associated with severe injury and with increased morbidity and mortality.[3] Displaced rib fractures occasionally may result in thoracic or abdominal injury. In infants, rib fractures have a high specificity for child abuse. The rib fractures in abused infants often are located posteriorly and may be difficult to identify in the acute setting.

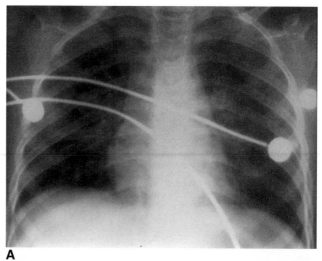

A

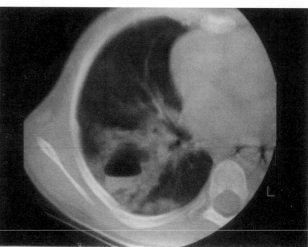

B

Fig. 14-2
Pulmonary laceration not visualized by chest radiography. **A**, Anteroposterior chest radiograph does not demonstrate any abnormalities. **B**, CT scan through the midthorax in same child shows a pulmonary laceration with surrounding parenchymal contusion.

Pulmonary Parenchymal Injury

Pulmonary parenchymal injury after blunt trauma results from a variety of mechanisms including (1) direct compression, (2) contrecoup compression, (3) shearing forces, or (4) laceration by fractured ribs.[4] Parenchymal injury previously was characterized as either pulmonary contusion or pulmonary laceration. It now is recognized that these entities represent a spectrum of injury, and parenchymal contusion and laceration commonly coexist.

Pulmonary contusion, which is characterized by areas of alveolar and interstitial hemorrhage and edema, appears on imaging as areas of ill-defined opacities that do not follow anatomic boundaries (Fig. 14-3). It results in disruption of the alveolar-capillary interface.

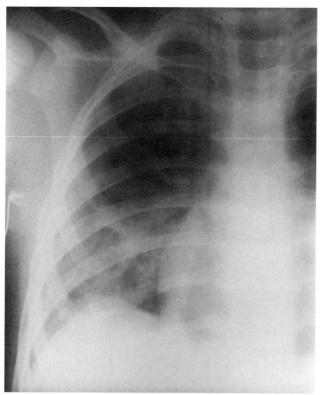

Fig. 14-3
Pulmonary contusion. Anteroposterior view of the right hemithorax demonstrates a focal area of ill-defined parenchymal opacity in the right middle and lower lung zones indicative of parenchymal contusion.

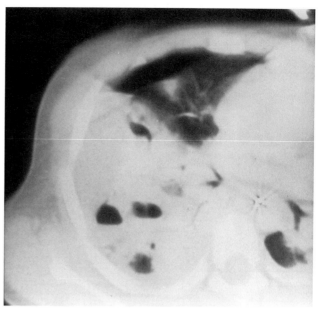

Fig. 14-4
Pulmonary laceration. CT scan through the lower thorax demonstrates multiple small air cavities in the right lung indicative of pulmonary laceration. Also note extensive parenchymal consolidation due to contusion, as well as associated hemopneumothorax.

Secondary edema is reported to peak at 24 to 36 hours after the injury.[5] Therefore, the radiographic appearance of the lungs may worsen over the first several days.

Pulmonary laceration is characterized by torn alveoli or bronchioles.[4] Imaging examination reveals parenchymal air cavities (see Fig. 14-2). The cavities may be small, partially filled with blood, or surrounded by adjacent parenchymal hemorrhage (Fig. 14-4). They may be difficult to visualize with chest radiography. Multifocal pulmonary contusion or laceration leads to extensive ventilation-perfusion mismatches and can result in respiratory failure.

Pneumothorax and Pneumomediastinum

Pneumothorax and pneumomediastinum most commonly occur following alveolar or small airway rupture. Less commonly, they may result from tears of the trachea, large bronchi, or esophagus. After small airway rupture, air dissects medially along peribronchial tissues toward the mediastinum or pleural space. If the air dissection is extensive, it produces a tension pneumothorax that can be life threatening. Because the mediastinum is flexible and mobile, increased air pressure shifts the mediastinum

away, compressing contralateral lung and twisting the great vessels. If the condition is not corrected emergently, venous return to the heart is decreased and shock may ensue. Even small pleural air collections can continue to accumulate and become life threatening, particularly among patients receiving mechanical ventilation.

Radiographic findings associated with pneumothorax include hyperlucency in the lower chest or along the cardiac border, depression of the ipsilateral diaphragm, or deepening of the lateral costophrenic sulcus (Fig. 14-5). The size of pneumothoraces often is missed or underestimated with supine chest radiography. CT is useful in the early detection of pleural and mediastinal air collections that may be missed with chest radiography.[1,2]

Thoracic air leak due to tracheal or main bronchial injury is rare in children. Imaging findings associated with such injury in addition to the air leak include subcutaneous air in the neck, discontinuity of the tracheal wall, abnormal endotracheal tube position, or the "fallen lung" sign, which is defined as *collapse of the involved lung away from the hilum.*[6]

Mediastinal Injury

Esophageal injury is also rare in children and typically is associated with major compressive injury. Common imaging findings include mediastinal air, mediastinal hemorrhage, and hemothorax. However, these findings are nonspecific. Therefore, patients with suspected esophageal injury should undergo esophagoscopy or an esophagram. The esophagram will demonstrate soft tissue extravasation of administered contrast (Fig. 14-6). CT is useful for monitoring for complications such as mediastinitis and abscess formation.

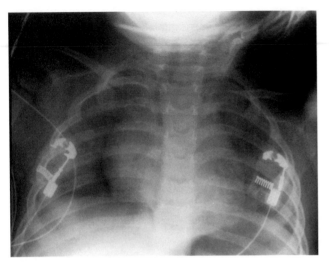

Fig. 14-5
Right-sided pneumothorax. Anteroposterior chest radiograph demonstrates an area of hyperlucency lateral to the right cardiac border indicative of a pneumothorax.

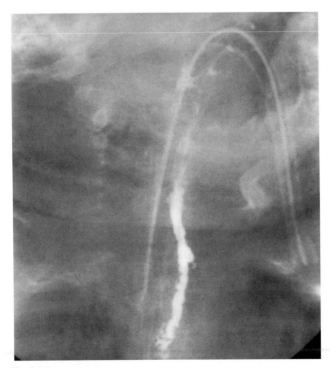

Fig. 14-6
Esophageal rupture. Spot film of the neck after administration of contrast into the upper esophagus demonstrates contrast extravasation into the soft tissues of the neck diagnostic of esophageal rupture.

Hemothorax

Hemothorax typically results from injury to low-pressure pulmonary veins or to larger, central pulmonary vessels. The former typically stops spontaneously or is managed successfully with tube thoracostomy. The latter can compress lung, interfere with gas exchange, and twist great vessels (Fig. 14-7). Additionally, hemothorax is the leading thoracic cause of shock after trauma.[7] Thus, hemothorax can be life threatening.

On supine chest radiographs, pleural fluid results in a generalized increased opacity over the involved hemithorax. Blunting of the costophrenic angle or elevation of a hemidiaphragm may be seen on semierect radiographs. CT is useful in the identification and quantification of small-to-moderate-sized hemothoraces that may be missed by chest radiography.[1,2]

Diaphragm Injury

Diaphragm rupture is another rare injury in children. The pathognomonic finding with chest radiography is intrathoracic bowel loops. Another highly suggestive finding is an elevated hemidiaphragm (Fig. 14-8). An early diagnosis may be difficult, because initial radiographs are normal or show nonspecific findings in nearly one half of patients.

Aorta and Great Vessels

Aortic and great vessel injury is rare in children, owing to the relatively greater elasticity of the great vessels when compared with those in adults. Chest radiography lacks specificity for the detection of mediastinal hemorrhage. If the mediastinal contour appears abnormal on a supine

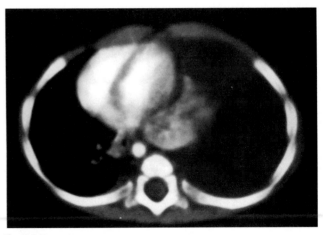

Fig. 14-7
Large hemothorax. CT scan through the midthorax demonstrates a large left-sided hemothorax. Note the left lung compression and mediastinal shift across the midline.

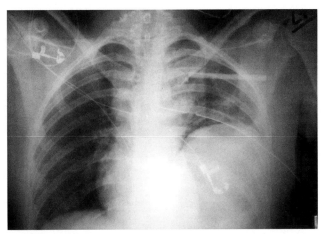

Fig. 14-8
Diaphragmatic rupture. Anteroposterior chest radiograph demonstrates abnormal elevation of the left hemidiaphragm secondary to diaphragm rupture.

chest radiograph, a repeat examination in a recumbent position should be obtained. Persistent mediastinal widening at radiography is an indication for CT or arteriography.

In summary, evaluation of thoracic injury in children requires a systematic diagnostic approach. Imaging plays a critical role in the evaluation. Awareness of important anatomic and physiologic differences between children and adults is important in the imaging evaluation of thoracic injury. Early and accurate diagnosis is imperative to facilitate expeditious management.

ABDOMINAL AND PELVIC INJURY

CT is the imaging modality of choice in the evaluation of abdominal and pelvic injury after trauma in hemodynamically stable children. Most injuries occur after blunt trauma. Penetrating injury is rare in childhood. Evaluation with CT allows for accurate detection and quantification of injury to solid and hollow viscera. CT also identifies and quantifies associated intraperitoneal and extraperitoneal fluid or blood. Additionally, CT demonstrates skeletal injury to the ribs, lumbar spine, and bony pelvis.

An important difference between children and adults with abdominal injury relates to the smaller size of blood vessels and enhanced vasoconstrictive response in the pediatric population. Therefore, bleeding in injured solid viscera usually stops spontaneously, even with severe injury. Consequently, most solid viscus injury in children can be managed successfully without surgery.

Technique

Various imaging considerations should be considered when imaging the pediatric abdomen with CT in order to

minimize the examination time and maximize the diagnostic information obtained. Monitoring devices and metallic leads should be removed from the scanning plane, because they will cause artifacts. Gastric distension should be relieved, because that also may cause streak artifacts. Important differences in the CT technique between children and adults were discussed in the section on thoracic injury. The only difference in imaging the abdomen relative to what was described for the chest is the use of a slightly higher mA. An mA of 100 is used in children under the age of 6 years, 125 in children 6 to 12 years of age, and an mA of 175 in children over 12 years.

Solid Organ Injury

Solid viscus abnormalities seen with CT include contusion, laceration, hematoma, or infarction. A contusion is a region of delayed contrast enhancement that may be focal or diffuse (Fig. 14-9) and rapidly resolves, demonstrated by follow-up imaging. A laceration is a parenchymal tear (Fig. 14-10) and may be simple or complex. A hematoma shown by CT appears as a focal lesion that does not enhance. It may be intraparenchymal, subcapsular, or adjacent to injured viscus (sentinel clot) (Fig. 14-11).[8] Variations in the appearance of the hematoma relate to the time since injury and density of surrounding tissues. An infarct is recognized as parenchymal nonenhancement resulting from major vascular injury (Fig. 14-12).

The liver is the most frequently injured viscus. Most injury occurs in the posterior segment of the right lobe.[9] The effects of trauma are enhanced in this location owing to fixation of the posterior right lobe by the coronary

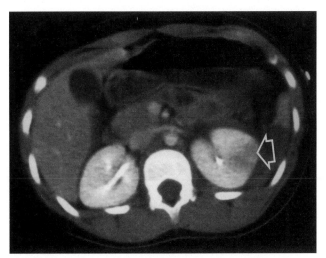

Fig. 14-9
Renal contusion. Contrast-enhanced CT scan through the midabdomen demonstrates focally decreased enhancement in the left kidney (*arrow*) indicative of renal contusion.

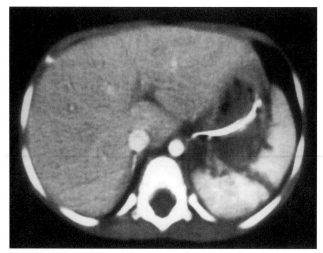

Fig. 14-10
Splenic laceration. Contrast-enhanced CT scan through the upper abdomen demonstrates a linear low-attenuation defect through the spleen representing a laceration.

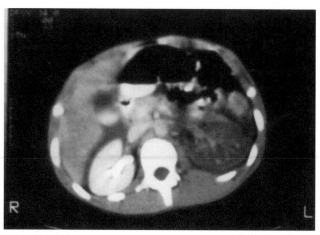

Fig. 14-12
Devascularizing injury of the left kidney. Contrast-enhanced CT scan through the midabdomen demonstrates nonenhancement of the left kidney indicating devascularizing injury.

ligament. Intraperitoneal hemorrhage may not be present if the injury does not extend to the surface of the liver, if the hepatic capsule is not disrupted, or if there is extension to the bare area of the liver, which is devoid of peritoneal reflections (Fig. 14-13).[10] Hemoperitoneum is absent in over one third of children with hepatic injury.[11]

Injury extending to the bare area of the liver may lead to associated retroperitoneal hemorrhage, with blood often surrounding the adrenal gland or extending into the anterior pararenal space.

Most hepatic injury, including parenchymal lacerations and hematomas, resolve without complications over weeks to months. Operative management rarely is required for hepatic injury in the pediatric population,

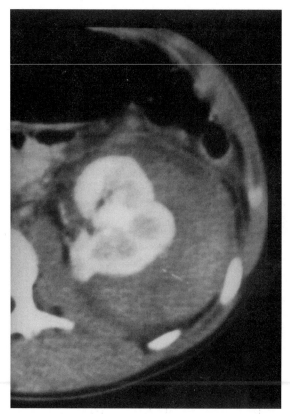

Fig. 14-11
Perinephric hematoma. Contrast-enhanced CT scan through the midabdomen shows a large perinephric hematoma.

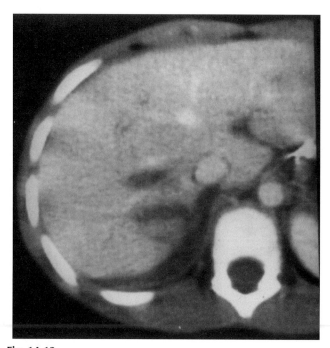

Fig. 14-13
Hepatic injury through the bare area. Contrast-enhanced CT scan through the upper abdomen shows a hepatic laceration extending through the bare area.

even with extensive organ injury.[12] Complications of injury are rare and include infection in devitalized tissue and pseudoaneurysm formation.[13] Therefore, imaging findings rarely affect the decision for operative intervention.[12] Injury characterization with CT does play a useful role in guiding various interventions, including restriction of physical activity and determining the intensity of inpatient care.

Circumferential zones of periportal low attenuation may be seen in the liver after trauma (Fig. 14-14).[14,15] They may be focal or diffuse. The presence of periportal low attenuation on CT should not be confused with hepatic injury. The portal tracts form a natural tissue plane within the liver, along which any fluid can dissect. In the trauma setting, these zones typically result from third-space fluid losses after fluid resuscitation, resulting in distention of lymphatics along the portal triads.[14]

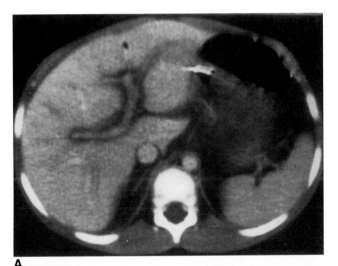

A

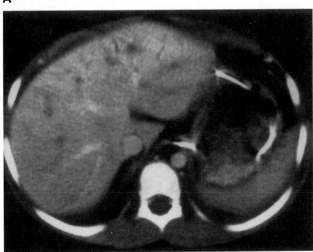

B

Fig. 14-14
Periportal low-attenuation zones. **A** and **B**, Contrast-enhanced CT scans through the upper abdomen demonstrate diffuse periportal low-attenuation zones.

When hepatic injury is coexistent, blood may also track along this region.

Splenic injury in children is also common after trauma. Because the spleen is much smaller than the liver, complex injury results in shattering or fragmentation of the organ (Fig. 14-15). As with hepatic injury, associated intraperitoneal hemorrhage is not always present.[11] Most children with splenic injury can be managed successfully without surgery as was noted with hepatic injury.[12] Pitfalls that may result in false-positive diagnosis of splenic injury include heterogeneous enhancement early during the bolus and splenic lobulations and clefts that may mimic laceration. Splenic lobulations and clefts typically have smooth contours, whereas lacerations have irregular contours.

Renal injury is common after trauma in children, although not as common as hepatic or splenic injury. Renal parenchymal injury results from direct impact of the blunt force, whereas vascular and collecting system injury typically results from deceleration. Renal parenchymal injury ranges from parenchymal contusion to complex laceration. Parenchymal contusion is the most common renal injury. Extensive renal injury is often associated with subcapsular or perinephric hematoma.

Injury extending to the renal collecting system may result in urinary extravasation of intravenous contrast medium (Fig. 14-16). Urine leakage typically remains encapsulated in the perirenal space and is referred to as a *urinoma*. Urinary extravasation may extend into the pelvis, as a result of direct communication between the perirenal space in the abdomen and the prevesical extraperitoneal space in the pelvis in some individuals. Urine leakage occasionally also may extend into the greater peritoneal cavity.

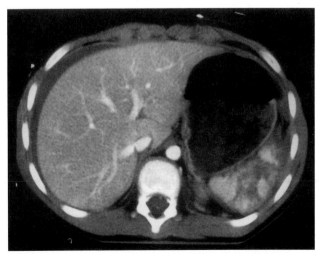

Fig. 14-15
Shattered spleen. Contrast-enhanced CT scan through the upper abdomen demonstrates a complex splenic injury with multiple fracture fragments.

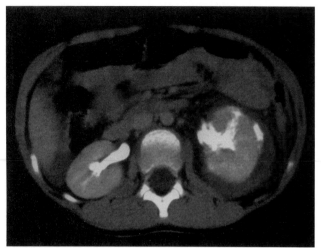

Fig. 14-16
Renal collecting system injury. Contrast-enhanced CT scan through the midabdomen shows a deep renal laceration extending into the collecting system. Note the contrast-opacified urine tracking through the laceration into the perirenal space.

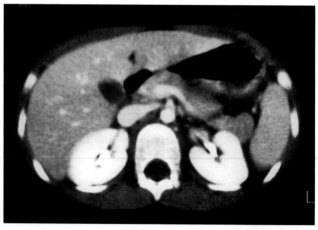

Fig. 14-17
Pancreatic laceration. Contrast-enhanced CT scan through the upper abdomen shows a linear laceration through the body of the pancreas.

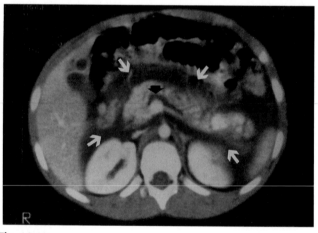

Fig. 14-18
Peripancreatic fluid associated with pancreatic injury. Contrast-enhanced CT scan through the upper abdomen in a child with pancreatic injury demonstrated intraoperatively reveals peripancreatic fluid in the anterior pararenal space (*white arrows*). Also note fluid tracking between the splenic vein and pancreas (*black arrow*).

Pancreatic injury is relatively uncommon in children. Injury to the pancreas typically results from direct compression of the organ against the vertebral column secondary to blunt-force injury. Direct signs of injury may be difficult to identify because of the small size of the gland, paucity of surrounding fat, and minimal separation of fracture fragments (Fig. 14-17). Indirect signs of injury are usually due to associated pancreatitis and include focal or diffuse gland enlargement, extraperitoneal or intraperitoneal fluid, infiltration of peripancreatic fat, and thickening of the anterior renal fascia. The best indicator of injury shown by CT is peripancreatic fluid, consisting of anterior pararenal space or lesser sac fluid (Fig. 14-18).[16,17] Such fluid may also track between the splenic vein and pancreas.[17]

Injury to the main pancreatic duct is a principal determinant in the development of significant complications after pancreatic injury. As a result, major ductal laceration is recognized as an indication for prompt surgical intervention. Peripancreatic fluid is not pathognomonic for major ductal injury. It may be seen as a result of hemorrhage with a partial thickness parenchymal injury or secondary to posttraumatic pancreatitis.

Hollow Viscus Injury

Bowel injury is uncommon after trauma in childhood. Injury can result in intramural hematoma, bowel rupture, or bowel ischemia. Most injuries are noted in children with linear, lower abdominal or flank ecchymoses, also referred to as *lap-belt ecchymoses*.[18,19]

An intramural bowel hematoma results from a partial thickness tear. The most common location for an intra-

mural hematoma is the duodenum. Large hematomas appear dumbbell shaped on CT and can result in proximal small bowel obstruction (Fig. 14-19). These injuries usually can be managed without surgery, although patients may require gastric decompression and no oral intake for a week or more, depending on the severity of intraluminal obstruction.

Bowel rupture occurs most commonly in the mid-to-distal jejunum.[20] The most specific CT findings for bowel rupture include extraluminal air, discontinuity of bowel wall, and extravasation of administered oral contrast material (Fig. 14-20). However, these findings are not seen in most cases.[20-22] Extraluminal air is present in only one third to one half of cases. Oral contrast extrava-

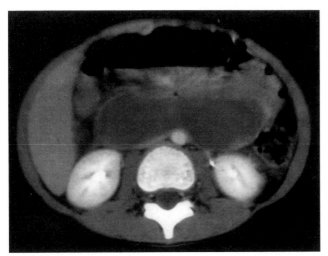

Fig. 14-19
Duodenal hematoma. Contrast-enhanced CT scan through the upper abdomen shows a large dumbbell-shaped duodenal hematoma.

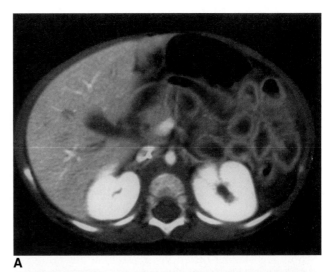

A

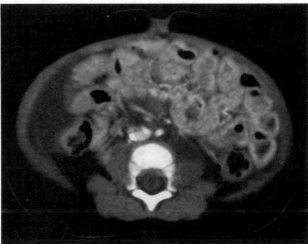

B

Fig. 14-21
Bowel rupture with "unexplained" free peritoneal fluid. CT scans through the upper (**A**) and midabdomen (**B**) in a child with jejunal rupture demonstrates free peritoneal fluid in both paracolic spaces. Also note small bowel wall thickening and abnormally intense enhancement of small bowel wall.

sation and direct evidence of bowel wall discontinuity are relatively uncommon. The most common associated CT finding has been moderate to large "unexplained" peritoneal fluid collections, defined as *peritoneal fluid in the absence of solid visceral injury or pelvic fracture* (Fig. 14-21).[20-22] Additional findings include abnormally intense bowel wall enhancement, bowel wall thickening, and bowel dilation.[20-22]

Devascularizing bowel injury often follows injury to mesenteric vessels supplying a bowel segment, resulting in bowel ischemia. Acutely, CT findings may include bowel wall thickening, bowel dilation, or peritoneal fluid. Clinical symptoms may be delayed, and patients may later experience bowel obstruction as fibrosis develops within the ischemic segment, resulting in stricture and luminal narrowing.[23]

Bladder injury is also uncommon in children. Injury may be intraperitoneal, extraperitoneal, or a combination of both. Intraperitoneal bladder rupture typically is caused by shearing of the bladder dome by a lap belt, while extraperitoneal rupture often results from laceration of the bladder base by a bony spicule associated with pelvic fracture.[24] The latter injury may be associated with injury to the posterior urethra. Distinction between intraperitoneal and extraperitoneal bladder rupture is important, because management of the two types of injury differs. Intraperitoneal rupture typically requires emergency

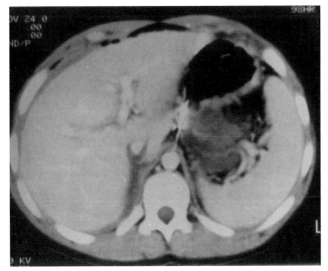

Fig. 14-20
Bowel rupture with extraluminal air. Contrast-enhanced CT scan through the upper abdomen demonstrates two small collections of peritoneal air anterior to the liver.

laparotomy owing to the increased risk for peritonitis. Conversely, extraperitoneal rupture usually can be managed successfully without surgery.

Differentiation between intraperitoneal and extraperitoneal bladder rupture is made on the basis of the location of extravasated fluid.[24] Intraperitoneal fluid in the pelvis will be located in the lateral perivesical spaces superior to the bladder and in the midline pouch of Douglas, posterior to the bladder and anterior to the rectosigmoid colon.[25] Extraperitoneal pelvic fluid will be localized in the perivesical space that surrounds the bladder and the prevesical space that extends above the bladder superiorly and anteriorly to the umbilicus and posteriorly behind the rectum.[26] CT is a highly sensitive modality for the detection of bladder rupture in children.[24] Proper attention to maximizing bladder distention is essential, including the use of a 3- to 5-minute scanning delay with CT, before imaging the pelvis to demonstrate extravasation of contrast-enhanced urine (Fig. 14-22). Additionally, if a Foley catheter is present, it should be occluded prior to intravenous contrast administration.

Active Hemorrhage and Hypoperfusion Complex

Children typically are excluded from undergoing CT if they are hemodynamically unstable. Occasionally, CT may demonstrate active hemorrhage in children who appear hemodynamically stable.[27,28] The only CT sign of active hemorrhage is the presence of focal or diffuse high-attenuation areas (>90 HU) (Fig. 14-23). The CT identification of ongoing hemorrhage depends on brisk extravasation of contrast-enhanced blood. Thus, vascular enhancement with dynamic scanning is essential. This finding is useful not only in indicating ongoing hemorrhage that is likely to require prompt surgical attention but in localizing the site of hemorrhage. The amount of hemoperitoneum noted with CT is not a measure of ongoing hemorrhage. It simply reflects the cumulative amount of bleeding that occurred between the time of injury and the time that CT was performed.

Because of advances in trauma care and the primary role of CT in the evaluation of injured children, more seriously injured children are being evaluated with CT. A characteristic hypoperfusion complex associated with hypovolemic shock may be seen in severely injured young children.[29,30] It was reported initially in children under the age of 2 years, likely due to their smaller circulating blood volume, but has since been reported in older children and adults. Most children with the hypoperfusion complex have arterial hypotension on admission.[30] This hypotension may be corrected transiently, and the children may be thought to be hemodynamically stable enough to undergo CT. However, arterial pressure can be maintained at or near normal levels after severe hemor-

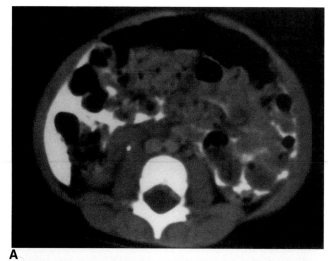

A

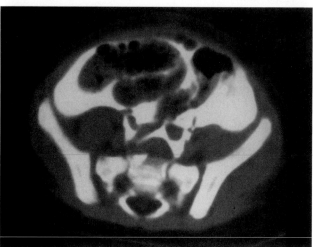

B

Fig. 14-22
Intraperitoneal bladder rupture. Contrast-enhanced CT scans through the lower abdomen (**A**) and upper pelvis (**B**) demonstrate diffuse intraperitoneal high-attenuation fluid representing extravasated contrast-enhanced urine.

rhage longer than can cardiac output. As a result, these children subsequently may develop rapid hemodynamic decompensation. The hypoperfusion complex is a marker for severe injury and a high-risk indicator for a poor outcome.[29,30] The reported mortality in children demonstrating the complex has been 85%, compared with an overall mortality rate of 2% in children with blunt trauma studied with CT.[30]

CT findings in all children with the hypoperfusion complex include diffuse intestinal dilation with fluid and abnormally intense contrast enhancement of bowel wall, mesentery, kidneys, aorta, and inferior vena cava (Fig. 14-24).[29,30] The inferior vena cava often appears flattened. Variable findings associated with systemic hypoperfusion include abnormally intense contrast enhancement of the adrenal glands, decreased splenic or

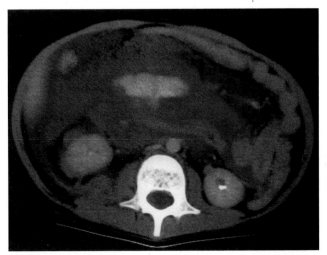

Fig. 14-23
Active hemorrhage. Contrast-enhanced CT scan through the midabdomen demonstrates an oval high-attenuation collection representing active hemorrhage from a mesenteric vessel.

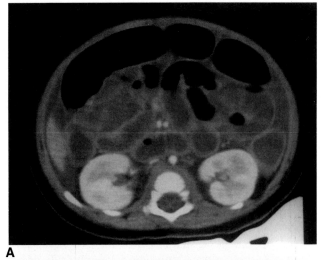

A

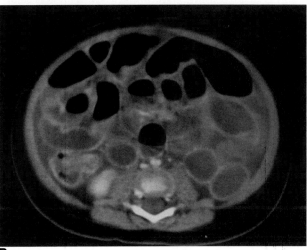

B

Fig. 14-24
Hypoperfusion complex. Contrast-enhanced CT scans through the midabdomen (**A**) and lower abdomen (**B**) show diffuse intestinal dilation with fluid, abnormally intense bowel wall enhancement, intense renal and great vessel contrast enhancement, and small-caliber great vessels including flattened inferior vena cava. This constellation of findings is seen with systemic hypoperfusion.

pancreatic enhancement, periportal low-attenuation zones, peritoneal or extraperitoneal fluid collections, and bowel wall thickening.

In summary, CT provides the primary means of evaluating abdominal and pelvic injury in children. CT imaging findings play an important role in guiding patient management. CT diagnosis and quantification of solid viscus injury assist primarily in guiding nonoperative management decisions. CT primarily impacts surgical decision making in the diagnosis of hollow viscus injury.

SKELETAL INJURY

Conventional radiography is the primary method for the initial evaluation of skeletal injury in children. CT with image reformatting in the coronal and sagittal planes plays an important role in the characterization of complex bony injury. Magnetic resonance imaging also plays a role in the evaluation of bony injury, particularly in the follow-up evaluation of growth plate injuries. There are several important differences in children relative to adults with respect to skeletal injury. First, extremity fractures occur more frequently in children than they do in adults. Second, children have increased bone flexibility; therefore, bone is more likely to bend and deform rather than break. This results in plastic bowing (Fig. 14-25), greenstick, and torus fractures. A third difference is that fractures heal more rapidly in children.[31] Therefore, radiographic evidence of fracture healing, including the initial appearance of periostitis, soft and hard callous formation, and loss of fracture definition, will be seen earlier in children. The differences in fracture healing are more pronounced in infants and young children. Periostitis and soft callous formation may be seen as

early as 7 days after injury in infants and young children. This compares with 10 to 14 days in older children and adults. Hard callous may be seen initially between 3 and 6 weeks after injury in infants and young children, compared with between 2 and 3 months in older children and adults. Another difference is that children have stronger and more active periosteum than adults. Therefore, the periosteal reaction is usually more pronounced. Finally, ligament injuries occur less commonly in children than in adults. This is because children's ligaments are relatively stronger than bone.

The weakest area in the pediatric extremity is the chondroosseous junction, or growth plate. The developing skeleton has cartilaginous growth plates and cartilaginous epiphyses. Therefore, the growth plate is relatively

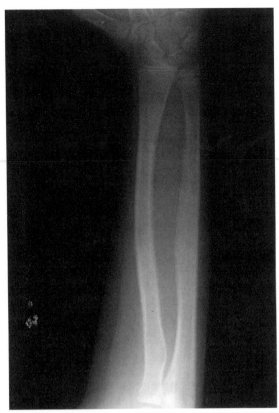

Fig. 14-25
Plastic bowing fracture. Anteroposterior view of the right forearm demonstrates bowing deformity of the radius secondary to a plastic bowing fracture.

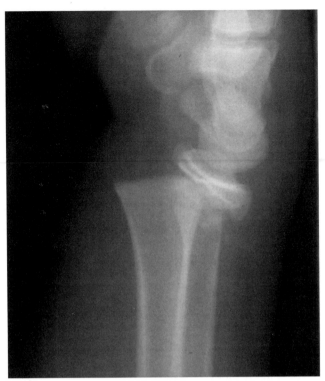

Fig. 14-26
Salter-Harris type II fracture. Lateral view of the right wrist shows a fracture extending through the metaphysis into the growth plate. Note the small metaphyseal avulsion fracture and the posteriorly displaced epiphysis.

weak when loaded with torsion or shear, leading to a high prevalence of growth plate injury in childhood. Approximately one third of skeletal injury in children involves the growth plate. The most common sites are the wrist and ankle. Growth plate injuries are classified according to the Salter-Harris classification. The proper characterization of growth plate injury is important, because management and prognosis vary with the different injury types. A Salter-Harris type I fracture extends through the growth plate without involving bone. It results in widening of the growth plate. Salter-Harris type II fractures extend through the metaphysis and growth plate (Fig. 14-26). Salter-Harris type III fractures extend through the epiphysis and growth plate. A Salter-Harris type IV fracture extends through the metaphysis, epiphysis, and growth plate. Salter-Harris type V fractures represent a crush injury to the growth plate. They are rare and are difficult to diagnose. Comparison with the contralateral extremity would show an asymmetric decrease in diameter of the growth plate at the injury site.

The growth plate is an important area because, during growth, cartilage proliferation and enchondral bone formation occur in this region. The healing process is complex for various reasons. First, a dual blood supply is present. Second, after injury, callous formation occurs concurrently with continued enchondral bone formation. Finally, there is potential for premature growth plate closure after injury, secondary to bone bridge formation through the growth plate. The diagnosis of bone bridge formation is important in children with injury to the lower extremity growth plate, because it can lead to leg length discrepancy that can be very debilitating. Bone bridge formation is best demonstrated with magnetic resonance imaging.[32] Bone bridge formation primarily is seen after Salter-Harris type IV fractures. Additional complications associated with growth plate injury include extremity deformity and avascular necrosis. The complication rate is higher for lower extremity injury than for upper extremity injury. The highest complication rate is seen with proximal femoral injuries. All proximal femoral growth plate injuries carry an unfavorable prognosis.

Child Abuse

The identification of skeletal injury plays a critical role in the diagnosis of child abuse. Although skeletal injury is rarely life threatening in these children, the skeletal system often is injured first, and such injury is central to documentation of abuse.[33] Skeletal injury associated with child abuse is seen more commonly in younger children. Based on the nature, location, and chronicity of injury, skeletal injury can be divided into three group levels of specificity for suggesting abuse. Higher specificity lesions are seen most commonly in children under the age of 1 year. They generally relate to indirect forces inflicted by shaking, pulling, twisting, or swinging. High-specificity injuries include metaphyseal lesions, posterior rib fractures, scapular fractures, spinous process fractures, and sternal fracture.[33] The metaphyseal lesions are seen most frequently in the tibia, distal femur, and proximal humerus. They have been characterized as *corner* (Fig. 14-27) or *bucket-handle* fractures based on their radiographic appearance. They are virtually pathognomonic of child abuse. Rib fractures are unusual in infants after unintentional trauma and generally require significant force. Beyond infancy, rib fractures may be seen more commonly with unintentional trauma but should still raise the possibility of abuse.

Moderate-specificity injuries should raise the suspicion of abuse but will be seen more frequently with unintentional trauma. They include fractures of different ages, epiphyseal separations, vertebral body fractures and subluxations, and complex skull fractures (Fig. 14-28).[33]

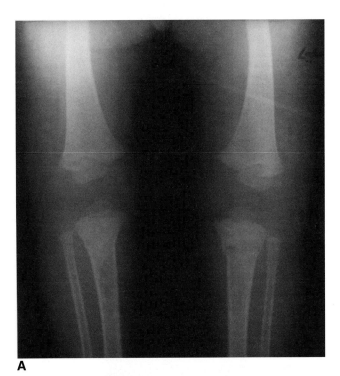

A

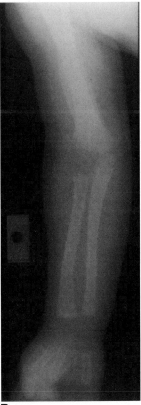

B

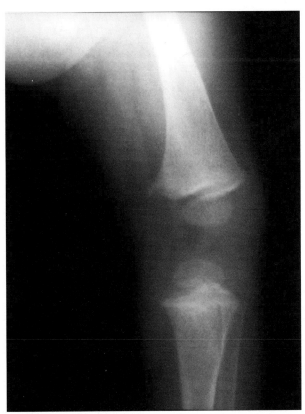

Fig. 14-27
Metaphyseal corner fracture in child abuse. Anteroposterior view through the left knee demonstrates a metaphyseal avulsion fracture off the medial aspect of the distal left femur representing a corner fracture.

Fig. 14-28
Multiple fractures of different ages in child abuse. **A**, Anteroposterior view of the lower extremities demonstrates acute fractures of both proximal tibias. **B**, Oblique view of the right upper extremity in the same child demonstrates a prior fracture of the right humerus, with associated hard callus formation.

Low-specificity injuries include clavicular fractures, long bone diaphyseal fractures, and linear skull fractures. It should be noted that the low-specificity injuries are the most frequent injuries in abused children, particularly those older than 1 year. However, the low-specificity injuries commonly are associated with unintentional trauma, and care should be taken in interpreting their significance.

In summary, children demonstrate different patterns of skeletal injury than adults. The differences in the type and pattern of injury are based on differences in the immature, developing skeletal system. Additionally, the healing process after bony injury differs from that of adults, particularly in infants and younger children. Finally, the spectrum of skeletal injury associated with child abuse often differs from injury associated with unintentional trauma, particularly in children under the age of 1 year. The type and pattern of skeletal injury play an important role in documenting potential child abuse.

REFERENCES

1. Sivit CJ, Taylor GA, Eichelberger MR: Chest injury in children with blunt abdominal trauma: evaluation with CT, *Radiology* 171:815, 1989.
2. Manson D, Babyn PS, Palder S, et al: CT of blunt chest trauma in children, *Pediatr Radiol* 23:1, 1993.
3. Garcia VF, Gotschall CS, Eichelberger MR, et al: Rib fractures in children: a marker of severe trauma, *J Trauma* 30:6975, 1990.
4. Wagner RB, Crawford WO, Schimpf PP: Classification of parenchymal injuries of the lung, *Radiology* 167:77, 1988.
5. Cohn SM: Pulmonary contusion: review of the clinical entity, *J Trauma* 42:973, 1997.
6. Unger JM, Schuchmann GG, Grossman JE, et al: Tears of the trachea and main bronchi caused by blunt trauma: radiologic findings, *AJR Am J Roentgenol* 153:1175, 1989.
7. Tocino I, Miller MH: Computed tomography in chest trauma, *J Thorac Imaging* 2:45, 1987.
8. Orwing D, Federle MP: Localized clotted blood as evidence of visceral trauma on CT: the sentinel clot sign, *AJR Am J Roentgenol* 153:747, 1989.
9. Stalker HP, Kaufman RA, Towbin R: Patterns of liver injury in childhood: CT analysis, *AJR Am J Roentgenol* 147:1199, 1986.
10. Patten RM, Spear RP, Vincent LM, et al: Traumatic laceration of the liver limited to the bare area: CT findings in 25 patients, *AJR Am J Roentgenol* 160:1019, 1993.
11. Taylor GA, Sivit CJ: Posttraumatic peritoneal fluid: is it a reliable indicator of intraabdominal injury in children? *J Pediatr Surg* 30:1644, 1995.
12. Ruess L, Sivit CJ, Eichelberger MR, et al: Blunt hepatic and splenic trauma in children: correlation of a CT severity scale with clinical outcome, *Pediatr Radiol* 25:321, 1995.
13. Basile KE, Sivit CJ, Sachs PB, et al: Hepatic arterial pseudoaneurysm: a rare complication of blunt abdominal trauma in children, *Pediatr Radiol* 29:306, 1999.
14. Patrick LE, Ball TI, Atkinson GO, et al: Pediatric blunt abdominal trauma: periportal tracking at CT, *Radiology* 183:689, 1992.
15. Sivit CJ, Taylor GA, Eichelberger MR, et al: Significance of periportal low-attenuation zones following blunt trauma in children, *Pediatr Radiol* 23:388, 1993.
16. Sivit CJ, Eichelberger MR, Taylor GA, et al: Blunt pancreatic trauma in children: CT diagnosis, *AJR Am J Roentgenol* 158:1097, 1992.
17. Sivit CJ, Eichelberger MR: CT diagnosis of pancreatic injury in children: significance of fluid separating the splenic vein and pancreas, *AJR Am J Roentgenol* 165:921, 1995.
18. Taylor GA, Eggi KD: Lap-belt injuries of the lumbar spine in children: a pitfall in CT diagnosis, *AJR Am J Roentgenol* 150:1355, 1998.
19. Sivit CJ, Taylor GA, Newman KD, et al: Safety-belt injuries in children with lap-belt ecchymosis: CT findings in 61 patients, *AJR Am J Roentgenol* 157:111, 1991.
20. Sivit CJ, Eichelberger MR, Taylor GA: CT in children with rupture of the bowel caused by blunt trauma: diagnostic efficacy and comparison with hypoperfusion complex, *AJR Am J Roentgenol* 163:1195, 1994.
21. Jamieson DH, Babyn PS, Pearl R: Imaging gastrointestinal perforation in pediatric blunt abdominal trauma, *Pediatr Radiol* 26:188, 1996.
22. Strouse PJ, Close BJ, Marshall KW, et al: CT of bowel and mesenteric trauma in children, *Radiographics* 19:1237, 1999.
23. Shalaby-Rana E, Eichelberger MR, Kerzner B, et al: Intestinal stricture due to lap-belt injury, *AJR Am J Roentgenol* 158:63, 1992.
24. Sivit CJ, Cutting JP, Eichelberger MR: CT diagnosis and localization of rupture of the bladder in children with blunt trauma: significance of contrast extravasation in the pelvis, *AJR Am J Roentgenol* 16:1243, 1995.
25. Meyers MA: Intraperitoneal spread of infections. In Meyers MA, ed: *Dynamic radiology of the abdomen: normal and pathologic anatomy*, New York, 1994, Springer-Verlag.
26. Korobkin M, Silverman PM, Quint LE: CT of the extraperitoneal space: normal anatomy and fluid collections, *AJR Am J Roentgenol* 159:933, 1992.
27. Sivit CJ, Peclet MH, Taylor GA: Life threatening intraperitoneal bleeding: demonstration with CT, *Radiology* 171:430, 1989.
28. Taylor GA, Kaufman RA, Sivit CJ: Active hemorrhage in children after thoracoabdominal trauma: clinical and CT features, *AJR Am J Roentgenol* 162:401, 1994.
29. Taylor GA, Fallat ME, Eichelberger MR: Hypovolemic shock in children: abdominal CT manifestations, *Radiology* 182:723, 1987.
30. Sivit CJ, Taylor GA, Bulas DI, et al: Post traumatic shock in children: CT findings associated with hemodynamic instability, *Radiology* 182:723, 1992.
31. Salter RB: Special features of fractures and dislocation in children. In Heppenstall RB, ed: *Fracture healing: fracture treatment and healing*, Philadelphia, 1980, WB Saunders.
32. Jaramillo D, Hoffer FA, Shapiro F, et al: MR imaging of fractures of the growth plate, *AJR Am J Roentgenol* 155:1261, 1990.
33. Kleinman PK, ed: *Diagnostic imaging of child abuse*, Philadelphia, 1998, Mosby.

15 Thoracic Imaging in the Intensive Care Unit

Charles S. White and Robert D. Pugatch

Imaging in the intensive care unit (ICU) plays a major role in the evaluation of the status of the patient with trauma and contributes significantly to recommendations for treatment. This type of imaging may be used to confirm the positioning of support tubes and lines or to identify conditions that may impede recovery.[1-3] A substantial proportion of ICU imaging of the thorax consists of bedside radiography. However, computed tomography (CT) scanning is increasingly being used to assess patients with complex disease in which the radiographic appearance is confusing. This chapter reviews these techniques and the major thoracic abnormalities encountered in the ICU.

CHEST RADIOGRAPHY

Bedside chest radiography differs from standard erect radiography in several critical respects. Standard erect radiography is generally consistent from patient to patient and among different examinations for the same patient. In contrast, bedside radiography is characterized by far greater variability in positioning and technique.

Unlike patients receiving standard upright chest radiography, the ICU patient is rarely in a truly erect position.[4] Most studies that are designated by the technologist as being erect are in fact acquired with the patient in a semierect position. In many instances, only a supine radiograph can be obtained. The lack of upright positioning has important effects on the interpretation of the study. In contrast to erect studies, air-fluid levels on semierect or supine films are usually not in tangent with the x-ray beam and thus may not be visible. Likewise, small quantities of air in the peritoneal space beneath the diaphragm may be difficult to detect (Fig. 15-1).

A second, related factor with bedside radiography is the great variability in patient position.[4] Day-to-day variations in the extent of patient rotation can have profound effects on radiographic appearance. A patient with a clear costophrenic angle on a well-centered frontal radiograph may falsely appear to have a pleural effusion on a rotated examination. Rotation may also cause a uniform increase in one hemithorax, which may be misinterpreted as pneumonia or a posteriorly layering pleural effusion.

Lordotic or reverse lordotic positioning is much more likely to occur on bedside radiography than on standard radiography. Variations in lordosis can cause a substantial alteration in radiographic appearance, which may be interpreted as reflecting true changes in pulmonary status. On lordotic projections, the anterior portions of the diaphragm are in tangent with the x-ray beam, and the interface between the heart and medial left hemidiaphragm is lost. This loss of silhouette is frequently misinterpreted as left lower lobe atelectasis or pneumonia.

Patient factors, such as body habitus or the extent of lung inspiration, may influence the appearance of the radiograph.[4] In large patients, underexposure of the radiograph may occur because of insufficient output by the portable unit or improper phototiming, leading to a light appearance of the pulmonary parenchyma, which mimics pulmonary edema. The phase of respiration during

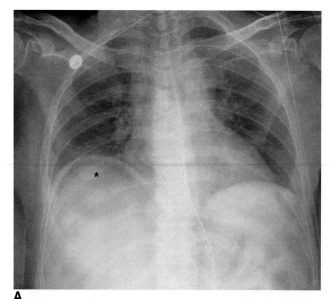

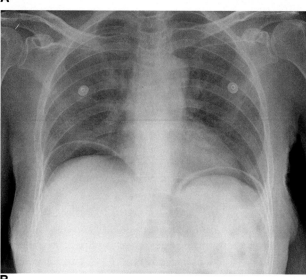

Fig. 15-1
A and **B,** A portable supine chest film shows lucency in the right upper quadrant (*asterisk*). On a repeat upright exam, the large pneumoperitoneum is easily recognized as air outlines the diaphragm. Positioning plays an important role in portable ICU radiography, and air-fluid levels and collections of air are often difficult to observe.

intrathoracic structures. The apparent heart size is particularly affected by portable radiography. In upright radiography, posteroanterior positioning is used, and the heart is located adjacent to the cassette. The requirement for anteroposterior positioning with portable radiography causes substantial magnification of the heart because of both the shorter source-to-receptor distance and the increased distance from the cassette.

Difficulties in interpretation of portable radiographs are often introduced by variability in radiographic technique.[5] Day-to-day variation in factors such as kVp, exposure timing, ventilator settings, and source-to-patient distance can cause marked change in the appearance of radiographs. It is often difficult to distinguish differences caused by technical factors from true alterations in cardiopulmonary status. Thus consistency in choosing radiographic technique is paramount.

Unlike standard upright radiography, most bedside radiography is performed without an antiscatter grid. Reasons for this include the additional weight of the grid in the portable setting and the difficulty in obtaining proper alignment at the bedside. The failure to use a grid leads to increased scatter of radiation and noise. Even if a grid is used, misalignment may cause "grid cutoff," in which the primary beam is partially blocked by the lead strips of the grid. Grid cutoff may cause increased opacity over a portion of the film, which can mimic parenchymal disease.

Digital Radiography

Digital radiography is increasingly being adopted in the ICU.[4,5] This technique employs a photostimulable phosphor plate that permits wide exposure latitude and is more forgiving of exposure errors than is film-screen radiography. Thus the need for repeat imaging is reduced, and day-to-day variation in the appearance of the radiographs is decreased. The images can be digitally archived and displayed on a workstation. With the use of a picture archiving communications system (PACS), old and new images can be quickly retrieved for interpretation on a workstation.

Digital radiography addresses many of the issues of portable radiography, but pitfalls can occur. The algorithm used to produce digital radiographs may cause edge enhancement, which in the lungs may be misinterpreted as interstitial lung disease. Although digital radiography algorithms can compensate for erroneous exposure factors, severe underexposure leads to mottling of the images. Unlike the film-screen system, in which an underexposed film appears light, a digital system adjusts the image to its standard opacity level. Thus the brightness of the image appears appropriate, but mottling occurs because the image is composed of an inappropriately low number of photons.

exposure often cannot be controlled in ICU patients because of frequent requirement for ventilatory support. Pulmonary edema may be falsely suspected if lung inflation is diminished.

Several other important deleterious effects are related to technical considerations of portable radiography.[4] In standard radiography, the source-to-image-receptor distance is typically 180 cm (72 in). In portable radiography, the distance between the source and the cassette is often less than 120 cm. The shorter distance creates greater beam divergence and increased magnification of

SUPPORT DEVICES IN THE INTENSIVE CARE UNIT

Support devices in the ICU serve a variety of purposes.[6,7] Central venous catheters (CVC) and pulmonary artery (Swan-Ganz) catheters permit access to the vascular system and allow pressure monitoring. Endotracheal tubes provide ventilatory support, and nasogastric tubes allow feeding and administration of medicines. Chest tubes facilitate drainage of air and fluid collections. More advanced devices, such as intraaortic balloon pumps, pacemaker wires, and ventricular assist devices, may occasionally be used. Imaging in the ICU helps to ensure correct placement of these devices and facilitates rapid detection of complications.

Central Venous Catheters

Central venous catheters are usually inserted from a subclavian or internal jugular vein approach. The most common complications are malposition and pneumothorax.[7] In one study, vascular perforation was responsible for 94% of fatalities due to CVC placement.[8] Ideally, a CVC should be positioned within the superior vena cava.

The CVC may be improperly placed in many venous structures, reflecting the complex mediastinal venous anatomy. A common anomalous placement of internal jugular CVCs is in the ipsilateral subclavian or axillary vein. The reverse may also occur, with positioning of a subclavian CVC in the internal jugular vein. A CVC also may be placed across the midline into the contralateral brachiocephalic or subclavian vein. Although insertion of a catheter into the right atrium previously has been reported to risk right atrial rupture, dialysis catheters are routinely placed in this location without significant reports of complications.

Unusual venous positioning does not necessarily require repositioning, particularly if the tip of the CVC is in a large vein. If accurate central venous pressure monitoring is desired, the catheter must be medial to the most central venous valves, which are typically located within the internal jugular and subclavian veins approximately 2.5 cm before their junction to form the brachiocephalic vein.

Less often, the CVC tip may be inserted into the azygos vein and small tributaries such as the left superior intercostal vein, internal mammary vein, or pericardiophrenic vein. The catheter may also be placed into anomalous venous structures. The most common such anomalous positioning is in a persistent left superior vena cava (SVC) (Fig. 15-2). More than 50% of patients with a left SVC have absence of a left brachiocephalic vein. In these patients, a catheter placed into the left subclavian or internal jugular vein is often directed into the

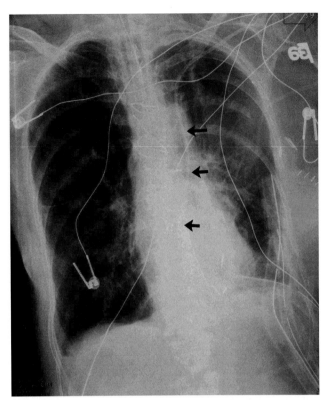

Fig. 15-2
The left subclavian catheter never crosses the anatomic midline as it descends on the left and curves medially at its termination (*arrows*). This is the typical course of a persistent left-sided vena cava. The catheter will eventually reach the right atrium by coursing through the coronary sinus.

left SVC. Occasionally, a CVC may be deflected into an anomalous pulmonary vein.

Extravenous malposition may occasionally occur, with placement of the catheter into an artery or in an extravascular location (Fig. 15-3). Positioning of the CVC in the aorta may be difficult to detect on an anteroposterior radiograph but can be suspected if the catheter overlies the aortic shadow and is clearly outside the expected location of the major venous structures. Extravascular positioning with vascular laceration may cause formation of an extrapleural or mediastinal hematoma.

Pneumothorax accounts for 30% of complications of CVC placement and is usually recognized on the immediate postplacement film. Many pneumothoraces are small and self-limited, but larger collections may require chest tube placement for evacuation (Fig. 15-4). Catheter-related venous thrombosis occasionally complicates CVC placement but is typically associated with more chronic placement. Infection of indwelling lines occurs in as many as 10% of cases and is associated with duration of catheter placement. Rare complications of CVC insertion include knotting of the catheter or shearing of a portion of the tubing, injury to nerves or the thoracic duct, and venous air embolism.

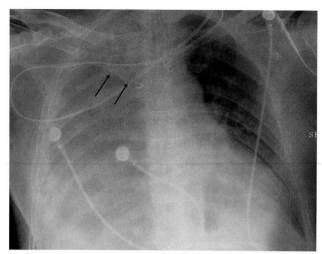

Fig. 15-3
The "right subclavian line" does not approximate the inferior aspect of the clavicle (*arrows*). The right hemithorax is opacified. The line had directly entered the right pleural space, where its contents were being infused. Knowledge of the anatomy of the central venous system should ensure appropriate identification and placement of lines and tubes on portable radiographic studies.

Pulmonary Artery Catheters

Flow-directed Swan-Ganz catheters have several ports and an inflatable balloon at the tip. Measurement

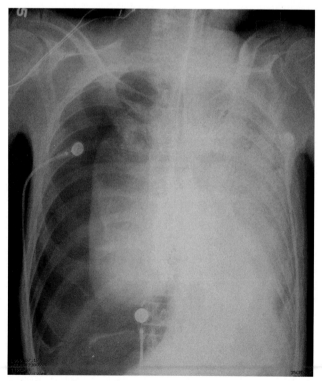

Fig. 15-4
A large right-sided tension pneumothorax shifts the heart and mediastinum to the right and depresses the right hemidiaphragm in this patient with barotrauma from positive pressure ventilation.

through a distal port with the balloon inflated and wedged allows determination of the pulmonary capillary wedge pressure, which reflects left ventricular filling pressures. Pressure tracings can also be obtained from the SVC, right atrium, right ventricle, and pulmonary artery. Cardiac output can be determined using the thermodilution technique. Thus the Swan-Ganz catheter plays an important role in assessing the hemodynamic status of critically ill patients. Intravenous fluid or medications can also be instilled using these ports.

The Swan-Ganz catheter is inserted into the internal jugular or subclavian vein or, less commonly, the femoral vein.[6] The tip should be positioned in the central pulmonary arteries. Placement within either the right main, interlobar, or left main pulmonary arteries is acceptable. If the tip is positioned too distally in the pulmonary arteries, the balloon cannot be inflated safely. Placement of the tip proximal to the pulmonary valve is suboptimal and causes inaccurate pressure measurements.

Insertion of a Swan-Ganz catheter is accompanied by the same complications that occur in CVC insertion, because a similar approach is used. However, there are several additional risks that are specific to the use of a Swan-Ganz catheter.[9] Threading of the catheter through the right atrium and ventricle may induce arrhythmias, which can sometimes be serious. Occasionally, a portion of the Swan-Ganz catheter may be coiled in the right atrium, and irritation may cause an atrial arrhythmia.

Placement of the balloon tip in a distal pulmonary artery is associated with additional complications. Occlusion of the vessel may occur, particularly if the balloon is not deflated after each wedge measurement. In one study, 9 (7.5%) of 125 patients with a Swan-Ganz catheter developed catheter-related pulmonary ischemia or infarction.[10] Inflation of the balloon in a distal vessel may lead to perforation and life-threatening pulmonary hemorrhage. Alternatively, the rupture may be contained in a pulmonary artery pseudoaneurysm, which may later rupture if not recognized (Fig. 15-5). Typically, a pseudoaneurysm manifests as a solitary nodule in an area where previously there was airspace consolidation adjacent to the tip of the Swan-Ganz catheter.[11]

Endotracheal Tubes

The position of the endotracheal tube should be checked daily in ventilated patients.[7,12] The endotracheal tube is recognized by a radiopaque marker on one side of the tube, and the inflated tracheal balloon may be seen just above the endotracheal tube tip. The tip is ideally placed approximately 5 to 7 cm above the carina (an inappropriately low placement leads to intubation of the bronchi). This positioning is also optimal because of neck movement. With flexion, the tip may advance up to 2 cm more inferiorly; neck extension may produce

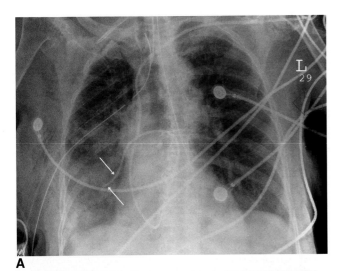

A

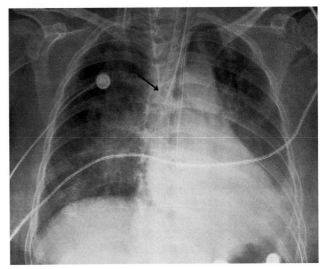

Fig. 15-6
Right main stem intubation is identified as the tip of the endotracheal tube begins to enter the right main stem bronchus (*arrow*).

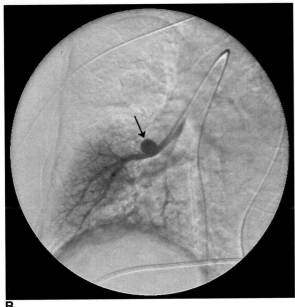

B

Fig. 15-5
A and **B**, The Swan-Ganz catheter (*arrows*) lies much too peripherally in this patient who developed hemoptysis. A selective pulmonary arteriogram identified the pulmonary artery pseudoaneurysm (*arrow*), which was successfully embolized. While this is a rare complication of Swan-Ganz line placement, peripheral locations need to be identified and corrected.

movement of 2 cm superiorly. If the tube is too high, the vocal cords may be traumatized.

On the portable chest film, the carina can be identified by tracing the left main bronchus to its junction with the right main bronchus. Most commonly, the carina is located at the level of the T6 vertebral body. The diameter of the endotracheal tube should be about two thirds that of the tracheal air column. The tracheal balloon should not significantly expand the trachea.

The most common complication of endotracheal tube placement is malposition in the bronchi.[13] The right

main bronchus is most often affected because of its straighter course relative to the trachea. Intubation of a main bronchus may cause collapse of the contralateral lung (Figs. 15-6 and 15-7). Less commonly, intubation may be associated with tracheal perforation. This complication often manifests with subcutaneous emphysema or pneumomediastinum.

An infrequent but important complication of intubation is inadvertent placement of the endotracheal tube into the esophagus.[14] Esophageal intubation may be difficult to recognize because of the frequent superimposition of the trachea over the esophagus on an anteroposterior

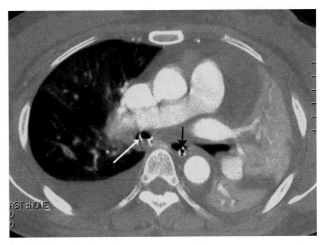

Fig. 15-7
CT clearly shows the endotracheal tube in the right main stem bronchus (*white arrow*). The left lung has collapsed. A nasogastric tube is also seen malpositioned in the left main stem bronchus (*black arrow*).

radiograph. A slightly oblique radiograph may show the tracheal air column distinct from the endotracheal tube. Other findings that suggest the diagnosis include distension of the gastric bubble and an endotracheal tip that projects below the carina but not over the main bronchi. Additional complications related to endotracheal intubation are aspiration of gastric contents, tracheoesophageal fistula, and dislodgement of teeth.

Chronic intubation may lead to tracheal stenosis or tracheomalacia. In patients who are intubated for more than 2 weeks, tracheostomy tube placement is advisable. The frontal radiograph is useful to demonstrate appropriate positioning of the tip of the tracheostomy tube over the air column.

Feeding Tubes

Nasogastric and feeding tubes should be positioned with their sidehole beyond the lower esophageal sphincter, at the level of the diaphragm.[6] The most common complication of nasogastric tube placement is malposition. Improperly inserted tubes may coil in the hypopharynx and lie entirely above the field of view of the radiograph. Another potentially serious malposition is unintentional placement of the nasogastric tube in the airway. This complication may occur even in the presence of an endotracheal tube and may lead to aspiration of tube feedings. Vigorous application of pressure in this situation may lead to perforation of the airway with pneumothorax.

Chest Tubes

Chest tubes are frequently used in the setting of trauma in the ICU to evacuate collections of pleural fluid, blood, and air. Optimal placement is in the posterior pleural space for collections of fluid and in the anterior space for collections of air. Nevertheless, because chest tubes are generally inserted without imaging guidance, there is little assurance that optimal placement will be achieved. If inadequate drainage is achieved with blind insertion, placement of a chest tube or smaller-bore pigtail catheter can be undertaken with CT or ultrasound guidance.

A properly positioned chest tube should overlie the pleural space and lung, with the sidehole medial to the inner margin of the ribs.[15] The sidehole is recognized by an interruption of the radiopaque marker that extends along the length of the chest tube. Even if the chest tube overlies the pleura on a posteroanterior radiograph, it may be located in the anterior or posterior chest wall. If the tube is properly located within the pleural space, adjacent air will outline and allow visualization of the nonradiopaque margin of the tube. If this interface is absent, chest wall placement should be suspected.

In addition to placement in the chest wall, the tube may be inadvertently positioned in the fissure or lung parenchyma or, on occasion, below the diaphragm in the upper abdomen. Intrafissural placement leads to a higher rate of nonfunctioning of the chest tube.[16] An intrafissural location may be confirmed on a lateral radiograph or CT scan. Intraparenchymal placement of a chest tube is a potentially serious complication that may cause hemorrhage or laceration of the lung or a bronchopleural fistula.

Other Support Devices

Numerous other support devices are employed in the ICU. Intraaortic balloon pumps and pacemakers are commonly used in the setting of myocardial infarction. In the trauma setting, such devices may be necessary for patients with cardiac contusions or injury to the coronary arteries.

Intraaortic balloon pumps are inserted through the groin into the proximal descending aorta. In diastole, the balloon inflates and augments coronary artery perfusion. In systole, the balloon deflates, decreasing afterload and improving peripheral perfusion. The radiopaque tip of the balloon pump should project over the proximal descending aorta, just distal to the left subclavian artery.[17] When inflated in diastole, the balloon may produce a sausage-shaped lucency over the descending aorta. Aside from cranial or cephalic malposition, complications of balloon pump insertion include pseudoaneurysm at the site of insertion, traumatic aortic dissection or rupture, and distal embolization of thrombus.

A temporary pacing wire may be required for patients with arrhythmias.[18] These wires are generally inserted through the internal jugular or subclavian vein. Occasionally, a femoral vein approach may be used. The tip of the pacemaker should ideally be placed in the apex of the right ventricle. Sharp angulation of the wire should be avoided. Complications of temporary pacemaker insertion are similar to those of a central venous catheter. In addition, the wire may be malpositioned in the coronary sinus. Myocardial perforation and lead fracture are less common complications.

ACUTE CARDIOPULMONARY DISEASE

Patients who are transferred to the intensive care unit after traumatic injury often have cardiopulmonary disorders due to the traumatic event. Pulmonary edema or contusion, pneumonia, pleural hematoma or pneumothorax, and other abnormalities are common at presentation. In addition, many patients who are initially free of cardiopulmonary disease develop complications during a prolonged hospital stay. Distinction among the different entities is often difficult on portable ICU radiographs. In general, erect and semierect positioning permits the most optimal visualization of cardiopulmonary pathology and is preferred to supine positioning.

Pulmonary Edema

Pulmonary edema may be due to cardiac failure, overhydration, or increased cardiac permeability. The distinction among types of edema can present a challenge in the ICU setting, but certain findings may be valuable.

In cardiac failure, the heart is typically enlarged, and pleural effusions are common.[19] On upright radiographs, diversion of blood flow to the upper lobes is common. On supine examinations, flow diversion to the upper lobes is physiologic, and this important finding cannot be used. Cardiogenic edema typically manifests as diffuse airspace disease with interstitial lines (Kerley lines), peribronchial cuffing, and an enlarged vascular pedicle (Fig. 15-8). The vascular pedicle measurement is the width of the mediastinum just above the aortic arch and is a reflection of circulating blood volume.[20]

Overhydration edema is usually caused by fluid overload or renal failure.[21] Overhydration edema has similar features to cardiogenic edema and may not be distinguishable radiographically. As compared with cardiogenic edema, overhydration edema features a more central distribution of edema, balanced but not upwardly diverted blood flow, and a somewhat wider vascular pedicle. Both types of edema may respond rapidly to therapy.

Increased capillary permeability edema is usually due to a noxious insult and is common in trauma patients. In this form of edema, the gas-exchanging membrane is disrupted, allowing protein-rich fluid to leak into the interstitium and ultimately into the alveoli. Patients may develop hypoxemia, lung infiltrates, and the adult respiratory distress syndrome (ARDS) (Fig. 15-9). Among patients treated in the trauma ICU, the site of the initiating insult varies and includes alveolar damage from smoke inhalation or near-drowning and toxic effects on the capillaries from such causes as sepsis or fat embolism.

The radiographic appearance of increased vascular permeability edema is usually distinct from other types of edema.[22] The heart is typically normal in size, and the vascular pedicle is not widened. Diversion of flow, bronchial cuffing, Kerley lines, and pleural effusions are uncommon. A peripheral pattern of airspace disease may occur, and air bronchograms may be evident. If substantial positive end-expiratory pressure (PEEP) is used, the radiographic appearance may demonstrate a more interstitial pattern. The onset of the airspace disease is progressive but gradual, and resolution of lung infiltrates is usually slow, often extending over several weeks.

Fat embolism is an uncommon condition that occurs 12 to 72 hours after multiple fractures are sustained.[23] Numerous fat droplets are deposited in the capillaries and lead to occlusion and chemical capillaritis. Fever, petechiae, hypoxemia, and lung infiltrates develop. The radiographic appearance is typical of ARDS, with delayed clearing of infiltrates.

Atypical patterns of pulmonary edema occur in patients with underlying lung disease. In chronic obstructive pulmonary disease, the edema may be nonuniform and display an interstitial appearance. Asymmetric edema may also manifest in association with interstitial lung fibrosis and after lung injury from radiation therapy. A pattern of predominantly right upper lobe edema has been recognized in mitral regurgitation, presumably because of the

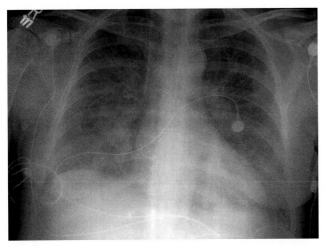

Fig. 15-8
Diffuse lung disease is a common finding on portable radiographs, and its exact cause is often difficult to determine. The presence of Kerley lines should suggest left ventricular failure with pulmonary edema.

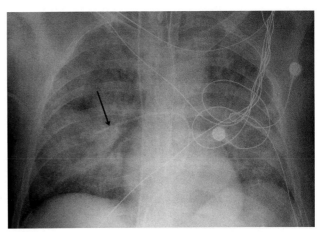

Fig. 15-9
Diffuse airspace disease with consolidation and air bronchograms is the hallmark of ARDS on a chest film. Note the peripherally situated Swan-Ganz catheter (*arrow*).

vector of the regurgitant jet.[24] Unilateral pulmonary edema may result from decubitus positioning, aspiration, or lung reexpansion after pneumothorax.[25]

Pulmonary Hemorrhage

In the setting of trauma, pulmonary hemorrhage causes lung opacification that may mimic other conditions.[26] Pulmonary contusion permits fluid and blood into the interstitium and alveoli; it manifests as an area of parenchymal consolidation similar to pneumonia. The consolidation typically occurs at presentation or shortly thereafter and resolves over the course of several days or a week. A disruption of lung architecture results in pulmonary laceration, which may take several weeks or even months to resolve. In its earliest stages, a pulmonary laceration may be obscured by associated contusion or other lung consolidation. The architectural disruption leads to formation of a cavity or hematoma that is radiographically visible. The cavity may eventually thin to form a pneumatocele. Pneumatoceles and hematomas are most often solitary and range in size from 2 to 5 cm.

Atelectasis

Atelectasis is the most common radiographic abnormality in the ICU. Multiple etiologies may work in combination to produce atelectasis. Hypoventilation due to a depressed sensorium or anesthesia, posttraumatic splinting, and obstruction due to secretions may each contribute to atelectasis.

Bandlike or subsegmental atelectasis can be found in a majority of ICU patients. Lobar atelectasis carries greater clinical significance and was reported in 8.5% of surgical ICU patients in a study by Shevland et al.[27] (Fig. 15-10). Regardless of the cause of ICU admission, the left lower lobe is the most common location of atelectasis (Fig. 15-11). In the aforementioned study, left lower lobar atelectasis accounted for 66% of cases, followed by the right lower lobe (22%) and the right upper lobe (11%). It is speculated that the left lower lobe may be more prone to compression by the heart in supine, critically ill patients.

Proper attention to radiographic technique is critical in avoiding overdiagnosis of atelectasis in the left lower lobe. Underpenetration may lead to the perception of opacity in the retrocardiac area, which may be misinterpreted as left lower lobe collapse. Zylak and others have shown that cranial beam angulation (lordotic) as small as 10% causes "pseudoconsolidation" of the left lower lobe, with loss of the diaphragmatic contour.[28]

Atelectasis can be recognized by parenchymal opacification, with associated signs of volume loss.[7] Ipsilateral shift of the mediastinum, elevation of the diaphragm, and crowding of the bronchovascular markings and ribs

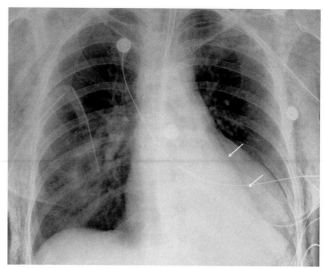

Fig. 15-10
A triangular area of density is present as the left lower lobe collapses because of retained secretions. The sharp demarcation (*arrows*) represents reorientation and visualization of the left major fissure.

are all indicative of volume loss. Atelectasis may or may not be associated with air bronchograms. The absence of air bronchograms suggests the likelihood of central obstruction from mucous plugging or other cause. Bronchoscopy may be beneficial in such patients. Conversely, the presence of air bronchograms suggests more distal obstruction or nonobstructive atelectasis and indicates that supportive therapy may be more valuable.

Atelectasis and pneumonia may be difficult or impossible to distinguish at times, particularly when localized in the left lower lobe. Atelectasis is more likely to show

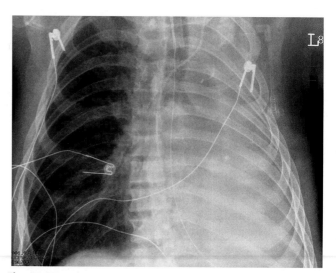

Fig. 15-11
The left hemithorax is opacified, and the heart and mediastinum are shifted to the left because of mucous plugging in the immediate postoperative period.

signs of volume loss and to exhibit rapid resolution. Pneumonia more frequently demonstrates air bronchograms or a cavitary component.

Pneumonia

Nosocomial, or hospital-acquired, pneumonia is estimated to occur in approximately 10% of ICU patients and may be fatal in one third of cases. Unlike outpatient pneumonias that are usually due to viruses, *Mycoplasma* species, or *Streptococcus pneumoniae*, nosocomial pneumonia is often caused by gram-negative or fungal organisms.

Pneumonia in the ICU patient may be difficult to diagnose. The patients are often critically ill and may not develop a fever, leukocytosis, or sputum production, which often are associated with outpatient pneumonia. Conversely, symptoms such as fever, which are usually associated with pneumonia, may be due to other causes in the ICU patient. In one study of patients who died of ARDS, only 61% of patients with pneumonia were correctly diagnosed premortem.[29]

The radiographic appearance of pneumonia is nonspecific.[30-33] Pneumonia may manifest as lobar or segmental patchy consolidation containing air bronchograms. Consolidation in the absence of volume loss, particularly in the mid- or upper lung zones, is suggestive of pneumonia. However, lower lobe pneumonia may be indistinguishable from lobar or sublobar atelectasis. Frequently, pneumonia in the ICU patient manifests as bilateral areas of consolidation containing air bronchograms that may be symmetric or asymmetric. In this situation, a distinction from pulmonary edema may not be possible.

Complications of pneumonia in the ICU patient may facilitate diagnosis.[34] Development of a cavity in an area of consolidation indicates the likelihood of a necrotic pneumonia or abscess. An air-fluid level may be visible within the cavity. An effusion may occur in association with pneumonia and may be parapneumonic. However, a loculated effusion should raise suspicion of an empyema. A loculated effusion can be distinguished from an abscess by its obtuse margins and tendency to displace lung markings away from the ribs (Fig. 15-12). An abscess usually demonstrates acute margins with the ribs. Rarely, pneumonia may be complicated by a pneumothorax from a bronchopleural fistula.

Infection may also spread to the lung hematogenously and cause septic embolism. In the ICU patient with trauma, a wound infection or indwelling catheter is often the source of infection. The radiographic appearance of septic embolism consists of multiple rounded areas of consolidation that are typically peripheral and basilar. Cavitation of some of the rounded densities is typical. Unfortunately, this characteristic picture is often difficult to appreciate on portable ICU radiographs and is more easily diagnosed on CT (Fig. 15-13). However, a

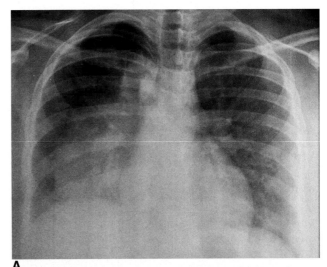

A

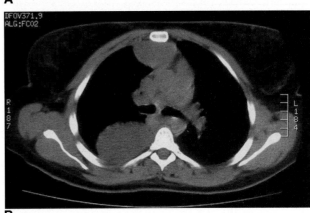

B

Fig. 15-12

A, Anteroposterior (AP) chest film shows increased density over the right hemithorax, which does not conform to lobar anatomy. The recognition of pleural fluid collections may be difficult to make on portable films, and ultrasound or CT (**B**) may be required to further define the abnormality.

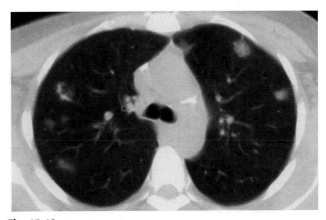

Fig. 15-13

Multiple peripheral cavitary and noncavitary nodules are present in this patient with right-sided endocarditis and staphylococcal septic emboli.

peripheral distribution of infiltrate should raise suspicion of the diagnosis.

ICU patients typically have a decreased level of consciousness and an impaired gag reflex and are prone to pulmonary aspiration of gastric contents.[35] Insertion of support tubes may further predispose the patient to aspiration. The severity of the pneumonitis that develops depends on the toxicity of the aspirated materials. Aspiration of bland substances such as blood may occur with minimal effect; aspiration of infected secretions may cause frank pneumonia; and aspiration of substances such as gastric acid or water-soluble contrast material may lead to fulminant pulmonary edema. An initial chemical pneumonitis may be complicated by superinfection.

Aspiration typically occurs into dependent parts of the lung. Thus the radiographic appearance of aspiration pneumonitis often consists of basilar infiltrates or infiltrates in the superior segments of the lower lobes. However, the appearance may be variable or mimic pulmonary edema in cases of massive aspiration.

Abnormal Air Collections

Abnormal air collections in the ICU patient may be due to direct trauma but are often caused by instrumentation. Mechanical ventilation is a common cause of pneumomediastinum and pneumothorax. Accidental traversal of the pleural space during insertion of central venous or pulmonary arterial catheters may lead to pneumothorax. Pneumomediastinum may occasionally occur after endotracheal intubation or nasogastric tube insertion.

Pneumothorax is particularly common among patients who undergo mechanical ventilation for ARDS, occurring in 4% to 17% of such patients.[36] High peak inspiratory pressures and the use of positive endexpiratory pressure contribute to the development of pneumothorax in this setting. It is postulated that alveolar rupture occurs with extension of air into the interstitium. The air dissects through the bronchovascular space peripherally to cause subpleural blebs that rupture into the pleural space. In addition to mechanical ventilation and line insertion, other causes of pneumothorax include surgical procedures of the chest or abdomen, chest tube insertion, pneumonia, and bronchopleural fistula.

The radiographic appearance of pneumothorax in the ICU patient is often distinct from that in an otherwise healthy individual who can be examined with erect radiography.[37] On an upright radiograph, a pneumothorax is recognized as a visceral pleural line accompanied by apical and lateral lucency due to pleural air. In the supine or semierect position more often encountered in the ICU patient, air collects atypically, particularly in an anteromedial or subpulmonic location. A discrete pleural edge

may not be visualized, and relative lucency may provide the only diagnostic clue to the presence of a pneumothorax. In an anteromedial pneumothorax, air outlines the heart border, and the pericardial fat pad on the affected side may become more apparent. In a subpulmonic pneumothorax, air collects in the lateral costophrenic sulcus and causes lucency in this region, a finding termed the *deep sulcus sign*. A lateral decubitus or cross-table lateral radiograph or CT scan may be valuable to confirm the diagnosis. Air from pneumothorax may occasionally collect in a posteromedial or intrafissural location.

Tension pneumothorax is a clinical diagnosis that can be suggested radiographically if the heart border is flattened, the mediastinum is shifted, or the ipsilateral diaphragm is flattened.[38,39] However, tension pneumothorax may occur in the mechanically ventilated patient in the absence of any of these findings. The poorly compliant lungs may not fully collapse in such patients. Thus a more aggressive therapeutic approach to pneumothorax is mandatory in the ICU setting.

Skin folds cause line shadows that can be particularly difficult to distinguish from a pneumothorax in the supine patient. This mimic can often be recognized by extension of the skin fold beyond the edge of the lung, as well as lack of lucency and presence of vascular structures beyond the line shadow.

Pneumomediastinum is frequently due to barotrauma from mechanical ventilation.[40] In this instance, air dissects through the interstitium toward the hilum and enters the mediastinum. Other causes include traumatic or iatrogenic rupture of the trachea or esophagus and mediastinitis. Air may also dissect into the mediastinum from the neck or retroperitoneum. Pneumomediastinum can be recognized radiographically by outlining of mediastinal structures such as the trachea as well as the great vessels and their branches. Pneumomediastinum typically extends into the neck and ultimately may progress to subcutaneous emphysema in severe cases. Mediastinal air often collects along the left heart border and may mimic a medial pneumothorax or pneumopericardium. Because the left and right sides of the mediastinum are contiguous, air may collect above the central tendon of the diaphragm, giving rise to the continuous diaphragm sign. Pneumomediastinum may be complicated by unilateral or bilateral pneumothoraces.

Dissection of air in the interstitium may be a precursor of a pneumothorax or pneumomediastinum and is termed *pulmonary interstitial emphysema*. While this finding is more often recognized in infants, it occasionally can be visualized in adults who are undergoing mechanical ventilation. The radiographic appearance is that of linear lucencies that occur in a mechanically ventilated patient, usually with severe ARDS.[41] The lungs may develop a mottled appearance, and pneumatoceles or subpleural blebs may form. Early recognition of and intervention for pulmonary interstitial emphysema may prevent pneumothorax and pneumomediastinum.

Pneumopericardium is caused by violation of the pericardial space by penetrating trauma or surgery. Radiographically, air collects along the left heart border but may surround the heart in more severe cases (Fig. 15-14). In contrast to pneumomediastinum, the air does not extend from the left heart border to the trachea and neck because it is confined by the pericardial reflection approximately 3 cm above the root of the great vessels.

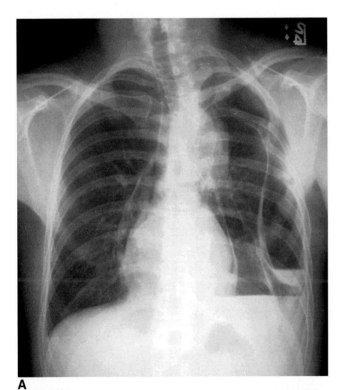

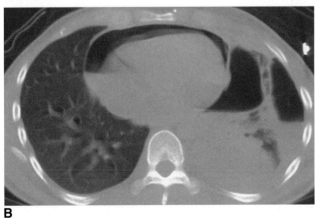

Fig. 15-14
A and **B**, Complicated postoperative air and fluid collections are difficult to analyze on plain films. This patient has a left-sided hydropneumothorax that communicates with a hydropneumopericardium. The CT scan clearly defines the anatomy and allows for appropriate guidance for drainage.

Abnormal Fluid Collections

Pleural effusions are extremely common in the ICU setting and may be due to congestive heart failure, fluid overload, pneumonia, pulmonary edema, or surgery, in addition to trauma. Because of the semierect or recumbent position of ICU patients, pleural effusions are often not recognized.[42]

In an erect patient, a pleural effusion manifests as blunting of the costophrenic angles, with basilar density that obscures the diaphragm and lower lung structures. In a supine or semierect patient, a free-flowing effusion collects in a posterobasal distribution.[43] Radiographically, the appearance is that of hazy, homogeneous opacity over the lower lungs, without loss of bronchovascular markings. The fluid often collects in a subpulmonic location, giving rise to apparent elevation of the ipsilateral hemidiaphragm. If the effusion is unilateral, the only finding may be a uniformly diffuse increase in hazy density of the affected hemithorax.

Patients may also present with or develop pleural hemorrhage or empyema.[44] In such cases, the fluid may become loculated and collect in the lateral pleural space or over the lung apices. Intrafissural collections of fluid may mimic a lung mass. The presence of air within the pleural space in the absence of instrumentation suggests an empyema.

Several approaches are valuable to diagnose pleural effusion in difficult cases. A lateral decubitus radiograph may show layering of the effusion along the lateral chest wall. In patients who are immobilized, either ultrasound or CT scanning can be useful to diagnose and characterize the effusion.

In addition to trauma, a variety of conditions can cause pericardial effusion, including congestive heart failure, infection, surgery, myocardial infarction, and uremia. The radiographic appearance in the ICU patient is nonspecific and may consist of a somewhat enlarged heart. The diagnosis typically relies on echocardiography, although pericardial effusion is well visualized on CT or MRI.[45]

CHEST CT IN THE INTENSIVE CARE UNIT

CT scanner technology has improved dramatically over the past 2 decades. Currently, multislice spiral scanners permit coverage of the entire chest in 10 seconds or less. The ICU setting presents special difficulties for CT imaging, since many patients are unable to breath-hold because of respiratory compromise and mechanical ventilation. Nevertheless, the ability of newer scanners to obtain images in less than 0.5 sec permits substantial reduction in motion artifacts. In the near future, the availability of scanners with a large number of detectors and improved temporal resolution will facilitate clearer imaging. CT development has also occurred in other directions. Newer technologies include portable CT and CT fluoroscopy.

An important consideration in treatment of the ICU patient is the appropriate use of CT imaging.[46-48] In most instances, portable radiography provides adequate assessment of the location of support devices, as well as the patient's cardiovascular status. A major limitation of CT is that the patient must be removed from the monitored setting of the ICU. CT is also more expensive than mobile radiography and delivers a higher radiation dose. Often, little incremental information is gained from CT. Thus careful patient selection is mandatory to maximize the benefits of CT. Despite these caveats, CT plays an important ancillary role in the critically ill patient.

Lung

CT is occasionally useful to delineate an occult cause of respiratory failure. CT may show an area of pneumonia that is not visible on chest radiography, either because the portable film is not of optimal quality or because the opacification is present in a part of the lung that is typically not well visualized on portable radiography.[48] Moreover, in the trauma ICU setting, subcutaneous emphysema may obscure the underlying lung parenchyma. The tomographic format of CT permits separation of chest wall from lung structures.

CT may demonstrate areas of necrosis within the lung or frank cavitation, which suggest lung abscess. In patients with suspected pulmonary emboli, chest radiography often shows nonspecific areas of consolidation. CT can be valuable in this setting and shows multiple rounded peripheral nodules, some of which are cavitary. CT may occasionally be useful to ascertain the position of support lines or tubes when their location is uncertain on radiography.

Pleura

Complex pleuroparenchymal disease often presents a confusing appearance on radiography. In particular, it may occasionally be difficult to distinguish a lung abscess from an empyema.[49] A lung abscess is typically round with acute margins in relation to the chest wall. An empyema is ovoid because it conforms to the pleural space and has obtuse margins. CT demonstrates these findings optimally and may add further information. On CT, an abscess wall appears irregular, whereas the pleural layers marginating an empyema are smooth. With contrast injection, the separated visceral and parietal pleural layers of an empyema may enhance substantially, giving rise to the split pleura sign (Fig. 15-15).

In the trauma setting, CT permits characterization of a pleural collection. The demonstration of a multilocu-

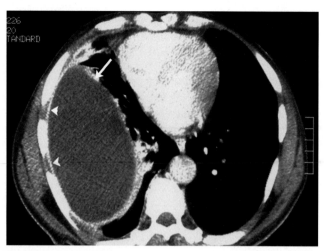

Fig. 15-15
A low-density, homogeneous fluid collection occupies the posterior pleural space. On this contrast-enhanced CT scan, the visceral (*arrow*) and parietal layers (*arrowheads*) of the pleura are split. Note the enhancement of the parietal pleura in this proven empyema.

lated collection suggests that drainage may be difficult. A split pleura sign indicates the likelihood of an empyema. If the collection contains high-density material, pleural hemorrhage is an important consideration (Figs. 15-16 and 15-17).

CT is also useful to detect subtle pneumothoraces that are not evident on radiographs. In a series of 25 patients with head trauma, 21 pneumothoraces were found among 15 patients by CT. Of the pneumothoraces, 11 were detected by CT alone, 9 of which required chest tube placement.[50]

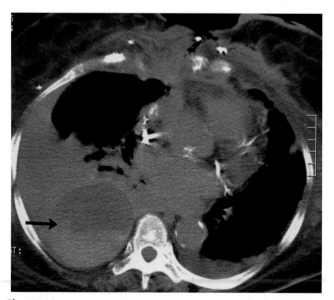

Fig. 15-16
Patient with hemothorax and complicated pleural fluid collections is shown. Note the fluid-fluid level (*arrow*), with denser blood products seen marginating with less dense fluid.

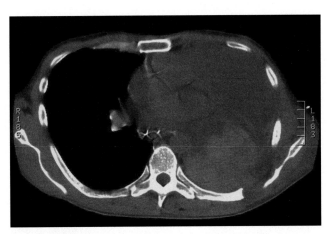

Fig. 15-17
Another patient with a hemothorax and complicated pleural fluid collection.

Pleural collections can be drained blindly, but smaller or loculated collections of fluid or air are more optimally evacuated with image guidance. In general, ultrasound is valuable to guide percutaneous drainage of free-flowing fluid collections; it is rapid, uses nonionizing radiation, provides real-time imaging, and is portable. An 8 to 14 French pigtail catheter is inserted, depending on the size and viscosity of the collection. In patients with an empyema, urokinase can be instilled through the catheter. A CT scan is more valuable to guide drainage of air collections or fluid collections that contain loculations. Occasionally, CT can be used to assist drainage of a lung abscess, particularly if the abscess abuts the pleural space.

Mediastinum

The mediastinum is often difficult to evaluate on portable radiography. CT plays a critical role in the trauma setting in assessing for vascular, esophageal, and airway injuries. Even after initial evaluation, CT may be useful in the ICU setting to detect pneumomediastinum or mediastinal abscess, which may not be apparent on plain films.

Vascular

Pulmonary embolism is the third leading cause of death and is a major cause of morbidity and mortality in the ICU. Trauma patients are particularly vulnerable to pulmonary embolism because of the frequency of surgical procedures and long-term immobilization. The clinical signs of the disorder, pleuritic chest pain and shortness of breath, are nonspecific. Chest radiography, ventilation-perfusion radionuclide scanning, and pulmonary angiography are the traditional methods of evaluating for pulmonary embolism. More recently, CT scanning has come into widespread use.

The chest radiograph is of limited value in detecting pulmonary embolism. In the study by Greenspan et al.,[51] sensitivity and specificity of 33% and 59%, respectively, were reported. Most often, the radiograph is normal or shows nonspecific findings of subsegmental atelectasis. Pleural effusions are present in as many as 50% of cases. Rarely, more specific findings of a wedge-shaped subpleural area of consolidation corresponding to infarction (Hampton's hump) or regional oligemia (Westermark's sign) may suggest the diagnosis. These findings are particularly difficult to visualize on portable radiography. The main indication for radiography is to suggest an alternative cause such as pneumonia.

Ventilation-perfusion scintigraphy is sometimes used to evaluate pulmonary embolism.[52] The diagnosis is confirmed by demonstration of multiple ventilation-perfusion mismatches. The main limitation of this technique is the high rate of nondiagnostic studies, which may exceed 40%. This shortcoming is particularly problematic in the ICU patient, who may have several concurrent diseases and a markedly abnormal radiograph.

Pulmonary angiography remains the definitive diagnostic test for pulmonary embolism. The finding of an intraluminal filling defect is considered confirmatory. However, pulmonary angiography is invasive and is associated with morbidity and a low but well-defined mortality. The test is also limited by interobserver disagreement as well as technical challenges that may lead to a suboptimal study.

Computed tomography has emerged recently as an important technique in the evaluation of pulmonary embolism.[53] When a spiral CT technique and rapid bolus injection of contrast material (3 to 4 ml/sec) are used, the central pulmonary arteries are well delineated. On CT pulmonary angiography, pulmonary embolism is visualized as one or more filling defects within the contrast-filled vessels (Figs. 15-18 and 15-19). With the use of multislice technology, subsegmental pulmonary arteries to the fifth order can be analyzed.

Several studies have indicated sensitivity and specificity for diagnosis of central pulmonary embolism that approach or exceed 90%, using catheter-based pulmonary angiography or a diagnostic ventilation-perfusion scan as the reference standard.[54,55] These statistics are somewhat lower for more peripheral vessels. CT pulmonary angiography has also proved valuable in excluding pulmonary embolism. A negative predictive value of 99% was reported by Garg et al., as compared with values of 96% and 100% for low probability and normal ventilation-perfusion scanning, respectively.[56] Recent success has been reported with a technique that involves a continuation of the contrast bolus used for CT pulmonary angiography to acquire CT venography of the pelvis and legs, allowing concurrent assessment for deep venous thrombus (Figs. 15-20 and 15-21).

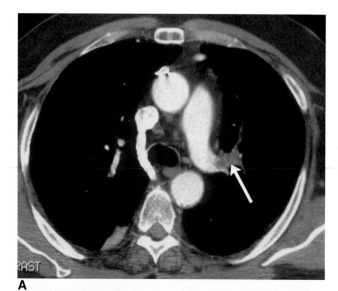

A

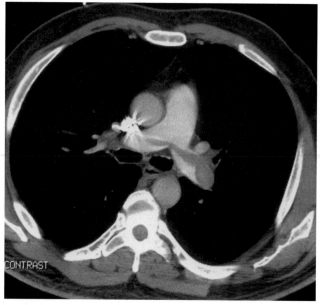

Fig. 15-19
At many institutions, multislice CT has become the procedure of choice for diagnosing pulmonary embolism. A large filling defect straddles the midline in this patient with an acute saddle embolism.

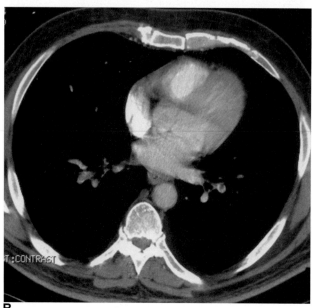

B

Fig. 15-18
A and **B**, Segmental and subsegmental pulmonary emboli are identified as intraluminal filling defects (*arrows*).

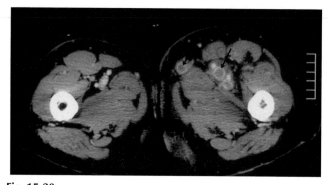

Fig. 15-20
A CT study of the lower extremities performed after a chest examination for pulmonary embolus shows deep venous thrombosis (*arrows*).

Performance of CT pulmonary angiography in ICU patients presents many of the same obstacles previously described for other techniques. Substantial shortness of breath may cause blurring of the CT image and produce a suboptimal study. Parenchymal opacity may interfere with visualization of distal emboli in adjacent small vessels. The better temporal resolution and thin-slice capability of multislice CT may overcome these limitations. In addition, CT is superior to ventilation-perfusion scanning and pulmonary angiography in detecting etiologies other than pulmonary embolism, such as pneumonia or heart failure, which might explain the patient's symptoms. In the study by Kim et al.,[57] CT pulmonary angiog-

raphy suggested an alternative diagnosis in 67% of patients who did not have pulmonary embolism.

Newer Techniques

Portable CT is a recently developed technique that allows the patient to remain in the monitored ICU environment while imaging is performed. The University of Maryland uses a Philips Tomoscan that consists of three components—an operator's console, gantry, and table—which can be wheeled independently to the bedside. The scanner is battery-powered, has a weight limit of 350 lb, and provides a temporal resolution of 2 sec. In a study at the University of Maryland, portable CT provided images of

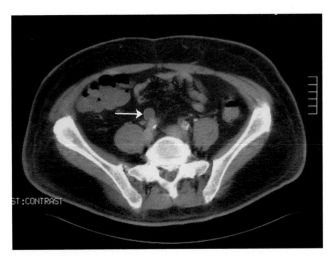

Fig. 15-21
A CT scan performed with a CT pulmonary angiogram shows bilateral thrombus in the right common iliac vein (*arrow*).

diagnostic quality in the ICU setting.[58] Moreover, drainage procedures of complicated air collections were performed successfully at the bedside. The development of spiral capability for the portable CT scanner will likely extend indications for its use, including assessment for pulmonary embolism in the ICU.

CT fluoroscopy is a technique that uses a rapid-array processor and real-time reconstruction to display six or more images per second, generating a "real-time" effect. This technique has been found to be valuable in performing drainage of fluid collections because of the rapid feedback that CT fluoroscopy provides, permitting optimal coordination of catheter insertion with respirations.[59] This capability is particularly helpful in ICU patients, who are often short of breath. An in-room control panel and monitor allow the operator to remain in the room to closely monitor both the patient and the course of the procedure.

REFERENCES

1. Henschke CI, Pasternack GS, Schroeder S, et al: Bedside chest radiography: diagnostic efficacy, *Radiology* 149:23, 1983.
2. Janower ML, Jennas-Nocera Z, Mukai J: Utility and efficacy of portable chest radiographs, *AJR Am J Roentgenol* 142:265, 1984.
3. Bekemeyer WB, Crapo RO, Calhoon S, et al: Efficacy of chest radiography in a respiratory intensive care unit: a prospective study, *Chest* 88:691, 1985.
4. MacMahon H: Pitfalls in portable chest radiology, *Resp Care* 44:1018, 1999.
5. Wandtke JC: Bedside chest radiography, *Radiology* 190:1, 1994.
6. Goodman LR, Putman CE: *Critical care imaging*, ed 3, Philadelphia, 1992, WB Saunders.
7. Swensen SJ, Peters SG, LeRoy AJ, et al: Radiology in the intensive-care unit, *Mayo Clin Proc* 66:396, 1991.
8. Scott WL: Complications associated with central venous catheters: a survey, *Chest* 94:1221, 1988.
9. McLoud TC, Putman CE: Radiology of the Swan-Ganz catheter and associated pulmonary complications, *Radiology* 116:19, 1975.
10. Foote GA, Schabel SI, Hodges M: Pulmonary complications of the flow-directed balloon-tipped catheter, *N Engl J Med* 290:927, 1974.
11. Dieden JD, Friloux LA 3rd, Renner JW: Pulmonary artery false aneurysms secondary to Swan-Ganz pulmonary artery catheters, *AJR Am J Roentgenol* 149:901, 1987.
12. Goodman LR, Conrardy PA, Laing F, Singer MM: Radiographic evaluation of endotracheal tube position, *Am J Roentgenol* 127:433, 1976.
13. Rashkin MC, Davis T: Acute complications of endotracheal intubation: relationship to reintubation, route, urgency, and duration, *Chest* 89:165, 1986.
14. Smith GM, Reed JC, Choplin RH: Radiographic detection of esophageal malpositioning of endotracheal tubes, *AJR Am J Roentgenol* 154:23, 1990.
15. Cameron EW, Mirvis SE, Shanmuganathan K, et al: Computed tomography of malpositioned thoracostomy drains: a pictorial essay, *Clin Radiol* 52:187, 1997.
16. Maurer JR, Friedman PJ, Wing VW: Thoracostomy tube in an interlobar fissure: radiologic recognition of a potential problem, *AJR Am J Roentgenol* 139:1155, 1982.
17. Hyson EA, Ravin CE, Kelley MJ, Curtis AM: Intraaortic counterpulsation balloon: radiographic considerations, *AJR Am J Roentgenol* 128:915, 1977.
18. Jafri SM, Kruse JA: Temporary transvenous cardiac pacing, *Crit Care Clin* 8:713, 1992.
19. Aberle DR, Wiener-Kronish JP, Webb WR, Matthay MA: Hydrostatic versus increased permeability pulmonary edema: diagnosis based on radiographic criteria in critically ill patients, *Radiology* 168:73, 1988.
20. Milne EN, Pistolesi M, Miniati M, Giuntini C: The vascular pedicle of the heart and the vena azygos. I. The normal subject, *Radiology* 152:1, 1984.
21. Milne EN, Pistolesi M, Miniati M, Giuntini C: The radiologic distinction of cardiogenic and noncardiogenic edema, *AJR Am J Roentgenol* 144:879, 1985.
22. Gurney JW, Goodman LR: Pulmonary edema localized in the right upper lobe accompanying mitral regurgitation, *Radiology* 171:397, 1989.
23. Smith RC, Mann H, Greenspan RH, et al: Radiographic differentiation between different etiologies of pulmonary edema, *Invest Radiol* 22:859, 1987.
24. Feldman F, Ellis K, Green WM: The fat embolism syndrome, *Radiology* 114:535, 1975.
25. Calenoff L, Kruglik GD, Woodruff A: Unilateral pulmonary edema, *Radiology* 126:19, 1978.
26. Wagner RB, Crawford WO Jr, Schimpf PP: Classification of parenchymal injuries of the lung, *Radiology* 167:77, 1988.
27. Shevland JE, Hirleman MT, Hoang KA, Kealey GP: Lobar collapse in the surgical intensive care unit, *Br J Radiol* 56:531, 1983.
28. Zylak CJ, Littleton JT, Durizch ML: Illusory consolidation of the left lower lobe: a pitfall of portable radiography, *Radiology* 167:653, 1988.
29. Andrews CP, Coalson JJ, Smith JD, Johanson WG Jr: Diagnosis of nosocomial bacterial pneumonia in acute, diffuse lung injury, *Chest* 80:254, 1981.
30. Lipchik RJ, Kuzo RS: Nosocomial pneumonia, *Radiol Clin North Am* 34:47, 1996.
31. Winer-Muram HT, Jennings SG, Wunderink RG, et al: Ventilator-associated *Pseudomonas aeruginosa* pneumonia: radiographic findings, *Radiology* 195:2472, 1995.
32. Mock CN, Burchard KW, Hasan F, Reed M: Surgical intensive care unit pneumonia, *Surgery* 104:494, 1988.
33. Schachter EN, Kreisman H, Putman C: Diagnostic problems in suppurative lung disease, *Arch Intern Med* 136:167, 1976.
34. Rubin SA, Winer-Muram HT, Ellis JV: Diagnostic imaging of pneumonia and its complications in the critically ill patient, *Clin Chest Med* 16:45, 1995.

35. Khawaja IT, Buffa SD, Brandstetter RD: Aspiration pneumonia: a threat when deglutition is compromised, *Postgrad Med* 92:165, 1992.

36. Rankine JJ, Thomas AN, Fluechter D: Diagnosis of pneumothorax in critically ill adults, *Postgrad Med J* 76:399, 2000.

37. Tocino IM, Miller MH, Fairfax WR: Distribution of pneumothorax in the supine and semirecumbent critically ill adult, *AJR Am J Roentgenol* 144:901, 1985.

38. Zwillich CW, Pierson DJ, Creagh CE, et al: Complications of assisted ventilation: a prospective study of 354 consecutive episodes, *Am J Med* 57:161, 1974.

39. Gobien RP, Reines HD, Schabel SI: Localized tension pneumothorax: unrecognized form of barotrauma in adult respiratory distress syndrome, *Radiology* 142:15, 1982.

40. Cyrlak D, Milne EN, Imray TJ: Pneumomediastinum: a diagnostic problem, *Crit Rev Diagn Imaging* 23:75, 1984.

41. Woodring JH: Pulmonary interstitial emphysema in the adult respiratory distress syndrome, *Crit Care Med* 13:786, 1985.

42. Woodring JH: Recognition of pleural effusion on supine radiographs: how much fluid is required? *AJR Am J Roentgenol* 142:59, 1984.

43. Ruskin JA, Gurney JW, Thorsen MK, Goodman LR: Detection of pleural effusions on supine chest radiographs, *AJR Am J Roentgenol* 148:681, 1987.

44. Muller NL: Imaging of the pleura, *Radiology* 186:297, 1993.

45. Breen JF: Imaging of the pericardium, *J Thorac Imaging* 16:47, 2001.

46. Gross BH, Spizarny DL: Computed tomography of the chest in the intensive care unit, *Crit Care Clin* 10:267, 1994.

47. Mirvis SE, Tobin KD, Kostrubiak I, Belzberg H: Thoracic CT in detecting occult disease in critically ill patients, *AJR Am J Roentgenol* 148:685, 1987.

48. Snow N, Bergin KT, Horrigan TP: Thoracic CT scanning in critically ill patients: information obtained frequently alters management, *Chest* 97:1467, 1990.

49. Stark DD, Federle MP, Goodman PC, et al: Differentiating lung abscess and empyema: radiography and computed tomography, *AJR Am J Roentgenol* 141:163, 1983.

50. Tocino IM, Miller MH, Frederick PR, et al: CT detection of occult pneumothorax in head trauma, *AJR Am J Roentgenol* 143:987, 1984.

51. Greenspan RH, Ravin CE, Polansky SM, McLoud TC: Accuracy of the chest radiograph in diagnosis of pulmonary embolism, *Invest Radiol* 17:539, 1982.

52. The PIOPED Investigators: Value of the ventilation/perfusion scan in acute pulmonary embolism: results of the prospective investigation of pulmonary embolism diagnosis (PIOPED), *JAMA* 263:2753, 1990.

53. Remy-Jardin M, Remy J, Baghaie F, et al: Clinical value of thin collimation in the diagnostic workup of pulmonary embolism, *AJR Am J Roentgenol* 175:407, 2000.

54. Goodman LR, Curtin JJ, Mewissen MW, et al: Detection of pulmonary embolism in patients with unresolved clinical and scintigraphic diagnosis: helical CT versus angiography, *AJR Am J Roentgenol* 164:1369, 1995.

55. Mayo JR, Remy-Jardin M, Muller NL, et al: Pulmonary embolism: prospective comparison of spiral CT with ventilation-perfusion scintigraphy, *Radiology* 205:447, 1997.

56. Garg K, Sieler H, Welsh CH, et al: Clinical validity of helical CT being interpreted as negative for pulmonary embolism: implications for patient treatment, *AJR Am J Roentgenol* 172:1627, 1999.

57. Kim KI, Muller NL, Mayo JR: Clinically suspected pulmonary embolism: utility of spiral CT, *Radiology* 210:693, 1999.

58. White CS, Meyer CA, Wu J, Mirvis SE: Portable CT: assessing thoracic disease in the intensive care unit, *AJR Am J Roentgenol* 173:1351, 1999.

59. White CS, Meyer CA, Templeton PA: CT fluoroscopy for thoracic interventional procedures, *Radiol Clin North Am* 38:303, 2000.

16 Abdominal Imaging in the Intensive Care Unit

Jade J. Wong-You-Cheong and Barry Daly

The critically ill patient with clinical features of sepsis, such as fever, leucocytosis, and hypotension, presents a diagnostic challenge. Other conditions, such as vascular thrombosis or ischemia, hemorrhage, and bowel obstruction or perforation, are causes of serious morbidity and mortality in the intensive care unit (ICU) also. Physical signs may be unhelpful, and laboratory tests may be nonspecific. This chapter reviews common acute problems occurring in the setting of the intensive care unit and outlines the important role of diagnostic imaging in diagnosis and treatment.

IMAGING MODALITIES

By definition, patients in the ICU are not mobile or easily moved around the hospital. Imaging studies must be tailored with consideration to the individual patient's condition and, whenever practical, the imaging service must be brought to the bedside rather than the patient being brought to the radiology department. Moving unstable and critically ill patients may further compromise their condition and is usually a very labor-intensive process requiring medical, nursing, and ventilatory support personnel. For these reasons, mobile radiography and ultrasound machines have advantages over other imaging modalities and are often the diagnostic studies of first choice in the ICU.

Plain radiography of the abdomen is often used as a screening tool in critically ill patients with abdominal distension or abnormal bowel sounds; its major role is in the diagnosis of perforation and bowel dilatation. Small amounts of free intraperitoneal gas may be occult on supine abdominal films. Because critically ill patients cannot be elevated, decubitus (right-side-up) or semi-erect views may be necessary. It should be noted that mobile radiography units have limited x-ray–generation capacity and may be unable to adequately penetrate the abdomen in large patients without long exposure times, resulting in respiratory or bowel motion artifact on the image.

Plain radiographs are limited for evaluation of infection; however, pneumatosis intestinalis (Fig. 16-1) or large abscesses may be detected as linear or bubbly collections of gas, respectively. In the presence of sepsis, pneumatosis is usually considered an ominous sign, indicating necrotizing infection or bowel infarction, but sometimes may have a benign etiology. Chronic obstructive pulmonary disease, positive pressure ventilation, transplantation (Fig. 16-2), peptic ulceration, bowel obstruction, collagen vascular disease (in particular, scleroderma), and steroid treatment have all been reported to cause benign pneumatosis.[1,2] Computed tomography (CT) is superior to radiography for the detection of pneumatosis and, given the appropriate clinical picture, can usually distinguish benign pneumatosis from the more serious causes[3,4] (Figs. 16-3 and 16-4).

Bowel dilatation may be found in septic patients as a result of obstruction or paralytic ileus. The distinction between obstruction and ileus is based upon the presence and distribution of gas in the bowel lumen. In small

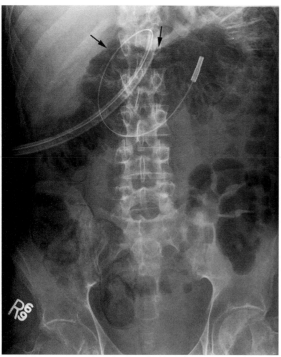

Fig. 16-1
Pneumatosis coli. Asymptomatic 68-year-old diabetic recipient of a pancreas transplant. Plain abdominal film shows linear gas within the wall of the ascending and transverse colon, as well as extraluminal gas (*arrows*).

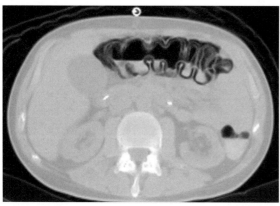

Fig. 16-2
Pneumatosis coli. Asymptomatic 68-year-old recipient of a pancreas transplant. The CT scan shows pneumatosis and extraluminal gas adjacent to the transverse colon.

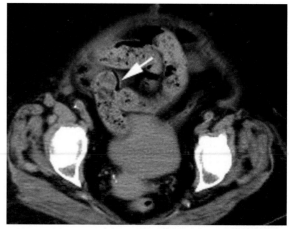

Fig. 16-3
Adynamic ileus. CT scan in a postoperative patient with abdominal distension and lack of bowel movement. There is stool in the small bowel. The curvilinear gas (*arrow*) and mottled fecal contents could be mistaken for pneumatosis.

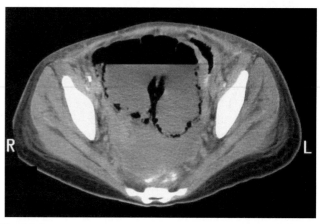

Fig. 16-4
Infarcted cecum. Septic 25-year-old patient. The cecum is dilated and fluid-filled, with intramural gas.

bowel obstruction, there is a transition between the dilated proximal small bowel and the nondistended distal small bowel and the colon (Fig. 16-5), with emptying of colonic gas within 24 to 48 hours.[5] In adynamic ileus, there is no such transition zone (Fig. 16-6).

Water-soluble iodine contrast studies may be used at the bedside to confirm the position of feeding gastrostomy tubes or suspected leaks at tube insertion sites. Small and large bowel contrast studies are occasionally required to confirm or exclude obstruction or leaks and to localize the site of an obstruction (Fig. 16-7).

Enterocutaneous fistulae (Fig. 16-8) are relatively common sequelae of major trauma and often are associated with breakdown of abdominal wounds and/or bowel obstruction. Fistulogram studies with direct injection of contrast into the fistula using a sterile feeding tube or Foley catheter are used to identify the source and course of the fistula and to look for evidence of associated bowel obstruction or infection. Such investigations are best deferred until the patient's condition allows transfer to the radiology department without difficulty.

For patients with sepsis of possible abdominal origin, sonography may be used as the initial imaging modality, especially if the liver or gallbladder is the suspected source. Sonography is a relatively inexpensive imaging

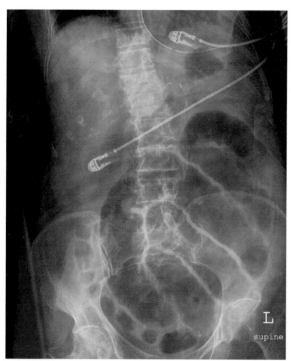

Fig. 16-5
Adhesive small bowel obstruction. Plain abdominal film in an 80-year-old patient, post-left nephrectomy. There is a dilated small bowel with undilated distal ileum and colon.

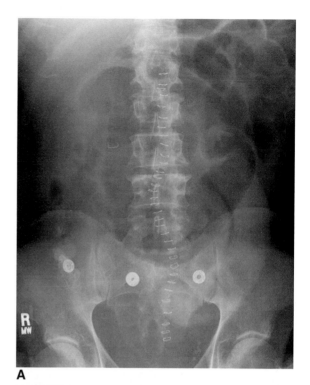

A

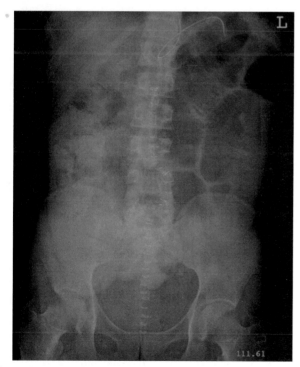

Fig. 16-6
Adynamic ileus after laparotomy. Plain abdominal film shows dilated small and large bowel containing gas and fluid. There is contrast medium within the colon for a CT scan.

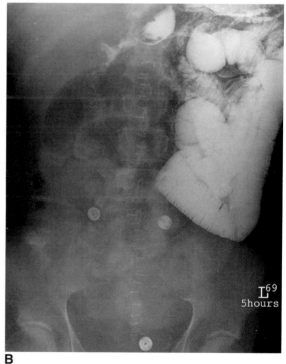

B

Fig. 16-7
Internal hernia and small bowel obstruction. **A,** Plain abdominal film in a 55-year-old patient with abdominal pain and distension after a pancreas transplant. There is dilated proximal small bowel with distal decompression and an undilated colon. **B,** Small bowel series. Film taken at 5 hours shows high-grade obstruction in the midabdomen secondary to an internal hernia.

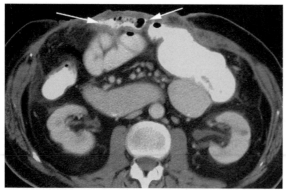

Fig. 16-8
Ileocutaneous fistula. Enhanced CT shows spillage of oral contrast (*arrows*) onto the defective anterior abdominal wall. This is diagnostic of a fistula from the bowel, but the exact origin of the fistula cannot always be determined.

modality and can be performed at the patient's bedside. Major applications include the detection of hepatobiliary and renal disease, ascites, and subphrenic or pelvic abscess. However, sonography is of limited value in the assessment of retroperitoneal or bowel pathology. Bowel gas, obesity, and bone all reflect or absorb the ultrasound beam, making this imaging modality unsuitable for evaluation of the entire abdomen. If fluid collections are visible by sonography, it is the preferred technique for bedside guidance of percutaneous drainage in critical care patients (see below).

CT is a very sensitive modality for the detection of abdominal pathology; it is not operator-dependent and is less limited by body habitus than is sonography. CT does require transport of the patient to the scanner suite and may not be feasible in unstable patients. Furthermore, an optimal study requires the use of enteric and iodinated intravenous contrast, and the latter may be contraindicated in patients who have established renal failure or progressively worsening renal function.

The role of abdominal magnetic resonance imaging (MRI) is limited in critically ill patients but may include evaluation of the viscera and vascular tree in patients with renal failure, because magnetic resonance contrast (gadolinium chelates) is not associated with nephrotoxicity. Magnetic resonance studies may be particularly useful for detection of microabscesses of the liver and spleen and evaluation of the major pancreatic and biliary ducts for occlusion, injury, or calculus disease. For good technical studies, a high degree of patient cooperation and periodic suspended respiration is required, which is difficult for the typical ICU patient.

Nuclear scintigraphic studies commonly used for the abdomen in the ICU setting consist mainly of hepatobiliary imaging and gastrointestinal bleeding studies. Portable scanning is usually unavailable, necessitating transfer of the patient to the nuclear medicine depart-

ment. For selected clinical diagnoses (which are discussed later), nuclear medicine studies are the primary or secondary imaging test indicated.

COMMON ABDOMINAL PATHOLOGIES IN THE CRITICAL CARE UNIT
Acute Acalculous Cholecystitis

Acute acalculous cholecystitis (AAC) is a serious complication in critically ill patients following trauma, surgery, burns, sepsis, or extended hospitalization in the ICU. AAC occurs in up to 18% of surgical ICU patients[6] but is less common in medical ICU patients (1% to 4% if on total parenteral nutrition).[7] Clinical and biochemical signs are nonspecific, and mortality rates as high as 66% have been reported, resulting mainly from delayed diagnosis.[6] Potential predisposing factors for the development of AAC include prolonged fasting and parenteral nutrition, use of narcotic medications and vasoconstrictive agents, infection, ventilatory support, shock, transfusions, and metabolic disturbances.[6,8] Cholestasis, mucous secretion, and biliary sludge develop in a previously normal gallbladder, followed by superimposed infection and ischemia.

Because most of these patients are receiving ventilatory support, are paralyzed, and may have multiple coexisting medical problems, the clinical manifestations of AAC may be masked or nonspecific. Laboratory findings are also nonspecific but include leukocytosis and elevation of bilirubin, alkaline phosphatase, and other hepatic enzymes. In a septic patient with hepatic function abnormality, sonography is the first-choice imaging modality for gallbladder evaluation. Sonographic features of acalculous cholecystitis include gallbladder wall thickening (>3 mm), distension (width >4 cm and length >8 cm), intramural lucencies/striated wall edema, pericholecystic fluid, luminal sludge, and the sonographic Murphy's sign[9-12] (Fig. 16-9). In one study, sonography was found to have a sensitivity of 36% and a specificity of 89% if sludge, wall thickening, and distension were all present concurrently.[7] Less stringent criteria for diagnosing AAC improve sensitivity but decrease specificity.[7]

The high prevalence of sonographic abnormalities in the general ICU population adversely affects the diagnostic accuracy of sonography for AAC.[13-15] In a prospective study of 44 ICU patients, Boland et al. found that a majority (84%) had at least one of the sonographic criteria associated with acalculous cholecystitis, and 57% had three signs.[15] The most common signs were sludge (59%) and distension (33%) (Fig. 16-10). Gallbladder wall lucencies and thickening were found in 13% and 19% of scans, respectively[15] (Fig. 16-11). These authors did not find clinical parameters to be more discriminatory than sonography in the diagnosis of AAC. Their findings have been corroborated by other authors, who noted

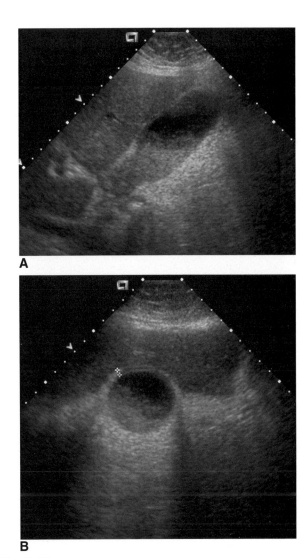

A

B

Fig. 16-10
Nonspecific ultrasound findings. **A**, Ultrasound scan of a distended gallbladder filled with sludge. **B**, There was mild wall thickening (4 mm). This was not acute cholecystitis.

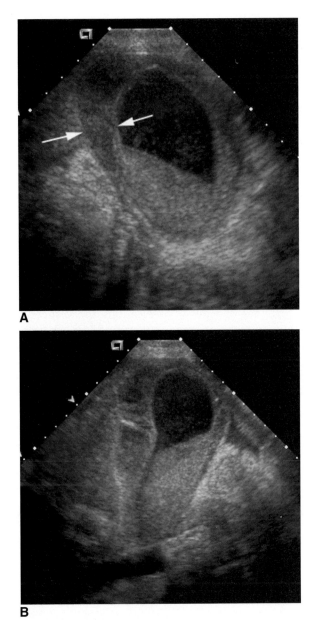

A

B

Fig. 16-9
Acute acalculous cholecystitis. **A**, Ultrasound of a markedly thickened gallbladder wall (*arrows*) with sludge and debris. Gangrenous cholecystitis was found at surgery. **B**, There are linear echo lucencies within the gallbladder wall.

wall thickening in 86% of patients, distension in 75%, sludge in 61%, pericholecystic fluid in 45%, and striated thickening in 39%.[14]

Gallbladder sludge may resolve spontaneously or progress to the development of stones or acute cholecystitis.[16] Sludge has been found more likely to be associated with gallbladder pathology than is wall thickening, assuming a normal serum amylase and liver function.[17] For indeterminate cases, serial sonography may be valuable, particularly if combined with a sonographic scoring system. Changing scores can guide clinical management

as can the detection of complications such as gallbladder perforation. In one series of medical ICU patients, 61% had gallbladder abnormalities detected by sonogram, but none developed acute cholecystitis.[13] Follow-up sonography may also be of value in patients with inconclusive findings.[18] Development of wall thickening on surveillance should be considered suspicious for acute cholecystitis if other causes of wall thickening have been excluded (Fig. 16-12). Diagnostic percutaneous procedures, such as cholecystostomy or aspiration (Fig. 16-13), may be necessary, given a lack of specific sonographic findings. These procedures provide a sample of bile for culture and allow decompression of the gallbladder.

Cholescintigraphy with technetium 99m (Tc 99m)-labeled analogues of iminodiacetic acid (IDA compounds) offers complementary anatomic and functional information to sonography (see Chapter 13). These

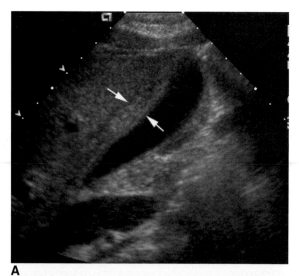

A

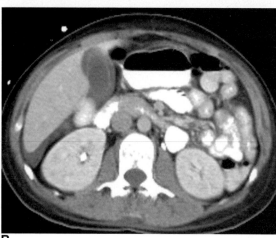

B

Fig. 16-11
False-positive ultrasound scan. **A,** Sonogram of a thick-walled gall-bladder with mural edema in an immunosuppressed patient with right upper quadrant pain. **B,** CT also shows wall thickening and ascites. The HIDA scan (Fig. 16-14) was negative for acute chole-cystitis.

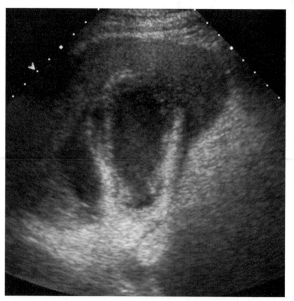

Fig. 16-12
Cholecystitis in a 45-year-old patient with necrotizing pancreatitis and suspected acalculous cholecystitis. On sequential ultrasound scans, the gallbladder developed a very thick, irregular wall with intramural fluid. There is a pericholecystic fluid collection. Despite percutaneous cholecystostomy, the gallbladder remained thickened, and the patient did not improve.

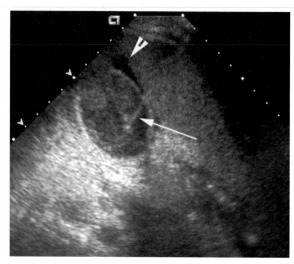

Fig. 16-13
Acute acalculous cholecystitis with infected bile at aspiration. The needle (*arrow*) is seen traversing the liver into a distended gallbladder with sludge. There is some pericholecystic fluid (*arrowhead*).

injected tracers are metabolized exclusively by the liver and excreted into the biliary tree. In a normal study (Fig. 16-14), common hepatic duct filling precedes gallbladder and duodenal filling. In acute acalculous cholecystitis, because of the functional obstruction of the cystic duct, the gallbladder fails to accumulate tracer within 60 minutes, despite bile duct patency and adequate bowel filling (Fig. 16-15). These criteria can achieve a high sensitivity of 97% and specificity of 93%.[19] Additional signs of acute cholecystitis include increased blood flow to the area surrounding the gallbladder on the early phase and the "rim sign," denoting increased activity in the liver, adjacent to the inflamed gallbladder on delayed images. The rim sign is reported to have a positive predictive value for acute cholecystitis of 90%.[20] Potential sources of false-positive results include fasting for more than 24

hours, resulting in thick, inspissated bile; severe intercurrent illness; liver failure; chronic cholestasis; and hyperalimentation.

In some centers, routine delayed imaging at 2 to 4 hours is performed to ensure that the delay in gallbladder filling is not simply due to chronic cholecystitis or stasis.[21] However, delayed scans may not be feasible in a critically ill patient, and they can be substituted with morphine-

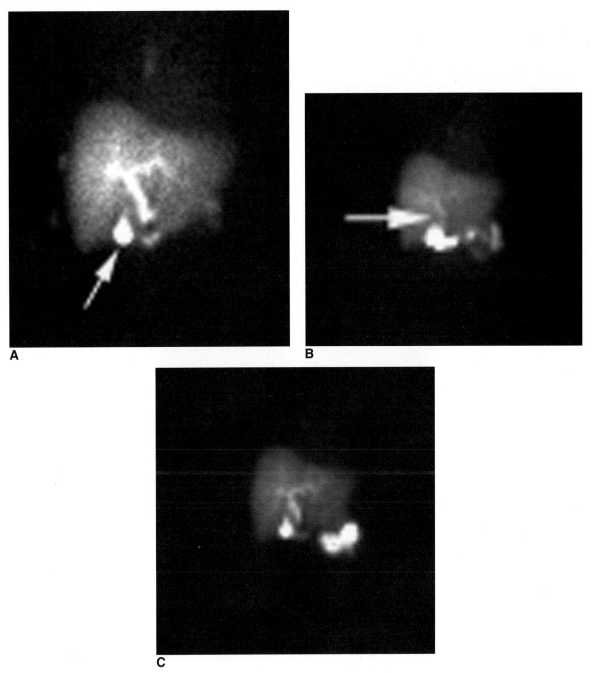

Fig. 16-14
A, Normal HIDA scan. Right upper quadrant pain in immunosuppressed patient. Ultrasound and CT showed gallbladder wall thickening, and there was local tenderness (Fig. 16-11). The HIDA scan was normal, with prompt filling of the gallbladder (*arrow*). **B,** Early phase with parenchymal uptake and prompt filling of the common bile duct and gallbladder (*arrow*). **C,** Concentration of activity in the gallbladder and excretion into the small bowel.

augmented cholescintigraphy.[22,23] Intravenous injection of morphine sulfate causes constriction of the sphincter of Oddi, increasing intraluminal pressure in the common bile duct and allowing preferential flow of tracer into the cystic duct and gallbladder. This approach effectively

decreases the study duration, because filling of a normally functioning gallbladder should occur within 5 to 10 minutes. Cholecystokinin causes contraction of the functioning gallbladder and is injected before the radioisotope to empty the gallbladder, also shortening the study and

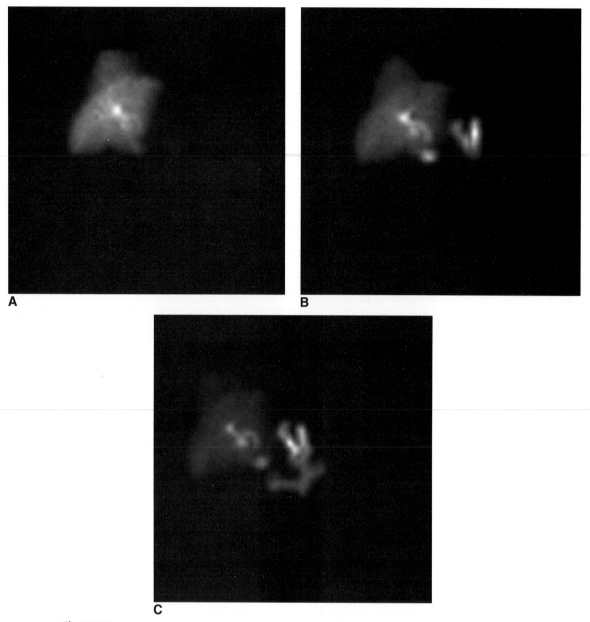

Fig. 16-15
Acute acalculous cholecystitis on HIDA scan. **A,** Early phase with parenchymal uptake and filling of the common bile duct. The gallbladder is not seen. **B,** Excretion of isotope into the common bile duct and duodenum. **C,** Nonfilling of the gallbladder on delayed phase, consistent with acute cholecystitis.

decreasing the number of false-positive results. Morphine and cholecystokinin can be used together.[22,23]

In the overall evaluation of acute cholecystitis, the sensitivity of cholescintigraphy with pharmacologic enhancement is as high as 99%, with specificity of 91%.[24] However, in critical care patients with multisystem disease and AAC, the sensitivity of cholescintigraphy is less, at 67% to 79%.[7,25,26] In a prospective study comparing cholescintigraphy with bedside sonography for the diag-

nosis of AAC in critically ill patients, cholescintigraphy with morphine augmentation achieved a sensitivity of 79% and a specificity of 100%, compared with 36% and 89%, respectively, for sonography.[7] The combination of dimethyl iminodiacetic acid (HIDA) scans and sonographic imaging provided the highest overall diagnostic accuracy. In another series of intensive care patients, the positive predictive value of cholescintigraphy was found to be 100%.[26] The low false-positive rate of <5% could be further reduced by morphine augmentation.[7,24,26] False negatives can occur in partial cystic duct obstruction. Disadvantages of cholescintigraphy include the relatively longer time required to perform the study, as compared with sonography, higher cost, and the need to move the patient.

CT findings of AAC include wall thickening, pericholecystic stranding or fluid, distension, subserosal edema, and high-attenuation bile[27,28] (Figs. 16-16 and 16-17). Sensitivities and specificities of 100% have been reported, and CT is superior for the assessment of pericholecystic fluid and inflammation.[27,29] CT may also readily detect other intraabdominal processes responsible for a patient's condition, providing a more thorough general screening of the abdomen and pelvis than is possible with sonography. CT can serve as a useful study if the source of the patient's septic or febrile state is not clearly related to the gallbladder or when bedside sonography does not provide sufficient diagnostic information and patient movement is possible.

Acute Calculus Cholecystitis

Gallstones may be associated with acute cholecystitis, obstructive jaundice, biliary colic, or acute pancreatitis. In the critically ill patient, acute calculous cholecystitis (ACC) may present in a nonspecific manner, with unexplained sepsis or abnormal liver function tests. Sonography is the primary modality for the diagnosis of gallstones, with sensitivity and accuracy greater than 95% and a specificity of 99%.[30,31] Gallstones are hyperechoic, shadowing, mobile, nondependent intraluminal masses (Fig. 16-18). A contracted gallbladder filled with stones is referred to as the "wall echo shadow" complex.[32] Features suggesting ACC are the same as those associated with

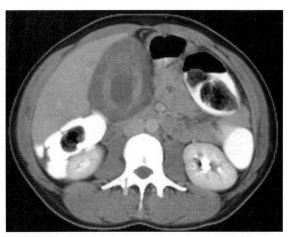

Fig. 16-17
Acute calculous cholecystitis. Enhanced CT shows a markedly thickened, distended gallbladder with prominent mucosal enhancement. The gallbladder was gangrenous at surgery.

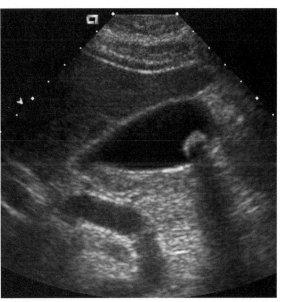

Fig. 16-18
Gallstone. Ultrasound scan of gallstone without cholecystitis. Acoustic shadowing is seen deep to the echogenic calculus.

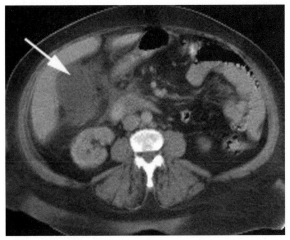

Fig. 16-16
Acute acalculous cholecystitis. Enhanced CT of an abnormally thickened gallbladder (*arrow*) with extensive pericholecystic inflammatory change.

acute acalculous cholecystitis: namely, wall thickening >3 mm, a positive sonographic Murphy's sign, pericholecystic fluid, and distension[9,11,12,33] (Fig. 16-19). The positive predictive value of these signs is 99%.[12] While the sonographic Murphy's sign, together with gallstones, has a positive predictive value of 92%, the sign may be difficult to elicit in intubated, paralyzed, or mentally obtunded patients.[12] It should be noted also that gallbladder wall thickening in the setting of stones and a critically ill patient could be due to many factors other than acute cholecystitis. These conditions include hypoproteinemia, cardiac or renal failure, adjacent inflammatory conditions such as pancreatitis and hepatitis, or portal

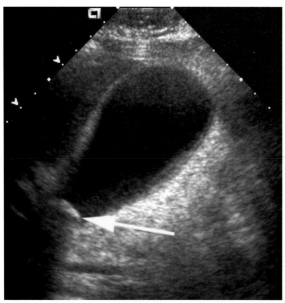

Fig. 16-19
Acute calculous cholecystitis with gangrene at surgery. Ultrasound scan of a markedly distended gallbladder with a calculus impacted in the neck (*arrow*). Layering sludge and mild wall thickening are noted.

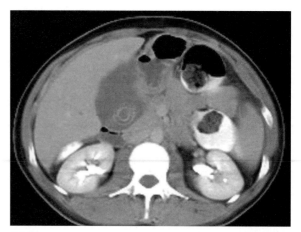

Fig. 16-20
Acute calculous cholecystitis. Enhanced CT shows a distended gallbladder containing a laminated calculus.

hypertension. Pericholecystic fluid may also be part of generalized ascites and may develop secondary to numerous other pathologic conditions. Gallbladder sludge develops in patients with biliary stasis from intravenous hyperalimentation or prolonged fasting and may predispose to stones, acute cholecystitis, and pancreatitis[16,17] (see Fig. 16-10).

Cholescintigraphy is equivalent to sonography for the diagnosis of acute calculous cholecystitis (sensitivity of 90% to 95%).[25] In many centers, HIDA scanning is used as an adjunct to indeterminate sonography. Impaired liver function adversely impacts the performance of scintigraphy.

CT is less sensitive than sonography for the diagnosis of stones but is equivalent in sensitivity and specificity for the diagnosis of ACC.[28] CT may be a useful adjunct to sonography if findings are equivocal. CT signs include wall thickening with mucosal enhancement (Fig. 16-20) and hyperemia in the surrounding liver manifested by increased attenuation.[28] CT is particularly useful in the diagnosis of complications resulting from acute calculous cholecystitis.

Complications of Acute Cholecystitis

Complications of acute cholecystitis include emphysematous cholecystitis (Fig. 16-21), hemorrhage, perforation (Fig. 16-22) with abscess formation, acute pancreatitis, and gallstone ileus. Gallbladder perforation results in localized simple or complex pericholecystic fluid collections that may be detected by CT or sonography.[34] Emphysematous cholecystitis is more accurately detected with CT.[35] CT is the modality of choice for gallstone ileus, but plain radiography may be highly suggestive if

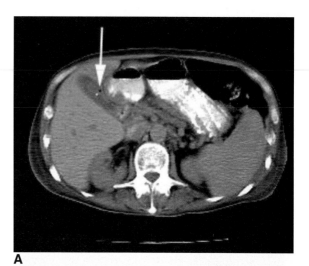

A

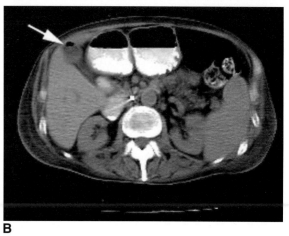

B

Fig. 16-21
Gas in gallbladder in acute cholecystitis. **A,** CT shows a small bubble of gas and a calcified calculus (*arrow*) within the thickened gallbladder. **B,** More gas is seen inferiorly (*arrow*).

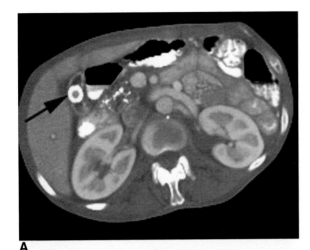

A

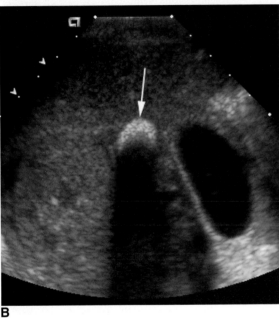

B

Fig. 16-22
Gallbladder perforation. **A,** Enhanced CT shows a calcified gallstone (*arrow*) in a normal gallbladder. **B,** Ultrasound scan 2 months later when the patient had right upper quadrant pain. The stone (*arrow*) has been extruded from the gallbladder, which is not thickened.

gas is seen in the biliary tree in the presence of small bowel obstruction.

Treatment of Acute Cholecystitis

The preferred treatment for acute calculous or acalculous cholecystitis has been open surgical or laparoscopic cholecystectomy. However, coexisting injuries or multisystem organ failure in the critical care patient may result in unacceptably high morbidity and mortality and preclude surgery. In the general population, mortality for surgical or laparoscopic cholecystectomy is less than 0.8% but in very sick patients increases to 14% to 30%.[36] This factor has led to the development of percutaneous cholecystostomy as both a therapeutic and diagnostic

tool for acute cholecystitis. Aspiration of bile from the gallbladder can produce a sample for bacteriologic evaluation and can decompress a tense gallbladder filled with inspissated sludge (see Fig. 16-13). These procedures can be performed at the bedside, using sonographic guidance and local anesthesia.

Percutaneous placement of a self-retaining drainage pigtail or balloon catheter can be achieved by a transhepatic (Fig. 16-23) or transperitoneal route. Either a "single stick" trocar catheter assembly (6–10 French) or

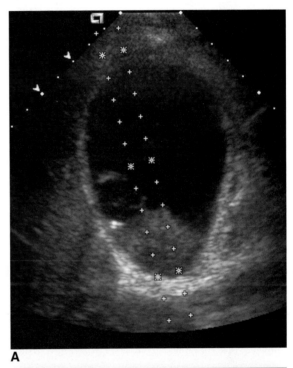

A

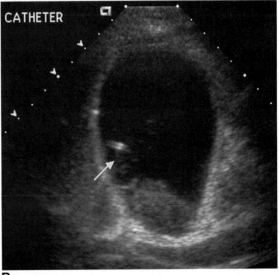

B

Fig. 16-23
Percutaneous cholecystostomy. **A,** Ultrasound guides (*vertical lines*) for catheter placement into a distended gallbladder containing sludge. **B,** Catheter (*arrow*) coiled in the gallbladder.

a Seldinger technique (starting with an 18- to 20-gauge needle) can be used. Coagulopathy should be corrected, and broad-spectrum antibiotics should be administered intravenously before or during the procedure. Intravenous sedation and systemic analgesia with additional local anesthesia are usually required. Imaging guidance depends on local preference and patient condition, but the procedure is most commonly performed using sonography, with CT being reserved for obese patients. Generally, a transhepatic route, avoiding pleura and colon, is selected. Traversing liver tissue usually assists with immobilization of the catheter and avoids a bile leak into the peritoneal cavity. However, some centers have adopted a transperitoneal approach.[37] The needle or catheter assembly is advanced under real-time guidance into the gallbladder, and bile is aspirated for culture. The catheter is coiled in the gallbladder and fixed to the skin. The gallbladder is manually decompressed. Catheters should be kept in situ for a minimum of 10 days to allow a tract to form and prevent bile leakage upon catheter removal. Prior to removal of the drainage tube, a cholangiogram should be performed to ensure patency of the cystic and common bile ducts. Patients with calculous cholecystitis will eventually need a cholecystectomy when improved or may undergo dissolution therapy or percutaneous stone removal if appropriate.[38]

Patients with acalculous cholecystitis typically improve within 1 to 12 hours, and the majority will do so within 48 hours.[39,40] Response rates in ICU patients (55% to 59%) are lower than those in mixed populations (73% to 90%).[36,37,40] In one series of 24 patients with selection criteria of unexplained sepsis and a distended gallbladder on sonography, there was a 58% response rate to a trial of percutaneous cholecystostomy, despite negative bile cultures in 10 of the 14 patients who had a favorable clinical response.[41] No serious complications occurred in this series, although two minimal bile leaks developed on removal of the tubes after 10 days.

Technical success rates for percutaneous catheter drainage are very high, ranging from 97% to 100%.[36,39] Complication rates range from as low as 2% to 25% in some series.[36,37,42] Procedure-related mortality rates are lower than those for open cholecystectomies.[43] These deaths have largely been due to hemorrhage from liver lacerations and exacerbation of sepsis.[36,43] Morbidity from the procedure includes bile leaks, tube dislodgement, sepsis, hemorrhage, and incorrect tube placement in the colon.[36,43] In one series, use of a transperitoneal route for drainage was not associated with an increase in complications.[37]

Failure to respond may be due to either an inaccurate diagnosis of acute cholecystitis or a coexisting disease or may indicate gangrene of the gallbladder wall with perforation (Fig. 16-24). This last group of patients will

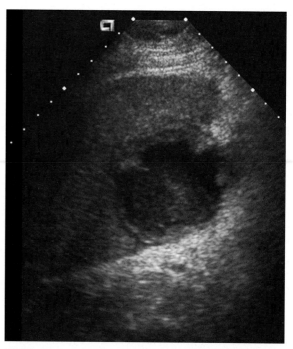

Fig. 16-24
Failure of response to percutaneous cholecystostomy. Irregular, thick-walled gallbladder with sludge. Same patient as Fig. 16-12.

require surgical cholecystectomy. Focal pericholecystic fluid, a sign of focal perforation, correlates with a lack of response to percutaneous drainage.[44] In a series by England et al.,[36] which was not limited to critical care patients and included both calculous and acalculous cholecystitis, pain and tenderness in the right upper quadrant and gallstones with pericholecystic fluid correlated with a favorable clinical response to drainage. Clearly, pain and tenderness may not be elicited in ventilated ICU patients and are poor predictors in this group. Favorable response rates did not appear to correlate with positive bile cultures but did rise with an increased number of radiologic signs.[35] Indeed, percutaneous aspiration and culture have been reported to be less than 50% sensitive for the diagnosis of acalculous cholecystitis.[27,45]

Another approach to the management of acute acalculous cholecystitis has been percutaneous aspiration alone. In a series of noncritically ill but high-risk patients, both aspiration and cholecystostomy drainage achieved success rates of 97%.[46] More patients responded in the drainage group, but this was not statistically significant, and a 12% complication rate occurred after drainage, compared with none after aspiration alone. Aspiration is less expensive and better tolerated but may not be technically possible when the bile is very viscid. Patients who fail to respond within 48 hours can then undergo catheter drainage.

GASTROINTESTINAL TRACT PATHOLOGY
Pseudomembranous Colitis

Pseudomembranous colitis (PMC) and other types of antibiotic-associated diarrhea are increasing in incidence secondary to the widespread use of antibiotics. The normal colonic flora is disrupted, resulting in an overgrowth of pathogens causing an acute colitis. The most common organism is *Clostridium difficile* accounting for 90% to 99% of antibiotic-associated colitis.[47] *C. difficile* produces watery diarrhea, fever, abdominal pain, and leucocytosis and is a significant cause of infection in critically ill patients. Atypical presentations include a picture simulating an acute abdomen in 5% to 20% of patients, potentially leading to unnecessary laparotomy.[47]

Antibiotics given orally have the greatest propensity to cause PMC, but intravenous and topical antibiotics have also been implicated. Typically, these are broad-spectrum antibiotics; however, nearly all types of antibiotics can be involved. Abdominal surgery is also reported as an additional risk factor. Complications include toxic megacolon, perforation, peritonitis, sepsis, renal failure, and metabolic disturbances. Mortality from toxic megacolon and perforation ranges from 2% to 8%.[48]

The diagnosis of PMC is made from a combination of the clinical picture, positive stool cultures, *C. difficile* toxin in the stool, and the finding of pseudomembranes at colonoscopy. The diagnosis may be suggested by the plain radiographic findings of colonic distension and wall thickening with thumbprinting (Figs. 16-25 and 16-26). Associated small bowel ileus is not uncommon. However, these are all nonspecific findings and may be insensitive. Serial films are very useful for evaluation of response to therapy or deterioration in clinical status. Abdominal radiography may reveal polypoidal mucosal thickening, toxic megacolon, perforation, or pneumatosis. Contrast enema studies show the nodular plaques of inflamed mucosa (Fig. 16-27) but are to be avoided because of the risk for perforation in severe infection. Furthermore, the findings are nonspecific, and these patients may not be able to tolerate the procedure.

CT is commonly used as a screening test in undiagnosed sepsis and may show bowel abnormalities suggesting previously unsuspected PMC. The major findings in PMC are colonic wall thickening (>3 mm) (Fig. 16-28) with pronounced mucosal enhancement.[49] The juxtaposition of the edematous low-density submucosa and the enhanced mucosa in cross section results in a "target" sign. Trapping of oral contrast between the thick haustral folds results in alternating high- and low-density bands and is known as the "accordion" sign[49] (Fig. 16-29). The accordion sign has not proved to be specific for PMC and has been detected in cirrhosis with severe colonic edema, other infectious colitides, and ischemic colitis.[50] PMC

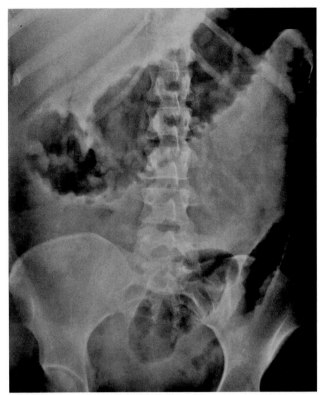

Fig. 16-25
Toxic megacolon and thumbprinting. Note the colonic distension and the nodular mucosa.

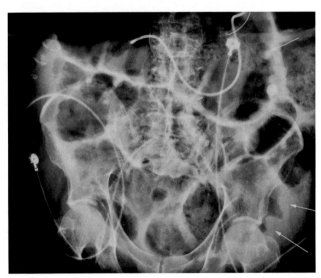

Fig. 16-26
Pseudomembranous colitis. Plain abdominal film shows colonic dilatation with mucosal thickening and "thumbprinting" (*arrows*), especially in the sigmoid colon.

can involve the whole colon or may be segmental, with sparing of the rectum. Pericolonic stranding and ascites are additional findings. On CT, increasing thickness of the colonic wall and ascites are poor prognostic signs.[51] CT has a sensitivity of 70%, a specificity of 93%, and a positive predictive value of 88%.[52] If the CT is suggestive,

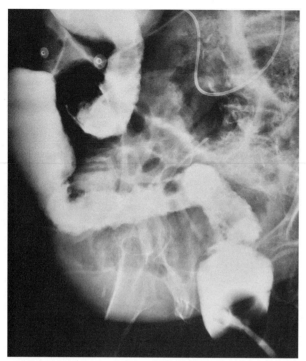

Fig. 16-27
Pseudomembranous colitis. Contrast enema demonstrates diffuse mucosal abnormality with a shaggy contour.

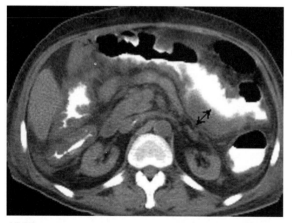

Fig. 16-28
Pseudomembranous colitis. Unenhanced CT demonstrating the thickened colon, most markedly the distal transverse colon (*two-headed arrow*).

some authors advocate starting antibiotic treatment before results of stool assays.[52] However, CT may be normal in up to 39% of patients with PMC.[53]

Radiologic evaluation is of major use in the detection of complications, such as perforation, that are treated surgically. No CT criteria have been able to separate patients that require surgery from the nonsurgical group.[54] Sonography is not used widely for this diagno-

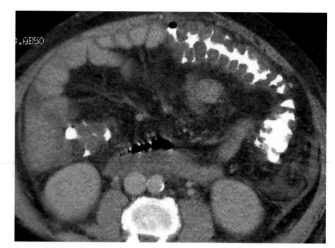

Fig. 16-29
Pseudomembranous colitis. Unenhanced CT demonstrating the "accordion sign" of thickened mucosa protruding into the colonic lumen with intervening contrast.

sis in the United States but may show wall thickening and effacement of the bowel lumen.[55,56]

The differential diagnosis of PMC includes colitis from any other cause, including granulomatous drug-mediated inflammatory bowel disease, ischemic colitis, or acute bacterial or viral infection (e.g., cytomegalovirus). Metronidazole is the first-line drug for treatment of PMC, with vancomycin being reserved for failure of response or for early pregnancy.

Hemorrhage and Gastrointestinal Bleeding

Bleeding may originate in the gastrointestinal tract or may occur in the retroperitoneum, abdominal wall, or peritoneal cavity. Spontaneous nongastrointestinal hemorrhage is usually related to a bleeding diathesis or anticoagulation. In the acute setting, hemorrhage may be detected on unenhanced CT as a hyperattenuating collection, such as in the psoas or rectus muscles (Fig. 16-30), intraperitoneal hemorrhage, or as high density intraperitoneal fluid. Dynamic arterial phase–enhanced scans can show the bleeding vessel and provide useful information for subsequent angiography and embolization.

Stress-related mucosal damage from splanchnic hypoperfusion is the most common cause of gastrointestinal bleeding in patients being ventilated. Endoscopic abnormalities are detected in 74% to 100% of patients receiving mechanical ventilation within 24 hours of admission to the ICU. Mucosal damage produces detectable bleeding in up to 25% of cases, of which 5% are clinically significant.[8] Contributory factors include decreased cardiac output, increased vascular resistance, and splanchnic hypoperfusion.[8] Effects are most prominent in the fundus and body of the stomach, causing gastritis and gastric ulcers. The distal esophagus, antrum, and duodenum

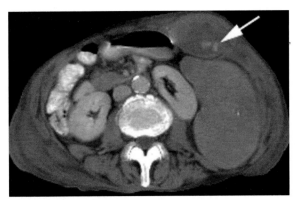

Fig. 16-30
Spontaneous bleeding into the rectus muscle. Enhanced CT shows a bleeding vessel (*arrow*) and hematoma in the left rectus abdominis.

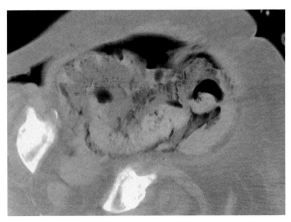

Fig. 16-31
Perforated, necrotic bowel. Enhanced CT shows widespread pneumatosis intestinalis with pneumoperitoneum.

may also be involved. Endoscopy is the diagnostic method of choice, although plain radiographs and contrast studies are of value if perforation is suspected. Cross-sectional imaging is of limited use in the evaluation of acute gastrointestinal bleeding. Prophylaxis contributes significantly to decreased morbidity and mortality. Nuclear scintigraphy with Tc 99m–labeled red cells is highly sensitive and can detect bleeding rates as low as 0.1 ml/min[57] (see Chapter 13) Angiography is of value both for diagnosis and immediate treatment with embolization or vasoconstrictors (see Chapter 12).

Perforation

Perforation of a viscus may be secondary to such entities as stress ulcers, duodenal ulcers, infarcted bowel, closed loop obstruction, or diverticulitis. Plain abdominal radiographs with erect or decubitus views are the first-line imaging choice for the detection of perforation. However, small amounts of free intraperitoneal gas may be missed on abdominal radiography, particularly if erect and decubitus films are suboptimal or cannot be performed. CT is highly sensitive and superior to radiography for the detection of free gas and is the modality of choice when patients have signs of peritonitis[58-60] (Fig. 16-31). The exact source of the perforation may be difficult to establish, but signs of local inflammation, such as fluid, extraluminal gas, and infiltration, may suggest the origin[60] (Fig. 16-32).

Paralytic Ileus

Paralytic or adynamic ileus results from loss of peristalsis of the gut, with distension of the entire gastrointestinal tract from stomach to colon. This most commonly occurs in the week following abdominal surgery but may also result from narcotic and anticholinergic medications, generalized or abdominal sepsis, trauma, and electrolyte imbalance.[8,61] Nearly 50% of patents with respiratory

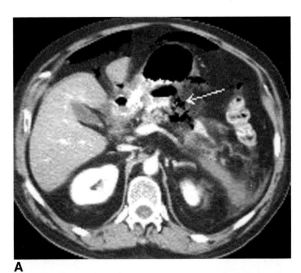

A

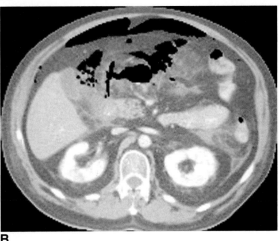

B

Fig. 16-32
Perforated duodenal ulcer. **A**, Enhanced CT shows pneumoperitoneum anteriorly, secondary to a perforated duodenal ulcer. Gas and oral contrast in the lesser sac (*arrow*) indicate the location of the perforation. **B**, CT at extended window levels better shows the free intraperitoneal gas.

failure develop paralytic ileus.[8] Patients typically develop a distended abdomen with few bowel sounds, intolerance to enteral feeds, and increased nasogastric tube output.

Imaging reveals distension of the stomach and the small and large bowel with air-fluid levels on radiographs obtained in the erect or decubitus position (see Fig. 16-6). This appearance can be distinguished from true obstruction by the pattern of distension and lack of a transition point on abdominal radiographs obtained in the supine, decubitus, or prone positions. Differential air-fluid levels (air-fluid levels at different vertical heights) on erect views or a width of an air-fluid level greater than 25 mm suggest obstruction rather than ileus.[62] CT is superior to plain radiographs in differentiating postoperative ileus from small bowel obstruction[63] (Fig. 16-33). CT was found to be 100% sensitive and specific in a series of 36 patients evaluated within 10 days of laparotomy.[63] In the same group, the sensitivity of plain radiographs was 19%.[63] Contrast studies may occasionally be required to exclude a partial small bowel or distal colonic obstruction.

Isolated colonic ileus (distension without obstruction), also commonly known as pseudo-obstruction or Ogilvie's syndrome, represents colonic atony secondary to an imbalance between sympathetic and parasympathetic stimulation. This condition is a variant of adynamic ileus confined to the colon, where persistent peristalsis within the small intestine may produce increased bowel sounds suggestive of obstruction. Risk factors include recent surgery or abdominal trauma, sepsis, shock, metabolic abnormalities, and steroid use. Plain radiographs may be inconclusive, but the presence of rectal gas and colonic distension suggests the diagnosis (Fig. 16-34). Prone radiographs, if feasible, may be

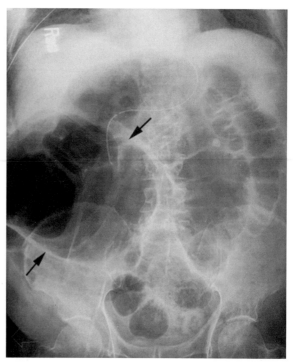

Fig. 16-34
Ogilvie's syndrome. Plain abdominal film shows pancolonic distension with more pronounced dilatation of the cecum (*arrows*). Colonic decompression was performed.

helpful in the exclusion of colonic obstruction by allowing gas to move into the rectum. Serial assessment with abdominal radiographs can detect an enlarging cecum, which puts the patient at risk for perforation when it becomes larger than 10 cm.[64] Contrast studies and CT can be used to confirm the lack of obstruction or evaluate for complications such as perforation and infarction.

Bowel Obstruction

Bowel dilatation in ICU patients may be secondary to obstruction. The most common cause (50% of cases) of bowel obstruction is adhesions.[65] Other causes include internal and external hernias (15% of cases) (Figs. 16-35 and 16-36), neoplasms (15% of cases), abscesses, gallstone ileus, intussusception, and inflammatory conditions. Bowel obstruction is traditionally evaluated with erect and supine abdominal radiographs. Small bowel loops greater than 2.5 cm in width are considered distended. Differential air-fluid levels greater than 20 mm or a mean width of an air-fluid level greater than 25 mm on an erect projection are most predictive of higher grades of small bowel obstruction.[62,66] In the ventilated or paralyzed patient who cannot be elevated, decubitus films can be substituted for the erect view but are technically less satisfactory. Plain radiographs are diagnostic in 50% to 60% of patients and equivocal in another 20% to

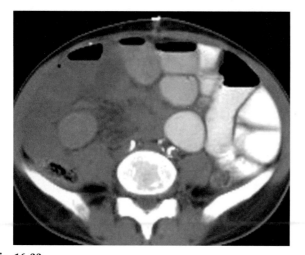

Fig. 16-33
Postoperative adynamic ileus. There is dilatation of the small bowel and lack of a transition zone on CT.

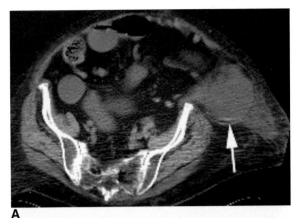

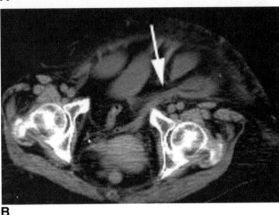

Fig. 16-35
Strangulated inguinal hernia. **A,** CT of the hernia sac containing fluid with a debris level (*arrow*). The bowel was gangrenous at surgery. **B,** CT of the neck of the hernia (*arrow*) with two adjacent collapsed loops. The proximal bowel is dilated.

30%.[65] While enteroclysis is often considered the study of choice, it is not feasible in ICU patients. CT has been found superior to plain radiographs in the diagnosis of small bowel obstruction, but abdominal radiography may still be used to screen patients for further workup.[63] CT scans can be performed with or without enteric contrast. Fluid-filled bowel loops provide excellent intrinsic contrast and obviate the need for enteric contrast. Furthermore, enteric contrast may obscure intramural hemorrhage due to small bowel ischemia. Intravenous contrast is, however, essential for the evaluation of bowel wall perfusion and patency of major vessels. CT can accurately show the presence, cause, and level of obstruction, as well as the presence of secondary changes such as bowel wall thickening and mesenteric stranding or fluid and major complications such as perforation or strangulation.[67-70]

Bowel obstruction can be simple or incarcerated (closed-loop). In simple obstruction, the diagnostic features are a dilated bowel with a transition zone into normal caliber or decompressed bowel. The transition zone should be carefully examined to determine the level and cause of obstruction. Pathologic entities such as internal and external hernias, masses, abscesses, gallstone ileus, and intussusception are well demonstrated by CT. The absence of such a definitive cause or the finding of angulated or beaklike loops suggests adhesions as the cause[67] (Fig. 16-37).

Closed-loop obstructions produce a dilated, U-shaped, fluid-filled loop of bowel with a radial distribution of mesenteric vessels in the concavity of the loop. At the apex of the closed loop, there are two collapsed adjacent loops (see Fig. 16-35, *B*) and a beak or whirl sign.[71] Incarceration of the bowel predisposes to strangulation. Plain radiographs are of little value in the diagnosis of ischemia, but CT is 90% to 96% sensitive for the diagnosis.[72,73] CT signs include bowel wall thickening with a target appearance from submucosal edema, increased wall density from hemorrhage on unenhanced scans, decreased or absent enhancement compared with adjacent normal loops (Fig. 16-38), and congestion of mesenteric veins.[71-73] Ischemia may progress to infarction with pneumatosis intestinalis and portal venous gas[72] (Figs. 16-39 and 16-40). Secondary hemorrhage into the lumen may be seen as well as stranding and fluid in the mesentery or peritoneal cavity.[60,65] The high specificity of enhanced helical CT without enteric contrast (93%) and the negative predictive value of 99% support its use in this clinical setting.[73]

CT has a high sensitivity of 90% to 100% and an accuracy of 90% to 95% for the diagnosis of high-grade or complete small bowel obstruction.[60,63,67,68,70] In low-grade obstruction, the sensitivity of CT drops to 48%.[74] Prior gut decompression with nasogastric suction or lack of a distinct transition zone decreases sensitivity. Another diagnostic pitfall is the presence of gas and fluid-filled ascending and transverse colon and collapsed descending colon, which is often seen in adynamic ileus and should not be diagnosed as colonic obstruction unless there is definite splenic flexure pathology.[67] Fluoroscopic contrast studies are useful in this situation. Patients from the ICU who are postoperative or who have signs of abdominal inflammation should undergo CT examination for a suspected diagnosis of small bowel obstruction.[75]

Mesenteric Thrombosis

Thrombosis of either the mesenteric arteries or venous system may occur in the intensive care unit setting. In the posttraumatic or postsurgical state, hypotension, hypovolemia, and preexisting circulatory disease may contribute to the onset of this acute complication. Mesenteric arterial thrombosis is most often seen in the superior mesenteric artery (SMA) territory. Patients commonly have underlying disseminated atherosclerotic disease with preexisting stenosis of the SMA. The onset of arterial thrombosis is usually characterized by a sudden

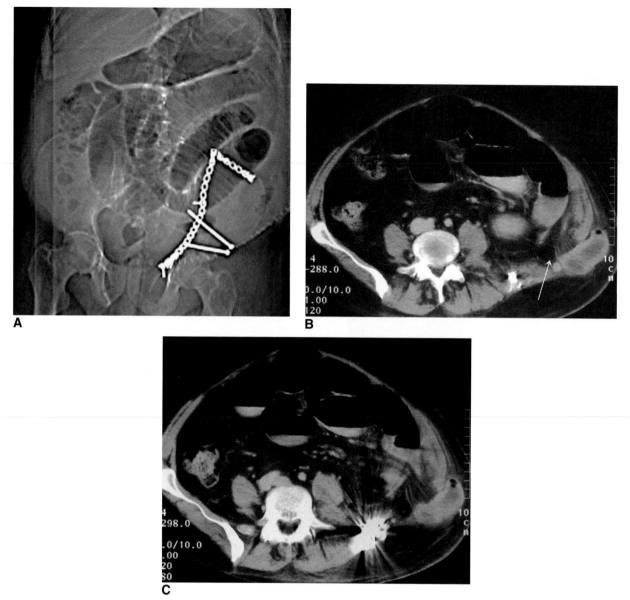

Fig. 16-36
Iatrogenic lumbar hernia. Abdominal distension 2 weeks after pinning of a pelvic fracture. **A,** The scout view from the CT shows proximal small bowel dilatation. **B,** There is a peritoneal defect in the lateral abdominal wall through which the small bowel has herniated (*arrow*). There is bowel thickening, but it was viable at surgery. **C,** Lumbar defect with herniation of the bowel.

onset or increase in generalized abdominal pain, abdominal wall tenderness, paralytic ileus, elevated white cell count, or metabolic acidosis. Superior mesenteric artery thrombosis is treated surgically, and early diagnosis is essential. In untreated SMA thrombosis, extensive bowel ischemia may progress to bowel infarction that is likely to be fatal if untreated.[76] Mesenteric venous thrombosis is more indolent at onset but otherwise shares many of the clinical features of arterial mesenteric thrombosis; it is more likely to occur in hypercoagulable states.[76]

Mesenteric vein thrombosis may, on occasion, lead to infarction of the bowel also.

Plain radiographs may show dilation of the affected small bowel or colon, with mucosal edema leading to a thick-walled appearance or "thumbprinting." CT imaging with dynamic contrast enhancement is the most appropriate imaging investigation in suspected mesenteric arterial or venous thrombosis. Oral contrast is often unnecessary, because fluid is usually present within the bowel lumen secondary to the thrombosis and the

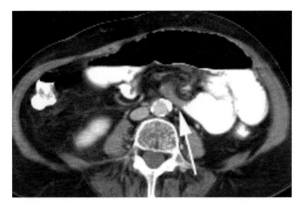

Fig. 16-37
Adhesive small bowel obstruction. CT shows a transition zone to the left of midline (*arrow*) with beaking of the small bowel secondary to adhesions.

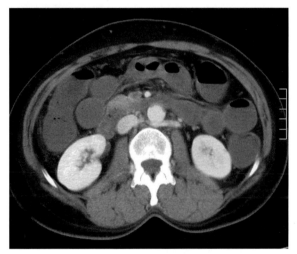

Fig. 16-38
A 44-year-old patient with aortic dissection and small bowel ischemia. There is small bowel dilatation and poor mural enhancement, especially in the right-sided loops.

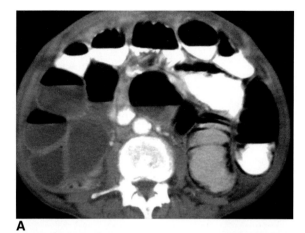

A

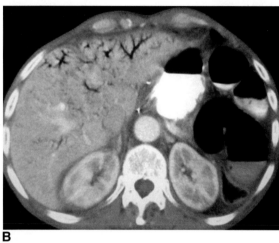

B

Fig. 16-39
Small bowel infarction. **A**, Infarcted small bowel with dilatation and pneumatosis. **B**, Portal venous gas in the liver. Note the peripheral-branching low density, a distinguishing feature from biliary gas, which tends to be more central.

ensuing ileus. Absence of contrast within the arterial branches and poor or nonenhancement of the bowel wall are indicative of arterial thrombosis (see Fig. 16-38). Pneumatosis or gas within the mesenteric or hepatic blood vessels usually indicates the presence of bowel necrosis and/or gangrene[77] (see Figs. 16-39 and 16-40). In mesenteric venous thrombosis, thrombus may be identified within the superior mesenteric vein or its main branches (Fig. 16-41). Bowel wall thickening or mesenteric edema may also be present.[78] Severe infection of the gastrointestinal tract (most often acute appendicitis or diverticulitis) may cause septic thrombosis of the mesenteric and portal veins, which carries a high mortality if untreated. In addition to mesenteric vein thrombus, CT may demonstrate intraabdominal abscess formation and gas in the mesenteric veins, portal vein, and liver. Infection may seed the liver with resultant abscess formation.[79]

Shock Bowel

Shock bowel describes the generalized abnormality noted within the small bowel in patients who have undergone sustained periods of systemic hypotension with resultant hypoperfusion of the bowel and secondary ischemic changes.[80,81] This typically occurs in the setting of major trauma or other causes of major acute blood loss. Manifestations on CT typically include dilated, fluid-filled loops of bowel that have thickened walls (Fig. 16-42), and increased contrast enhancement of the bowel wall is usually noted.[81] The findings are usually confined to the small bowel, with sparing of the stomach and colon. Associated CT features of hypoperfusion are diminished calibers of the aorta and inferior vena cava (see Fig. 16-42). Diffuse bowel wall thickening from shock bowel may persist and be detected in the ICU setting after the patient has been resuscitated and circulating blood volume has been restored. Shock bowel should be

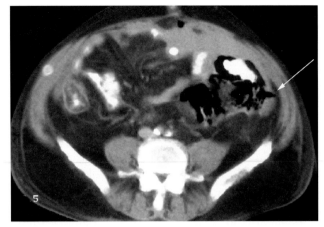

Fig. 16-40
Colonic infarction with perforation. Pelvic CT shows a thickened sigmoid colon with pneumatosis and focal perforation (*arrow*).

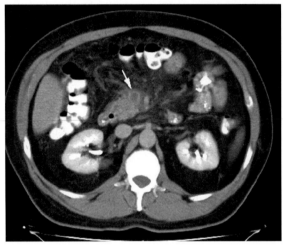

Fig. 16-41
Idiopathic superior mesenteric vein thrombosis in a 54-year-old patient with abdominal pain. The superior mesenteric vein is distended with intraluminal thrombus (*arrow*). There are perivascular inflammatory changes in the mesentery.

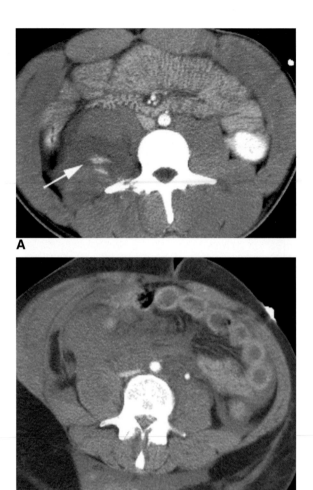

Fig. 16-42
Shock bowel. **A**, There is pronounced small bowel wall thickening. Active bleeding (*arrow*) is seen in the right paravertebral area from a transverse process fracture. **B**, The inferior vena cava and aorta are small, secondary to volume loss. Marked small bowel enhancement is also seen.

differentiated from other causes of bowel wall thickening, such as infection or hemorrhage. Typically, hemorrhage is not as diffusely distributed as shock bowel. The findings of shock bowel are usually reversible, with restoration of normal bowel appearance on CT over time.

Acute Pancreatitis

Patients in the critical care unit may be more susceptible to developing acute pancreatitis because of drug therapy and mechanical ventilation.[8] Acute pancreatitis has a variable clinical course but may be a cause of serious morbidity and mortality, with death occurring in approximately 10% of all cases. Complications of acute pancre-

atitis include pancreatic necrosis, abscess formation, acute renal failure, respiratory distress syndrome, septicemia, metabolic acidosis, disseminated intravascular coagulation, or hypotension.

Imaging studies may be initially directed to the detection of underlying etiologic factors such as gallstones or biliary obstruction, and sonography is frequently used for this purpose. The pancreas may appear enlarged and diffusely hypoechoic. Peripancreatic edema and fluid collections may also be detected with sonography.[82] Unfortunately, in the setting of acute pancreatic inflammation, the pancreas and its surrounding tissues are often inadequately imaged by sonography because of obesity or the presence of paralytic ileus and excessive bowel gas. Therefore, evaluation of clinically severe acute pancreatitis or detection of related complications is best achieved with enhanced CT. This requires transfer of the patient to the CT scanner suite, but no bedside test can reliably detect important complications such as pancreatic necrosis, peripancreatic fluid collections or pseudocysts (Fig. 16-43, A), and abscess formation. Infected pancreatic necrosis and abscess formation are serious complications that have high associated mortality rates and may require percutaneous or surgical drainage. Fluid collections arising from the pancreas spread most commonly into the lesser sac, transverse mesocolon, and anterior pararenal spaces but may also migrate far from the pancreas; therefore, the patient should be scanned from the chest through the pelvis. No imaging criteria are specific for superinfection of necrosis or fluid collections, though the presence of gas bubbles within fluid is suspicious. Percutaneous needle aspiration of fluid under ultrasound or CT guidance is recommended to reliably detect infected fluid and, if practical, imaging-guided drainage may be undertaken also. The presence of a hemorrhagic fluid collection in severe acute pancreatitis is a concern because of the possible development of a pseudoaneurysm of the gastroduodenal or splenic artery (Fig. 16-43). This rare complication occurs because of erosion of vessel walls by pancreatic enzymes and, if left untreated, is associated with a high mortality.[83] Enhanced CT with a good contrast bolus or Doppler ultrasound of fluid collections allows differentiation of a pseudoaneurysm from other fluid collections in acute pancreatitis. Angiographic embolization allows a minimally invasive and effective means of repair that avoids open surgery.

GENITOURINARY
Acute Pyelonephritis

In the ICU, patients are at increased risk for renal infection because of the use of urinary catheters for bladder drainage. Infection of the lower urinary tract may subsequently extend to the kidney. Seeding of infection into the kidney may also occur as a result of systemic bacteremia. The symptoms of renal infection may be less easily identified if the patient has suffered major trauma or is sedated and the diagnosis depends on urine analysis and microbiologic culture. In pyelonephritis, the kidney is often normal in appearance but may be enlarged. The process may be unilateral or bilateral. Sonography at the bedside may show renal swelling with diffuse or focal regions of decreased or increased echogenicity, and hydronephrosis may be present.[84,85] On enhanced CT, single or multiple round or wedge-shaped areas of poorly enhancing tissue can be seen within the enlarged kidney[86] (Fig. 16-44). In severe cases, renal abscess may develop, and perinephric spread of infection may occur. These complications are best imaged with enhanced CT.[87]

Acute Renal Failure

Patients in the ICU frequently develop acute renal failure (ARF) as a complication of major underlying pathologies. These pathologies include the common prerenal causes of hypotension and hypovolemia after major trauma or surgery and intrarenal causes such as acute tubular necrosis secondary to medications or rhabdomyolysis.[88] Such factors may exacerbate underlying chronic renal insufficiency, and intravenous or intraarterial iodinated contrast may have a similar effect (Fig. 16-45).

Postrenal failure is caused by urinary tract obstruction and is potentially the most treatable form of ARF. Causes

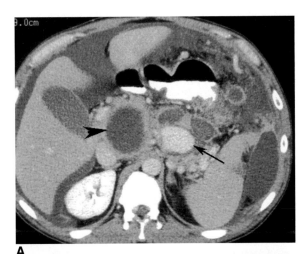

A

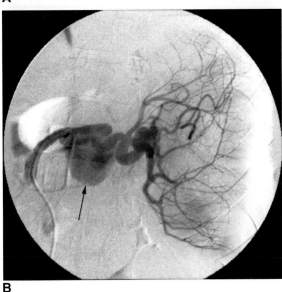

B

Fig. 16-43
Acute pancreatitis. **A,** Enhanced CT demonstrating multiple fluid collections within the pancreatic head and body (*arrowhead*). There is peripancreatic stranding and ascites. There is a rounded vascular structure (*arrow*) posterior to the pancreatic body, corresponding to a splenic artery pseudoaneurysm. **B,** Corresponding arteriogram confirming the pseudoaneurysm (*arrow*).

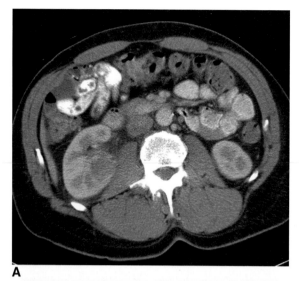

A

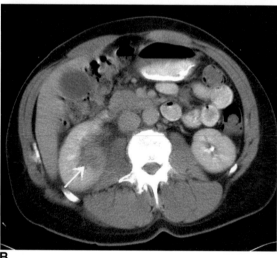

B

Fig. 16-44
Acute pyelonephritis. 46-year-old patient with fever, pyuria, and right flank pain. **A**, Enhanced CT in corticomedullary phase. The right kidney is enlarged, and there is a focal hypoattenuating area in the medial aspect. Perinephric stranding is also present. **B**, On excretory-phase images there is persistent poor enhancement of the area of focal acute pyelonephritis (*arrow*).

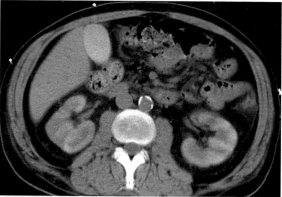

Fig. 16-45
Contrast nephropathy. CT performed without intravenous contrast 2 days after cardiac catheterization. There is retention of contrast in the renal cortices in a patchy distribution without excretion. There is vicarious excretion of contrast into the gallbladder.

include bilateral ureteric or bladder outlet obstruction, and patients with urinary stone disease or recent pelvic trauma or major pelvic surgery are at increased risk. Abdominal radiographs may allow detection of more than 90% of urinary stones, but sonography at the bedside is the imaging investigation of choice to look for dilation of the renal collection systems, ureters, or bladder and to discover the presence of renal stones. If obstruction of the ureters is detected, sonography may be used to guide percutaneous nephrostomy drainage at the bedside if necessary.

Specific prerenal causes of ARF, such as thrombosis of the renal arteries or veins, may be detected by the use of

sonography.[89] The kidneys are often diffusely enlarged (>12 cm length), and Doppler ultrasound may demonstrate absence of flow and specific spectral waveform features. Even where no acute cause for renal failure is demonstrable, sonography may be of value in the detection of underlying chronic renal failure. Findings such as small kidney size (<9 cm length), cortical thinning, and diffuse hyperechoic cortical echo texture are likely to reflect longstanding renal dysfunction.

NON-ORGAN-SPECIFIC PATHOLOGY
Abscess Formation

Patients who are admitted to the intensive care unit following major trauma are at risk for abscess formation from several causes. Hematoma, tissue necrosis, organ perforation, pulmonary laceration, or aspiration pneumonia may all lead to the development of abscess formation. Contamination of the peritoneum during emergent surgical procedures is another important etiology. Clinical features include fever, tachycardia, metabolic acidosis, or elevated white cell count. Imaging evaluation is best performed with CT scanning following the administration of both oral and nonionic intravenous iodinated contrast.[90] The necessity of oral contrast administration to differentiate normal bowel from focal fluid collections such as abscess should be emphasized. Signs of abscess formation on CT include low-attenuation fluid collections with thick enhancing walls, often with surrounding inflammatory reaction in the connective tissues. Gas may be present within the abscess because of the growth of gas-forming organisms (Figs. 16-46 to 16-48). These signs are not always present, and gas also may be present in the setting of noninfected tissue necrosis.

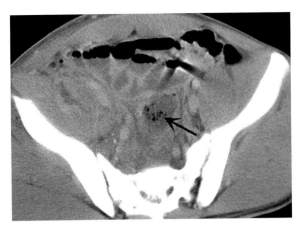

Fig. 16-46
Abscess. CT scan of pelvic fluid collection containing gas (*arrow*).

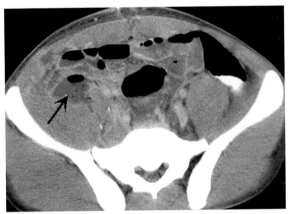

Fig. 16-47
Abscess. CT scan of fluid collection containing gas (*arrow*) in the right iliopsoas muscle.

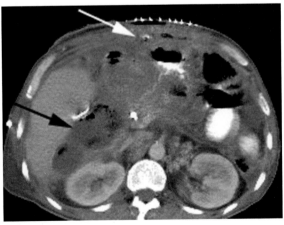

Fig. 16-48
Abscess and enteric leak. Enhanced CT of an abscess (*black arrow*) in Morison's pouch containing gas bubbles. There is also a subfascial collection of contrast (*white arrow*) from an enteric leak.

Sonographic examination at the bedside may be appropriate where a more focal source of infection is suspected, for example, acalculous cholecystitis or empyema. Abscess formation is variable in appearance on sonography, which may reveal a collection containing anechoic, hypoechoic, or complex-appearing fluid. Abscesses may have a very echogenic appearance if the contents are semisolid or contain gas. The bowel may appear similar and may be differentiated from a gas-containing abscess by the presence of peristalsis. Unfortunately sonography is less reliable than CT for abscess diagnosis and is usually ineffective in evaluating the entire abdomen because of the inability to image gas-filled bowel. If a suspicious fluid collection is identified on CT or sonographic imaging, fluid aspiration and, if appropriate, catheter drainage may often be possible at the bedside, using sonographic guidance.[91]

Drainage Techniques. Gallbladder drainage for suspected acute (usually acalculous) cholecystitis is one of the most commonly performed percutaneous interventions in the ICU patient and has been addressed earlier in this chapter. In general, drainage procedures may be performed using sonographic or CT guidance. Sonography has the major advantage of being portable, thereby allowing percutaneous procedures to be performed at the bedside in the ICU.[91,92] Sonography also allows real-time imaging during aspiration needle or catheter placement, of great importance if the target lesion or adjacent organs move during the procedure because of patient inability to suspend respiration. Catheter drainage may require intravenous conscious sedation for pain management, although this may impair patient cooperation during the procedure. Sonography can be used only if the fluid collection and the access pathway for percutaneous catheter placement are clearly visible. Many sonographic scanners have needle guide attachments that allow easier visualization of the aspiration needle or catheter during insertion and are recommended for all but very large or superficial targets[93] (see Fig. 16-23, *A*). Broad-spectrum antibiotics are usually given prior to catheter drainage of an abscess to reduce the risk for septicemia.

Catheter insertion may be performed as a single-step trocar technique for very large or superficial targets, but for all other situations, the authors favor a multistep Seldinger technique, with initial aspiration needle placement under direct sonographic guidance, followed by guidewire, dilator, and catheter placement as multiple, separate steps. Following completion of each step, the guidewire, dilator, and catheter positions may be easily checked by sonography. Catheter size selection depends upon the nature of the fluid being aspirated—thin fluid may be drained effectively with an 8 French diameter catheter, whereas more viscous fluid (e.g., thick, purulent fluid) usually requires a 12 to 14 French drain. Important catheter management includes regular irrigation of the catheter at least twice daily with a brisk injection of 10 ml of normal saline. The purpose of irrigation is to prevent blocking of the catheter lumen and side holes, a frequent cause for failure of percutaneous catheter drainage. Irrigation must be maintained until drainage is judged to be successful, usually by follow-up imaging with sonography or CT. Complications associated with sonographic-guided catheter drainage include inadvertent transgression of the bowel, contamination of a noninfected collection, bacteremia, hemorrhage, and pneumothorax.[94] Persistent high volume drainage through a

catheter is suggestive of the presence of a fistula between the fluid collection and adjacent bowel.

CT may be a superior guidance technique for deep collections or those close to bowel gas, lung, or bone, but this technique requires transport of the critically ill patient to the CT scanner suite. Conventional CT does not allow for continuous imaging during interventional procedures, though CT fluoroscopy scanners that have real-time CT capability are now available in some centers.[95]

Deep Venous Thrombosis

The true incidence of deep venous thrombosis (DVT) in high-risk hospitalized patients is unknown but estimated to be as high as 30%.[96] In the ICU, prophylactic measures may be effective to reduce the risk for DVT in immobilized at-risk patients but are unlikely to abolish it. Deep venous thrombosis may be symptomatic or asympto-

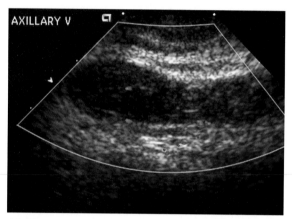

Fig. 16-49
Axillary vein thrombosis. Color Doppler image of an axillary vein that is distended with thrombus. There is minimal flow.

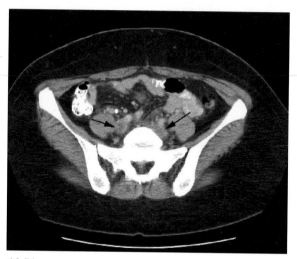

Fig. 16-51
Iliac vein thrombosis. Enhanced CT showing unsuspected bilateral iliac vein thrombus (*arrows*).

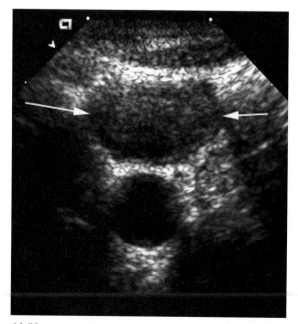

Fig. 16-50
Internal jugular vein thrombus. The internal jugular vein (*arrows*) is distended with intraluminal thrombus. It was noncompressible.

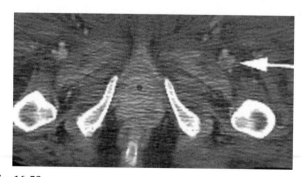

Fig. 16-52
Deep venous thrombosis. Enhanced CT in a ventilated patient with anasarca. There is a filling defect in the left common femoral vein (*arrow*).

matic. Typically, the symptomatic DVT causes occlusion of major lower limb deep veins, leading to pain, edema, or swelling of the affected limb. Asymptomatic DVT is often nonocclusive and clinically silent. Deep venous thrombosis may propagate from the calf vessels to the popliteal and femoral veins if untreated.[97] Upper limb DVT (Fig. 16-49) may also occur in association with central venous catheter placement, especially if the line becomes infected.

Doppler ultrasound, utilizing spontaneous color flow and graded compression techniques, is a sensitive test for the detection of DVT in the lower limb, though it is limited in evaluation of the adductor canal region and the area above the inguinal ligament.[96] On ultrasound, venous thrombus is typically an echogenic mass within the major veins, but it may be very hypoechoic or anechoic in its early phase, an appearance that simulates normal blood. Compression over the affected veins will fail to occlude the lumen when thrombus is present (Fig. 16-50), a reliable finding with sensitivity of 95% and specificity of 98% in the popliteal and femoral veins.[98] As is the case with all other ultrasound techniques, Doppler venous sonography can be readily performed in the ICU and may be easily repeated in the event of uncertain findings or recurrent symptoms. Because DVT in the iliac veins and inferior vena cava is more difficult to detect by sonography, patients at high risk or the suspicion of central DVT may be evaluated further by contrast-enhanced CT (Figs. 16-51 to 16-53) or MRI. In the authors' experience, it is not rare to encounter DVT in the deep pelvic veins or inferior vena cava as a serendipitous finding on enhanced CT studies performed for other reasons.

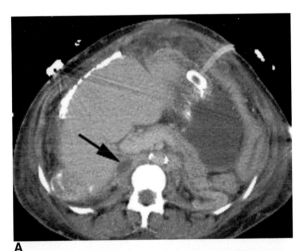

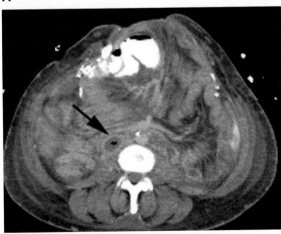

Fig. 16-53
Multisystem failure with venous access complications and extensive caval thrombosis. **A,** Enhanced CT shows a filling defect within the inferior vena cava. **B,** At a lower level there is gas within the clot from intravenous injection.

REFERENCES

1. Jones B, Fishman EK, Siegelman SS: Ischemic colitis demonstrated by computed tomography, *J Comput Assist Tomogr* 6:1120, 1982.
2. Heng Y, Schuffler MD, Haggitt RC, et al: Pneumatosis intestinalis: a review, *Am J Gastroenterol* 190:1747, 1995.
3. Federle MP, Chun G, Jeffrey RB, et al: Computed tomographic findings in bowel infarction, *AJR Am J Roentgenol* 142:91, 1984.
4. Kelvin FM, Korobkin M, Rauch RF, et al: Computed tomography of pneumatosis intestinalis, *J Comput Assist Tomogr* 8:276, 1984.
5. Teplick SK, Brandon JC, Shah HR, et al: Acute gastrointestinal disorders. In Goodman LR, Putnam CE, eds: *Critical care imaging*, ed 3, Philadelphia, 1992, WB Saunders.
6. Raunest J, Imhof M, Rauen U, et al: Acute cholecystitis: a complication in severely injured intensive care patients, *J Trauma* 32:433, 1992.
7. Prevot N, Mariat G, Mahul P, et al: Contribution of cholescintigraphy to the early diagnosis of acute acalculous cholecystitis in intensive-care-unit patients, *Eur J Nucl Med* 26:1317, 1999.
8. Mutlu GM, Mutlu EA, Factor P: GI complications in patients receiving mechanical ventilation, *Chest* 119:1222, 2001.
9. Marchal GJ, Casaer M, Baert AL, et al: Gallbladder wall sonolucency in acute cholecystitis, *Radiology* 133:429, 1979.
10. Herlin P, Jonsson PE, Karp W: Postoperative acute acalculous cholecystitis—an assessment of diagnostic procedures, *Gastrointest Radiol* 5:147, 1980.
11. Laing FC, Federle MP, Jeffrey RB, et al: Ultrasonic evaluation of patients with acute right upper quadrant pain, *Radiology* 140:449, 1981.
12. Ralls PW, Colletti PM, Lapin SA, et al: Real-time sonography in suspected acute cholecystitis: prospective evaluation of primary and secondary signs, *Radiology* 155:767, 1985.
13. Molenat F, Boussuges A, Valantin V, et al: Gallbladder abnormalities in medical ICU patients: an ultrasonographic study, *Intensive Care Med* 22:356, 1996.
14. Helbich TH, Mallek R, Madl C, et al: Sonomorphology of the gall bladder in critically ill patients: value of a scoring system and follow up examinations, *Acta Radiol* 38:129, 1997.
15. Boland GWL, Slater G, Lu DSK, et al: Prevalence and significance of gallbladder abnormalities seen on sonography in intensive care unit patients, *AJR Am J Roentgenol* 174:973, 2000.
16. Janowitz P, Kratzer W, Zemmler T, et al: Gallbladder sludge: spontaneous course and incidence of complications in patients without stones, *Hepatology* 20:291, 1994.
17. Jennings WC, Drabek GA, Miller KA: Significance of sludge and thickened wall in ultrasound evaluation of the gall bladder, *Surg, Gynecol Obstet* 147:394, 1992.

18. Brooke Jeffrey R, Somner FG: Follow-up sonography in suspected acalculous cholecystitis, *J Ultrasound Med* 4:183, 1993.

19. Samuels BI, Freitas JE, Bree RL, et al: A comparison of radionuclide hepatobiliary imaging and real-time ultrasound for the detection of acute cholecystitis, *Radiology* 147:207, 1983.

20. Aburano T, Yokoyama K, Taniguchi M, et al: Diagnostic values of gallbladder hyperperfusion and the rim sign in radionuclide angiography and hepatobiliary imaging, *Gastrointest Radiol* 15:229, 1990.

21. Drane WE, Nelp WB, Rudd TG: The need for routine delayed radionuclide hepatobiliary imaging in patients with intercurrent disease, *Radiology* 151:763, 1984.

22. Kim CK: Pharmacologic intervention for the diagnosis of acute cholecystitis: cholecystokinin pretreatment or morphine, or both? *J Nucl Med* 38:647, 1997.

23. Chen CC, Holder LE, Maunoury C, et al: Morphine augmentation increases gallbladder visualization in patients pretreated with cholecystokinin, *J Nucl Med* 38:644, 1997.

24. Flancbaum L, Choban PS, Sinha R, et al: Morphine cholescintigraphy in the evaluation of hospitalized patients with suspected acute cholecystitis, *Ann Surg* 220:25, 1994.

25. Shuman WP, Rogers JV, Rudd TG, et al: Low sensitivity of sonography and cholescintigraphy in acalculous cholecystitis, *AJR Am J Roentgenol* 142:531, 1984.

26. Mariat G, Mahul P, Prevot N, et al: Contribution of ultrasonography and cholescintigraphy to the diagnosis of acute acalculous cholecystitis in intensive care unit patients, *Intensive Care Med* 26:1658, 2000.

27. Mirvis SE, Vainwright JR, Nelson AW, et al: The diagnosis of acute acalculous cholecystitis: a comparison of sonography, scintigraphy, and CT, *AJR Am J Roentgenol* 147:1171, 1986.

28. Fidler J, Paulson EK, Layfield L: CT evaluation of acute cholecystitis: findings and usefulness in diagnosis, *AJR Am J Roentgenol* 166:1085, 1996.

29. Blankenberg F, Wirth R, Jeffrey RB Jr, et al: Computed tomography as an adjunct to ultrasound in the diagnosis of acute acalculous cholecystitis, *Gastrointest Radiol* 16:149, 1991.

30. McIntosh DM, Penney HF: Gray-scale ultrasonography as a screening procedure in the detection of gallbladder disease, *Radiology* 136:725, 1980.

31. Cooperberg PL, Burhenne HJ: Real-time ultrasonography: diagnostic technique of choice in calculus gall bladder disease, *N Engl J Med* 302:1277, 1980.

32. MacDonald FR, Cooperberg PL, Cohen MM: The WES triad: a specific sonographic sign of gallstones in the contracted gall bladder, *Gastrointest Radiol* 6:39, 1981.

33. Ralls PW, Halls J, Lapin SA, et al: Prospective evaluation of the sonographic Murphy sign in suspected acute cholecystitis, *J Clin Ultrasound* 10:113, 1982.

34. Madrazo BL, Francis I, Hricak H, et al: Sonographic findings in perforation of the gall bladder, *AJR Am J Roentgenol* 139:491, 1982.

35. Gill KS, Chapman AH, Weston MJ: The changing face of emphysematous cholecystitis, *Br J Radiol* 70:986, 1997.

36. England RE, McDermott VG, Smith TP, et al: Percutaneous cholecystostomy: who responds? *AJR Am J Roentgenol* 168:1247, 1997.

37. van Overhagen H, Meyers H, Tilanus HW, et al: Percutaneous cholecystostomy for patients with acute cholecystitis and an increased surgical risk, *Cardiovasc Intervent Radiol* 19:72, 1996.

38. Boland GW, Lee MJ, Mueller PR, et al: Gallstones in critically ill patients with acute calculous cholecystitis treated by percutaneous cholecystostomy: nonsurgical therapeutic options, *AJR Am J Roentgenol* 162:1101, 1994.

39. Lo LD, Vogelzang RL, Braun MA, et al: Percutaneous cholecystostomy for the diagnosis and treatment of acute calculous and acalculous cholecystitis, *JVIR* 6:629, 1995.

40. Boland GW, Lee MJ, Leung J, et al: Percutaneous cholecystostomy in critically ill patients: early response and final outcome in 82 patients, *AJR Am J Roentgenol* 163:339, 1994.

41. Lee MJ, Saini S, Brink JA, et al: Treatment of critically ill patients with sepsis of unknown cause: value of percutaneous cholecystostomy, *AJR Am J Roentgenol* 156:1163, 1991.

42. Goodwin SC, Bansal V, Greaser LE, et al: Prevention of hemobilia during percutaneous biliary drainage: long term follow up, *JVIR* 8:881, 1997.

43. Chang L, Moonka R, Stelzner M: Percutaneous cholecystostomy for acute cholecystitis in veteran patients, *Am J Surg* 180:198, 2000.

44. Teplick SK, Harshfield DL, Brandon JC, et al: Percutaneous cholecystostomy in critically ill patients, *Gastrointest Radiol* 16:154, 1991.

45. McGahan JP, Lindfors KK: Acute cholecystitis: diagnostic accuracy of percutaneous aspiration of the gall bladder, *Radiology* 167:669, 1988.

46. Chopra S, Dodd GD, Mumbower AL, et al: Treatment of acute cholecystitis in non-critically ill patients at high surgical risk, *AJR Am J Roentgenol* 176:1025, 2001.

47. Klingler PJ, Metzger PP, Seelig MH, et al: Clostridium difficile infection: risk factors, medical and surgical management, *Dig Dis* 18:147, 2000.

48. Surawicz CM, McFarland LV: Pseudomembranous colitis: causes and cures, *Digestion* 60:91, 1999.

49. Fishman EK, Kavuru M, Jones B, et al: Pseudomembranous colitis: CT evaluation of 26 cases, *Radiology* 180:57, 1991.

50. Macari M, Balthazar EJ, Megibow AJ: The accordion sign at CT: a nonspecific finding in patients with colonic edema, *Radiology* 211:743, 1999.

51. Prendergast TM, Marini CP, D'Angelo AS, et al: Surgical patients with pseudomembranous colitis: factors affecting progress, *Surgery* 116:768, 1994.

52. Kirkpatrick IDC, Greenberg HM: Evaluating the CT diagnosis of Clostridium difficile colitis: should CT guide therapy? *AJR Am J Roentgenol* 176:635, 2001.

53. Boland GW, Lee MJ, Cats AM, et al: Antibiotic-associated diarrhea: specificity of abdominal CT for the diagnosis of Clostridium difficile disease, *Radiology* 191:103, 1994.

54. Kawamoto S, Horton KM, Fishman EK: Pseudomembranous colitis: can CT predict which patients will need surgical intervention? *J Comput Assist Tomogr* 23:79, 1999.

55. Downey DB, Wilson SR: Pseudomembranous colitis: sonographic features, *Radiology* 180:61, 1991.

56. Ros PR, Buetow PC, Pantongrag-Brown L, et al: Pseudomembranous colitis, *Radiology* 198:1, 1996.

57. Thrall JH, Ziessman HA: Gastrointestinal system. In Thrall JH, Ziessman HA, eds: *Nuclear medicine: the requisites*, ed 1, St Louis, 1995, Mosby.

58. Jeffrey RB, Federle MP, Wall S: Value of computed tomography in detecting occult gastrointestinal perforation, *J Comput Assist Tomogr* 7:825, 1983.

59. Seltzer SE: Abnormal intraabdominal gas collections visualized on computed tomography: a clinical and experimental study, *Gastrointest Radiol* 9:127, 1984.

60. Gore RM, Miller FH, Pereles FS, et al: Helical CT in the evaluation of the acute abdomen, *AJR Am J Roentgenol* 174:901, 2000.

61. Neitlich JD, Burrell MI: Drug-induced disorders of the colon, *Abdom Imaging* 24:23, 1999.

62. Lappas JC, Reyes BL, Maglinte DDT: Abdominal radiography findings in small-bowel obstruction: relevance to triage for additional diagnostic imaging, *AJR Am J Roentgenol* 176:167, 2001.

63. Frager DH, Baer JW, Rothpearl A, et al: Distinction between postoperative ileus and mechanical small bowel obstruction: value of CT compared with clinical and other radiographic findings, *AJR Am J Roentgenol* 164:891, 1995.

64. Johnson CD, Rice RP, Kelvin FM, et al: The radiologic evaluation of gross cecal distension: emphasis on cecal ileus, *AJR Am J Roentgenol* 145:1211, 1985.

65. Balthazar EJ: CT of small bowel obstruction, *AJR* 162:255, 1994.

66. Harlow CL, Stears RLG, Zeligman BE, Archer PG: Diagnosis of bowel obstruction on plain abdominal radiographs: significance of air-fluid levels at different heights in the same loop of bowel, *AJR Am J Roentgenol* 161:291, 1993.

67. Megibow AJ, Balthazar EJ, Cho KC, et al: Bowel obstruction: evaluation with CT, *Radiology* 180:313, 1991.

68. Fukuya T, Hawes DR, Lu CC, et al: CT diagnosis of small-bowel obstruction: efficacy in 60 patients, *AJR Am J Roentgenol* 158:765, 1992.

69. Gazelle GS, Goldberg MA, Wittenberg J, et al: Efficacy of CT in distinguishing small-bowel obstruction from other causes of small-bowel dilatation, *AJR Am J Roentgenol* 162:43, 1994.

70. Frager D, Medwid SW, Baer JW, et al: CT of small-bowel obstruction: value in establishing the diagnosis and establishing the degree and cause, *AJR Am J Roentgenol* 162:37, 1994.

71. Balthazar EJ, Birnbaum BA, Megibow AJ, et al: Closed-loop and strangulating intestinal obstruction: CT signs, *Radiology* 185:769, 1992.

72. Frager D, Baer JW, Medwid SW, et al: Detection of intestinal ischemia in patients with acute small bowel obstruction due to adhesions or hernia: efficacy of CT, *AJR Am J Roentgenol* 166:67, 1996.

73. Zalcman M, Sy M, Donckier V, et al: Helical CT signs in the diagnosis of intestinal ischemia in small-bowel obstruction, *AJR Am J Roentgenol* 175:1601, 2000.

74. Maglinte DT, Gage SN, Harmon BH, et al: Obstruction of the small intestine: accuracy and role of CT in diagnosis, *Radiology* 188:61, 1993.

75. Maglinte DDT, Balthazar EJ, Kelvin FM, et al: The role of radiology in the diagnosis of small-bowel obstruction, *AJR Am J Roentgenol* 168:1171, 1997.

76. Nolan D, Herlinger H: Vascular disorders of the small bowel. In Gore R, Levine M, eds: *Textbook of gastrointestinal radiology*, ed 2, Philadelphia, 2000, WB Saunders.

77. Scott J, Miller W, Urso M, et al: Acute mesenteric infarction, *AJR Am J Roentgenol* 113:269, 1971.

78. Vogelzang R, Gore R, Anscheutz S, et al: Thrombosis of the splanchnic veins: CT identification, *AJR Am J Roentgenol* 150:93, 1988.

79. Balthazar E, Gollapundi P: Septic thrombophlebitis of the mesenteric and portal veins: CT imaging, *JCAT* 24:755, 2000.

80. Taylor GA, Fallat M, Eichelberger M: Hypovolemic shock in children: abdominal CT manifestations, *Radiology* 164:479, 1987.

81. Mirvis S, Shanmuganathan K, Erb R: Diffuse small bowel ischemia in hypotensive adults after blunt trauma (shock bowel): CT findings and clinical significance, *AJR Am J Roentgenol* 163:1375, 1994.

82. Jeffrey RB: Acute hepatobiliary and pancreatic disease. In Goodman LR, Putnam CE, eds: *Critical care imaging*, ed 3, Philadelphia, 1992, WB Saunders.

83. Balthazar E: Pancreatitis. In Gore R, Levine M, eds: *Textbook of gastrointestinal radiology*, ed 2, Philadelphia, 2000, WB Saunders.

84. Morehouse H, Weiner S, Hoffman-Tretin J: Inflammatory disease of the kidney, *Semin Ultrasound CT MR* 7:246, 1986.

85. Piccirillo M, Rigsby C, Rosenfield A: Sonography of renal inflammatory disease, *Urol Radiol* 9:66, 1987.

86. Rosenfield RT, Glickman MG, Taylor KJW, et al: Acute focal bacterial nephritis, *Radiology* 132:553, 1979.

87. Papanicolaou N, Pfister RC: Acute renal infections: advances in uroradiology volume 1, *Radiol Clin North Am* 34:965, 1996.

88. Dunnick N: Acute genitourinary disease. In Goodman LR, Putman CE, eds: *Critical care imaging*, ed 3, Philadelphia, 1992, WB Saunders.

89. Kriegshauser J, Carroll B: The urinary tract. In Rumack C, Wilson S, Charboneau J, eds: *Diagnostic ultrasound*, St Louis, 1991, Mosby.

90. Ryan J, Mueller P: Abdominal abscess. In Gore R, Levine M, eds: *Textbook of gastrointestinal radiology*, ed 2, Philadelphia, 2000, WB Saunders.

91. Jeffrey R, Wing V, Laing F: Real-time sonographic monitoring of percutaneous abscess drainage, *AJR Am J Roentgenol* 144:469, 1985.

92. McGahan J: Aspiration and drainage procedures in the intensive care unit: percutaneous sonographic guidance, *Radiology* 154:531, 1985.

93. McGahan J: Ultrasound-guided aspiration and drainage. In Rumack C, Wilson S, Charboneau J, eds: *Diagnostic ultrasound*, St Louis, 1991, Mosby.

94. Lambiase R, Deyoe L, Cronan J, et al: Percutaneous drainage of 335 consecutive abscesses: result of primary drainage with one year follow-up, *Radiology* 184:167, 1992.

95. Daly B, Krebs T, Wang S, Wong-You-Cheong J: Percutaneous abdominal and pelvic interventional procedures utilizing CT fluoroscopic guidance, *AJR Am J Roentgenol* 173:637, 1999.

96. Polak J: The peripheral vessels. In Rumack C, Wilson S, Charboneau J, eds: *Diagnostic ultrasound*, St Louis, 1991, Mosby.

97. Kakkar V, Howe C, Flanc C, et al: Natural history of post-operative deep venous thrombosis, *Lancet* 2:230, 1969.

98. Comerota A, Katz M, Greenwald L, et al: Venous duplex imaging: should it replace hemodynamic tests for deep venous thrombosis? *J Vasc Surg* 11:53, 1990.

17 The Future of Trauma Imaging: A Clinical Perspective

Thomas M. Scalea and Stuart E. Mirvis

The current sophistication available in imaging has linked trauma radiologists and trauma surgeons both tightly and symbiotically. It is interesting to remember that this is a relatively recent phenomenon. The diagnostic algorithm for the evaluation of the injured patient up until the early 1980s was based on a belief that identifying the presence of an injury was all that was necessary. Surgeons believed that virtually all injuries were best served by direct exploration. For instance, nonoperative management of solid visceral injuries or expectant management for penetrating torso trauma was extremely unusual. The simple presence of abdominal pain or tenderness or aspirations of blood on diagnostic peritoneal lavage were considered absolute indications for exploratory laparotomy. Diagnostic imaging of the abdomen was relatively crude. Nuclear medicine scanning of the abdomen, via liver-spleen scanning, and intravenous pyelography were all that were available to help make the diagnosis of organ-specific injury.

The advent of CT scanning was perhaps the greatest advance in modern trauma care in the last 25 years. Once adequate experience was gained, CT allowed trauma specialists to make the diagnosis of organ-specific injury. It also facilitated the recognition of the wide range of injuries that existed. For instance, asymptomatic, low-grade liver injuries are now seen on CT scans. Previously, many of these injuries were not diagnosed, and virtually all of them healed spontaneously. CT categorization of these clinically insignificant injuries supplied the impetus for nonoperative management of solid visceral injuries. The paradigm was reversed. It was rapidly realized that CT provided the ability to explore without surgery. The number of truly diagnostic laparotomies began to fall precipitously. Still, CT was a static examination that furnished information at only one point in time. It allowed the physician to view the inside of the organ but did not provide the same perspective that a surgeon had when viewing an organ during surgical exploration. Thus it should have come as no surprise when reports began to detail the lack of correlation between CT grading and operative grading of visceral injuries.[1,2]

CT became more sophisticated, and its resolution improved. Correspondingly, the ability to characterize organ injury likewise increased. At the same time, interventional radiologists were becoming far more important in the care of the injured patient. Angiographic embolization was routinely used to treat bleeding from blunt pelvic fractures.[3] Diagnostic algorithms for abdominal visceral injury began to evolve, where screening tests could be performed using either ultrasound or diagnostic peritoneal lavage. Patients without injury could be observed. Those patients at high risk or with proven injury could then have diagnostic tests such as CT that could confirm the diagnosis of organ-specific injury. Because CT still could not successfully predict outcome of observation, angiography became part of the diagnostic algorithm. Patients with vascular injury seen on angiography could then potentially be treated by coil embolization.[4]

Angiographic embolization was first popularized for the management of splenic injuries and increased splenic salvage to more than 98% in the first large series.[5] This technique has now been much more widely applied to other areas of the body. Angiographic embolization is now commonplace for liver injuries as well as vascular structures that are surgically inaccessible, such as arterial injuries deep within the hypogastric circulation or lumbar artery injuries.[6,7]

Perhaps most important, it became clear that the surgeon and radiologist have both complementary and important roles to play. The question was no longer whether patients needed surgery or imaging; it became a discussion regarding what benefits could be gleaned from each specialty. Damage control, a philosophy of care, was first described in 1993 by Rotondo et al.[8] Using damage control, only immediately life-threatening injuries were cared for at the time of initial exploration. Nonimmediately life-threatening injuries, such as gastrointestinal injuries, were treated with resection without anastomosis. The patients were taken to the intensive care unit and could be more fully resuscitated. These nonimmediately life-threatening injuries could then be dealt with several days later when the patient was more stable. This new technique cemented the relationship between radiology and trauma surgery. These desperately ill patients could go to the operating room for control of main vessel bleeding. Ancillary hemostasis was almost always better accomplished via transcatheter techniques. This also provided time for additional diagnostic evaluation with CT. Each specialty brought unique talents to the table.

With a look to the future, this relationship should continue to evolve. The ideal diagnostic imaging strategy is noninvasive, rapid, portable, and accurate. Many of the current diagnostic modalities have some of these attributes. Very few have all of them. Virtually all invasive tests come with some degree of complication. Admittedly, this risk is small in the typically young trauma patient. However, trauma patients are aging, as is the rest of society. Elderly patients tolerate complications poorly. Invasive techniques often require specialized equipment such as an angiography suite, which exists only in certain areas of the hospital. This requires transporting the patient to the resources. Portable technology, particularly if hand-held, has the distinct advantage of being able to be applied quickly in the resuscitation area. Ideally, this technology would be able to be used to image more than one area of the body.

Ultrasonography has already assumed a far greater role in trauma evaluation. Directed ultrasound is now commonly used to diagnose hemoperitoneum, hemopericardium, or hemothoraces. The reported accuracy is quite good.[9,10] One could anticipate this technology becoming only more advanced and more available. In addition, a wide variety of physicians must become proficient in its use. Ultrasonography cannot be the domain of a single specialty, particularly because these specialists may not be present at the time of patient presentation. Physician training and credentialing and quality assurance must be very prominent as this technology evolves.

Proven accuracy must be an important part of the future of imaging. Perhaps most important, whereas false positives are a concern, false negatives can be devastating. Surgical exploration for a presumed injury that is found to be negative is not as potentially catastrophic as the failure to recognize that an injury exists. All new advances in imaging must be held to this standard.

Several years ago CT scanning of the thorax was useful only to exclude aortic injury. CT scanning now can make the diagnosis of aortic injury, and therapy can be based solely on CT.[11] This limits the time from injury to therapy. Although there is concern that CT alone may miss anatomic abnormalities, a congenital mediastinal vascular abnormality in a patient with an aortic injury was recently diagnosed on CT. This type of sophisticated imaging should only continue to evolve.

The presence of contrast blush in the spleen, liver, or pelvis on spiral CT correlates with failure of simple observation.[12] Future-generation CT scanning should allow more complete characterization of vascular abnormalities. Already CT angiography is becoming commonplace for the diagnosis of vascular injuries in the neck. Technical improvement should continue, permitting better prediction of those patients who would benefit from angiography or surgery based on CT findings.

The greatest advances are likely to be in the diagnosis and management of traumatic brain injury (TBI). Magnetic resonance imaging (MRI) can demonstrate areas of abnormality that are not possible to detect on routine computerized tomography. Functional MRI is another application of this technology, which promises far greater understanding of deficits related to TBI and perhaps potential for recovery of cerebral tissue. Secondary brain injury from ischemia almost certainly occurs around the areas of acutely traumatized brain. Imaging of the future should not only be able to identify areas of ischemia but also estimate the precise degree of that ischemia on a real-time basis as interventions are made. This approach would be a step toward optimizing therapy to limit the extent of neurologic damage. Early and prompt treatment of areas "at risk" from TBI would almost certainly result in a decrease in mortality and disability so common with severe TBI. CT perfusion imaging is a developing technique to measure total and regional brain perfusion, which may contribute to better understanding of cerebral blood flow at various stages of brain trauma.

These same issues apply to spinal cord injury as well. Final neurologic performance is not always predicted by the level of spinal column injury seen at the time of patient presentation. Once again, secondary cord injury is almost certainly a function of ongoing ischemia. Directed resuscitation strategies aimed at optimizing both cerebral and spinal cord perfusion offer hope for improving prognosis, particularly if the results of interventions can be quantified in a noninvasive, nondestructive manner.

Perhaps the greatest current deficit in trauma imaging is the limited ability to correlate anatomic images with physiologic function. For instance, CT scanning of the brain is able to make the structural diagnoses of epidural or subdural hematoma but is not able, other than at the extremes of injury, to estimate neurologic function or likelihood of recovery. CT scanning of the abdomen can make the diagnosis of hemoperitoneum in addition to organ injury and can quantify the amount of lost blood, yet it cannot reveal how the patient has tolerated the blood loss in physiologic terms.

In injury, critical care must be a concept and not a location. Trauma imaging would certainly follow along those lines. The era when CT scanners are based in a fixed location in the hospital will almost certainly end. Portable CT scanning is currently available in helical form. All imaging technologies should also be adapted for portability. Imagine a trauma patient presenting to the resuscitation unit with hypotension and neurologic injury. Simultaneous resuscitation and imaging could be performed if the CT were portable. The diagnosis of brain injury and a rapid search for areas of blood loss could be undertaken simultaneously. Patients with visceral injury or perivascular hematoma could undergo CT with fast multiplanar reformation to allow for diagnosis and characterization of vascular injury. Cervical spine trauma could be fully assessed, including the ligaments, using a specialized, portable, low-field magnetic resonance unit. Instead of having the patient undergo a series of static radiographs as part of the "radiographic survey," potentially, using digital technology, a tailored device could scan the entire body in one sweep, providing a one-shot "survey" of injured regions, with detailed studies acquired later as appropriate. Thus a full diagnostic evaluation could be performed within the period of initial physical assessment and stabilization, assuming appropriate concern for radiation safety and magnetic field issues. Perhaps the most sophisticated imaging techniques would still require transport to a specialized location once the patient is stabilized.

In this paradigm, the differences between the trauma surgeon, the trauma imager, and the trauma interventionalist begin to blur. Trauma surgery has become more correctly termed *trauma medicine*. In the future, the resuscitation area, imaging area, operating room, and interventional radiology suite will begin to merge. Patients will be immediately evaluated and stabilized and have investigations performed simultaneously. The next step, of course, is to begin to be able to intervene and provide nonoperative hemostasis once the diagnosis is made. Some patients will still require open surgical techniques to stem life-threatening blood loss. However, operating rooms are already equipped with biplanar angiography capabilities. The ability to perform both of these techniques nearly simultaneously will continue to evolve.

The relationship between trauma imaging and trauma surgery has been the impetus for much of the improvement in American trauma care. As the twenty-first century continues, this relationship will only be further developed. However, technology becomes more expensive each year, and medical resources are becoming more limited. It will be the responsibility of all who care for injured patients to critically evaluate any application of new technology to assess if that technology does more than just provide nicer pictures and in fact improves care and ultimately saves lives.

REFERENCES

1. Becher DC, Spring P, Glatti A, Schweizer W: Blunt splenic trauma in adults: can CT findings be used to determine the need for surgery? *AJR Am J Roentgenol* 162:343, 1994.
2. Mirvis SE, Whitley NO, Gens DR: Blunt splenic trauma in adults: CT-based classification and correlation with prognosis and treatment, *Radiology* 171:33, 1989.
3. Evers BM, Cryer HM, Miller FB: Pelvic fracture hemorrhage: priorities in management, *Arch Surg* 124:422, 1989.
4. Baron BJ, Scalea TM, Sclafani SJ, et al: Non-operative management of blunt abdominal trauma: the role of sequential diagnostic peritoneal lavage, computed tomography, and angiography, *Ann Emer Med* 22:1556, 1993.
5. Scalfani SJ, Shaftan GW, Scalea TM, et al: Nonoperative salvage of computed tomography-diagnosed splenic injuries: utilization of angiography for triage and embolization for hemostasis, *J Trauma* 39:818, 1995.
6. Velmahos GC, Chahwan S, Hanks SE, et al: Angiographic embolization of bilateral internal iliac arteries to control life-threatening hemorrhage after blunt trauma to the pelvis, *Am Surg* 66:858, 2000.
7. Roberts LH, Demetriades D: Vertebral artery injuries, *Surg Clin North Am* 81:1345, 2001.
8. Rotondo MF, Schwab CW, McGonigal MD, et al: `Damage control': an approach for improved survival in exsanguinating penetrating abdominal injury, *J Trauma* 35:375, 1993.
9. Rozycki GS, Ballard RB, Feliciano DV, et al: Surgeon-performed ultrasound for the assessment of truncal injuries: lessons learned from 1540 patients, *Ann Surg* 228:557, 1998.
10. Udobi KF, Rodriguez A, Chiu WC, Scalea TM: Role of ultrasonography in penetrating abdominal trauma: a prospective clinical study, *J Trauma* 50:475, 2001.
11. Downing SW, Sperling JS, Mirvis SE, et al: Experience with spiral computed-tomography as the sole diagnostic method for traumatic aortic rupture, *Ann Thoracic Surg* 72:495, 2001.
12. Davis KA, Fabian TC, Croce MA, et al: Improved success in nonoperative management of blunt splenic injuries: embolization of splenic artery pseudoaneurysms, *J Trauma* 44:1008, 1998.

Index